D1765478

Advanced Monitoring and Procedures for Small Animal Emergency and Critical Care

BISHOP BURTON LRC
WITHDRAWN

ACCESSION No _____

CLASS No. _____

Advanced Monitoring and Procedures for Small Animal Emergency and Critical Care

Editors

Jamie M. Burkitt Creedon, DVM, DACVECC

Chief, Emergency and Critical Care Service
Red Bank Veterinary Hospital, Cherry Hill
Cherry Hill, New Jersey

Harold Davis, BA, RVT, VTS (ECC) (Anesth)

Manager, Emergency and Critical Care Service
William R. Pritchard Veterinary Medical Teaching Hospital
University of California, Davis
Davis, California

WILEY-BLACKWELL

A John Wiley & Sons, Inc., Publication

This edition first published 2012 © 2012 by John Wiley & Sons, Inc.

Wiley-Blackwell is an imprint of John Wiley & Sons, formed by the merger of Wiley's global Scientific, Technical and Medical business with Blackwell Publishing.

Registered office: John Wiley & Sons Ltd, The Atrium, Southern Gate, Chichester, West Sussex, PO19 8SQ, UK

Editorial offices: 2121 State Avenue, Ames, Iowa 50014-8300, USA
The Atrium, Southern Gate, Chichester, West Sussex, PO19 8SQ, UK
9600 Garsington Road, Oxford, OX4 2DQ, UK

For details of our global editorial offices, for customer services and for information about how to apply for permission to reuse the copyright material in this book please see our website at www.wiley.com/wiley-blackwell.

Authorization to photocopy items for internal or personal use, or the internal or personal use of specific clients, is granted by Blackwell Publishing, provided that the base fee is paid directly to the Copyright Clearance Center, 222 Rosewood Drive, Danvers, MA 01923. For those organizations that have been granted a photocopy license by CCC, a separate system of payments has been arranged. The fee codes for users of the Transactional Reporting Service are ISBN-13: 978-0-8138-1337-0/2012.

Designations used by companies to distinguish their products are often claimed as trademarks. All brand names and product names used in this book are trade names, service marks, trademarks or registered trademarks of their respective owners. The publisher is not associated with any product or vendor mentioned in this book. This publication is designed to provide accurate and authoritative information in regard to the subject matter covered. It is sold on the understanding that the publisher is not engaged in rendering professional services. If professional advice or other expert assistance is required, the services of a competent professional should be sought.

Library of Congress Cataloging-in-Publication Data
Advanced monitoring and procedures for small animal emergency and critical care / editors, Jamie M. Burkitt Creedon, Harold Davis.
      p.   ;   cm.
  Includes bibliographical references and index.
  ISBN 978-0-8138-1337-0 (pbk. : alk. paper)
  I. Creedon, Jamie M. Burkitt.   II. Davis, Harold, 1958–
  [DNLM: 1. Emergency Treatment–veterinary.   2. Critical Care–methods.   3. Monitoring, Physiologic–veterinary.   4. Therapeutics–veterinary.   SF 778]
  636.089'6028–dc23

                                                                        2011036425

A catalogue record for this book is available from the British Library.

Wiley also publishes its books in a variety of electronic formats. Some content that appears in print may not be available in electronic books.

Set in 10.5/12.5 pt Minion by Toppan Best-set Premedia Limited
Printed and bound in Malaysia by Vivar Printing Sdn Bhd

1   2012

To Dr. Janet Aldrich, who taught me that thinking and knowing are different, and that the former is far more important.

To Dr. Steve Haskins, who showed me that listening is the teacher's most important skill.

To my parents, Robbie and Mike, who taught me that caring is always worth it.

And to my husband Mike, who gives selflessly over and over and over again.

I love and thank you all.

–Jamie M. Burkitt Creedon

First and foremost this book is dedicated to my parents, Dr. Harold Davis, Sr., and Barbara Davis, and my sister, Deborah Davis-Gillespie, for their love, support and guidance. To Thomas J. Bulgin, DVM, for giving me my start as a veterinary assistant and Gary L. Reinhardt, DVM, and Steve C. Haskins, DVM, DACVECC, for their mentorship. To each current and past member that I have served with on the board of directors for the Veterinary Emergency and Critical Care Society. To the veterinary technicians and nurses that I have talked to around the world and former veterinary students of U.C. Davis: I have enjoyed sharing my knowledge and experiences with you. Finally, to the co-founding and charter members of the Academy of Veterinary Emergency, and Critical Care Technicians: it was an honor, pleasure, and a joy to work with you in developing the first veterinary technician speciality academy.

–Harold Davis

Contents

This book has a companion website including images and protocols from the book available at www.wiley.com/go/burkittcreedon.

Contributors

Amanda Adams, LVT, VTS (ECC)
Critical Care/Dialysis Technician
VCA Veterinary Specialty Center of Seattle
Seattle, Washington

Janet Aldrich, DVM, DACVECC
Formerly Clinical Veterinarian
Veterinary Medical Teaching Hospital
University of California
Davis, California

Lori Baden Atkins, AAS, LVT, VTS (ECC)
Small Animal ICU/ER Coordinator
Veterinary Medical Teaching Hospital
Texas A&M University
College Station, Texas

Devon A. Ayres, RVT, BS
Intensive Care Unit Technician
Veterinary Specialty Hospital
San Diego, California

Linda S. Barter, MVSc, BSc (Vet), PhD, DACVA
Assistant Professor of Veterinary Anesthesiology
University of California
Davis, California

Linda Barton, DVM, DACVECC
Staff Veterinarian
Department of Critical Care
VCA Veterinary Specialty Center
Lynnwood, Washington

Elana Moss Benasutti, CVT
Critical Care Nurse
Intensive Care Unit
Matthew J. Ryan Veterinary Hospital
University of Pennsylvania
Philadelphia, Pennsylvania

Amanda K. Boag, MA, VetMB, DACVIM, DACVECC, FHEA, MRCVS
Clinical Director
Vets Now
Scotland, United Kingdom

Jennifer Boyle, RVT, VTS (ECC)
CE Relationships Manager
Veterinary Information Network
Davis, CA

Benjamin M. Brainard, VMD, DACVA, DACVECC
Associate Professor, Critical Care
Department of Small Animal Medicine and Surgery
College of Veterinary Medicine
University of Georgia
Athens, Georgia

Yekaterina Buriko, DVM, DACVECC
Staff Doctor
Animal Medical Center
New York, New York

Jamie M. Burkitt Creedon, DVM, DACVECC
Chief, Emergency and Critical Care Service
Red Bank Veterinary Hospital, Cherry Hill
Cherry Hill, New Jersey

Christopher G. Byers, DVM, DACVECC, DACVIM
Faculty Internist / Criticalist
MidWest Veterinary Specialty Hospital
Omaha, Nebraska

Mary Tefend Campbell, CVT, VTS (ECC)
Nursing Manager
Carriage Hills Referral Hospital
Montgomery, Alabama

Scott Campbell, BVSc (Hons), MACVSc, DACVN
Senior Lecturer in Clinical Nutrition
Clinical Nutrition Support Service
School of Veterinary Science
University of Queensland
Brisbane, Australia

Vicki L. Campbell, DVM, DACVA, DACVECC
Assistant Professor
Clinical Care Unit
Department of Clinical Sciences
Colorado State University
Fort Collins, Colorado

Daniel L. Chan, DVM, DACVECC, DACVN, FHEA, MRCVS
Senior Lecturer in Emergency and Critical Care
Clinical Nutritionist
Department of Veterinary Clinical Sciences
The Royal Veterinary College
University of London
Hertfordshire, United Kingdom

Rosalind S. Chow, VMD, DACVECC
Criticalist
Veterinary Medical and Surgical Group
Ventura, California

Monica C. Clare, VMD, DACVECC
Director of the ICU
Intensive Care Unit
Veterinary Specialty Hospital
San Diego, California

Edward Cooper, VMD, MS, DACVECC
Assistant Professor, Small Animal Emergency
and Critical Care
Department of Veterinary Clinical Sciences
Ohio State University
Columbus, Ohio

Stacey Cooper, RVT, VTS (ECC)
Veterinary Medical Center
Ohio State University
Columbus, Ohio

Craig Cornell, BA, RVT, VTS (ECC) (Anesthesia)
Department of Small Animal Anesthesia
University of California
Davis, California

Meredith L. Daly, VMD, DACVECC
Bluepearl Veterinary Partners
New York, New York

Harold Davis, BA, RVT, VTS (ECC) (Anesthesia)
Manager, Emergency and Critical Care Service
William R. Pritchard Veterinary Medical Teaching
Hospital
University of California
Davis, California

Julie Denton-Schmiedt, CVT, BA
Large and Small Animal Anesthesia Veterinary
Technician
Hull, Georgia

Jennifer Devey, DVM, DACVECC
Department Head, Emergency and Critical
Care Service
Director of Education
Lauderdale Veterinary Specialists
Fort Lauderdale, Florida

Pamela Dilley, RVT, CCRA
Veterinary Medical and Surgical Group
Ventura, California

Katherine Dobbs, RVT, CVPM, PHR
interFace Veterinary HR Systems, LLC
Appleton, Wisconsin

Jeni Dohner, CVT, VTS (ECC)
Emergency Service
Matthew J. Ryan Veterinary Hospital
School of Veterinary Medicine
University of Pennsylvania
Philadelphia, Pennsylvania

Julie A. Eveland-Baker RVT, VTS (ECC)
Shift Supervisor, Small Animal Intensive Care Unit
Veterinary Medical Teaching Hospital
University of California
Davis, California

Mary M. Flanders, RVT, VTS (ECC)
Veterinary Medical Teaching Hospital
University of Missouri
Columbia, Missouri

Daniel J. Fletcher, PhD, DVM, DACVECC
Assistant Professor of Emergency and Critical Care
Department of Clinical Sciences
College of Veterinary Medicine
Cornell University
Ithaca, New York

Adrian Ford, BS, LVT, VTS (ECC)
Chief Operations Officer, Hospital Administrator
Emergency Pet Center Hospitals
Emergency Pet Clinic INC
San Antonio, Texas

Sharon Fornes, RVT, VTS (Anesthesia)
Program Director
Veterinary Technology
Carrington College California
San Leandro, California

Robert Goggs, BVSc, DACVECC, MRCVS
Wellcome Trust Research Training Fellow
School of Physiology and Pharmacology
University of Bristol
Bristol, United Kingdom

Sarah Gray, DVM, DACVECC
Criticalist
Veterinary Medical and Surgical Group
Ventura, California

Rebecca J. Greer, DVM, MS, DACVECC
Staff Criticalist
Veterinary Specialty Services
Manchester, Missouri

Sarah L. Haldane, BVSc, BAnSc, MACVSc, DACVECC
Senior Lecturer
Department of Emergency and Critical Care
University of Melbourne
Melbourne, Victoria, Australia

Natalie Harvey, BApSc (VT)
Nutrition Technician
Clinical Nutrition Support Service
School of Veterinary Science
University of Queensland
Brisbane, Australia

Steve C. Haskins, DVM, MS, DACVA, DACVECC
Professor Emeritus
University of California
Davis, California

Cindy Hauser, MBA, CVT, VTS (ECC)
Wheat Ridge Animal Hospital
Wheat Ridge, Colorado

Marie K. Holowaychuk, DVM, DACVECC
Assistant Professor, Emergency and Critical Care
Medicine
Department of Clinical Studies
Ontario Veterinary College
University of Guelph
Guelph, Ontario, Canada

Kate Hopper, BVSc, PhD, DACVECC
Assistant Professor, Small Animal Emergency and
Critical Care
Department of Veterinary Surgical and Radiological
Sciences
University of California
Davis, California

Katherine Jayne Howie, VN, VTS (ECC)
Senior Veterinary Nurse
Vets Now Farnham
Farnham, United Kingdom

Karl E. Jandrey, DVM, MAS, DACVECC
Assistant Professor of Clinical Small Animal
Emergency and Critical Care
Department of Surgical and Radiological Sciences
William R. Pritchard Veterinary Medical Teaching
Hospital
University of California
Davis, California

**Michael S. Kent, DVM, DACVIM (Oncology),
DACVR (Radiation Oncology), MAS**
Assistant Professor
Department of Surgical and Radiological Sciences
School of Veterinary Medicine
University of California
Davis, California

Lesley G. King, MVB, DACVECC, DACVIM
Department of Clinical Studies
Matthew J. Ryan Veterinary Hospital
School of Veterinary Medicine
University of Pennsylvania
Philadelphia, Pennsylvania

Casey J. Kohen, BA
Research Assistant, Mellema Lab
School of Veterinary Medicine
University of California
Davis, California

Timothy Koors, DVM
Resident
Veterinary Specialty Services
Manchester, Missouri

Mary Anna Labato, DVM, ACVIM
Clinical Professor
Section Head, Small Animal Medicine
Cummings School of Veterinary Medicine
Tufts University
North Grafton, Massachusetts

Michael S. Lagutchik, DVM, MS, DACVECC
Medical Director
Emergency Pet Center Hospitals
San Antonio, Texas

Cathy Langston, DVM, DACVIM
Staff Veterinarian, Head of Nephrology, Urology,
and Hemodialysis Unit
Department of Renal Medicine and Hemodialysis
Animal Medical Center
New York, New York

Carine Laporte, VMD
School of Veterinary Medicine
University of Pennsylvania
Philadelphia, Pennsylvania

Jennifer Larsen, DVM, PhD, DACVN
Assistant Professor of Clinical Nutrition
Department of Molecular Biosciences
School of Veterinary Medicine
University of California
Davis, California

Stephanie Leone, BS, RVT
Emergency Service Manager
Pet Emergency & Specialty Center
La Mesa, California

Rosemary Lombardi, CVT, VTS (ECC)
Director of Nursing
Matthew J. Ryan Veterinary Hospital
School of Veterinary Medicine
University of Pennsylvania
Philadelphia, Pennsylvania

Bridget Lyons, BA, CVT
ICU Nurse, VHD Candidate
Intensive Care Unit
University of Pennsylvania School of
Veterinary Medicine
Philadelphia, Pennsylvania

Elisa M. Mazzaferro, MS, DVM, PhD, DACVECC
Director of Emergency Services
Wheat Ridge Animal Hospital
Wheat Ridge, Colorado

Douglass K. Macintire, DVM, MS, DACVECC
Professor of Acute Medicine and Critical Care
Department of Clinical Sciences
College of Veterinary Medicine
Auburn University
Auburn, Alabama

F. A. (Tony) Mann, DVM, MS, DACVS, DACVECC
Director of Small Animal Emergency
and Critical Care Services
Small Animal Soft Tissue Surgery Service Chief
Veterinary Medical Teaching Hospital
University of Missouri
Columbia, Missouri

Margo Mehl, DVM, DACVS
San Francisco Veterinary Specialists
San Francisco, California

Megan Patterson Melcher, RVT
ICU Technician
VCA Veterinary Referral Associates
Gaithersburg, Maryland

Matthew S. Mellema, DVM, PhD, DACVECC
Assistant Professor, Small Animal Emergency
and Critical Care
School of Veterinary Medicine
University of Califronia
Davis, California

Martin D. Miller
Operations Manager
AVETS
Monroeville, Pennsylvania

Elizabeth Olmstead, CVT, BS
Blood Donor Supervisor, ICU Technician
Department of Small Animal Medicine
College of Veterinary Medicine
University of Minnesota
St. Paul, Minnesota

Joao Orvalho, DVM, DACVIM (Cardiology)
Veterinary Medical Center
School of Veterinary Medicine
University of California
San Diego, California

Carl A. Osborne, DVM, PhD, DACVIM
Professor of Veterinary Internal Medicine
College of Veterinary Medicine
University of Minnesota
St. Paul, Minnesota

Sara M. Ostenkamp
Veterinary Technician
ICU Department
North Carolina State University
Raleigh, North Carolina

Romain Pariaut, DVM, DACVIM (Cardiology), ECVIM CA (Cardiology)
Assistant Professor of Cardiology
Department of Veterinary Clinical Sciences
School of Veterinary Medicine
Louisiana State University
Baton Rouge, Louisiana

Sally C. Perea, DVM, MS, DACVN
Senior Nutritionist
Department of Research and Development
P&G Pet Care
Mason, Ohio

Karen Poeppel, BS, LVT
Head Technician, Hemodialysis Unit
Department of Internal Medicine
Animal Medical Center
New York, New York

David J. Polzin, DVM, PhD, DACVIM
Professor of Veterinary Internal Medicine
College of Veterinary Medicine
University of Minnesota
St. Paul, Minnesota

Lisa L. Powell, DVM, DACVECC
Clinical Professor, Emergency and Critical Care
Small Animal ICU Director
College of Veterinary Medicine
University of Minnesota
St. Paul, Minnesota

Paul Primas, RVT
Supervisor, Radiation and Medical Oncology
William R. Pritchard Veterinary Medical Teaching Hospital
University of California, Davis
Davis, California

Jennifer E. Prittie, DVM, DACVIM, DACVECC
Criticalist
Department of Emergency and Critical Care
Animal Medical Center
New York, New York

Jane Quandt, DVM, MS, DACVA, DACVECC
Associate Professor in Anesthesia
Department of Small Animal Medicine
College of Veterinary Medicine
University of Georgia
Athens, Georgia

Marc R. Raffe, DVM, MS, DACVA, ACVECC
Associate Director
Pfizer Animal Health

Louisa J. Rahilly, DVM, DACVECC
Medical Director of Emergency and Critical Care
Cape Cod Veterinary Specialists
Buzzards Bay, Massachusetts

Erica L. Reineke, VMD, DACVECC
Assistant Professor, Emergency and Critical Care Medicine
Department of Clinical Studies
Matthew J. Ryan Veterinary Hospital
School of Veterinary Medicine
University of Pennsylvania
Philadelphia, Pennsylvania

Angel Rivera, AHT, VTS (ECC)
Animal Emergency Center and Specialty Services
Glendale, Wisconsin

Joris H. Robben, PhD, DECVIM CA
Assistant Professor
Head of the ICU
Department of Clinical Sciences of Companion Animals
Faculty of Veterinary Medicine
Utrecht University
Utrecht, The Netherlands

Amy Rodriguez, CVT, VTS (Anesthesia)
Anesthesia Nurse
Department of Anesthesia
Colorado State University
Fort Collins, Colorado

Elizabeth Rozanski, DVM, DACVECC, DACVIM
Associate Professor
Section of Critical Care
Cummings School of Veterinary Medicine
Tufts University
North Grafton, Massachusetts

Elke Rudloff, DVM, DACVECC
Director of Education
Animal Emergency Center and Specialty Services
Glendale, Wisconsin

Emily Savino, BA, AAS, CVT, VTS (ECC)
ICU Nursing Supervisor
Matthew J. Ryan Veterinary Hospital
School of Veterinary Medicine
University of Pennsylvania
Philadelphia, Pennsylvania

Jessica Schavone, BS, CVT
Blood Bank Technician Supervisor and Emergency and
Critical Care Technician
Section of Critical Care
Department of Clinical Sciences
Cummings School of Veterinary Medicine
Tufts University
North Grafton, Massachusetts

Connie M. Schmidt, CVT
Training/Education Coordinator, Senior Technician
Fox Valley Animal Referral
Appleton, Wisconsin

Lila K. Sierra, CVT, VTS (ECC)
Assistant Nursing Supervisor/Intensive Care Unit
Matthew J. Ryan Veterinary Hospital
School of Veterinary Medicine
University of Pennsylvania
Philadelphia, Pennsylvania

Deborah Silverstein, DVM, DACVECC
Assistant Professor of Critical Care
Matthew J. Ryan Veterinary Hospital
School of Veterinary Medicine
University of Pennsylvania
Philadelphia, Pennsylvania

Carolyn A. Sink, MS, MT(ASCP)
Supervisor, Diagnostic and Support Services
Veterinary Teaching Hospital
Virginia Maryland Regional College of Veterinary
Medicine
Blacksburg, Virginia

Sean D. Smarick, VMD, DACVECC
Hospital Director
Emergency and Critical Care Specialist
AVETS
Monroeville, Pennsylvania

Lisa Smart, BVSc (Hons), DACVECC
Senior Lecturer in Veterinary Emergency and Critical
Care
Department of Veterinary Clinical Sciences
School of Veterinary and Biomedical Sciences
Murdoch University
Murdoch, WA, Australia

Michelle Storay, CVN DipECC
Animal Emergency Centre Nursing Director
Mount Waverley, Australia

Rebecca S. Syring, DVM, DACVECC
Staff Criticalist
Veterinary Specialty and Emergency Center
Levittown, Pennsylvania

Chiara Valtolina, DVM, DACVECC
Department of Clinical Sciences of Companion
Animals
Faculty of Veterinary Medicine
Utrecht University
Utrecht, The Netherlands

Lori S. Waddell, DVM, DACVECC
Adjunct Assistant Professor, Critical Care
Department of Clinical Studies
School of Veterinary Medicine
University of Pennsylvania
Philadelphia, Pennsylvania

Nicole M. Weinstein, DVM, DACVP
Assistant Professor, Clinical Pathology
Department of Biomedical Sciences and Pathobiology
Virginia Maryland Regional College of Veterinary
Medicine
Blacksburg, Virginia

Diane M. Welsh, CVT
Cummings School of Veterinary Medicine
Tufts University
North Grafton, Massachusetts

Janelle R. Wierenga, DVM, DACVECC
Seattle, Washington

Jill A. Williamson, DVM, DACVECC
Animal Internal Medicine and Specialty Services
San Francisco, California

Monika L. Wright, CVT
Intensive Care Unit Staff
Matthew J. Ryan Veterinary Hospital
School of Veterinary Medicine
University of Pennsylvania
Philadelphia, Pennsylvania

Brian C. Young, VMD, DACVIM, DACVECC
Staff Criticalist
Department of Emergency and Critical Care
Animal Specialty Group
Los Angeles, California

Preface

The disciplines of small animal emergency medicine and critical care have grown significantly in the past decade. There are many references available that describe the diagnosis and medical treatment of problems encountered in small animal emergency and critical care practice. However, none is dedicated specifically to the daily hands-on practice of the specialties: for instance, the placement and maintenance of arterial catheters and the interpretation of direct pressure waveforms they provide, or the nursing care required to maintain a patient on long-term mechanical ventilation (what do all those buttons on the ventilator do, anyway?). We believe the veterinary community would benefit from a single reference written by informed, experienced people to improve and expand the standard of care, and we hope this textbook serves that purpose. The experienced veterinarian and veterinary technician contributors to *Advanced Procedures and Monitoring for Small Animal Emergency and Critical Care* have provided herein a well-referenced textbook that we believe contains useful information on the "non-medicine" aspects of ECC practice, from practice design to technical procedures and nursing care to interpretation of monitoring results.

There is no small animal specialty in which cooperation between all healthcare team members is more important than in emergency and critical care. Thus, some chapters are authored by a veterinarian, others by a veterinary technician, and some by pairs. The interdependence of all members of the ECC healthcare team requires that veterinary technicians understand why clinicians ask them to do what they do, and that veterinarians understand proper ECC nursing care and technical procedures. The book's contributors come from around the world, from both university and private practice. We aimed to provide the best-referenced, highest-quality textbook that we could. Contributors congenially answered our frequent "Do you have a reference for this?" inquiries and high-quality image requests, so that the reader could have confidence in the recommendations contained herein and see illustrations of how to perform procedures or interpret results. When high-quality references or guidelines were unavailable, these qualified authors made recommendations based on their experience; in such cases, such personal recommendation is noted in the text for transparency.

The textbook is organized roughly by organ system or general topic, but there is considerable overlap in some areas. For instance, some authors of device insertion chapters included a maintenance section, and maintenance of that device may also be covered in another chapter specifically on insertion site maintenance or artificial airway maintenance, and so on. **Standardized protocols** are included for procedures for which they were deemed useful and appropriate. These protocols are based on best-available evidence and guidelines, and where such citations were unavailable or inappropriate, they are based on author experience. We hope these protocols will help raise and equalize the standard of care across our profession, and serve as the backbone for a protocol book to use in your emergency or critical care practice.

We welcome corrections and ideas for future versions of this textbook. Should further editions follow, we are committed to their currency and relevancy, and thus will continue to push for best-practice, evidence- and guideline-based recommendations. Lastly, we would like to thank each contributor; we believe they did an amazing job stepping up to the challenges that this unique textbook posed.

Jamie M. Burkitt Creedon
Harold Davis

Advanced Monitoring and Procedures for Small Animal Emergency and Critical Care

SECTION I

Introduction

1

Triage

Harold Davis

The concept of triage finds its origin in the French military. The word comes from the French verb *trier*, meaning to sort. In human medicine the goals of triage have varied over the years depending upon the situation. After World War II triage came to mean the process of identifying those soldiers most likely to return to battle after medical care. Following the Korean and Vietnam conflicts the goals of triage came to mean the greatest good for the greatest number of wounded.[1] In times of disaster, the goals of triage are similar to the military. Daily human emergency room triage began in the 1960s and has evolved into a method to separate efficiently those patients stable enough to wait for treatment from those who require immediate medical attention. In veterinary medicine we have adopted the goals of our counterparts in the human emergency room. Thus, we prioritize cases by medical urgency when presented with multiple emergencies at the same time.

Triage occurs both by telephone and in the hospital. A client often calls the hospital seeking advice for the care of his or her pet; the receptionist or veterinary technician must ascertain useful information about the pet in a short period of time. In addition the receptionist or technician should have the knowledge required to provide the appropriate advice. The information obtained during the telephone conversation will also be useful in preparing for patient arrival. On initial presentation to the hospital the veterinary technician is usually first to receive the patient and therefore to perform basic triage. This person must determine whether the patient needs immediate care and, in the case of simultaneous patient arrivals, prioritize treatment based on medical need.

Telephone triage

In theory, telephone triage requires clinic staff to determine the urgency of a pet's problem and to provide advice based on that determination. However, because the client may not possess the training to give an accurate account of the pet's problem(s), it is generally safest to recommend the client take the pet to a veterinarian for evaluation. Particularly, any patient experiencing breathing difficulty, seizures, inability or unwillingness to rise, or traumatic injury should be seen by a veterinarian without question.

At the beginning of the telephone conversation staff should establish the animal's signalment (breed, sex, age, and weight) if possible. Questions asked of the owner should be basic and straightforward. They should address the patient's level of consciousness, whether or not the patient is breathing, experiencing seizures, or has obviously broken or exposed bones (see Table 1.1). Based on the owner's responses, advice can be given on first aid, assuming that the problem can be clearly defined and is simple. See Table 1.2 for a list of problems requiring attention by the veterinary health care team without delay.

Information gathered during the phone conversation can aid the veterinary technician in preparation for the arrival of the patient at the hospital. Simply knowing the animal's breed or approximate weight can enable the technician to pre-select appropriate sizes for vascular catheters, fluid bags, and endotracheal tubes.

Owners should be instructed on safe transport for the animal. Animals that have suffered trauma are often in pain, and owners should be instructed on how to

Advanced Monitoring and Procedures for Small Animal Emergency and Critical Care, First Edition. Edited by Jamie M. Burkitt Creedon, Harold Davis.
© 2012 John Wiley & Sons, Inc. Published 2012 by John Wiley & Sons, Inc.

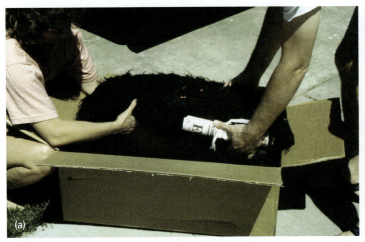 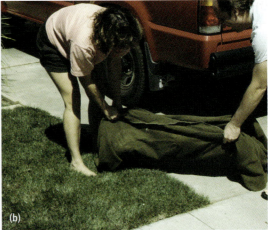

Figure 1.1 (a) Placing a dog in a box for transport. (b) Using a blanket as a stretcher. The animal is placed on a blanket and the edges of the blanket used to lift the patient.

Table 1.1 Questions useful in telephone triage, and suggested responses

1. Is the animal breathing and conscious?
   a. If neither, institute mouth-to-snout; if yes to either of these, do not.
2. Is the animal actively experiencing a seizure?
   a. If yes, remove from danger of falling or any sharp objects. Take to veterinarian immediately after seizure ends, or if it lasts longer than 1–2 minutes, bring during seizure. Watch out for the mouth; don't get bit.
3. For people who live a distance from medical assistance or cannot/will not come in: Has the animal ingested something that you know or suspect is poisonous in the last 2 hours?
   a. In some situations, at–home emesis may be recommended.
4. Is there active bleeding, an obvious fracture, or exposed bone?
   a. Recommend clean towel over the site, pressure if spurting blood. Warn clients to be VERY CAREFUL not to get bitten.

Table 1.2 Problems requiring immediate attention by the veterinary health care team

Respiratory distress	Bleeding from body orifices
Pale mucous membranes	Weakness
Neurological abnormalities	Rapid abdominal distension
Protracted vomiting	Inability to urinate
Severe coughing	Ingestion of toxins

Hospital triage

Three major body systems are assessed during the initial triage: respiratory, cardiovascular, and neurological. Triage begins when approaching the patient. Visually assess breathing effort and pattern; presence of blood or other foreign material on or around the patient; and the patient's posture and level of consciousness (LOC). Note if there are airway sounds audible without a stethoscope. Note whether or not the animal responds as you approach. If the animal is conscious, ask the owner about the patient's temperament and take the appropriate precautions regarding physical restraint or muzzling. The veterinary technician cannot rely on the client's statement that an animal "never bites," but if he or she is told that the patient is aggressive, the patient should definitely be muzzled. Physical restraint and muzzling should be performed with extreme caution in patients with respiratory distress, as such steps can cause acute decompensation and respiratory arrest. If time permits, a brief history should be obtained.

The ABCDEs

A reasonable and systematic approach to triage is the use of the ABCDEs of emergency care, which are: (A) airway,

approach the pet and place a makeshift muzzle using a neck tie, belt, or strips of cloth. If the animal is nonambulatory, owners may be told to place the animal in a box or carrier, or to use a blanket or towel as a stretcher (see Fig. 1.1). The use of a blanket stretcher makes it easier to get an animal in and out of a car.

When the caller is not a regular client of the facility, the staff member should obtain the client's phone number in case of disconnection and make the caller aware of the address, location, or easiest directions to the clinic. The client should be informed of the clinic's payment policy.

(B) breathing, (C) circulation, (D) dysfunction of the central nervous system, and (E) examination (see Fig. 1.2). Patients with respiratory distress or arrest, signs of hypovolemic shock or cardiac arrest, altered LOC, or ongoing seizure activity should be immediately taken to the treatment area for rapid medical attention. Conditions that affect other body systems are generally not life-threatening in and of themselves, but their effects on the three major body systems may be life-threatening. For example, a fractured femur bleeding into a limb can lead to life-threatening hypovolemia. The following is a list of problems that also require immediate medical attention:

- Exposure to toxins (ingested or topical)
- Excessive bleeding
- Open fractures
- Snake bite
- Burns
- Prolapsed organs
- Wound dehiscence
- Dystocia
- Trauma

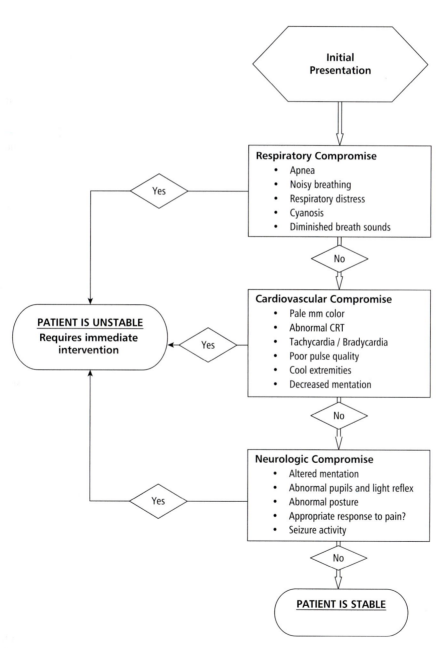

Figure 1.2 Triage Algorithm.

Airway and breathing

Expedient respiratory system assessment and rapid correction of abnormalities is critical. First, patency of airway and breathing effort should be assessed. This is done by visualization, auscultation, and palpation. When looking at the animal, an experienced individual can determine if the animal has increased breathing rate or effort. Some animals with respiratory distress may assume a posture with the head and neck extended and the elbows abducted (held away from the body). Additional concerning signs include absent chest wall motion, exaggerated breathing effort, flaring of the nares, open mouth breathing and paradoxical breathing. When sustained high breathing effort leads to respiratory fatigue, paradoxical breathing can occur, which is characterized by opposing movements of the chest and abdominal walls during inspiration and expiration. Cyanosis, a blue or purplish tint to the mucous membranes, usually indicates hypoxemia and warrants immediate medical intervention. The chest wall may be palpated to assess chest wall integrity. Crepitus about the body may indicate subcutaneous emphysema, which can be caused by tracheal tears or chest wall defects.

Some assessment questions the triage technician should consider:

- Is the patient having difficulty breathing?
- Are breath sounds auscultable?
- Are facial injuries interfering with the airway?
- Has a bite wound disrupted the larynx or trachea?
- Is subcutaneous emphysema present?
- What color are the mucous membranes?
- Does respiratory distress get worse with patient position change?
- Is there evidence of thoracic penetration or a flail chest?

Circulation

Many of the signs suggestive of decreased cardiac output are a result of a compensatory sympathetic reflex, which helps maintain arterial blood pressure. Clinical signs suggestive of decreased cardiac output include: tachycardia, pale or gray mucous membranes, prolonged capillary refill time, poor pulse quality, cool extremities, and decreased mentation. Decreased cardiac output may be due to hypovolemia as a result of blood or other fluid loss (internally or externally; active or historical), trauma, or cardiac disease.

Circulation is assessed by visualization, palpation, and auscultation. The focus of the cardiovascular assessment is the six perfusion parameters (see Table 1.3).

Table 1.3 The six perfusion parameters

- Mucous membrane color
- Capillary refill time
- Heart rate
- Pulse quality
- Extremity temperature
- Mentation

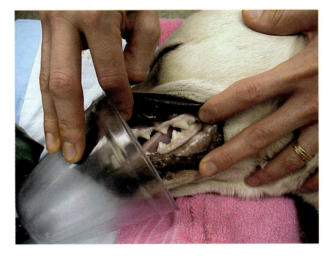

Figure 1.3 Assessing a patient's mucous membrane color.

Mucous membrane color

After assuring it is safe to do so, evaluate the mucous membranes by examining the color of the gums (see Fig. 1.3). As an alternative in the fractious animal or patients with pigmented gums examine the conjunctiva, penis, or the vulva. The normal color of pink is a result of oxygenated hemoglobin in red blood cells in the capillary bed. Mucous membrane color may vary with circulatory related problems. Mucous membrane color may be pale or white due to blood loss anemia or vasoconstriction. Brick red or injected mucous membranes are a result of vasodilation and can be seen with hyperthermia or sepsis. Cyanotic or blue mucous membranes are an indicator of severe hypoxemia. The absence of cyanosis does not rule out hypoxemia. Icteric or yellow mucous membranes are due to the breakdown of red cells (hemolysis) or liver disease. Methemoglobinemia results in brown or chocolate-colored mucous membranes.

Capillary refill time (CRT)

Evaluation of CRT is done by applying digital pressure to the surface of the mucous membranes and forcing the blood from the capillary bed and observing the return of color. Normal CRT is 1–2 seconds. A shortened CRT (<1/2 second) is suggestive of vasodilation. A prolonged capillary refill time (>2 seconds) is also a result of peripheral vasoconstriction and causes decreased peripheral perfusion.

Heart rate

Heart rate is a nonspecific parameter. It is usually measured by auscultation of the heart, palpation of the apex beat, or palpation of an artery. Increase in heart rate (tachycardia) may be caused by hypovolemia (the tachycardia is a compensatory mechanism), hypoxemia, hypotension, drugs, fever, excitement, exercise, and pain. Tachycardia is generally defined as a heart rate >160 beats per minutes (bpm) in the dog or 200 bpm in the cat. Decrease in heart rate (bradycardia) may be caused by increased vagal tone, severe electrolyte disturbances and hypothermia, drugs, or disturbances of the cardiac conduction system. Bradycardia is generally defined as a heart rate <60 bpm in the dog and 140 bpm in the cat. Auscultation of the heart also provides information about rhythm and murmurs. Auscultation of the heart and palpation of an artery should occur simultaneously, so that pulse deficits (the difference between heart and pulse rate; they should be the same) can be determined. Pulse deficits are suggestive of arrhythmias.

Pulse quality

Palpation of the artery provides information about the animal's heart rate and rhythm. The femoral or dorsal pedal arteries are the commonly palpated arteries. In addition, pulse quality is an indicator of stroke volume, the amount of blood pumped out of the heart with each beat. Palpating a peripheral pulse is feeling the difference between the systolic and diastolic pressures and duration of the waveform. Ideally, the pulse should be full, regular, and strong, indicating a normal stroke volume. A thready pulse is defined as a narrow waveform and a weak pulse refers to a small amplitude pulse difference, both of which are indicative of a decreased stroke volume. Bounding pulses have a large pulse pressure difference and wide waveforms usually associated with increased stroke volume and vasodilation.

Extremity temperature

The paws, limbs, or ears should normally feel warm to the touch. Cool extremities are a result of vasoconstriction.

Mentation

As previously mentioned, evaluation of mentation starts from afar. Observe the attitude of the patient without stimulation. If the patient has an altered mental state, it is assessed for its response to touch, sound, and painful stimuli. An inappropriate mental state can be a result of inadequate perfusion or a primary brain problem.

Some assessment questions the triage technician should consider:

- Is the patient's mentation normal?
- Is there evidence of hemorrhage?
- Is there swelling associated with an extremity or evidence of a fracture?
- Are the mucous membranes pale?
- Is the capillary refill time prolonged?
- Are the pulses weak and rapid?
- Is the heart rate abnormal?
- Are the extremities cold?

Dysfunction or disability of the neurological system

Dysfunction or disability refers to the neurological status of the patient. This may be assessed through visualization and palpation. A cursory neurologic exam is performed focusing on the patient's LOC, pupillary light reflex, posture, and response to pain (superficial and deep). Depressed mentation may be a result of poor oxygen delivery or trauma to the brain. Seizure activity may be due to intra- or extracranial causes.

A patient that is recumbent, has an abnormal posture, or is not seen to ambulate or make voluntary movements should be assumed to have spinal trauma and stabilized on a backboard (see Fig. 1.4) until proven otherwise.

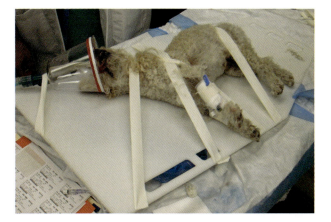

Figure 1.4 A patient with suspected head and spinal trauma restrained on a backboard. The cranial end of the board is elevated slightly because of suspected increased intracranial pressure.

Some assessment questions the triage technician should consider:

- Is the animal bright, alert, and responsive or obtunded (depressed but rousable), stuporous (roused only with painful stimulation), or comatose?
- Are the pupils dilated, constricted, of equal size, and responsive to light?
- What is the posture of the animal?
- Are there any abnormal breathing patterns?
- Does the animal respond to painful stimuli?
- Is there obvious seizure activity?

Examination

Finally, a rapid whole-body examination is performed. The goal is to determine and address any additional problems.

Some assessment questions the triage technician should consider:

- Are there lacerations, wounds, or punctures?
- Is there bruising and is it getting worse?

- Are there any fractures?
- Is the abdomen painful or distended?
- Is there evidence of debilitation or other signs of disease?

Summary

In some emergencies, minutes count. The triage performed by the veterinary technician should be rapid and efficient. The goal is rapid recognition of and intervention for life-threatening conditions such as hypoxemia and inadequate perfusion. A systematic approach to patient assessment is essential for the best possible patient outcome.

Reference

1. Bracken JE. Triage. In: Newberry L, ed. Sheehy's Emergency Nursing Principles and Practice. St. Louis: Mosby 1998;105–111.

2

The small animal emergency room

Martin D. Miller and Sean D. Smarick

Emergency medicine can be defined as "the diagnosis and treatment of unforeseen illness or injury."[1] The practice of emergency medicine takes place in primary care clinics during regular business hours or when veterinarians are on call, in dedicated "after-hours" free-standing emergency clinics, and in multispecialty referral hospitals. No clinical veterinary practice is immune to the realms of emergency medicine, as vaccines can cause anaphylactic reactions, anesthesia-related cardiopulmonary arrests can occur, and without warning clients may present a pet with a traumatic injury or critical illness.

The Veterinary Emergency and Critical Care Society (www.veccs.org), whose mission includes "To promote the advancement of knowledge and high standards of practice in veterinary emergency medicine and critical patient care," provides guidelines for emergency practice.[2] In looking to these standards along with applicable state board regulations, a practice should define for its patients, clients, the public, and for itself expectations for its *emergency* practice.

The practice of emergency medicine differs from primary care and other specialty practices by the urgency and breadth of the patients' conditions. Depending on the degree a practice wishes to diagnose and treat unforeseen illnesses and injuries, varying degrees of adaptations in the physical plant, equipment, inventory, staffing, and hospital systems are needed.

Physical plant

The facility requirements for an emergency practice at the most basic level do not differ significantly from a modern primary care practice. The differences between a dedicated emergency practice and that of primary care or specialty practice can be found in the layout and organization of space and equipment. The space needed ranges from a minimum of 2000–3000 square feet for a free-standing off-hours emergency clinic compared with 5000–10,000 square feet for a 24-hour emergency and critical care center either as a stand-alone facility or part of a multispecialty hospital (see Tables 2.1 and 2.2).

Hospital design and flow

When creating a floor plan concept for an emergency facility, a great deal of thought should be given to the specific aspects of the emergency practice. Good "flow" is essential to good design. Flow represents the natural movements of patients, clients, doctors, and staff in the daily activity of the practice;[3] arranging for such movement is almost like choreographing a dance. Thought should be given to dynamic situations such as how best to move clients from the lobby to examination rooms to discharge, and how most efficiently to move a large dog from x-ray to a surgical preparation area and then into a surgical suite.

In larger facilities the idea of a hub and spoke concept[4] can be applied to the flow of a practice. The hub can be a centralized space such as the treatment area. The spokes from the hub may be clinical areas such as the in-house laboratory, radiology, surgery, patient wards, isolation ward, and pharmacy. In even larger facilities, multiple hub and spoke areas may exist, such as one for the intensive care unit (ICU) and one for the emergency service. Industry-specific publications such as *Veterinary Economics* commonly address veterinary and emergency facility design.

Advanced Monitoring and Procedures for Small Animal Emergency and Critical Care, First Edition. Edited by Jamie M. Burkitt Creedon, Harold Davis.
© 2012 John Wiley & Sons, Inc. Published 2012 by John Wiley & Sons, Inc.

Table 2.1 Area approximation for a small dedicated emergency clinic

Space	Dimensions	Area (Sq Ft)
Lobby	15′ × 20′	300
Client bathroom	8′ × 8′	64
Reception area	10′ × 10′	100
Triage area	8′ × 10′	80
Exam room 1	10′ × 11′	110
Exam room 2	10′ × 11′	110
Exam room 3	10′ × 11′	110
Treatment room	30′ × 20′	600
Isolation ward	10′ × 10′	100
Surgical suite	15′ × 10′	150
Radiology	10′ × 8′	80
Staff bathroom	10′ × 9′	90
Staff break area	12′ × 10′	120
Administrative office	12′ × 10′	120
Utility/laundry room/storage	14′ × 8′	112
Total		**~2200 sq.ft.**

Table 2.2 Area approximation for a 24-hour emergency practice

Space	Dimensions	Area (Sq Ft)
Lobby	35′ × 25′	875
Client bathroom	8′ × 8′	64
Reception area	15′ × 10′	150
Check out area	10′ × 12′	120
Check out lobby	12′ × 15′	180
Triage area	8′ × 10′	80
Exam room 1	10′ × 11′	110
Exam room 2	10′ × 11′	110
Exam room 3	10′ × 11′	110
Exam room 4	10′ × 11′	110
Exam room 5	10′ × 11′	110
Consultation room	12′ × 12′	144
Treatment room	30′ × 40′	1200
Wards	15′ × 25′	375
Isolation ward	12′ × 12′	144
Laboratory	15′ × 20′	300
Surgical suite	15′ × 10′	150
Surgical preparation area	20′ × 12′	240
Radiology	12′ × 11′	121
Staff break area	12′ × 10′	120
Staff bathroom	10′ × 10′	100
Administrative office 1	10′ × 10′	100
Administrative office 2	10′ × 10′	100
Administrative office 3	10′ × 10′	100
Conference room	25′ × 15′	375
Doctors' office/library	15′ × 20′	300
Server room	8′ × 8′	64
Utility/laundry room	14′ × 12′	168
Storage room	10′ × 12′	120
Total		**~6250**

Lobby

Accessible to the (emergency) entrance of the facility, the client waiting area must be large enough to accommodate a simultaneous influx of many clients and their pets. While benches or more utilitarian styles of seating may work well in a primary care practice where wait times are short, the client presenting a pet for an emergency may spend hours in the emergency practice lobby. Comfortable, well-padded chairs, a beverage service in the form of a water cooler or vending machine, and a restroom that is easily accessible to the client should be considered (see Fig. 2.1).

Reception area

This is the area where clients are initially received and usually discharged. Ideally, some degree of privacy should exist for the discharge area where financial or sensitive communication is taking place.

Security

Emergency practices have more security concerns than day practices because they are open during non-business hours and may be perceived to be rich in cash and narcotics. To provide a safe environment for staff and clients, enhanced security measures should be considered.

An alarm system can be installed in the facility that can notify a monitoring service or the police if the alarm is triggered. In continuous operations, "panic" buttons can be placed, whereas door, window, motion, and other

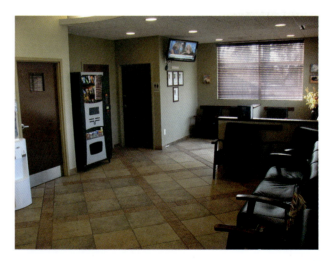

Figure 2.1 Lobby. Since clients may spend hours in an emergency practice lobby, it should be furnished with comfortable, well-padded chairs, beverage service, and an easily accessible restroom.

sensors can be used in off-hour practices. Cameras can be placed in critical areas such as the reception and check-out areas, and at exterior doors. These cameras can be viewed on a monitor that can be placed in a well-staffed area such as the treatment room or the doctors' and technicians' stations. Additionally, these cameras can be connected to a secure recorder or monitored by off-site services.

To allow for efficient traffic flow but provide some security, doors can be fitted with mechanical, electric, or magnetic locks. A mechanical door lock often utilizes a push-button combination lock to avoid the need for keys while maintaining relative security. Magnetic or electric strike locks are commonly found in combination with a proximity card reader close to the door or a remote release switch located in a secure area.

Triage area

The area where patients can be taken to establish their medical priority is referred to as a triage area (for further explanation of triage, see Chapter 1, Triage). The triage area may be a (dedicated) examination room or a specifically designed space easily accessible from the lobby. This space serves as a private area for a technician to greet clients and their pets while observing the presenting complaint and performing a triage physical examination (also called the primary assessment), which may include a rectal temperature and body weight if the pet is stable (see Fig. 2.2).

Usually, triage areas are simple spaces that include a surface such as an exam table or a gurney on which to

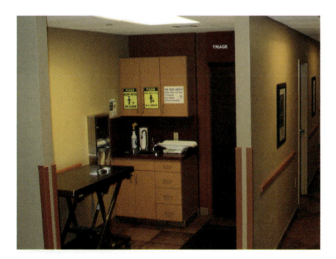

Figure 2.2 Triage. The triage area should be a specifically designed, private space easily accessible from the lobby that allows a technician to obtain the presenting complaint and perform a triage examination.

examine the pet. The space should also include a walk-on scale for larger dogs, an infant scale for cats and smaller dogs, and a gram scale for neonates or small exotics. It is also advisable to have a hand-washing sink in this area for both staff and pet owners who may have transported a soiled pet. Also, a mop sink close to this location is helpful to facilitate rapid cleaning of the area for the next patient.

Preferably a gurney and minimally a stretcher should be available to transport a nonambulatory patient. A portable oxygen tank (with a regulator, tubing, and a mask) can be stored in this area if it is some distance to the treatment area. Other items to stock in the triage area may include registration and critical or immediate care estimate forms, muzzles and other personal protection equipment, and basic bandaging materials that can be used to cover a wound or control bleeding.

Examination rooms

Examination or consultation rooms can be quite simple or rather complex, depending on preference and flow of the emergency practice. Basic design choices include the number of entrances to the room (a single common entrance as opposed to separate client and staff entrances), the size of the room, the types of examination surfaces (stationary, fold down, lift or elevator table), and whether to include a hand-washing sink, a hand sanitizer dispenser, or both.

While some practices may prefer stationary examination tables made of stainless steel or plastic laminate, an alternative with space efficiency advantages is the stainless steel ironing board–like fold-down tables. These tables provide flexibility for an unpredictable caseload, as small and medium patients can be examined on the table while larger breed dogs can remain standing on the floor with the table in the upright position. For a basic room with a standard folding, wall-mounted examination table, a room size of 10 feet × 11 feet is adequate.

The ability and desire to integrate technology into emergency practice exists, and electrical, networking, and hardware needs must be considered. Medical record keeping, review of diagnostic images such as digital radiographs, visual aid display, and website review can be accomplished with fixed computers with monitors in each room, a laptop computer on a roll cart, or a computer "tablet" with the appropriate (i.e., Internet) capabilities. Despite advances in technology, even practices with digital imaging in-house will need illuminated viewing boxes to review radiographic films.

To help comfort pet owners, especially those visiting their hospitalized pets, receiving difficult news, or having a pet euthanized, a hospital may provide consultation

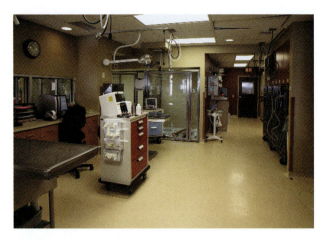

Figure 2.3 Treatment room. The treatment room is the heart of an emergency facility, and is home to treatment tables or stations, animal cages, in-house laboratory equipment, pharmacy, surgical preparation area, and doctor and technician workstations.

room(s) with a less clinical feel. Such rooms include comfortable furniture, extra floor space to accommodate an entire family, noncommercial lighting, and home-like interior appointments. Having an exit from the hospital in close proximity facilitates a private departure for a deceased pet or for emotional owners.

Treatment area

In a dedicated emergency practice, the treatment area is the heart of the facility (see Fig. 2.3). This space is home to treatment tables or stations, animal cages, in-house laboratory equipment, a pharmacy, a surgical preparation area, and doctor and technician workstations. As the size of the practice increases, some of these areas can be designed as separate spaces.

Emergency practice usually involves performing a number of procedures on each patient; therefore, an adequate number of quality work areas is needed. A vast array of treatment tables is available to outfit the emergency facility with a wide range of cost depending on features and materials. As with tables in examination rooms, a "dry" table would consist of a solid laminate or stainless steel surface; stainless steel dry tables may be on casters or wheels. A wet sink treatment table is a stainless steel tub ranging from a few inches to 18 inches deep and often topped with a grate and a removable solid stainless steel cover. These tables offer the opportunity to address procedures often associated with bodily and other fluids so often encountered in emergency practice. In a practice with no lack of debilitated patients, a hydraulic or electric lift table is recommended. Such a table may be fixed or may be on casters or wheels. Larger dogs can be placed on the tabletop at floor level and then

raised to an appropriate height for treatment or examination. A docking area for the electric lift tables should be available to keep the unit charged when not in use. Some manufacturers have combined features in their treatment tables such as the "wet sink" lift table or tables with integrated scales. It is important to account for the space surrounding these tables to accommodate the people and equipment often needed in addressing emergent and critical patients.

Adequate lighting is crucial in the treatment area and starts with high-quality overhead space lighting. This is then supplemented with mounted or portable examination lights to cover the treatment tables.

With the practice of emergency medicine comes an increase in the number of patient-side infusion pumps, heating devices, and monitors. Integrating the equipment in close proximity to the patient calls for utilizing door or pole clamps, adjacent cages, the tops of cages, or custom-built shelving or cabinetry between, above, or below the patient space. Electrical needs are met with an increased number of outlets strategically placed and having calculated the anticipated electrical load of the equipment. Adequate storage for this equipment in the form of shelving, cabinetry, or a closet should be considered along with the energy needs of charging internal batteries. Some practices have integrated "charging" closets with many electrical outlets and much shelving space.

Special treatment area consideration: The isolation ward

Emergency practices should have (or if dictated by state regulations, may be required to have) an isolation ward distinctly separate from the treatment area and other hospital areas[5] to house patients with communicable diseases. A consultation room may be incorporated into or adjacent to the space. These spaces are not only physically separate from other patient housing areas of the hospital but also have dedicated heating, ventilation, and air conditioning (HVAC) systems. Dedicating cageside equipment such as heat support and infusion pumps limits the potential for disease transmission to the general hospital population. Stocking the isolation ward with treatment supplies limits foot traffic and increases efficiency when treating patients in the ward (see Fig. 3.7).

The in-house laboratory

A dedicated area in the treatment room or a specific space near the treatment room should be planned for laboratory equipment and activities. The laboratory machines take up a good amount of counter space and deserve electrical considerations such as surge suppression, line conditioning, and potentially battery back-up. A dedicated sink in the proximity of the laboratory is useful for dealing with contaminated samples and is sometimes needed to drain laboratory equipment. A refrigerator and freezer will also most likely be necessary in the laboratory or in close proximity to store fluid samples and certain laboratory testing materials.

Radiology suite

The radiology suite in an emergency practice does not differ tremendously from a primary care practice: space is needed for an x-ray machine along with adequate distance or physical shielding as required by state regulations to protect the staff and patients from ionizing radiation. The image processing and storage considerations will differ tremendously between digital and film systems with the latter requiring space and mechanicals for a processor, and storage for unexposed and developed film. As more advanced imaging and related medical procedures may take place in an emergency practice, additional consideration for space and equipment should be given.

The surgical suite

As with the radiology suite, a surgical suite in an emergency practice is similar to that of any other veterinary practice with consideration given to the types of procedures being performed. Work flow and available space will dictate whether a separate surgical patient preparation area is needed adjacent to the surgical suite(s), along with a dedicated or shared storage area for surgical supplies, packs, and sterilization equipment. The incorporation of anesthesia and monitoring equipment, proper lighting, positive pressure HVAC, separate spaces for surgeon's scrub sink, and gowning area is an additional but not unique design consideration for this area.

Nonclinical areas

The size and scope of the nonclinical spaces can vary depending on the size of the practice and the makeup of the organization, but are nevertheless an important aspect in an emergency practice.

Staff spaces

Because emergency practice often involves a larger staff that work long shifts during which leaving the premises is often unrealistic, the design of the staff area should include a place for the staff to store, prepare, and enjoy a meal while on break. Water fountains or coolers should be available so that staff can remain hydrated through-

out their shifts. The size of the area and its complement of amenities, such as a refrigerator, microwave, stovetop, seating, and tables are determined by shift staff size and by other purpose(s) of the space (e.g., if the area also serves as a meeting or locker room). Lockers provide an efficient and secure option for storage of coats and a secure place for personal items. Adequate restrooms for the staff and clients should not be overlooked. The addition of a staff shower in a restroom may be a welcome amenity.

Office space

A designated space for doctors and technicians to use the telephone to communicate with clients, to prepare medical records, and to consult with each other should be contemplated. In an emergency practice, this area is often situated either adjacent to or as part of the treatment area; however, some practices also incorporate traditional office space distant from the clinical areas.

Meeting space

To address day-to-day administrative and management needs, facilitate staff education, and house all-staff meetings or referring veterinarian functions, meeting space is often incorporated into an emergency practice. The desired functions of the space and resources will dictate the size and amenities such as computer and Internet access, white boards, projectors, and seating.

Utility spaces

Throughout the facility, many spaces are needed for utility purposes. "Janitor's closets" are small spaces that include a mop sink, floor cleaning, and other cleaning supplies. These should be strategically located to allow for easy access and quick cleanup of any area in or around the hospital. A designated space for a refrigerator or freezer to accommodate deceased pets waiting disposition should ideally be located near a private door that can allow a crematory service to discreetly remove the bodies from the facility. Emergency practices use towels and bedding, and laundry facilities must be adequate to handle large loads continually. Storage space for items such as medical records, medical supplies, and pet food needs to be considered in the design of the facility.

Advanced emergency practices may start to resemble small hospitals, with central oxygen storage and manifolds, fire suppression systems, centralized medical or maintenance vacuums, anesthetic gas scavenging systems, and computer servers that all require space and supporting mechanical systems.

Equipment

Due to the increased number and severity of critically ill patients encountered in an emergency practice, the amount and sophistication of equipment often exceeds that found in a primary care facility.

Imaging

Imaging plays an important role in many emergency cases. A high quality radiographic system is crucial for a dedicated emergency practice, as is an ultrasound capable of detecting cavity effusions. Computed tomography (CT) and magnetic resonance imaging (MRI) are in use in some emergency centers, and may be considered for larger practices.

Radiography

Choices exist in both film-based and digital radiography. Considerations when deciding between film-based and digital radiography include throughput, image acquisition time, and capital expenditure. While film-based systems can of course offer diagnostic images, digital systems have the advantages of decreased required mechanical space, digital storage and filing, decreased labor and increased throughput, and, with some systems, virtually immediate image viewing. In a high emergency caseload practice, these advantages are more pronounced.

Ultrasound

The choices for ultrasound to detect cavity effusion are many, and easy access, durability, dependability, and cost-effectiveness must be considered when selecting an ultrasound machine for the emergency department.

Advanced imaging

Advanced imaging to include "diagnostic" ultrasound, CT, and MRI is rarely supported solely by an emergency practice but can be utilized as a shared resource with other in-house specialties or with other referral practices.

The in-house laboratory

Many emergency practices house a fair amount of point-of-care or in-house laboratory equipment. The Veterinary Emergency and Critical Care Society has established a guideline for the minimum capacity of an emergency practice laboratory.[2] At minimum, emergency practice in-house laboratories should include a microscope, microhematocrit and tube centrifuges, blood chemistry analyzer, blood gas and electrolytes analyzer (either in combination or separate), coagulation analyzer, and a cell counter.

Patient monitors and equipment

Patient monitors are needed to screen for physiological abnormalities and to monitor ill patients for disease progression. These monitors may include electrocardiographs (ECGs, often with an incorporated defibrillator); pulse oximeters; Doppler, oscillometric, and direct blood pressure monitoring systems; side- or mainstream capnographs; and temperature monitors. Electrical needs, networking, and telemetry are considerations when selecting monitors. Monitoring equipment may be separate or bundled together into multiparameter monitors or networks with central viewing stations.

Fluid and drug administration

Fluid infusion pumps and syringe pumps are required to deliver fluids and medications at set rates. Many fluid infusion pumps and at least a few syringe pumps are likely to be required in even a smaller emergency practice.

Thermal support

Many emergency care patients require heat support to maintain adequate body temperature. Patient warming devices are machines that provide external thermal support to the hypothermic patient. They generally utilize circulating warm water, forced warm air, or electrically generated heat, and each system type has its own advantages based on cost, versatility, reliability, and effectiveness.

Oxygen

Emergent patients often require oxygen supplementation, positive pressure ventilation, or anesthesia necessitating oxygen. Thus, oxygen access is vital to emergency practice. Several options are available to deliver supplemental oxygen. The most simple and appropriate for primary care settings is the oxygen tank ("E" size for portable tanks, "H" for stationary tanks) equipped with a regulator and hose. This system is connected to an oxygen cage, directly to a nasal cannula, to a nonrebreathing system with a mask, or to an anesthesia machine. Central systems consist of copper piping (which resembles water supply piping) that delivers oxygen from a source to the point(s) of care.

Oxygen sources

A simple cascade system can be employed as an oxygen source. This system involves a series of high-pressure oxygen tanks (usually size "H") that are connected via flexible piping to a main pipe that acts as the system manifold. Other oxygen sources include liquid oxygen or an oxygen generator. Backup systems with high-pressure tanks are often employed.

Oxygen delivery points

Oxygen is piped from the source manifold to oxygen receptacles. These receptacles have a special fitting (the Diameter Index Safety System) to connect oxygen hosing or a regulator. Quick connects are available in different popular configurations such as Chemetron, Puritan-Bennett, and Ohmeda (available from suppliers such as Precision Medical, Northampton, PA, and Allied Healthcare Products, St. Louis, MO). Oxygen receptacles can be placed on walls or in ceilings and can be recessed or wall-mounted.

Several types of cages are designed to create an atmosphere of higher oxygen concentration. The most simple is a clear plastic cage door that replaces the standard cage door. This door has an opening for an oxygen supply line that can be placed either directly into the cage or through a humidifying bubbler. While this setup is a relatively inexpensive solution as an oxygen cage, it provides no temperature control and has no integrated oxygen meter. To assess the cage's oxygen concentration, the probe of an oxygen concentration meter must be placed in the cage, and temperature and humidity in the cage must be monitored closely. An animal in a nearly sealed cage can raise the cage's temperature and the humidity quickly and considerably, leading to a heat stroke hazard. These cages can usually attain a maximum fraction of inspired oxygen (FiO_2) of approximately 0.6 (i.e., a 60% oxygen environment). Technologically advanced oxygen cages can be programmed to achieve a desired oxygen concentration, have nearly airtight door seals to minimize gas leak, often have integrated oxygen sensors, and can condition the interior space with digital temperature and humidity controls. Such oxygen cages can often achieve FiO_2s in excess of 0.8 (see Fig. 2.4).

Patients that do not respond to oxygen administration require positive pressure ventilation, which can be provided at the most basic level with a bag-valve-mask device, nonrebreathing circuit, or anesthesia machine. An anesthetic ventilator or ideally a critical care ventilator is used for long-term (more than a few hours') ventilation.

Anesthesia waste gas scavenging

Some practices simply use a specially designed charcoal canister that connects to the exhaust port valve of the anesthesia machine to collect waste gas. In emergency

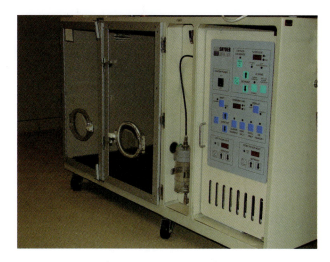

Figure 2.4 Critical care oxygen unit. Technologically advanced oxygen cages can be programmed to achieve a desired oxygen concentration, have nearly airtight door seals to minimize gas leakage, often have integrated oxygen sensors, and can condition the interior space with digital temperature and humidity controls.

practice, patients will undergo anesthesia in the radiology and other imaging areas, the treatment area, and the surgical and associated preparation areas. A centralized scavenging system can provide connections in strategic locations for anesthesia machines. When installed and maintained properly, centralized scavenge is one of the safest methods to deal with anesthetic waste gases.

Medical vacuum

Besides providing for suctioning of a body cavity in surgery, medical vacuum provides for airway suctioning and continuous thoracic drainage, all commonly used in emergency medicine. Minimally, a hand-powered device such as the Laerdal V-Vac Manual Suction Unit (Laerdal Medical Corporation, Wappingers Falls, NY) can be used for airway suctioning, while a central system similar to the oxygen and waste gas scavenging systems provides vacuum outlets in strategic areas. Portable, electrically powered suction units would be a compromise for a small practice.

Computer system

Practice management software saves time,[8] and allows for orderly storage of medical records, financial information, client database, and inventory information, all desirable attributes for an emergency practice. A networked computer system is needed for such software and includes a file server, a number of workstations, and printers. As medical records and financial data must be maintained as per regulation, appropriate data backup systems are strongly recommended.

In addition to being workstations equipped with practice management software, computers are a source of medical information. Searchable online or CD-ROM "textbooks" and access to veterinary Internet sites such as the Veterinary Information Network (www.vin.com) are invaluable when managing emergency cases, particularly when information is needed urgently or when there are no colleagues to consult.

Miscellaneous equipment

In a busy 24-hour emergency practice that uses towels and blankets for bedding, a large and near-constant flow of dirty laundry is the norm. Industrial laundry equipment is ideal for handling large loads on a continual basis. Due to the nature of the practice, an emergency hospital must be prepared to deal with deceased patients. A refrigerated cooler or freezer is necessary, which can range from a residential chest freezer to a walk-in cooler, depending on practice size and caseload. Many patients presented for an emergency require some fur removal, and a central, nonmedical vacuum system can provide efficient fur cleanup in addition to routine facility cleaning.

It is critical that an emergency practice provide continual care; therefore, a diesel or natural gas-fueled electrical generator is a consideration to power vital areas such as the treatment room, surgical suites, laboratory, security systems, computer networks, and the phone system in times of power outage.

Inventory

Providing high-quality care for the acutely ill patient requires a full inventory of supplies and drugs. Many emergencies can be treated with the inventory stocked by most primary care practices; however, due to the breadth and seriousness of disease encountered in emergency practice, an extensive inventory beyond that of a primary care clinic is required. The emergency caseload, resources allocated to inventory, and geographical location are relevant to the inventory. For instance, an emergency hospital that is near a 24-hour human community pharmacy or hospital may be able to take advantage of such resources and have fewer rarely used drugs in stock, while a practice without such resources will need a full complement of medications. Essential inventories for practices not routinely seeing emergencies and for dedicated emergency practices are shown in Table 2.3.

Medical supplies

Basic supplies to support the ABCs–airway, breathing, and circulation–should be stocked in every practice, while additional supplies may be found in more advanced emergency practices.

Airway management

A laryngoscope with multiple appropriate blade sizes, endotracheal tubes, and a bulb syringe for suctioning are basic emergency airway supplies that all practices should have. As a source of medical vacuum, a Yankauer suction tip and suction catheters are effective and should be considered for removing liquid from the pharynx and trachea, respectively. Lidocaine sprayed from an atomizer or directly instilled to a cat's larynx will help prevent laryngospasm. A polypropylene urinary catheter can act as a guide for the endotracheal tube during difficult tracheal intubation (see Chapter 23, Tracheal Intubation).

Ideally, supplies to perform a tracheostomy should be available in all practices; such supplies include self-retaining retractors, scalpels, sutures, needle drivers, and forceps. Many tracheostomy tubes are sold commercially, and a shortened endotracheal tube can be used if a tracheostomy tube is not available (see Chapter 23, Temporary Tracheostomy).

Breathing

Rescue breathing can be delivered with mouth-to-snout or endotracheal tube, but because such practice compromises caregiver safety, it is recommended only when no other option exists. Cost effective bag-valve devices are available through veterinary distributors (such as Jorgensen Laboratories, Loveland, CO). Practices that use general anesthesia usually have an anesthesia machine and nonrebreathing circuits that can be used to provide positive pressure ventilation.

Many emergency patients need oxygen supplementation even when they do not require endotracheal intubation. A practice should therefore have other equipment to deliver oxygen. Such items could include rigid plastic masks; hoods, which are commercially available or can be made from a plastic wrap-covered Elizabethan collar or a plastic bag; and nasal cannulas, which can be made from red rubber catheters or human bilateral nose prongs. Plastic wrap over the front of a cage or around a cat carrier with some area left for a vent can also be effective. See Chapter 20, Oxygen Therapy, for more detailed information.

Oxygenation and ventilation can be compromised by pleural space filling. Butterfly needles, peripheral intravenous (IV) catheters, extension tubing, three-way stopcocks, syringes, thoracostomy tubes, tubing connections, Heimlich valves, and three-bottle drainage systems are

Table 2.3 Emergency Practice Inventory

Emergency Medical Supplies*
  Bag-valve-mask e.g. Ambu bag
  Endotracheal tubes
  Feeding tubes, red rubber
  Heimlich valve
  Infusion needles, butterfly style
  Intraosseus cannula or spinal needles
  Intravenous catheters
  Intravenous drip and extension sets
  Laryngoscope with blades
  Lubricating jelly
  Oxygen mask(s) (hood)
  Pressure infusion bag
  Suction bulb (catheters and Yankauer tips)
  Three-way stop cock
IV Fluids
  0.9% sodium chloride for injection*
  Balanced and buffered electrolyte solution e.g. Lactated
  Ringers
  D5W for injection
Cardiac Drugs
  Atropine sulfate for injection*
  Lidocaine 2% for injection
  Nitroprusside for injection
  Propranolol
  Epinephrine 1:10,000 for injection*
  Sodium bicarbonate 8.4% for injection*
Sedatives/analgesia/anesthesia
  Acepromazine for injection
  Benzodiazepine*
  Dexmedetomidine
  Ketamine for injection
  Mixed and pure mu agonist narcotics for injection* (patch,
  tablets)
  Propofol
Reversal Agents (* if using relevant agents)
  Atipamezole
  Naloxone
Anti-infectives
  Aminoglycosides
  Anthelmintic
  Antiprotozoal
  Beta-lactam antibiotics
  Fluoroquinolone antibiotics
  Macrolides
  Metronidazole
  Tetracyclines

Miscellaneous
  Acetylcysteine
  Activated charcoal*
  Apomorphine*
  Calcium gluconate 10% for injection
  Chlorpromazine for injection
  Corticosteroid, quick acting* e.g., Dexamethasone sodium
  phosphate
  Dextrose 50% for injection*
  Diphenhydramine*
  Dopamine for injection
  Famotidine for injection
  Fomepizole or ethyl alcohol (* if ethylene glycol a potential
  toxin)
  Furosemide 5% for injection
  Methocarbamol for injection
  Metoclopramide for injection
  Misoprostol tablets
  NSAID for injection
  Oxygen*
  Oxytocin for injection
  Phenobarbital for injection
  Regular insulin
  Silver sulfadiazine cream 1%
  Sucralfate tablets
Ophthalmic
  Artificial tears ointment/drops
  Atropine 1% ophthalmic solution
  Eye wash (sterile buffered isotonic)
  Fluorescein stain ophthalmic strips
  Prednisone 1% ophthalmic solution
  Antibiotic solution (without steroid)
Transfusion supplies
  Donor dog or cat and donor supplies
  Blood administration set or in-line filter
  (Fresh) frozen plasma
  Packed red bloods cells or HBOC
  Blood typing cards
  Blood cross-match kit

*Essential.

supplies used to evacuate the pleural space. Such equipment should be on-hand and readily available at any emergency clinic. See Chapter 30, Pleural Space Drainage, for more details.

To evaluate for effective ventilation and oxygenation by measuring blood gases, the clinic must have syringes, needles, and heparin, or specialized pre-heparinized vented syringes, as discussed in Chapters 5 and 22.

Circulation

Maintaining effective circulating volume is crucial for the emergency patient, and every practice should have the ability to gain vascular access through intravenous catheters ranging from 24- to 16-gauge for peripheral placement. "Butterfly" needles offer a short-term alternative to IV catheters and are preferred to standard hypodermic needles for infusions. A pressure infusion bag can assist in delivering large volumes of fluids in a short amount of time. Intraosseous cannulation, an often overlooked vascular access technique, can be accomplished with hypodermic needles, spinal needles, or purpose-designed or mechanically placed intraosseous needles. See Chapter 4, Catheterization of the Venous Compartment, for more specific information.

The goal of maintaining effective circulating volume is to deliver oxygen to the tissues. When anemia is severe, an oxygen-carrying fluid must be provided. Disposables required for transfusion include equipment for blood typing and cross-match, blood administration sets, in-line filters, and collection supplies such as anticoagulant and blood collection bags for collecting donor blood in the clinic.

Advanced emergency practices may include long-term single or multilumen central intravenous catheters to obtain central venous pressure measurements, administer multiple infusions simultaneously, and obtain repeated venous blood samples, all of which provide a continuum from emergent to critical care.

Additional supplies

The emergency practice should have supplies available to cannulate any patient orifice or cavity. While red rubber catheters are cost-effective and versatile, a dedicated emergency practice should stock purpose-specific feeding tubes, urinary catheters (and collection bags), and wound drains, as these tend to cause less tissue reactivity and are more effective for the intended purpose. Orogastric tubes to address gastric dilatation and perform gastric lavage should be stocked in all but the most basic of practices. With each tube comes the need for specific connector(s), so appropriate adapters should not be overlooked.

Pharmacy

Any practice must minimally be able to address shock and cardiopulmonary arrest; dedicated emergency practices need to have a pharmacy to address infections, analgesia, sedation and anesthesia, intoxications, and emergencies of the gastrointestinal, endocrine, urogenital, ophthalmologic, and neurological systems.

Shock and cardiopulmonary arrest

Shock, defined as inadequate cellular energy production, is usually the result of hypovolemia, hypoglycemia, hypoxemia, sepsis, or cardiac failure and is the primary acute condition every practice should be prepared to address. Cardiopulmonary cerebral resuscitation (CPCR) minimally requires oxygen, a vasopressor (namely, epinephrine and justifiably vasopressin), atropine, and sodium bicarbonate as a buffer (and for treatment of hyperkalemia). See Chapter 16, Cardiopulmonary Cerebral Resuscitation, for more information.

Oxygen, not often thought of as a drug, should be the first one administered to all patients presenting in shock due to its ease of administration and high therapeutic index (ratio of therapeutic to toxic dose). Oxygen can be supplemented while an IV catheter is being placed.

The most common cause of shock is hypovolemia, and restoration of effective circulating volume with crystalloids, artificial colloids, and blood products may be needed. There is no universally ideal solution for resuscitation, so the more emergencies a practice sees, the more bags and types of fluids and blood products are warranted. Minimally, isotonic saline (0.9% NaCl) and a buffered, balanced electrolyte solution such as lactated Ringer's solution should be stocked. If blood products are not stocked, donors and blood collection supplies (or, if available, a hemoglobin-based oxygen carrier) are alternatives. More advanced emergency practices should also stock synthetic colloids and hypertonic saline.

Diuretics, antiarrhythmics, afterload reducers, and inotropes may be needed to address cardiac emergencies. For disturbances in electrical rhythm that may compromise cardiac output, atropine and at least one antiarrhythmic drug, each from the sodium channel blocking, beta-blocker, and calcium channel blocker classes, are recommended. Bronchodilators and corticosteroids may be needed to improve oxygenation in the patient with severe allergic bronchitis. A high percentage dextrose solution should be stocked as an emergency energy source.

Patients in septic shock, by definition, are not responsive to intravenous fluids alone and require vasopressors and possibly positive inotropes. Many inotropes and vasoactive medications require constant rate infusions (CRI). Infusion or syringe pumps to deliver these medications along with appropriate diluents, that is, D5W (dextrose 5% in water) are required for their administration.

The treatment for anaphylactic shock includes IV fluids, epinephrine, antihistamines, and glucocorticoids.

Anti-infectives

Antibiotics are used to treat, and in very specific situations to prevent, bacterial infections. Parenteral antibiotics effective against the organisms encountered in the emergent setting requires stocking antibiotics to address gram-positive and gram-negative, aerobic, and anaerobic organisms. Beta-lactam, fluoroquinolone, and aminoglycoside antibiotics are basic requirements, and metronidazole, macrolides, and tetracyclines play important roles. Antiprotozoal and anthelmintic medications round out the anti-infective inventory, with consideration given to the organisms and parasites encountered in the practice.

Analgesics

With a growing body of evidence supporting the benefits of effective pain control, the essential emergency pharmacy should have drugs for parenteral administration that interfere with the transduction, transmission, modulation, and perception of pain. Local anesthetics, alpha-2 agonists, NMDA antagonists, nonsteroidal anti-inflammatory drugs (NSAIDs), and opioids are classes of drugs to stock for analgesia. Chapters 42–44 provide more specific information on analgesia.

Sedation and anesthesia

Patients with an acute presentation usually raise cardiopulmonary concerns beyond those of a healthy patient; the drugs stocked for sedation and anesthesia in emergency practice should reflect this. Balanced anesthetic techniques with cardiovascular sparing drugs are most appropriate, and such drugs include opioids, benzodiazepines, and NMDA antagonists. Propofol, barbiturates, alpha-2 agonists, and promazines still play important roles in the emergent setting, despite their more profound cardiovascular effects.

Intoxications

Intoxications always warrant supportive care, which may tap into the essential emergency pharmacy, and every practice should carry gut decontaminant drugs such as activated charcoal. Dedicated emergency practices should have specific antidotes in stock as well. Either fomepizole or ethyl alcohol can be life-saving as an antidote for ethylene glycol. At least one form of vitamin K_1 (phytonadione) must be on-hand for anticoagulant rodenticide intoxication, and if the patient is already bleeding, fresh frozen plasma may also be required. Despite efforts at client education, acetaminophen and NSAID intoxications are still seen; such toxicities necessitate keeping acetylcysteine and misoprostol on the shelf. Based on geography and other factors, other antidotes also warrant consideration, such as crotalid polyvalent antivenin for crotalid snake envenomation, methocarbamol for metaldehyde-based snail baits or other tremoragenic toxins, and lipid solutions for fat-soluble intoxications.

Gastrointestinal (GI) medications

A patient presenting with signs referable to the gastrointestinal tract is one of the most common presenting emergencies. The emergency practice should probably carry at least one each of the proton pump inhibitors and H_2 antagonists as antacids; parenteral forms are often useful. Sucralfate should also be considered for local gut protection. Parenteral antiemetics affecting the chemoreceptor trigger zone or the vomiting center, such as NK-1 receptor antagonists, phenothiazines, metoclopramide, and 5-HT_3 antagonists, are the best antiemetics for the emergent patient. Antiemetics that decrease gut motility, such as aminopentamide, are contraindicated in many causes of vomiting.

Endocrine emergencies

Endocrine emergencies include hypoadrenocortism, diabetic ketoacidosis, and aberrations in calcium homeostasis. For Addison's disease, injectable dexamethasone is an important drug, as it will not interfere with ACTH stimulation testing. Due to dexamethasone's lack of mineralcorticoid activity, hydrocortisone or prednisone will be required for subsequent doses if a mineralcorticoid (such as desoxycorticosterone pivalate or fludrocortisone) is not available. Diabetic ketoacidosis requires intramuscular or intravenous administration of regular insulin. Hypercalcemia can be treated with IV fluids, a loop diuretic, an alkalinizing agent, and, in certain instances, a corticosteroid. Hypocalcemia requires parenteral calcium supplementation.

Urogenital emergencies

Urogenital emergencies amenable to pharmacologic intervention include dystocia, oliguria, and hyperkalemia. After ensuring adequate vascular volume, loop and osmotic diuretics may be required in an attempt to restore adequate urinary output. Hyperkalemia's affect on the heart may be antagonized by a slow IV push of calcium, while insulin and alkalinizing agents shift the potassium into the intracellular space.

Oxytocin, along with dextrose and calcium supplementation, is used to treat uterine inertia.

Ophthalmologic emergencies

Ophthalmologic examinations require a topical anesthetic for the cornea, fluorescein stain, and sterile, buffered saline eye rinse. Artificial tears and ointment are needed to prevent exposure keratitis in patients with decreased tear production or blinking, and in those under sedation or anesthesia, even for a short time. Glaucoma in the acute setting requires lowering the intraocular pressure with a topical and/or systemic carbonic anhydrase inhibitor, an osmotic diuretic, and/or prostaglandin analogues. Inflammatory diseases use a topical steroid product in the absence of corneal ulceration, and most bacterial infections can be addressed with a few choices in antibiotic ointments or drops. A dilating agent such as topical atropine offers relief from ciliary spasm and prevents synechia formation in corneal lesions.

Neurological emergencies

Medications to control seizures and lower intracranial pressure round out the drugs recommended for the emergency pharmacy. They include medications already presented: osmotic diuretics to address increases in intracranial pressure, and benzodiazepines, propofol, and pentobarbital for treatment of active seizures. Additionally, a long-term anticonvulsant such as phenobarbital is recommended for emergency drug loading.

Staffing the emergency practice

Depending on caseload variations of the season, day of the week, and time of the day; the scope of the practice; and the population serviced, staffing of a dedicated emergency practice can range from a single veterinarian and assistant to multiple veterinarians supported by a plethora of support staff.

Typical veterinary staffing (Certified Veterinary Technicians or Registered Veterinary Technicians, assistants, kennel aides, and receptionists) have roles in an emergency practice as they would in primary care. It is ideal to have a high ratio of technicians to veterinarians with the support staff in dedicated positions.[6] This can be accomplished with consistent and high case loads; however, case loads in emergency practice can vary tremendously and both veterinarians and support staff may be called upon to assume multiple or nontraditional roles.

The specialized skills and knowledge of the emergent practice staff will often find even Registered or Certified Veterinary Technicians and employees with years of experience in other practices needing additional training. In-house training programs are crucial at the basic level. The Academy of Veterinary Emergency and Critical Care Technicians offers an avenue to become a Veterinary Technician Specialist and gain recognition in the field by pursuing advanced training.

Due to the nature of emergency practice, a number of other unique staffing considerations exist. Scheduling for a practice operating off-hours or continuously 24 hours a day has challenges of shift transitions and continuing education, performance review, and staff meetings. The highly emotional environment of an emergency practice may also lead to compassion fatigue,[7] a detailed discussion of which can be found in Chapter 65.

Hospital systems

As discussed, facility, equipment, supplies, pharmacies, and staffing of an emergency practice are often larger and more complex than those for primary care practice. The off-hours, continuous operating nature of the emergency practice makes communication among coworkers and between management and staff difficult, yet it is crucial for the successful delivery of emergency care. The hospital systems in an emergency practice must address these challenges to keep operating smoothly.

Checklists

A continuously operating hospital must still be cleaned, stocked, and maintained. Managing these issues requires planning, implementation, and monitoring beyond that of a practice operating during more traditional hours. Checklists can be employed at regular intervals to allow for continuous operation and preparedness. To be effective, these checklists and the intended results must be reviewed by a supervisor or manager at regular intervals. For example, a checklist can be used at the beginning of every shift and after each use to ensure the proper stocking of a "crash cart." A daily supervisor spot check and an avenue for staff feedback are required to ensure that the system is effective.

Inventory

As discussed, the limiting factor of emergency care that can be provided may depend on a drug or supply. Due to the inconsistent nature of an emergency practice's usage of inventory items and the inability to obtain such supplies on a moment's notice during off-hours, a robust inventory system is needed. Inventory item usage can be tracked through physical markers signaling an item has been depleted, daily physical inspections, or utilizing practice management software that includes inventory control or a supply management system such as the computer-controlled bank of drawers often found in human hospitals.

Practice management software

A powerful tool in veterinary practice management is industry-specific software. This software can include client and patient databases, medical records, inventory control, invoicing, accounting, and even treatment orders. An emergency practice should seek a software vendor that provides features specifically for referral practices such as tracking the source of referrals, referring veterinarian information, and referral letter generation and distribution.[8] In addition to helping manage referring veterinarian relationships, computerized invoicing and medical records provide easy access to information from a patient's previous visits.

Medical records

Medical records contain the history of each patient and a chronology of the approach to the medical care given to the patient, and represent a critically important link to the patient.[9] Their contents may be regulated by the state veterinary board and the Veterinary Emergency and Critical Care Society (VECCS) recommends that the Problem Oriented Medical Record as outlined by the American Veterinary Medical Association be followed and be kept at the emergency facility.[2]

It is imperative that such records are legible and organized, because another veterinarian in the emergency, primary care, or other specialty practice must be able to continue care based on them. As discussed above, there are practice management software products that include medical record keeping and are therefore ideally suited for use in an emergency practice.

However, a "paperless" emergency practice is a challenge as not all the components of the medical record can be computerized. For example, paper "treatment sheets" are still commonly used in the dynamic environment of emergency practice despite the availability of computerized options. The system of treatment orders is an important one in emergency practice, and Chapter 64 provides a detailed discussion on medical charting. Other forms in emergency practice that are often kept on paper include authorization and estimate forms (especially for those patients in critical condition requiring immediate care), CPCR documentation forms, and certain lab reports.

Summary

While emergency practice shares many features with other types of veterinary practices, facility design, equipment, inventory, staffing, and hospital systems become more specialized to provide care for patients with unforeseen illness and injuries. Every clinical practice should have a minimal set of tools to treat common emergencies that are likely to be experienced in any practice.

References

1. American College of Emergency Physicians. Policy Statement approved 2008 for the definition of emergency medicine. Available at: http://www.acep.org/content.aspx?id=29164&terms=definition
2. Recommendations for Emergency and Critical Care Facilities. Available at: http://veccs.org/guidelines.php.
3. Hospital Design Planning Workbook. June 2008. Veterinary Economics. 49(6):S25–S31.
4. Hill, P. 2006 Renovating vs. Building New. Proceedings of the International Veterinary Emergency and Critical Care Symposium.
5. Murtuagh, R., Kaplan, P. 1992. Veterinary Emergency and Critical Care Medicine, p. 3. Mosby-Year Book.
6. Fanning J, Shepherd A. April 15, 2010. Contribution of veterinary technicians to veterinary business revenue, 2007. Journal of the American Veterinary Medical Association 236(8):846–846.
7. Huggard, P.K. & Huggard, E.J. 2008. When the Caring Gets Tough: Compassion fatigue and veterinary care. VetScript, May, 14–16.
8. Harper J. July 2005. Apples to apples: Comparing your software options. Veterinary Economics 46(7):66–82.
9. Principles of Veterinary Medical Ethics of the AVMA. Available at: http://www.avma.org/issues/policy/ethics.asp.

Further information

Academy of Veterinary Emergency and Critical Care Technician website: http://avecct.org.
Hospital design articles: http://veterinaryhospitaldesign.dvm360.com/.

3

ICU design

Joris H. Robben and Julie A. Eveland-Baker

The primary objective of an intensive care facility is to provide a high level of continuous patient care. A well-designed intensive care unit (ICU) is necessary for the creation of a safe, efficient, and, not the least, pleasant environment for patients, personnel, owners, and other visitors. In order to design an ICU effectively, it is necessary to define its requirements in terms of staffing and operations.

In veterinary medicine no consensus or standards exist regarding what should constitute an ICU for companion animals. Currently, there is a wide variety of ICU types in various clinical settings. Considering this variety, a description of current practices or effective design options can never be complete. Nevertheless, as in human intensive care medicine, veterinary medicine should strive for unification and basic, general guidelines for ICU design to ensure a predefined and, preferably, centrally guided, high quality of intensive patient care. The topics that are addressed here are intended to constitute a basis for such future guidelines.

In smaller practices with a variable need for intensive care it may be most economically viable to combine the ICU facility with the emergency service (ES) and recovery room.[1] Although these facilities are closely related, they should be considered separate units with different operational patterns. Physical separation is particularly important for the ICU as it helps to prevent unnecessary commotion and traffic, which may help to reduce the introduction of infection and improve patient comfort. This discussion will focus on intensive care medicine only, and the ICU will be considered as an independent, functional unit.

A well-designed ICU should not only have the correct floor plan, interior design, and equipment, but should also take into account staffing and have proper operating procedures as described in protocols and guidelines. For a successful design all these aspects have to be considered and put into context with one another. However, for reasons of constraint and in accordance with the intention of this text, this chapter will not discuss the important aspect of staffing. Most equipment used in the ICU will be discussed in other chapters of this book and the reader will be directed to those chapters for a more in-depth discussion. The aspect of operations will be discussed in general overview.

The design process

Development

Intensive care unit design has significant impact on daily patient care. The extensive investment of time and effort in the long and complicated design process will be rewarded when one experiences its positive impact on the day-to-day operations. A stepwise approach helps to organize the development from initial concept to completed structure (Table 3.1). The planning and design process should include research that leads to evidence-based recommendations for materials in compliance with local legislation directives. A major step in the development process is the description of ICU program goals and objectives. These can be best defined by a planning team that includes ICU veterinarians and technicians, pet owners, administrators, and design professionals.

Advanced Monitoring and Procedures for Small Animal Emergency and Critical Care, First Edition. Edited by Jamie M. Burkitt Creedon, Harold Davis.

© 2012 John Wiley & Sons, Inc. Published 2012 by John Wiley & Sons, Inc.

Table 3.1 Steps in planning and Designing a Veterinary ICU

1. Review of articles on practice, team building, and planning
2. Education in the change process
3. Visits to new and renovated units
4. Vendor fairs
5. Legislation and local directives relating to the build
6. Vision and goals
7. Development planning
8. Space planning, including methods to visualize 3-dimensional space if available
9. Operations planning including traffic patterns, functional locations, and relationship to ancillary services
10. Interior planning
11. Surface materials selection
12. Review of blueprints, specifications, other documents, and mock-ups
13. Building and construction
14. Post-construction verification and remediation

Based on White RD, 2007.[2]

The intensive care facility and all its contents should support, and be a logical extension of, the manner in which the ICU is operated. Therefore, the design should creatively reflect the vision and spirit of ICU staff and pet owners. It is important to allow everyone involved in the development process to comment, as design aspects have to be judged from different perspectives. A close interaction between external experts in hospital construction and an internal interdisciplinary team is mandatory to reach a professional design that agrees with user requirements.

Location in the hospital

The unit has to be situated within the hospital in relation to other facilities such as ES, anesthesia induction and recovery room, intermediate or general wards, and ancillary services. Close proximity to the surgical theaters, recovery room, and ES reduces the distance to move critically ill patients and enables the easy transfer of staff, equipment sharing, and the common use of ancillary functions. Furthermore, the sharing of engineering services can more easily be accomplished during the building process. The ICU should be located with consideration for other services that receive ICU patient or personnel traffic. Such services include the diagnostic imaging facilities, pathology, and the clinical laboratories if limited or no point–of–care testing is available in the ICU. In the absence of imaging technicians and laboratory staff, ICU personnel should be able to use these facilities in a swift and easy manner.

Facility configuration

An ICU can be divided into three major areas: staff work area, patient area, and ancillary services. The last is either part of the facility or located elsewhere in the hospital and shared with other services. As with the location of the ICU within the hospital, the topographic positioning of areas within the ICU should be considered and defined early in the design process. The value of the relationships between different rooms, areas, and functions can be *prioritized* by a system of grading. It helps in this conceptual phase to think of the ICU as a group of concentric circles with the patient modules at the center. (For the purpose of this discussion, each individual patient care area, i.e., cage and direct surroundings, will be considered a *patient module.*) By positioning the different rooms, areas, and functions within the smaller and larger concentric circles surrounding the patient modules, relations can be discussed and adjusted accordingly.

The *character* of the relationship between areas, rooms, and functionalities must also be described, and is based on the need for visual or auditory contact with patients, and the patterns of physical movement of patients, people, and materials (being either clean or dirty, small or large) through the space.

Based on the priorities for ICU positioning within the hospital, the priorities for situating areas and functionalities within the ICU, the need for shared engineering services, and design considerations from other services, the configuration of the facility can be drawn within the limitations of the building.

ICU size

Several aspects must be taken into consideration when deciding on ICU size (Table 3.2). A facility that can accommodate 6 to 12 patients with a mean occupancy of 60%–70% is often considered a practical and viable companion animal ICU size. Smaller units may not benefit from economy of scale, and may garner an insufficient caseload to maintain skills and expertise. Larger units may present problems of clinical management.[3] Larger units should only be considered when the facility admits patients to the ICU that need less intensive care, such as when a facility combines intensive care with a medium care function. Larger institutions could consider the design of subunits that manage patient care independently.

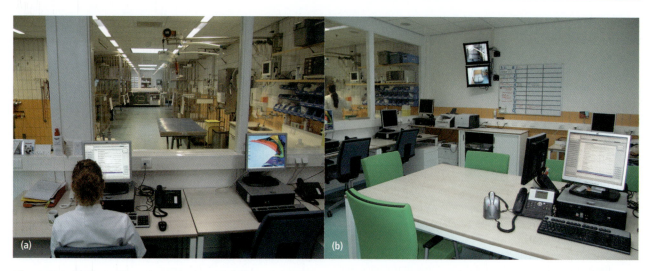

Figure 3.1 (a) The entire patient area can easily be surveyed from the technicians' station through large glass windows. (b) With the use of cameras in the isolation ward and wall-mounted monitors in the technicians' station, the isolation ward can be monitored from within the station. Auditory surveillance is possible through the installation of microphones and speakers.

Table 3.2 Considerations to determine the size of the intensive care facility

Historical information	Size of previous ICU facility
	History of patient refusals at prior size
Regional influence	Role in the regional veterinary community
Size of hospital/practice	
Size and type of other specialties and facilities	Presence, size, and level of the emergency service
	Presence, size, and level of other in-hospital specialties
	number of surgical theatres, surgical case load
Organizational restrictions	Space available
	Staffing available
	Type of patients (admittance policy)
	Level of care
	Number of elective (planned) admissions
	Financial restrictions

The ground plan

Staff work areas

Technicians' station

A central technicians' station can improve organization and efficiency of patient care and improve comfort and convenience for technical staff. Such a station should be an area of sufficient size to accommodate all necessary staff functions. The station should be situated such that it offers a clear, unobstructed view of the patient area. Sliding glass doors and glass partitions function to separate the technicians' station and the patient area acoustically (both ways) (Fig. 3.1a).[4] If an isolation ward is part of the ICU, visual and audible contact should be available from the station (Fig. 3.1b).

The station should contain an area or desk with computer terminals for patient record maintenance and Internet access. This setup facilitates more detailed record compilation, completion of requisitions, and in- and out-of-hospital telephone communications. The station could also accommodate storage facilities for protocols, patient chart material, request forms, and other medical stationery. Depending on the space available a medical book collection, printers, fax, photocopier, and a table to perform patient rounds can be made part of the station. Anything that makes work efficient and the working experience attractive should be considered for this area.

If the technicians' station cannot provide enough room for all these facilities and functions, a separate medical or administrative office should be available in close proximity to the patient area.

Staff break room

Work in an intensive care unit can be physically demanding, and staff should have the opportunity to step back from the environment when necessary and as part of scheduled breaks. A staff lounge should provide a private, comfortable, and relaxing environment with external windows, comfortable seating and distractions such as magazines, radio, and television. Kitchen facilities such as a sink, microwave, food refrigerator, and dishwasher may be integrated or directly adjacent. Lockers for safekeeping of personal belongings can be installed. The room should be equipped with communication systems such as telephones, computers, intercom, and emergency call buttons.

Conference or multipurpose room

This room facilitates staff meetings, teaching sessions, and other group meetings. For this purpose it should contain proper seating, projection facilities, a white board, and illuminated viewing box. It can also be used as a library by equipping it with journals, reference books, internet-connected computer terminals and printers. Both the staff break room and the conference room should be in close proximity to the ICU so that staff are not dispersed during their absence.

Patient area

The patient area should be compact and offer close, unobstructed visual (and audible) contact with all patients. The number of staff in a veterinary ICU is often limited, and one staff member should be able to monitor multiple patients at once. This factor should play a major role in the positioning of the different patient modules in the area. However, the requirement for a relatively small unit must be balanced with the need for increasing numbers of cage-side monitors and therapeutic equipment, the growing awareness of the importance of hygiene, and the need for a pleasant, comforting and ergonomically designed environment for patients, staff, and owners.

The patient area should allow unobstructed movement of staff, owners, visitors, patients, and equipment. Therefore, doors, aisles, and corridors should be designed such that stretchers, patient carts, and large equipment can easily be moved around within the unit and into and out of the facility.

Besides the presence of patient modules and a treatment area for specialized procedures, the patient area is often used for storage of disposables, smaller (surgical) equipment, and larger medical equipment for monitoring and treatment. However, the storage of such disposables and equipment in the patient area should be minimized, as it contributes to the impression of chaos and limited space.

Patient modules

Patient modules consist of the patient's cage and its direct surroundings, the "bedside." The modules should be arranged and designed in such a fashion that observation of *all patients* by direct or indirect (e.g., by video monitor) visualization is possible from many locations in the ICU. Such an arrangement permits the monitoring of patient status during both routine and emergency circumstances.

Patient modules should be designed to support all necessary healthcare functions. Nursing staff spend considerable time monitoring, supporting, and treating patients. Therefore, patients should be easily accessible, and ergonomics and hygiene should be considered. The more complex the care rendered, the more "bedside" space should be available to position the supporting and monitoring equipment. Equipment should not impede access and nursing care to the patient.

These considerations force us to rethink the design of the patient area with special attention to the concept of the patient module. Different frequencies and intensities of care may warrant different types of patient modules to cater to different types of patients. The admittance policy should be considered when deciding on the baseline patient module. A well-balanced mix of different patient module types to include moderate, advanced, and intensive one-on-one patient care options probably serves needs best. This variety allows more economic use of the limited available space.

"Bedside" utilities

One of the most valuable resources to have at the "bedside" is space. Open space maximizes access for caregivers, reduces cross-contamination between patients, and provides the most private and comfortable environment for visiting owners.

Every patient module should have its own light. This enables the staff to care for one animal during quiet, nightly hours without having to use the main light that illuminates the whole patient area. Preferably, every cage is equipped with one or more devices for warming the patient, such as floor heating or a heating lamp.

Light switches, electrical power sockets, and other outlets must be organized to ensure safety, easy access, flexibility, and maintenance. Depending on the type of cage, outlets can be mounted on the wall above or on both sides of the enclosure. Alternately, they may be brought from the wall or ceiling in a more free-standing arrangement to a boom or trunk over the cage, via a "stalactite" structure from the ceiling or via a "stalagmite" structure from the floor. The number and location of the power sockets depend on the amount of electrical equipment, but a minimum of eight per patient module seems reasonable for most patient modules, especially with the routine use of infusion pumps (Fig. 3.2). The

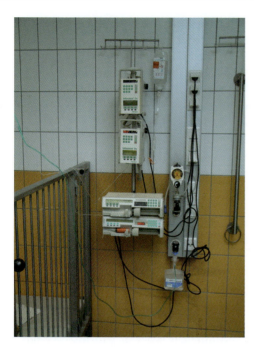

Figure 3.2 With the ever-increasing use of infusion pumps and other medical equipment, the need for power outlets increases. A number of 8 per patient module seems sufficient in most instances but up to 16 may sometimes be necessary.

current standard in human medicine is as many as 16 power sockets per bed.[4]

The number of outlets for vacuum, oxygen, and compressed air may vary with the type of patient module, but every cage should have easy access to at least one of each. Patient modules designed for mechanical ventilation need more service outlets and may need an extra outlet for evacuation of anesthetic gases.

Equipment may be supported on wall-mounted rails, shelves, the top of the cage, or on mobile service stands ("drip poles"). When equipment is too heavy, too bulky, or is shared between patient modules, it can be mounted on a trolley. A combination of these arrangements may be suitable. Bedside monitoring equipment should be located to permit easy access and viewing, and should not interfere with the visualization of, or access to, the patient. The status of each patient should be readily observed at a glance. This goal can also be achieved by a central monitoring station (telemetry) that permits the observation of more than one patient simultaneously, preferably from within the technicians' station.

Storage units (cupboards, baskets, shelves) could be placed in more advanced patient modules to provide for easy access to specific drugs, disposable materials for specific patient care procedures such as mouth care, and emergency resuscitation equipment.

The patient's daily record and flow sheet can be located in the patient module or at the central technicians' station. Their position should be easily accessible to the nursing and medical staff (Fig. 3.3). A move toward paperless bedside recording as is now the custom in human medicine is not expected soon in veterinary medicine.

Cage designs

As care and treatment of patients is the core duty of an ICU and is primarily performed in and around patients, the design of the cages is of the utmost importance. Many different "cage" designs can be found in veterinary ICUs today (Fig. 3.4).

A kennel or run can be described as a small fenced space with a door at the front (Fig. 3.4a); such a space is often used to enclose larger dogs. When the patient is recumbent, care and treatment must be performed on the floor of the kennel, often with the patient positioned on padded bedding or a mattress. Runs make it difficult to position equipment, and often drip poles are used in or in front of the run. From the perspective of hygiene, practicality, and working conditions for the staff this is less than ideal for the treatment for most types of ICU patients.

"Stacked" cages can be made of stainless steel, fiberglass, or plastic and can be stacked in different arrangements (Fig. 3.4b). The cages have a wire or plastic front with a door and all other sides closed. This setup of cages appears most widely used in companion animal ICUs. Such a conformation uses limited space, which is often important in an ICU. Although the construction is more elevated than a run, the close contact between patients is not ideal for maintaining hygiene and reducing cross-contamination. Cages that are positioned in the second or third row from the bottom offer an ergonomic advantage. Patient visibility is not optimal, as one must stand directly in front of the cage to be able to see clearly inside. Equipment, wires, and infusion lines can only reach the patient from the front. With several patients housed directly next to and on top of each other, this arrangement often makes the whole situation chaotic and difficult to oversee. Additionally, banks of cages such as these make procedures that require two or more veterinary technicians difficult (or impossible) to perform with the animal in the cage. Considering added equipment and lines, this setup makes patient care challenging.

Ideally, oxygen cages control not only the oxygen concentration in the closed environment of the cage, but also temperature, humidity, and carbon dioxide levels. Many ICUs are fitted with one or two oxygen cages, as they are an easy way to administer oxygen with minimal

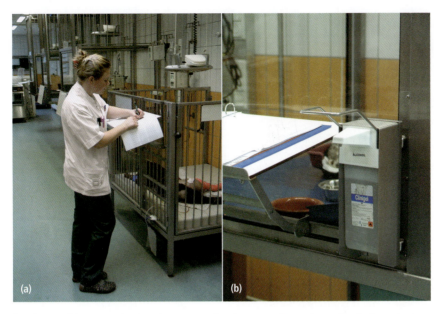

Figure 3.3 (a) A small writing tableau attached to the cage makes it easy to keep the patient's flow sheet current. The tableau can be folded away when not in use to increase space for maneuvering carts and equipment. (b) An alcohol dispenser is placed conveniently alongside some tableaus so staff can disinfect hands and forearms between patients.

patient stress. Some ICUs have made the oxygen cage their standard cage, mainly because they are convenient. The oxygen cage makes it difficult to have frequent, direct physical contact with the patient without sacrificing oxygen supplementation, and current oxygen cage designs sometimes fail to maintain the environment at preset values. Although the smooth inner surface of many designs makes cleaning the cage easy, disinfection of the cages' internal gas delivery systems can be cumbersome. Some oxygen cage designs provide more space for the patient and service openings on the cage's side; such designs make visual contact with and approach to the patient easier than with stacked cages. Auditory contact is often hampered by the closed environment and the noise of the air conditioning.

Wall-mounted or free-standing singular cages are designed such that the bottom of the cage is at table height (Fig. 3.4c). The design as shown in Figure 3.4c originates from combining the characteristics of a metabolic cage with those of a fume cabinet. Three or all sides of the cages are made out of glass windows or bars that give ideal visualization of the patient. These cages can be opened from two sides, which makes it possible for two or more people to handle the patient at once. Equipment and lines can easily be organized around the cage. Of course such a cage takes up more space, but it is ideal for dealing with ICU patients that need elaborate intensive care.

The "playpen" type cage is an excellent alternative for large dogs (Fig. 3.4d). Its bottom is conveniently lifted about 40 cm from the floor: easy for the patient to step into and raised enough to ensure hygiene. The whole construction is made of stainless steel, and the doors and bottom can easily be taken out for proper cleaning and disinfection. The bottom is lined with a watertight cushion. The playpen height is more comfortable for staff than a floor-level run. Equipment and lines can be easily organized around the cage.

"Mechanical ventilation" station

An ICU that has the resources to perform long-term mechanical ventilation should have one to three stations specifically designated for this task (Fig. 3.5). Rather than being restrained by a cage, patients are immobilized by anesthesia or neuromuscular disease. Ventilated patients need intensive care with frequent contact with caregivers and connection to many monitoring devices and other equipment such as infusion pumps. An open area with a table for the patient in the center serves these needs best. The ventilator and most supporting equipment can be arranged at the head of the table.

It is ideal to be able to change the height and tilt of the patient table. Patients that are immobile over a long period need special attention to prevent pressure lesions. The table surface should be padded and large enough for the patient to lie comfortably without its legs extending beyond the edge of the tabletop. For most hydraulic tables this means the top must be extended beyond the standard size.

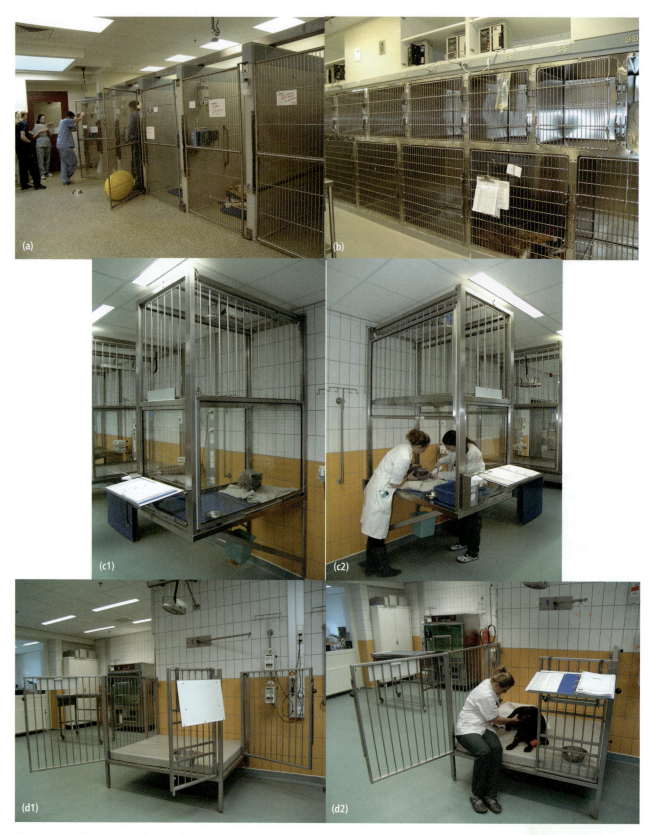

Figure 3.4 Different cage designs that are used currently in companion animal ICUs. See the text for additional information. (a) Kennel/run (ICU, Cummings School of Veterinary Medicine at Tufts University); (b) stacked cages (ICU, Cummings School of Veterinary Medicine at Tufts University); (c1, c2) wall-mounted singular type; (d1, d2) "playpen" type.

Procedure area

A procedure area is often included in the patient area because many minor interventions such as catheter placement and wound management are performed in the ICU (Fig. 3.6), and a different room would separate staff from the patients for too long. The treatment area is organized around one or two procedure tables. A hydraulic table with a tiltable top offers advantages for some medical interventions. A wet table enables patient bathing and wound care; however, close attention to hygiene is imperative when considering such a construction in the ICU.

One or two high-intensity lights should be mounted above every table. The table should be easily accessible

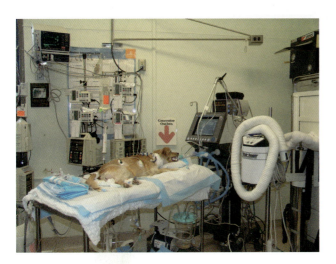

Figure 3.5 Mechanical ventilation station.

by multiple staff from different directions. On one or two sides, the procedural table can be surrounded by countertops on which to arrange and prepare disposables and equipment. A hands—free hand-washing station should be available in this area. Positioning of rails or shelves for support of monitoring equipment above the countertop permits easy access and viewing. Light switches, electrical power, oxygen, compressed air, vacuum, and gas evacuation outlets must be easy to access. They can be mounted on the wall above the counters. The number and location of the power sockets depend on the number of electrical appliances present on the shelves or counter. A free-standing, ceiling-mounted, or floor-mounted utility column directly adjacent to the procedural table improves access and flexibility; the column can also contain controls for the lighting. The use of mobile devices such as poles, carts, and trolleys should be limited, as they often hinder patient and staff mobility. However, there should be room to place the crash cart, mechanical ventilator equipment, or other larger equipment that may be required near the procedural table(s). Some storage facilities such as cupboards, drawers, refrigerator, freezer, and incubator for fluids can be positioned under the counters or above them. As the treatment area is often centrally located in the patient area, this is a suitable place to park a fully equipped crash cart.

Isolation ward

The isolation ward is ideally maintained as a separate facility in close proximity to the ICU. The entrance to the isolation ward should consist of a separation

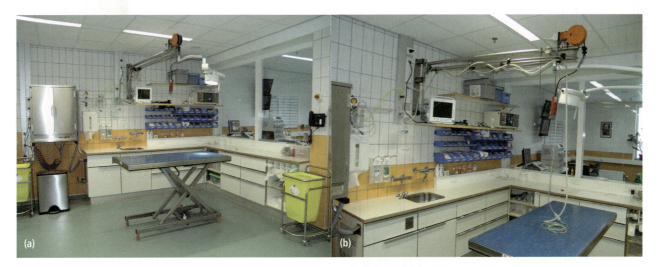

Figure 3.6 (a) The procedure area contains all the necessary equipment to perform small surgical interventions. (b) When the ceiling is not available for a service unit, a mobile arm mounted on the adjacent wall can bring all necessary wires and tubes to the table, which prevents people from tripping over them.

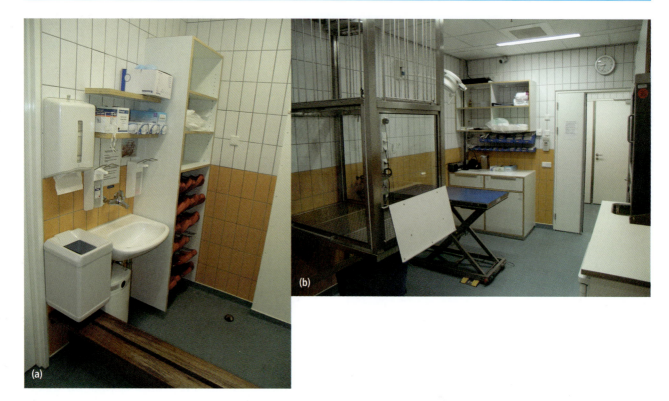

Figure 3.7 (a) The isolation ward can be accessed via a separation corridor, which enables staff to change clothing and wash and disinfect hands. (b) As much as possible, the isolation ward should function stand-alone. Therefore a small treatment area is part of the isolation ward.

corridor (Fig. 3.7a). This area should make it possible to prepare to enter the ward with appropriate protection, and to leave it with minimal risk of breaching the isolation. The corridor should be divided in two separate areas, potentially separated with a shower. The corridor should enable the change from regular hospital clothing to protective gowning, hair cap, footwear, and gloves, and should include a hands–free hand-washing station. When a completely separate facility is not feasible, a closed room adjacent to the ICU with a large glass window for easy observation of patients can be effective. Sometimes the only practical and cost–effective alternative is to isolate patients in part of the main ICU patient area; however, this puts the general ICU population at much higher risk. Besides dedicated personnel, design considerations such as temporary physical barriers should be considered.

The isolation ward should be designed to function independently as much as possible without needing to introduce disposables or equipment (Fig 3.7b). Ideally, the isolation area is a smaller version of the main patient area with storage facilities, refrigerator, a procedure area, and patient area. As this room is to isolate patients, only a limited number of cages (two to four) are necessary.

Very rarely do pets have to be isolated as a group and probably not many facilities can provide for that in a cost-effective manner. Any disposables or contaminated equipment should leave the isolation area in sealed containers for further processing.

Ventilation systems for isolation rooms should be independent of other systems in the hospital with 100% exhaust to the outside. Ideally, the system should have the capacity to create negative or positive air pressure (relative to the open area). If the room is designed to control airborne infections, all walls, ceilings, and floors, including doors and windows, should be sealed tightly.

Separate isolation facilities should have electronic means of communication. Remote patient monitoring capability via cameras and microphones with a central viewing location in the ICU is necessary (Fig. 3.1b).

Outside runs

ICU patients often have limited mobility. However, for a successful recovery the incentive of a small outside area close to the ICU can be important. The use of patches of (artificial) grass invites patients to relieve themselves more easily, but hygiene is more difficult to maintain compared with a concrete area. As there is constant risk of cross-contamination, this outdoor area is dedicated to ICU patients alone and not shared with other hospitalized animals, and (as much as possible) these areas should be cleaned and disinfected after every patient visit.

Ancillary rooms

Laboratory facilities

The ICU should have easy access to a laboratory facility which supplies emergency–directed 24–hour clinical laboratory services. When such services cannot be provided by the central hospital laboratory, a satellite laboratory within the ICU must serve this function. It is advantageous to have the laboratory facility close to the patient area so that technicians are never far away in case of an emergency in the ICU.

At a minimum, it is ideal to have 24-hour capability to measure blood gas and electrolytes, blood glucose, packed cell volume, total protein, activated clotting time, blood urea nitrogen, and creatinine, and to have a microscope to evaluate cytology and blood smears.[5] The laboratory bench should offer enough space and be equipped with a sufficient number of power outlets for all the necessary equipment. Network connections may be necessary to link laboratory equipment with the hospital network and download laboratory results directly into the patient's medical record.

Fume hoods may be advantageous or even legally required if stains for cytological preparations are used. A sink and water tap can sometimes be fitted with a device to produce laboratory quality deionized water. There should be enough room to store instruction manuals and administrative records, and to stock laboratory disposables and reagents, in a refrigerator or freezer if necessary. Also a refrigerator, freezer, and heating incubator dedicated to the temporary storage of biological specimens must be readily available. Connections and space for a computer terminal and a communication system may be considered. Local regulations may demand emergency shower or eye wash installation.

Pharmacy

Guided by local considerations and organization, a satellite pharmacy can be part of the ICU. A separate room is warranted if the ICU is serviced by its own pharmacy. The air–conditioned pharmacy should have room for storage of medications including a lockable cabinet for controlled substances, a refrigerator for pharmaceuticals, storage for intravenous (IV) fluids, and a refrigerator and a freezer for the storage for blood products. A

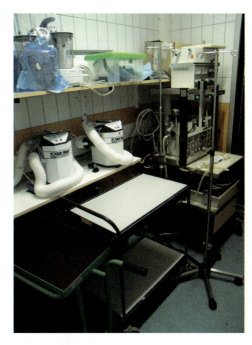

Figure 3.8 A separate room for storage of medical equipment helps keep the patient area organized and uncluttered. The walls of the room can be fitted with shelves and rails. Part of the wall should be kept clear to accommodate free-standing items. Shelving should be shallow for easy location of desired equipment.

small counter with storage cabinets, drawers, a sink, and water tap must be provided to prepare medications. A glassed wall can be used to permit visualization of patients and ICU activities while preparing medications if this area is enclosed.

Medical equipment storage

Unused drip stands, trolleys, gurneys, pediatric incubators, portable suctioning devices, ultrasound machines, and so on cannot stand in the patient area, as they contribute to a cluttered, disorganized appearance of the ICU. This equipment is best stored in a separate room with easy access for retrieval (Fig. 3.8). Appropriate, grounded electrical outlets should be provided within the storage area in sufficient numbers to permit recharging of battery-operated items. Lockable storage should be provided for small but valuable items and fiber–optic equipment.

Consumable supply storage

Any ICU depends heavily on a multitude of disposables and recyclable equipment, like sterile minor surgery packages. Depending on the size of the practice or hospital, a three–stage storage management system may be desirable. The central supply of the hospital/clinic constitutes the first storage area. The second storage area consists of a utility room adjacent to the ICU. Storage can be organized on open scaffolding, on shelves, in cupboards, and in drawers. A desk with a computer and sufficient room for administrative papers allows for convenient management of inventory. The third and final storage space is situated in the patient area itself for items frequently used. Attempts to stock everything in the ICU itself causes overcrowding, as needs always grow over time.

Soiled bedding and waste disposal storage

There should be a dedicated area for storing soiled bedding, waste materials, and material for recycling until collection. This material should not be kept in the main ICU patient care area. The size and nature of this space will depend on the arrangements for collection. If the practice or hospital has a central facility, this can also be used.

Facilities outside the ICU complex

What should be part of the ICU complex and what should be supplied in the rest of the hospital or clinic is somewhat arbitrary. In addition to the numerous previously mentioned requirements, other functions and rooms that have to be considered are a kitchen for preparation of patient food, a doctor's room for any onsite overnight watch, a medical office including a library, individual office space, a storage area for patient records, a receptionist's office and area, a waiting area, an owner visiting room, a patient groom room, and a linen room. Furthermore, ICU staff require ready access to facilities for changing with showers, toilets, and lockers. Both the changing room and lockers must be individually lockable.

Environmental services

Gas supply

The ICU patient areas should be fitted with connections for central oxygen, compressed air, and vacuum. Gas scavenge systems should be implemented at the design stage if sedation with use of nitrous oxide or volatile anesthetic gases in the ICU is planned.

Service of the systems can be made easier by leading the pipes through wall- or ceiling-mounted, water-resistant conduits. The choice of service location (e.g., wall, stalactite, stalagmite) will have a major impact on the service arrangements and on operational use. The outlets must consist of keyed plugs to prevent accidental interchanging. For detailed requirements for pressures and flows, human guidelines can be applied with specific local guidelines taken into account (see Recommended Reading).

Lighting, electrical power, network, and communication cables

Ambient lighting should be available throughout the ICU, and especially around the cages and in the treatment areas. Diurnally cycled lighting has potential benefit in the recovery of infants.[6] Therefore it seems prudent to have adjustable lighting in the patient area, from both natural and electrical sources. The lights should dim without flicker. If windows or skylights are present, shading devices should be in place and easily controlled. It may also benefit the unit to have tinted glass panes in the exterior windows. During the night the main lights in the facility should be dimmed or turned off completely.

The patient modules and treatment areas should have spotlighting that can be controlled independently to prevent increased lighting for other patients, especially during periods of rest or at night (Fig. 3.9). Mobile spotlighting and lighting at low level under the cages or tables to illuminate drains and underwater seals (i.e., for thoracostomy drainage systems) may be added. Treatment areas should have separate procedure lighting with adjustable intensity, field size, and direction in order to properly evaluate patients or perform procedures. Independent lighting of support areas, such as the hand-washing stations, medication preparation area, and charting areas, can be beneficial.

Consideration should be given to provide a space easily accessible to all staff that will provide an opportunity for exposure to higher–intensity light levels for at least 15 minutes per shift in order to ameliorate the effects of working at night and "seasonal affective disorder."[7] The presence of natural daylight is also considered beneficial to staff and owners.

Electrical power, network, and communication cables should be routed via easily accessible conduits that are wall-mounted or located above the ceiling to make additional cabling relatively simple. The power supply must be single–phase with a single common safety ground. Supply lines must not cause interference with monitoring or computer equipment. Standard multiplex electrical outlets may not be suitable, since some outlets may not be accessible when oversized equipment plugs are in use.

It is critical that the ICU staff have immediate access to the main electrical panel if power must be interrupted or restored in case of an electrical emergency. A set of lights in the ICU and several power outlets supported by a backup generator should be available in case of a power outage.

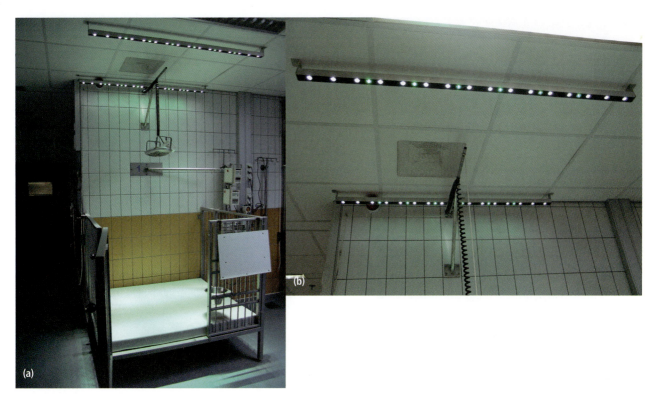

Figure 3.9 (a) Every patient module should have its own light. (b) Each module is lit by bright LED lights that can be dimmed stepwise and do not emit unwanted heat.

Ambient temperature and ventilation

The air conditioning system to the ICU patient area should provide a thermo–neutral temperature of 16–27°C (60–80°F) and a relative humidity of about 30%–60%, while avoiding condensation on wall and window surfaces. Control of humidity and condensation can be a challenge, as regular cleaning of cages and floors requires abundant amounts of water. System capacity and room air change frequencies should take this into account. Ventilated air delivered to the ICU should be filtered and the ventilation pattern should inhibit particulate matter from moving freely in the space. The air-conditioning system should be accessible such that regular monitoring and maintenance services may easily be performed.

Noise reduction

Reduction of both incoming noise and internally generated noise should be considered. Background noise produced by equipment and mechanical systems such as air conditioning should be minimal and absorbed as much as possible. Floor coverings that absorb sound should be used, keeping infection control, maintenance, and equipment movement needs under consideration. Walls and ceilings should be constructed of materials with high sound absorption capabilities. Especially in smaller rooms such as the isolation ward, special attention should be paid to unacceptable noise levels as a result of barking.

Water supply and plumbing

Sinks with hot and cold running water supplies must be located throughout the ICU. Depending on local regulations, heating boilers that reduce the risk of bacterial growth in the plumbing system must be installed directly adjacent to each water supply. Sinks are used either as hand-washing stations (see the special section on this topic) or for disposal of (contaminated) organic liquid materials and cleaning of equipment. The sinks should be large, and deep enough to ensure that the direct surroundings are not soiled. The installation of shower-heads can help with cleaning both equipment and the sink itself.

Sinks, water taps, and their direct surroundings are notorious for harboring bacteria that can cause nosocomial infections. Therefore, it is important to have different stations for hand washing, disposal of bodily fluids, and cleaning of equipment. Separate water fountains for drinking should be supplied.

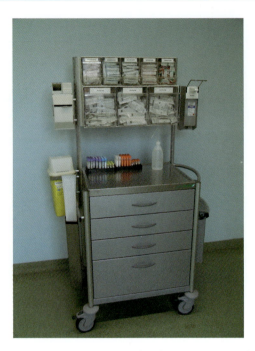

Figure 3.10 Furniture that is used in the patient area and ancillary rooms should be easily cleanable, with the fewest possible seams.

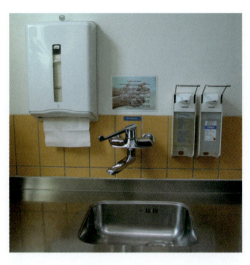

Figure 3.11 Hand washing and disinfection facilities should be strategically and conveniently positioned throughout the ICU.

Floors, walls, and ceilings

There are many things to consider regarding the surfaces in the patient area. Floor surfaces should be easy to clean and should minimize the growth of microorganisms. They should be highly durable and dense to withstand frequent cleaning and heavy traffic. They should keep their new appearance and glossiness, have acceptable acoustical properties, and give enough grip for staff and patients to walk upon safely, even when wet. In addition, the floors should be aesthetically pleasing to the eye. To choose an appropriate floor for the patient areas is certainly a challenge. It helps in the design phase to pay special attention to floors when visiting other facilities, with a focus on durability. See the section on Control of Infection below, under Operational Considerations, for more information regarding the floor's impact on hygiene and infection control.

The walls should be easy to clean, noise-reducing, and durable with extra protection provided at points where contact with movable equipment is likely to occur. Some walls may need to be reinforced if wall–mounted cages, rails, or shelves are used.

Ceilings should also be easy to clean, noise-absorbing, and invulnerable to dust accumulation, both on the ceiling itself and on ceiling-mounted light fixtures. The ceiling structure in the patient module or procedure area should be strong enough to carry the weight of any suspended equipment.

Furnishings

In the patient area the use of cabinets with doors and drawers is preferred over shelves, as closed cabinets contribute to an uncomplicated environment. Designs specific for use in medical facilities are ideal, as they have standardized sizes and take into account unique requirements of the medical field.

Chairs and free-standing furnishings such as cabinets and carts in the patient area and ancillary rooms should be easily cleanable with minimal seams (Fig. 3.10). Countertops in particular should have few or no seams. Furnishings should be of durable construction.

Special design considerations

Hand washing and disinfection facilities

Stations for clinical hand washing and disinfection should be strategically positioned at every entrance to the ICU (Fig. 3.11). Depending on the size of the unit, additional hand washing stations should be provided. The stations should be used only for hand washing and not to clean dishes or other equipment or to dispose of organic materials such as bodily fluids. The stations should have hot and cold running water that can be turned on and off by hands—free controls, and the basins should be large enough for surgical hand washing. To dry one's hands, disposable towels or hot air dryers can be used. An antimicrobial hand rub (often alcohol–based) dispenser should be present at every hand-washing facility. The setup should be complemented with clear instructions on when and how to wash and disinfect hands and lower arms correctly. For ease of access, additional antimicrobial hand rub dispensers should be placed strategically throughout the ICU (Fig. 3.3b).

Safety and security measures

Depending on the hospital situation, it may be necessary to have areas of the ICU that can lock from the inside to secure the safety of personnel and patients, particularly after regular office hours. Areas or storage units that contain valuable equipment should be locked. However, ICU staff should have use of all essential equipment and areas; therefore, a key cabinet available to all personnel can be located centrally in the ICU to allow such access.

The safety of patients, personnel, and visitors can be related to fire hazards, other hazards caused by failure or malfunction of services or equipment, and chemical or biohazards. Local fire safety regulations determine certain aspects of ICU design, and the consultation of fire safety officials should be part of the design process. At least two independent escape routes should be available, both accessible for personnel, mobile patients, and those on gurneys. Most local regulations will require installation of a sprinkler system.

Low-pressure warning systems for the gas services must be visible and audible in the ICU. Shut—off valves or switches for the ICU should be located adjacent to the unit where their operations can be controlled by the staff.

The main electrical panel should preferably be located with easy access to ICU personnel. Each outlet cluster within an ICU should be serviced by its own circuit breaker in the main panel. The electrical panel should be connected to an emergency power source that will quickly resupply power in the event of power interruption. If capacity of the backup power source is limited, special attention should be paid during the design process to identify which operations need backup. Emergency power source sockets should be distinguishable, for example, by color coding.

Access to positive distractions

Everybody remembers the classic gloomy, white appearance of hospitals. However, when patients are monitored, treated, and cared for around the clock, special attention should be paid to alleviate this strenuous working environment. The ambient atmosphere can have an enormous and positive effect on potentially stressed staff, owners, and sick animals away from their familiar homes. Words like soothing, relaxed, bright, calm, organized, pleasant, and familiar should apply. Not only visual but also auditory input, such as from audio equipment, helps to create this pleasant environment for both staff and patients. White or gray should not be the dominating color in the ICU. Natural daylight with an outside view is essential for both patients and staff. Visual distractions such as pictures and other features such as plants should not be reserved for the owner visiting room, but should be strategically placed throughout the ICU to enhance a positive atmosphere.

Medical equipment

Introduction

A comprehensive list of required equipment is beyond the scope of this chapter; Table 3.3 gives an abbreviated outline of ICU equipment possibilities. Furthermore, since many pieces of equipment are discussed throughout this book, the discussion here has been limited to some specific ICU-related considerations.

Specific considerations

Laboratory equipment

Equipment in an ICU laboratory must provide results quickly. Furthermore, as nonspecialized personnel often need to make use of these machines, they should also be easy to use, maintain, and calibrate.

Monitoring equipment

While in human ICUs the bedside monitoring setup is complete and committed to one bed only, this is seldom financially feasible in veterinary medicine. To make more economic use of the expensive equipment, extensive monitoring is either limited to those cages that are intended for the most critically ill patients; monitoring devices are positioned in such a way they can service multiple cages; or the equipment is mobile and can be moved between patient modules as necessary. In some situations every cage can be set up with monitoring modules that deliver a basic set of monitoring parameters (see Table 3.3). The setup chosen is based on the design of the ICU, the type of patients admitted to the ICU, the clinician's preferences, and financial constraints. The introduction of a modular setup for multiparameter monitoring devices is a very attractive development.

Of special interest are telemetry monitors, which offer several advantages. Mostly telemetry is used for the electrocardiogram, but larger setups can be used for multiple parameters. When used for one or two parameters the transmitter device is often small enough to tape onto the patient. This allows more free movement and minimizes the patient getting caught in wires and leads. Second, all collected data can be sent to a central monitor in the technicians' station, which supports continuous monitoring of the parameter(s).

Table 3.3 General overview of type and location of equipment in the intensive care unit

General Use	Location	Group	Apparatus/Function
Diagnostic/ monitoring	Laboratory	Sample preparation and storage	Blood tube centrifuge
			Microtube centrifuge
			Cytospin centrifuge
			Freezer
			Refrigerator
			Heating incubator
			Ice-making machine
		Measurement	Microscope
			Hematology
			Coagulation
			Biochemistry
			Blood gas machine
	Patient module and procedure area		Electrocardiograph
			Blood pressure monitors (invasive and non-invasive)
			Pulse oximeter
			Capnograph
			Continuous body thermometers
			Etc.
Therapeutic	Patient module	Infusion pumps	Syringe pump
			Standard volume fluid pump
		Mechanical ventilation	Mechanical ventilator
			Heating humidifier (oxygen/air blender)
	Patient area	CPCR	Crash cart
Other	Patient area	Patient care	Central supply cart
	ICU	Temperature controllers	Refrigerator
			Freezer
	Procedure area		Laboratory heating incubator
	ICU	Waste and soiled materials	Nonbiohazardous waste receptacle
			Biohazardous waste receptacle
	Laboratory, pharmacy, and patient area		Sharp safe
	soiled utility/holding room		Receptacle for soiled fleeces and blankets
			Receptacle for surgical instruments

Mechanical ventilation

Patients receiving mechanical ventilation constitute the "high end" of patient care in the companion animal ICU. A mechanical ventilator for the ICU should have an easy-to-use interface, give a wide array of options for different ventilation settings, and should be able to ven-tilate a wide range of patient sizes. Mechanical ventila-tors designed for use in anesthesia generally do not suffice. Equipment that specifically monitors respiratory parameters related to tidal volume, gas flow, and airway pressures should be part of the ventilation unit. The ventilator should be equipped with a humidifier and heating unit, as a heat and moisture exchanger

(HME) device does not work in all patients. Though they are built into modern critical care ventilators, some older units may need an ancillary oxygen and air blender.

Crash cart

In settings such as the emergency room and ICU where cardiopulmonary arrest is anticipated, it is important to have a complete set of equipment and supplies for cardiopulmonary cerebral resuscitation (CPCR) available and ready for use at all times. As an arrest can occur anywhere in the ICU, a mobile cart or trolley is preferred over a fixed CPCR station. However, the arrest cart should be placed in a designated, clearly indicated area to retrieve it without delay in case of an emergency (see Chapter 16, Cardiopulmonary Cerebral Resuscitation, for more details).

Central supply cart

Although the patient area may have enough room to stock all necessities for direct patient care, it is often convenient to have one or two central supply carts that contain the commonly used equipment and disposables. A limited range of frequently used drugs such as potassium chloride, heparin to prepare the heparin lock solution, sterile water or sodium chloride 0.9% to use as diluent for patients' medications or flushing fluid lines, eye lubrication, and xylocaine jelly can be stocked in this cart. The cart can be moved to anywhere in the patient area as needed. If the top of the cart is kept free, it offers an extra area to place, prepare, and organize equipment and disposables prior to the intervention.

Disposal of waste

Separate receptacles for biohazardous and nonbiohazardous waste, according to local regulation, should be available throughout the ICU (Fig. 3.12; see Chapter 54, Minimizing Nosocomial Infection, and Chapter 57, Personnel Precautions for Patients with Zoonotic Disease, for more details). Sharp disposal containers should be present on or near every counter to facilitate quick and easy disposal.

Operational considerations

Introduction

The discussion so far has addressed the physical components ("hardware") of the companion animal ICU. However, the organization or "software" is also an essential aspect of ICU design. Intensive care staff constitutes a large organization, and intensive care medicine requires a team approach. The team consists of different groups

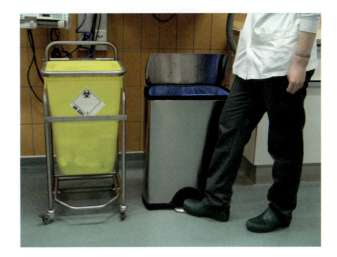

Figure 3.12 Separate disposal bins should be available for biohazardous and nonbiohazardous waste throughout the ICU according to local legislation. The use of a foot control limits the contact of hands with the waste bin.

such as managers, veterinarians, technicians, and cleaning staff. Staffing of the ICU with regard to number, qualifications, individual job descriptions, and appropriate training is the cornerstone of the ICU organization. As in any larger organization, cooperation and effective communication between the different groups determines the quality of the final product. In recent years several directives have been published by critical care organizations in human medicine to define optimal staffing and operational requirements.[8–11] Such directives have identified written communications and infection control as important management aspects that contribute to the performance of a facility.

Patient record keeping

Proper record keeping is an important part of patient management and serves a specific purpose. Primarily, it ensures and improves communication among ICU personnel regarding the patient. But it is also important for retrospective evaluation of the care given to the patient, both for internal quality control and research and for external scrutiny.

Medical record

The medical record is mainly kept by the veterinary staff and is often performed in digital form. The medical record describes the complete time period of the patient's hospitalization until discharge. The record should contain at least the initial information (signalment, history, physical examination), problem list, rule-outs, additional diagnostic and therapeutic plans and

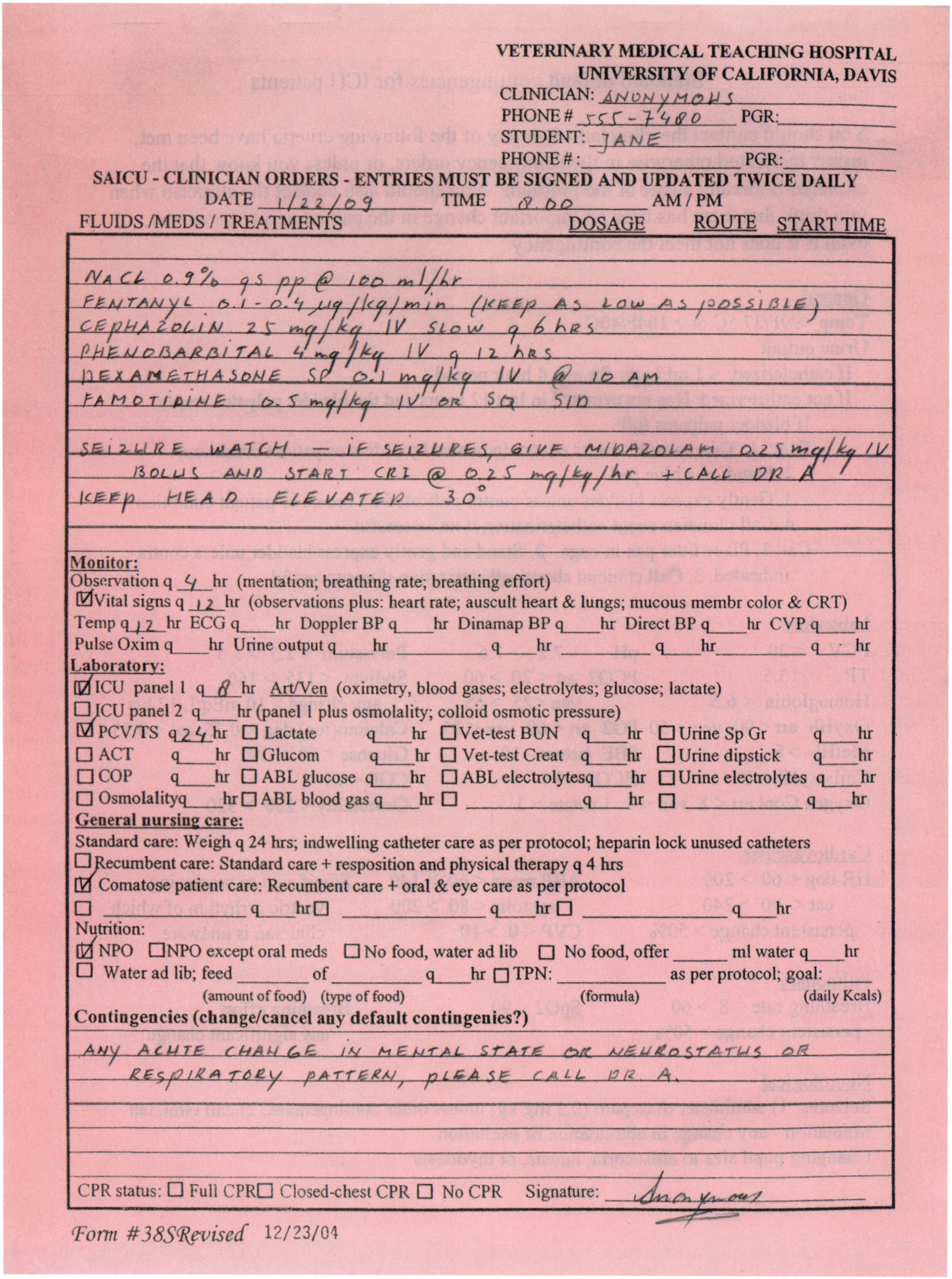

VETERINARY MEDICAL TEACHING HOSPITAL
UNIVERSITY OF CALIFORNIA, DAVIS

CLINICIAN: _ANONYMOUS_

PHONE # _555-7480_ PGR:_____

STUDENT: _JANE_

PHONE #:_____ PGR:_____

SAICU - CLINICIAN ORDERS - ENTRIES MUST BE SIGNED AND UPDATED TWICE DAILY

DATE _1/22/09_   TIME _8.00_   AM / PM

FLUIDS /MEDS / TREATMENTS   DOSAGE   ROUTE   START TIME

NaCl 0.9% qs pp @ 100 ml/hr
FENTANYL 0.1 - 0.4 µg/kg/min (KEEP AS LOW AS POSSIBLE)
CEPHAZOLIN 25 mg/kg IV SLOW q 6 hrs
PHENOBARBITAL 4 mg/kg IV q 12 hrs
DEXAMETHASONE SP 0.1 mg/kg IV @ 10 AM
FAMOTIDINE 0.5 mg/kg IV OR SQ SID

SEIZURE WATCH — IF SEIZURES, GIVE MIDAZOLAM 0.25 mg/kg IV
    BOLUS AND START CRI @ 0.25 mg/kg/hr + CALL DR A
KEEP HEAD ELEVATED 30°

Monitor:
Observation q _4_ hr (mentation; breathing rate; breathing effort)
☑Vital signs q _12_ hr (observations plus: heart rate; auscult heart & lungs; mucous membr color & CRT)
Temp q_12_ hr ECG q___hr Doppler BP q___hr Dinamap BP q___hr Direct BP q___hr CVP q___hr
Pulse Oxim q___hr Urine output q___hr   q___hr   q___hr   q___hr

Laboratory:
☑ICU panel 1 q _8_ hr Art/Ven (oximetry, blood gases; electrolytes; glucose; lactate)
☐ICU panel 2 q___hr (panel 1 plus osmolality; colloid osmotic pressure)
☑PCV/TS q_24_hr ☐ Lactate   q___hr ☐Vet-test BUN   q___hr ☐Urine Sp Gr   q___hr
☐ ACT   q___hr ☐Glucom   q___hr ☐ Vet-test Creat q___hr ☐Urine dipstick   q___hr
☐ COP   q___hr ☐ABL glucose q___hr ☐ABL electrolytesq___hr ☐Urine electrolytes q___hr
☐ Osmolalityq___hr☐ABL blood gas q___hr ☐_____q___hr ☐_____q___hr

General nursing care:
Standard care: Weigh q 24 hrs; indwelling catheter care as per protocol; heparin lock unused catheters
☐Recumbent care: Standard care + resposition and physical therapy q 4 hrs
☑Comatose patient care: Recumbent care + oral & eye care as per protocol
☐ _____ q___hr☐ _____ q___hr☐ _____ q___hr

Nutrition:
☑NPO ☐NPO except oral meds ☐ No food, water ad lib ☐ No food, offer _____ ml water q___hr
☐ Water ad lib; feed _____ of _____ q___hr ☐TPN: _____ as per protocol; goal: _____
         (amount of food) (type of food)   (formula)   (daily Kcals)

Contingencies (change/cancel any default contingenies?)

ANY ACUTE CHANGE IN MENTAL STATE OR NEUROSTATHS OR
RESPIRATORY PATTERN, PLEASE CALL DR A.

CPR status: ☐ Full CPR☐ Closed-chest CPR ☐ No CPR   Signature: _Anonymous_

Form #38S Revised 12/23/04

Figure 3.13 Daily order sheet with written instructions for the patient's care.

interventions, and progress notes, including (presumptive) diagnosis, treatment, and prognosis.[12]

Daily ICU orders

It is the responsibility of the overseeing veterinarian to write orders that describe diagnostic, therapeutic, monitoring, and care instructions for the next 24 hours for each patient (Fig. 3.13). These orders can be written directly onto the patient treatment or "flow" sheet, but given the complexity of ICU patient orders and the frequency with which critically ill patients' orders change in a day, a separate order sheet is much more useful. It is the task of the technician to be able to read, interpret, and evaluate the orders, and to clarify with the clinician what is not understood.

A special sheet with patient-specific information related to the event of CPCR—such as owner's resuscitation wishes, drug dosages, and owner and primary veterinarian contact information—may be part of the daily ICU orders.

Flow sheet

The essence of critical care is continuous patient monitoring, which is beneficial only if the data are collected and recorded in a useful manner. A patient flow sheet is the traditional method for recording all information relevant to an ICU patient for a 24-hour period. Maintaining the flow sheet is primarily the responsibility of the nursing staff caring for the patient (Fig. 3.14a). The flow sheet is used to document the results of "bedside" diagnostic, therapeutic, monitoring, and care instructions, and to document that the orders have been carried out and at what time.[13] Flow sheets are helpful in registering subtle trends, and as such, their design should include tables or graphs (Fig. 3.14b). The flow sheet can contain both subjective and objective assessments. However, subjective assessments are best communicated verbally with the attending veterinarian and others involved in the patient's care.

Protocols

In a complicated environment such as an ICU, having consistent protocols for procedures and techniques is essential. The development of protocols should include the close cooperation between all hospital groups, both within and outside the ICU, that are involved in patient care or the organization of the ICU. Protocols are necessary for several reasons.

- To improve, support, and reduce unnecessary repetition of oral communications and instructions among the staff.

- To standardize patient care, organization, hygiene, and other strategies among staff members.
- To disseminate the best available knowledge so that it may be implemented when appropriate (evidence—based veterinary medicine). Protocols should contain references if available.
- To record and describe in clear detail any actions that need to follow legal instructions or legislation, for example, the use of controlled drugs in the ICU.
- To scrutinize constantly the strategies that are described in the protocols.

Every protocol should contain the following information: title, classification or subject group, names of author(s), date of compilation, names of author(s) who made changes, dates of amendments, and the persons to whom the protocol is of interest. For administrative purposes it may be helpful to introduce a coding system.

Protocols are often written by different people, with the ICU staff often performing the initial writing. It is a challenge to keep the protocols as effective as possible by keeping them concise, informative, and complete without becoming too elaborate. Proper referencing can help the interested reader to find more background information if necessary. The ICU protocol book is constantly under construction and never finished as a result of rigorous scrutiny and improvements, adaptation to the latest information, and adjustments to changes in

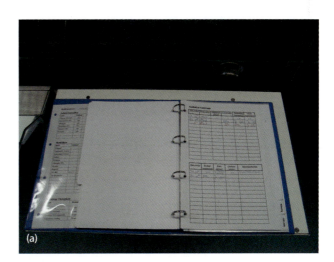

(a)

Figure 3.14 (a) At the ICU at the Department of Clinical Sciences of Companion Animals of the Utrecht University, the flow sheet consists of a folder with divider sheets for different aspects such as patient particulars, problem list, monitoring, fluid therapy, and medications. (b1, b2) Tables and graphs are important ways to present the collected information in an orderly fashion that facilitates the interpretation of data.

ICU LABORATORY

TIME	1752	1820	2202	0208	0606	0810
PCV (%)	37			46	45	
TP (Gm/dl)	4.7			5.6	5.5	
Plasma color	CLR			CLR	CLR	
Plasma transparency	CLR			CLR	CLR	
Arterial/Venous	A	A	A	A	A	A
Body temperature (C/F)	99.5	98.4	98.5	99.2	99.5	99.5
Inspired oxygen (%)	21	74m	21	30	21	25
Hemoglobin (Gm/dl)	12.1	12.2	13.0	14.6	14.0	13.7
Oxyhemoglobin (%)	91.6	98.8	91.9	97.4	99.5	96.0
Methemoglobin (%)	0.1	0.2	0.6	0.0	0.0	0.2
Carboxyhemoglobin (%)	0.4	0.3	0.6	0.7	0.6	0.6
Oxygen content (ml/dl)	15.3	16.7	16.5	19.6	17.8	18.1
Potassium (mEq/L)	3.9	4.0	3.9	3.8	4.1	4.1
Sodium (mEq/L)	148	147	146	148	150	149
Calcium(ionized) (mM/L)	1.34	1.39	1.38	1.41	1.40	1.41
Chloride (mEq/L)	120	118	117	120	124	121
Glucose (mg/dl)	130	125	150	140	139	137
Lactate (mM/L)	0.9	0.6	0.5	0.3	0.2	0.2
pH tc (units)	7.207	7.199	7.225	7.243	7.229	7.233
PCO2tc (mmHg)	54.1	56.7	54.4	49.5	52.3	50.5
PO2tc (mmHg)	86.1	192	83.6	123	85.2	109
A-a pO2 (mmHg)						
SBE c (mEq/L)	-6.1	-5.6	-4.8	-5.6	-5.4	-5.8
HCO3c (mEq/L)	20.5	21.3	21.7	20.5	20.9	20.4
COP (mm Hg)						
Osmolality (mOsm/Kg)						
Creatinine (Vet-test)						
BUN (Vet-test)						
Azostick						
Glucometer						
Activ Clotting Time (sec)						

Urinalysis Time	1800	2200	0200	0600
Collection method	UCS	UCS	UCS	UCS
Color	YELL	YELL	YELL	YELL
Transparency	CLR	CLR	CLR	CLR
Specific Gravity	1.016	1.013	1.010	1.014
Osmolality (mOsm/Kg)				
Sodium (mEq/L)				
Potassium (mEq/L)				
Chloride (mEq/L)				
Protein	TRACE			
pH	7			
Blood	+++			
Ketones	NEG			
Bilirubin	1			
Glucose	NEG			

(b1)

Figure 3.14 (*Continued*)

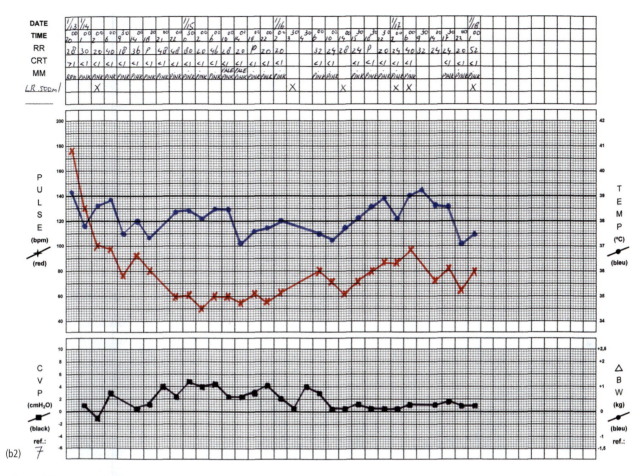

(b2)

Figure 3.14 (*Continued*)

Figure 3.15 A strategically placed patient board containing accurate, current information gives anyone who requires it a quick and complete overview of ICU patient status.

the ICU organization. Protocol books published in recent years can be very helpful in setting up one's own ICU protocol book.[14] Many protocols are available throughout this textbook to serve as a starting point for protocols in veterinary ICUs.

Bulletin boards

There is always a need for brief communications among the staff. Bulletin boards are most often used to communicate in this fashion and have the additional advantage of being available to everyone with one quick glance.

A strategically placed patient board (Fig. 3.15) contains the numbers of the patient modules, the patients' names that occupy them, their problems and/ or diagnosis, their therapies, the current plans, and the name of the staff member who bears primary responsibility. Additional patient identification numbers and telephone number or other contact information of owner and staff can be helpful. This is of benefit during busy times to keep overview of all patient—related activities.

Bulletin boards can be used to facilitate quick and important communication among ICU staff or between ICU staff and other hospital staff, such as the pharmacy or those responsible for ordering and stocking. This information is limited to current topics on staffing and organization and is especially helpful in maintaining communication among staff on different shifts. With the use of different bulletin boards, different groups or topics within the ICU organization can be targeted on each board.

Control of infection

Community acquired infections are one of the main reasons patients end up in the ICU. But nosocomial infections, that is, those acquired in—hospital, are becoming of increasing importance, as they often burden resources and extend patient hospital stay. Medicine, including veterinary medicine, has traditionally focused on antimicrobials to treat infections. However, a change in approach is warranted because of the growing number of multidrug–resistant microbe strains and because of the trend to treat patients that are sicker. The situation is exacerbated by the increase in invasive actions on debilitated patients, such as surgical interventions and the placement of catheters, tubes, and drains that circumvent many natural defense mechanisms. As a result the balance between host defenses and microbial propensity for invasion becomes more and more disturbed. Improvement and refinement of our antimicrobial strategy no longer appears to suffice, and additional measures that prevent these infections from developing in the first place are becoming a major focus.

Increased incidence of multidrug resistant microbe infections such as methicillin–resistant *Staphylococcus* species, *Clostridium difficile*, *Acinetobacter* species, *Escherichia coli* and vancomycin–resistant *enterococci* has improved the awareness of the risk of nosocomial infections (although strictly speaking they may have also been community acquired).[15,16] The risk of infection may be relevant not only to patients but also to the caretakers, as some of these microbes have the potential to be zoonotic.

An infection can be community-acquired or hospital-acquired.[17] Hospital-acquired infections occur by direct and indirect contact with people, other patients, instrumentation, or the environment. The focus here is on the measures that can be taken in general to prevent the establishment and dissemination of infections in the ICU. These measures may need drastic expansion the moment an infection with a nosocomial or multiresistant infection has been established. Furthermore, necessary additional measures vary depending on the microbe involved and epidemiologic characteristics that differ not only geographically but even among facilities.[18] Although the prevention of nosocomial infections is still subject to debate and study, more disturbing is the notion that implementation of effective measures to reduce the number of nosocomial, and particularly mul-

tiresistant, infections into veterinary hospital policies appears to lag behind reality.[19]

With the introduction of infection control measures to the ICU another problem may become apparent: the lack of compliancy of personnel in the ICU. This aspect is a great concern and a challenge for anyone who is responsible for developing hygiene measures in the ICU. The establishment of infection control teams can be very beneficial, not only to prepare policies and to initiate interventions to reduce the spread of pathogens but, more important, to educate and continually encourage staff to follow these policies in their daily duties.[15] The infection control team should enforce procedures such as antibiotic policy, clothing of staff and visitors, hand washing, sterilization, aseptic precautions for invasive procedures, use of disposables, filtering of patients' respired air, changing of catheters, humidifiers, ventilator tubing and other equipment, isolation of at—risk or infected patients, and cleaning of the unit. Furthermore, design significantly affects discipline and behavior as, for example, the absence of proper facilities reduces the possibility of hand washing. However, an abundance of sinks will not necessarily ensure that this behavior is adopted.[3] No single measure will be effective on its own, and packages of measures known as "care bundles" have been demonstrated to be a more effective preventive method.[15]

Personal hygiene

Staff and visitors should be aware that they may act as a reservoir for nosocomial microbial species, and should understand their roles in the possible introduction of these microbes to the ICU. They can also play a role in the spread of nosocomial infections *within* the ICU.

The first measure to reduce the introduction and spread of nosocomial infections is to reduce any unnecessary contact. Therefore, it is important to reduce unnecessary traffic in and out of the ICU and to reduce contact of unauthorized persons with patients. If possible, staff and especially veterinary technicians who have frequent patient contact should be restricted to the care of a limited number of patients. If multiple patients are treated consecutively, it is necessary to determine the order in which patients can best be contacted. Moving to another patient should be a trigger to address hand hygiene measures and barrier change.

The measures for personal hygiene dictate that long hair be tied back, fingernails be trimmed short, skin lesions be covered with waterproof dressings, and a change of working clothes be available during one's shift. There is an essential and growing awareness that nosocomial infections originate and are spread primarily by those parts of the body that make the most contact with the patient: lower arms and hands of owners and personnel.[20] Therefore, extensive instructions have been described for proper hand and lower arm sanitation.[21] As the lower arms are part of the protocol, sleeves of uniforms should end at the elbow or otherwise be rolled up. However, the risk of microbial spread is not limited to lower arms and hands. Signs of affection such as kissing and nose rubbing can have the same results. Also, personal equipment such as thermometers and stethoscopes should be cleaned and disinfected between patients.

The intensive care unit should be designed to facilitate any attempt of personnel to maintain a high level of hygiene. Therefore, hand-washing and disinfection facilities should be strategically placed outside the entrance and within the ICU. Additional containers with an antimicrobial rub or gel (often alcohol—based) should be present at strategic points throughout the ICU. The use by the staff of alcohol containers attached to uniforms for quick use between patient contacts should be considered. Hand-rub dispensers are a visual cue for cleanliness and can be quickly used before and after handling an animal and before touching pens, keyboards, and so on.[15,18]

Everyone should be aware that disinfection is not a replacement for hand washing—dirty hands reduce the effectiveness of any antiseptic. Also, visitors should be made aware of their roles in spreading infections by the use of informational brochures and posters.

Barriers such as examination gloves and gowns are most effective in the event of contact with soiled materials and during the disposal of bodily fluids. Face and eye protection should be worn if aerosols are likely to be generated.[18] The primary role of barriers is personal protection and to reduce contact and soiling of one's own hands and clothes. In combination with proper hand washing and disinfection, this reduces the risk of contamination. Barriers may also be used when handling patients or equipment. However, in this respect they are no replacement for hand washing and disinfection. The use of barrier materials can give the user the false assumption of improved protection. However, the prolonged use of gloves or gowns while in contact with different surfaces and multiple patients eliminates their effectiveness.

Patient-related considerations

Infected or colonized animals may act as reservoirs for further transmission to humans or other patients; this is an important reason to limit interpatient contact. In the situation of a known nosocomial and/or multidrug-resistant microbial infection, additional isolation measures may be warranted. But the main focus should be the awareness that an infection with all its detrimental consequences can only develop *after* contamination.

Many microbes do not cause infection in a healthy individual and are considered "opportunistic" pathogens. As a result, healthy individuals can act as reservoirs for such microbes. But the defense mechanisms in ICU patients are reduced by their illness and the multiple interventions that circumvent the natural host defenses. The best way to improve the patient's resistance is to resolve its primary disease processes. While doing so, there are certain measures that can support or improve the immune system of the patient. Besides the improvement and refinement of antimicrobial strategies, the implementation of a well—balanced and patient-specific diet is important to maintain the patient's defenses. Also the prevention and care of wounds, either surgical or nonsurgical, should be addressed by evidence—based protocols and their proper execution. Though it has not yet been widely applied in veterinary medicine, selective decontamination of the digestive tract has been used to help prevent nosocomial infections in human ICU patients.[22] Furthermore, extremely immunocompromised animals may need additional measures; preemptive isolation may even be necessary.

If the first measure to reduce nosocomial infections is to minimize contact, the second measure is to reduce the number of indwelling devices or procedures used to treat and care for the patient. The risks of contamination and the way to reduce them are well known in relation to intravascular catheters, urologic catheters, and mechanical ventilation.[21,23] Every ICU should have protocols that address the proper application and standard care of these devices or procedures, with emphasis on the prevention of contamination with "opportunistic" microbes, especially the ones that originate from the same patient. For example, most ventilator-associated pneumonias (VAPs) are a result of gastrointestinal bacteria from the same patient that contaminate the upper airway and tracheal tube. Protocols may recommend the location where the intervention should take place (cage, ICU treatment area, surgical theater); the surgical preparation of the procedure site, hand hygiene and the use of sterile gloves, gowns, hats, and masks; the use of sterile equipment and single-use disposable equipment; and the proper disposal of contaminated material.

Environmental considerations

Decontamination of the environment should be an integral extension of the cleaning protocols that are applied in the ICU. Proper cleaning with removal of all (biological) dirt must precede disinfection efforts, as many disinfectants are inactivated prematurely if in contact with biological material. It is important to screen the cleaning protocols and address the effectiveness of the disinfectants to eradicate pathogens. For example, a detergent does not eradicate spores of *Clostriduim difficile*, and thus chlorine—releasing agents are essential.

A range of disinfectants should be used for different materials, furniture, equipment, and surfaces, and their specific uses should be described in the hygiene protocols. A predetermined cleaning and disinfection roster should be used to reach an effective interruption of environmental contamination. In particular it is important to address surfaces that are in regular contact with personnel and patients. These can be difficult surfaces to clean, such as computer keyboards, monitoring equipment, infusion pumps, telephones, doorknobs, patient cages, and the handles of cabinets and drawers. Also in the design process the choice of materials should be explicitly directed by this consideration, for example, by the introduction of waterproof and flat keyboards. The main contact area for a patient is its cage. Cages and their bedding should be cleaned regularly, at least once a day. Disinfection should be performed between patients or whenever sensible, such as during a long patient stay. All these measures have proven less effective if not combined with adequate numbers of staff and suitable space and facilities.[24] Therefore, this entire chapter should be considered in the light of infection control.

Decontamination measures are not the only strategy that must be applied. The trafficking of people and patients makes long-lasting decontamination of the floor an impossible task. Therefore, the floor should always be considered "contaminated," and any contact with it should be followed by stringent cleaning and disinfection measures. This strategy relates to equipment, disposables and other materials, patients, and persons. If it is not possible to clean and disinfect, the object (such as a blanket or a syringe that is accidently dropped) that has been in contact with the floor should be discarded. The floor should not be considered a convenient "table," and nothing should be stored on it without additional precautions.

Routine culturing of persons, patients, and the environment

It is important to realize that routine microbial screening of staff is not necessary in most circumstances. Screening is not a substitute for rigorous infectious disease control measures, particularly hand hygiene and cleaning.[18] In any individual, differentiation between transient carriage to colonization and persistent carriage has to be considered. For example, transient carriage is more common and is most effectively controlled by hand decontamination and other hygienic measures. Only in continuing outbreaks after appropriate infection control measures have been introduced can staff screening be advised by infection control staff. The issues of consent, confidentiality, and any additional consequences must be carefully addressed.

As the epidemiology of certain pathogens can have temporal and geographical variations, routine culturing of patients can be used to obtain important insights in the local situation, such as the prevalence of colonization in the hospital patient population.[25] Active surveillance of patients may reveal higher numbers of positive samples when compared with the sole use of clinical specimens, and appears to improve the control of infections if combined with early and appropriate isolation measures.[24] However, the latter appears impractical in many veterinary hospitals, since preemptive isolation (i.e., before the result of the culture is known) seems warranted.

An infection control team or infection control experts should be consulted to advise on the use and sense of environmental sampling. Routine culturing may have some merit to establish potential risk sites in the ICU. Results should be used to guide and improve cleaning and disinfection procedures.

While much can be done within the ICU itself, multidrug-resistant infections in the ICU often reflect difficulties elsewhere in the hospital and in veterinary health service generally, in terms of the control and prevention of healthcare—associated infection.[24]

References

1. Recommendations for veterinary emergency and critical care facilities. San Antonio, TX: Veterinary Emergency and Critical Care Society. Available at: http://www.veccs.org/index.php?option=com_content&view=article&id=75:recommendations-for-veterinary-emergency-and-critical-care-facilities&catid=38:about-veccs&Itemid=187. Accessed December 29, 2010.
2. White RD. Recommended standards for newborn ICU design. Report of the Seventh Consensus Conference on Newborn ICU Design February 1, 2007. Clearwater Beach, FL. Available at: http://www.nd.edu/~nicudes/. Accessed December 29, 2010.
3. Standards for intensive care units (1997). Standards, Safety and Quality Committee. London: The Intensive Care Society. Available at: http://www.ics.ac.uk/intensive_care_professional/standards_and_guidelines/standards_for_intensive_care_2007. Accessed December 29, 2010.
4. Guidelines for intensive care unit design. Guidelines/Practice Parameters Committee of the American College of Critical Care Medicine, Society of Critical Care Medicine. Crit Care Med 1995;23(3):582–588.
5. Moses L, Curran A. Basic Monitoring of the Emergency and Critical Patient. In: Battaglia A, ed. Small animal emergency and

critical care for veterinary technicians. 2nd ed. St Louis, MO: Saunders Elsevier, 2007;9–32.

6. Rivkees SA. Emergence and influences of circadian rhythmicity in infants. Clin Perinatol 2004;31(2):217–228.

7. Glickman G, Byrne B, Pineda C, et al. Light therapy for seasonal affective disorder with blue narrow—band light—emitting diodes (LEDs). Biol Psychiatry 2006;59(6):502–507.

8. Depasse B, Pauwels D, Somers Y, et al. A profile of European ICU nursing. Intensive Care Med 1998;24:939–945.

9. Galley J, O'Riordan B. Guidance for nurse staffing in critical care. London: Royal College of Nursing, 2003. Available at: http://www.rcn.org.uk/__data/assets/pdf_file/0008/78560/001976.pdf. Accessed December 29, 2010.

10. Haupt MR, Bekes CE, Brilli RJ, et al. Guidelines on critical care services and personnel: recommendations based on a system of categorization of three levels of care. Crit Care Med 2003;31(11): 2677–2683.

11. Gunning K, Gillbe C. Standards for consultant staffing of intensive care units. London: Intercollegiate Board for Training in Intensive Care Medicine (IBTICM) and the Intensive Care Society 2007. Available at: http://www.ics.ac.uk/intensive_care_professional/standards_and_guidelines/standards_for_consultant_staffing_2007. Accessed December 29, 2010.

12. Van Sluijs FJ, van Nes JJ. Medical records. In: Rijnberk A, van Sluijs FJ, eds. Medical history and physical examinations in companion animals. 2nd ed. Edinburgh, United Kingdom: Saunders Elsevier, 2009;27–39.

13. McGee ML, Spencer CL, Van Pelt DR. Critical care nursing. In: Bonagura JD, Twedt DC, eds. Kirk's current veterinary therapy XIV. Philadelphia: WB Saunders, 2008;106–110.

14. Matthews K. Veterinary emergency and critical care manual. 2nd ed. Guelph, Ontario, Canada: Lifelearn, 2006.

15. Wilson APR. Hospital acquired infections—which lessons can be learned from the human health services? In Proceedings 18th Annual ECVIM—CA Congress 2008;46–48.

16. Weese JS, van Duijkeren E. Methicillin—resistant *Staphylococcus aureus* and *Staphylococcus pseudintermedius* in veterinary medicine. Vet Microbiol 2009; doi:10.1016/j.vetmic.2009.01.039.

17. Ogee—Gyles JS, Mathews KA, Boerlin P. Nosocomial infections and antimicrobial resistance in critical care medicine. J Vet Emerg Crit Care 2006;16(1):1–18.

18. BSAVA MRSA Practice Guidelines, 2007. Available at: http://www.bsava.com/Advice/MRSA/tabid/171/Default.aspx Accessed December 29, 2010.

19. Benedict KM, Morley PS, Van Metre DC. Characteristics of biosecurity and infection control programs at veterinary teaching hospitals. J Am Vet Med Assoc 2008;233:767–773.

20. Simmons B, Bryant J, Neiman K, et al. The role of handwashing in prevention of endemic intensive care unit infections. Infect Control Hosp Epidemiol 1990;11:589–594.

21. Centers for Disease Control and Prevention. Guideline for hand hygiene in health—care settings: recommendations of the Healthcare Infection Control Practices Advisory Committee and the HICPAC/SHEA/APIC/IDSA Hand Hygiene Task Force. Morb Mort Weekly Rep 2002;51(No.RR—16):1–45.

22. Silvestri L, van Saene HKF, Milanese M, et al. Selective decontamination of the digestive tract reduces bacterial bloodstream infection and mortality in critically ill patients. Systematic review of randomized, controlled trials. J Hosp Infect 2007;65: 187–203.

23. Smarick SD, Haskins SC, Aldrich J, et al. Incidence of catheter—associated urinary tract infection among dogs in a small animal intensive care unit. J Am Vet Med Assoc 2004;224: 1936–1940.

24. Humphreys H. Can we do better in controlling and preventing methicillin—resistant *Staphylococcus aureus* (MRSA) in the intensive care unit (ICU)? Eur J Clin Microbiol Infect Dis 2008;27(6):409–413.

25. Heller J, Armstrong SK, Girvan EK, et al. Prevalence and distribution of meticillin—resistant *Staphylococcus aureus* within the environment and staff of a university veterinary clinic. J Small Anim Pract 2009;50:168–173.

Recommended reading

These website pages and the documents on them provide insight to the approach in human medicine to define and design intensive care facilities. Although far from the reality of companion animal intensive care medicine, the information certainly gives a lot to consider when designing a companion animal ICU, and stimulates "out—of—the—box" thinking necessary to explore design options to the max.

The ESICM guidelines and recommendations. Brussels, Belgium: The European Society of Intensive Care Medicine. Available at: http://www.esicm.org/Data/ModuleGestionDeContenu/PagesGenerees/06-publications/0D-guidelines-recommendations/92.asp. Accessed December 29, 2010.

Learn ICU. Des Plaines, IL: Society of Critical Care Medicine. Available at: http://www.learnicu.org/Pages/default.aspx. Accessed December 29, 2010.

Standards, Safety and Quality Committee. London: The Intensive Care Society. Available at: http://www.ics.ac.uk/intensive_care_professional/standards__safety_and_quality. Accessed December 29, 2010.

White RD. Recommended standards for newborn ICU design. Report of the Seventh Consensus Conference on Newborn ICU Design February 1, 2007. Clearwater Beach, FL. Available at: http://www.nd.edu/~nicudes/ Accessed December 29, 2010.

BISHOP BURTON COLLEGE

SECTION II

Cardiovascular

4

Catheterization of the venous compartment

Mary Tefend Campbell and Douglass K. Macintire

Intravascular catheter placement is the most common method used to gain access to the vasculature to allow for fluid therapy, medication administration, serial blood sampling, and hemodynamic monitoring. Correct anatomic selection and precise placement of an intravascular catheter are essential whether performing a single intravenous injection or providing long-term vascular access in an ill or injured patient.

Selection of catheter insertion site and type

Many factors will influence the type of intravenous catheter used and the site chosen for its placement (summarized in Tables 4.1 and 4.2). The length and diameter of the catheter selected must be appropriate for its intended use. In emergency patients, large-bore peripheral catheters are ideal for rapid fluid resuscitation; however, placement can be problematic in patients with hypotension, hypovolemia, vascular collapse, trauma, and skin stiffness. Therefore, central line catheters may be preferable in some severely hypovolemic patients, or if serial blood sampling is indicated. A central venous catheter is required in order to measure central venous pressure.

In general, although smaller diameter catheters may be easier to place and can be less traumatic to a vessel, rapid fluid administration through small-bore catheters can be difficult because of high resistance to fluid flow. Larger, more rigid catheters are typically easier to advance through the skin but have the potential to cause more damage to vessel walls compared with the smaller diameter catheters. The authors recommend placing the largest bore catheter possible without causing significant vascular trauma or stress in any patient requiring intravenous access. This recommendation applies particularly to emergency patients and to any patient that will undergo a surgical or anethestic event, because these patients are most likely to experience a hypotensive crisis requiring rapid fluid administration or life-saving intravenous medication. The most common vascular access sites are the peripheral veins such as the cephalic and accessory cephalic of the thoracic limb, and the lateral saphenous of the pelvic limb. The medial saphenous vein may also be used and is an easy port of entry in the feline patient, though securing the catheter at this site can be challenging for long-term use. Auricular veins may be used in dogs with large ears such as Basset Hounds or Cocker Spaniels. External jugular and saphenous veins are typically used for the placement of centrally situated catheters in both the canine and feline patient. When the pelvic limb is the site of catheter insertion, the medial saphenous vein is preferred in the cat and the lateral saphenous vein is generally preferred in the dog.

There is a vast market of intravenous catheters (Fig. 4.1). Catheters are generally categorized as over-the-needle, through-the-needle, or winged ("butterfly"), and as either single or multilumen catheters. The structural material of the catheter can influence rigidity, ease of placement, and the potential for thrombosis or phlebitis of the vessel. Common materials for intravenous catheters include Teflon, polypropylene, polyurethane, and silicone. Also available are specialty catheters impregnated with radiopaque metal salts for radiographic confirmation of correct anatomic placement, or to locate accidentally freed catheter fragments. In addition, intravenous catheters coated with antimicrobial substances marketed to decrease the incidence of infection are now commercially available.

Advanced Monitoring and Procedures for Small Animal Emergency and Critical Care, First Edition. Edited by Jamie M. Burkitt Creedon, Harold Davis.
© 2012 John Wiley & Sons, Inc. Published 2012 by John Wiley & Sons, Inc.

Table 4.1 Catheter insertion site location considerations

- Patient size and species
- Venous accessibility
- Presence of physical barriers (wounds, fractures, neoplasia, neurologic insufficiencies)
- Restraint requirements
- Temperament of patient
- Hemodynamic stability
- Coagulation abnormalities

Table 4.2 Catheter selection considerations

- Length of hospitalization
- Frequency of blood sampling
- Coagulation abnormalities
- Nutritional delivery
- Hemodynamic monitoring plan

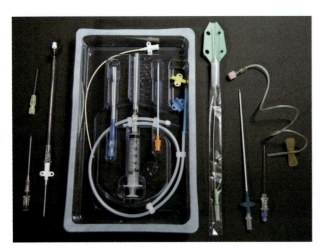

Figure 4.1 There are many different venous catheters available. Catheter selection should be based on patient need and length of hospital stay.

Peripheral catheter placement

Peripheral venous catheters are the most commonly used tool for obtaining **vascular access** in the small animal patient. Ease and speed of insertion, low cost, and versatility of access in different anatomical locations make peripheral catheters advantageous over other catheter types. Most peripheral catheter types are categorized as over-the-needle, meaning that the catheter is fitted outside or over a steel needle (Fig. 4.2). The steel needle extends slightly beyond the catheter tip to facilitate venous entry. Once venipuncture is accomplished, the catheter is slid off the needle into the targeted vessel.

Anatomical locations for placement of peripheral catheters include the cephalic, accessory cephalic, or

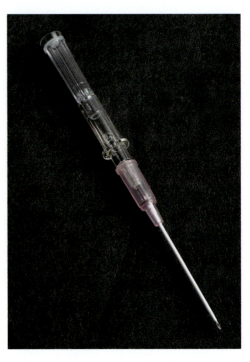

Figure 4.2 The most common peripheral catheter is the over-the-needle type, meaning that the catheter is fitted outside or over a steel needle. Such catheter types are very versatile and can be placed in many different anatomical locations.

even the jugular vein during triage. Other easily accessible sites for placement include the lateral saphenous vein in the dog or medial saphenous vein in the cat. Less common placement sites include the dorsal common digital vein, auricular vein, or lingual vein. Rapid administration of fluids can be easily accomplished through a large-bore (14- to 16-gauge) catheter regardless of placement site, although catheters placed centrally or in the cephalic regions may reach the heart more rapidly. Other common uses for the over-the-needle catheter type include pericardiocentesis, abdominocentesis, and thoracocentesis.

Peripheral catheters are available in a variety of both gauges and lengths, typically ranging from 24 gauge to 12 gauge and from 1.25 inches (3.1 cm) to 12 inches (30.5 cm) in length. Longer catheters used for pericardiocentesis or abdominocentesis are typically fenestrated for optimum fluid collection.[1]

Peripheral catheters are prone to insertion mishaps, such as frayed or burred tips that can develop if the catheter is aggressively pushed through tough skin during placement. Anchoring the catheter can also be problematic in saphenous vessels, as the catheter may slide in and out of the skin, increasing the chance of bacterial contamination or extravasation. Because their most common insertion sites are in jointed limbs, peripheral catheters can also be "positional," meaning that flow through the catheter may change based on limb movement or position. A positional catheter can create deleterious effects on flow rate and patency. However, overall ease of insertion and low costs associated with placement and maintenance make the peripheral intravenous catheter ideal for initial venous access in the emergency patient. Peripheral over-the-needle catheterization is the most common venous access technique in veterinary medicine.

If possible, placement of the peripheral catheter should be avoided around a moving joint (e.g., elbow), in order to avoid positional (flow) complications. After placement of the peripheral catheter, it is important that the catheter not move within the vein, as damage to the vessel may occur and increase the risk of thrombus formation and phlebitis. If the patient is to be administered intravenous fluids, anchoring a small portion of the tubing line directly to the bandage will help reduce catheter migration and movement.

Protocol 4.1 Peripheral catheter placement

Items Required
- Clippers
- Examination gloves
- Surgical scrub
- 2-inch porous medical tape
- T-port
- Infusion cap
- Saline flush
- Bandage material
- Appropriate work surface and at least one assistant

Procedure
1. Select best placement site, taking into consideration patient comfort, ease of accessibility, and anticipated catheter dwell time. If chemical restraint is necessary, allow adequate time for optimum results.
2. Collect necessary supplies.
3. Closely clip a generous area (2–2.5 inches—approximately 5 cm) around the intended insertion site and remove any loose fur.
4. Aseptically prepare the area. Alternate cleansing scrub with isopropyl alcohol; prepare in circular motions, starting from the center and finishing at the periphery with each swab.
5. Perform hand hygiene and don examination gloves; if the patient is immunocompromised, it is recommended to wear sterile gloves.
6. Restrain patient; avoid excessive stress to patient. Restrainer should occlude the vessel manually and proximally to ensure maximum visualization.
7. Palpate or visualize targeted vessel; point of entry should be directly on top of intended vessel.
8. Introduce catheter into the skin with bevel side up, ensuring that the catheter length does not contact the operator or the patient's fur during insertion.
9. After a "flash" of blood is visualized in the stylet hub (Fig. 4.3), slide the catheter off the needle and into the vessel.
10. Attach a sterile, preflushed T-port to the catheter hub.
11. Flush catheter with saline to ensure patency.
12. Anchor catheter with adhesive tape, or suture in place to avoid migration. Adequate adhesive tape should be pulled from the roll to circumnavigate the limb 1.5–2 times. One end of this tape should be applied directly to the catheter hub with the "sticky side" up and folded around the hub first. This tape should then be wrapped sticky side down around the entire circumference of the limb to provide a firm anchor. Additional pieces of tape should be applied sticky side down both above and below the initial anchored tape. Apply a light, protective bandage.

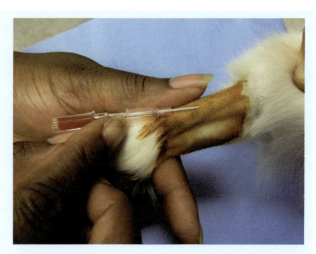

Figure 4.3 The catheter is slid off the needle and into the vessel after a "flash" of blood is visualized in the stylet hub.

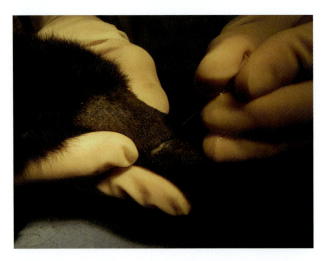

Figure 4.4 A sterile 18- to 22-gauge hypodermic needle can be used to create a mini "cutdown" when venous visualization is difficult.

Peripheral cutdown techniques

In emergency situations, if traditional peripheral catheterization attempts are unsuccessful and the patient is in peril, venous catheterization may require a cutdown procedure (e.g., exposing the vein surgically). Cutdowns allow quick vessel visualization and ensure catheterization on the first attempt. In addition, cutdowns can allow placement of a larger catheter than what can typically be placed percutaneously. Aseptic technique should be followed except in dire situations. The veterinarian performing the cutdown procedure should wear sterile gloves.

Mini cutdown

The mini cutdown technique is performed in order to gain access to either the cephalic or lateral saphenous vessel that may be collapsed and is difficult to enter. This procedure often creates a less traumatic skin blemish than is typically made during traditional catheter placement, particularly if the skin is tough and previous catheterization attempts have resulted in catheter burring.

Procedure

Using a sterile 18- to 22-gauge hypodermic needle, hold the needle with the bevel up and use the needle tip to cut the skin directly over and parallel to the targeted vessel (Fig. 4.4). Infusion of subcutaneous lidocaine prior to the mini cutdown is rarely needed. Once the incision has been made, the skin defect can be moved directly over the vessel. Tearing of the skin will release skin tension without damaging the underlying vessel,

Protocol 4.2 Mini cutdown

Items Required
- Clippers
- Surgical scrub
- 20- or 18-gauge hypodermic needle
- Peripheral catheter
- Saline flush
- T-port
- Catheter cap
- 2-inch medical tape
- Bandage material

Procedure
1. Select best placement site, taking into consideration patient comfort, ease of accessibility, and anticipated catheter dwell time. If chemical restraint is necessary, allow adequate time for optimum results.
2. Collect necessary supplies.
3. Closely clip a generous area (2–2.5 inches– approximately 5 cm) around the intended insertion site and remove any loose fur.
4. Aseptically prepare the area. Alternate cleansing scrub with isopropyl alcohol; prepare in circular motions, starting from the center and finishing at the periphery with each swab.
5. Perform hand hygiene and don examination gloves; if the patient is immunocompromised, it is recommended to wear sterile gloves.
6. Restrain patient; avoid excessive stress to patient. Restrainer should occlude the vessel manually and proximally to ensure maximum visualization.
7. Palpate or visualize targeted vessel.
8. Use edge of bevel of 20- or 18-gauge hypodermic needle as a "scalpel" to cut the skin in a distal-to-proximal direction adjacent and directly parallel to the targeted vessel.
9. Dissect around vessel further as needed, using needle as a mini scalpel with bevel directed parallel to vein.
10. Visualize vein and insert catheter.
11. Secure catheter as usual and place sterile dressing.

allowing for better visualization necessary for rapid catheter placement. A small incision can also be made adjacent to the vein with a number 11 scalpel blade, using caution to avoid incising the vessel and subcutaneous tissue. Blunt dissection with mosquito forceps may be required to visualize the vein; minimal dissection is usually required for the placement of an over-the-needle or through-the-needle catheter.

Surgical cutdown

A surgical cutdown is sometimes necessary to obtain vascular access in patients with hypovolemic shock or if central venous access is needed for hemodynamic monitoring, parental nutrition, or hemodialysis. Surgical cutdowns can be used to access the external jugular, cephalic, or lateral saphenous veins, with similar technique for all venous sites. Complications of a surgical cutdown can include perforation of the vascular wall, hematoma, thrombosis, venous transection, infection, and cellulitis.

Cutdown incisions should be made (a) in the middle to cranial portion of the jugular groove for catheterizing the external jugular vein or (b) on the dorsal antebrachium or lateral aspect of the distal tibia,

Protocol 4.3 Surgical venous cutdown

Items Required
- Clippers
- Surgical scrub
- Sterile gloves
- Sterile mosquito forceps
- Sterile thumb forceps
- Sterile sharp-ended scissors
- Sterile needle holder
- Sterile catheter
- Sterile syringes filled with heparinized saline
- Sterile injection plug and T-port
- Sterile absorbable monofilament suture
- Sterile scalpel blades (#10, #11, #15)
- Sterile 4×4-inch gauze squares
- Bandage material
- Optional: catheter introducer, towel clamps

Procedure
1. Select best placement site, taking into consideration patient comfort, ease of accessibility, and anticipated catheter dwell time. If chemical restraint is necessary, allow adequate time for optimum results.
2. Collect necessary supplies.
3. Closely clip a generous area (2–2.5 inches—approximately 5 cm) around the intended insertion site and remove any loose fur.
4. Aseptically prepare the area. Alternate cleansing scrub with isopropyl alcohol; prepare in circular motions, starting from the center and finishing at the periphery with each swab.
5. Perform hand hygiene and don sterile gloves.
6. Restrain patient; avoid excessive stress to patient. Restrainer should occlude the vessel manually and proximally to ensure maximum visualization, but should release occlusion during incision to avoid accidental vessel laceration.
7. If chemical sedation or general anesthesia is not feasible, infuse lidocaine (0.2–0.5 mL) into the subcutaneous region around the intended insertion site.
8. Prepare skin with a final surgical scrub and maintain a sterile field.
9. Make a skin incision over the vessel with a #10 or #15 scalpel blade.
10. Use blunt dissection to expose vein; dissect vein with curved hemostats so minimal fascia remains attached.
11. Slide hemostats under vein to level of handles in order to create a platform.
12. Tie off vein distally (or cranially if jugular vein is used) using absorbable monofilament suture; keep ends long to use for traction.
13. Place second suture around vein proximally, but do not tie.
14. Insert #11 scalpel blade parallel to vessel length, through center of vessel; turn 90° and cut outward.
15. Using catheter introducer or blunt end of curved needle, open vessel and slide in largest bore catheter possible.
16. Tie second suture trapping vein to catheter; ensure at least 3-mm tissue bumper.
17. Secure catheter to fascia of neck or thigh muscles as appropriate for location.
18. Suture incision (leave partially open if not performed under aseptic conditions).
19. Towel clamps can be used for temporary closure of incision.
20. Place sterile dressing.

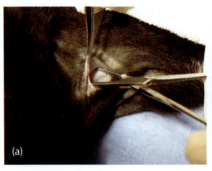
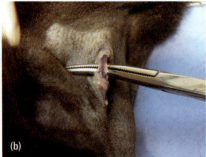
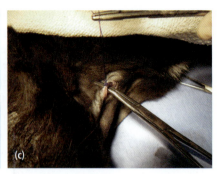

Figure 4.5 (a) The isolation of the vessel can be accomplished by blunt dissection of the subcutaneous tissue adjacent to the vein. (b) A hemostat can be slid underneath the vessel to create a "platform" to facilitate venous entry. (c) Tie off the vessel proximally using absorbable suture.

respectively, for the cephalic and lateral saphenous catheterization.

After clipping and performing an aseptic preparation of the targeted area, a scalpel blade is used to incise the skin directly over or adjacent to the vein. Either a transverse or a parallel skin incision can be made, using caution to incise only the full thickness of the skin. If the vessel is not immediately identified, it may be necessary to bluntly dissect with mosquito forceps adjacent to the vein (Fig. 4.5a). The vein can be identified as a blue-to-purple tubular structure within the subcutaneous tissue. Thumb forceps can be used to retract the subcutaneous tissues to expose the vessel. Dissection of adventitial tissue adjacent to the vein can be accomplished by the use of sharp-ended scissors dorsally and ventrally to the vein; dissecting in a parallel fashion will minimize vessel trauma or rupture.

Once the vessel is isolated from the subcutaneous tissue, a blunt hemostat is slid beneath the vessel through tissue as a type of "platform" for the vessel to lie on top of the instrument (Fig. 4.5b). A silk suture is then clasped by the hemostat and drawn beneath the vessel. The suture can be used to retract the vein distally to provide adequate tension for catheterization in the case of peripheral vessels. Alternately, the jugular vein may be sacrificed by ligating it cranially and using the ligature to retract the vessel. A second suture is placed beneath the vessel proximally (Fig. 4.5c). The vein is then cannulated through a venotomy (or by venipuncture) between the two ligatures. Following catheterization, the distal suture is tied, securing the catheter in the vein.[1]

The catheter should be replaced once the patient is resuscitated and hemodynamically stable. Remove the catheter by using gentle traction and applying direct pressure over the insertion site for several minutes. Allow the incision to heal by second intention if it was not placed under aseptic conditions.

Central venous access

Central venous catheters have many advantages over peripheral catheters, including that they allow for longer dwell time, safer administration of hyperosmolar solutions such as total parental nutrition, measurement of central venous pressure, and blood sampling with minimal stress to the patient. The central venous catheter is typically introduced via the jugular vein, but it can be readily inserted into the caudal vena cava via the lateral saphenous in the dog or the medial saphenous vein in the cat. Central venous catheters are available with either a single lumen or with multiple lumens, which allows for the simultaneous delivery of incompatible fluid types as is often needed in the critical patient. Central venous catheters are less likely to be affected by both patient positioning and motion at the point of insertion than peripheral catheters. Centrally situated catheters also allow for cannulation of larger vessels.

Disadvantages of central venous catheters include a longer placement time, greater expense, slight patient discomfort during placement, and the longer length may make rapid fluid administration problematic. Monitoring for extravasations with the central venous catheter can also be more difficult than in the peripheral over-the-needle catheter; veterinary technicians should monitor the patient for edema of the neck or sternum, pain with administration of medication, sluggish flow through the catheter, or inability to aspirate blood back from the catheter. It may be prudent to avoid central venous catheters in patients at risk of thrombosis (e.g., immune-mediated hemolytic anemias) or in animals with known or suspected coagulopathy. In addition, occlusion of the jugular vein may increase intracranial pressure during insertion, which is a relative-to-absolute contraindication in patients with head trauma or other central nervous system disturbances. In patients requiring central venous access and whose intracranial pressure may be elevated, a peripherally inserted central catheter (PICC) can instead be placed via the medial saphenous or lateral saphenous vein.

Catheter types for central veins

Central venous catheter types include long over-the-needle, through-the-needle, and guide-wire catheters; all types can be placed via a peripheral or central vessel. **Long over-the-needle** types of central venous catheters are inexpensive and come in a variety of diameters and lengths, ranging from 22 to 16 gauge and from 6 to 12 inches (approximately 15–30 cm) in length. These catheters can be placed into a central vessel via the jugular or a peripheral vein, and are often also used for pericardial or abdominal centesis (i.e., Milacath, Mila International, Erlanger, KY). Shorter over-the-needle catheters are used primarily for peripheral vein catheterization but can be centrally placed in pediatric patients. One disadvantage of centrally located over-the-needle catheters is patient discomfort, as these items tend to be stiff and can malfunction due to kinking. In addition, most over-the-needle long catheters are made of Teflon material, and should be replaced after 72 hours if possible.[2]

Guide-wire central venous catheters are placed by the Seldinger technique and include single and multilumen catheter systems (i.e., Arrow central venous catheter, Teleflex Medical, Research Triangle Park, NC; see Fig. 4.6). Catheters placed by the Seldinger technique—a common term for placing a catheter over a guide wire—are typically soft and flexible and are made of a polyurethane material, which is antithrombogenic and can

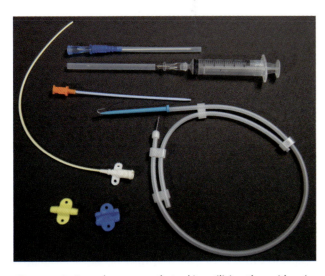

Figure 4.6 Central venous catheter kits utilizing the guide-wire (Seldinger) technique; such catheters range from single to multilumen devices.

dwell in the patient for longer periods. These catheters are available in a multitude of gauge, length, and lumen-number combinations. Certain guide-wire central venous catheters are impregnated with antimicrobial substances that may reduce the likelihood of catheter-related sepsis. Disadvantages of the Seldinger central venous catheter types are expense, increased risk of local hemorrhage during insertion, procedure time, and expertise needed for placement. It is the authors' opinion, however, that the risks and expense of such central venous catheters are far outweighed by the advantages in many critical patients.

Through-the-needle long catheters are passed through the needle and are typically longer than over-the-needle catheters (8–12 inches, approximately 20–30 cm) and are available in various diameters. Multiple varieties are commercially available (e.g., BD Intracath, BD Medical, Sandy, UT; BD L-cath, BD Medical, Sandy, UT; see Fig. 4.7a). Primarily used in the jugular vein, placement is typically quick and uncomplicated. A plastic sleeve around the catheter prevents its contamination during placement (Fig. 4.7b). The needle remains with the catheter while the catheter is in place, and it is protected by a plastic guard to avoid trauma to the animal or the catheter itself (Fig. 4.7c). Through-the-needle catheters can be placed in a peripheral vessel (canine lateral saphenous or feline medial saphenous) when the jugular vein is not a feasible option, such as in patients with coagulopathy or severe bite wounds to the cervical region. Advantages to the through-the-needle catheter include low cost, and speed and ease of placement. Disadvantages include the potential of shearing of the catheter, excessive bleeding (the hole made by the needle is slightly larger than the catheter that remains), and the bulky bandage required to anchor the catheter.

Central venous catheter placement techniques

Guide-wire central venous catheter technique

Guide-wire catheters utilize the **Seldinger technique**, and can be placed percutaneously or via a mini or surgical cutdown. Commercially available in single, double, or triple lumen, sizes range from 22- to 16-gauge catheters for peripheral use, and from 14- to 24-gauge catheters for central use; lengths range from 16 to 55 cm. Most guide-wire catheters come in kits containing the percutaneous introductory short catheter, the central venous catheter, guide wire (typically encased in a protective plastic case for sterile insertion), dilator, flush syringe, and anchoring device (Fig. 4.6). The authors recommend using a short, large-bore over-the-needle catheter as the percutaneous, introductory catheter,

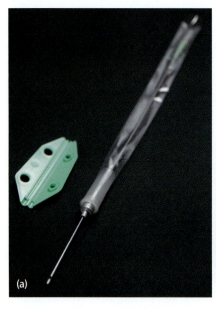
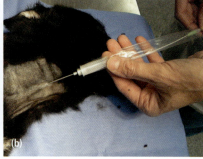
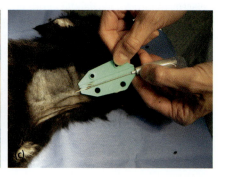

Figure 4.7 (a) A through-the-needle long catheter. (b) A plastic sleeve around the catheter prevents contamination during placement of the through-the-needle catheter. (c) Once the through-the-needle catheter has been fed entirely into the vessel, the needle is backed out of the skin and a protective guard is snapped over the needle. Ideally, the operator should practice aseptic technique during this procedure, to include donning sterile gloves.

and not the catheter or needle included in most kits, as the provided catheters are stiff and longer than is necessary in veterinary patients. Most central catheters are made of polyurethane to help prevent thrombosis, and can also be purchased with silver sulfadiazine, chlorhexidine (ArrowEVOLUTION with Chlorag+ard, Teleflex Medical, Research Triangle Park, NC), or heparin coating. With correct placement and care these catheters can stay in place for longer times, usually for the duration of hospitalization. (Table 4.3 summarizes the indications for the different catheter types.)

Care of central venous catheters is critical to maintain patency and patient comfort and to prevent infection (see Chapter 55, Care of Indwelling Device Insertion Sites, for more information). The central venous catheter bandage should be monitored frequently as it may tighten with neck movement and rehydration; the patient should be monitored for airway compromise and facial edema. When the catheter is removed, apply direct pressure to the insertion site for 5 minutes followed by application of a neck bandage to prevent hemorrhage. The neck bandage may be removed after 1–2 hours.

Through-the-needle catheters

Placement of a through-the-needle catheter requires standard fur clipping and aseptic site preparation. With either the neck or limb extended, the needle is inserted with the bevel side up, over the targeted vessel, taking care not to drag the needle over fur or nonprepared skin. The insertion site should be close to, but not directly on, the targeted vessel. After the needle is passed through the skin, the vein is then punctured directly from the top. Blood will usually flash back into the catheter, which confirms that the catheter is situated within the vessel; the catheter is then advanced into the vein. Resistance to advancement should be minimal. Once the catheter has been fed entirely into the vessel, the needle is backed out of the skin and either a guard is snapped in place over the needle (see Fig. 4.7c) or the needle is peeled away, depending on catheter design. If present, the stylet is then removed and the catheter is aspirated, to ensure blood flow, and flushed with either 0.9% saline or heparinized saline. The catheter should be anchored with either skin sutures or sterile bandaging. As the needle guard stays with the catheter, secure bandaging is important to avoid catheter migration. In addition to skin sutures, the catheter should be anchored with surgical tape around the neck or limb (being careful not to place the tape too tight) followed by cast padding and Vetwrap (3M Animal Care Products, St. Paul, MN). If the catheter is placed in the jugular vein, the authors recommend that a "bumper" of rolled cotton or gauze be placed outside the wrap and up against the upright guard to protect the catheter from migrating or bumping against the cage or other objects.

Table 4.3 Indications for different catheter types

Peripheral through-the-needle long catheter
- Jugular vein not accessible
- Coagulopathy
- Severe bite wounds or edema to the cervical region
- Frequent blood sampling needed
- Aggressive cat; restraint often easier for medial saphenous placement than for jugular placement
- Cervical disease or pain (AA luxation or cervical disk disease)
- Increased intracranial pressure; desire to avoid increasing intracranial pressure through occlusion of jugular vein
  Potential complications
  - Catheter shearing by introducer needle
  - Excessive bleeding

Central venous catheter
- Central venous pressure monitoring indicated
- Infusion of total parenteral nutrition or other hyperosmotic fluid
- Prolonged hospitalization expected
- Frequent blood sampling required
- Multiple ports required for simultaneous delivery of various fluids and medications
  Relative or potential contraindications
  - Thromboembolic disease
  - Coagulopathic disease
  - Respiratory disease (increased placement time)
  - Immune-mediated hemolytic anemia (due to thromboembolic disease potential)
  - Increased intracranial pressure (actual or suspected)
  - Cervical disease or pain (AA luxation or cervical disk disease)

Vascular access port
- Chemotherapy
- Delivery of sedation for repeated radiation therapy treatments
- Long-term delivery of intravenous medications or fluids
- Repeated blood sampling
- Blood donation
- Total parenteral nutrition
  Potential complications
  - Sepsis
  - Thrombosis

Intraosseous catheterization
- Severe hypotension
- Severe dehydration
- Extremely small body size (neonates, exotic animals, pocket pets)
- Inaccessible venous access (e.g., edema, thrombosis, severe burns)
  Contraindications
  - Pneumatic bones
  - Metabolic or infectious bone disease
  - Skin infection around proposed catheter insertion site

Protocol 4.4 Seldinger technique–placing a vascular catheter over a guide wire

Items Required
- Clippers
- Surgical scrub
- Sterile gloves
- 2 sterile drapes
- Large-bore, short, over-the-needle catheter
- #11 scalpel blade
- Guide-wire catheter kit
- Sterile gauze squares
- Heparinized saline
- T-port(s)
- Suture material
- Needle holders
- Thumb forceps
- Bandage scissors
- Bandage material
- At least one assistant

(Continued)

Procedure

1. Collect necessary supplies. If chemical restraint is necessary, allow adequate time for optimum results.
2. Patient should be placed in lateral recumbency with neck extended and thoracic limbs gently pulled caudally. It is recommended that two persons restrain the animal, one occluding the vessel and restraining the cranial end of the patient, the other restraining the patient's caudal end. Chemical restraint is typically not necessary.
3. Clip a wide area of fur to avoid contamination of insertion site, at least 2–2.5 inches (at least 5 cm) around intended insertion site.
4. Aseptically prepare the area. Alternate cleansing scrub with isopropyl alcohol; prepare in circular motions, starting from the center and finishing at the periphery with each swab.
5. Perform hand hygiene and don sterile gloves.
6. If chemical sedation or general anesthesia is not feasible, infuse lidocaine (0.2–0.5 mL) into the subcutaneous region around the intended insertion site.
7. Prepare skin with a final surgical scrub and maintain a sterile field.
8. Sterilely drape the area cranial and caudal to insertion site
9. Using sterile technique, premeasure the guide wire from the intended insertion point to the third or fourth intercostal space (ICS), with the tip of guide wire not beyond the fourth ICS. It is not necessary to premeasure the guide wire if placed via a saphenous vessel.
10. Premeasure the central catheter length from the intended insertion site to the intended catheter tip resting point. For jugular catheters, the ideal resting point is in the cranial vena cava at approximately the level of the 3rd–4th ICS. The tip of the jugular catheter should rest in the cranial vena cava just cranial to the right atrium if central venous pressure monitoring is anticipated.
11. Place a large-bore, short, over-the-needle catheter into the vein, with the tip pointing in the direction of the heart; ensure a "clean" stick with adequate blood flow.
12. Insert the straight end of the guide wire into the vessel through the over-the-needle catheter to the premeasured length (Fig. 4.8a).
13. Remove over-the-needle catheter; ensure that the wire does not inadvertently back out or touch a nonsterile field.
14. Insert the plastic dilator into the vessel by placing the wire through it and guiding it into the vessel. Passage of the dilator may be facilitated by "tenting" the skin and gently rotating the dilator into the vessel (Fig. 4.8b). A cut into the skin with a #11 scalpel blade next to the wire may ease insertion and prevent "burring." Insert one-half the length of the dilator into the vessel, hold for a few seconds, and then remove the dilator from the guide wire. Expect bleeding from the insertion site, and use sterile gauze to apply pressure if needed while transitioning to the next steps.
15. Insert the catheter over the wire and guide it into the vessel to predetermined length (Fig. 4.8c). Ensure the end of the wire is projecting out the distal end of the catheter before advancement; the wire should be held as the catheter is advanced into the vessel. If multilumen catheters are used, the wire should exit the distal port. Remember to remove the cap from the distal port so that the wire is able to emerge. Remove the wire and leave the catheter in place.
16. Aspirate catheter with a small syringe; blood should easily flow into the syringe. Flush the catheter with sterile saline and cap port(s) with a T-port or injection plug. Repeat procedure for each port if a multilumen catheter is used. It is important to always aspirate the catheter first, before flushing, so as not to create an air embolus, even if the catheter port(s) were preflushed.
17. If entire length of catheter is not used, secure excess catheter with plastic catheter holders provided. Secure the catheter in place with sutures between the skin and the designated grooves or holes on the catheter hub and/or the plastic catheter holders (Fig. 4.8d). Place a sterile dressing over the insertion site, such as a sterile cotton ball or a small sterile gauze square.
18. Apply a loose neck wrap containing cast padding or stretch bandaging followed by a water-resistant bandage. Tape T-port or multilumen ports onto top of the bandage for easy access (Fig. 4.8e). Ensure the bandage is not tight; several fingers should easily slide under the bandage. Recheck patency of the catheter by aspirating blood once the bandage is in place.

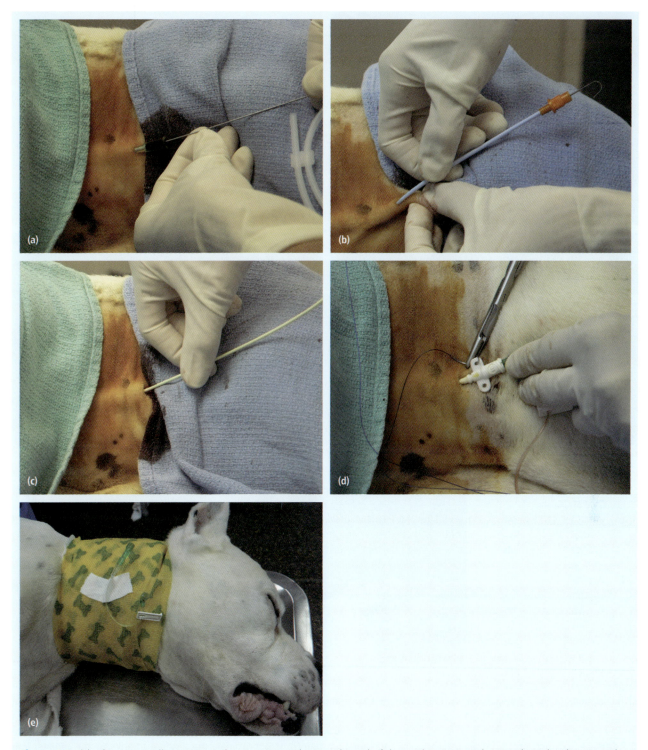

Figure 4.8 (a) After aseptically preparing the area, insert the straight end of the guide wire into the vessel via the short over-the-needle catheter. (b) Passage of the dilator may be accomplished by "tenting" the skin and gently but firmly rotating the dilator into the vessel. (c) Insert the catheter over the wire and guide into the vessel. (d) The catheter is secured in place with skin sutures attached to the wings of the plastic applicator. (e) A bandage is applied around the central catheter; a T-port is anchored on top of the bandage for easy access.

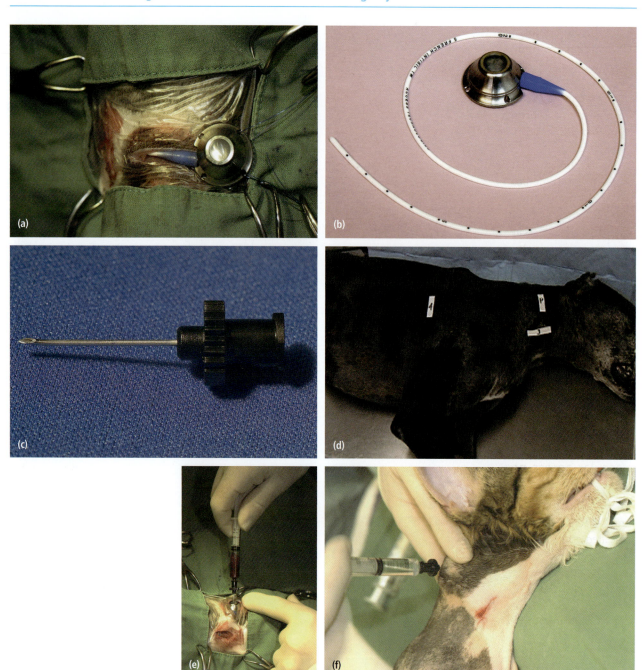

Figure 4.9 (a) Vascular access ports are subcutaneous delivery systems that allow serial blood sampling or intravenous administration of medications or fluid (CompanionPort, Mila International, Erlanger, KY). (b) The vascular access port (VAP) consists of a compact injection reservoir, self-sealing septum, and attached catheter. (c) A Huber point needle is necessary to access the VAP percutaneously. (d) The port should be implanted in a pocket lateral to and level with the lateral spine of the 3d–4th cervical vertebrae (P). Measure the distance from port pocket location to the vena cava–atrial junction (J), to approximate the distance to advance the catheter into the vasculature. (e) Port patency is confirmed by using a Huber needle attached to a syringe of sterile saline. (f) The port should be placed in the subcutaneous port pocket such that the septum does not lie directly beneath the skin incision.

Alternate vascular access options

Vascular access ports

Vascular access ports (VAPs), or implantable vascular access systems, are subcutaneous delivery systems, which allow serial blood sampling or intravenous administra-

tion of medications or fluid (i.e., CompanionPort, Mila International, Erlanger, KY). Vascular access ports are surgically placed subcutaneously (typically dorsal to the shoulder) in order to provide long-term venous access to chronically ill patients (Fig. 4.9). The catheter and port can be accessed without patient discomfort or sedation; therefore, most patients with VAPs can be treated intermittently on an outpatient basis. Clinical indications for the use of VAPs include delivery of chemotherapy, delivery of sedation for long-term radiation therapy, chronic diseases requiring medication or fluid administration (chronic renal failure), serial blood sampling, or blood donation. Vascular access ports are unobtrusive, creating only a slight bump under the skin. Other advantages of VAPs include reduction in patient stress, reduced medication administration time, and the "rest" of peripheral vessels, which allows peripheral veins to remain intact for future use.

CompanionPorts are available in three sizes to accommodate various pets. The port itself is biocompatible and will not degrade over time. A Huber point needle must be used at all times to access the CompanionPort in order to maintain integrity of the septum.

Complications associated with VAP systems are similar to those seen with other types of intravenous devices, including local infection, sepsis, thrombosis, or extravasation. Nursing care required for VAPs includes daily insertion site inspection, mild antiseptic cleansing, and intermittent heparinized flushes to prevent clogging or occlusion. Minimal maintenance is required every 3–4 weeks.

Vascular access port implantation procedure

The VAP is a totally implantable access system consisting of a compact injection reservoir, self-sealing septum, and attached catheter (Fig. 4.9b). It is designed for repeated entry to the vascular system or body cavity for drug delivery or withdrawal of venous blood samples. The port is accessed percutaneously with a Huber point needle (Fig. 4.9c). Once the port is accessed, fluid and/or medication delivery is through the skin, via the needle, into the port reservoir.

Patient preparation

Place the patient in lateral recumbency with a towel under the neck to increase access to surgical site. Mark the target area of the port and catheter placement with a permanent marker; the port should be implanted lateral to and level with the lateral spine at the level of the 3rd–4th cervical vertebrae (Fig. 4.9c). Place the patient under general anesthesia.

Clip and aseptically prepare a surgical field 2–2.5 inches (approximately 5–7 cm) around intended placement site of the port, as well as the jugular site. Approximate the distance the VAP's catheter must be tunneled to reach the jugular by measuring the distance from the port pocket location (insertion site) to the vena-cava–atrial junction using the centimeter markers on the distal end of the catheter (Fig. 4.9d).

Surgical procedure

Note: Aseptic technique is critical in preventing premature catheter occlusion or port failure. Techniques listed below follow protocols intended for use of the CompanionPort (Mila International, Erlanger, KY), a vascular device designed specifically for the veterinary patient.

Step 1: Incisions

While the patient is awake and upright, mark the areas of the planned port and catheter placement with a marker. The port should be implanted lateral to and level with the lateral spine at the level of the 3rd–4th cervical vertebrae directly over the supraspinatus muscle. Ensure that the placement area will not interfere with normal neck motion. Place the patient in lateral recumbency; a towel under the neck may facilitate access to the surgical site. Anesthetize and intubate the patient; clip and aseptically prepare the area. It is recommended that the patient be transported to a sterile operating room with the final prep on the surgical table. Sterile procedure, including surgical gown, cap, mask, sterile gloves, and drape, is necessary before the start of the procedure.

Make a small skin incision over the jugular vein ventral to the port pocket site; use blunt forceps to expose the vessel. Place a wet sponge over the site. Next, make a skin incision at the port placement site and create a pocket in the SQ tissue large enough to bury the port, about 6 cm. Place a wet sponge over the site.

Step 2: Tunneling the VAP

Create a tunnel from the port pocket incision site to the jugular incision site using forceps. Remove the protective sleeve from the catheter and grasp the boot (proximal end of the catheter) with the forceps. Then, pull the catheter through the tunnel from the jugular incision site to the port pocket incision (pulling "backward" feeding outward to the port site). A hollow trocar may be used to help create a tunnel, although such a device is not included with the port kit and would need to be ordered separately. Clamp the port end of the catheter to prevent backflow of blood once the catheter is inserted into the jugular vein.

Step 3: Placing the catheter into the vessel

Puncture the vessel with the needle introducer; ensure blood flashback in the flush chamber. Next, withdraw the introducer needle, leaving the "T" handle peel-away sheath portion in the vessel (some bleeding may be expected).

Slide the rounded tip (distal end) of the catheter through the introducer sheath; depth markings on the catheter can help determine desired length of the catheter advancement. Recommended placement length rests the catheter tip at the vena-cava–atrial junction. As the catheter is advanced into the vessel, simultaneously withdraw the introducer sheath, advancing the catheter as the introducer is pulled out.

Grasp the "T" handle of the introducer sheath and pull outward and up, peeling the sheath apart and freeing the catheter. Use the depth markings to verify optimal placement of catheter tip. Correct tip location is important as the junction of the vena cava and right atrium is an area of high blood flow, reducing the incidence of VAP catheter occlusion.

Step 4: Connecting the port to the catheter

Trim the catheter to the length necessary for attachment to the barbed outlet pin on the port; it is usually necessary to leave a little "wiggle" room for normal neck movement. Using a 22-gauge Huber point straight needle (provided in the kit), flush the port with sterile saline prior to connecting port and catheter. Replace the boot (or clear sleeve) onto the catheter; the wide end of the boot should face the port and the pointed end should face the catheter. Slide the catheter over all the barbs on the connector pin of the port; slide and screw the boot over the catheter–port connection. Confirm patency by using the Huber needle attached to a syringe of sterile saline; flush and prime the port prior to suturing (Fig. 4.9e). If blood cannot be aspirated, manipulate the catheter until blood can be withdrawn. At all points in the procedure, take care not to introduce air into the patient's vascular system.

Step 5: Completing VAP placement

Place the port in the subcutaneous port pocket off to one side, so that the septum will not lie directly beneath the skin incision (Fig. 4.9f). Secure the port in place with nonabsorbable suture; all of the port's anchor holes should be utilized to prevent port migration. Confirm port patency by sterile aspiration; close skin incision routinely and flush the port well with sterile saline followed by a sterile heparin–saline lock solution.

Intraosseous catheterization

Intraosseous catheterization is a procedure in which a needle is placed into a bone, typically when the need for vascular access is urgent and venous catheterization cannot be performed quickly. The intraosseous space is easily accessible even in the most dehydrated or hypovolemic animal. Advantages of intraosseous catheter placement include speed and ease of placement, minimal complication rates, ease of fluid administration, and minimal cost of supplies.

Clinical indications for intraosseous catheterization include severe vascular collapse (e.g., hypovolemic shock), severe vascular trauma, peripheral edema, thrombosis, small patient size (e.g., neonates, exotics), or even obesity. Mastering intraosseous catheterization, which is simple to perform, can prevent patient death when timely vascular attempts are not feasible or practical. Locations for intraosseous catheter placement include the trochanteric fossa of the femur, the wing of the ileum, the proximal humerus, and the tibial tuberosity (Fig. 4.10a). Potential complications are minimal; fracture of the bone at the catheter site, infection, osteomyelitis, edema, and patient discomfort associated with rapid fluid infusion are the reported complications to intraosseous catheterization.[3] The most common complication is dislodgement of the catheter due to animal movement. When this technique is applied to other species, care must be taken never to introduce fluids into pneumatic bones. Medications targeted for intravenous administration can be used via the intraosseous catheter or needle. Rate of maximal fluid administration is related to the diameter of the catheter or needle.

Swan–ganz catheters

A special balloon-tipped catheter called a Swan–Ganz catheter is used to measure pulmonary vascular pressures and to gather data used to calculate cardiac output. A Swan–Ganz catheter can be used to measure cardiac output, right atrial pressure, pulmonary arterial pressure (systolic, diastolic, and mean), and pulmonary arterial occlusion pressure (also called wedge pressure). Some Swan–Ganz catheters are also equipped with an oximeter to measure mixed venous oxygen saturation. The Swan–Ganz catheter has several ports that can be utilized for fluid or medication administration. For more information on Swan–Ganz catheters, see Chapter 12, Cardiac Output Monitoring.

Placement of a Swan–Ganz catheter for assessment of pulmonary arterial pressures, cardiac output, and oxygen extraction ratios requires specialized training and often expensive equipment; consequently, use of this particular catheter is typically limited to advanced critical care units. Risks associated with the placement of Swan–Ganz catheters include cardiac valvular damage, catheter migration, pulmonary artery rupture, arrhythmias, and pulmonary infarction.[4]

Maintenance and care of intravenous catheters

Catheter care is important in order to avoid complications and to ensure patency for the desired length of

Protocol 4.5 Intraosseous catheterization (Fig. 4.10)

Items Required
- Clippers
- Surgical scrub
- 2% lidocaine in a 1-mL syringe with a 23- to 25-gauge needle
- Suture material
- Saline flush
- T-port
- Hypodermic needle appropriate for patient size (e.g., 22-gauge, ¾ or ½ inch long) for small patients or neonates, or spinal needles
- Bone marrow needles for adult patients whose bones have already ossified

Note. Spinal needles, containing an outer needle and an inner stylet, are preferred in the authors' opinion because the shafts of hypodermic needles used on the neonate can become clogged during placement. Many veterinary companies also manufacture intraosseous catheters that can be used in adult patients, including intraosseous drills to facilitate insertion.

Procedure
1. Select best placement site, taking into consideration patient comfort, ease of placement, and anticipated catheter dwell time.
2. Collect necessary supplies.
3. Closely clip a generous area (2–2.5 inches–approximately 5 cm) around the intended insertion site and remove any loose fur.
4. Aseptically prepare the area. Alternate cleansing scrub with isopropyl alcohol; prepare in circular motions, starting from the center and finishing at the periphery with each swab.
5. Perform hand hygiene and don examination gloves; if the patient is immunocompromised, it is recommended to wear sterile gloves.
6. Restrain patient; avoid excessive stress to patient.
7. Administer a small amount of lidocaine to the level of the periosteum.
8. Prepare skin with a final surgical scrub and maintain a sterile field.
9. Place a finger on the long axis of the bone in which the catheter will be placed, to determine the bone's axis and location.
10. If using the femoral trochanteric fossa, adduct the limb slightly (toward ventral midline) and rotate trochanteric fossa laterally to avoid the sciatic nerve.
11. Insert the catheter distally lengthwise into the medulla of the femur or humerus cortex parallel to the finger held alongside the bone, aiming for the trochanteric fossa if the femoral trochanteric fossa is the insertion site. Simultaneously push and twist the needle in a single line (i.e., avoid movement in the third dimension). Expect initial resistance as the needle passes through the cortex. If resistance is felt as the needle passes through the cortex into the medulla, the bevel of the needle may be seated incorrectly, causing blockage. Gently turn the needle 90°–180° to dislodge and attempt placement again.
12. Once the needle is in place, push the hub of the needle back and forth, simultaneously moving the limb; the hub of the needle should be seated securely in the shaft of the bone and move along with the bone when the limb is moved.
13. Aspirate needle or catheter; aspiration of bone marrow confirms placement. A radiograph can also confirm the correct anatomical location.
14. Flush gently with a small amount heparinized saline; little resistance should be felt.
15. Check surrounding tissue for fluid leakage; if leakage is evident, the catheter may need to be removed and another bone tried.
16. Attach a T-port.
17. Anchor the catheter either by placing a stay suture through the skin near the catheter hub and attaching that suture to the tubing of the T-port, or by stapling a small butterfly tape anchor from the catheter hub to the skin.
18. Check for displacement of the catheter at least twice daily.

(Continued)

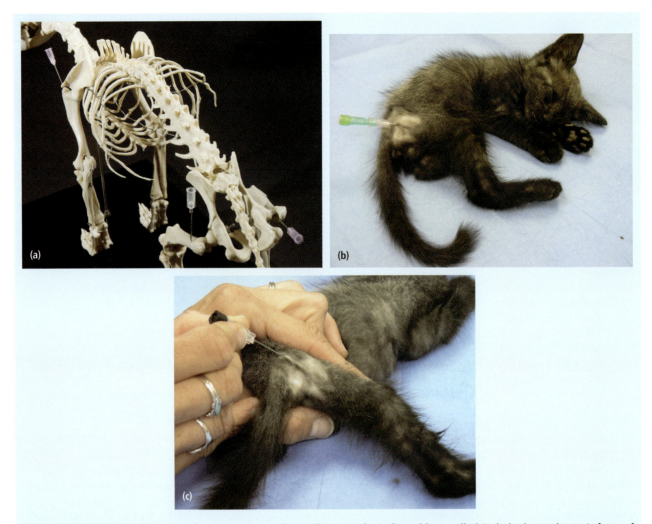

Figure 4.10 (a) Potential locations for intraosseous catheter placement (as indicated by needles) include the trochanteric fossa of the femur, the wing of the ileum, the proximal humerus, and the tibial tuberosity. (b) A hypodermic or spinal needle appropriate for patient size or a bone marrow needle can be used as an intraosseous catheter. Ideally, the catheter should be inserted with gloved hands through an aseptically prepared site. (c) The catheter or needle is inserted into the medullary cavity of the femur or humerus along the long axis of the bone.

time. Any indwelling intravenous device predisposes a patient to nosocomial infection. All personnel involved with the placement or handling of the catheter should use aseptic technique when changing bandages, administering fluids or medications, withdrawing blood, or while using monitoring devices attached to the catheter. Infection may occur as a result of contaminated intravenous solutions, contaminated injection ports, catheter caps, or T-ports, poor skin preparation or insertion techniques, or failure to routinely change the catheter bandage. Monitoring equipment should be cleaned and disinfected between patients. Multiple ports and lines

should be labeled appropriately and handled with aseptic technique. Ports should be swabbed with alcohol prior to introduction of a needle. Insertion sites should be routinely monitored for thrombosis, which causes a "ropey" feel to the vessel; for patient discomfort, redness, heat, or swelling around the insertion site; for catheter migration either into or out of the skin, compared with its depth at initial insertion; and for subcutaneous extravasation, which can lead to discomfort upon injection and accumulation of fluids or medications under the skin.

Catheter bandages should be removed fully to allow inspection of the catheter site at least once daily. Adhesive tapes must be examined for tightness and dryness; bandages contaminated with body fluids should be replaced immediately.

While sterile technique should be maintained for any vascular device intervention, nursing management of catheters used for parenteral nutrition (PN) warrants special focus, since nutritional formulae are excellent media for bacterial colonization. Proper catheter care of a PN catheter includes strict aseptic technique during insertion, including proper skin preparation, placement of a sterile underwrap over the insertion site, and strict aseptic technique when handling PN administration tubing and bags. The intravenous (IV) lines should not be disconnected; if diagnostic testing or frequent walking is necessary, PN administration lines and bags should accompany the patient after clamping lines to avoid accidental rapid infusion. If a multilumen catheter is placed, proper identification of each port is necessary, with one line dedicated to the PN solution only.

Catheter flushing

Catheters should be flushed with a small volume of sterile saline (0.5–2 mL, depending upon catheter length and size of patient) at least every 8–12 hours.[5] Judicious use can also be made of a heparinized saline solution, paying particular attention to the heparin dose given to small patients or those with coagulopathies. The authors recommend flushing any unused central venous catheters or ports every 4 hours with 3–5 mL of flush using sterile technique. See Chapter 55, Care of Indwelling Device Insertion Sites, for more detailed information.

Peripheral intravenous catheters

A **peripheral intravenous catheter** should be replaced every 72–96 hours, or immediately if it is suspected to be the source of an infection or phlebitis.[2] Minimizing tape use and anchoring with suture to secure catheters will aid in insertion site inspection and patient comfort. Any cutdown incision made during placement can increase the potential for infection; these catheters should be replaced or removed as soon as possible. Any catheter should be removed when no longer needed.[2] Intraosseous catheters are similar to IV catheters and it has been suggested that they can stay in place for over 3 days in veterinary patients if no signs of infection are found.[5]

Central intravenous catheters

Central intravenous catheters may dwell for the length of patient hospitalization as long as there is no suspicion of catheter-related infection,[2] but they require daily insertion-site inspection for signs of thrombosis or leakage, and daily site maintenance. Central venous

catheter care also requires daily inspection as indicated above for peripheral catheters. As central catheters are significantly longer than peripheral catheters, signs of extravasation may not be as apparent. The midsternal region should be examined for edema related to any jugular venous catheter, and the proximal aspect of the pelvic limb should be examined for edema related to lateral or medial saphenous venous catheter placement. Patency can be evaluated by ensuring blood can be aspirated. Note that neck bandages should follow the "two finger rule," wherein the bandage is loose enough to slide two fingers underneath to help ensure patient comfort. If it is necessary to change a central catheter and catheter-related infection is not suspected, replacement can sometimes be done by passing a sterile guide wire through the existing catheter, removing the catheter, and aseptically placing a new one over the wire.[2]

Complications

Bacterial contamination of catheter sites can result from skin contamination at insertion, contamination from patient interference, soiled bandages, improper handling, contaminated injectates, blood left inside an injection port or T-port, and from the tops of multiuse intravenous medication bottles. Personnel should practice proper hygiene protocols, including washing hands frequently, swabbing ports and medication bottles with antiseptics, and frequent bandage changes for any catheter in any anatomic location. The authors recommend that flush solution be changed every 48 hours to avoid microbial contamination. Any patient with an unexplained fever, pain upon injection, or inflammation at a catheter insertion site should be investigated for a catheter-related infection. Suspicious catheters must be removed in an aseptic manner and submitted for bacterial culture and susceptibility. See Chapter 54, Minimizing Nosocomial Infection, for in-depth discussion.

Phlebitis is another commonly encountered complication of indwelling vascular catheterization. Phlebitis can occur due to inflammation associated with movement of the catheter in the vessel, or due to bacterial infection, which can lead to sepsis.

Air embolism can occur if lines become disconnected or a significant volume of air is present within an administration set. Central venous catheters have the highest risk of incidence as air can be sucked in due to negative pressure within the thorax.[2] Central venous catheters and large-bore catheters pose the risk of exsanguination if patient interference or disconnection goes undetected. Catheter embolism can occur if a fragment of the catheter becomes free within the vessel either due to placement error or patient interference. Radiopaque catheters can allow radiographic investigation to locate any such fragments and aid in planning for surgical retrieval.

Thrombus formation can occur with any venous or arterial cannulation, particularly if there is endothelial damage within the vessel. Smaller veins with slower blood flow, the use of rigid catheters, insertion over a joint, or pre-existing conditions such as immune-mediated hemolytic anemia, glomerulonephritis, or vasculitis may increase the risk of thrombus formation. Severe thrombus formation could lead to pulmonary thromboembolism.

Acknowledgment

A special thanks to Dr. James S. Wohl, for materials referenced throughout this chapter.

References

1. Wohl J, Tefend M. Vascular access techniques. In: Bonagura JD, ed. Kirk's Current Veterinary Therapy XIV. 8th ed. Philadelphia: WB Saunders; 2007:38–43.
2. Centers for Disease Control website. Guidelines for the prevention of intravascular catheter-related infections. Available at: www.cdc.gov/mmwr/preview/mmwrhtml/rr5110a1.htm. Accessed January 2, 2001.
3. Mazzaferro EM. Intraosseous catheterization: an often underused, life-saving tool. Clinician's Brief 2009;7:9–12.
4. Waddell L. Advanced vascular access options. Proceedings. 20th Annu Amer Coll Vet Int Med Forum 2004;719–722.
5. Cave C. High dependency nursing. In: Aspinall V, ed. The Complete Textbook of Veterinary Nursing. 1st ed. St. Louis, MO: Elsevier; 2006:545.

Recommended reading

Hadaway L. Technology of flushing vascular access devices. J Infus Nurs 2006;29(3):137–145.

5

Arterial puncture and catheterization

Elisa M. Mazzaferro and Cindy Hauser

Arterial puncture and catheterization are among the most important techniques required for monitoring the critically ill small animal patient. Arterial puncture is most commonly performed to obtain arterial blood samples for blood gas analysis. If repeated arterial blood sampling is required, or if the patient requires continuous direct blood pressure monitoring, the placement of an arterial catheter is necessary.

Arterial puncture

To perform an arterial puncture, clip and clean (i.e., with isopropyl alcohol) the area over the artery, particularly if the animal is immunosuppressed and at risk of infection. In most cases, a full surgical scrub is unnecessary unless an indwelling catheter is going to be introduced into the artery. Prefabricated syringes that contain a pellet of lithium heparin can be purchased from a variety of manufacturers (i.e., Smith Medical; Vital Signs, Inc.; Becton Dickinson; Cardinal Health). A simpler and less expensive technique, however, is to use equipment that is already stocked in the emergency room (ER) or intensive care unit (ICU).

Procedure

The supplies required to perform arterial puncture for blood sample collection are heparin and a 3-mL syringe with a 22- or 25-gauge needle attached—or a lithium heparin arterial blood gas syringe with its needle attached—as well as pressure bandaging supplies appropriate for the sampling site.

If using a standard 3-mL syringe and needle, pull a small amount of liquid heparin into the syringe, and pull the plunger to the 3-mL mark to coat the entire inner surface of the syringe with the heparin. Expel all the heparin and air from the syringe. Pull air back into the syringe to the 3-mL mark and forcibly expel all the heparin and air from the syringe again; repeat this forced air expulsion procedure three times.[1] This syringe evacuation procedure minimizes sample dilution with liquid heparin, which would cause significant preanalytical error in blood gas and electrolyte values. Even using this technique, ionized calcium concentration should not be measured on heparinized samples.[1]

Arterial puncture is most commonly performed on the dorsal pedal artery (or one of its metatarsal branches) or the femoral artery. Following aseptic preparation of the proposed needle insertion site, palpate for the dorsal pedal pulse over the second and third metatarsal bones, or for the femoral pulse over the cranial aspect of the proximal femoral diaphysis. Insert the needle at a 15°–20° angle with respect to the skin over the point where the pulse is most easily palpable. It is easiest to feel the pulse with the nondominant hand. Advance the needle very slowly in 1- to 2-mm increments; after each movement, look at the syringe hub carefully for a flash of blood. If the needle has been advanced to what seems a sufficient depth and a flash of blood has not been encountered, the needle should be slowly withdrawn in the plane of entry. As the needle is withdrawn, watch closely for a blood flashback. In some cases, the needle has punctured through the deep portion of the vessel wall and blood will enter the needle and syringe during withdrawal. If the needle must be redirected, pull it to the superficial subcutaneous tissues before redirecting.

Advanced Monitoring and Procedures for Small Animal Emergency and Critical Care, First Edition. Edited by Jamie M. Burkitt Creedon, Harold Davis.
© 2012 John Wiley & Sons, Inc. Published 2012 by John Wiley & Sons, Inc.

Protocol 5.1 Arterial puncture for blood sample collection

Items Required
- Clean clippers and blade
- Skin-cleaning supplies: isopropyl-alcohol-soaked cotton, or full surgical scrub as appropriate
- Prefabricated lithium heparin arterial blood gas (ABG) syringe
-or-
- 3-mL syringe, liquid heparin, and a 25- or 22-gauge needle
- Pressure bandage for postpuncture wrap
- An assistant (usually only one is required)

Procedures
If using a prefabricated ABG syringe, begin at step 6.
1. Collect necessary supplies.
2. Equip the 3-mL syringe with the needle.
3. Pull a small amount of the heparin into the syringe, then pull the plunger back to coat the entire inner surface of the syringe.
4. Expel all the heparin and air from the syringe.
5. Pull air into the syringe to the 3-mL mark and forcibly expel contents from the syringe; repeat three times. The syringe and needle hub should appear evacuated of liquid heparin.
6. Closely clip a generous area (2–2.5 inches—approximately 5 cm) around the intended insertion site and remove any loose fur.
7. Aseptically prepare the area. Alternate cleansing scrub with isopropyl alcohol; prepare in circular motions, starting from the center and finishing at the periphery with each swab.
8. Perform hand hygiene and don examination gloves.
9. Restrain patient; avoid excessive stress to patient.
10. Palpate for the pulse: over the 2nd and 3rd metatarsal bones for the dorsal pedal artery, or over the cranial aspect of the proximal femoral diaphysis for the femoral artery.
11. Insert needle at 15°–20° angle with respect to the skin where the pulse is most easily palpable.
12. Advance needle very slowly, checking frequently for a "flash" of blood. If the needle has been advanced a sufficient depth and no flash has been encountered, slowly withdraw the needle in the plane of entry, watching closely for a flash.
13. Once the needle tip enters the artery, gently pull the plunger or allow arterial pressure to fill the syringe.
14. Gently withdraw the needle from the skin and apply pressure with a bandage for many minutes to an hour.

Once the needle tip is seated in the artery, gently pull the plunger of the syringe to withdraw blood, or allow arterial pressure to fill the syringe. The latter technique confirms that the blood is arterial rather than venous. Gently withdraw the needle from the skin when an adequate sample has been withdrawn. Apply pressure with a bandage for many minutes to an hour. When a pressure bandage is applied with tape and left on the patient for a period of time, it may be useful to write "Remove Pressure Bandage" on the patient's order sheet so the bandage is not left in place for a prolonged time. (See Protocol 5.1.)

Sublingual venipuncture

Sublingual veins are also used for sampling in anesthetized patients because oxygenation in this vascular bed closely approximates arterial blood. Thus, samples from this site can be used for arterial blood gas analysis. These superficial, soft-walled vessels are usually punctured with a 25-gauge needle. Firm pressure on the vessel must be performed for a minimum of 5 minutes to prevent hematoma formation after puncture. The sublingual veins are not usually used for catheterization in clinical patients.

Special considerations for arterial catheter placement

Although the placement of an arterial catheter can be more technically difficult than placement of a peripheral venous catheter, the equipment necessary and the procedures performed are largely the same. The materials and supplies required to attach an arterial catheter to a transducer for continuous blood pressure monitoring are discussed elsewhere in this text (see Chapter 8, Fluid-Filled Hemodynamic Monitoring Systems, for more details). Special considerations for arterial catheter placement follow here.

Arterial catheter site selection

A variety of arteries can be used for arterial catheter placement, including the dorsal metatarsal artery (commonly called the dorsal pedal artery) and the radial, coccygeal, femoral, or auricular artery. When selecting a site for placement, it is important to consider the patients' mobility and activity level, and whether the patient has access to the site and could potentially remove the catheter. As mentioned below, one should also consider risk of contamination and practicality of keeping the area clean when selecting an arterial catheterization site. More-peripheral arteries may be preferable in patients with hemostatic concerns. Finally, the operator's experience and expertise with different anatomic sites may impact catheter site selection.

Aseptic technique

The most important aspect of minimizing the risk of catheter-related infection is strict adherence to aseptic technique when placing an arterial catheter.[2] Therefore, an important consideration when placing an arterial catheter is whether the location has a high risk of contamination. For example, although the dorsal pedal arteries are perhaps the most simple to catheterize, consider whether the patient has diarrhea that could potentially contaminate the arterial catheter site. It is generally recommended that no catheter be placed into an area of damaged skin, abrasion, or pyoderma.[3]

One of the most common causes of hospital-acquired infection is the transmission of disease-causing bacteria on the hands of hospital personnel. Therefore a very basic, and extremely important, tenet of infection control and antiseptic technique is for the operator to thoroughly wash his or her hands before placing an arterial catheter. The Centers for Disease Control has published hand-washing guidelines that instruct on proper hand hygiene techniques for healthcare workers.[4] Additionally, the reader may see Chapter 54, Minimizing Nosocomial Infection, for detailed information. For arterial catheter placement, after carefully scrubbing the hands the operator should don examination gloves, unless the patient is immunocompromised, in which case sterile gloves should be worn.

Once an acceptable artery has been identified, carefully clip all fur over the artery and circumferentially around the patient's extremity, leaving at least 5 cm (~2 in.) between the fur margin and the proposed insertion. Next, perform a surgical preparatory scrub on the area over and around the catheter insertion site.

Analgesia

Placement of an arterial catheter can be uncomfortable, so some patients benefit from sedation or a local anesthetic during placement.

Percutaneous facilitation

The placement of the arterial catheter through a small hole in the skin helps prevent the tip of the catheter from becoming burred. If a burr develops, catheter insertion will be difficult and there exists increased risk of thrombus formation.[5]

The concept of percutaneous facilitation involves making a small nick in the skin surface over a proposed site of catheter placement in animals that are extremely dehydrated or have very thick or tough skin. Percutaneous facilitation is most commonly performed with the bevel of an 18- or 20-gauge hypodermic needle. Tent the skin over the catheter insertion site and make a nick through the skin with the needle's sharp bevel, taking care to avoid underlying vessels. If the bevel of the needle nicks the underlying artery, the artery will spasm and the pulse will wane or disappear. When an artery spasms, it is very difficult to cannulate until a palpable pulse returns.

Securing the Arterial Catheter

If an arterial catheter accidentally becomes disconnected, excessive blood loss can quickly occur, which may increase morbidity in an already critical patient. As such, it is recommended that the infusion plug and T-port have Luer lock connections (e.g., Luer-Lok [Becton, Dickinson and Company, Franklin Lakes, NJ]). Any attached fluid-filled monitoring system should likewise have Luer lock connections. When securing the arterial catheter itself, some clinicians prefer to use surgical glue to adhere the catheter hub to the patient's skin. However, skin glue can be difficult and painful to remove. If the catheter hub and patient's skin are dry and free of debris, the catheter can usually be secured adequately with standard white medical tape as described below.

Dorsal pedal artery catheterization

The dorsal pedal artery and its metatarsal arterial branches are located over the metatarsal bones. The most prominently palpable is usually found on the dorsomedial aspect of the foot between the second and third metatarsal bones, just distal to the tarsus (the hock).

Place the patient in lateral recumbency on the side in which the catheter is to be placed (i.e., if the proposed

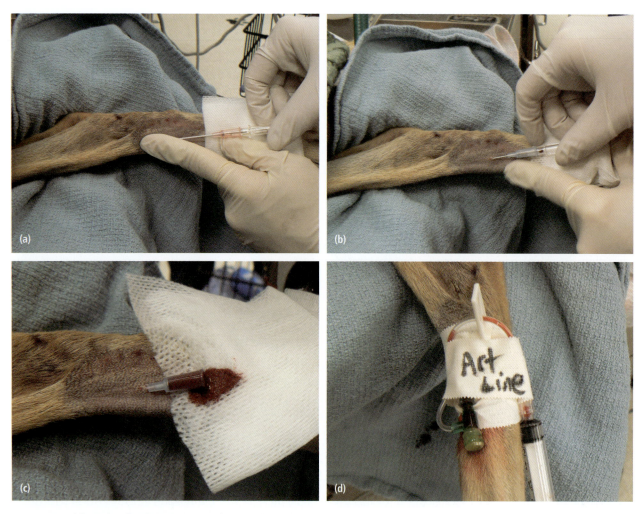

Figure 5.1 (a) Angle of catheter insertion for dorsal metatarsal artery. Note that the operator palpates for the pulse between the second and third metatarsal bones. (b) Watch for blood in the hub of the catheter. (c) Once a catheter is in place, pulsatile blood will flow from the catheter hub. (d) Securing the catheter involves wrapping pieces of tape around the catheter hub, under the catheter hub, and around the limb. The catheter should be labeled as an arterial catheter so it is not inadvertently used for infusion.

insertion is the right dorsal pedal artery, the patient should be positioned in right lateral recumbency). The limb should be extended comfortably for the patient, and the distal limb gently rotated such that the dorsal pedal artery is palpable and on the nondependent, medial surface of the limb. Some people tape the digits to the table or a heavy sandbag to keep the limb in place during catheter placement. This positioning will help the operator introduce the catheter into the artery. Palpate the foot between the second and third metatarsal bones distal to the tarsus to locate the pulse.

Once the artery has been located, clip the fur at least 5 cm (~2 in.) in all directions from the proposed catheter insertion site, as patient size allows. One may choose to clip fur circumferentially from the metatarsal region to maximize tape adhesion when securing the catheter.

Following aseptic preparation, feel again for the dorsal pedal pulse over the second and third metatarsal bones. Remember to palpate the artery gently, so as to not occlude the vessel and obscure the pulse. Once the pulse is located, a nick can be made in the skin to facilitate catheter placement (see "Percutaneous facilitation" above). Insert an over-the-needle catheter through the nick or directly through the skin, at a 15°–20° angle with respect to the skin over the point where the pulse is most easily palpable. It is easiest to feel the pulse with the nondominant hand, then insert the catheter through the skin under the gloved fingertip (see Fig. 5.1a). Direct the catheter through the skin and into the artery, taking care to advance the needle and catheter very slowly in 1- to 2-mm increments. After each movement, one should inspect the catheter hub carefully for a flash of

Protocol 5.2 Dorsal pedal (dorsal metatarsal) arterial catheterization

Items Required
- Clean clippers and blade
- Sandbag for limb positioning, if desired
- Surgical scrub preparation supplies
- Examination or sterile gloves for operator
- Sterile gauze squares
- Surgical tape (½- and 1-inch widths)
- Cotton roll gauze
- Water-resistant bandaging material, if desired
- 22- to 20-gauge needle
- Over-the-needle or over-the-wire intravascular catheter
- Luer lock T-port or Luer lock infusion plug
- Preservative-free heparinized saline flush syringes
- "Not for IV Infusion" label or indelible marker
- One or two assistant(s)

Procedure
1. Collect necessary supplies, prepare tape, and prepare and flush the T-port or male adapter with preservative-free heparinized saline.
2. Place patient in lateral recumbency, with limb of proposed catheter insertion adjacent to the table.
3. Assistant should restrain the animal in lateral recumbency.
4. Secure patient's digits to a sandbag or the table's edge with medical tape.
5. Palpate gently for arterial pulse over 2nd and 3rd metatarsal bones to determine proposed insertion site.
6. Clip fur over dorsal aspect of the metatarsus at least 5 cm (~2 inches) from the proposed catheter insertion site. Wipe clipped fur away with a gauze square.
7. Aseptically prepare the proposed catheter insertion site using surgical scrub technique. Allow a minimum of appropriate contact time of the cleanser with the skin, according to manufacturer's instructions.
8. Perform hand hygiene and don examination gloves (sterile gloves if the patient is immunocompromised).
9. Gently remove residual scrub with sterile gauze moistened with sterile water or saline.
10. Place sterile gauze square over the fur on the distal limb, to avoid contamination of the catheter.
11. Use gloved index finger to palpate dorsal metatarsal pulse in the surgically scrubbed area.
12. Once pulse is found, perform percutaneous facilitation with bevel of a 20- to 22-gauge needle, if needed.
13. Gently insert over-the-needle catheter through the skin, directing the catheter at a 15° angle with respect to the skin toward the pulsing artery.
14. Advance the stylet–catheter apparatus in 1- to 2-mm increments into the area of the pulse. Observe catheter hub for a flash of blood.
15. Once a flash is observed in the hub, insert the stylet 1–2 mm more and push the catheter off the stylet into the artery.
16. Before removing the stylet from the catheter, place sterile gauze squares beneath catheter hub to absorb blood.
17. Remove the stylet, and quickly place the male adapter or T-port into the catheter hub. Take care to avoid removing the catheter from the skin.
18. With sterile gauze squares, wipe away excess blood, making sure that the skin under the catheter hub and around the limb is dry.
19. Secure a length of ½-inch medical adhesive tape around the catheter hub, then around the limb.
20. Secure a length of 1-inch medical adhesive tape under the catheter hub, around the limb, finishing with the tape over the catheter hub.
21. Secure a third length of tape around the male adapter or T-port and then around the limb as described for step 20.
22. Bandage the catheter with cotton gauze and an outer layer.
23. Secure a "Not for IV Infusion" sticker over the catheter bandage, or make a note with indelible marker.

blood (see Fig. 5.1b). If the catheter has been advanced to what seems a sufficient depth and a flash of blood has not been encountered, the catheter system should be slowly withdrawn. While withdrawing the catheter system, watch closely for a blood flashback. In some cases, the catheter system has punctured through the deep portion of the vessel wall. If there is blood in the catheter hub, advance the needle and catheter another 1–2 mm in the plane of the artery, then gently push the catheter off of the stylet into the vessel. If the catheter does not easily advance into the artery, gently withdraw the catheter back over the stylet, and redirect the catheter system in small increments to replace it into the artery. If the catheter does not easily withdraw back over the stylet, it should not be forced back over, as the stylet may perforate the catheter; rather, if the catheter is difficult to pull back over the stylet, the whole system should be removed from the patient's skin and evaluated. In some cases, it is necessary to leave the original catheter and stylet in place and start over, attempting catheterization again proximal to the original site of catheter insertion. If the original catheter system is removed after it has disturbed the artery but before the catheter has been advanced into the vessel, the artery can spasm or bleed and thus complicate further attempts at catheter placement.

Once the catheter is inserted completely into the artery, be careful! Once the stylet is removed, blood should pulse readily from the catheter hub, which helps confirm placement in the artery rather than a vein. Prepare ahead of time by placing several sterile 4×4-inch gauze squares under the catheter hub to prevent contamination of the site with blood (see Fig. 5.1c). Once the stylet is removed, quickly secure a Luer lock male adapter or T-port (preflushed with preservative-free heparinized saline) to the catheter hub, taking care not to inadvertently dislodge the catheter from the artery.

Carefully wipe any blood from the area, then place a length of ½-inch white surgical tape around the catheter hub. Squeeze the tape securely around the hub to ensure the hub of the catheter does not spin within the tape, as spinning catheters fall out easily. Once the tape is secured to the catheter hub, wrap it snugly around the limb. Place a second length of 1-inch tape under the catheter hub, and wrap it around the limb. This piece of tape should be snug, but not so snug that it constricts the limb and impairs venous return. Secure a third piece of tape over the Luer lock T-port or male adapter and around the limb, such that it also encompasses the catheter hub. The distal limb and catheter can now be wrapped with gauze rolls of choice. The entire apparatus should be labeled as an arterial catheter to help avoid accidental medication infusion (see Fig. 5.1d).

Femoral artery catheterization

Percutaneous placement of a femoral arterial catheter is almost identical to placement of a dorsal pedal arterial catheter, except for anatomic location. Percutaneous facilitation is required less frequently at this site.

Place the patient in lateral recumbency, with the medial aspect of the patient's limb exposed. The person performing the restraint can pull the nondependent limb proximally, cranially, or caudally, depending on patient comfort. The limb should be clipped and aseptically scrubbed over its medial aspect from the inguinal region to the stifle. The femoral pulse is usually palpable on the cranial aspect of the femur near the inguinal region. The operator should palpate the femoral pulse with his or her nondominant hand, then insert an over-the-needle catheter at a 15°–20° angle with respect to the skin, directing the stylet–catheter apparatus toward the point where the pulse is palpable. Watch carefully for a flash of blood in the catheter hub and redirect the stylet with incremental 1- to 2-millimeter changes in direction. Once a flash of blood is observed in the catheter hub, the catheter angle should be dropped so that the catheter is in a good plane with the artery before attempting to feed the catheter into the vessel. Once the catheter is seated into the femoral artery, the stylet is removed. Then quickly place a flushed, Luer lock T-port or male adapter onto the catheter hub. Tape the catheter in place as described for dorsal pedal catheters, and flush it again with preservative-free, sterile heparinized saline solution. Depending on patient size and limb conformation, the operator may choose to reinforce the catheter hub's security by suturing the hub's tape to the patient's skin. See Protocol 5.3. See Table 5.1 (Advantages and disadvantages of various sites of arterial catheter placement).

Auricular artery catheterization

Auricular arterial catheters can sometimes be placed in dogs with large, pendulous ears. This technique is generally reserved for patients that are anesthetized, as the pinna is very sensitive to touch and has a twitch reflex that makes its artery difficult to catheterize when the animal is awake. The auricular artery is located on the dorsal aspect of the pinna (see Fig. 5.2a). Palpate the pulse on the pinna surface and trace it to the ear tip to determine the artery's location. Clip and aseptically prepare the entire dorsal surface of the ear pinna as previously described, while supporting the pinna with four fingers of the nondominant hand; fold the ear tip with the thumb so that it is perpendicular to the main portion of the pinna. Perform percutaneous facilitation if needed, and insert the catheter system through the skin directly into the artery in 1- to 2-mm increments. Once a flash of blood is visible in the catheter hub, gently advance the catheter into the auricular artery. Quickly remove the catheter stylet and replace it with a preflushed Luer lock male adapter or T-port. Wipe the area clean; then secure a length of ½-inch medical tape to the catheter hub and wrap it around the pinna (see Fig. 5.2b). Because the ear is floppy and can fold on itself, use several folded 4×4-

Protocol 5.3 Femoral artery catheterization

Items Required
- Clean clippers and blade
- Surgical scrub preparation supplies
- Examination or sterile gloves for operator
- Sterile gauze squares
- Surgical tape (½- and 1-inch widths)
- Cotton roll gauze
- Water-resistant bandaging material, if desired
- Suture material, needle driver, thumb forcep, and suture scissors, if desired
- Over-the-needle or over-the-wire intravascular catheter
- Luer lock T-port or Luer lock infusion plug
- Preservative-free heparinized saline flush syringes
- "Not for IV Infusion" label or indelible marker
- One or two assistants

Procedure
1. Collect necessary supplies, prepare tape, and prepare and flush the T-port or male adapter with preservative-free heparinized saline.
2. Place patient in lateral recumbency, with limb of proposed catheter insertion adjacent to the table.
3. Assistant should restrain the animal in lateral recumbency. The patient should be immobile, and top limb should be well out of operator's field.
4. Palpate gently for arterial pulse on cranial aspect of proximal femoral diaphysis (near inguinal region) to determine proposed insertion site.
5. Clip fur over the femoral artery, from inguinal area to stifle, on medial aspect of dependent limb. If the patient's fur is long, clip limb circumferentially.
6. Aseptically prepare the proposed catheter insertion site using surgical scrub technique. Allow a minimum of appropriate contact time of the cleanser with the skin, according to manufacturer's instructions.
7. Perform hand hygiene and don examination gloves (sterile gloves if the patient is immunocompromised).
8. Gently remove residual scrub with sterile gauze moistened with sterile water or saline.
9. Place sterile gauze square over the fur on scrubbed area's distal margin, to avoid contamination of the catheter.
10. Use gloved index finger to palpate femoral pulse in the surgically scrubbed area.
11. Gently insert over-the-needle catheter through the skin, directing the catheter at a 20° angle with respect to the skin toward the pulsing artery.
12. Advance the stylet–catheter apparatus in 1- to 2-mm increments into the area of the pulse. Observe catheter hub for a flash of blood.
13. Once a flash is observed in the hub, drop catheter angle to align with vessel and push catheter off the stylet into artery.
14. Before removing the stylet from the catheter, place sterile gauze squares beneath catheter hub to absorb blood.
15. Remove the stylet, and quickly place the male adapter or T-port into the catheter hub. Take care to avoid removing the catheter from the skin.
16. With sterile gauze squares, wipe away excess blood, making sure that the skin under the catheter hub and around the limb is dry.
17. Secure a length of ½-inch medical adhesive tape around the catheter hub, then around the limb.
18. Secure a length of 1-inch medical adhesive tape under the catheter hub, around the limb, finishing with the tape over the catheter hub.
19. Secure a third length of tape around the male adapter or T-port and then around the limb as described for step 18.
20. Suture catheter hub in place, if desired, by suturing the hub's tape to the patient's skin.
21. Bandage the catheter with cotton gauze and an outer layer.
22. Secure a "Not for IV Infusion" sticker over the catheter bandage, or make a note with indelible marker.

inch gauze squares or a roll of cotton gauze to softly splint the underside of the pinna such that the lateral aspects of the pinna are folded around the rolls (see Fig. 5.2c). The catheter and rolls of gauze or cotton are taped in place in a manner similar to that used for dorsal metatarsal catheters. Often, the weight of the bandage becomes too cumbersome in an awake patient and stimulates head shaking. This can cause the catheter to become dislodged. Also, the pinna has a relatively high risk of ischemia with prolonged arterial

Table 5.1 Advantages and disadvantages of various sites for arterial catheter placement

Location	Advantages	Disadvantages
Auricular	Easy to visualize Easy to catheterize Not affected by obesity	Easily dislodged with patient motion Can create thrombosis Best used for anesthetized patients Not for long-term use
Coccygeal	Easy to palpate Easy to secure	Easily dislodged with movement Easily contaminated with fecal material Smaller catheters necessary Not for long-term use
Dorsal metatarsal	Easy to palpate Easiest to cannulate Less danger of hemorrhage in patients with coagulopathies	May be affected by obesity
Radial	Easy to palpate	Metacarpal pad may interfere with placement May easily become thrombosed Not for long-term use
Femoral artery	Easy to palpate	Risk of hemorrhage, particularly if coagulopathy present Affected by obesity Easily dislodged with movement

occlusion. Therefore, auricular artery catheterization is often used only in extremely subdued, obtunded, or anesthetized patients for a limited time. See Protocol 5.4.

Radial artery catheterization

Catheterization of the radial artery is technically more difficult than for other anatomic locations because the radial artery is small. This technique can be performed in larger dogs while the patient is under general anesthesia. To place a radial arterial catheter, the patient is placed in lateral recumbency with the target limb adjacent to the table, and the palmar aspect of the patient's paw is clipped just proximal to the metacarpal footpad. After the aseptic scrub, the patient's paw is held in the operator's hand and the radial pulse palpated with the forefinger. Percutaneous facilitation is often helpful in this location. With the dominant hand, an over-the-needle catheter is inserted through the skin at a 15°–20° angle, while the operator observes closely for a flash of blood. The size and length of catheter depends on the size of the patient and the artery. Longer catheters (e.g., 1½ inch) should be chosen for larger dogs, as skin movement in this area can dislodge shorter catheters. Once a blood flash is visible in the catheter hub, the catheter is

inserted and a flushed Luer lock T-port or male adapter is attached in place of the stylet. It is the author's recommendation that radial arterial catheters not remain in place for longer than 24 hours, particularly in cats and smaller dogs, because of the risk of arterial thrombosis and inhibition of perfusion to the distal extremity. See Protocol 5.5.

Coccygeal artery catheterization

The coccygeal artery can be catheterized in patients under general anesthesia. For coccygeal arterial catheter placement, the patient is positioned in either dorsal or lateral recumbency, and the ventral aspect of the tail base is clipped. Circumferential clips of the tail base should be considered in patients with long fur that could potentially contaminate the catheter site. After an aseptic scrub and proper hand hygiene, the coccygeal pulse is palpated on the tail's ventral midline. The pulse is palpable between coccygeal vertebrae. Once the pulse is felt, an over-the-needle catheter is inserted at a 15°–20° angle with respect to the skin, into the artery, while the catheter hub is observed for blood. Once a blood flash is visible in the catheter hub, the catheter is inserted and a flushed Luer lock T-port or male adapter is attached in place of

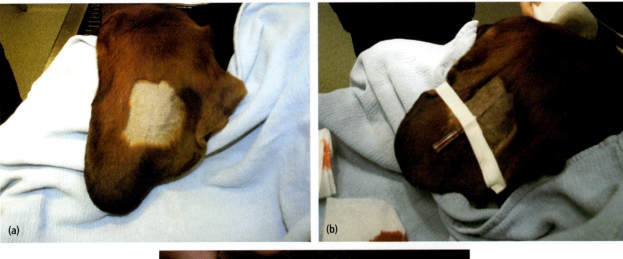

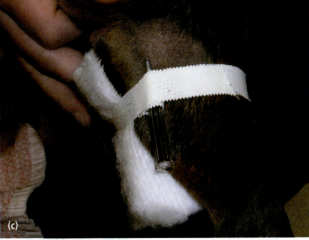

Figure 5.2 (a) The auricular artery is located approximately on the midline of the pinna's dorsal surface. (b) Once the catheter is in place, the hub should be secured by applying adhesive tape around the hub and extending the tape circumferentially around the pinna. (c) Folded 4 × 4-inch gauze squares or rolls of gauze should be used to splint the pinna with the arterial catheter in place, to enhance security.

the stylet. The catheter is secured to the tail with medical tape and gauze as previously described. See Protocol 5.6 for details. Coccygeal arterial catheters usually clot within 24 hours, so they must be watched very closely and flushed carefully. Also, because of the risk of contamination by fecal material, and also because the catheters tend to become dislodged with patient movement, coccygeal arterial catheters should be removed after general anesthesia and/or surgery has been completed.

Arterial catheter care

Because significant hemorrhage can occur quickly if an arterial catheter is dislodged, it is important that the catheter be securely placed. The catheter should be labeled appropriately to avoid intra-arterial infusion of drugs, intravenous fluids, or blood products. Except for small amounts of preservative-free, heparinized or non-

heparinized flush, no other drugs, blood products, or solutions should be administered through the arterial catheter.[5–7] In human patients, complications have been associated with inadvertent intra-arterial administration of vasopressors, dextrose, potassium chloride, antibiotics, and insulin.[7] Arterial catheters should be flushed with preservative-free heparinized saline every 1–4 hours to maintain patency. Care must be taken in small patients not to overheparinize or cause intravascular volume overload. If the arterial catheter is being used for continuous blood pressure monitoring, it can be attached to a pressure transducer attached to a bag of heparinized saline under pressure. Most pressure transducers contain a continuous flush system that delivers approximately 3 mL/hour of flush solution. In addition, most pressure transducer systems are equipped with a fast flush valve that allows for a rapid flush of the catheter whenever necessary.

Protocol 5.4 Auricular artery catheterization

Items Required
- Clean clippers and blade
- Surgical scrub preparation supplies
- Examination or sterile gloves for operator
- Sterile gauze squares
- 4 × 4-inch gauze squares, or 3-inch roll gauze
- Surgical tape (½- and 1-inch widths)
- Cotton roll gauze
- 22- to 20-gauge needle
- Over-the-needle or over-the-wire intravascular catheter
- Luer lock T-port or Luer lock infusion plug
- Preservative-free heparinized saline flush syringes
- "Not for IV Infusion" label or indelible marker
- An assistant, if needed

Procedure
1. Collect necessary supplies, prepare tape, and prepare and flush the T-port or male adapter with preservative-free heparinized saline.
2. Place the patient in sternal or lateral recumbency.
3. If the patient is not anesthetized, an assistant should restrain so the patient is immobile.
4. Clip the dorsal pinna surface on midline, 5 cm (~2 inches) from proposed insertion site in all directions.
5. Aseptically prepare the proposed catheter insertion site using surgical scrub technique. Allow a minimum of appropriate contact time of the cleanser with the skin, according to manufacturer's instructions.
6. Perform hand hygiene and don examination gloves (sterile gloves if the patient is immunocompromised).
7. Gently remove residual scrub with sterile gauze moistened with sterile water or saline.
8. Hold pinna in the nondominant hand, folding the ear over the fingers.
9. The auricular artery should be visible on dorsal midline of the ear pinna.
10. Perform percutaneous facilitation, if desired. Insert the catheter into the auricular artery.
11. Watch for a flash of blood in the catheter hub.
12. Once a flash of blood is visible in the catheter hub, advance the catheter and stylet an additional 1–2 mm.
13. Feed catheter off the stylet into the artery.
14. Before removing the stylet from the catheter, place sterile gauze squares beneath catheter hub to absorb blood.
15. Remove the stylet and quickly place the flushed male adapter or T-port into the catheter hub. Take care to avoid removing the catheter from the skin.
16. With sterile gauze squares, wipe away excess blood, and make sure that the skin under the catheter hub and around the ear is dry.
17. Secure a length of ½-inch medical tape around the catheter hub, then around the ear.
18. Secure a length of 1-inch medical tape under the catheter hub, around the ear, finishing with the tape over the catheter hub.
19. Secure a third length of tape around the male adapter or T-port and then around the pinna as described for step 18.
20. Place a roll of gauze or rolled up gauze squares under the ventral aspect of the ear.
21. Tape the gauze roll in place with several lengths of surgical tape.
22. Secure a "Not for IV Infusion" sticker over the catheter bandage, or make a note with indelible marker.

The catheter and bandage should be assessed frequently for evidence of moisture, soiling, or blood staining. The catheter bandage should be removed and the catheter evaluated at least once a day for evidence of redness, swelling, or discharge from the catheter insertion site. If there is pain when the catheter is flushed, or if any of the above abnormalities consistent with inflammation are observed, the catheter should be removed and a pressure bandage secured over the catheter insertion site for at least an hour, to decrease the risk of hemorrhage from the arterial puncture site. See Chapter 55, Care of Indwelling Device Insertion Sites, for more information on regular maintenance of arterial catheters.

Complications associated with arterial puncture or catheter placement

Artery puncture or inadvertent dislodgment of a catheter can result in arterial hemorrhage and hematoma

Protocol 5.5 Radial artery catheterization

Items Required
- Clean clippers and blade
- Surgical scrub preparation supplies
- Examination or sterile gloves for operator
- Sterile gauze squares
- Surgical tape (½- and 1-inch widths)
- Cotton roll gauze
- Water-resistant bandaging material, if desired
- 22- to 20-gauge needle
- Over-the-needle or over-the-wire intravascular catheter
- Luer lock T-port or Luer lock infusion plug
- Preservative-free heparinized saline flush syringes
- "Not for IV Infusion" label or indelible marker
- An assistant, if needed

Procedure
1. Collect necessary supplies, prepare tape, and prepare and flush the T-port or male adapter with preservative-free heparinized saline.
2. Position patient in lateral recumbency, with limb of proposed catheter insertion adjacent to the table.
3. If patient is not anesthetized, have assistant restrain.
4. Palpate gently for arterial pulse on caudomedial aspect of limb, just proximal to metacarpal footpad, to determine proposed insertion site.
5. Clip fur proximal to metacarpal footpad, at least 5 cm (~2 inches) from the proposed catheter insertion site in all directions. Wipe clipped fur away with a gauze square.
6. Aseptically prepare the proposed catheter insertion site using surgical scrub technique. Allow a minimum of appropriate contact time of the cleanser with the skin, according to manufacturer's instructions.
7. Perform hand hygiene and don examination gloves (sterile gloves if the patient is immunocompromised).
8. Gently remove residual scrub with sterile gauze moistened with sterile water or saline.
9. Place sterile gauze square over the metacarpal pad and the fur on the distal limb, to avoid contamination of the catheter.
10. Use gloved index finger to palpate radial pulse in the surgically scrubbed area.
11. Once pulse is found, perform percutaneous facilitation with bevel of a 20- to 22-gauge needle.
12. Gently insert over-the-needle catheter, directing the catheter at a 20° angle with respect to the skin toward the pulsing artery.
13. Advance the stylet–catheter apparatus in 1- to 2-mm increments into the area of the pulse. Observe catheter hub for a flash of blood.
14. Once a flash is observed in the hub, insert the stylet 1–2 mm more and push the catheter off the stylet into the artery.
15. Before removing the stylet from the catheter, place sterile gauze squares beneath catheter hub to absorb blood.
16. Remove the stylet, and quickly place the male adapter or T-port into the catheter hub. Take care to avoid removing the catheter from the skin.
17. With sterile gauze squares, wipe away excess blood, making sure that the skin under the catheter hub and around the limb is dry.
18. Secure a length of ½-inch medical adhesive tape around the catheter hub, then around the limb.
19. Secure a length of 1-inch medical adhesive tape under the catheter hub, around the limb, finishing with the tape over the catheter hub.
20. Secure a third length of tape around the male adapter or T-port and then around the limb as described for step 19.
21. Bandage the catheter with cotton gauze and an outer layer.
22. Secure a "Not for IV Infusion" sticker over the catheter bandage, or make a note with indelible marker.

formation at the puncture or insertion site. While severe hemorrhage from an arterial catheterization is rare, caution should be exercised with the femoral artery in particular. Basic precautions include inserting a catheter only as large as necessary to avoid premature clotting of the catheter, to obtain adequate blood samples, to obtain a good pressure waveform, and to avoid lacerating the artery during puncture.[8]

Contamination or soilage of the catheter bandage can result in local or catheter-associated bloodstream infection. For this reason, consider anatomic location of catheter placement carefully, to avoid contamination

Protocol 5.6 Coccygeal arterial catheterization

Items Required
- Clean clippers and blade
- Surgical scrub preparation supplies
- Examination or sterile gloves for operator
- Sterile gauze squares
- Surgical tape (½- and 1-inch widths)
- Cotton roll gauze
- Water-resistant bandaging material, if desired
- 22- to 20-gauge needle, if desired
- Over-the-needle or over-the-wire intravascular catheter
- Luer lock T-port or Luer lock infusion plug
- Preservative-free heparinized saline flush syringes
- "Not for IV Infusion" label or indelible marker
- An assistant, if needed

Procedure
1. Collect necessary supplies, prepare tape, and prepare and flush the T-port or male adapter with preservative-free heparinized saline.
2. Place the patient in lateral or dorsal recumbency.
3. Clip fur circumferentially from tail base, at least 5 cm (~2 inches) from the proposed catheter insertion site in all directions. Wipe clipped fur away with a gauze square.
4. Aseptically prepare the proposed catheter insertion site using surgical scrub technique. Allow a minimum of appropriate contact time of the cleanser with the skin, according to manufacturer's instructions.
5. Perform hand hygiene and don examination gloves (sterile gloves if the patient is immunocompromised).
6. Gently remove residual scrub with sterile gauze moistened with sterile water or saline.
7. Using a gloved index finger, palpate ventral midline of tail base, between coccygeal vertebrae.
8. Perform percutaneous facilitation with bevel of a 20- to 22-gauge needle, if desired.
9. Place sterile gauze square distal to the insertion site, to avoid contamination of the catheter.
10. Insert the catheter at a 20° angle with respect to the skin, between coccygeal vertebrae, toward the palpable pulse.
11. Advance the stylet–catheter apparatus in 1- to 2-mm increments into the area of the pulse. Watch the catheter hub for a flash of blood.
12. Once a flash of blood is observed, align catheter angle with the artery, then push the catheter off the stylet, into the artery.
13. Before removing the stylet from the catheter, place gauze squares under the catheter hub to absorb blood.
14. Remove the stylet, and quickly place the male adapter or T-port into the catheter hub. Take care to avoid removing the catheter from the skin.
15. Wipe away excess blood, and make sure that the skin under the catheter hub and around the tail is dry.
16. Secure a length of ½-inch medical tape around the catheter hub, then around the tail.
17. Secure a length of 1-inch medical tape under the catheter hub, around the tail, finishing with the tape over the catheter hub.
18. Secure a third length of tape around the male adapter or T-port and then around the tail as described for step 17.
19. Secure a "Not for IV Infusion" sticker over the catheter bandage, or make a note with indelible marker.

whenever possible. If an animal develops a fever, and the cause of the fever cannot be explained by the patient's disease, all catheters, including arterial catheters, should be removed and the tips cultured for bacterial growth.

Monitor the extremity distal to the catheter site for poor perfusion. If the limb distal to the catheter feels cool or cold to the touch, if the limb is painful, if the catheter is not working well or is no longer patent, or if the arterial pulse cannot be palpated, the artery may be thrombosed and perfusion to the limb may be compro-

mised. In such cases, remove the catheter immediately. Ischemic complications of arterial catheterization are especially common in cats, which generally have poorer collateral circulation than dogs.

Contraindications to arterial puncture and catheterization

Arterial puncture and catheterization can be problematic in patients with hemostatic abnormalities. For example, if an animal has severe thrombocytopenia with a platelet count less than 40,000 platelets/μL,[6] or if an animal has vitamin K antagonist rodenticide intoxication, arterial puncture or catheterization can result in hemorrhage from the arterial puncture or catheter site. In the presence of these conditions, placement of an arterial catheter is relatively contraindicated until the platelet count increases or until the coagulopathic toxicity has been resolved. The risk of hemorrhage must be outweighed by the need for direct arterial catheterization in very critical patients.

Hypercoagulable states, such as those associated with immune-mediated hemolytic anemia or a protein-losing nephropathy or enteropathy, can have an increased risk of thrombosis; embolism of the artery distal to the catheter site also may be an increased risk.[6] This complication is uncommon, so a prothrombotic state is a relative contraindication to catheter placement. One must weigh the benefits of catheter placement in a prothrombotic animal carefully with respect to the risks involved with its placement. If an animal has a pulmonary thromboembolism and will require numerous arterial blood gas analyses during the course of hospitalization, an arterial catheter may be necessary. However, if a catheter is placed simply to obtain continuous blood pressure monitoring, the use of an indirect method such as Doppler plethysmography or use of an oscillometric monitor may be preferable.

It is the author's opinion that arterial puncture or catheterization should not be performed if the skin and tissue overlying the artery are compromised in any manner.[3] Shearing injuries, pyoderma, burns, and even small abrasions potentially pose an increased risk of infection and, as tissue heals, an increased risk of thrombosis and wound contracture. For this reason, alterna-tive anatomic locations should be considered for arterial puncture or catheterization.

Troubleshooting

The arterial catheter should be assessed frequently for patency and cleanliness. If the catheter is not patent, the first step should be to unwrap the catheter to see if the catheter has slipped or is no longer in the artery. It is not uncommon for the catheter to kink at the insertion site, so this should be investigated before aggressively flushing the catheter. Because embolism is a possibility, an arterial catheter that is not flushing easily should always be evaluated. See Chapter 55, Care of Indwelling Device Insertion Sites, for more detail.

References

1. Hopper K, Rezende ML, Haskins SC. Assessment of the effect of dilution of blood samples with sodium heparin on blood gas, electrolyte, and lactate measurements in dogs. Am J Vet Res 2005;66:656–660.
2. Scheer BV, Perel A, Pfeiffer UJ. Clinical review: complications and risk factors of peripheral arterial catheters used for haemodynamic monitoring in anaesthesia and intensive care medicine. Crit Care 2002;6:199–204.
3. Mazzaferro EM. Arterial catheterization. In: Hopper K, Silverstein D, eds. Small Animal Critical Care Medicine. St. Louis, MO: Saunders Elsevier; 2009;206–208.
4. Handwashing video and recommendations by the CDC. Available at: http://www.cdc.gov/handhygiene
5. Beal MW, Hughes D. Vascular access: theory and techniques in the small animal emergency patient. Clin Tech Sm Anim Pract 2002;15:101–109.
6. Hughes D, Beal MW. Emergency vascular access. Vet Clin North Amer Sm Anim Pract 2000;30:491–507.
7. http://www.npsa.nhs.uk/patientsafety/alerts-and-directives
8. Bajaj L. Measurement of arterial blood gases and arterial catheterisation in children. Available at: http://www.uptodate.com/patients

6

Principles of electrocardiography

Joao Orvalho

Cardiac electrical activity

The main function of the heart is to pump blood; in order to accomplish that, a well-coordinated contraction is required. The myocardium is composed of muscle fibers linked by conduction system cells. A synchronized electrical stimulation of the muscle cells (myocytes) is necessary for an appropriate contraction. The myocytes are responsible for the contractile function, whereas the conduction cells deliver the electrical impulse that leads to myocyte contraction.[1]

The heart's electrical stimulus originates at the sinus node (also called the sinoatrial or SA node), which is the primary pacemaker of the heart and is located in the right atrium. The three internodal tracts (anterior, medial, and posterior) and Bachmann's bundle transmit the impulse to the atrioventricular node (AV node) and the left atrium, respectively.[2] Conduction is slowed through the AV node, and then proceeds to the bundle of His, which is the only conductive pathway between the atria and the ventricles. At the level of the aortic valve, the conduction pathway bifurcates into the left bundle branch and right bundle branch. (See Fig. 6.1.) Both bundles divide into a network of Purkinje fibers that are distributed to both ventricles.[3]

The wave of contraction follows the electrical impulse. Starting in the right atrium, continuing to the left atrium, and then to the ventricles.

The wave of depolarization

Cardiac myocytes are electrically charged and maintain an electrical gradient across the cell membrane, called the **resting membrane potential**. This gradient is main-

tained by multiple systems of active ion transport, including the sodium–potassium pump (Na^+–K^+ pump), which pumps sodium out of and potassium into the cell. The concentration of potassium (K^+) inside the cells is thus significantly higher than its concentration in the extracellular fluid.

A myocyte's resting membrane potential is considered negative because its intracellular fluid is more negatively charged than the extracellular fluid. When the myocyte is stimulated by the conduction system or by a neighboring myocyte, its polarity is reduced (the myocyte's interior becomes more positive). The less-negative membrane potential significantly alters the sodium and potassium permeability through the membrane. Sodium ions rush into the myocyte and K^+ ions move to the outside. This change in the cell's membrane polarity is called **depolarization**. As soon as a myocyte depolarizes, it stimulates the depolarization of adjacent cells, and the depolarization continues cell-to-cell throughout the myocardium. This chain reaction of cardiac myocyte depolarization is called the **wave of depolarization**.

Coordinated cardiac myocyte depolarization is responsible for the coordinated cardiac contraction.[4] An electrocardiogram is a graphic representation of the summation of all the action potentials of the heart over a period of time (Fig. 6.2).

The electrocardiogram

The **electrocardiograph** is a galvanometer or voltmeter, which is able to record the electrical impulses between nearby negative and positive electrodes placed in or on the body. A system of two points between which

Advanced Monitoring and Procedures for Small Animal Emergency and Critical Care, First Edition. Edited by Jamie M. Burkitt Creedon, Harold Davis.
© 2012 John Wiley & Sons, Inc. Published 2012 by John Wiley & Sons, Inc.

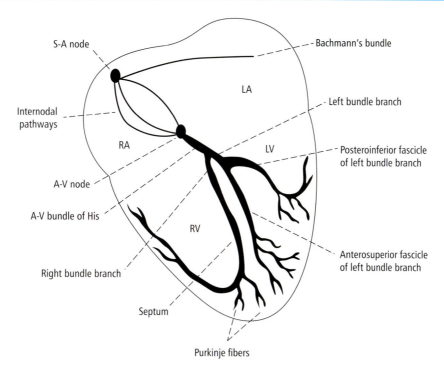

Figure 6.1 Conduction system of the heart (from Bruce NP, Flynn JM, Roberts F. ECG interpretation. In: Flynn JM, Bruce NP, eds. *Introduction to Critical Care Skills*. St. Louis, MO: Mosby; 1993:107).

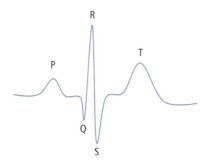

Figure 6.2 Idealized graphic representation of an electrocardiogram from a dog, with the P, QRS, and T waves labeled. The P wave is the result of atrial muscle depolarization. The QRS complex is the result of ventricular muscle depolarization. The T wave occurs as a result of ventricular muscle repolarization; T wave appearance can differ significantly from individual to individual, but it should generally be uniform within the same animal. More information is available in Chapter 7, Electrocardiogram Interpretation.

electrical impulses are conducted is called a **lead**. The electrodes are usually positioned on the animal's limbs (for standard leads), but they can also be placed on the thorax (for precordial chest leads) or in the heart (for intracardiac leads). The graphic representation of the information gathered from an electrocardiographic lead is the **electrocardiogram** (ECG [EKG is also used sometimes]).

The first electrocardiogram

Waller first demonstrated that the electrical changes of the heart during the cardiac cycle could be recorded and that this constituted a graphic representation, which he named the electrocardiogram. Later, Einthoven introduced the classification of P, QRS, and T for the standard electrocardiogram deflections.[5,6]

Recording the wave of depolarization

If a negative electrode is placed in the vicinity of the right atrium and a positive electrode is placed at the apex of the heart, the normal wave of depolarization travels toward the positive electrode and by convention is represented by a positive (upward) deflection on the ECG.[1,4,7] The electrical impulse of a normal cardiac cycle starts at the SA node. (See Fig. 6.1.) The atrial depolarization originates at the SA node, travels through the internodal tracts and Bachmann's bundle and terminates at the AV node. On the ECG, atrial muscle depolarization is represented by the P wave, which is the first positive deflection on the ECG before the QRS complex.[8] The atrial muscle depolarization also leads to atrial muscle contraction, and consequently to pumping of the blood from the atria to the ventricles.

There is a physiologic delay in impulse conduction at the AV node that allows time for the blood to flow from the atria to the ventricles prior to ventricular systole.

This physiologic delay is the origin of the P-R interval, or the electroneutral period between the P and QRS waves. Ventricular depolarization starts in the interventricular septum and is represented by a slight negative deflection on the ECG, called the Q wave. When the majority of the ventricular muscle depolarizes, it generates the R wave, a large-magnitude positive deflection. The last parts of the ventricles to depolarize are the basilar portions, which create a negative deflection on the ECG that follows the R wave, called the S wave.

After the S wave has occurred, the cardiac depolarization phase is complete. Cardiac repolarization, or the myocytes' regeneration of their resting membrane potentials, is necessary for another cardiac cycle to start. Ventricular repolarization is represented by the T wave, which in health can be positive, negative, or biphasic.[1–9] For information on ECG waveform interpretation, see Chapter 7, Electrocardiogram Interpretation.

Einthoven's triangle and the principle of leads

A bipolar lead is the result of the difference in electrical activity between electrodes when a negative electrode is paired with a positive electrode. Each lead "sees" and registers a different view of a single electrical event (such as a cardiac depolarization wave), which allows a more comprehensive understanding of the heart's electrical activity. Imagine that the P–QRS–T complex is an event such as a motor vehicle accident, and that each lead is a witness located in a different position in relation to the event. The witness in the two-story building has a different view than the person across the street, which is again different than that of the witness seated in the coffee shop. All the witnesses saw the same event, but each from a different angle. Thus we make our interpretation of the event with the advantage of combined observations and not just a single point of view.

Standard leads

In 1902 Willem Einthoven proposed the first fixed ECG lead system. Einthoven's equilateral triangle illustrates the three standard bipolar leads (see Fig. 6.3). To obtain these leads, electrodes are placed on the right thoracic limb or "arm" (RA; all ECG limb terminology is in arms and legs, by convention), the left thoracic limb or "arm" (LA) and left pelvic limb or "leg" (LL). The right pelvic limb (RL) is the connection to the ground.

As depicted in Figure 6.3, lead I detects the difference in electrical activity between the right thoracic limb (negative electrode) and the left thoracic limb (positive electrode); lead II detects the difference between the right thoracic limb (negative electrode) and the left

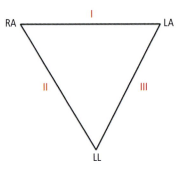

Figure 6.3 Equilateral triangle of Einthoven, illustrating standard leads I, II, and III (RA, right arm; LA, left arm; LL, left leg).

Table 6.1 Electrode position for standard bipolar and augmented unipolar leads: arm, thoracic limb; leg, pelvic limb

Lead	Positive	Negative/Neutral
I	Left arm	Right arm
II	Left leg	Right arm
III	Left leg	Left arm
aVR	Right arm	Left arm, left leg
aVL	Left arm	Right arm, left leg
aVF	Left leg	Right arm, left arm

pelvic limb (positive electrode); and lead III detects the difference between the left thoracic limb (negative electrode) and the left pelvic limb (positive electrode).[8] Standard leads are by far the most commonly used leads in the emergency room and intensive care unit.

Augmented unipolar leads

The unipolar, augmented leads use the same electrode placements as the standard leads and are generated by comparing a positive electrode and a neutral reference point. The neutral reference point is a result of the average of the other two electrodes, instead of using a negative electrode. Unipolar leads only record half the voltage of the standard leads; therefore, the ECG deflections must be amplified in order to obtain equivalent voltage of the standard leads.[9,10] For the augmented leads, an "*a*" precedes the designation, and all designations contain a "V," which identifies them as unipolar leads by convention. Lead aVR has its positive electrode at the **R**ight thoracic limb; lead aVL has its positive electrode at the **L**eft thoracic limb; and lead aVF has its positive electrode at the left pelvic limb (toward the **F**oot of a human). Electrode placement for the standard bipolar leads and augmented unipolar leads is shown in Table 6.1.

Table 6.2 Electrode position for unipolar precordial chest leads with analogous human lead designation in parentheses

Lead	Chest Location
CV$_5$RL (V$_1$)	Fifth intercostal space, near sternum, right side
CV$_6$LL (V$_2$)	Sixth intercostal space, near sternum, left side
CV$_6$LU (V$_4$)	Sixth intercostal space, costochondral junction, left side
V$_{10}$ (V$_6$)	Seventh thoracic vertebra, over spinous process

Table 6.3 Electrocardiograph color-coded cables

Cable Color	Limb
White	Right arm (RA), right thoracic limb
Black	Left arm (LA), left thoracic limb
Red	Left leg (LL), left pelvic limb
Green	Right leg (RL), right pelvic limb

Unipolar precordial chest leads

The unipolar precordial chest leads require different electrode placement than standard and augmented leads. Unipolar precordial chest leads record the electrical activity from the dorsal and ventral surfaces of the heart. These leads allow the operator to record the electrical activity of a specific cardiac region. A positive electrode is placed on the chest and, as with unipolar augmented leads, is paired with a neutral electrode that generates a "V" (unipolar) lead. The neutral electrode is the result of all the limb electrodes combined, and thus has a net voltage of zero volts. The positive exploring electrode can be moved on the chest to different positions, or multiple exploring electrodes can be used at the same time.

Six different types of V leads are commonly used in humans (V$_1$ through V$_6$), which have been modified for veterinary medicine into four chest leads (CV$_5$RL, CV$_6$LL, CV$_6$LU, and V$_{10}$). These leads are especially useful for detecting P waves and ventricular enlargement, and for identifying bundle branch blocks. (See Table 6.2.)

Procedures for diagnostic ECG measurement

Lead placement and patient position

The patient should be positioned in right lateral recumbency on a nonconductive surface. The handler should rest the right arm over the patient's neck and the left arm over the hindquarters, so the limbs are perpendicular to the body, still and separated (see Fig. 6.4).[9,10] An ECG can also be recorded with the patient in sternal or standing position, but this recording should only be used for rate measurement and detection of rhythm abnormalities. Fortunately, rhythm investigation is the most common use for ECG measurement in emergency and intensive care settings. Standing technique is especially useful in a dyspneic or tachypneic patient. More information about continuous ECG monitoring of acutely and critically ill animals is available in Chapter 7, Electrocardiogram Interpretation.

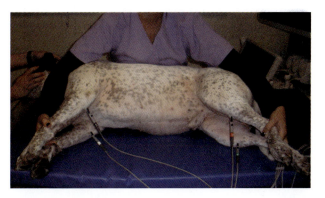

Figure 6.4 Standard patient position for recording an electrocardiogram (right lateral recumbency). Note the four standard electrocardiographic color-coded electrodes (RA, right arm, white; LA, left arm, black; RL, right leg, green; LL, left leg, red).

The thoracic limb electrodes are usually placed close to the olecranon (elbow) and the pelvic limb electrodes in the area of the patellar ligament (stifle). However, the electrodes may be placed at any point distal to the limb's junction with the trunk without significantly affecting the ECG. The limb electrodes are color coded by industry standard, and they should be placed as indicated in Table 6.3 and Figure 6.4. The chest leads are placed over the patient's thorax as indicated in Table 6.2 and Figure 6.5. The cables should not be twisted or placed over the patient's body, as this is likely to cause significant artifacts on the ECG.

Types of electrodes

The electrodes are attached directly to the skin with alligator clips, electrode patches, or metal plates (see Fig. 6.6).

Alligator clips are the most commonly used electrodes in veterinary medicine, since they are relatively simple to apply, are durable, and do not disconnect easily when the patient moves.[11] Before placing the electrode, a small skin fold should be made in the appropriate location. Isopropyl alcohol or electrocardiographic conducting gel must be applied to the area as a conduction medium; hair clipping is rarely necessary. Alcohol should be avoided in critical patients that may be candidates for defibrillation, since it is a very combustible substance. Electrocardiographic gel is also preferred when ECG recording will be required for longer than 10 minutes. It is preferable to apply the chosen conduction medium before placing the electrodes, as this will minimize interference from the patient's hair. Self-adhesive electrodes are also available (see Fig. 6.6b), which usually must be secured with a bandage to stay in place. They can be applied directly to the footpads or in an area of shaved skin.

Electrocardiogram recording

The electrocardiograph (galvanometer) control settings vary with the manufacturer, but there should be an option for paper speed, calibration, and filter settings.

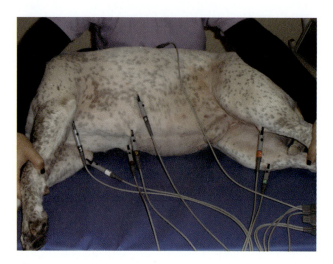

Figure 6.5 Standard position of the unipolar chest leads.

Paper speed

An ECG can be recorded at any paper speed, but the most commonly used speeds in veterinary medicine are 25 mm/sec and 50 mm/sec. This means that at a speed of 50 mm/sec, 50 mm of paper (10 large boxes) is recorded in 1 second. Therefore, the same patient's QRS complex appears wider on a 50-mm/sec recording than on 25-mm/sec because it is recorded faster, which corresponds to more space on the ECG paper.

When performing ECG wave and complex measurements, a lead II recording at 50 mm/sec should be used. For rhythm recordings 25 or 50 mm/sec can be used, with the choice largely dependent on the patient's heart rate and the desired ECG complex definition. A slower speed will allow a longer recording with the same amount of paper, which saves ECG paper. A minimum of three complexes should be recorded for each standard lead, and a longer recording is recommended when dysrhythmias are present. Augmented leads aVR, aVL, and particularly aVF can be useful when standard limb leads do not answer the operator's questions about ECG rhythm, wave, and complex appearance.

Sensitivity

Standard electrocardiographic calibration is 10 mm/mV, which means that a 1-mV electrical signal generates a 10-mm deflection from baseline on the ECG paper. The operator can recalibrate the electrocardiograph to produce larger (double sensitivity: 1 mV corresponds to 20 mm) or smaller (half sensitivity: 1 mV corresponds to 5 mm) ECG complexes. This feature is especially useful when the ECG complexes are very small, as is common in cats, or are very large, as ventricular premature complexes can be.

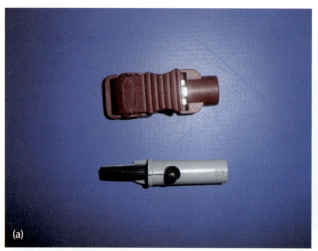

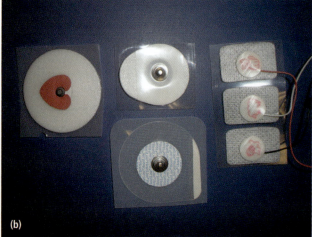

Figure 6.6 (a) An example of an alligator electrode clip (bottom) and a modified metal plate (top). (b) Different types of adhesive electrodes.

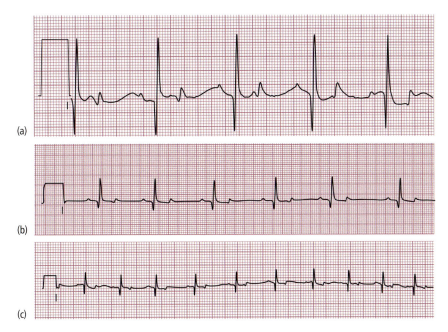

Figure 6.7 Electrocardiographic recordings of the same dog's ECG at (a) double, (b) standard, and (c) half sensitivities.

The calibration mark is a graphic representation of a selected recording voltage, which is used to gauge the amplitude of the ECG waves. It should appear automatically at the beginning of the recording in the form of a rectangle that represents the machine's current calibration (i.e., 10 mm high for standard calibration). The calibration mark precedes the first recorded complex (see Fig. 6.7).

Filter settings

Internal electrocardiographic filters are used to reduce baseline artifacts, but they are not necessary for a good electrocardiographic recording. In dogs, 50-Hz filters are usually appropriate, and 150-Hz filters can be used in cats. Filtering can reduce the amplitude of the complexes on an ECG; therefore, all complex measurements should be performed on an unfiltered tracing.

Ambulatory continuous electrocardiogram monitoring and ECG telemetry

Ambulatory continuous electrocardiogram monitoring (Holter monitoring)

Ambulatory continuous electrocardiogram monitoring is an electrocardiographic method that allows recording for longer periods of time, such as 24–48 hours. It is used for the diagnosis, monitoring, and therapeutic evaluation of arrhythmias. Most of these ECG monitors are powered by batteries and provide a digital recording with multiple channels.[10]

Since most dysrhythmias have a significant day-to-day variation, there is a considerable advantage to obtaining this longer diagnostic sample. The technique is also useful in the evaluation of syncope and collapse. The patient can go home with the recording device in place, and very limited monitoring is required.[10,12,13]

ECG telemetry

Electrocardiographic telemetry is a monitoring technique that helps in the supervision of hospitalized patients, with digital ECG tracings obtained through a wireless method. This technique allows the patient to move freely in the cage without the inconvenience of wires. These methods utilize a precordial lead system, which usually uses adhesive electrodes that are placed on a shaved area of the thorax.

Equipment problems leading to ECG artifacts

Artifacts can lead to incorrect ECG interpretation. Therefore, it is very important to minimize potential artifacts, such as electrical interference, muscle tremor, patient and system movement, and inappropriate patient or electrode positioning.[14] Incorrect electrode placement causes one lead to take on the appearance of another. Many possible lead misplacements can occur, but the most common mistake is switching the electrodes of the thoracic limbs, which will cause negative P waves in lead I and inverted leads II and III. This is the result of lead II becoming lead III, and vice-versa (see Fig. 6.8).

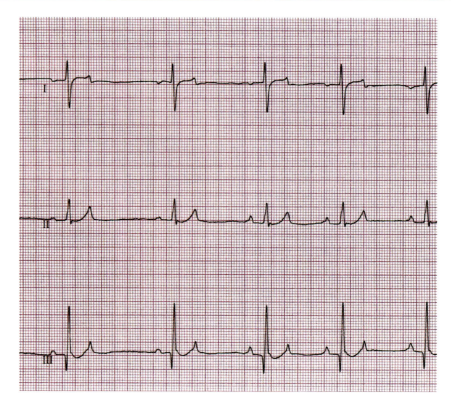

Figure 6.8 Electrocardiogram performed with electrodes placed incorrectly. Top tracing is "lead I"; middle tracing is "lead II"; and bottom tracing is "lead III." The electrodes of the front limbs were switched (the black electrode is on the right and the white on the left thoracic limb). Therefore, the P waves are negative in "lead I" and the readings for leads "II" and "III" are switched.

Information about other causes of ECG artifacts is found in Chapter 7, Electrocardiogram Interpretation.

References

1. Kittleson MD, Kienle RD. Small Animal Cardiovascular Medicine. St. Louis, MO: Mosby; 1998.
2. James TN. Anatomy of the conduction system of the heart. In: Hurst JW, ed. The Heart. New York: McGraw-Hill; 1974.
3. Racker DK. Atrioventricular node and input pathways: a correlated gross anatomical and histological study of the canine atrioventricular junctional region. Anat Rec 1989;224:336.
4. Cunningham JG. Textbook of Veterinary Physiology. Philadelphia: WB Saunders; 1991.
5. Waller AD. A demonstration on man of electromotive changes accompanying the heart's beat. J Physiol 1887;8:229.
6. Waller AD. The electrocardiogram of man and dog as shown by Einthoven's string galvanometer. Lancet 1909;1:1448.
7. Katz AM. Physiology of the Heart. New York: Raven Press; 1977.
8. Lauer MR, Sung RJ. Anatomy and physiology of the conduction system. In: Podrid PJ, Kowey PR, eds. Cardiac Arrhythmia— Mechanisms, Diagnosis & Management. 2nd ed. Philadelphia: Lippincott Williams & Wilkin; 2001.
9. Tilley LR. Essentials of Canine and Feline Electrocardiography. 3rd ed. Philadelphia: Lippincott Williams & Wilkin; 1992.
10. Miller MS, Tilley LR, Fox PR, et al. Electrocardiography. In: Fox PR, Sisson DD, Moise NS, eds. Textbook of Canine and Feline Cardiology. 2nd ed. Philadelphia: WB Saunders; 1999:67–105.
11. Detweiler DR. The dog electrocardiogram: a critical review. In: MacFarlane PW, Lawrie TDV, eds. Comprehensive Electrocardiography: Theory and Practice in Health and Disease. New York: Pergamon Press; 1988.
12. Tilley LR, Miller MS, Smith FW. Canine and Feline Cardiac Arrhythmias. Philadelphia: Lippincott Williams & Wilkin; 1993.
13. Fox PR, Harpster NK. Diagnosis and management of feline arrhythmias. In: Fox PR, Sisson DD, Moise NS, eds. Textbook of Canine and Feline Cardiology. 2nd ed. Philadelphia: WB Saunders; 1999:386–399.
14. Pipberger HV, et al. Report of committee on electrocardiography, American Heart Association. Recommendations for standardization of leads and of specifications for instruments in electrocardiography and vectorcardiography. Circulation 1967 Mar;35(3):583–602.

7

Electrocardiogram interpretation

Matthew S. Mellema and Casey J. Kohen

Introduction

Electrocardiography is an incredibly valuable diagnostic and monitoring tool in veterinary emergency and critical care. It provides continuous real-time information about the state of the cardiovascular and autonomic nervous systems in a noninvasive fashion. There are very few other tools that provide the quantity and quality of clinical information that electrocardiography can provide. It is both a cost-effective and a sensitive tool for monitoring cardiovascular status. No emergency room (ER) or intensive care unit (ICU) should be without one (or better yet, several). Electrocardiography is the gold standard for the detection and classification of arrhythmias and for the assessment of treatment responses. The emergency and critical care technician plays a vital role in the proper utilization of electrocardiography both in the acquisition of data and in the monitoring and screening for arrhythmias.

This chapter focuses on how to optimize the acquisition of a diagnostic electrocardiogram (ECG [EKG is sometimes used]) and on specific skills that veterinary emergency and critical care nursing staff should strive to master. A comprehensive discussion of electrocardiogram interpretation and all possible arrhythmias is beyond the scope of this chapter (or book) and interested readers are directed to several excellent texts on those topics. Also, see Chapter 6, Principles of Electrocardiography.

Acquisition of an electrocardiogram

Electrocardiography is a method of displaying or recording the heart's electrical activity using electrodes placed on the surface of the body. Electrocardiography performed in the ER or ICU is "surface" electrocardiography and thus measures changes in the overall electrical potential of the myocardium from the surface of the body. This technique can be used to assess changes in chamber size and conduction pathway function as well as to monitor heart rate and rhythm. Simultaneous monitoring of rate and rhythm is a common indication for ECG use in the emergency and ICU setting. With the widespread availability of radiography and echocardiography, the assessment of chamber size based solely on electrocardiography is rarely required.

Electrocardiography can be used as either a diagnostic or a monitoring tool. The proper use of electrocardiography depends on which of those roles the electrocardiogram is meant to serve. To obtain a diagnostic ECG that allows determination of complex amplitude, complex or interval duration, and mean electrical axis for comparison with normal values, the operator must apply standardized methodology (see below). These same standards are not generally applied when electrocardiography is used as a continuous monitoring tool.

Electrocardiography—the diagnostic ECG

Patient positioning

For short-term recording of a diagnostic ECG, it is standard to position the patient in right lateral recumbency. This position is used by convention to assess multiple leads, measure amplitudes of specific wave deflections, and calculate the mean electrical axis. If the animal is to be placed on a metal table or other conducting surface, a blanket or rubber pad should be placed between the

Advanced Monitoring and Procedures for Small Animal Emergency and Critical Care, First Edition. Edited by Jamie M. Burkitt Creedon, Harold Davis.
© 2012 John Wiley & Sons, Inc. Published 2012 by John Wiley & Sons, Inc.

patient and the surface used, to avoid conduction interference and artifacts.

Electrodes—options and proper placement

There are several methods of connecting ECG electrodes to a patient. Alligator clips are a common method for short-term recording and require very little patient preparation. To minimize patient discomfort, the teeth on the alligator clips should be flattened or filed and recording time should be limited. The clips should be placed on the caudal aspect of each elbow, proximal to the olecranon, and on each stifle at the level of the patellar ligament. Some ECG machines provide only three electrodes for connection to the patient. The white electrode should be placed at the right elbow, black at the left elbow, and red at the left stifle. If a fourth (green) electrode is present, it should be placed on the right stifle (see Fig. 6.4). Conducting medium should be placed between the electrode and the patient's skin. A gel designed for ECG electrodes is preferred as these gels are formulated for high inherent conductance, to reduce skin resistance, and they are generally hypoallergenic. Alcohol and many quaternary ammonia compounds are flammable substances and *should not* be applied if there is a chance a defibrillator will be used on the patient in the near future.

Adhesive pads are also available and can be applied for longer times if ECG monitoring is planned following the diagnostic ECG. Electrodes are available with snap adapters to connect to the pads. If pads are used, the patient's fur must be clipped and the skin cleaned and dried to maximize adhesion. The adhesive pads can be placed so that two are on opposite sides of the thorax just caudal to the scapulae, and the third and fourth are placed in the inguinal regions (see Fig. 7.1). The electrodes are connected in the orientation described previously (i.e., right thorax = white, right inguinal = green, left thorax = black, left inguinal = red).

If the waveform is difficult to interpret due to a patient's exaggerated breathing efforts, the cranial electrodes can be moved to the thoracic limbs; likewise, the caudal electrodes can be moved to the pelvic limbs. Once the electrodes are connected to the patient, the ECG waveform is assessed for quality and absence of artifacts (see below). Although any lead can provide information on heart rate and rhythm, lead II is routinely used to determine rate and rhythm and to measure waveform amplitude, as well as waveform and interval duration. The determination of mean electrical axis (although rarely done in the ER setting) requires that at least two leads be recorded for analysis.

Recording

A diagnostic ECG should include brief recordings of the three standard leads (I, II, and III) as well as the three augmented leads (aVR, aVL, and aVF) at 25 mm/sec paper speed. In addition 1–2 minutes of lead II at 50 mm/sec should be recorded to allow for rhythm and rate analysis. The ECG should be evaluated for the presence of artifacts (see below) and measures taken to remove any artifact noted. See Chapter 6, Principles of Electrocardiography, for more information about leads and diagnostic ECG acquisition.

Electrocardiography: continuous monitoring

Commonly in the ER and ICU setting, the electrocardiograph is used for longer term monitoring, and maintaining the patient in a standard position (i.e., right lateral recumbency) is not feasible or humane. Emergency and ICU patients are monitored primarily for changes in heart rate and rhythm, where specific positioning is less important. In this setting, the lead that

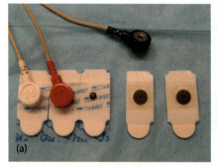
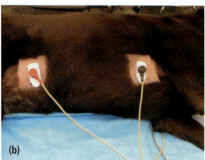
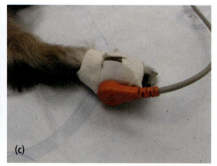

Figure 7.1 (a–c) Color-coded lead system using adhesive pads rather than alligator clips. (c) Adhesive pads can be placed on metacarpal or metatarsal footpads if needed.

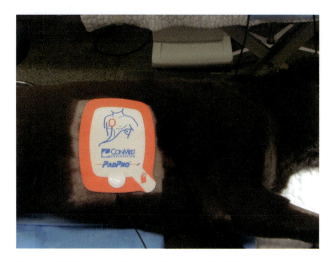

Figure 7.2 Using pacing-capable pads for ECG monitoring.

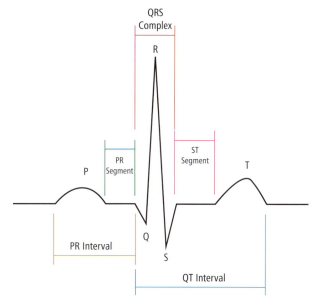

Figure 7.3 ECG waves as seen in lead II.

produces the most readily identifiable complexes is used. One must bear in mind that the optimal lead often changes as patient position is altered.

For continuous monitoring, adhesive pad electrodes offer substantial advantages over alligator clips (see Electrodes—Options and Proper Placement). If the patient's hair coat cannot be clipped or the patient requires ECG monitoring only temporarily during anesthesia, the adhesive pads can be applied to the metacarpal and metatarsal pads on the feet (see Fig. 7.1). Tape can be applied circumferentially to better secure the pads and electrodes. Some pads can adhere tightly to the skin after time and care should be taken when removing them, using adhesive remover as needed to prevent skin irritation and trauma. In patients with ventricular arrhythmias, which are prone to deteriorate into ventricular fibrillation, the placement of larger electrode pads that can be utilized for defibrillation is advisable (see Fig. 7.2).[1] These pads may also be used for external cardiac pacing in patients with complete heart block or who are symptomatic for other bradyarrhythmias (see Chapter 19, Temporary Cardiac Pacing, for more details).[2] If the patient is active in the cage, the electrode wires can be gathered and secured to the patient with a stockinette fitted over the thorax to avoid tangling. Regardless of the electrode placement method used, the ECG tracing should be inspected for artifacts after placement and measures taken to reduce any artifact present.

Continuous ECG monitoring often uses a combination of auditory and visual data. Most modern monitors are capable of producing an audible signal synchronized to the QRS complex. This feature allows for qualitative monitoring of rate and rhythm and can alert the clinic

staff to substantial alterations in either parameter. When auditory alterations are noted, it should prompt a visual inspection of the ECG display. Abnormalities noted after visual inspection should be recorded for analysis and documentation in the medical record. While recordings made at 25 mm/sec allow for more complexes to be recorded on a given length of paper, the authors recommend 50-mm/sec recordings, as they are generally easier to interpret.

Electrocardiogram waveforms

As noted in Chapter 6, Principles of Cardiography, the process of myocardial depolarization and repolarization (the re-establishment of resting membrane potential) leads to a series of deflections that are generally recognizable when displayed in sequence over time. Each portion of the typical ECG is associated with a specific portion of the myocardial depolarization–repolarization cycle. See Figure 7.3.

In a sinus rhythm, the **P wave** is the first deflection noted and reflects depolarization of the atria. As an impulse emerges from the area of the sinoatrial (SA) node, atrial depolarization begins and progresses from the right atrial myocardium to that of the left atrium. The direction of this wave of depolarization is such that a small positive deflection lasting less than 0.05 second is observed on lead II. The **P-R interval** is measured from the beginning of the P wave to the beginning of the QRS complex and represents the time required for the sinoatrial impulse to travel from the SA node to the ventricles. A substantial portion of this time is taken up by conduction through the atrioventricular (AV) node. Slower AV node conduction (e.g., when vagal tone is increased) results in a prolonged P-R interval.[3,4] When the AV node is bypassed (e.g., ventricular pre-excitation) the P-R interval is substantially shortened, and the atria and ventricles depolarize nearly simultaneously; thus, the P wave and QRS complex are closer together or begin to merge.[5] A P wave with increased duration or increased amplitude may indicate left or right atrial enlargement, respectively.[6]

The **QRS complex** is produced as a result of ventricular depolarization. The typical appearance of the QRS is due to the sequential depolarization of different portions of the ventricles such that the wave of depolarization is moving away from a given lead at times (e.g., negative Q and S deflections on lead II) and toward it at others (e.g., positive R deflection on lead II). The duration of the QRS complex indicates how long ventricular depolarization took to occur. Ventricular depolarization typically occurs quite rapidly (<0.06 second) due to the presence of specialized conducting tissue (the Bundle of His and its branches; see Figure 6.1) that rapidly conducts the signal to depolarize and distributes it throughout the ventricles. Prolongation of the QRS complex can indicate a conduction disturbance (e.g., bundle branch block), an ectopic origin of the complex (e.g., a ventricular premature complex [VPC]), ventricular hypertrophy, or some combination thereof.[5] Increases in the amplitude and duration of the QRS can be seen with ventricular hypertrophy in some cases.[7]

The **ST segment** is a period of relative electrical inactivity. In the healthy myocardium the ST segment is electrically silent and no differences in potential are detected on any lead. However, in the injured and/or ischemic myocardium an "injury current" may occur between adjacent diseased and healthy sections of myocardium (although recent studies suggest a more complex pathophysiology).[8] On the ECG this injury current manifests as either elevation or depression of the ST segment (see ECG Skill Set 9 at the end of this chapter); ST segment alterations can be important indicators of myocardial injury and should always be further investigated when noted.

The **QT interval** is measured from the beginning of the QRS to the end of the T wave. It represents the combined duration of the depolarization and repolarization processes for the ventricular myocardium as a whole. Although QT intervals vary inversely with heart rate (i.e., longer QT interval when heart rate slows), they are typically less than 0.25 second in duration at normal canine heart rates. Hypercalcemia can result in shorten-

ing of the QT interval; hypocalcemia results in prolongation of the QT interval. Hypomagnesemia and hypokalemia can also result in QT interval prolongation. While there are many reported associations of QT abnormalities with electrolyte disturbances such as those just mentioned, a recent study has suggested the associations are not particularly robust.[9]

The **T wave** is associated with ventricular repolarization and the re-establishment of resting membrane potential. The conformation of the T wave is highly variable in populations of normal, healthy dogs and may be positive, negative, or biphasic.[10] However, in an individual patient the appearance of their T wave is generally consistent. An abrupt alteration in the appearance of a patient's T wave should prompt evaluation of serum electrolytes and arterial blood gases (or pulse oximetry). Overly large T waves can herald hypoxemia or hyperkalemia.

Stepwise interpretation of the electrocardiogram

Correct interpretation of electrocardiographic data can be enhanced by taking a stepwise approach and consistently apply it in the same manner every time. While the steps may be taken in any order, there is some benefit to following a specific sequence such that the largest number of possible rule-outs is removed with each step. For example, determining heart rate first has the advantage of excluding a very large number of possible rhythms and allows one to focus further on the remaining possibilities (e.g., if heart rate is lower than normal, all the tachyarrhythmias may be excluded). The stepwise approach used by the authors is shown in Protocol 7.1 (at the end of this section) and further details of each step are provided here.

Instantaneous heart rate may be determined by measuring the time between successive P waves or QRS complexes. Mean heart rate may be calculated by determining the number of cardiac cycles over a given length of time (e.g., 3–6 seconds) and multiplying that number to give an average per minute. Dysrhythmias involving AV block or ectopic complexes and rhythms may create an overall rhythm in which the atrial heart rate and the ventricular heart rate are *not equal*. It is recommended that both an atrial rate (based on P wave frequency) and a ventricular rate (based on QRS frequency) be determined separately. An example of a situation in which this approach may prove beneficial is given in ECG Skill Set 2 at the end of this chapter.

Next, one may attempt to evaluate the overall cardiac rhythm by inspecting the entirety of the recorded study. Are there specific complexes appearing at unexpected

Protocol 7.1 Stepwise approach to electrocardiogram interpretation

- See accompanying text (in the section Stepwise Interpretation of the Electrocardiogram) for details of each step.

Procedure
1. Determine the heart rate(s):
   a. Atrial rate (frequency of the P waves)
   b. Ventricular rate (frequency of the QRS complexes)
   c. Are they the same?
2. Evaluate the overall cardiac rhythm:
   a. Is the rhythm regular or irregular?
      i. If irregular, is the rhythm regularly irregular or irregularly irregular?
      ii. Are there specific complexes appearing at unexpected intervals or with QRS morphology that is different than the rest?
3. Identify the complexes and the intervals; determine their amplitude and/or duration:
   a. P wave
   b. P-R interval
   c. QRS complex
      i. Assess morphology of the Q, R, and S deflections.
   d. QT interval
   e. T wave
   f. Inspect the ST segment for evidence of elevation or depression
4. Compare the amplitudes, durations, and morphology to normal values (see Table 7.1) for this species as well as to previous values for this individual (if available).

Table 7.1 Normal canine and feline ECG values

	Canine	Feline
Heart rate	Puppy: 70–220 beats/min Toy breeds: 70–180 beats/min Standard: 70–160 beats/min Giant breeds: 60–140 beats/min	120–240 beats/min
Rhythm	Sinus rhythm Sinus arrhythmia Wandering pacemaker	Sinus rhythm
P wave		
Amplitude	Maximum: 0.4 mV	Maximum: 0.02 mV
Duration	Maximum: 0.04 sec (Giant breeds 0.05 sec)	Maximum: 0.04 sec
PR interval	0.06–0.13 sec	0.05–0.09 sec
QRS		
Amplitude	Small breeds: 2.5 mV	Maximum: 0.9 mV
Duration	Large breeds: 3 mV Small breeds: 0.05 sec maximum Large breeds: 0.06 sec maximum	Maximum: 0.04 sec
ST segment		
Depression	<0.2 mV	None
Elevation	<0.15 sec	None
QT interval	0.15–0.25 sec at normal heart rate	0.12–0.18 sec at normal heart rate
T wave	May be positive, negative, or biphasic No more than 25% of the R wave amplitude	Typically positive

intervals or with P or QRS morphology that is different than the rest? This may indicate ectopic activity such as atrial or ventricular premature complexes (APCs, VPCs). The rhythm should be evaluated for whether it is regular or irregular. If the QRS complexes are evenly spaced, then the rhythm is considered regular; if the spacing is variable, then the rhythm is termed irregular. However, there may at times be a *pattern* to the irregularity; this is a "regularly irregular rhythm." An example of a regularly irregular rhythm is respiratory sinus arrhythmia wherein the heart rate varies with the phases of respiration (faster during inspiration and slower during expiration). In contrast, an "irregularly irregular" rhythm is one for which there is no discernible pattern to the irregularity. Atrial fibrillation is a classic example of an irregularly irregular rhythm.

Next, identify the complexes and the intervals, and determine their amplitude and/or duration. Prolongation of a given parameter indicates that whatever process that parameter represents is taking longer than normal. An example is a prolonged P-R interval. The P-R interval is the length of time it takes a signal to travel from the sinus node to the ventricle. The bulk of that time is spent traveling through the AV node, so a prolonged P-R interval indicates slowed AV node conduction (termed first-degree AV block). Increased amplitude of a complex may also carry important information (e.g., increased P wave amplitude indicating right atrial enlargement), but this information is generally more heavily scrutinized during a multilead diagnostic ECG study than when electrocardiography is being used as a continuous monitoring tool. Decreased amplitude may occur in a number of settings. Those most relevant to the emergency and critical care setting include pleural space filling disorders and pericardial effusion.[11]

The normal QT interval varies inversely with heart rate, but may be altered pathologically in electrolyte disturbances (most often those involving alterations in calcium or potassium). Normograms relating QT intervals and heart rates are available but are seldom used in our practice.[12]

The T wave arises from ventricular repolarization. The process of repolarization is a reflection of how depolarization occurred. If depolarization occurs slowly and atypically, then repolarization will occur abnormally as well. In clinical practice, this relationship is most often manifested in the wide and prominent T waves associated with VPCs. Electrolyte disturbances may also alter T wave morphology as evidenced by the tall peaked T waves seen in some hyperkalemic patients.[13] It should be noted that there is a vast array of T wave morphologies observed in normal patients.[10] T waves may be positive, negative, or biphasic in normal

animals.[10] What *is* important to note is when a patient's T wave morphology *changes* relative to what had been observed in that same patient previously, as the change may herald the development of myocardial injury.[14]

The ST segment should be inspected for evidence of elevation or depression. The significance of these findings is explained further in ECG Skill Set 9 at the end of this chapter.

Lastly, it is important to note that one should compare measurements not only with established normal values for this species, but also with previous recordings made from *this patient*. For example, has the QRS amplitude increased relative to the last visit, suggesting progressive left ventricular hypertrophy? Or is this elevation in heart rate something that has been observed every time this patient visits your clinic (e.g., white coat syndrome)?[15]

In all cases, abnormalities in rate, morphology, rhythm, or interval durations should be noted in the patient record and brought to the attention of the clinician on duty so that a treatment or monitoring plan can be constructed in a timely fashion.

Recognizing ECG artifacts

Electrocardiography is prone to a number of common artifacts that can interfere with interpretation, including respiratory artifact, poor-contact artifact, 60-cycle interference, muscle-activity artifact, and stylus-temperature artifact.

Respiratory artifact is due to lead motion during exhalation and inhalation. It results in a baseline that cyclically rises and falls rather than remaining stable (see Fig. 7.4a). Moving the cranial leads from the chest wall to the thoracic limbs usually reduces or eliminates this type of artifact. Poor-contact artifact results in the loss of recognizable complexes and coarse, ultra-high-frequency oscillations (see Fig. 7.4b). Using contact gel or applying tape to secure the electrode pads more firmly can help reduce poor-contact artifact.

In most parts of the world, alternating current is used to power devices plugged into outlets. This current alternates polarity (direction) 60 times each second. This alternating current results in an electrical field that can be picked up by electrocardiographic equipment. This type of artifact is termed 60-cycle interference and produces a baseline that has fine, persistent oscillations (see Fig. 7.4c); 60-cycle interference can be reduced by making sure that ECG equipment is plugged into a properly grounded outlet and that other devices plugged into this circuit are turned off or unplugged (if possible). Clippers are common sources of 60-cycle interference.

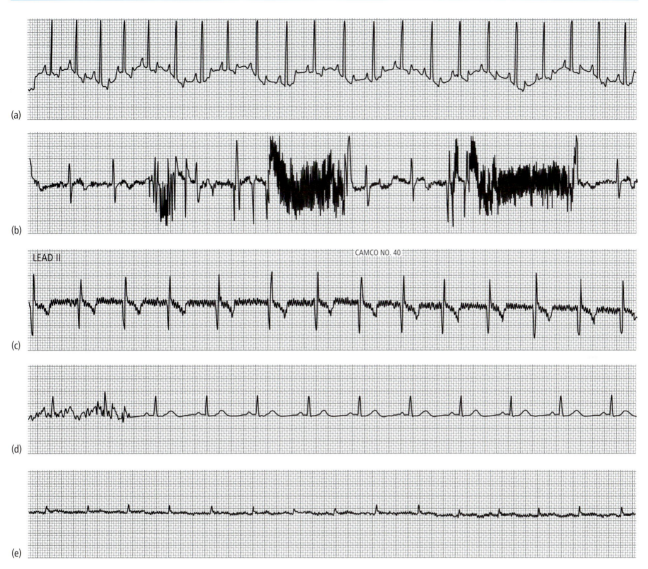

Figure 7.4 ECG recordings showing different types of artifact: (a) respiratory motion artifact; (b) poor lead contact artifact; (c) 60-cycle interference, lead II ECG at 50 mm/sec; (d) probable muscle-tremor artifact; (e) excessive stylus heat artifact.

Fluorescent overhead lighting should also be turned off if possible. Moving the patient and equipment away from walls containing electrical wiring may also help reduce 60-cycle interference.

Muscle activity can also produce an unstable, oscillating baseline that limits one's ability to interpret the ECG (see Fig. 7.4d). Muscle tremors and shivering commonly produce muscle-activity artifact, as can purring in cats. Removing muscle-activity artifact often requires that one address the underlying cause of the muscle activity (e.g., warm a patient that is shivering) or move the leads to a different location, or both.

Most ECGs are recorded on thermal paper that darkens when heat is applied to it. The heated stylus moves up and down while the paper is advanced at a predetermined speed (e.g., 50 mm/sec). Stylus temperature should be adjusted to provide a tracing with optimal clarity. A stylus that is set at too low a temperature will yield a very faint tracing while an overheated stylus produces a tracing that is overly wide and dark (see Fig. 7.4e). Either type of artifact can hamper interpretation efforts.

Conclusion

Electrocardiography is one of the most valuable monitoring tools available to the emergency and critical care (E/CC) staff. It provides continuous, real-time

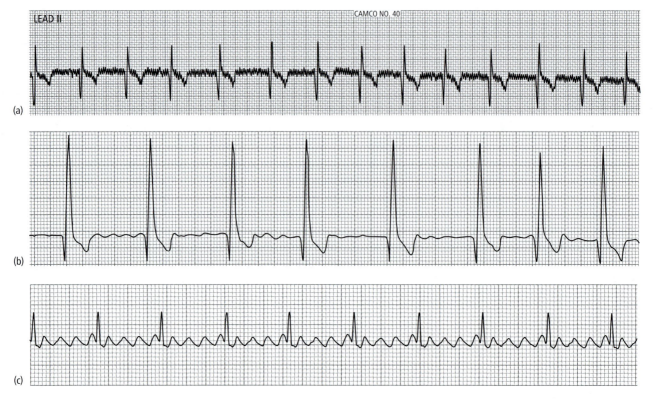

Figure 7.5 (a) Sixty-cycle interference, lead II ECG at 50 mm/sec; (b) atrial fibrillation, lead II ECG at 50 mm/sec; (c) atrial flutter, lead II ECG at 50 mm/sec.

information regarding cardiovascular status and auto-nomic tone. It defines the nature of cardiac arrest. The E/CC technician plays a vital role as a front-line inter-preter of ECG data. Ten essential skills for the E/CC technician to master are discussed in the final portion of this chapter.

Skill sets

Skill set 1: distinguishing 60-cycle interference from atrial fibrillation or atrial flutter—Figure 7.5a–c

The ICU and ER environments are frequently busy, crowded places with a great deal of equipment. The pace of clinical practice and the requisite instrumentation all too frequently lead to poor-quality ECG recordings. One common cause of poor-quality ECG recordings is inter-ference due to the transmission of power to electrical devices via alternating current in power lines, wires, and cords. In the United States, alternating current operates at a frequency of 60 Hz (also known as 60-cycle, meaning 60 cycles per second). In many other parts of the world, an operating frequency of 50 Hz is used. Signals from nearby alternating current can produce a rapid, repeti-

tive, oscillating artifact on an ECG that interferes with interpretation of the baseline and with P waves in par-ticular. Sixty-cycle interference is demonstrated in the first ECG (Fig. 7.5a). Note the extreme rapidity with which the baseline oscillates. A key difference between atrial flutter and 60-cycle interference is the rate at which the oscillations occur. The repetitive depolariza-tion of the atrial myocardium that occurs in atrial flutter can be quite rapid at times, but it does not approach the 3600 oscillations per minute found with 60-cycle inter-ference (60-cycle or 60 Hz equals 60 oscillations per second, which is 3600 per minute).

Atrial fibrillation and atrial flutter can also result in a baseline with an undulating or oscillating appearance. There are, however, key features that allow the techni-cian to distinguish these dysrhythmias from 60-cycle interference. Atrial fibrillation is demonstrated in the second ECG (Fig. 7.5b). Atrial fibrillation results in uncoordinated atrial electrical activity and thus the baseline undulations do not follow a repetitive pattern as is seen in 60-cycle interference. An example of atrial flutter is shown in the third ECG (Fig. 7.5c). One may note that this dysrhythmia also produces a baseline with a repetitive, oscillating appearance, just not as rapid and

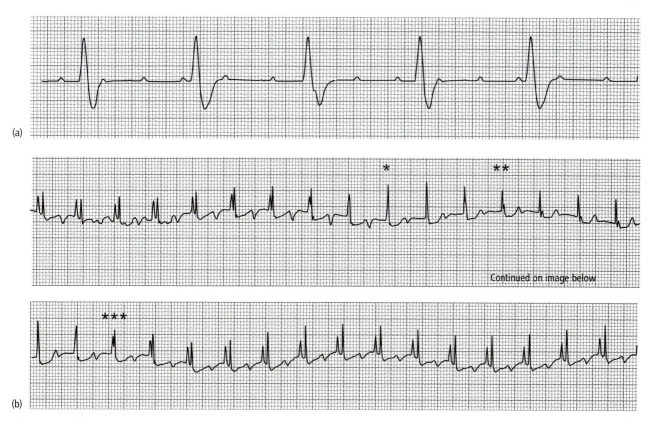

Figure 7.6 (a) Third-degree AV block, lead II ECG at 50 mm/sec; (b, top and bottom) an example of isorhythmic dissociation, lead II ECG at 25 mm/sec.

with a less uniform morphology than 60-cycle interference. Also note that with both atrial fibrillation and atrial flutter the R-R interval typically is irregularly irregular, which is not expected if 60-cycle interference is superimposed on a sinus rhythm.

Skill set 2: distinguishing third-degree AV block from isorhythmic dissociation—Figure 7.6a,b

Disorders of conduction through the atrioventricular (AV) node can result in many different types of dysrhythmia, including the many forms of AV block. Many of these are easily distinguished from one another based on the nature of the P-R interval and its relation to the QRS complex. However, a complete lack of AV node conduction can result from many causes, including AV nodal pathology, drugs, excessive vagal tone (though this typically results in less-severe AV conduction disturbances), or physiologic refractoriness of the AV node due to the activation of non-sinus-node pacemaker activity. The AV junction contains cells capable of intrinsic pacemaker activity similar to the sinus node cells. However, the activity of the AV junction site is usually suppressed by the higher intrinsic rate of the sinus node. On occasion, the discharge rate of the AV junctional pacemaker site can become increased to the point that its rate is nearly equal to that of the sinus node. When this happens, AV dissociation may occur. AV dissociation is a class of dysrhythmia wherein the atria and ventricles are controlled by separate and independent rhythms. On a surface ECG, these two independent rhythms are superimposed on one another and may appear to represent a single disorganized rhythm. When the rate of the junctional pacemaker site is close to that of the sinus node, the sinus node may be unable to pace the ventricles, as the AV node is refractory to conduction because it has already been depolarized by the ectopic pacemaker site. This represents a form of *functional* AV block. No AV node pathology is required for this type of conduction disorder to occur.

The first ECG (Fig. 7.6a) is an example of complete heart block (also known as third-degree [3°] AV block). The atria are being depolarized by the sinus node and thus regular P waves are noted. The QRS complex is wide, indicating that ventricular depolarization is atypically prolonged. In 3° AV block, the QRS complexes

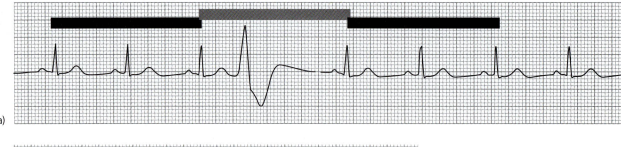

(a)

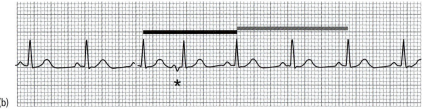

(b)

Figure 7.7 (a) VPC, lead II ECG at 50 mm/sec; (b) APC, lead II ECG at 50 mm/sec.

are the result of a ventricular escape rhythm, and ventricular depolarization frequency (and thus heart rate) is typically slower than normal. This form of AV dissociation is most commonly due to pathology of the AV nodal tissue.

The second ECG (Fig. 7.6b) is an example of iso-rhythmic dissociation, which is a category of dysrhythmia rather than a specific rhythm diagnosis, much like *tachycardia* is a category not a specific rhythm diagnosis. In the case example provided, one should note that, at the beginning of the strip, P waves and QRS complexes are distinct and appear as expected. However, in the center of the upper portion of Figure 7.6b one can see the P waves and QRS complexes merging (*) and summating (QRS amplitude appears increased). The P waves then begin to reappear in the downstroke of the R wave (**) and then ultimately reappear just to the left of the QRS complexes where they are usually found (***). In this case, there are two wholly independent rhythms present: a *sinus rhythm* depolarizing the atria and an *accelerated junctional rhythm* depolarizing the ventricles. An important distinguishing factor between the two ECGs (Fig. 7.6a and Fig. 7.6b) is that in 3° AV block there are many more P waves than QRS complexes, whereas in isorhythmic dissociation rhythms there are typically a few more QRS complexes than P waves. Also, in iso-rhythmic dissociation rhythms the most common source of ectopic pacemaker activity is the AV junction, and the QRS complexes are most often narrow and normal in appearance. Third-degree AV block is typically a significant clinical problem whereas isorhythmic dissociation rhythms may be an incidental finding with less-adverse effects on cardiovascular performance.

Skill set 3: distinguishing apcs from vpcs— Figure 7.7a,b

Ectopic depolarizations (often called *premature complexes*) may arise from supraventricular or ventricular foci. They represent paroxysmal depolarizations arising from sites other than the sinus node. Atrial premature complexes (APCs) could more correctly be termed *supraventricular ectopic depolarizations*, which more correctly describes them because (a) APCs may arise from ectopic sites other than the atria, such as the AV junction, (b) they are not always particularly premature, and (c) although APCs do result in depolarization they may not always result in myocardial contraction. *Ventricular premature complexes* (or ventricular ectopic depolarizations) arise from ectopic sites in the ventricles.

Both APCs and VPCs may be identified in small animal patients in the ER and ICU setting. In dogs, APCs are believed to result more often from primary cardiac disease than are VPCs, which frequently occur due to systemic disease and may be identified in normal dogs on occasion. In contrast, APCs are thought to arise most often due to underlying myocardial disease and less often due to extracardiac problems in canine patients.

Since APCs originate from foci at or above the AV junction, their transmission to the ventricle is typically via the Bundle of His and its branches. This normal path of impulse transmission means that ventricular depolarization occurs in the same manner as with a sinus depolarization. Thus, the QRS morphology and duration with APCs *should be comparable to the sinus complexes observed* (see the second ECG, Fig. 7.7b). In contrast, VPCs originate from foci within the ventricles; thus, ventricular depolarization is slower and less organized since the Bundle of His does not distribute the impulse as it does with a depolarization that originates from a supraventricular focus. This pattern of depolarization leads to the *wide and bizarre* morphology typical of VPCs. As repolarization reflects the pattern of depolarization, the T wave is also typically wide and prominent after a VPC. Repolarization of some portions of the ventricle may begin before more distant portions of the ventricle have completed depolarization, leading to slurring of the QRS and T wave together. See the first ECG (Fig. 7.7a) for an example of a VPC and note that the ectopic complex both lacks a P wave and has a wide and bizarre morphology.

APCs typically result in atrial depolarization and therefore generate a premature P wave (termed P′ wave) preceding the normal-appearing QRS. An APC with a P′ wave (*) is depicted in Figure 7.7b. P′ waves may have a different morphology than P waves on the same ECG due to different patterns of atrial depolarization. This feature along with the normal QRS morphology is most helpful in distinguishing APCs from VPCs.

APCs and VPCs also differ in that APCs may depolarize and therefore reset the sinus node, whereas VPCs generally do not. When an APC depolarizes and resets the sinus node, that APC is then followed by a "noncom-

pensatory pause" (see Fig. 7.7b: the grey bar is longer than the black bar)—the complex following the APC occurs after a normal-length R-R interval. Conversely, VPCs are almost always followed by a "compensatory pause," in which the next sinus complex occurs right on schedule (as if the VPC did not occur) because the VPC did not depolarize the SA node (see Fig. 7.7a: the grey bar is the same length as the black bars). The nature of the pause following an ectopic complex can on occasion assist in proper classification–in cases when the two types of ectopic depolarizations cannot be distinguished readily based on morphology, the differences in the types of pauses that follow them may allow proper characterization.

Skill set 4: distinguishing ventricular tachycardia from supraventricular tachycardia—Figure 7.8a,b

Distinguishing supraventricular from ventricular tachyarrhythmias accurately is an important skill for anyone performing ECG interpretation. These types of tachyarrhythmias need to be distinguished not only to guide proper antiarrhythmic drug selection, but also because of their different prognoses. Many drug agents that are effective for terminating supraventricular

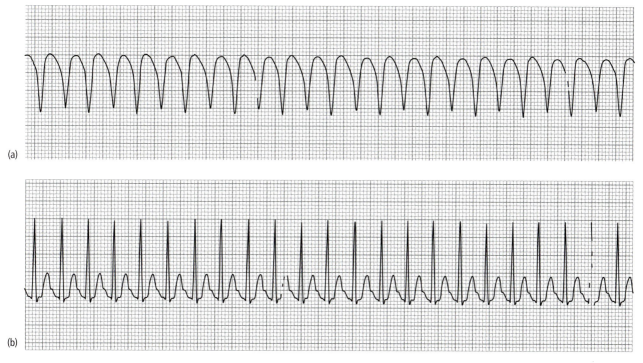

(a)

(b)

Figure 7.8 (a) Example of a ventricular tachyarrhythmia, lead II ECG at 25 mm/sec; (b) example of a supraventricular tachyarrhythmia, lead II ECG at 25 mm/sec.

tachyarrhythmias (e.g., calcium channel blockers) are less effective at addressing ventricular tachyarrhythmias. Moreover, rapid ventricular tachyarrhythmias carry greater risk of degenerating into ventricular fibrillation or flutter, which are associated with cardiac arrest. Rapid supraventricular tachyarrhythmias also need to be addressed promptly, as they compromise diastolic filling and can result in markedly reduced stroke volumes and poor cardiac output.

Supraventricular tachyarrhythmias (SVT) are usually associated with a QRS morphology that is narrow and normal in appearance (unless a conduction disturbance such as bundle branch block is *also* present). Supraventricular tachycardias include atrial and junctional tachyarrhythmias and this class of dysrhythmias is also referred to as *narrow QRS tachycardias* (this term therefore also includes atrial fibrillation and atrial flutter when ventricular rates are rapid). P′ waves (see Skill Set 3) may be identified or may be superimposed or merged with the T wave of the preceding complex (see the second ECG, Fig. 7.8b). The heart rate is rapid and often regular.

Ventricular tachycardia and ventricular flutter are tachyarrhythmias originating from within the ventricular myocardium. The Bundle of His and its branches do not distribute the impulse throughout the myocardium, which results in slower wave propagation and widening of the QRS complex as seen in the first ECG (Fig. 7.8a). These tachyarrhythmias may be referred to as *wide QRS tachycardias*. The occasional P wave may be identified if there is any baseline available for inspection (not usually the case when heart rate is rapid), but they do not have a predictable relationship to the QRS complexes.

The widened appearance of the QRS and the lack of P (or P′) waves is usually sufficient to distinguish SVT from ventricular tachyarrhythmias. However, there are times when the QRS seems only slightly widened and P waves are not identifiable; the classification of tachyarrhythmias becomes more challenging in this setting. Response to a trial intravenous dose of an antiarrhythmic agent (e.g., lidocaine, diltiazem) and/or response to a vagal maneuver may be required in some cases in order to accurately identify the nature of the rhythm disturbance.

Skill set 5: distinguishing vpcs from ventricular escape beats—Figure 7.9a,b

Ventricular ectopic activity is best assessed when considering the *context* in which it is seen. Ectopic ventricular activity may be pathologic (e.g., VPCs, ventricular tachycardia) or physiologic (e.g., ventricular escape beats, ventricular escape rhythms). VPCs and ventricular tachycardia are discussed in Skill Sets 3 and 4, respectively. Ventricular escape beats are ventricular depolarizations that also arise from a ventricular focus, but under very different circumstances than VPCs. There are cells within the ventricles capable of pacemaker activity at slow rates (20–40 per minute), but their activity is usually suppressed by the more rapid pacing activity of other sites (i.e., sinus node and/or AV junction). However, when the heart rates initiated by these other

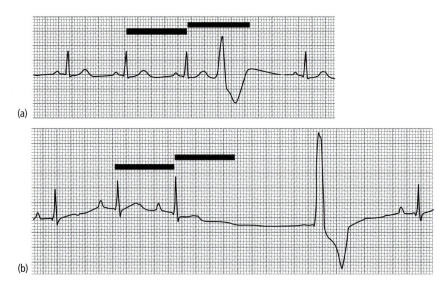

(a)

(b)

Figure 7.9 (a) Ventricular premature complex (VPC), lead II ECG at 50 mm/sec; (b) ventricular escape complex (ventricular escape beat), lead II ECG at 50 mm/sec.

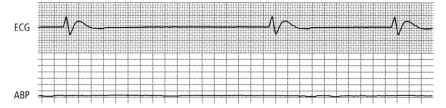

Figure 7.10 Pulseless electrical activity, lead II ECG at 25 mm/sec with arterial blood pressure (ABP).

sites fall below the intrinsic rate of the ventricular pacing cells, ventricular escape complexes or rhythms should occur. Once the rate of the sinus node or AV junction again exceeds that of the ventricles, the escape complexes will be suppressed once again.

The pacemaking sites in the AV junction and ventricle provide an important "safety net" and likely developed to ensure that a minimum heart rate will be maintained when the sinus node pauses, temporarily arrests, or fails altogether. A similar role is served when AV node conduction disturbances prevent the sinus node's depolarization signal from reaching the ventricles (e.g., complete or "third-degree" heart block; see Skill Set 2).

In the first ECG (Fig. 7.9a), a ventricular premature complex (VPC) is present following the third sinus complex. The lower black bar indicates the R-R interval between two successive sinus beats. The upper black bar indicates the time interval until the next sinus complex would be expected to occur based on this established R-R interval. The wide and bizarre complex lacking a P wave that occurs before the next sinus complex is expected (i.e., occurs prematurely) is a VPC. This ectopic beat does not reset the sinus node and a compensatory pause follows it (see Skill Set 3). VPCs may be due to cardiac or extracardiac disease in dogs, but they often indicate myocardial disease in cats. Frequent or multiform VPCs may require antiarrhythmic therapy.

In the second ECG (Fig. 7.9b), a ventricular escape complex (also called ventricular escape *beat*) is present following the third sinus complex. Once again, the lower black bar indicates the R-R interval between two successive sinus beats. In this case, the wide and bizarre complex lacking a P wave occurs *after* the next sinus complex is expected to occur. Escape beats occur after pauses in the activity of the sinus node as is shown here. Escape beats are important to help maintain adequate cardiac output in the face of inadequate pacemaker activity from the sinus node or disruption of AV node conduction and *should not* be suppressed with antiarrhythmic therapies.

Skill set 6: recognition of pulseless electrical activity (PEA)—Figure 7.10

Pulseless electrical activity (PEA) is a rhythm associated with cardiac arrest in small animal patients. It was previously termed electromechanical dissociation (EMD), which is a less correct term: EMD indicates that myocardial depolarization is not leading to myocardial contraction; although this can occur, there are also situations when depolarization causes contraction but no effective stroke volume is ejected, which is still effectively cardiac arrest. A clinically relevant example of this latter scenario is cardiac tamponade due to pericardial effusion. The importance of recognizing the many causes for pulselessness when ECG activity is still present has led to preference of the more general term pulseless electrical activity.

Figure 7.10 shows the simultaneous electrocardiogram (upper tracing, ECG) and arterial blood pressure (lower tracing, ABP) from a veterinary patient with PEA. The upper tracing demonstrates that repetitive (but not regular) cardiac depolarization (QRS complex, which is widened) and repolarization (T waves) are occurring. The absence of P waves suggests atrial electrical activity may be absent, but precordial-lead recordings ("chest leads") should be obtained before this conclusion is made. Regardless of the exact rhythm diagnosis, one should note the complete absence of an arterial pulse wave associated with any of the three QRS complexes.

The identification of PEA should prompt the immediate initiation of cardiopulmonary cerebral resuscitation (CPCR) measures in the unconscious patient while *other* personnel check for a pulse and determine if the arterial pressure monitoring system is working properly (see Chapter 16, Cardiopulmonary Cerebral Resuscitation). It is advised that, if ultrasonography is available, the thorax be inspected for evidence of pericardial tamponade or tension pneumothorax (which may require rapid, diagnostic thoracocentesis). The other setting in which PEA is commonly identified is after euthanasia with barbiturate or potassium solutions. Electrical

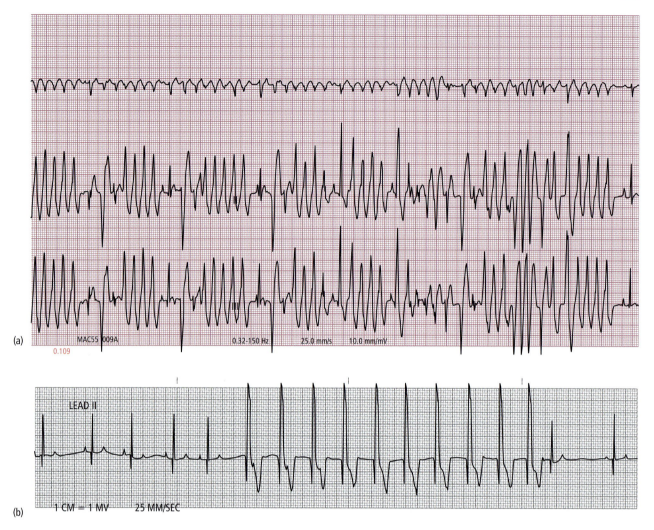

Figure 7.11 (a) An example of ventricular tachycardia, leads I, II, and III ECG at 25 mm/sec; (b) accelerated idioventricular rhythm (AIVR), lead II ECG at 25 mm/sec.

activity often persists for several minutes after pulse generation has ceased.

Skill set 7: distinguishing ventricular tachycardia from accelerated idioventricular rhythm—Figure 7.11a,b

Ventricular dysrhythmias may be due to a number of different mechanisms (e.g., re-entry, enhanced automaticity) and may represent a finding that (a) must be treated (e.g., ventricular flutter), (b) often should be treated (e.g., ventricular tachycardia), (c) may not require treatment (e.g., accelerated idioventricular rhythm), or (d) should *not* be treated (e.g., ventricular escape rhythms). The decision to treat or not treat a ventricular dysrhythmia is often subjective and based on clinical judgment; however, some general guidelines are outlined in Box 7.1.

Box 7.1

Ventricular dysrhythmias likely **should** be treated if:

- The rate is rapid (>160–180 bpm).
- The dysrhythmia is sustained.
- Cardiovascular performance appears depressed (e.g., poor perfusion parameters, hypotension) as a result of the dysrhythmia.
- The ectopic activity has a polymorphic appearance.
- "R-on-T" is identified.
- Risk associated with leaving it untreated appears greater than the risks associated with the treatment selected.

Excessively rapid heart rates reduce diastolic filling of the ventricles and can reduce stroke volume and cardiac output while increasing myocardial workload. As such, ventricular tachyarrhythmias with rates greater than 160–180 beats per minute (bpm) are more likely to require treatment than those exhibiting slower rates. Similarly, sustained dysrhythmias are more likely to compromise cardiovascular performance than those that are brief and intermittent. Patients whose cardiovascular parameters are normal may not require treatment of mild, intermittent dysrhythmias. When the ectopic complexes have varying morphology, this may suggest more widespread ventricular myocardial injury and is more likely to prompt the initiation of therapy. In the "R-on-T" phenomenon the QRS complex of one beat occurs before the T wave of the preceding beat has been completed. Ventricular dysrhythmias exhibiting R-on-T behavior are at greater risk of deteriorating into ventricular fibrillation and warrant therapy. Lastly, one must always consider that all antiarrhythmic agents are also pro-arrhythmic and needlessly treating a benign dysrhythmia with these types of drugs may result in a more dangerous dysrhythmia developing.

The first ECG (Fig. 7.11a) shows a simultaneous recording of leads I, II, and III from a veterinary patient. Paroxysmal ventricular tachycardia is present. The rapid rate, polymorphic appearance, and R-on-T appearance all indicate that treatment is warranted.

The second ECG (Fig. 7.11b) shows a monomorphic, intermittent ventricular dysrhythmia that is termed accelerated idioventricular rhythm (AIVR). This dysrhythmia typically occurs at a rate that is too slow to be classified as a true tachyarrhythmia (as is the case in the example shown). Further, it often causes little impairment in cardiovascular performance and rarely progresses to a more life-threatening form. This dysrhythmia is frequently identified in canine patients presenting for splenic masses, hemoabdomen, postoperative gastric dilatation–volvulus (GDV), or intracranial disease. Emergency and critical care technicians play an important role in recognizing that this dysrhythmia rarely requires treatment other than general supportive care and treatment of the primary problem. Experienced clinicians may opt to terminate ECG monitoring rather than let this generally benign dysrhythmia become a distraction that actually impairs patient care.

Skill set 8: recognition of ventricular flutter and fibrillation—Figure 7.12a,b

Ventricular flutter and fibrillation represent two of the most immediately life-threatening dysrhythmias that the veterinary patient may develop. It is essential that the emergency and critical care technician be able to recognize these rhythms. Once it is recognized that ventricular flutter or fibrillation has developed, one should immediately alert the clinician on duty—without

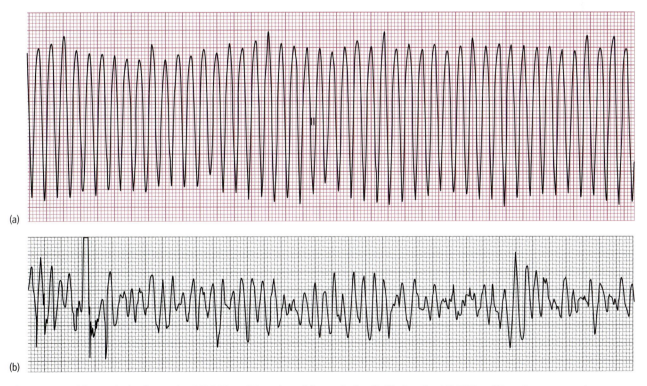

(a)

(b)

Figure 7.12 (a) Ventricular flutter, lead II ECG at 25 mm/sec; (b) ventricular fibrillation, lead II ECG at 25 mm/sec.

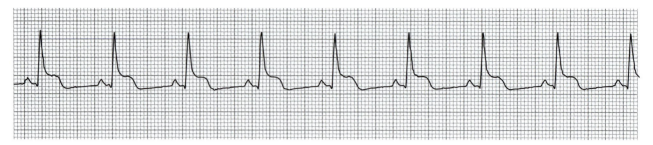

Figure 7.13 ST segment elevation, lead II ECG at 25 mm/sec.

delay—and preparations for cardiopulmonary cerebral resuscitation (CPCR) should be initiated.

Ventricular flutter (see the first ECG, Fig. 7.12a) is a rapid, often regular-appearing rhythm with wide and bizarre QRS complexes that slur into the T waves. The ST segment and other portions of the ECG that typically appear flat are absent and a sinusoidal appearance to the rhythm is generally noted. Treatment options are similar to those for ventricular tachycardia (i.e., D/C cardioversion, Class I antiarrhythmics [e.g., lidocaine], ultrashort-acting Class II agents [e.g., esmolol], Class III agents [e.g., amiodarone], and/or magnesium sulfate). However, the authors would note that in many cases ventricular flutter deteriorates into ventricular fibrillation by the time intravenous antiarrhythmic agents can be administered, and defibrillation equipment should be readied once ventricular flutter is recognized.

Ventricular fibrillation (see the second ECG, Fig. 7.12b) represents a chaotic ventricular dysrhythmia wherein organized electrical activity of the ventricular myocardium as a whole is absent. The lack of organized electrical activity results in the absence of effective myocardial contraction, and cardiac output basically ceases. Ventricular fibrillation is a more common arrest rhythm in humans than in veterinary patients, presumably due to the greater human predisposition to myocardial infarction. However, ventricular fibrillation is identified in many cardiac arrest events in dogs and cats. The key features of ventricular fibrillation on an ECG are the lack of recognizable P–QRS–T complexes and the rapid rate coupled with irregular, bizarre waveforms. The example provided in Figure 7.12b is an example of *coarse* ventricular fibrillation. However, it is important to note that *fine* ventricular fibrillation can also occur, in which the waves are quite small in amplitude. Fine ventricular fibrillation may be mistaken for asystole at times. The only effective therapy for ventricular fibrillation is electrical defibrillation, which should be performed without delay once this dysrhythmia is recognized (see Chapter 18, Defibrillation). Coarse ventricular fibrillation is

thought to respond more readily to electrical defibrillation than fine ventricular fibrillation. Epinephrine may be given prior to defibrillation in an attempt to convert fine ventricular fibrillation to the coarse form before performing defibrillation.

Skill set 9: recognition of ST segment elevation or depression—Figure 7.13

The ST segment on an ECG is a portion that is typically electrically silent and has a flat appearance. The ST segment encompasses the period of time after ventricular depolarization but prior to the initiation of repolarization. Little or no electrical potential difference is detectable on any surface lead. However, in the injured myocardium an "injury current" may occur as current flows between diseased myocardium and adjacent, healthier myocardium. This injury current can result in an electrical potential difference being detectable during the ST segment that shifts its position above or below baseline (see Fig. 7.13). Whether the ST segment becomes shifted upward (elevation) or downward (depression) depends on the relative orientation of the diseased and healthier tissue to one another (e.g., epicardial injury vs. endocardial injury). Myocardial hypoxia can result in ST segment elevation or depression. ST segment changes should always be noted and brought to the clinician's attention when they develop. Investigation of myocardial injury (e.g., echocardiography, arterial blood gas analysis, arterial blood pressure assessment, biomarker assessment [NT-proBNP, troponin], thoracic radiography) may be warranted once this finding has been detected.

Skill set 10: distinguishing bundle branch block (BBB) from ventricular rhythms—Figure 7.14a–c

The QRS complex may appear wide on an ECG for a number of reasons. Slight QRS widening may occur with left ventricular or biventricular hypertrophy (i.e.,

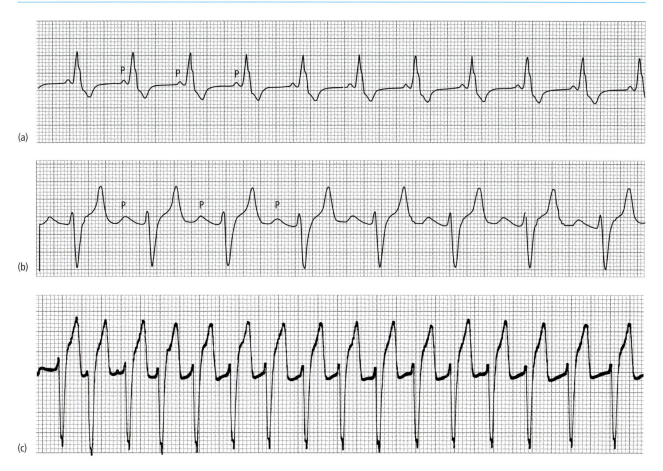

Figure 7.14 (a) Left bundle branch block (LBBB), lead II ECG at 25 mm/sec; (b) right bundle branch block (RBBB), lead II ECG at 50 mm/sec; (c) a ventricular rhythm that lacks evident P waves, lead II ECG at 25 mm/sec.

depolarization takes a bit longer because there is more ventricular tissue to depolarize). Marked QRS widening is typically due to either (a) dysfunction of one or more of the branches of the Bundle of His ("bundle branch block" [BBB]) or (b) the process of depolarization bypassing the Bundle of His entirely (e.g., ventricular escape beats, premature ventricular complexes). It is important that the emergency and critical care technician not assume that all QRS complexes with a "wide and bizarre" appearance are ventricular in nature. One needs to stop and inspect the ECG tracing for evidence of aberrant conduction (e.g., BBB).

The first two ECGs (Fig. 7.14a,b) show examples of block of the left and right branches of the Bundle of His (LBBB and RBBB), respectively. The most notable difference between LBBB and a normally conducted sinus beat is the widening of the QRS complex. With RBBB, the QRS appearance on lead II exhibits a deep, slurred S wave (the complex appears "upside down" in lead II) in addition to the widened appearance of the QRS

complex. If a six-lead ECG study is available, a right-axis deviation of the mean electrical axis may be noted. It must be noted that with both LBBB and RBBB the rhythm originates from sinus-node pacemaker activity. Since atrial depolarization precedes ventricular depolarization, P waves are present and the P-R interval is regular and normal (see labeled P waves in Fig. 7.14a and 7.14b).

Acknowledgments

The authors thank Craig Cornell and Dr. Bill Thomas in particular for contributing many interesting ECGs to our collection over the years.

References

1. Link MS, et al. Part 6: electrical therapies: automated external defibrillators, defibrillation, cardioversion, and pacing: 2010 American Heart Association Guidelines for Cardiopulmonary

Resuscitation and Emergency Cardiovascular Care. Circulation 2010;122(18 Suppl 3):S706–719.

2. DeFrancesco TC, et al. Noninvasive transthoracic temporary cardiac pacing in dogs. J Vet Intern Med 2003;17(5):663–667.

3. Bexton RS, Camm AJ. First degree atrioventricular block. Eur Heart J 1984;5(Suppl A):107–109.

4. Bexton RS, Camm AJ. Second degree atrioventricular block. Eur Heart J 1984;5(Suppl A):111–114.

5. Alzand BS, Crijns HJ. Diagnostic criteria of broad QRS complex tachycardia: decades of evolution. Europace 2011;13(4):465–472.

6. Tsao CW, et al. Accuracy of electrocardiographic criteria for atrial enlargement: validation with cardiovascular magnetic resonance. J Cardiovasc Magn Reson 2008;10:7.

7. Nakayama H, Nakayama T, Hamlin RL. Correlation of cardiac enlargement as assessed by vertebral heart size and echocardiographic and electrocardiographic findings in dogs with evolving cardiomegaly due to rapid ventricular pacing. J Vet Intern Med 2001;15(3):217–221.

8. Yan GX, et al. Ventricular repolarization components on the electrocardiogram: cellular basis and clinical significance. J Am Coll Cardiol 2003;42(3):401–409.

9. Golzari H, et al. Prolonged QTc intervals on admission electrocardiograms: prevalence and correspondence with admission electrolyte abnormalities. Conn Med 2007;71(7):389–397.

10. Detweiler DK. The dog electrocardiogram: a critical review. In: MacFarlane PW, Lawrie TDV, eds. Comprehensive Electrocardiography: Theory and Practice in Health and Disease. New York: Pergamon Press; 1998.

11. Rush JE, Hamlin RL. Effects of graded pleural effusion on QRS in the dog. Am J Vet Res 1985;46(9):1887–1891.

12. Tattersall ML, et al. Correction of QT values to allow for increases in heart rate in conscious Beagle dogs in toxicology assessment. J Pharmacol Toxicol Methods 2006;53(1):11–19.

13. Feldman EC, Ettinger SJ. Electrocardiographic changes associated with electrolyte disturbances. Vet Clin North Am 1977;7(3): 487–496.

14. Rosen KG. Alterations in the fetal electrocardiogram as a sign of fetal asphyxia—experimental data with a clinical implementation. J Perinat Med 1986;14(6):355–363.

15. Crowell-Davis SL. White coat syndrome: prevention and treatment. Compend Contin Educ Vet 2007;29(3):163–165.

8

Fluid-filled hemodynamic monitoring systems

Jamie M. Burkitt Creedon and Marc R. Raffe

Intravascular pressures are commonly measured in acute and critical illness. Intravascular or "blood" pressure is the physical pressure that blood exerts on the vessel wall. This pressure is important because the difference in intravascular pressure at any two points in the vascular network is the driving force for blood circulation. The pressure at the root of the aorta is much greater than the pressure in the vena cava so that blood flows from the arterial to the venous side, delivering oxygen and other nutrients to cells along its path. Intravascular pressures commonly measured in small animals are peripheral arterial blood pressure (ABP) and central venous pressure (CVP). Pulmonary arterial pressure (PAP) and pulmonary arterial occlusion pressure (PAOP; also called pulmonary capillary wedge pressure or "wedge pressure") are also directly measured; however, these measurements are less commonly performed in the veterinary patient.

Peripheral arterial blood pressure may be directly evaluated by measuring intraluminal pressure following placement of an intravascular catheter measurement system, or it can be indirectly measured by surface-applied cuff pressure and flow-detection methods such as Doppler ultrasound or oscillometry. Central venous pressure can only be measured directly by measuring pressure transmitted from the central vein into a catheter-associated measuring system. This chapter deals specifically with the technical aspects of the direct measurement of intravascular pressure using fluid-filled monitoring systems.

Basic pressure principles

Pressure is defined as a force per unit area:

$$P = F/A \qquad (8.1)$$

where P is pressure, F is applied force, and A is the cross-sectional area over which force is applied. To interpret measured pressure, it must be compared with a known pressure standard. For instance, one can only appreciate the effect of pressure applied to the surface of a rubber band if one knows the pressure the rubber band exerts back on the operator—whether or not the band will distort (stretch) depends on the difference between these pressures. In medicine, the accepted standard pressure against which physiologic pressures are compared is barometric pressure (P_B), or the pressure in the earth's atmosphere, which is approximately 760 mm Hg (1031 cm H_2O) at sea level. Clinically, we often are more interested in knowing the intravascular pressure at a given site compared with P_B (i.e., "What is the ABP as measured in the femoral artery of this cat?") than in knowing the difference in pressure between two different sites.

To understand the physiologic determinants and importance of intravascular pressure, one must also understand Ohm's law of hydrodynamics, which is expressed as follows:

$$\Delta P = Q \times R \qquad (8.2)$$

Advanced Monitoring and Procedures for Small Animal Emergency and Critical Care, First Edition. Edited by Jamie M. Burkitt Creedon, Harold Davis.
© 2012 John Wiley & Sons, Inc. Published 2012 by John Wiley & Sons, Inc.

where ΔP is the pressure difference between an upstream and a downstream measurement site, Q is the flow of blood between those sites, and R is the resistance between those sites. The ΔP may be referred to as the **driving pressure**. Blood flow (Q) is the volume of blood movement per unit time and is directly correlated with ΔP. Resistance to flow, R, is the force opposing forward fluid movement. In very basic terms, the higher the driving pressure (the pressure differential between the arterial and venous sides of a blood vessel), the more likely blood will flow through that blood vessel; the higher the resistance across the blood vessel, the less likely blood will flow through that vessel. An important concept herein is that blood flow through a blood vessel or to an organ is not guaranteed by a "normal" driving pressure if high resistance is present; conversely, blood flow through an organ may be adequate at low driving pressure if the resistance through that blood vessel or organ is also low.

Determinants of intravascular pressure

Determinants of systemic arterial pressure

Systemic ABP is the product of cardiac output (CO) and systemic vascular resistance (SVR) such that

$$ABP = CO \times SVR \tag{8.3}$$

This equation is derived from Ohm's law, where CO is blood flow (Q), SVR is vascular resistance (R), and ABP is driving pressure (ΔP).

Systemic ABP is determined by cardiac factors such as heart rate and contractility, by blood volume, and by systemic (also called peripheral) vascular tone. Blood pressure is under tight minute-to-minute and long-term control by an integrated neural, endocrine, and paracrine system. Full discussion of these physiologic influences is outside the scope of this chapter, and details can be found elsewhere.[1,2]

Determinants of central venous pressure

Central venous pressure is frequently used as a surrogate for right atrial (RA) pressure under conditions of no flow obstruction into the RA and normal tricuspid valve function. CVP is very close to right ventricular end diastolic pressure; this value represents the filling pressure of the right side of the heart. Factors determining central venous (RA) pressure include effective blood volume at the site of measurement, pleural pressure (which influences transmural pressure across the great veins and right heart), venous vascular resistance, and right heart "function." Changes in CVP are commonly used to estimate blood volume in critically ill veterinary patients.

Despite its widespread use for this purpose, there is evidence from human literature that there is no relationship between fluid responsiveness and either CVP or a change in CVP.[3]

Determinants of pulmonary arterial pressure

Pulmonary arterial pressure (PAP) is analogous to ABP, but is measured in the pulmonary circulation. Pulmonary arterial pressure is the product of CO and pulmonary vascular resistance (PVR):

$$PAP = CO \times PVR \tag{8.4}$$

Pulmonary vascular resistance is affected by multiple factors such as pleural pressure variation (in disease or secondary to the respiratory cycle) and pulmonary venous pressures. A thorough review of these factors is available elsewhere.[4]

Indications for direct monitoring

Direct intravascular pressure measurement is an integral part of the critically ill patient's monitoring plan. Central venous pressure must always be directly measured. Indications for CVP monitoring are discussed elsewhere (see Chapter 11, Central Venous Pressure Monitoring). Pulmonary arterial pressure is commonly estimated in small animals via Doppler echocardiographic evaluation using modified Bernoulli equation rather than measured directly. However, any time precise, continuous, or frequent measurements of PAP are desirable, it must be measured directly with a pulmonary arterial catheter (see Chapter 12, Cardiac Output Monitoring).

Systemic ABP can be measured either by a direct method using a peripheral arterial catheter system or by an indirect method using surface-applied pressure from an inflatable cuff partnered with flow-detection methodology (sphygmomanometry). The most common methods of indirect ABP measurement in dogs and cats are Doppler ultrasonic or oscillometric techniques, which are discussed in Chapter 10, Noninvasive Arterial Blood Pressure Monitoring.

Most human intensive care references consider direct pressure monitoring the "gold standard" against which indirect methods are compared.[5–8] Direct pressure measurement is generally more accurate because detection and measurement of arterial pressure occurs directly in the vessel lumen. Cuff measurement techniques depend on blood *flow* to provide pressure measurement. Cuff methods are particularly poor in patients with low blood pressure secondary to myocardial failure or in cases where significant alteration in vascular resistance occurs (shock).[5,7] In these cases, there can be large differences between values provided by indirect methods versus

> **Box 8.1** Indications for continuous direct arterial blood pressure measurement[7,8]
>
> - Hypotensive states with actual or potential tissue malperfusion
> - Significant peripheral vasoconstriction
> - Severely hypertensive states
> - Vasodilator therapy
> - Intraoperative and postoperative monitoring of critically ill patients

direct measurement. The Association for the Advancement of Medical Instrumentation (AAMI) has set performance standards for indirect ABP monitors in humans.[9] Multiple veterinary studies have found that commonly used indirect methods fail to meet these standards in dogs and cats, though study methods did not match those of the AAMI.[10–13] Therefore, continuous invasive pressure monitoring is indicated in many critically ill patients, and particularly those in shock states (see Box 8.1).

Despite the advantages noted with direct intravascular pressure measurement, this technique is more technically challenging and measurement errors are noted even when equipment is properly calibrated, leveled, and zeroed. The potential for inaccuracy is high for directly measured systolic and diastolic ABP. Directly measured mean arterial blood pressure (MAP) is more consistent and is a useful value to monitor, as it is the mean (continuous) pressure the organs "see." The inherent pitfalls of even the gold standard of pressure monitoring underscore the importance of evaluating the whole patient—reported values that do not fit the whole clinical picture should be considered suspect, and the monitoring system investigated for sources of error. System inaccuracy and sources of error will be addressed specifically later in the chapter.

Both central venous and arterial pressure monitoring require large venous and arterial catheterization, respectively, and therefore carry the risks of these techniques. Complications, troubleshooting, and contraindications for central venous and arterial catheterization are discussed in Chapters 4 and 5, respectively.

Types of direct intravascular pressure monitoring systems

Direct pressure monitoring systems in veterinary practice are usually (normal saline) **monitoring systems** consisting of fluid-filled tubing that connects a vascular catheter at or near the site of interest to a measuring device. Pressure waves move from the area of interest within the body (such as the cranial vena cava for CVP measurement), through the catheter and fluid-filled tubing either to a water manometer or to a pressure-transducer–processor–display system. Fluid must completely fill the system because fluid is relatively noncompressible and therefore transmits pressure waves well; air is too compressible to accurately transmit pressure waves. The fluid column between the site of interest and the measurement system must be unobstructed for the measuring system to provide accurate information.

The **water manometer** is the simpler of the two common measurement systems. The intravascular catheter is attached to a fluid-filled system of tubing and a manometer (see Fig. 8.1). There is a continuous fluid column between the catheter tip within the patient's body and the manometer. The pressure at the catheter tip supports a column of fluid within the manometer; the pressure is then reported as the height of the fluid within the column. Therefore, when used properly, this technique allows for direct measurement of the pressure at the catheter tip. Measurements are manually performed intermittently. Water manometers are calibrated in centimeters of water (cm H_2O) and are generally only used for CVP measurement in veterinary practice. Peripheral ABP is too high to allow for practical measurement with a water manometer (ABP is higher than the pressure produced by the standard fluid column, so arterial blood would shoot out the top of the water

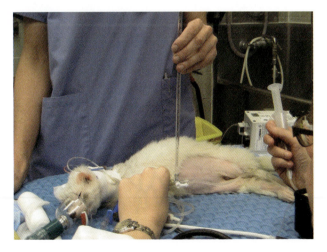

Figure 8.1 A water manometer being used to measure central venous pressure (CVP) in a ferret. Note the bottom of the manometer, at 0 cm in height, is being leveled with the ferret's right atrium, establishing the right atrium as the zero reference point to which the CVP will be compared.

manometer). Water manometers generally report a single value, which is considered the mean intravascular pressure in the cavity (vessel, cardiac chamber) of interest at the reference height (more regarding reference height, leveling, and zeroing below).

For direct arterial blood pressure measurement, a fluid-filled catheter system attached to a pressure-transducer–processor–display system. This system is commonly used for systemic blood pressure because it is designed to accommodate the higher pressures generated in arterial blood vessels and permits continuous monitoring. There is a continuous fluid column between the catheter tip within the patient's body and a pressure transducer, which changes (transduces) the physical pressure wave into an electronic signal (see Fig. 9.1). The electronic signal is transmitted via a cable to a processor where the signal is amplified and processed into a real-time display of graphic waveform and numeric pressure values. Digital monitors generally display pressure in millimeters of mercury (mm Hg), and report systolic, mean, and diastolic pressures. Transducer–processor–display systems are often one component of patient monitors designed to simultaneously report multiple physiologic parameters (such as temperature, respiratory rate, electrocardiogram, multiple pressures, pulse oximetry; see Fig. 8.2). Blood pressure waveforms are displayed on the monitor screen in addition to the numerical pressure values that are displayed.

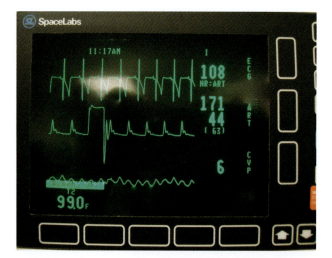

Figure 8.2 The screen of a multiparameter monitor displaying a simultaneous lead I ECG, heart rate, arterial blood pressure waveform, arterial blood pressure values, central venous pressure waveform, mean central venous pressure, and rectal temperature.

Measurement system components

Both the manometer system and the pressure-transducer–processor–display system begin with an intravascular catheter and specialized fluid-filled tubing. Beyond the tubing, the manometer system consists of a three-way stopcock, a water manometer, and a fluid reservoir (source). Beyond the tubing, the electronic system consists of at least one stopcock, a pressure transducer, a pressurized fluid reservoir, a flush device, cable connecting the transducer to a processor, and the processor–display, which is generally a single unit.

For the pressure (and waveform, with an electronic system) to be reported faithfully, each of the system components must meet certain physical and technical criteria. Even if each of the system components meets the required criteria, combining the components alters the physical properties such that the system as a whole may not provide accurate information. Therefore, the operator should be able to do the following: appropriately set up the system; recognize waveform patterns in electronic systems consistent with system malfunction; and test the electronic system for fidelity.

Intravascular catheter

The catheter's gauge, length, insertion site, orientation, and proximity to the vessel wall all affect reported pressures. Frictional resistance to fluid movement within the system increases as the catheter's inner diameter decreases or the catheter lengthens. Therefore, the ideal catheter for pressure-wave transmission would be short with a large bore. However, because the catheter itself increases resistance within the vessel at the insertion site and thus alters pressure, the catheter should ideally occupy no more than 10% of the vessel lumen.[5] The reality for dogs and cats is somewhere in the middle: in general, the catheter selected should be one that reasonably fits within the vessel while minimizing the likelihood of vascular occlusion.

The catheter insertion site should be chosen for cleanliness, ease of placement, and maintenance. If a "stiff" catheter is used, it should remain straight along its entire path to minimize occlusion. Catheters for CVP monitoring are most commonly inserted into the external jugular vein in both dogs and cats and threaded into the cranial vena cava. Alternately, a long, flexible catheter may be placed into a saphenous vein and threaded cranially into the thoracic vena cava. Because saphenous-inserted thoracic caval catheters yield similar values as those placed through the external jugular vein,[14] this is common practice in dogs and cats. Venous catheter insertion is discussed in detail in Chapter 4, Catheterization of the Venous Compartment.

Common insertion sites for arterial catheters in dogs are the perforating metatarsal artery (commonly called the dorsal pedal artery) and the radial, coccygeal, femoral, and auricular arteries. In cats, the femoral artery is most commonly used; the perforating metatarsal artery can also be used in larger cats for short durations (hours). Information regarding arterial catheter insertion can be found in Chapter 5, Arterial Puncture and Catheterization. Mean pressure is lower in distal portions of the arterial tree compared with the aorta because pressure-wave energy is lost as heat generated by frictional flow resistance along the vessel length. The pressure difference along the arterial tree is not considered a significant factor when selecting measurement sites.

Catheter tip orientation in relation to direction of blood flow affects the measured pressure value in both arterial and venous systems. A catheter tip facing into the blood flow (upstream) will measure a slightly higher pressure value than the actual intravascular pressure; a catheter tip facing away from the flow of blood (downstream) will measure a pressure value slightly lower than actual pressure. These differences are due to alteration in kinetic and potential energy at the catheter tip; these differences are relatively small in the vascular catheters commonly placed in veterinary practice.

Noncompliant tubing

The tubing that connects the intravenous catheter and pressure transducer must be made of specialized material to prevent pressure-wave energy from being absorbed (or "dampened") by the tubing wall. This tubing is called rigid, noncompliant, or high-pressure tubing. The tubing must be completely filled with fluid without any air bubbles present. Use of standard fluid extension tubing between the vascular catheter and the pressure transducer will lead to significant error in the pressure and waveform measurement. Noncompliant tubing is less important for CVP measurement as the pressure values are significantly lower than systemic arterial pressure.

Water manometer

Water manometers are used for intermittent measurement of CVP, which is detailed in Chapter 11, Central Venous Pressure Monitoring. The water manometer is a plastic tube that is marked in centimeters along its length and has a "zero," or reference, mark near the bottom of the column height (sometimes the bottom *is* the zero mark, as in Fig. 8.1). The zero mark is used as a reference site for aligning the manometer at the level of the right atrium prior to CVP measurements (see Zeroing the Transducer, below). If a commercially produced water manometer is unavailable, one can create a water manometer from standard fluid extension tubing hand-marked with centimeters indicated along its length. The base of the water manometer fits into a three-way stopcock with the noncompliant-tubing–catheter system on the second port and the fluid reservoir on the third.

Although it is called a "water" manometer, the tubing column is filled with a biologically compatible crystalloid fluid to perform the measurement. The fluid reservoir for the water manometer is usually a 20-mL syringe filled with isotonic crystalloid. Full details regarding assembly and use of the water manometer pressure measurement system are available in Chapter 11, Central Venous Pressure Monitoring, specifically in Protocol 11.1, Intermittent Central Venous Pressure Measurement.

Pressure transducer

When an electronic pressure monitoring system is used, the noncompliant tubing is attached to a pressure transducer (see Fig. 9.1). The transducer has a pressure-sensitive membrane that distorts in response to pressure changes that are created when pressure waves strike it. The transducer converts the membrane distortion into an electronic signal using an integral electronic circuit that functions by the "Wheatstone bridge" principle.[5] The generated electrical signal is transmitted to the processor–display unit by a shielded electrical cable. Most pressure transducers used in an integral veterinary medicine are classified as "disposable," meaning that they are intended for single use in humans. Disposable transducers are sterile in their packaging and electronically precalibrated; some models come with high-pressure tubing attached.

Pressure transducers have a female adapter for connection to the fluid reservoir. The fluid reservoir is a bag of sterile isotonic crystalloid and administration set attached to the transducer. The bag of isotonic crystalloid is held under constant pressure such that a small volume of fluid continuously flushes through the system, preventing blood from flowing back and contaminating the monitoring system. The infused volume is generally 2–4 mL/hour (read manufacturer's specifications for more precise value). Most transducers have a pigtail or lever protruding from the housing that activates an integrated "flush valve" that allows rapid infusion ("fast flush") of fluid from the pressurized fluid bag through the system to clean the transducer "head."

Handled with care, "disposable" transducers may be cleaned and reused following ethylene oxide

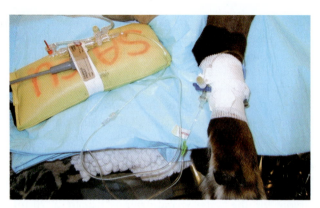

Figure 8.3 Part of a direct arterial pressure monitoring system in a dog. The dog's perforating metatarsal (dorsal pedal) arterial catheter is attached to a T-port, which is connected to noncompliant, fluid-filled tubing by a three-way stopcock. This stopcock is optional to the system and is in place here for serial arterial blood sampling. The noncompliant tubing is attached to the pressure transducer, which is secured to a yellow sandbag with medical tape; the sandbag provides a stable base for the transducer and helps raise the transducer's zero point (top of the transducer's stopcock) to the level of the patient's right atrium. The red pigtail on the transducer can be used to provide rapid system flush from the pressurized fluid bag (not pictured; its tubing leads from the pigtail to the fluid bag out the top of the frame). The grey cable runs from the transducer to the electronic processor and display monitor (not pictured).

resterilization. Resterilization can lead to damage of the pressure-sensitive membrane, which can lead to inaccurate pressure reporting. When a resterilized transducer is used, the operator should always perform a calibration prior to performing clinical measurements (see below for information about calibration).

Assembling the electronic direct pressure measurement system

A full list of supplies and step-by-step instructions required to assemble the electronic direct pressure measuring system are available in Protocol 8.1. Figure 8.3 shows a portion of a direct arterial pressure monitoring system in use.

Technical aspects of the electronic direct pressure measurement system

Direct pressure monitoring is relatively complex and far from foolproof. There are many technical points that must be carefully followed for accurate measurement. It

is extremely important that the operator understand the technical principles that affect its fidelity, how to properly configure and test the system for fidelity, and how to recognize and correct for system error.

Zeroing the transducer

To interpret measured pressure, it must be compared with a known pressure standard. The standard pressure against which direct intravascular pressure measurements are compared is barometric pressure (P_B), which is approximately 760 mm Hg (1031 cm H_2O) at sea level.

The electronic pressure measurement system is calibrated to standard pressure, or "**zeroed**," by opening the transducer's stopcock port (see Fig. 9.1) to the atmosphere and depressing the "zero" button on the electronic pressure monitor (see Protocol 8.2 for instructions on zeroing a transducer). Zeroing the transducer to atmospheric pressure makes discussion of physiologic pressures easier (i.e., "The patient's MAP is 98 mm Hg" rather than "The patient's MAP is 760 + 98 = 858 mm Hg"). Transducer zeroing should be done at initial system setup, any time system components are removed or replaced, or if any problems occur with system readings. If a transducer system fails to zero, the transducer, the monitor, or the connecting cable may be faulty (most often it is the transducer, especially when using a resterilized disposable transducer). These items should be sequentially changed until the faulty component is identified and replaced.

Water manometers are always open to the atmosphere and are thus inherently "zeroed" to atmospheric pressure. Therefore, no zeroing actions need to be performed on a water manometer, but its top must always remain open to the air or readings will be inaccurate.

Calibrating the system

After the system is zeroed to the atmosphere, it must be calibrated prior to use. To calibrate a measuring instrument is to compare and align its readings with known standards so that the measuring instrument can provide accurate readings. Calibrating a water manometer device simply involves comparing the markings on the manometer against those on a centimeter ruler. Such calibration is unnecessary on commercially available manometers, since they come premarked, but is required if regular fluid extension tubing is used to contain the fluid column.

Calibration is required for electronic systems each time the system is assembled and again any time problems arise. The transducer must be calibrated to confirm that when standard pressure is applied to the transducer,

Protocol 8.1 Assembling the electronic direct pressure measurement system for CVP or ABP monitoring

Items Required
- Indwelling vascular catheter at the appropriate site
- ≤2 lengths of high-pressure tubing with locking fittings—keep as short as feasible
- Stopcocks with locking fittings—2 or fewer
- 1–2 sterile infusion plugs with locking fittings
- Sterile pressure transducer with integrated fast flush device
- Sandbag and medical tape, or other stabilizing device to fix the transducer
- Bag of isotonic crystalloid flush solution with standard administration set attached; standard extension set(s) as needed
  - Most commonly the flush solution is heparinized—ask clinician for any special considerations.
- Pressure bag of appropriate size for fluid bag used
- Monitor, with its power cord and transducer-to-monitor cable
- Power source

Procedure
1. Collect necessary supplies.
2. Plug the monitor in, turn it on, and attach the transducer-to-monitor cable to the monitor. Configure the monitor per manufacturer's instructions to display pressure from the socket into which you have inserted the transducer-to-monitor cable.
3. Perform hand hygiene and don clean examination gloves.
4. Aseptically prepare the patient's catheter port onto which the monitoring system will be attached. Flush the patient's catheter gently to ensure patency.
5. Heparinize the flush solution unless the clinician instructs otherwise. Standard dilution is 1 unit heparin per milliliter of flush. Mark the fluid bag to indicate its additives. Remove all air from the fluid bag by inserting a 22-gauge needle into the medication port and withdrawing gas until none remains. This minimizes the risk of air embolism from the pressurized system.
6. Attach a standard fluid administration set, with the roller clamp closed, to the heparinized fluid bag and squeeze the drip chamber until it is approximately half-full. Prime the fluid line with flush using gravity flow, then reclamp the fluid line. Handle fluid line aseptically such that the end remains sterile.
7. Insert the fluid bag into a pressure bag and inflate to approximately 300 mm Hg. Hang the pressurized bag and fluid line near the patient's area.
8. Remove the pressure transducer (see Fig. 9.1) from its packaging and manipulate all moving parts to ensure they move as intended. Handle aseptically such that all ports remain sterile. Inspect for any evidence of damage, particularly if the unit has been resterilized.
9. Attach the primed flush fluid line to the transducer. If necessary, attach one length of high-pressure tubing to the transducer on the patient side. If necessary, add more high-pressure tubing to reach the patient, to a maximum of two lengths total. Place a sterile, locking injection port to the transducer's zeroing (air) port.
10. The vented cap on a new transducer's stopcock should be thrown away, as its vents may allow contaminants to enter the system.
11. If blood sampling from the catheter is desired, place a stopcock between the high-pressure tubing and the catheter or catheter's T-port. The unused port should have a sterile, locking injection port attached.
12. Use the fast flush device on the transducer to prime the entire system until fluid drips from the end of the high-pressure tubing. Flush slowly to avoid air bubble formation in the tubing.
13. Attach the monitoring system to the patient's vascular catheter or the catheter's T-port.
14. Tighten all connections and engage all fitting locks to prevent inadvertent disconnection and subsequent blood loss.
15. Plug the monitor cable into the transducer and fix the transducer to its stabilizing device (i.e., sandbag with tape) such that the transducer's zeroing (air) port is at the appropriate height (at the level of the right atrium).
16. Zero and level the system. (See the sections Zeroing the Transducer and Leveling the Transducer, for more information.)
17. Turn all stopcocks in the system open to the patient.
18. Perform a fast flush test and make any necessary adjustments to the system to optimize the system's dynamic response. (See text for more information about dynamic response.)

Protocol 8.2 Zeroing a pressure transducer

Items Required
- An assembled electronic direct pressure measurement system, attached to its monitor via the transducer cable

Procedure
1. Plug in and turn on the monitor. Configure the monitor such that the screen displays an option to zero the transducer (see manufacturer's instructions for specific steps).
2. Perform hand hygiene and don clean examination gloves.
3. Turn the transducer's stopcock "off" to the patient's side of the system so there is a continuous fluid column between the stopcock's injection cap and the transducer's pressure diaphragm.
4. Remove the injection cap from the stopcock, maintaining system asepsis.
5. Depress the "zero" button on the monitor.
6. The pressure tracing should be a flat line at the zero mark on the display.
7. If the pressure reads a number other than 0, or if the pressure tracing is not a flat line at the zero mark on the graph, the transducer may be faulty, in which case it must be replaced with another flushed, sterile transducer. If this does not remedy the issue, the transducer cable or monitor itself may be faulty and may need to be replaced.
8. Once the monitor displays "0" with the transducer's fluid interface open to the atmosphere via the stopcock, aseptically replace the injection cap and turn the stopcock "off" to the injection cap, opening the fluid column between the transducer and the patient end of the system.

---

the correct pressure is reported. Calibration should be conducted with the transducer attached to the monitor, as instructed by the monitor's manufacturer. Alternately, a water manometer filled with fluid to a set height may be attached to the transducer's stopcock and the display's reading compared with the known applied pressure from the fluid column, remembering that 1.36 cm H_2O exerts the same pressure as 1 mm Hg. Calibration problems can be due to transducer, monitor, or connecting-cable problems.

Leveling the transducer

A transducer is both zeroed, to eliminate the influence of atmospheric pressure from vascular pressure readings, and **leveled,** to eliminate the influence of *gravity.* For both CVP and ABP, the "level" reference point is the right atrium (RA); thus the RA is called the **zero reference point**. To level the measuring system, the transducer should be placed at the height of the RA and zeroed at that point by opening the three-way valve to air. This step should be performed *prior to every measurement* (see Protocol 8.3). An external anatomic landmark that correlates well with the RA reference point is the sternum of the cat or dog lying in lateral recumbency. As stated in Chapter 11, Central Venous Pressure Monitoring, in a sternally recumbent animal the RA lies at a point roughly 40% the height of a vertical line that extends from the sternum to the top of the dorsal spinous process just caudal to the shoulder.

Once the transducer is zeroed at RA height, it must remain at RA height for every measurement. The reason for this requirement may best be explained by example. In a patient undergoing CVP monitoring, if the transducer falls below RA level by 10 cm (approximately 4 inches), a 10-cm blood fluid column is exerting pressure on the transducer in addition to the actual CVP. Though this additional pressure is not a change in CVP, the transducer will "see" both the actual CVP and the additional 10-cm blood column and will report a value equal to the CVP plus 10 cm H_2O. The opposite is true if the transducer ends up higher than its zero reference point— the pressure reported will be falsely low in such cases (see Fig. 8.4). For peripheral ABP monitoring, such changes are less likely to create clinical confusion because as a proportion of the pressure of interest, the error is smaller. For instance, while a difference of 10 cm H_2O (7.4 mm Hg) in CVP can greatly influence a clinician's decision-making process, that same 7.4 mm Hg difference in MAP is less likely to cause an error in clinical judgment. This example underscores the importance of evaluating the whole clinical picture before making decisions, and the importance of proper transducer leveling at the zero reference point (the RA) prior to *every measurement*, particularly when monitoring CVP.

Dynamic response of the system

Intravascular pressures are pulsatile in nature. Reflection of pressure waves through the vessel creates multiple

Protocol 8.3 Leveling a pressure transducer at the zero reference point (the right atrium)

Items Required
- An electronic direct pressure measurement system, attached to a powered-on monitor and to the patient
- Carpenter's level
- Piece of string

Procedure
1. Configure the monitor such that the screen displays an option to zero the transducer (see manufacturer's instructions for specific steps).
2. Perform hand hygiene and don clean examination gloves.
3. Turn the transducer's stopcock "off" to the patient's side of the system so there is a continuous fluid column between the stopcock's injection cap and the transducer's pressure diaphragm.
4. Remove the injection cap from the stopcock, maintaining system asepsis.
5. Ensure the transducer's fluid–air interface is at the height of the right atrium. Assess this level using the string and carpenter's level for accuracy—this will enhance accuracy and repeatability from one operator to the next for repeated measures.
   a. With the patient in lateral recumbency, RA height is approximately the height of the sternum.
   b. For a dog or cat in sternal recumbency, the RA is approximately 40% the distance from the sternum to the dorsal spinous process just caudal to the scapula.
6. Secure the monitor at this height if performing continuous monitoring and the patient is immobile.
7. Depress the "zero" button on the monitor.
8. The pressure tracing should be a flat line at the zero mark on the display.
9. If the pressure reads a number other than 0, or the pressure tracing is not a flat line at the zero mark on the graph, the transducer may be faulty, in which case it must be replaced with another flushed, sterile transducer. If this does not remedy the issue, the transducer cable or monitor itself may be faulty and may need to be replaced.
10. Once the monitor displays "0" with the transducer's fluid–air interface open at RA height, aseptically replace the injection cap and turn the stopcock "off" to the injection cap, opening the fluid column between the transducer and the patient end of the system.
11. Allow the system to equilibrate and record the measured value.

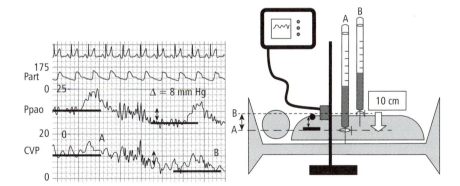

Figure 8.4 Illustration of what happens when the patient's right atrium (RA; level shown by dashed line A) falls below the transducer's zero reference point (at the level of dotted line B) as the bed is lowered: (left) change in recorded pressures (P_{art}, peripheral arterial; P_{pao}, pulmonary arterial occlusion [wedge]; CVP, central venous pressure); (right) water manometers (tubes A and B) that demonstrate how lowering the RA relative to the transducer lowers the measured pressures. In this example, the bed was lowered by 10 cm, which means that the patient's RA (the proper level) is 10 cm lower than the current zero reference point (B), which translates to a pressure drop of 10 cm H_2O, or approximately 8 mm Hg. Figure reprinted and legend adapted from Magder S, Invasive intravascular hemodynamic monitoring: technical issues, *Critical Care Clinics*, Vol. 23, pp. 401–414, 2007, with permission from Elsevier.

oscillating waves of different amplitude and frequency (Fourier series) that summate to create the observed waveform. An intravascular pressure monitoring system must have the physical properties required to measure pressures within the expected range and must be able to respond adequately to physiologic pressure pulsations. The ideal system would report the pressure waves of interest and no others. The ability of a system to accurately display the shape and amplitude of the pulse pressure waveform is determined by the system's **dynamic response**, also called the system's frequency response. The system's dynamic response is determined by its physical properties, specifically its mass, elasticity, and friction.[15] Dynamic response is discussed in terms of natural frequency and damping coefficient, both of which are measurable and have significant impact on a waveform's appearance.

Effect of a system's natural frequency

When stimulated, every structure naturally vibrates at a characteristic frequency, which is expressed in cycles per second or hertz (Hz). This frequency is called the structure's **natural frequency**, fundamental frequency, or resonant frequency. Adding components together (as in connecting a catheter, noncompliant tubing, and transducer) alters a system's natural frequency. It is important that the natural frequency of a fluid-filled monitoring system not coincide with the frequency of physiologic pressure waves, because frequency overlap causes summation (from the patient and the system) and results in exaggerated waveforms and numerical values. Exaggerated results are due to *too low a system natural frequency*, and such exaggeration leads to what is often called overshoot, **ringing**, or resonance of the waveform.[15] Ringing causes pointy, spiked waveforms, falsely high systolic pressure readings, and falsely low diastolic pressure readings.

A fluid-filled monitoring system will have optimal responsiveness if its natural frequency is as high as possible. Though individual materials made for intravascular pressure monitoring are designed with this principle in mind, once a catheter–tubing–transducer system is assembled, the natural frequency drops to minimal requirements for humans.[5] Because dogs and cats generally have pulse rates that exceed humans', their pulse pressure waveforms have a higher frequency than people's, and thus almost certainly overlap the natural frequency of most measurement systems. This overlap means that without correction through damping (see below), our patients' pulse pressure waveforms will almost always ring, systolic pressures will be falsely high, and diastolic pressures will be falsely low. One way to maximize a system's natural frequency is to keep the system as simple as possible, for instance with as short a tubing length and as few components as possible.

Effect of a system's damping coefficient

Damping is loss of the pulse pressure energy between the catheter tip and the transducer. Damping is due to frictional resistance along the system's length, absorption of energy by the tubing and other materials, and air bubbles, which are more compressible than fluid. The more damped a system is, the more quickly it returns to "zero" after an applied stimulus due to this energy loss.

Damping in a pressure system is measured and expressed as the **damping coefficient**; the higher the coefficient, the more significant the damping. An **overdamped** pressure waveform has slurred upstrokes and downstrokes, loss of detail, and a generally flattened appearance; overdamped systems cause a falsely narrowed pulse pressure with falsely low systolic and falsely high diastolic pressure readings (see Fig. 9.7). Conversely, **underdamped** waveforms contain nonphysiologic points and spikes, extra waves, and appear exaggerated—they are overshot or have excessive ringing, as discussed previously regarding natural frequency. Underdamping causes falsely high systolic and falsely low diastolic pressure readings. A system with an infinitely high natural frequency does not require damping to produce accurate results (see Fig. 8.5), but because available systems have natural frequency overlap as noted previously, they usually require some operator-implemented damping.

Determining the system's dynamic response

Many catheter–tubing–transducer systems have weak natural frequencies to faithfully reproduce physiologic pressure data; thus, these systems are inherently underdamped. Within a certain range, adjusting the system's damping can help produce more accurate values and waveforms (Fig. 8.5). To know whether a system has adequate dynamic response, its natural frequency and damping coefficient should be determined and plotted onto a graph such as Figure 8.5. These properties are measured by performing a fast flush or **"square wave" test** on the system. When the transducer's fast flush device is activated, the transducer–tubing–catheter system is exposed to the high pressure in the flush fluid bag (300 mm Hg). To perform the test, the fast flush device should be opened briefly (<1 second) and released quickly several times to produce multiple square waves for analysis. The high pressure should appear on the recorder as a square waveform as shown in Figure 8.6. A normal square wave has a nearly 90° upstroke, a flat

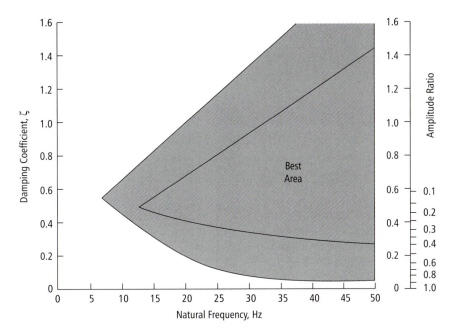

Figure 8.5 Use of natural frequency and damping coefficient to determine if the catheter–tubing–transducer system is producing accurate pressure waveforms and values. Plot the system's frequency and damping coefficient; the intersection falls in the gray area for an adequately responsive system. Overdamped readings will fall above the gray area and underdamped readings will fall below the gray area. This figure and its legend were altered and used here with permission from *Hemodynamic Waveform Analysis*; Ahrens RS, Taylor LA; Technical considerations in obtaining hemodynamic waveform values, pp. 209–258, copyright Saunders 1992.

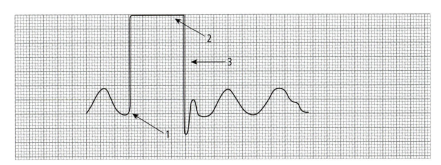

Figure 8.6 Performing a square wave test. The fast flush device is activated at point 1. Squaring of the waveform occurs as the transducer is exposed to 300 mm Hg pressure from the flush fluid bag and has a flat plateau (2) with right angles on both sides. A rapid downstroke occurs as the fast flush device is released (3). This test should be performed several times and the square waves analyzed to determine the system's natural frequency and damping coefficient. These values can then be plugged into the graph in Figure 8.5 to determine whether the system has adequate dynamic response. This figure used with permission from *Hemodynamic Waveform Analysis*; Ahrens RS, Taylor LA; Technical considerations in obtaining hemodynamic waveform values, pp. 209–258, copyright Saunders 1992.

plateau at 300 mm Hg, and a rapid downstroke as the fast flush device is released. The top is squared, as the test's name implies. Protocol 8.4 describes how to determine a system's natural frequency and damping coefficient, and thus the system's dynamic response, using waveforms from square wave tests.

A square wave test should be performed when the system is initially assembled and any time there are questions about the fidelity of measurement results.

Optimizing dynamic response by altering a system's natural frequency and damping coefficient

There are many steps one can take to optimize a system's dynamic response by either increasing the natural frequency or altering the damping coefficient. Underdamping is far more common in dogs and cats than overdamping. An example from a ringing, underdamped

Protocol 8.4 Determining the dynamic response of a fluid-filled monitoring system (Figs. 8.7–8.9)

Items Required
- An electronic direct pressure measurement system, attached to a powered-on monitor (with printer) and to the patient
- Calculator
- Straightedge (i.e., ruler)
- Pen and paper

Procedure
1. Ensure the pressure bag containing the flush fluid is pressurized to 300 mm Hg.
2. Perform hand hygiene and don clean examination gloves.
3. Perform a square wave test during diastole by activating the transducer's fast flush device briefly (for <1 second) and quickly releasing the device. A square wave should appear on the monitor—print this waveform with 1–2 seconds of strip on either side. Repeat this process 3–5 more times and collect the square waves for analysis.
4. Evaluate the square waves to determine the system's natural frequency. The natural frequency is the frequency with which the waveform oscillates after the fast flush device is released. For example: The paper speed in Figure 8.7 is 25 mm/sec. Note the number of blocks between oscillation peaks—in this case just over 2 blocks between oscillations. Divide the paper speed by the number of blocks to determine the system's natural frequency: (25 mm/sec) ÷ (2 mm) = 12.5 cycles/sec = 12.5 Hz, which is a minimally acceptable natural frequency for measurements in humans.
5. Determine the frequency on all of the square waves collected, and average the values to reach the mean natural frequency. Use this mean natural frequency in the dynamic response graphic plot (see step 8).
6. Evaluate the square wave to determine the system's damping coefficient. This is done by comparing the length of two successive oscillations and dividing the second (smaller) oscillation by the first (see Fig. 8.8). The number generated is called the amplitude ratio. For example: The paper speed in Figure 8.8 is 25 mm/sec. Measure the length of two successive oscillations (i.e., from peak to valley, and from that same valley to the next peak). Divide the smaller oscillation by the larger to determine the amplitude ratio. Here, 6 mm ÷ 28 mm = 0.21, which is the amplitude ratio.
7. Determine the amplitude ratio on all of the square waves collected and average the values to reach the mean amplitude ratio. Use the graph in Figure 8.9 to determine the damping coefficient from the amplitude ratio.
8. Use a straightedge to plot the mean natural frequency against the damping coefficient on the graph in see fig 8.5 above. If the intersecting point falls into the gray area, the system is adequately responsive. Overdamped readings will fall above the gray area and underdamped readings will fall below the gray area.

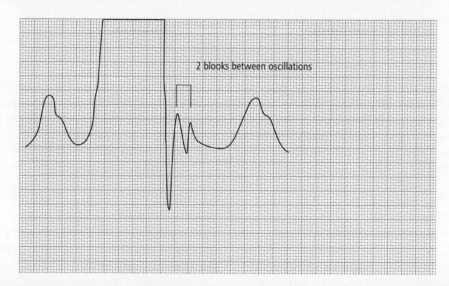

Figure 8.7 Step 4, determine system's natural frequency. Paper speed 25 mm/sec. First, note the number of blocks between oscillation peaks—in this case just over 2 blocks between oscillations. Then divide the paper speed by the number of blocks to determine the system's natural frequency: (25 mm/sec) ÷ (2 mm) = 12.5 cycles/sec = 12.5 Hz, which is a minimally acceptable natural frequency for measurements in humans. Figure altered and used with permission from *Hemodynamic Waveform Analysis*; Ahrens RS, Taylor LA; Technical considerations in obtaining hemodynamic waveform values, pp. 209–258, copyright Saunders 1992.

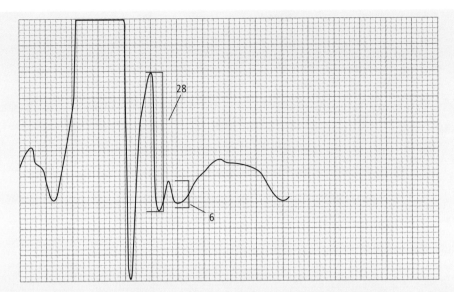

Figure 8.8 Step 6, calculating the amplitude ratio to determine damping coefficient. Paper speed 25 mm/sec. First measure the length of two successive oscillations (i.e., from peak to valley, and from that same valley to the next peak). Then divide the smaller oscillation by the larger to determine the amplitude ratio. Here, 6 mm ÷ 28 mm = 0.21, which is the amplitude ratio. Figure altered and used with permission from *Hemodynamic Waveform Analysis*; Ahrens RS, Taylor LA; Technical considerations in obtaining hemodynamic waveform values, pp. 209–258, copyright Saunders 1992.

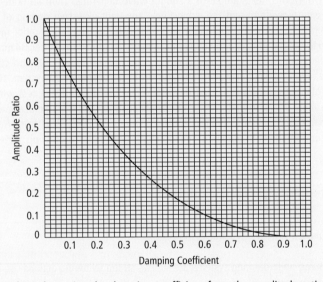

Figure 8.9 Step 7, Use this graph to determine the damping coefficient from the amplitude ratio. Figure altered and used with permission from *Hemodynamic Waveform Analysis*; Ahrens RS, Taylor LA; Technical considerations in obtaining hemodynamic waveform values, pp. 209–258, copyright Saunders 1992.

system and one from an overdamped system are shown in the square wave tests in Figure 8.10 Further discussion of the effects of underdamping and overdamping on ABP waveforms and values is found in Chapter 9, Direct Systemic Arterial Blood Pressure Monitoring. Measures

to take that may help optimize the system's dynamic response are listed in Box 8.2.

Though it is important for accurate pressure readings and interpretation, it is unclear that the systems in clinical use today commonly have adequate dynamic

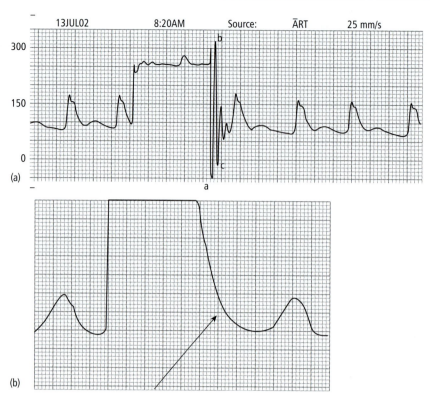

Figure 8.10 Square wave test waveforms: (a) Example of a square wave generated from an underdamped system. Note the spiky, pointy nature of the arterial pressure waveform and the subjectively apparent excessive ringing of the square wave test compared with the normal example in Figure 8.6. To confirm underdamping, calculate the amplitude ratio: measure vertically from point a to point b, 37 mm; then from point b to point c, 34 mm; then divide the smaller length by the larger, 34 mm ÷ 37 mm = 0.92. An amplitude ratio of 0.92 corresponds to a damping coefficient of less than 0.1, which is extremely low and corroborates the impression of an underdamped waveform. (b) Example of a square wave generated from an overdamped system. Note the slurred arterial pressure waveform with no apparent dicrotic notch, and the slurred downstroke of the square wave test with lack of oscillations at baseline (arrow). It is very difficult to determine damping coefficient in the absence of any measurable oscillations, but the damping coefficient here is high, probably greater than 0.6.[16] Part (b) is altered and used here with permission from *Hemodynamic Waveform Analysis*; Ahrens RS, Taylor LA; Technical considerations in obtaining hemodynamic waveform values, pp. 209–258, copyright Saunders 1992.

Box 8.2 Measures to help optimize a system's dynamic response

The corrections for overdamped and underdamped systems are similar, so the following actions can be tried in the case of either problem.[16,17]
- Simplify the system as much as possible to increase its natural frequency:
  - Remove as many lengths of tubing between the catheter and the patient as possible such that the tubing does not exceed 3–4 feet in length.
  - Remove any unnecessary stopcocks.
  - Consider removing any T-ports or other connections.
- Ensure only noncompliant tubing is present between the catheter and the transducer, particularly for arterial pressure monitoring.
- Check for and remove any visible clots or air bubbles.
- Check tubing for kinks or occlusions.
- Gently aspirate and flush the catheter to assess for occlusion.
- If the catheter is <18-gauge (or 7 Fr), compliant, or long, consider replacement with a shorter, larger-bore, stiffer catheter.
- If the waveform is underdamped, consider insertion of a damping device into the system.

response.[15] It is important to remember both this source of inaccuracy and that *pressure waveforms and pressure values are altered by simple changes the operator makes to the system* such as alterations in system components and damping. Thus, the gold-standard invasive pressure monitoring system is also inherently flawed by inevitable operator manipulations.

Summary

Fluid-filled monitoring systems provide important information in patients with cardiovascular instability. Though they are more complicated than noninvasive measurement techniques, they can provide continuous monitoring. As with any technique, one becomes more proficient with practice and use. A solid understanding of the principles behind fluid-filled monitoring systems allows the clinician to make the most of these systems' capabilities and avoid common technical errors. It is important to remember that there is a potential for technical error if equipment is incorrectly configured, inaccurately zeroed, uncalibrated, or poorly leveled. It is also important to remember that actions we take to optimize the dynamic response of a system (altering natural frequency and damping) can change the reported pressure results and mislead the clinician.

References

1. Boulpaep EL. Regulation of arterial pressure and cardiac output. In: Boron WF, Boulpaep EL, eds. Medical Physiology. Philadelphia: Saunders; 2003:534–557.
2. Kittleson MD, Kienle RD. Normal clinical cardiovascular physiology. In: Kittleson MD, Kienle RD, eds. Small Animal Cardiovascular Medicine. St. Louis, MO: Mosby; 1998:11–35.
3. Marik PE, Baram M, Vahid B. Does central venous pressure predict fluid responsiveness?: a systematic review of the literature and the tale of seven mares. Chest 2008;134(1):172–178.
4. Boron WF. Ventilation and perfusion of the lungs. In: Boron WF, Boulpaep EL, eds. Medical Physiology. Philadelphia: Saunders; 2003:686–711.
5. Fessler HE, Shade E. Measurement of vascular pressure. In Tobin MJ, ed. Principles and Practice of Intensive Care Monitoring. New York: McGraw-Hill; 1998:91–106.
6. Lodato RF. Arterial pressure monitoring. In: Tobin MJ, ed. Principles and Practice of Intensive Care Monitoring. New York: McGraw-Hill; 1998:733–749.
7. Shoemaker WC, Parsa MH. Invasive and noninvasive monitoring. In: Grenvik A, Ayres AM, Holbrook PR, Shoemaker WC, eds. Textbook of Critical Care, 4th ed. Philadelphia: W.B. Saunders; 2000:74–91.
8. Vincent J-L. Arterial, central venous, and pulmonary artery catheters. In: Parrillo JE, Dellinger RP, eds. Critical Care Medicine: Principles of Diagnosis and Management in the Adult. Philadelphia: Mosby Elsevier; 2008:53–64.
9. Prisant LM, Alpert BS, Robbins CB, et al. American national standards for nonautomated sphygmomanometers. Am J Hypertens 1995;8:210–213.
10. Binns SH, Sisson DD, Buoscio DA, et al. Doppler ultrasonographic, oscillometric sphygmomanometric, and photoplethysmographic techniques for noninvasive blood pressure measurement in anesthetized cats. J Vet Intern Med 1995;9:405–414.
11. Haberman CE, Kang CW, Morgan JD, et al. Evaluation of oscillometric and Doppler ultrasonic methods of indirect blood pressure estimation in conscious dogs. Can J Vet Res 2006;70:211–217.
12. MacFarlane PD, Grint N, Dugdale A. Comparison of invasive and non-invasive blood pressure monitoring during clinical anesthesia in dogs. Vet Res Commun 2010;34:217–227.
13. Bosiack AP, Mann FA, Dodam JR, et al. Comparison of ultrasonic Doppler flow monitor, oscillometric, and direct arterial blood pressure measurements in ill dogs. J Vet Emerg Crit Care 2010;20(2):207–215.
14. Machon RG, Raffe MR, Robinson EP. Central venous pressure measurements in the caudal vena cava of sedated cats. J Vet Emerg Crit Care 1995;5(2):121–129.
15. Mark JB. Technical requirements for direct blood pressure measurement. In: Mark JB, ed. Atlas of Cardiovascular Monitoring. New York: Churchill Livingstone; 1998:100–126.
16. Ahrens TS, Taylor LA. Technical considerations in obtaining hemodynamic waveform values. In: Ahrens TS, Taylor LA, eds. Hemodynamic Waveform Analysis. Philadelphia: W.B. Saunders; 1992:209–258.
17. Darovic GO, Zbilut JP. Fluid-filled monitoring systems. In: Darovic GO, ed. Hemodynamic Monitoring: Invasive and Noninvasive Clinical Application, 3rd ed. Philadelphia: Saunders; 2002:113–131.

9

Direct systemic arterial blood pressure monitoring

Edward Cooper and Stacey Cooper

Arterial blood pressure (ABP) measurement is one of the major hemodynamic monitoring tools used in patient assessment because adequate systemic blood pressure is required to perfuse vital organs. Arterial blood pressure, or more specifically mean arterial blood pressure (MAP), is a function of cardiac output (CO) and systemic vascular resistance (SVR). This relationship is represented by the following equation:

$$MAP = CO \times SVR \tag{9.1}$$

While ABP is often measured to assess whether systemic blood pressure is adequate to perfuse vital organs, as Equation 9.1 indicates, a normal blood pressure value does not guarantee adequate blood flow, as MAP is affected by vascular tone. The body's compensatory response to homeostatic insult, largely mediated by the sympathetic nervous system, results in tachycardia and vasoconstriction and serves to sustain blood pressure at all costs. Increasing SVR through vasoconstriction can actually diminish flow to peripheral tissues, even when ABP is maintained. Therefore, just because the blood pressure is normal does not mean blood flow is normal or that tissue perfusion is adequate. Hypotension occurs only when sympathetic compensatory mechanisms have failed after an insult.

Other monitoring techniques, such as serial physical examination, the determination of cardiac output, assessment of blood lactate concentration or central venous hemoglobin saturation, or even direct imaging of the microcirculation, potentially offer greater insight into blood flow and tissue perfusion. However, with the exception of serial physical examination and blood lactate concentration, these techniques are of limited availability and largely impractical for most practitioners. Therefore, despite the limitations of the information provided by its measurement, arterial blood pressure is still used commonly to assess hemodynamic stability in veterinary medicine. As the level of care provided to veterinary patients continues to grow, especially in a critical care setting, the value and availability of direct arterial blood pressure (dABP) monitoring has increased significantly. This chapter explores the practical and technical aspects of dABP measurement in veterinary practice.

Indications for direct arterial pressure monitoring

Blood pressure measurements provide insight into the cardiovascular status of a patient. In patients that are critically ill or have cardiovascular compromise, it is generally accepted that dABP monitoring is more accurate than methods used to obtain blood pressure indirectly (e.g., Doppler or oscillometric monitors).[1-5] Direct ABP measurement is considered to be the "gold standard" for blood pressure monitoring. There are numerous clinical scenarios in which accurate and continuous dABP monitoring would be beneficial (see Table 9.1).[6] The information obtained using dABP measurement can be used to help tailor administration of medications affecting blood pressure (e.g., titration of vasopressors or antihypertensive medications) or to help guide fluid therapy (e.g., resuscitation of hypovolemic shock) on a

Advanced Monitoring and Procedures for Small Animal Emergency and Critical Care, First Edition. Edited by Jamie M. Burkitt Creedon, Harold Davis.
© 2012 John Wiley & Sons, Inc. Published 2012 by John Wiley & Sons, Inc.

Table 9.1 Clinical scenarios benefitting from dABP monitoring[6]

- Patients in shock with hypotension or cardiovascular collapse
- Patients requiring the use of vasopressors
- Titration of medications for afterload reduction in patients with severe congestive heart failure
- Patients receiving pharmacotherapy for severe hypertension
- Patients placed on mechanical ventilation
- Patients with high anesthetic risk

minute-to-minute basis.[6] To further understand why dABP measurement might be chosen over indirect blood pressure measurement methods, it is important to understand the benefits and limitations of each modality.

Advantages and disadvantages of indirect blood pressure monitoring

As indirect arterial blood pressure (iABP) monitoring is covered in depth in Chapter 10, Noninvasive Arterial Blood Pressure Monitoring, here it is only briefly discussed in the context of comparison with dABP monitoring. Indirect methods (such as Doppler ultrasound or oscillometry) are noninvasive to the patient and therefore do not require arterial catheterization or seting up a fluid-filled monitoring system. As such, indirect methods are generally less technically demanding. While there is cost associated with acquiring equipment for iABP monitoring, it is typically much less expensive than the equipment required for dABP measurement (e.g., pressure transducers, special hemodynamic monitors). For these reasons, iABP is measured much more commonly than dAPB in both human and veterinary medicine.

Perhaps the greatest limitation to the use of iABP monitoring is its accuracy. Direct ABP measurement has been shown to be more accurate in both dogs and cats, whether awake or anesthetized.[1 5] This appears to be especially true in hypotensive, hypothermic, and small patients.[7] There are factors such as cuff size, differences in technique, and the possibility of operator error that can further affect the reliability of iABP determination. In addition, iABP measurement provides less information than does dABP measurement. For example, Doppler ultrasound technique only measures systolic blood pressure whereas the direct method measures systolic, diastolic, and mean arterial pressures. While oscillometric machines provide all three pressures, standard oscillometry may be less reliable in cats and small dogs compared with dABP or Doppler ultrasound measurement techniques.[8–9]

Advantages and disadvantages of direct arterial pressure monitoring

The dABP measurement technique offers the benefit of beat-to-beat blood pressure monitoring. This allows clinicians and technicians to monitor trends in both blood pressure and arterial waveform, thus permitting rapid recognition of changes in status and more immediate intervention. Having blood pressure readings continuously available also allows the technician to perform other treatments and monitoring, rather than spending the time necessary to acquire frequent iABP measurements. The "hands-off" nature of dABP monitoring, once it is established, may also diminish the effect that patient handling can have on the arterial blood pressure values obtained. As the stress secondary to handling may iatrogenically elevate blood pressure, dABP could allow for more accurate assessment. In addition to its role in hemodynamic monitoring, placement and maintenance of an arterial catheter also allows for ease of arterial blood sampling to monitor acid–base status and blood-gas parameters, which are typically also of great interest in the critical care patient. For more information on arterial catheterization and sampling, please see Chapter 5, Arterial Puncture and Catheterization.

Though the technique may be more accurate in critically ill patients, dABP monitoring is not without drawbacks, risks, and complications. Obtaining and maintaining arterial access can be technically challenging. Further, the equipment necessary to monitor dABP, especially continuously, can be expensive (pressure transducers, hemodynamic monitors, etc.) compared with the techniques used for indirect determination. While it is considered to be the most accurate method for blood pressure determination, there are numerous factors (both technical and mechanical) that can interfere with blood pressure signal transduction and overall accuracy of the readings, making even this gold standard prone to error. Technical issues that contribute to inaccuracy (overdamping, underdamping, zeroing errors, etc.) are discussed in detail in Chapter 8, Fluid-Filled Hemodynamic Monitoring Systems. Potential complications associated with arterial catheterization include hematoma or bleeding at the catheter insertion site, infection, arterial thrombosis and associated tissue ischemia, and significant hemorrhage if the transducer system becomes disconnected.

Continuous dABP equipment and setup

Once the decision is made to measure dABP, all of the necessary equipment must be available (see Protocols 8.1–8.4).

The first step in establishing dABP monitoring is obtaining arterial access. Arterial catheter placement is discussed in depth in Chapter 5, Arterial Puncture and Catheterization; what follows here is a brief overview. Placement of an arterial catheter can be done percutaneously or by a cutdown method. The most common arteries used for dABP monitoring in small animals are the dorsal pedal and femoral, though coccygeal can also be used. It has been demonstrated in human patients that there is no significant difference in the accuracy of pressures obtained from a peripheral as opposed to a central arterial catheter, especially with regard to MAP.[10] Patient size often plays a role in catheter insertion site as dorsal pedal access can be very challenging in cats and very small dogs. Femoral or coccygeal arteries may be better options in these patients. The catheter site should be clipped and aseptically prepared. Local anesthetics such as 2% lidocaine can be injected locally prior to the procedure to decrease patient discomfort, especially if a cutdown is performed. Special arterial catheters are commercially available; they are generally more rigid, may contain a guide wire to facilitate placement, and are intended for longer-term use. These catheters are more typically used for femoral arterial access. Most commonly an over-the-needle peripheral intravenous (IV) catheter is used. Once the area has been prepared, the artery is palpated and the catheter advanced through the skin toward the pulse. Given the relatively small lumen of arteries compared to veins, it is important that only very small incremental advances are made until there is a flash of blood in the catheter hub. Once this occurs the catheter is advanced off the stylet and into the artery. The catheter is secured with tape and appropriate protective wrap, keeping the insertion site clean and dry. It is further important to label the catheter as "Arterial Line" so that intravenous injections are not inadvertently administered. The site should be inspected daily to ensure there are no signs of bleeding or infection. Warmth of the extremity distal to the insertion site should be assessed regularly to monitor for arterial thrombosis.

Once arterial access has been established, the pressure transducer and monitoring system can be attached to the catheter (see Protocols 8.1–8.4). At one end the pressure transducer is attached via an administration set to a pressurized 500-mL or 1.0-L bag of 0.9% NaCl to which heparin has been added (to achieve a 1–2 U/mL concentration). The pressure bag must be inflated to a pressure greater than the patient's systolic blood pressure or blood will flow back into the line. Typically a pressure between 250 and 300 mm Hg is adequate unless the patient has significant hypertension. Heparinized saline is flushed through the system to prime the tubing,

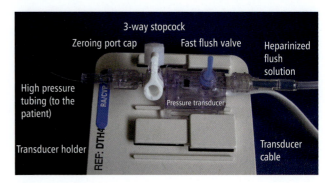

Figure 9.1 Pressure transducer for a fluid-filled hemodynamic monitoring system.

making sure to evacuate any air bubbles. When connected to the pressurized saline bag, the transducer will allow a slow forward flow of fluid through the system to decrease the risk of clot formation and catheter occlusion (check the manufacturer's materials for exact flow rates through a given transducer). Most pressure transducers also have a unidirectional flush valve ("fast flush valve") that can be used to prime the noncompliant tubing (see Fig. 9.1). At the other end of the transducer is rigid, noncompliant ("high-pressure") tubing that will be attached to the arterial catheter (see Fig. 9.1). If your transducer system does not come equipped with noncompliant tubing, you will need to supply your own and use it to complete the circuit. *It is important that standard extension tubing is not used for this purpose, as its compliant nature will result in signal distortion and affect the accuracy of blood pressure readings* (see Abnormal Arterial Pressure Waveforms below). Once the tubing is connected to the patient, the catheter is flushed to verify patency. The use of Luer lock adapters (such as Luer-Lok from Becton, Dickinson and Company, Franklin Lakes, NJ) throughout the system aids in safety and integrity. Finally, the pressure transducer is connected to the hemodynamic monitor via a transducer cable.

Before you can begin monitoring patient blood pressure you must zero the transducer. This sets a reference point (called a zero point) with which the pressure readings from the system are compared. To zero the system, the transducer should be placed at the level of the right atrium (RA) to best approximate central venous pressure. If peripheral pressures are preferred, the transducer should be placed at the level of the catheter. Once the transducer is positioned, the stopcock is closed to the patient and opened to the atmosphere, and the "zero transducer" or similar button on the monitor is engaged. The waveform line should flatten and the screen should read "0/0 (0)." When zeroing is complete the stopcock is closed to the atmosphere and opened to the patient and

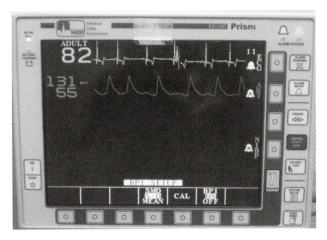

Figure 9.2 Hemodynamic monitor screen capture demonstrating standard output of arterial waveform with systolic and diastolic pressures displayed.

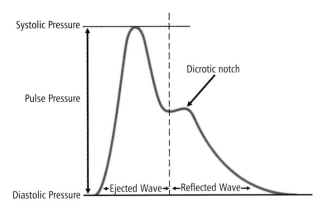

Figure 9.3 Idealized arterial pressure waveform.

the arterial waveform should appear on the screen, providing continuous arterial blood pressure measurements (see Fig. 9.2).

Normal arterial pressure waveforms

The waveform generated by the hemodynamic monitor is a reflection of the pressure changes transmitted along the arterial tree and sensed by the transducer. An idealized schematic of an arterial pressure waveform is depicted in Figure 9.3. The "baseline" of the waveform represents **diastolic arterial pressure** (DAP) and indicates the minimum blood pressure, which is present during ventricular relaxation (diastole). Diastolic arterial pressure is a function of blood viscosity, arterial distensibility, systemic vascular resistance, and the length of the cardiac cycle.[11,12] The initial upstroke in the waveform represents the rapid rise in arterial pressure from DAP to **systolic arterial pressure** (SAP), which occurs with opening of the aortic valve and stroke volume ejection. Systolic arterial pressure represents the peak blood pressure during ventricular contraction (systole), and its determinants are stroke volume, velocity of left ventricular ejection, systemic vascular resistance, arterial distensibility, and left ventricular preload.[12,13] The difference between DAP and SAP is called the **pulse pressure** and is responsible for the intensity of palpated peripheral pulses. As the stroke volume runs off into the arterial tree toward the end of systole, there is a decline in pressure (initial downslope). Once aortic pressure exceeds left ventricular pressure (with left ventricular relaxation), the aortic valve closes. Elastic recoil of the arterial tree in the presence of a closed aortic valve causes a slight rebound (or elevation)

of arterial blood pressure and results in the dicrotic notch, also called the incisura (see Fig. 9.3). This notch causes disruption in the downslope of the waveform as pressures return to diastolic values. The presence of the dicrotic notch is largely a function of arterial elasticity and can be significantly diminished to absent in the face of vasoconstriction.[14]

Although the arterial waveform tends to take on the appearance just described, there are changes that occur as the pressure wave moves from central arterial circulation out to the periphery. This phenomenon is referred to as **distal pulse amplification**. As such there can be slight differences in tracings obtained depending on where the catheter tip is located. In general, the initial upstroke becomes steeper, the systolic pressure increases, the dicrotic notch appears later, and the end-diastolic pressure decreases as the waveform moves from central to peripheral (Fig. 9.4).[15] Despite the higher systolic pressure and wider pulse pressure obtained peripherally, the lower peripheral diastolic pressure results in little net effect on the mean arterial pressure from central to peripheral measurement sites.

In addition to differences in arterial pressure and waveform referable to catheter location, there can also be normal, minor variations in blood pressure seen with spontaneous as opposed to mechanical ventilation. During spontaneous breathing, SAP is slightly lower during inspiration than it is during expiration. During mechanical ventilation the opposite is true: SAP slightly increases during inspiration and decreases during expiration (Fig. 9.5). Arterial pressure changes during the respiratory cycle because alterations in pleural pressure affect thoracic vasculature and cardiac function, which in turn cause changes in stroke volume. During mechanical inspiration, positive pleural pressure results in an increase in left ventricular preload and a decrease in left ventricular afterload. The net effect is an increase in

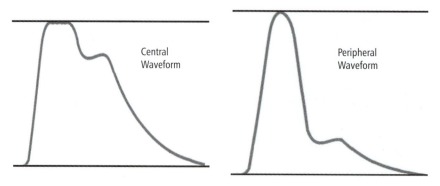

Figure 9.4 Comparison of idealized arterial waveforms from a catheter placed either centrally (left) or peripherally (right).

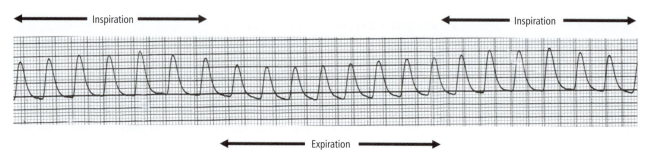

Figure 9.5 Respiratory-associated variation in arterial pressure for a patient undergoing mechanical ventilation.

left ventricular stroke volume and thereby SAP. However, pleural pressure changes also result in decreased stroke volume leading to decreased SAP during passive expiration in the mechanically ventilated patient. Under normal circumstances this pressure variation, which typically does not exceed 5 mm Hg, is not clinically significant.[16] However, as discussed later, there are certain pathological conditions that can lead to exaggeration of this respiratory cycle-related arterial pressure variation, making the variation more important both diagnostically and therapeutically.

Normal arterial blood pressures in dogs have been reported to range from 110 to 190 mm Hg for systolic and from 55 to 110 mm Hg for diastolic pressure, whereas cats have systolic pressures ranging from 120 to 170 mm Hg and diastolic pressures ranging from 70 to 120 mm Hg.[7] Mean arterial blood pressure normally ranges from 80 to 130 mm Hg in both species.

Calculations derived from the arterial pressure waveform

Mean arterial pressure is generally considered superior to systolic pressure as an indicator of true driving pressure for tissue perfusion.[17] In addition, MAP is much less susceptible to variability associated with catheter loca-

tion and transducer signal distortion. As such, determination of MAP is important for assessing clinical status as well as guiding therapeutic decisions. Using dABP measurement, most hemodynamic monitors calculate MAP by averaging the area under the arterial pressure waveform over several beats. It is also possible to approximate MAP through a calculation based solely on SAP and DAP. Based on the premise that approximately two-thirds of the cardiac cycle is spent in diastole, the equation

$$MAP = DAP + (SAP - DAP)/3 \qquad (9.2)$$

provides a good estimate of MAP. However, patients with tachycardia have decreased diastolic filling time, and thus this equation will underestimate MAP. In addition, this equation may overestimate MAP in patients with narrow arterial pulse pressure waveforms, as these waveforms have a smaller area under the curve (and thereby a lower true MAP), regardless of the SAP and DAP.

Calculations of arterial blood pressure variation

As previously stated, there are normally minor variations in systolic blood pressure during both spontane-

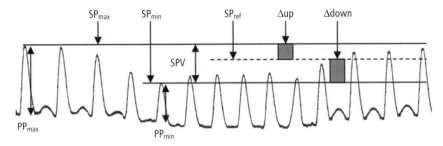

Figure 9.6 Variables used to determine volume responsiveness based on ventilation-associated variation in blood pressure: SPV, systolic pressure variation; SP_{max}, maximum systolic pressure; SP_{min}, minimum systolic pressure; SP_{ref}, reference systolic pressure; PP_{max}, maximum pulse pressure; PP_{min}, minimum pulse pressure.[16]

ous and mechanical ventilation. Hypovolemia magnifies this effect because, during hypovolemia, the heart and the thin-walled intrathoracic vessels (such as the vena cava and pulmonary veins) are more collapsible. Under such circumstances, the changes in pleural pressure that occur during the respiratory cycle can have more significant hemodynamic impact and thus result in greater pressure variation. This fact has led to the notion that respiratory cycle-associated arterial pressure variation could be used as an indicator of volume responsiveness for patients undergoing positive-pressure ventilation. Spontaneously breathing patients generally have wide variation in tidal volume, and thereby variable changes in intrathoracic pressures, which unfortunately makes respiratory effects on arterial pressure less consistent and interpretation very challenging. Systolic pressure variation (SPV), Δup/Δdown, and pulse pressure variation (PPV), all markers of respiratory cycle-associated arterial pressure variation, have been explored as indicators of volume responsiveness for patients undergoing positive-pressure ventilation and are discussed here briefly:

- *Systolic pressure variation*—Systolic pressure variation, very simply, is the difference between the maximum systolic pressure (SP_{max}) present during inspiration and the minimum systolic pressure (SP_{min}) present during expiration:

$$SPV = SP_{max} - SP_{min} \tag{9.3}$$

An SPV greater than 10 mm Hg has been shown to correlate fairly well to hypovolemia in human patients.[18] In addition, in people, SPV has been shown to correlate with pulmonary capillary wedge pressure and left ventricular end-diastolic area, both correlates of intravascular volume status.[19,20]

- *Δup and Δdown*—As an extension of SPV, some investigators have evaluated the utility of Δup and Δdown

as indicators of intravascular volume status and a patient's potential for fluid responsiveness (see Fig. 9.6). To use Δup and Δdown, one must first determine a reference systolic pressure (SP_{ref}) by measuring SAP during an end-expiratory pause. Δup is then the difference between SP_{max} and SP_{ref} and more specifically reflects the positive-pressure-inspiratory increase in SAP. Conversely, Δdown is the difference between SP_{ref} and SP_{min} and reflects the expiratory decrease in SAP:

$$\Delta up = SP_{max} - SP_{ref} \tag{9.4}$$

$$\Delta down = SP_{ref} - SP_{min} \tag{9.5}$$

Since it is thought that the expiratory decrease in systolic pressure contributes the majority of the SPV seen with hypovolemia, it stands to reason that Δdown might be a more useful calculation than SPV. However, Δdown has not been shown to offer any better correlation to hypovolemia or volume responsiveness when compared with SPV in human patients with sepsis-induced hypotension.[21]

- *Pulse pressure variation*—Pulse pressure variation (PPV) offers yet another way to quantify respiratory variation in arterial pressures associated with ventilation (see Fig. 9.6). Pulse pressure variation is obtained by dividing the difference between the maximum and minimum pulse pressures (PP_{max} and PP_{min}) over a single breath by the mean of the two values.[22] The PPV, expressed as a percentage, is given by the following equation:

$$PPV(\%) = 100 \times (PP_{max} - PP_{min})/[(PP_{max} + PP_{min})/2] \tag{9.6}$$

Compared with SPV, Δup, and Δdown, *PPV appears to have the strongest correlation to hypovolemia and volume responsiveness*, with higher PPVs correlating to greater degrees of volume responsiveness.[23,24]

There are several limitations to using these techniques. Perhaps the most significant is that, as previously mentioned, arterial blood pressure variation equations can only be used in patients undergoing positive-pressure ventilation. This limits the application to patients needing ventilatory support for hypoxemia, hypoventilation, or during anesthesia. In addition, factors such as technical issues, the presence of arrhythmias, effects of chest wall and lung compliance, or right or left ventricular failure could all interfere with the accuracy and utility of these values in determining volume responsiveness.[16]

Other uses for the arterial pressure waveform

In addition to use in assessment of volume status, arterial waveforms have also been used to determine cardiac output through pulse contour analysis. Pulse contour analysis provides beat-to-beat cardiac output values based on computation of the area under the systolic portion of the arterial pressure curve after calibration with a known cardiac output (typically determined by either lithium dilution or thermodilution). Cardiac output determination from the arterial pressure waveform requires additional equipment and software. Available systems include PulseCO (LiDCO Ltd, London, UK), PiCCO (Pulsion Medical Systems, Munich, Germany), and Flotrac (Edwards Lifesciences, Irvine, CA), all of which have been validated in a variety clinical scenarios in humans.[25–29] While potentially useful in clinical veterinary medicine, cardiac output determination by pulse contour analysis has been shown to have poor correlation compared with lithium dilution in patients with anesthesia or hypovolemia-induced hypotension, and frequent recalibration is required.[30,31]

Abnormal arterial pressure waveforms

Recognition of abnormal pressure waveforms is an essential component of utilizing dABP (see Protocol 9.1). Alterations in waveform morphology could reflect true changes in clinical condition, thereby warranting intervention for the patient. On the other hand, they could indicate a technical or mechanical issue that would require troubleshooting the system rather than the patient.

Technical problems that cause abnormal arterial pressure waveforms

One of the major technical issues that can arise with use of a dABP transducer system is pressure waveform overdamping or underdamping. Damping is the inherent

---

Protocol 9.1 Suggested step-by-step approach for assessing direct arterial blood pressure (dABP)

Procedure

1. Determination of arterial blood pressure:
   a. What is the reported systolic pressure?
   b. What is the reported diastolic pressure?
   c. What is the reported or calculated mean pressure?
   d. What is the calculated pulse pressure?
   e. Do these values reflect hypotension or hypertension?
   f. Do these values match the patient's clinical condition?
   g. Do these values coincide with palpated pulse quality?
   h. Is there significant ventilation-associated variation?
2. Assessment of pulse rate and rhythm:
   a. What is the pulse rate reported by the monitor?
   b. Does this value reflect bradycardia or tachycardia?
   c. Does the rate match the auscultated and ECG heart rate?
   d. Is the pulse rhythm regular or irregular? Does it match changes in the ECG (i.e., is there a pulse waveform for each QRS complex)?
3. Assessment of waveform morphology:
   a. Has the waveform morphology changed significantly?
   b. Is the morphology consistent from beat to beat?
   c. Is a dicrotic notch present?
   d. Has the waveform become muted (significant decrease in pulse pressure)?

---

tendency for the system itself to alter the pressure signal as it is transmitted from the patient to the transducer. Underdamping occurs when the resonant frequency of the monitoring system too closely matches the frequency of the pressure waveform. The result is a summation or resonance of the two frequencies, amplification of the signal, overestimation of SAP, and underestimation of DAP. *All dABP monitoring systems have some inherent underdamping effects and, as such, tend to report falsely high SAPs and falsely low DAPs.* The degree of inaccuracy can be minor or significant. The MAP reported is generally considered accurate. Normal arterial pressure waveforms have no "pointy" or jagged parts—waveforms with points or sharp peaks are therefore likely underdamped. The length of tubing connecting the arterial catheter to the transducer can contribute to underdamping in a direct relationship—increased length of tubing proportionally worsens underdamping.

Overdamping, on the other hand, results in attenuation or muting of the arterial pressure waveform, leading

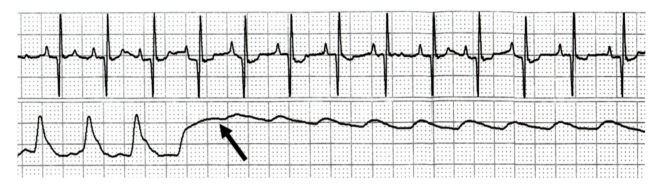

Figure 9.7 Arterial waveform from a patient with sudden and marked overdamping of the pressure signal (arrow) associated with catheter occlusion. Note the sudden loss of waveform morphology, slight decrease in systolic pressure, increase in diastolic pressure, and loss of dicrotic notch, all without any change in heart rate.

to falsely low SAP and falsely elevated DAP. The net effect is a significant reduction in the pulse pressure though the MAP generally remains relatively accurate. Overdamped waveforms are very smooth with loss of many of their defining characteristics, such as the systolic upstroke and dicrotic notch (see Fig. 9.7). Potential causes of overdamping include air bubbles in the line, line occlusion from kinking or clotting, or use of overly compliant tubing. More detail concerning system damping and technical issues of fluid-filled monitoring systems can be found in Chapter 8, Fluid-Filled Hemodynamic Monitoring Systems.

Patient problems that cause abnormal arterial pressure waveforms

Alterations in arterial waveforms can also manifest as a result of significant changes in patient hemodynamics. For example, various arrhythmias can have a significant impact on cardiac output and blood pressure, and can result in diminished to completely absent arterial waveforms despite the presence of electrical activity (see Fig. 9.8).

Significant hypotension secondary to low cardiac output (as from hypovolemic or cardiogenic shock) can result in markedly muted waveforms secondary to small stroke volumes combined with peripheral vasoconstriction. As such, pressure waveforms from patients with hypotension can be difficult to distinguish from those caused by overdamped systems. Clearly, recognizing the difference is essential to taking appropriate action if the patient is truly hypotensive. The patient's clinical status (mental responsiveness, heart rate, manual palpation of pulses) as well as the MAP (remembering that MAP is typically preserved with overdamping and will be low with hypotension) can be helpful in distinguishing between the two. Alternately, a fast flush test (described

in Chapter 8, Fluid-Filled Hemodynamic Monitoring Systems) can be performed to assess the system for damping.

Another manifestation of respiratory arterial pressure variation can occur in the form of pulsus paradoxicus, most commonly associated with pericardial effusion that has resulted in cardiac tamponade. Similar to hypovolemia, the effective decrease in venous return from increased pericardial pressure results in an exaggeration of the difference between the SAP during inspiration and the SAP during expiration. Provided the patient is breathing spontaneously, SAP will be higher on expiration and lower on inspiration (see Fig. 9.9a).

Finally, there are certain clinical scenarios whereby a patient has waveforms with increased pulse pressure ("tall") but are of fairly short duration ("narrow") (see Fig. 9.9b). This morphology is typically caused by an increased SAP and a very rapid falloff to DAP, the latter occurring either because of decreased blood viscosity or backward flow of blood. Potential causes of "tall and narrow" waveforms, also referred to as water hammer or Corrigan's pulses, include aortic regurgitation, patent ductus arteriosus, hypertension, and hemodilutional anemia.[32]

Thresholds of concern for arterial pressure value and waveform abnormalities

Significant changes in blood pressure or waveform morphology should prompt assessment of clinical condition and intervention as indicated (see Table 9.2). Onset or worsening of hypotension, generally defined as SAP less than 80 mm Hg or MAP less than 60 mm Hg, should be addressed as soon as possible to limit tissue ischemia and potential for cardiac arrest.[7] Along similar lines, marked hypertension, generally defined as SAP greater

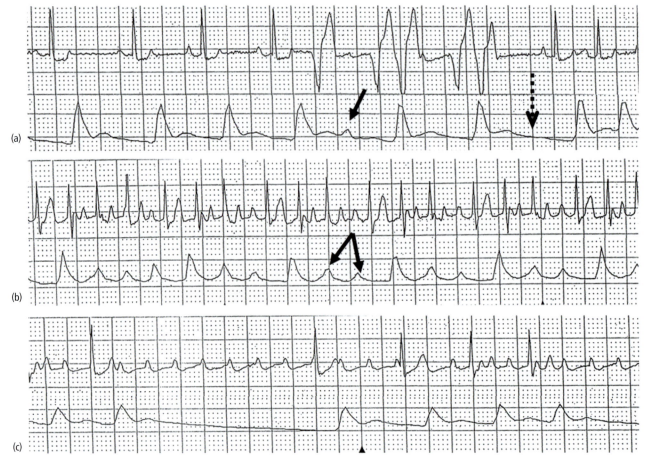

Figure 9.8 Examples of arrhythmia-associated changes in arterial waveform morphology. (A) Ventricular premature contractions associated with diminished (solid arrow) to absent (dashed arrow) pressure tracings. (B) Marked tachycardia (heart rate 210 beats per minute) resulting in progressively diminished waveforms and blood pressure (arrows). (C) Atrial flutter with prolonged periods of absent ventricular contraction resulting in absent arterial waveforms.

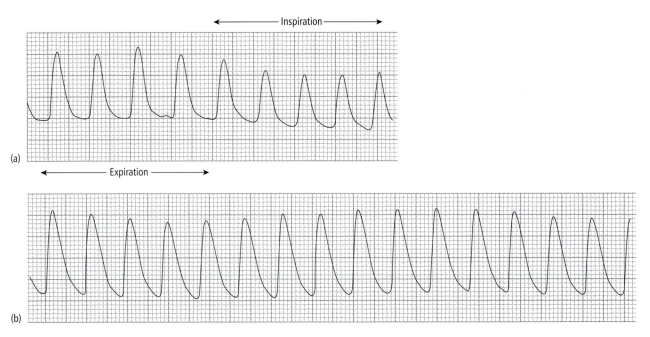

Figure 9.9 (a) Arterial waveforms from a patient with pulsus paradoxicus demonstrating respiratory-associated arterial pressure variation. (b) Arterial waveforms from a patient with hemodilutional anemia demonstrating "tall and narrow" morphology.

Table 9.2 Guidelines indicating need for clinician intervention based on dABP monitoring

- Hypotension[7]
  - SAP < 80 mm Hg
  - MAP < 60 mm Hg
- Hypertension[33]
  - SAP > 180–200 mm Hg
  - MAP > 140 mm Hg
- Arrhythmias[35]
  - Tachyarrhythmias
    - HR > 180–200 (dog)
    - HR > 240 (cat)
  - Bradyarrhythmias
    - HR < 60 (dog)
    - HR < 80–100 (cat)

than 180–200 mm Hg or MAP greater than 140 mm Hg, could cause significant end-organ injury and would require intervention.[33] The presence of ventilatory variation in systolic pressure greater then 10 mm Hg might suggest hypovolemia (prompting more aggressive fluid resuscitation) or pericardial effusion (prompting pericardiocentesis).[34] Arrhythmias that result in a sustained impact on blood pressure or even intermittent hypotension would need to be addressed with antiarrhythmic medications or a pacemaker. This could include tachycardia with heart rate greater than 180–200 beats per minute (bpm) in dogs or 240 bpm in cats, or bradycardia with heart rate less than 60 bpm in dogs and 80–100 bpm in cats.[35]

Troubleshooting abnormal waveforms

One of the primary objectives in troubleshooting abnormal waveforms is to determine whether changes in blood pressure or waveform morphology indicated by dABP monitoring are truly reflective of hemodynamic changes in the patient or if they are a function of technical or mechanical issues. These issues arise most commonly with the apparent presence of significant hypotension (and muting of the arterial waveform) or hypertension (and exaggeration of the waveform). Several steps can be followed to systematically work through the potential causes for these changes (see Protocol 9.2). When an abnormal waveform is detected, the first step is to determine if there are concurrent changes in the patient's clinical status such as alteration in responsiveness, heart rate, or palpable pulse quality that might require immediate intervention. In addition, if not already being continuously monitored, an ECG should be obtained to determine if an arrhythmia is

present. If there are not any readily discernable changes in clinical condition or ECG, the transducer setup should be assessed to make sure that the noncompliant tubing is not kinked and that there are no air bubbles present in the fluid column. It is also important to ensure the pressure bag is still inflated to at least 250 mm Hg. If there has been significant change in patient position, it may be beneficial to relevel and rezero the transducer. To assess patency of the arterial catheter, the catheter should be aspirated to ensure arterial blood is obtained; any air bubbles or clots should be removed. If the catheter does not readily aspirate, the system can be gently, manually flushed to assess patency and to evacuate any air bubbles or clots. A fast or forceful flush of an arterial catheter that does not readily aspirate carries the risk of introducing air or small thrombi into distal arterial circulation. If the system does not flush or aspirate readily, the arterial catheter should be closely inspected to confirm its position and functionality. If the catheter appears to be at least partially patent then a "fast flush test" (described in detail in Chapter 8, Fluid-Filled

Protocol 9.2 Troubleshooting abnormal arterial pressure waveforms

Procedure
- Assess patient for changes in clinical status to explain change in morphology:
  - Assess mentation, heart rate, pulse quality, mucous membrane color, capillary refill time, and extremity temperature.
  - Assess ECG for changes in rate and rhythm coinciding with changes in waveform.
- If patient parameters have not changed:
  - Assess transducer setup and make sure:
    - Noncompliant tubing is used between patient and transducer.
    - Noncompliant tubing is not kinked.
    - There are no air bubbles in the fluid column.
    - Pressure bag is inflated to at least 250 mm Hg.
  - Relevel transducer to level of the patient's heart base and rezero the transducer, if patient position has changed significantly.
  - Assess patency of arterial catheter:
    - Aspirate arterial catheter.
      - Ensure arterial blood is easily obtained.
      - Remove air bubbles and clots from line.
    - Flush arterial catheter.
      - Ensure catheter flushes easily—do not force.
      - Evacuate air bubbles or small clots from system.
- Perform "fast flush test" to assess for system overdamping or underdamping.

Hemodynamic Monitoring Systems) can be performed to assess for the presence of overdamping or underdamping. If underdamping is present, it may be necessary to use shorter noncompliant tubing between the pressure transducer and the arterial catheter. If overdamping is present and does not resolve with flushing, it may be necessary to confirm the presence of noncompliant rather than standard extension tubing between the catheter and the transducer, and to assess all system connections and the arterial catheter itself.

Conclusions

Despite the potential limitations and technical difficulties associated with its use, dABP monitoring offers valuable information regarding hemodynamic status. If equipment is available and a level of familiarity is obtained, dABP measurement could be used in any 24-hour veterinary hospital and is especially useful if critically ill patients are routinely seen.

References

1. Sawyer DC, Brown M, Striler EL, et al. Comparison of direct and indirect blood pressure measurement in anesthetized dogs. Lab Anim Sci. 1991;41:134–138.
2. Bodey AR, Michell AR, Bovee KC, et al. Comparison of direct and indirect (oscillometric) measurements of arterial blood pressure in conscious dogs. Res Vet Sci. 1996;61:17–21.
3. Meurs KM, Miller MW, Slater MR. Comparison of indirect oscillometric and direct arterial methods for blood pressure measurements in anesthetized dogs. J Am Anim Hosp Assoc. 1996;32:471–475.
4. Caulkett NA, Cantwell SL, Houston DM. A comparison of indirect blood pressure monitoring techniques in the anesthetized cat. Vet Anesth. 1998;27:370–377.
5. Stepien RL, Rapoport GS. Clinical comparison of three methods to measure blood pressure in nonsedated dogs. J Am Vet Med Assoc. 1999;215:1623–1628.
6. Lodato RF. Arterial pressure monitoring. In: Tobin MJ, ed. Principles and Practice of Intensive Care Monitoring, New York: McGraw-Hill, 1998.
7. Wadell LS. Direct blood pressure monitoring. Clin Tech Small Anim Pract. 2000;15(3):111–118.
8. Haberman CE, Morgam JD, Kang CW, et al. Evaluation of Doppler ultrasonic and oscillometric methods of indirect blood pressure measurement in cats. Intern J Res Vet Med. 2004;2(4):279–289.
9. Bodey AR, Young LE, Bartram DH, et al. A comparison of direct and indirect (oscillometric) measurements of arterial blood pressure in anaesthetized dogs, using tail and limb cuffs. Res Vet Sci. 1994;57:265–269.
10. Mignini MA, Piacentini E, Dubin A. Peripheral arterial blood pressure monitoring adequately tracks central arterial blood pressure in critically ill patient: an observational study. Critical Care. 2006;10:R43.
11. O'Rouke MF. What is blood pressure? Am J Hypertens. 1990;3:803–810.
12. Bridges EJ. The systemic circulation. In: Woods L, Motzer S, Sivarajan-Froelicher ES, eds. Cardiac Nursing. 4th ed. Philadelphia: LB Lippincott; 1999:51–71.
13. Nutter D. Measurement of the systolic blood pressure. In: Hurst J, ed. The Heart, Arteries, and Veins. 5th ed. New York: McGraw-Hill; 1982:182–187.
14. Dawber TR, Thomas HE Jr, McNamara PM. Characteristics of the dicrotic notch of the arterial pulse wave in coronary heart disease. Angiology. 1973;24(4):244–255.
15. Mark JB, Slaughter TF. Cardiovascular monitoring. In: Miller R, ed. Miller's Anesthesia. 6th ed, Philadelphia: Elsevier, 2005.
16. Michard F. Changes in arterial pressure during mechanical ventilation. Anesthesiology. 2005;103:419–428.
17. Marino PL. Arterial blood pressure. In: Marino P, ed. The ICU Book. 3rd ed. Philadelphia: Lippincott, Williams and Wilkins; 2006:143–153.
18. Rick JJ, Burke SS. Respirator paradox. South Med J. 1978;71:1376–1378.
19. Marik PE. The systolic blood pressure variation as an indicator of pulmonary capillary wedge pressure in ventilated patients. Anaesth Intensive Care. 1993;21:405–408.
20. Coriat P, Vrillon M, Perel A, et al. A comparison of systolic blood pressure variations and echocardiographic estimates of end-diastolic left ventricular size in patients after aortic surgery. Anesth Analg. 1994;78:46–53.
21. Tavernier B, Makhotine O, Lebuffe G, et al. Systolic pressure variation as a guide to fluid therapy in patients with sepsis-induced hypotension. Anesthesiology. 1998;89:1313–1321.
22. Michard F, Chemla D, Richard C, et al. Clinical use of respiratory changes in arterial pulse pressure to monitor the hemodynamic effects of PEEP. Am J Respir Crit Care Med. 1999;159:935–939.
23. Michard F, Boussat S, Chemla D, et al. Relation between respiratory changes in arterial pulse pressure and fluid responsiveness in septic patients with chronic circulatory failure. Am J Respir Crit Care Med. 2000;162:134–138.
24. Bendjelid K, Suter PM, Romand JA. The respiratory change in preejection period: a new method to predict fluid responsiveness. J Appl Physiol. 2004;96:337–342.
25. Hamilton TT, Huber LM, Jessen ME. PulseCo: a less-invasive method to monitor cardiac output from arterial pressure after cardiac surgery. Ann Thorac Surg. 2002;74(4):S1408–S1412.
26. Pitmann J, Bar-Yosef S, SumPing J, et al. Continuous cardiac output monitoring with pulse contour analysis: a comparison with lithium indicator dilution cardiac output monitoring. Crit Care Med. 2005;33(9):2015–2021.
27. Godje O, Hoke K, Goetz AE, et al. Reliability of a new algorithm for continuous cardiac output determination by pulse-contour analysis during hemodynamic instability. Crit Care Med. 2002;30(1):52–58.
28. Schuerholz T, Meyer MC, Friedrick L, et al: Reliability of continuous cardiac output determination by pulse-contour analysis in porcine septic shock. Acta Anaesthesiol Scand. 2006;50:407–413.
29. Button D, Weibel L, Reuthebuch O, et al. Clinical evaluation of the FloTrac/Vigileo system and two established continuous cardiac output monitoring devices in patients undergoing cardiac surgery. Br J Anaesth. 2007;99(3):329–336.
30. Cooper ES, Muir WW. Continuous cardiac output monitoring via arterial pressure waveform analysis following severe hemorrhagic shock in dogs. Crit Care Med. 2007;35(7):1724–1729.
31. Chen HC, Sinclair MD, Dyson DH, et al. Comparison of arterial pressure waveform analysis with the lithium dilution technique

to monitor cardiac output in anesthetized dogs. Am J Vet Res. 2005;66(8):1430–1436.

32. Vakil RJ, Golwalla AF, Golwalla SA. The cardiovascular system. In: Vakil RJ, Golwalla AF, Golwalla SA, eds. Physical diagnosis: a textbook of symptoms and physical signs. 9th ed. Mumbai, India: Media Promoters and Publishers Private Limited; 2001:277–341.

33. Brown S. Hypertensive Crisis. In: Silverstein D, Hopper K, eds. Small Animal Critical Care Medicine. St. Louis, MO: Saunders (Elsevier); 2009.

34. McGhee BH, Bridges ME. Monitoring arterial blood pressure: what you may not know. Crit Care Nurse. 2002;22(2):60–4, 66–70, 73.

35. Hackett TB. Physical examination. In: Silverstein D, Hopper K, eds. Small Animal Critical Care Medicine. St. Louis, MO: Saunders (Elsevier); 2009.

10

Noninvasive arterial blood pressure monitoring

Jill A. Williamson and Stephanie Leone

Blood pressure is the force that the flow of blood exerts on the wall of the blood vessels.[1] Blood pressure can be broken down into three components: the systolic arterial pressure (SAP), the diastolic arterial pressure (DAP), and the mean arterial pressure (MAP). The SAP and DAP correlate to respective phases of the cardiac cycle; MAP is the average of the arterial pressure measured millisecond by millisecond over a period of time. It is not equal to the average of SAP and DAP because more of the cardiac cycle is spent in diastole.[2] The following equation provides an estimate of MAP and demonstrates this principle:

$$MAP = [(SAP - DAP)/3] + DAP \qquad (10.1)$$

Systemic mean arterial blood pressure (MAP) is the product of systemic cardiac output (CO) and systemic vascular resistance (SVR). Cardiac output is blood flow provided by the heart and is the product of stroke volume (SV; the volume of blood ejected with each heartbeat) and heart rate (HR)[3]:

$$MAP = CO \times SVR \qquad (10.2)$$

$$CO = SV \times HR \qquad (10.3)$$

Systemic vascular resistance is affected by both vascular tone and blood viscosity. While increased SVR leads to increased blood pressure, this increased resistance decreases blood flow, as described by this modification of Ohm's law:

$$Q = \Delta P/R \qquad (10.4)$$

In this equation, Q is blood flow, ΔP is the driving pressure of blood from one point in the circulation to another, and R is resistance. The equation can be altered specifically for MAP as relates to CO and SVR:

$$CO = (MAP - RAP)/SVR \qquad (10.5)$$

where RAP is right atrial pressure. This concept underscores the notion that elevations in blood pressure do not guarantee improvements in blood flow.

When monitoring blood pressure, it is important to remember the determinants of MAP since therapy should target the aberrant underlying component, whether that be cardiac output, systemic vascular resistance, or both. For example, if a septic patient is hypotensive, one may need to address both cardiac output (due to hypovolemia or poor cardiac contractility) and systemic vascular resistance (due to systemic vasodilation).

Indirect blood pressure monitoring: background

Comparing direct and indirect blood pressure monitoring

Blood pressure monitoring in small animals has become a crucial part of clinical practice. The evolution of noninvasive blood pressure (NIBP) monitoring has led to easier monitoring and management of both hypertensive and hypotensive states. Invasive, direct blood pressure (dABP) monitoring is considered the gold standard in both veterinary and human medicine.[4–7] Direct blood pressure monitoring involves intra-arterial catheterization, a pressure transducer, and a monitor allowing continuous reporting of SAP, DAP, and MAP. While it is considered the most accurate method, dABP

Advanced Monitoring and Procedures for Small Animal Emergency and Critical Care, First Edition. Edited by Jamie M. Burkitt Creedon, Harold Davis.

© 2012 John Wiley & Sons, Inc. Published 2012 by John Wiley & Sons, Inc.

monitoring is considered invasive[4,8] and has several other drawbacks, including that it is relatively technically demanding (especially in small patients), catheterization can be painful, the catheter system increases the patient's risk of sepsis, system problems such as catheter occlusion prevent measurement, and more equipment and expertise are required than for NIBP measurement.[4] Another potential drawback of dABP monitoring is increased cost to the client, as the required equipment and advanced training of technical staff are more extensive and expensive than for NIBP measurement. Advantages of dABP monitoring include the following: it is continuous and has an optional auditory signal with each pulse for closer, moment-to-moment monitoring of the most critically ill patients; after initial setup, no patient intervention is performed to obtain a pressure reading; the dABP monitors display arterial pressure waveforms that can be helpful in monitoring and diagnosis; and it is generally considered more accurate than indirect methods.

Noninvasive blood pressure monitoring techniques depend on detection of flow that passes beneath an occluding cuff, though the sensor differs between methods. In general all NIBP techniques offer the advantages over direct techniques of being quicker, noninvasive, easier to perform, and requiring relatively minimal technical expertise.[9] The primary disadvantages of NIBP monitoring are that it has relatively poor accuracy during peripheral vasoconstriction (i.e., hypovolemia, shock), it is less accurate at extremely high and low pressures compared with dABP methods, and it is not truly continuous. Also, the Doppler method requires that an operator be physically involved during each measurement. However, given the technical requirements and costs associated with dABP monitoring, it has become commonplace to use NIBP methods to obtain blood pressure measurements.

Validation of NIBP

The ease and widespread availability of NIBP monitoring has made this method the most common for obtaining blood pressure measurements in veterinary medicine. Therefore, it is important to know the accuracy of NIBP monitoring devices compared with the dABP method. Given that direct blood pressure measurement is considered the gold standard, NIBP devices have been evaluated for accuracy primarily by comparing dABP and NIBP measurements in both human and veterinary patients.[10–12] The Association for the Advancement of Medical Instrumentation (AAMI) has developed guidelines for validation of NIBP measuring devices in people, which involve comparison of NIBP measurements versus dABP measurements.[13,14] Few indirect blood pressure measuring devices have met these criteria in people, and to date, no indirect blood pressure measuring devices have been validated by these criteria in conscious dogs or cats.[10,15]

Discrepancies between direct and indirect arterial blood pressure measurements can be attributed largely to the fact that the dABP technique measures blood pressure directly, whereas most indirect techniques measure some variable related to blood *flow*.[6,15,16] Noninvasive blood pressure measurement techniques estimate blood pressure by detecting return of blood flow by Doppler ultrasonic technology or by sensing arterial wall motion beneath or distal to an occlusive cuff as that cuff is slowly released. Indirect methods are somewhat limited by the fact that they require a large superficial artery on a distal extremity that can be occluded by a pressure cuff. The limited presence of these vessels, the variability in size and shape of the limbs, and the potential inaccessibility of these arteries due to trauma or peripheral venous catheters can all make it difficult to obtain reliable NIBP readings.[4]

Comparison with the dABP measurement method should not be the only way in which NIBP measurement devices are judged.[7,10,15] Inherent limitations such as patient noncompliance, significant differences in patient sizes and conformations, and lack of protocol standardization make NIBP measurements in dogs more difficult to obtain than in humans.[7] Thus, validation of veterinary devices should likely take into consideration these inherent difficulties in our unique clinical setting. In 2007, a panel of experts on systemic hypertension in the American College of Veterinary Internal Medicine (ACVIM) made recommendations for the validation of NIBP methods in veterinary patients.[15] These recommendations are based on the AAMI guidelines for humans and state that the tested NIBP monitoring device should be compared against a dABP measurement device or another NIBP measuring device for which validation has been published in a refereed journal; that a device is validated for only the species and condition in which the validation test was conducted; and that a device may be validated for systolic, diastolic, or both types of measurements. The ACVIM panel states that the investigational criteria and recommendations of the AAMI should be followed; criteria for validation of system efficacy are detailed and strict.[15] Although there are no validated NIBP measuring devices for use in veterinary patients, NIBP monitoring is nevertheless more commonly used than direct monitoring in clinical practice.[15,17–19] The ACVIM consensus statement advocates the use of receiver–operator curve characteristics to evaluate NIBP measurement method efficacy in dogs and cats until such methods are properly validated.[15,19]

Indications for noninvasive blood pressure monitoring

There are many indications for monitoring blood pressure in dogs and cats. Blood pressure should be measured in patients with known hypotension or hypertension, in patients with diseases or conditions that may lead to hypotension or hypertension, and in many undergoing anesthesia. Table 10.1 gives arterial blood pressure values that are considered normal for dogs and cats.

Hypotension, or low arterial blood pressure, is not a primary disease but is rather a clinical manifestation of another problem. There are multiple diseases that can lead to hypotension by various mechanisms. Potential conditions or disease processes include all types of shock (cardiogenic, distributive, hypovolemic, septic), trauma, anaphylaxis, and gastric dilatation–volvulus.[20] Anesthesia is a common cause of hypotension. Many injectable and all inhalant anesthetic agents can cause depression of cardiac output and peripheral vasodilation, either of which can result in hypotension.[20,21] The American College of Veterinary Anesthesiologists recommends blood pressure monitoring during anesthesia for all patients with moderate to severe systemic disease.[22] NIBP allows monitoring of trends and allows for appropriate therapeutic intervention.

Hypertension is a sustained increase in systemic blood pressure.[15] Systemic arterial hypertension is becoming more commonly recognized as a complication of several disease processes (see the end of this section). This increased index of suspicion for hypertension has made screening and monitoring with NIBP measurement devices invaluable in clinical practice. There are two clear indications for measuring blood pressure: evidence of end-organ damage consistent with a hypertensive episode and the presence of a disease or condition that is known to cause hypertension.[15] The four major organs affected by hypertension are the kidneys, eyes, brain, and heart. Sustained or acute rises in blood pressure can have detrimental effects on these organ systems. See Table 10.2 for specific clinical signs of end-organ damage.

Systemic arterial hypertension can be either primary (idiopathic) or secondary to another disease. Secondary

Table 10.1 Arterial blood pressure values commonly considered normal in dogs and cats[1]

	Dogs	Cats
Systolic arterial pressure	90–140 mm Hg	80–140 mm Hg
Diastolic arterial pressure	50–80 mm Hg	55–75 mm Hg
Mean arterial pressure	60–100 mm Hg	60–100 mm Hg

Table 10.2 Common end-organ damage secondary to hypertension

Organ or System	Effect of Hypertension	Effects More Likely	Comments
Kidneys	Enhanced rate of decline of renal function Nephron loss Enhancement of proteinuria or microalbuminuria	SAP>160 mm Hg	Renal disease may be a cause or an effect of hypertension.[15,23–25]
Eyes	Exudative retinal detachment Retinal or vitreal hemorrhage, hyphema Retinal vessel tortuosity or perivascular edema Secondary glaucoma Retinal degeneration	SAP>180 mm Hg	"hypertensive choroidopathy" or "hypertensive retinopathy"[15,26]
Brain	Disruption of blood flow due to failure of autoregulation Fibrinoid arteriolar necrosis Thrombosis with subsequent hypoxic damage Cerebral swelling or edema	SAP>180 mm Hg acutely	Clinical signs result from ischemic stroke and/or hemorrhage damage.[15,24]
Heart	Concentric LV hypertrophy, leading to increased wall stress and promoting ischemia Secondary murmur or gallop rhythms	Unknown	In cats cardiac changes may resolve with successful antihypertensive therapy.[15,26]

SAP, systemic arterial blood pressure; LV, left ventricular.

hypertension can also occur in response to therapeutic agents that are known to cause hypertension, such as erythropoietin, phenylpropanolamine, glucocorticoids, or nonsteroidal anti-inflammatory agents, among others.[15] Both dogs and cats are affected by certain diseases and conditions known to cause hypertension. In dogs, diseases commonly associated with hypertension include acute or chronic renal disease, hyperadrenocorticism, diabetes mellitus, obesity, hyperaldosteronism, pheochromocytoma, and hypothyroidism. In cats, chronic renal disease, diabetes mellitus, hyperthyroidism, and obesity are the common diseases and conditions associated with hypertension.[15] A clinician is likely to order blood pressure measurements in dogs and cats with these conditions, to screen and monitor them for hypertension.

Noninvasive blood pressure monitoring methods

There are several different ways to noninvasively monitor blood pressure, including Doppler ultrasound, oscillometric sphygmomanometry, photoplethysmography, and even crudely by physical examination.

Physical examination

Known as the "poor man's blood pressure monitor" pulse quality assessment during the physical examination may allow rough approximation of a patient's blood pressure. Palpation of dorsal pedal pulses generally correlates with SAP>90 mm Hg, while palpation of a femoral arterial pulse in the absence of a palpable dorsal pedal pulse roughly correlates with a SAP between 60 and 90 mm Hg. The inability to palpate a femoral pulse may indicate a SAP<60 mm Hg (see Table 10.3). These findings are based on the author's experience and are not meant to replace actual blood pressure monitoring of acutely or critically ill patients, but rather to serve as

Table 10.3 Physical examination findings

Estimated Systolic Blood Pressure	Physical Exam Findings
SAP > 60 mm Hg	Unable to palpate a femoral pulse
60 mm Hg > SAP > 90 mm Hg	Palpable femoral pulse, but no palpable dorsal pedal pulse
SAP > 90 mm Hg	Palpable dorsal pedal pulses

SAP, systemic arterial blood pressure.

guidelines for quick patient assessment. Pulse pressure is the difference between SAP and DAP:

$$Pulse\ pressure = SAP - DAP \qquad (10.6)$$

When blood pressure is normal, the difference between SAP and DAP tends to be greater than the difference between SAP and DAP at low blood pressures. Hence, patients with small pulse pressures may be more likely to have low blood pressure whereas those with normal pulse pressure may be more likely to have normal blood pressure. It is important to note that *no correlation* can be estimated regarding pulse pressures and hypertension.

Doppler ultrasound

Principles

Doppler ultrasonic blood pressure monitoring is one of the most common NIBP measurement methods. In this technique, a Doppler probe containing two piezoelectric crystals is placed against the skin overlying a peripheral artery, distal to a pressure cuff applied circumferentially to the animal's limb (see below). The Doppler probe emits ultrasonic waves into the tissue that are reflected back to the probe. The difference between the emitted and returning signals' frequencies, called the frequency shift, is detected at the transducer and converted to an audible signal emitted from the Doppler unit.[10,27] The SAP (only) is read from a sphygmomanometer connected to a pressure cuff placed proximal to the Doppler transducer. The cuff is inflated, which occludes the artery, until no sound is audible from the Doppler box. The cuff is then gradually deflated until the first audible arterial sound returns, which is documented as the SAP.[10,27] The Doppler technique cannot be used in dogs and cats to determine MAP or DAP. The Doppler ultrasonographic technique is inexpensive, easy to perform, and widely used in veterinary patients. The Doppler technique is a relatively sensitive NIBP measurement method in low-flow states and in smaller patients.[10,18,27]

The pressure cuff

The pressure cuff size is key to obtaining accurate results; the cuff's numerical size should be approximately 40% the circumference of the limb in centimeters in dogs (30%–40% in cats), at the point where the cuff will be placed. If the cuff size is too small, there can be erroneously high readings, whereas if the cuff is too large, the readings may be erroneously low—likely due to compression of a larger portion of the artery.[10,17,18,27–31] See Table 10.4 for appropriate pressure cuff sizing.

Table 10.4 Cuff selection for doppler ultrasonic or standard oscillometric blood pressure measurement

Cuff Size	Limb Circumference
1.0 cm	2.5–3.7 cm (1.0–1.5 in)
2.0 cm	3.8–6.2 cm (1.5–2.4 in)
3.0 cm	6.3–8.7 cm (2.5–3.4 in)
4.0 cm	8.8–11.2 cm (3.5–4.4 in)
5.0 cm	11.3–13.7 cm (4.5–5.4 in)
6.0 cm	13.8–16.2 cm (5.4–6.4 in)
7.0 cm	16.3–18.7 cm (6.4–7.4 in)
8.0 cm	18.8–21.2 cm (7.4–8.3 in)
9.0 cm	21.3–23.7 cm (8.4–9.3 in)
10.0 cm	23.8–26.2 cm (9.4–10.3 in)
11.0 cm	26.3–28.7 cm (10.4–11.3 in)

Table 10.5 Correction factors for a vertical distance of ≥10 cm (4 inches) between the RA and the pressure cuff

If the Cuff is . . .	Then . . .
≥10 cm *below* the RA	*Subtract* 0.8 mm Hg for every 1 cm the cuff is below the RA
≥10 cm *above* the RA	*Add* 0.8 mm Hg for every 1 cm the cuff is above the RA

RA, right atrium.

Systemic arterial blood pressure is generally referenced to the level of the right atrium (RA), which would require that the site of measurement (the cuff) be positioned at RA level. If the cuff is positioned lower than the RA, readings will be falsely elevated; the opposite is true if the cuff is positioned above the right atrium.[15,30] It is suggested that, if the vertical distance between the cuff and the RA is 10 cm (4 inches) or more, a correction factor be applied as in Table 10.5. Rather than applying correction factors, it is recommended that the cuff be as close as possible to the horizontal plane of the RA. However, these correction factors can be very helpful in animals with respiratory distress or in other situations that prevent the operator from repositioning the patient.

Performing Doppler ultrasonographic blood pressure measurement

Equipment required for Doppler ultrasonic blood pressure measurement includes clippers with blade, ultrasonic gel, medical adhesive tape, various size pressure cuffs, sphygmomanometer, and Doppler ultrasound machine. See Protocol 10.1 and Figure 10.1 for detailed instructions regarding performance of Doppler ultrasonic NIBP measurements.

The operator should perform several consecutive Doppler blood pressure measurements, discarding the first reading and averaging the following three to seven consecutive, consistent (<20% variability in value) readings.[15] This method appears to improve the reliability of NIBP measurements.[32]

Standard oscillometry (oscillometric sphygmomanometry)

Principles

The oscillometric sphygmomanometry technique is even less time consuming and requires less technical skill than the Doppler ultrasonic technique. Oscillometry involves the connection of a pressure cuff to a device that detects arterial wall oscillations during blood flow. Inflating the cuff occludes the artery. As the cuff is deflated, the arterial wall oscillations increase at SAP, reach a maximum at MAP, and decrease at DAP.[1,33] The oscillometric machines generally display MAP, SAP, DAP, and pulse rate. Many oscillometric machines calculate SAP and DAP from the MAP using proprietary algorithms; therefore, MAP is probably the most reliable reading obtained by standard oscillometry.

The pressure cuff

For oscillometry, the bladder of the cuff should be positioned over the artery for maximum sensitivity to oscillations. Other instructions regarding pressure cuff size and the pressure cuff position in relation to the right atrium are the same for standard oscillometry as for the Doppler method and are given in the preceding discussion of Doppler ultrasound.

Limitations of standard oscillometric blood pressure measurement

The oscillometric techniques measure pulse rate, which should always be compared with the patient's pulse rate as determined manually.[8] If the oscillometer's pulse rate estimate is inaccurate, the blood pressure results may be inaccurate as well. Although oscillometry is routinely used reliably in nonsedated dogs and for monitoring feline and canine blood pressures during anesthetic procedures,[5,6,34–36] this technique appears to be less reliable in nonsedated cats and small dogs. This is likely due to smaller peripheral artery size, which may not generate sufficient pulse pressure to generate detectable cuff pressure oscillations.[10,27] Additional reasons for invalid results using standard oscillometry include

Protocol 10.1 Doppler ultrasonic blood pressure measurement

Items Required
- Clippers with clean blade
- Ultrasonic conductance gel
- Medical adhesive tape
- Various size pressure cuffs
- Sphygmomanometer
- Charged (or plugged in) Doppler ultrasound machine, with headphones if desired
- Assistant, if required

Procedure
1. Collect necessary supplies.
2. Position patient in lateral or sternal recumbency while holding the planned cuff site at approximately the level of the right atrium (RA). (If this is not possible, see Note following the list of procedures.)
3. Clip hair from area over artery.
4. Secure a deflated cuff proximal to the artery and attach the sphygmomanometer. Cuff should be of a size that is approximately 40% of limb circumference in dogs or 30%–40% of limb circumference in cats. When measuring Doppler on the forelimbs, secure cuff on the radius. When measuring on the hind limbs, secure the cuff to proximal to the hock. Medical adhesive tape may be required to secure the cuff well.
5. Apply ultrasonic gel to concave surface of the Doppler probe.
6. Place gelled probe on the clipped skin overlying the artery, keeping the probe's cord parallel to the limb. Adjust with fine movements until the rhythmic "whooshing" arterial sound is audible.
7. Inflate sphygmomanometer to 30–40 mm Hg past the point at which the arterial sounds are no longer detectable.
8. Slowly deflate the cuff until the first sounds are detected, marking the systolic blood pressure.
9. Allow cuff to completely deflate, allowing blood flow to return to the limb.
10. The first measurement should be discarded and the average of three to seven consistent, consecutive readings recorded.
11. Record results, cuff size, and cuff location in patient record.

Note: If positioning the cuff at approximately the (vertical) level of the right atrium is not possible, use the following correction factors when recording measurements:

If the cuff is . . .	Then . . .
≥10 cm *below* the RA	*Subtract* 0.8 mm Hg for every 1 cm the cuff is below the RA.
≥10 cm *above* the RA	*Add* 0.8 mm Hg for every 1 cm the cuff is above the RA.

cardiac dysrhythmias, significant bradycardia or tachycardia, vasoconstriction, hypothermia, and patient movement. The Cardell (CAS Medical Systems INC, Branford, CT) oscillometric machine, unlike the Dinamap (Criticon Co., Tampa, FL), has been shown to be accurate in cats as well as dogs.[11,37]

Performing standard oscillometric blood pressure measurement

Equipment required for standard oscillometric blood pressure measurement includes various size pressure cuffs, adhesive medical tape, and the oscillometer. See Protocol 10.2 and Figure 10.2 for detailed instructions regarding performance of oscillometric NIBP measurements.

The operator should perform several consecutive blood pressure measurements, discarding the first reading and averaging the following three to seven consecutive, consistent (<20% variability in value) readings.[15] This method appears to improve the reliability of NIBP measurements.[32]

High-definition oscillometry

High-definition oscillometry (HDO) blood pressure monitors are relatively new to the veterinary world. The developers claim that HDO monitors have many advantages over conventional oscillometric blood pressure measurement devices. Contrary to standard oscillometry in which the MAP is measured and the SAP and DAP are calculated, HDO devices perform real-time analysis of arterial wall oscillations to obtain pressure wave amplitudes. Some additional putative benefits include electronically controlled valves that adapt to maintain linearity during cuff deflation, permitting accurate readings from 5 to 300 mm Hg; high-speed analysis that allows the detection of and accurate measurement of blood pressure in the face of dysrhythmias; and high sensitivity that allows measurements from minimal signals and during heart rates of up to 500 beats per minute.[38] There have been promising preliminary results in both the dog and the cat.[15,39–41] More recent studies following recommended validation guidelines unfortunately have not been able to officially validate the method, though as mentioned previously, no NIBP monitoring method has yet met these criteria for nonsedated dogs and cats. Recent studies of HDO in dogs and cats have not shown good correlation with other blood pressure measurement methods.[38,41] Since few peer-reviewed studies have been published evaluating HDO in clinical patients, its future role in small animal blood pressure monitoring remains unclear.

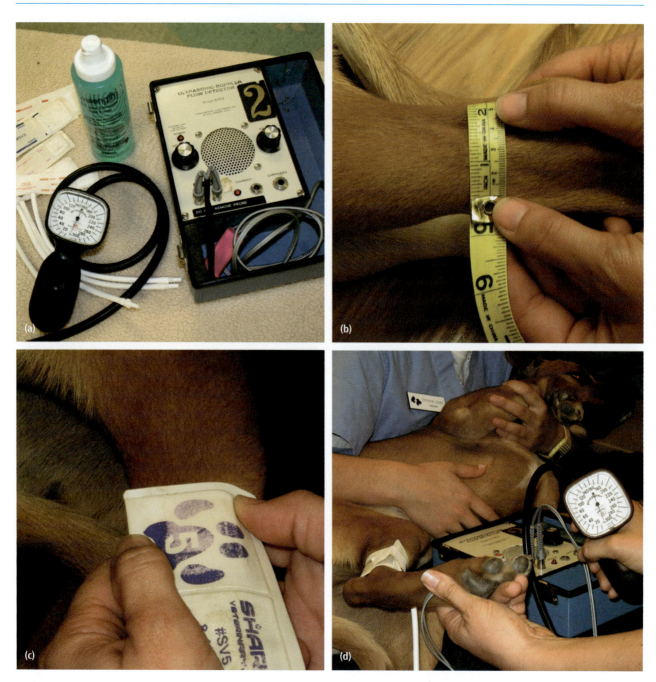

Figure 10.1 (a) Equipment required for Doppler blood pressure measurement: (clockwise from left) pressure cuffs of various sizes, ultrasonic gel, Doppler machine, sphygmomanometer. (b) Proper measurement technique for pressure cuff size. (c) Appropriate cuff size for this patient. (d) Proper patient and pressure cuff positioning (in relation to the patient's right atrium) for measurement of Doppler blood pressure in a dog.

Photoplethysmography

Photoplethysmography is a less frequently encountered NIBP measurement technique. The photoplethysmograph uses infrared radiation to measure blood volume.[1] This method is based on the "volume clamp" principle. The blood volume in an extremity varies in a cyclic fashion with the cardiac cycle. This variation is detected with a clamp attached to a finger in humans or on a foot or tail in veterinary patients. The pressure cuff is deflated and inflated rapidly to maintain a constant volume in the extremity; the cuff pressure will then equal intra-arterial pressure. This technique allows for real-time display of cuff pressure, and therefore intra-arterial

Protocol 10.2 Standard oscillometric sphygmomanometry blood pressure measurement

Items Required
- Various size pressure cuffs
- Oscillometer, with power cord
- Assistant, if required

Procedure
1. Collect necessary supplies.
2. Position patient in lateral or sternal recumbency while holding the planned cuff site at approximately the level of the right atrium (RA). (If this is not possible, see Note following the list of procedures.)
3. Secure a deflated cuff of a size that is approximately 40% of limb circumference in dogs or 30%–40% of limb circumference in cats.
4. The bladder of the cuff (the portion that fills with air) should be centered over the palpable pulse if possible.
   a. Cuff should be measured for and placed above the carpus in small dogs and in cats.
   b. Cuff should be measured for and placed over the metatarsal in larger dogs.
5. Push the button on the oscillometer that begins pressure readings. Discard the first reading and record the average of at least three to seven consecutive, consistent readings.
6. Record the average SAP, DAP, and MAP, and the cuff size and location in the patient record.

Note: If positioning the cuff at approximately the (vertical) level of the right atrium is not possible, use the following correction factors when recording measurements:

If the cuff is . . .	Then . . .
≥10 cm *below* the RA	*Subtract* 0.8 mm Hg for every 1 cm the cuff is below the RA
≥10 cm *above* the RA	*Add* 0.8 mm Hg for every 1 cm the cuff is above the RA

pressure, systolic and diastolic measurement.[8] This device is designed for use on the human finger and has the advantages of continuous monitoring ability, beat-to-beat assessment of blood pressure, and visualization of the pressure pulse waveform.[1,10,37] Disadvantages include its limited usefulness on awake animals and on larger animals, due to the clamp size.[1,10] Although it has been found to be accurate in both dogs and cats it has not come into favor as a commonly used clinical NIBP monitor.

Optimizing the reliability of noninvasive blood pressure measurement

The ACVIM consensus panel established some guidelines for optimizing the reliability of NIBP measurements. The panel cited operator experience as the most likely cause of inaccurate values; hence, an experienced operator should always perform measurements, and appropriately training staff cannot be overemphasized. The panel's recommendations also include the use of a standardized protocol (see Protocols 10.1 and 10.2), allowing the animal to acclimatize to its environment prior to measurement, proper and comfortable cuff placement, and performance of several readings as recommended previously. Although these recommendations are valid and should be followed when possible, some of them are not possible in the emergency room and the intensive care unit (ICU). Thus, it is important at the least that an experienced operator be measuring the blood pressure and to ensure appropriate cuff size and location. The consensus panel also recommends calibrating each NIBP device twice yearly for best accuracy.[15]

Acutely and critically ill patients are typically highly stressed and are often in shock; therefore, acquiring accurate and reliable NIBP measurements is very challenging even when using all recommended techniques. Hence, one should perform patient physical examination frequently and may consider additional monitoring such as electrocardiogram (ECG), which can help corroborate findings. The patient's pulse rate should correlate with the pulse rate on the NIBP device; lack of correlation raises concerns of inaccurate NIBP readings.

Conclusion

Hypotension and hypertension are both common findings in the emergency room and the ICU. Several disease conditions and clinical presentations warrant NIBP monitoring. Using blood pressure to help guide fluid resuscitation and specific pharmacologic interventions will help reduce both morbidity and mortality in these patients. Familiarizing the staff and clinicians with normal arterial pressure values, along with use of a standardized protocol for NIBP devices, will facilitate their use and optimize their reliability.

At this time there are no machines validated to perform NIBP measurement in dogs and cats, but that does not mean these methods are necessarily unreliable or unuseful in clinical practice. Stringent requirements for validation using the comparative gold standard of dABP monitoring should likely be re-evaluated. The

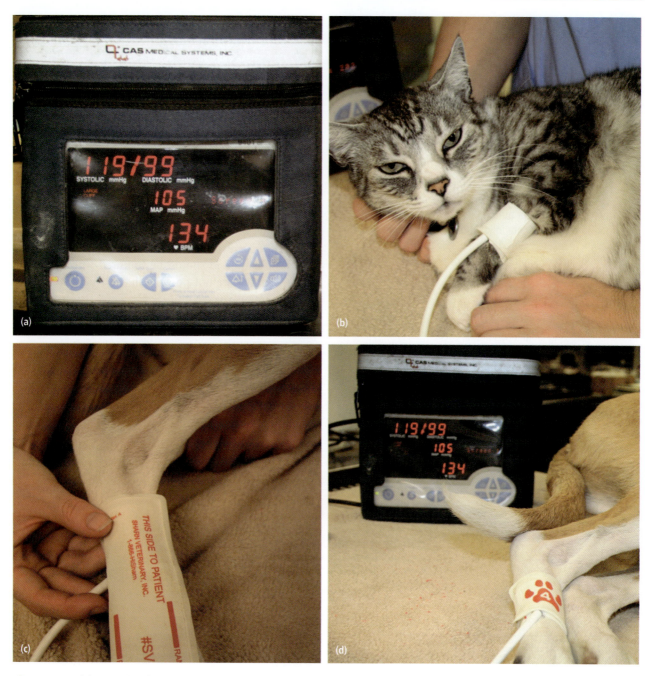

Figure 10.2 (a) Example of a standard oscillometric blood pressure monitor. (b) Proper pressure cuff and patient positioning for standard oscillometric blood pressure measurement in a cat. (c) Proper cuff size for standard oscillometric blood pressure measurement in this dog. (d) Proper positioning for standard oscillometric blood pressure measurement in a dog.

ACVIM consensus panel recommendations for validation should lead to some NIBP monitoring tools gaining validation in small animals.

Standardization of hospital protocols and staff training for use of NIBP devices is highly recommended. Following the ACVIM guidelines for blood pressure measurement is advised although in emergent and critical situations often it is not entirely possible. Adhering as closely as reasonably possible to standard protocols and using physical exam findings, along with other monitors, will improve the utility of NIBP devices and their measurement results.

References

1. Simmons JP, Wohl JS. Hypotension. In: Silverstein DC, Hopper K, eds. Small Animal Critical Care Medicine. Philadelphia: Saunders; 2009:27–33.

2. Guyton AC. Vascular distensibility and functions of the arterial and venous systems. In: Guyton AC, Hall JE, eds. Textbook of Medical Physiology. Philadelphia: Elsevier Saunders; 2006: 171–180.

3. Boulpaep EL. Organization of the cardiovascular system. In: Boron W, Boulpaep EL, eds. Medical Physiology. Philadelphia: WB Saunders; 2002:423–446.

4. Gains MJ, Grodecki KM, Jacombs RM, et al. Comparison of direct and indirect blood pressure measurements in anesthetized dogs. Can J Vet Res 1995;59:238–240.

5. Bodey AR, Young LE, Bartram DH, et al. A comparison of direct and indirect (oscillometric) measurements of arterial blood pressure in anaesthetized dogs, using tail and limb cuffs. Res Vet Sci 1994;57:265–269.

6. Stepien RL, Rapoport GS. Clinical comparison of three methods to measure blood pressure in nonsedated dogs. J Am Vet Med Assoc 1999;11:1623–1628.

7. Bosiack AP, Mann FA, Dodam JR, et al. Comparison of ultrasonic Doppler flow monitor, oscillometric, and direct arterial blood pressure measurements in ill dogs. J Vet Emerg Crit Care 2010;20(2):207–215.

8. Waddell, Brown JA. Hemodynamic monitoring. In: Silverstein DC, Hopper K, eds. Small Animal Critical Care Medicine. Philadelphia: Saunders; 2009:859–864.

9. Podell M. Use of blood pressure monitors. In: Kirk RW, Bonagura JD, eds. Kirk's XI Current Veterinary Therapy. Philadelphia: WB Saunders; 1992:834–837.

10. Binns SH, Sisson DD, Buoscio DA, et al. Doppler ultrasonographic, oscillometric sphygmomanometric, and photoplethysmographic techniques for noninvasive blood pressure measurement in anesthetized cats. J Vet Intern Med 1995; 9:405–414.

11. Pedersen KM, Butler MA, Ersboll AK, et al. Evaluation of an oscillometric blood pressure monitor for use in anesthetized cats. J Am Vet Med Assoc 2002;221:646–650.

12. MacFarlane PD, Grint N, Dugdale A. Comparison of invasive and non-invasive blood pressure monitoring during clinical anaesthesia in dogs. Vet Res Commun 2010;34:217–227.

13. Stokes DN, Clutton-Brock T, Patil C, et al. Comparison of invasive and noninvasive measurement of continuous arterial pressure using the Finapres. Br J Anaesth 1991;67:26–35.

14. Prisant ML, Alpert BS, Robbins CB, et al. American National Standard for non automated sphygmomanometer. Amer J Hypertension 1995;8:210–213.

15. Brown S, Atkins C, Bagley R, et al. ACVIM consensus statement: guidelines for the identification, evaluation, and management of systemic hypertension in dogs and cats. J Vet Intern Med 2007;21:542–558.

16. Henneman EA, Henneman PL. Intricacies of blood pressure measurement: reexamining the rituals. Heart Lung 1989; 18(3):263–271.

17. Valtonen MH, Eriksson LM. The effect of cuff width on accuracy of indirect measurement of blood pressure in dogs. Res Vet Sci 1970;11:358–362.

18. Sparkes AH, Caney SMA, King MCA, et al. Inter- and intraindividual variation in Doppler ultrasonic indirect blood pressure measurements in healthy cats. J Vet Intern Med 1999;12:314–318.

19. Stepien RL, Rapoport GS, Henik RA, et al. Comparative diagnostic test characteristics of oscillometric and Doppler ultrasonographic methods in the detection of systolic hypertension in dogs. J Vet Intern Med 2003;17:65–72.

20. Love L, Harvey R, Smith H, et al. Arterial blood pressure measurement: physiology, tools and techniques. Vet Learn.com 2006.

21. Haskins SC. Monitoring the anesthetized patient. In: Thurman JC, Tranquilli WJ, Benson GJ, eds. Lumb and Jones Veterinary Anesthesia and Analgesia. 4th ed. Philadelphia: Wiley-Blackwell; 2007:533–560.

22. ACVA American College of Veterinary Anesthesiologists. Anesthesiology guidelines developed. J Am Vet Med Assoc 1995;206(7):936–937.

23. Jacob F, Polzin DJ, Osborne CA, et al. Evaluation of the association between initial proteinuria and morbidity rate or death in dogs with naturally occurring chronic renal failure. J Am Vet Med Assoc 2005;226:393–400.

24. Jacob F, Polzin DJ, Osborne CA, et al. Association between initial systolic blood pressure and risk of developing a uremic crisis or of dying in dogs with chronic renal failure. J Am Vet Med Assoc 2003;222:322–329.

25. Jepson RE, Elliott J, Brodbelt D, et al. Effect of control of systolic blood pressure on survival in cats with systemic hypertension. J Vet Int Med 2007;21:402–409.

26. Maggio F, DeFrancesco TC, Atkins CE, et al. Ocular lesions associated with systemic hypertension in cats: 69 cases (1985–1998). J Am Vet Med Assoc 2000;217:695–702.

27. Henik RA, Dolson MK, Wenholz LJ. How to obtain a blood pressure measurement. Clin Tech Small Animal Pract 2005; 20:144–150.

28. Busch, SJ. Small Animal Surgical Nursing: Skills and Concepts. Philadelphia: Mosby; 2005;4:116–117

29. Stepien RL. Blood pressure measurement. In Coté E, ed. Clinical Veterinary Advisor. St. Louis: Mosby Elsevier, 2007: 1191–1192.Pickering TG. Principles and techniques of blood pressure measurement. Cardiol Clin 2002;20:207–223.

30. Glen JB. The accuracy of indirect determination of blood pressure in dogs. Res Vet Sci 1973;14:291–295.

31. Haberman CE, Kang CW, Morgan JD, et al. Evaluation of oscillometric and Doppler ultrasonic methods of indirect blood pressure estimation in conscious dogs. Can J Vet Res 2006;70:211–217.

32. Meldrum SJ. The principles underlying Dinamap—a microprocessor based instrument for the automatic determination of mean arterial pressure. J Med Eng Technol 1978;2:243–246.

33. Kallet AJ, Cowgill LD, Kass PH. Comparison of blood pressure measurements obtained in dogs by use of indirect oscillometry in a veterinary clinic versus at home. J Am Vet Med Assoc 1997;210:651–654.

34. McMurphy RM, Stoll MR, McCubrey R. Accuracy of an oscillometric blood pressure monitor during phenylephrine–induced hypertension in dogs. Am J Vet Res 2006;67: 1541–1545.

35. Deflandre CJA, Hellebrekers LJ. Clinical evaluation of the surgivet V60046, a non invasive blood pressure monitor in anaesthetized dogs. Vet Anaesth and Anal 2008;35:13–21.

36. Caulkett NA, Cantwell SL, Houston DM. A comparison of indirect blood pressure monitoring techniques in the anesthetized cat. Vet Surg 1998;27:370–377.

37. Wernick M, Doherr M, Howard J, et al. Evaluation of high-definition and conventional oscillometric blood pressure measurement in anaesthetized dogs using ACVIM guidelines. J Small Anim Pract 2010;51:319–324.

38. Muir W. Accuracy of a species and cuff site optimized oscillometric BP monitor in cats. Accuracy Study Abstracts 2008.

39. Muir W. Accuracy of a species and cuff site optimized oscillometric BP monitor in dogs. Accuracy Study Abstracts 2008.

40. Chetboul V, Tissier R, Gouni V, et al. Comparison of Doppler ultrasonography and high-definition oscillometry for blood pressure measurements in healthy awake dogs. Am J Vet Res 2010;71(7):766–772.

41. Petric AD, Petra Z, Jerneja A, et al. Comparison of high definition oscillometric and Doppler ultrasonic devices for measuring blood pressure in anaesthetised cats. J Feline Med Surg 2010;12:731–737.

11

Central venous pressure monitoring

Rosalind S. Chow and Pamela Dilley

Clinical management of the critically ill animal usually requires regular assessments of the adequacy of intravascular blood volume and cardiac preload. Hemodynamic instability may develop in many different ways. Excessive vomiting, diarrhea, polyuria, hemorrhage, or body cavity effusion can result in hypovolemia. Sepsis or systemic inflammatory response syndrome may alter vascular volume and tone. Central venous pressure (CVP) measurement can provide useful information in these and other situations. It represents the direct measurement of venous blood pressure from a catheter inserted into the cranial vena cava or, less commonly, into the caudal vena cava or the right atrium. When measured from the vena cavae, CVP is considered to be a close approximation of right atrial pressure,[1] which in turn is a determinant of right ventricular preload. As a result, CVP measurement is widely used as an index of circulating blood volume to help guide fluid resuscitation and diuretic therapy in veterinary patients.[2–5]

Determinants of central venous pressure

Central venous pressure is determined primarily by the interrelationship between venous return and right heart function.[6] In turn, venous return is affected by venous tone, venous wall compliance, and circulating blood volume, whereas right-sided cardiac output is determined by heart rate, preload, afterload, and contractility. Therefore any normal physiological process, disease, or medical intervention that alters one of these factors may affect CVP. This includes changes in sympathetic tone that occur during stress and illness, structural and func-

tional diseases of the heart, and vasoactive drugs such as vasopressors, sedatives, and general anesthetics.

While these factors affect CVP due to their influence on cardiovascular function or blood volume, in some cases, extravascular forces, such as increases in intrathoracic or intra-abdominal pressure, can also change the CVP.[7,8] High pressure within the thoracic cavity can develop secondary to a number of conditions, including effusion, presence of a space-occupying mass, a forced expiratory respiratory pattern, or positive end-expiratory pressure (PEEP) during mechanical ventilation. A sufficient rise in intrathoracic pressure will compress the vena cava and right atrium and raise the CVP. Similarly, elevations in intra-abdominal pressure can be seen with ascites, acute abdominal syndrome, neoplasia, active abdominal expiratory effort, and other conditions. When there is significant disease in the thoracic or abdominal cavities, it is important for the clinician to be aware of their potential influence on the CVP. In general, when interpreting CVP measurements to help with clinical decision-making, it is crucial to remember that many things other than circulating blood volume affect the CVP.

Indications for the measurement of central venous pressure

Monitoring CVP can help to guide fluid therapy in animals with abnormalities in circulating blood volume or abnormal right heart function. Central venous pressure cannot be used to make inferences about left ventricular preload or function, however.[9] Specific indications for CVP measurement include the presence of

Advanced Monitoring and Procedures for Small Animal Emergency and Critical Care, First Edition. Edited by Jamie M. Burkitt Creedon, Harold Davis.
© 2012 John Wiley & Sons, Inc. Published 2012 by John Wiley & Sons, Inc.

persistent hypotension despite fluid resuscitation, vasopressor therapy, extensive third space losses, oliguria or anuria, hemorrhage, trauma, sepsis, burns, and heart failure. Patients undergoing urgent or emergent surgical procedures, and those with multiple medical problems, can be predisposed to developing cardiovascular instability while anesthetized. In these animals it may be practical to insert a central venous catheter and begin monitoring preemptively to allow earlier detection of abnormalities in the perioperative period.

Risks

Central venous catheter use carries small but real risks of thrombosis, thromboembolism, carotid arterial puncture, infection, phlebitis, bleeding, and vascular erosion. Cardiac arrhythmias, or rarely cardiac wall perforation, can result if the catheter tip is accidentally advanced into the right atrium or right ventricle. There are fewer problems associated with CVP measurement itself. The main risk is accidental introduction of air or bacteria into the venous system, particularly if poor technique is practiced. The cranial vena cava is a low-pressure system, and opening the system to the atmosphere may result in air embolism formation. Fortunately, this is a rare occurrence with intermittent CVP measurement technique and even less common with continuous technique, as the system is closed to the outside environment. Additionally, several straightforward precautions will reduce the incidence of complications. These include following proper hand hygiene measures prior to handling the jugular catheter or CVP system, careful inspection of the tubing and transducer to assess for defects, the use of Luer lock connectors such as Luer-Lok (Becton, Dickinson and Company, Franklin Lakes, NJ), and periodic verification of the tightness of these connections, particularly in mobile patients.

Normal value

The most commonly used reference range for central venous pressure is around 0—5 cm H_2O,[3,10,11] although values of up to 10 cm H_2O can be normal.[2,12] The wide reference range reflects the inherent variability in normal resting CVP due to the impact of many factors on venous pressure, including blood volume, venous tone, and cardiac function.

The units of CVP measurement are millimeters of mercury (mm Hg) or centimeters of water (cm H_2O), depending upon the method of measurement. To convert from mm Hg to cm H_2O, multiply by a factor of 1.36:

$$CVP \text{ in } cm\,H_2O = CVP \text{ in } mm\,Hg \times 1.36 \qquad (11.1)$$

Measurement technique

Central venous pressure is typically measured from a specialized catheter that is inserted into the external jugular vein and advanced into the cranial vena cava or, less commonly, into the right atrium. Right atrial pressure can also be measured from the proximal lumen of a pulmonary artery catheter. Pressure measurements from the vena cava and the right atrium are generally considered interchangeable at rest,[13,14] although this is untrue if there exists an obstruction between these two sites, and their responses are not identical following fluid bolus or vasopressor therapy.[15] Several alternative techniques for obtaining the CVP have been described in animals, including catheter insertion into the omobrachial vein in dogs[16] with subsequent passage into the cranial vena cava, as well as placement into the femoral vein and caudal vena cava in dogs[17] and cats.[18] In human patients, peripheral venous pressure has also been used as an estimate of CVP due to the similarities between centrally and peripherally measured venous pressures.[19,20] Unfortunately, this technique has shown poor correlation in dogs and cats.[21]

Catheter selection and placement

Either single-lumen or multilumen vascular catheters can be used and should be of sufficient length to reach the thoracic vena cava from the point of insertion. Insertion of a multilumen catheter has the added advantage of allowing continued infusion of intravenous fluids and drugs through the proximal ports as the CVP is measured simultaneously from the catheter's distal port. The rate of fluid administration has been shown to have no affect on the CVP in humans, even during pressurized saline infusions of up to 9120 mL/hour via a double-lumen catheter and up to a combined rate of 14,340 mL/hour through the proximal ports of a triple-lumen catheter.[22] These results are likely similar in veterinary patients although similar experiments have not yet been published.

Prior to catheter placement, it is important to predetermine an appropriate depth of insertion. Before approaching the jugular vein, a good estimate of depth can be obtained by measuring the distance between the insertion site and the caudal aspect of the shoulder, which should position the tip within the cranial vena cava. Following placement, the catheter's position can be verified by radiography and by visualization of a characteristic central venous pressure waveform (as discussed in the Waveform Analysis section in this chapter). Radiographic confirmation is particularly important when alternative catheter insertion sites are used, such as the saphenous vein, as premeasurement is more difficult to perform with accuracy in such cases. Catheters advanced into the right atrium can occasionally generate arrhythmias and should be backed out slightly. Accidental advancement of the catheter tip into the ventricle should be avoided. However, if it occurs, it is not difficult to recognize once a pressure measurement is obtained, as peak right ventricular pressures approach 20–30 mm Hg in the normal animal.[2] They will be visible as extreme fluctuations of the fluid column of the water manometer (for intermittent CVP measurement) or of the displayed waveform on the electronic monitor (for continuous CVP measurement).

General principles

The two methods of obtaining the CVP are intermittent measurement and continuous measurement. In both methods, the catheter is connected via a fluid-filled tubing system to a pressure-measuring device that displays the venous pressure. Intermittent measurement involves connecting the catheter to a water manometer, infusing a predetermined volume of saline, and allowing the fluid level to equilibrate with the patient's central venous pressure. The height of the fluid column within the manometer is recorded in centimeters of water pressure (cm H_2O). Continuous CVP measurement is obtained by linking the catheter via noncompliant, fluid-filled tubing to a pressure transducer that converts the venous pressure wave to an electrical signal. The venous pressure waveform is displayed continuously and in real time on a monitor. The average venous pressure in millimeters of mercury (mm Hg) is also shown.

As is commonly the case where more than one method of measurement is available, there are advantages and disadvantages to each technique. The equipment needed to perform intermittent CVP monitoring is simple and inexpensive. However, repeated measurements are relatively time-consuming to obtain. In contrast, once the system for continuous CVP monitoring is assembled, moment-to-moment changes in CVP are displayed on the monitor without the need for additional intervention. The ability to view CVP continuously is particularly useful for unstable patients in the intensive care unit and in the operating room. Frequent measurements also permit better and more timely determination of a patient's response to therapy. However, a higher level of technical knowledge and skill is needed to set up and troubleshoot continuous CVP monitoring and it also requires purchase of a specialized monitor, which can be expensive. When available, refurbished and used monitors may represent a more economical solution for many hospitals.

Zeroing and leveling

To obtain reliable pressure measurements, two principles are important. First, atmospheric pressure, which measures approximately 760 mm Hg at sea level, is used as the standard reference point to which CVP is compared. Atmospheric pressure is created by the weight of air, which presses down on the body and everything within it, including the central veins. It also pushes on the transducer and the manometer fluid column. Since it exerts the same magnitude of pressure on each object, for simplicity it is cancelled out and atmospheric pressure is considered 0 cm H_2O (0 mm Hg) for purposes of CVP measurement. This allows a CVP of 770 mm Hg to be read as 10 mm Hg and eliminates the need to adjust CVP measurements for fluctuations in barometric pressure.[23] The process of correcting for atmospheric pressure is called **zeroing**. Pressure transducer systems have an integrated stopcock and port that can be opened to the atmosphere to calibrate, or *zero*, the transducer.

The second principle is the importance of aligning the transducer system (or manometer) with the vascular structure containing the pressure of interest, also known as the **zero reference point**, in order for the measurements to be accurate. In the case of CVP, the zero reference point is the center of the right atrium. The stopcock (for continuous CVP measurement) or the 0 cm H_2O mark on the manometer (for intermittent measurement) must be positioned or **leveled** on the same horizontal plane as the patient's right atrium during zeroing and thereafter during measurement, as demonstrated in Figure 11.1. See Chapter 8, Fluid-Filled Hemodynamic Monitoring Systems, for more information regarding zeroing and leveling transducers.

Due to species- and breed-related variability in thoracic conformation, there is no completely foolproof method of determining where the right atrium lies. However, as a general rule of thumb, the sternum is a good approximation for a dog or cat in lateral recumbency. For an animal in sternal recumbency, draw an imaginary vertical line at the caudal aspect of the shoulder that extends from the top of the dorsal spinous process to the sternum. The right atrium lies at a point that is roughly 40% of the height of this line.

Proper determination of the zero reference point is crucial, because *failure to level the transducer (or manometer) relative with it will result in an erroneous central venous pressure reading*. It will be falsely high if the transducer is resting below the right atrium and falsely low if the transducer is above the right atrium; if the error is not detected and the resulting measurements are used as the basis for fluid therapy decisions, harm to the patient could result. For this reason, the height of the

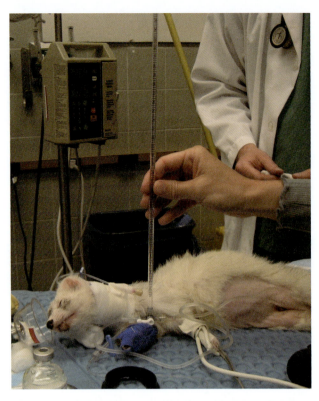

Figure 11.1 Leveling of the manometer with the zero reference point. Though this ferret's heart is far caudal of the manometer, note that the zero value must only be on the same horizontal plane as the patient's right atrium in order for measurements to be accurate.

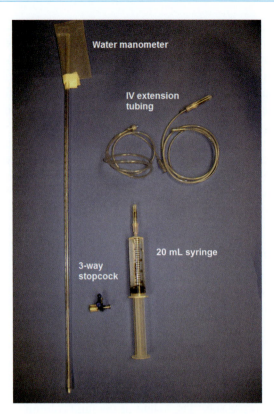

Figure 11.2 Equipment required for intermittent central venous pressure measurement.

transducer and stopcock system should always be evaluated prior to each pressure reading. Their position may need to be adjusted depending on whether the animal is recumbent, sitting, or standing. Gentle restraint may be needed with mobile patients to obtain accurate CVP readings. The transducer should also be periodically rezeroed—always at the level of the right atrium—due to the potential for drift.[24] Additionally, whenever possible, measurements should be taken by the same person to avoid inconsistent technique. The attending veterinarian should be notified if the CVP measurements are showing an upward or downward trend, particularly if they fall outside of expected or target values.

Intermittent central venous pressure measurement

Prior to initiating CVP measurement, it is important to verify the patient has a correctly positioned central venous catheter, as described earlier in this chapter. Two types of water manometers can be used for intermittent CVP measurement. The best one is a rigid, narrow, cylindrical tube made of glass or plastic specifically

manufactured for this purpose that has centimeter markings along its length. A simpler homemade alternative consists of a short section of IV fluid extension tubing that can be affixed to a ruler. Either standard fluid tubing or noncompliant tubing manufactured specifically for blood pressure monitoring can be used. The equipment required to perform intermittent CVP measurement is shown in Figure 11.2.

To ensure accuracy, the patient should rest in the same position for each measurement period and this position should be recorded on the patient's treatment sheet for future reference. Both lateral and sternal recumbencies are acceptable. It may be more difficult to obtain accurate readings from an animal that is sitting or standing. Whenever possible, use the same position for subsequent measurements. In some situations, it will be impractical or unsafe to position the patient in a certain way. If this is the case, it is important to adjust the height of the manometer so that the $0\,cm\,H_2O$ mark is level with the zero reference point (the right atrium) prior to recording the CVP. Alternatively, as CVP can occasionally fall below zero, it can be helpful to align the $10\,cm\,H_2O$ mark with the zero reference point to facilitate measurement of negative pressures. When this positioning is used, one must subtract $10\,cm\,H_2O$ from the height of the fluid column in the manometer to obtain the true CVP measurement.

The CVP is read at the bottom of the meniscus in the manometer (or at the center of the floating ball in the manometer, if present). Patient heartbeat or respiration may cause millimeter fluctuations in the meniscal level. In a spontaneously breathing animal, the CVP reading will decrease during inspiration and increase during expiration. The pressure reading should be obtained at end-expiration if the patient is breathing normally. If there is pronounced expiratory abdominal effort, the measurement should be obtained at the beginning of the expiratory phase, prior to the onset of active abdominal effort.[1,6] Detailed instructions on performing intermittent CVP measurement are available in Protocol 11.1.

The time interval between measurements will depend on the patient's cardiovascular status as well as personnel availability, but a reasonable place to start is to space readings 1–4 hours apart. If more frequent measurements are desired, continuous CVP measurement should be considered.

Protocol 11.1 Intermittent central venous pressure measurement

Items Required
- Indwelling central venous catheter (inserted to the proper depth)
- Disposable water manometer (calibration in centimeters), or a centimeter ruler and extension tubing
- 0.9% NaCl
- Three-way stopcock with locking fittings
- 20-mL syringe
- Noncompliant tubing or standard fluid extension tubing
- Heparinized saline flush
- One assistant

Procedure
1. Collect the necessary supplies.
2. Perform hand hygiene and don examination gloves.
3. The patient may lie in lateral or sternal recumbency. This position should be recorded on the patient treatment sheet for future reference.
4. If applicable and safe to do so, have the patient rest in the same position that was recorded in the treatment sheet for prior CVP measurements.
5. Flush the patient's central venous catheter with heparinized saline solution to ensure patency.
6. Assemble the CVP monitoring setup. First orient the manometer vertically. Then connect the three-way stopcock to the manometer, to the saline-filled syringe, and to the fluid tubing.
7. Orient the three-way stopcock valve so that it is closed to the manometer and open to the tubing and fluid-filled syringe. Then, prime (fill) the stopcock and fluid tubing with 0.9% NaCl from the syringe. Connect the fluid tubing to the central venous catheter. If a multilumen catheter is being used, connect the tubing to the central lumen.
8. Orient the stopcock valve so that it is closed to the patient's central venous catheter and open between the manometer and the fluid-filled syringe. Using the 20-mL syringe, fill the manometer with 0.9% NaCl to a level that is approximately $10–20\,cm\,H_2O$ greater than the patient's expected CVP. Do not allow the manometer to overflow while filling.
9. The manometer may be attached to an IV pole to facilitate height adjustments, held vertically in the operator's hand, or taped to the wall of the cage. Locate the $0\,cm\,H_2O$ mark and position the manometer so that it is level with the zero reference point (the patient's right atrium).
10. Close the stopcock valve toward the syringe, which will open a fluid column between the manometer and the patient. The fluid level in the manometer will initially fall as it flows into the patient and then stabilize as the fluid level equilibrates with the CVP.
11. The operator should ensure consistent readings by performing three or more consecutive measurements and calculating an average. Record the average pressure and patient position on the patient's treatment sheet.
12. When the measurements have been completed, turn the stopcock off to the manometer and disconnect the pressure tubing from the central venous catheter. If intravenous fluid therapy will not be immediately resumed, flush the central venous catheter with heparinized saline.

Continuous central venous pressure measurement

The list of supplies and equipment needed for continuous CVP measurement is more extensive than it is for intermittent measurement. To better familiarize the reader with the materials and monitoring technique, additional details are provided here.

Pressure transducer kits come presterilized and typically consist of a disposable pressure transducer, three-way stopcock with zeroing port cap, and a flush mechanism (see Fig. 9.1). Some also include noncompliant ("high-pressure") tubing that is needed to join the pressure transducer to the patient's central venous catheter. Additional tubing can be added between the transducer and the patient if more length is needed. Standard fluid extension tubing is soft and compliant, whereas noncompliant tubing made for blood pressure measurements is flexible but nondistensible. In theory, excessively long or compliant tubing could dampen transmission of the pressure waveform, resulting in waveform distortion.[25,26] Due to the low vascular pressures of the venous system, damping from overly compliant tubing is less of a concern with CVP measurement than it is with direct arterial blood pressure monitoring.[26] But optimization of the CVP waveform will be achieved with noncompliant tubing specifically manufactured for blood pressure monitoring. The reader is referred to Chapter 8, Fluid-Filled Hemodynamic Monitoring Systems, for more details regarding tubing characteristics.

The last element of the continuous monitoring setup is assembly of the flush system, which is pressurized and provides a simple method of flushing the catheter by pulling the rapid flush valve (usually referred to as a *pigtail* on the transducer). The flush solution consists of heparinized saline and it is prepared by adding unfractionated heparin to a bag of 0.9% NaCl to a final concentration of 1 U/mL.

Prior to beginning measurement, the transducer must be zeroed at the proper level by exposing it to atmospheric pressure in approximately the same horizontal plane as the right atrium (see Intermittent Measurement instructions for more details). The fluid-filled system is zeroed and leveled by turning the stopcock lever off toward the patient, removing (and saving) the zeroing port cap, and setting the monitor to zero. The reader should consult the reference manual for his or her specific monitor for additional details. Once this has been done, the monitor will display 0 mm Hg and the waveform tracing should overlap zero on the displayed scale. If the transducer does not zero, the transducer is the most likely culprit, and it should be replaced and the procedure reattempted. After the zeroing step, the

zeroing port cap is replaced and the stopcock is turned so it points off toward the port cap to create a continuous fluid column between the pressure transducer and the patient's central vein. Central venous pressure measurement may then begin.

As with intermittent CVP measurement, it is important to ensure the transducer is at the level of the zero reference point prior to zeroing or obtaining a reading. This is best achieved by having the patient lie in the same position for each measurement period. Specific instructions for assembling the continuous CVP measurement system are included in Protocol 11.2. Common issues and solutions that may be encountered during continuous CVP monitoring are summarized in Table 11.1.

Maintenance of the continuous CVP system

For the patient undergoing continuous CVP monitoring, certain maintenance procedures should be included in the patient's treatment orders, listed in Box 11.1. The patient can be disconnected from and reconnected to the CVP measurement system without the need to rezero the transducer as long as the disconnection occurs between the transducer and the central venous catheter. However, if the transducer cable is disconnected from the monitor, it will be necessary to rezero the transducer prior to obtaining a CVP reading.

CVP interpretation

Central venous pressure should never be used as the sole monitoring parameter to determine the adequacy of circulating blood volume. It must always be evaluated in conjunction with the patient's history, signalment, and physical examination, and ideally with knowledge of the animal's cardiac and renal function. Laboratory data

---

Box 11.1 Maintenance of the continuous CVP system

- The transducer and catheter system should be periodically flushed by pulling on the fast flush device. This should be performed at least once every 4 hours.
- The transducer should be rezeroed no less frequently than every 12 hours due to the potential for drift.
- Change the flush solution and tubing every 48 hours.
- Ensure there are no air bubbles in the fluid line at any time.
- Periodically inspect and reinflate the pressure bag to 300 mm Hg as necessary, and verify the heparinized saline bag is not empty.

Protocol 11.2 Continuous central venous pressure measurement

Items Required
- Indwelling central venous catheter inserted to the proper depth
- Pressure transducer kit
- Bag of 0.9% NaCl heparinized to a concentration of 1 U/mL
- Standard fluid administration set
- Pressure bag of appropriate size for heparinized saline bag
- Ideally, noncompliant fluid tubing; alternately, standard fluid extension tubing
- Electronic blood pressure monitor and its associated transducer cable

Procedure
1. Collect the necessary supplies.
2. Perform hand hygiene and don examination gloves.
3. The patient may lie in lateral or sternal recumbency. This position should be recorded on the patient treatment sheet for future reference.
4. Flush the patient's central venous catheter with heparinized saline solution to ensure patency.
5. Assemble the heparinized saline flush system by spiking the heparinized saline fluid bag with the standard fluid administration set and flushing fluid through the tubing. Clamp the tubing and cap the set's open end.
6. Place the pressure bag over the bag of heparinized saline, hang it on an IV pole placed next to the patient, and inflate the pressure bag to 300 mm Hg.
7. Assemble the transducer system by connecting it to the noncompliant tubing, to the assembled heparinized saline flush system, and to the transducer cable and electronic monitor, as shown in Figure 9.1.
8. Prime (fill) the transducer and noncompliant tubing system with heparinized saline by pulling the transducer's fast flush valve (pigtail).
9. Connect the pressure tubing to the central venous catheter. If using a multilumen catheter, the CVP measurement should be obtained from the most distal lumen, reserving the other lumens for IV fluid therapy, drug administration, or blood withdrawal. It is not necessary to discontinue IV fluid or drug administration through the other ports during CVP measurement.
10. Position the height of the transducer and stopcock system so that the stopcock is aligned at the same height as the zero reference point (the right atrium). The transducer may be attached to an IV pole, to the cage door, or taped to a stable support that is resting on the floor of the cage.
11. Flush the catheter by pulling on the pigtail and wait for the pressure to equilibrate.
12. The system must be calibrated (zeroed) before any measurements can be interpreted. To perform zero-calibration, with the stopcock at the height of the right atrium, turn the stopcock off toward the patient. Remove the zeroing port cap on the stopcock to open it to the atmosphere. Select the zeroing function on the display monitor and wait for it to read 0 mm Hg. Replace the zeroing port cap and turn the stopcock toward the zero port, which will allow the pressure to equilibrate between the patient's vena cava and the transducer.
13. Once the pressure has stabilized, record the CVP measurement.
14. For subsequent measurements, verify the transducer height is correctly positioned at the zero reference level before recording the CVP measurement.

and additional markers of hemodynamic status, such as arterial blood pressure and urine output, should also be factored into the clinical assessment.

Due to the number of potential factors that can influence CVP, an isolated value is difficult to interpret and is of minimal benefit. However, serial measurements over time may document trends in venous blood pressure that can provide useful information to assist in the assessment of circulating volume status. Apart from its usefulness as a diagnostic tool when hypovolemia is suspected, CVP measurement can also be used to monitor the effectiveness of fluid therapy to treat low circulating blood volume. However, in a similar manner, its success or failure should be determined by concurrently evaluating a combination of other clinical markers.

In hemodynamically unstable patients, the primary objective of fluid therapy is to optimize right ventricular preload in an effort to improve cardiac output and tissue perfusion. The rationale for performing CVP measurement is its ability to serve as an estimate of right atrial pressure, which is a major determinant

Table 11.1 Troubleshooting tips for continuous CVP measurement

Problem	Possible Cause
Pressure is displayed as a flat line rather than a waveform.	Complete occlusion of the catheter, stopcock, or fluid line (displayed pressure will be far above the normal reference range).
	Partial occlusion of the catheter, stopcock, or fluid line.
	Patient is small (cats and small dogs occasionally lack a visible waveform although the mean pressure can still be used for trending purposes).
	Air bubble or leak in the system.
No pressure is displayed on the monitor.	Monitor display settings are incorrect.
	Transducer was not zeroed.
	Transducer cable is broken or is not plugged into the monitor.
Pressure reading is higher than expected.	Intrathoracic or intra-abdominal pressure is significantly increased.
	Central venous catheter is clamped off or occluded.
	Transducer is below the level of the right atrium.
	Transducer is defective.
Pressure reading is lower than expected.	Transducer is above the level of the right atrium.
	Transducer is defective.
Waveform is "noisy."	Patient movement.
	Panting.
	Catheter tip is within the heart.
	Arrhythmia.
Sudden change in pressure.	Hemodynamic instability.
	Transducer position relative to the zero reference point (right atrium) has changed.
System does not flush.	Stopcock position is incorrect.
	Pressure bag is not sufficiently inflated.
	Heparinized saline bag is empty.
	Heparinized saline administration line is clamped off or occluded.
	Central venous catheter is clamped off or occluded.

of right ventricular end-diastolic pressure. Right atrial and right ventricular pressure are equal when the tricuspid valve is open and pressures have equilibrated at the end of ventricular diastole. Right ventricular end-diastolic pressure is in turn related to right ventricular end-diastolic volume, which determines end-diastolic myocardial wall stretch, or **preload.**

While the initial temptation would be to assume that low values of CVP correspond to hypovolemia and high values indicate volume overload, in reality, the association between CVP and preload is not always straightforward. Critics note that isolated values of CVP do not correlate well with intravascular blood volume, nor can CVP be used to predict stroke volume or cardiac output following a fluid challenge.[27] Despite these limitations, its proponents argue that CVP nevertheless provides useful information about preload and right-sided heart function and that these criticisms reflect misunderstanding and misuse of this monitoring tool.[14] A review of the physiological principles behind venous return and

venous pressure is useful here to highlight their reasoning.

Venous return describes the flow of blood from the systemic circulation back to the heart. Proper flow depends on the maintenance of an adequate pressure gradient, often referred to as the **driving pressure**, between the peripheral and central venous vasculatures. Driving pressure here is small. The pressure in the peripheral venous circulation averages only 5–10 mm Hg greater than the pressure within the central veins, and homeostatic adjustments ensure continued return blood flow as variables change.[7]

The dynamic properties of the venous system that allow it to regulate venous return also govern its other role, which is to serve as a blood reservoir. Veins contain approximately 65% of the systemic blood volume.[28] A major portion of that blood is contained within the splanchnic veins, which function as capacitance vessels capable of significant adjustments in wall compliance to accommodate changes in blood volume. When effective circulating volume is low, constriction of the splanchnic veins increases the circulating pool of blood to help support adequate venous return.[7] Central venous pressure may change minimally during this time despite the recruitment of additional volume, and clinically, the patient may appear to be coping quite well. However, once the blood reservoir has been depleted and other compensatory mechanisms have been exhausted, the patient will decompensate suddenly and CVP will fall.

The complex relationship between CVP and circulating blood volume may explain why a CVP within the normal reference range cannot distinguish the normovolemic patient from one with compensated hypovolemia or hypervolemia, due to homeostatic mechanisms that attempt to maintain an adequate pressure gradient for venous return. A severely elevated CVP may be due to normovolemia in the presence of severe cardiac dysfunction, or hypervolemia with adequate cardiac performance.[14] The complexity of these interactions may explain why studies have consistently failed to find a threshold CVP pressure below which fluid loading will always improve cardiac output.[27,29]

Despite these limitations, several generalizations about CVP interpretation can be made that ensure its continued usefulness in the ICU. First, CVP should be regarded as a probable, rather than an absolute, indicator of volume status. In other words, in the presence of normal cardiac function, patients with a low CVP are more *likely* to respond to volume than patients with a normal or high CVP. In human patients with severe circulatory dysfunction, a CVP less than 5 mm Hg has been shown to be an excellent positive predictor of fluid responsiveness.[30] In contrast, those with a CVP greater than 10–12 mm Hg are unlikely to benefit from a fluid bolus, although some still can.[1,14] Those that do respond may have a condition such as elevated intrathoracic or intra-abdominal pressure that is causing the CVP to overestimate the true transmural pressure.[1,8]

The second generalization that can be made is that rising or falling trends are clinically meaningful. A progressive drop in CVP should alert the clinician to the possibility of ongoing and excessive internal or external fluid losses, particularly if supported by the presence of other markers of hypoperfusion. In contrast, a rising CVP with concurrent evidence of worsening tissue perfusion may indicate declining cardiac function as the cause, and may suggest that additional fluid loading is unwise.[1] With the latter scenario, additional caution is warranted if hypoalbuminemia or vasculitis is present, as either of these conditions increases the risk of edema formation with intravenous fluid therapy. A summary of the possible clinical interpretations of rising or falling trends in CVP is provided in Table 11.2.

Potential sources of interpretation errors

As discussed earlier, extravascular forces, such as significant elevations in the pressure within the thoracic or abdominal cavities, can raise CVP. An increase in CVP of approximately 3 mm Hg was seen at PEEP levels of 10 cm H_2O in humans[31] and 15 cm H_2O in pigs.[32] However, in the absence of PEEP, an alteration of tidal volume alone (8 mL/kg versus 16 mL/kg) did not result in a similar effect.[31] Large elevations in intra-abdominal pressure, secondary to acute abdominal syndromes, ascites, or a forced expiratory respiratory pattern, can also lead to changes in the CVP due to transmission of the increased abdominal pressure across the diaphragm to the thoracic cavity.[8,29]

It is important to recognize that the higher CVP generated by an elevation in intrathoracic or intra-abdominal pressure *does not necessarily result in changes in driving pressure and venous return*. This is because the physiological variable that ultimately governs distension of the central veins is **transmural pressure**, not CVP.[1,6]

Table 11.2 Clinical interpretation of CVP measurement trend[21]

CVP Trend	Possible Cause
Low or falling	Shock Vasodilation
Normal	Normovolemia Compensated hypovolemia Compensated hypervolemia
High or rising	Volume overload Vasoconstriction or systemic hypertension Right-sided heart disease • Tricuspid regurgitation • Tricuspid stenosis Pericardial disease • Pericardial effusion • Constrictive pericarditis Vena caval obstruction Pulmonary disease • Pulmonary hypertension • Pulmonary thromboembolism Increased intrathoracic pressure • Pleural effusion • Intrathoracic mass • PEEP • Positive-pressure ventilation in the presence of hypovolemia • Pneumothorax Increased intra-abdominal pressure Occlusion of the catheter, fluid line, or stopcock

The concept of transmural pressure is best understood by recognizing that venous distension depends not only on the pressure exerted on the vascular wall from the inside (CVP), but also on the pressure exerted from the outside, and this is pleural pressure, not atmospheric pressure. The net difference (intravascular pressure minus extravascular pressure) is called transmural pressure. Due to the inherent difficulties in obtaining pleural or pericardial pressures in the clinical setting, transmural pressure is usually not directly determined. Fortunately, it corresponds fairly closely to CVP under most conditions. However, this relationship can unravel during certain situations, notably with increases in intrathoracic or intra-abdominal pressure.[7,8] In the PEEP example described above, the increased alveolar pressure generated by PEEP is transmitted to the heart and intrathoracic vessels and results in an elevation in CVP. However, PEEP is also transmitted to a similar extent to the pleural and pericardial spaces. As a result, central venous transmural pressure changes minimally.

However, as we have already mentioned, venous return depends ultimately on driving pressure, which is the difference between peripheral and central venous pressures. Driving pressure was previously defined as the difference between peripheral and central venous pressures. However, it is more accurately defined as the difference between peripheral and central *transmural* venous pressures. So in this example, although there has been an absolute increase in measured CVP, transmural central and peripheral venous pressures have remained steady. Therefore there is no change in the rate of return of blood to the heart.

Performing a fluid challenge

When CVP is extremely low or falling, the index of suspicion for hypovolemia should be high. Usually, an evaluation of other clinical markers will support an assessment of low circulating blood volume, and fluid resuscitation can be started immediately. However, on occasion, these findings will be unclear or contradictory; when this occurs, a fluid challenge is the classic method of verifying fluid responsiveness.

The idea is to give a small test volume as a rapid bolus and to monitor for an improvement in clinical perfusion parameters such as patient alertness, pulse quality, pulse rate, mucous membrane color, and capillary refill time. Faster administration reduces the volume needed to achieve an effect. If a beneficial response is seen following the volume challenge, additional fluid is given until the desired endpoint is reached. Under ideal monitoring circumstances this endpoint would be an increase in cardiac output. However, as cardiac output is difficult to measure without cardiac catheterization or other specialized techniques, several indirect indices are more commonly used, such as improved systemic arterial blood pressure, lower blood lactate concentration, increased urine production, and higher central venous oxygen saturation, as well as improvement in physical examination findings. See Chapter 15, Monitoring Tissue Perfusion: Clinicopathologic Aids and Advanced Techniques, for more information about many of these indirect perfusion indices.

A fluid challenge is performed by rapidly infusing a small volume of crystalloid or colloid using a pressure bag or fluid pump. Useful crystalloid test volumes are 15 mL/kg in the dog, or 5 mL/kg in the cat. If a colloid is used, 5 mL/kg in the dog or 2.5 mL/kg in the cat are reasonable. The fluid bolus is given over 10–15 minutes and the animal is monitored for signs of improved perfusion and CVP.

The classic response to a fluid challenge in the euvolemic animal is a rise in CVP of 2–4 cm H_2O, followed by a rapid return to the original value within 15 min.[33] However, if the starting CVP is low and it rises minimally or rapidly returns to baseline (within 5–15 minutes) following a fluid challenge, hypovolemia is likely,[33,34] particularly when corroborated by other findings as mentioned previously. The fall in CVP is due to the redistribution of fluid from the intravascular to the interstitial space, stress-induced relaxation of venous tone, and pooling of blood within the splanchnic vascular bed.[35] In contrast, a persistent, marked elevation in CVP following a fluid challenge, or a prolonged return to baseline (greater than 30 minutes) may support volume overload, decreased cardiac performance, or restrictive pericardial disease such as tamponade.[33]

It should be noted that these guidelines reflect general trends, not absolute rules. A low CVP will not always indicate that a patient has inadequate blood volume, just as a high CVP does not necessarily signify fluid excess or cardiac dysfunction.[14] Normovolemic animals may show a rise in CVP following a test bolus, even though they do not actually require fluid. Therefore, there is no substitute for careful patient assessment and clinical judgment when using CVP measurement to help guide fluid therapy.

The normal CVP waveform

Blood pressure in the central veins is pulsatile as a result of pressure changes in the right heart during the cardiac cycle. The baseline pressure also fluctuates from changes in intrathoracic pressure generated by the phases of respiration. Both intermittent and continuous CVP mea-

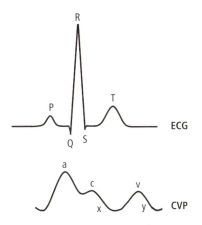

Figure 11.3 The relationship between the waves and descents of the CVP waveform and the electrocardiogram. Under normal circumstances, the mean of the *a* wave provides the best estimate of CVP because it corresponds to the venous pressure at the end of diastole. Ventricular systole begins immediately following the appearance of the QRS complex on the ECG.

surement techniques provide a mean CVP, although in the case of intermittent measurement, small pulsations are often evident in the fluid column.[33]

In a similar manner, the CVP reported during continuous measurement represents a mathematical average of this variable pressure. The pressure waveform is displayed on the monitor and classically consists of three "waves" (positive deflections from baseline: the *a* wave, *c* wave, and *v* wave) and two descents (negative deflections: the *x* descent and the *y* descent), which correspond to specific right atrial and right ventricular cardiac events (see Fig. 11.3).[36] Not all waves and descents will be evident in all CVP tracings and considerable individual variability in waveform appearance can be seen. Waveforms can be small or impossible to discern in cats and small dogs, and may be absent if the catheter lumen becomes partially occluded (such as by a blood clot).

The *a wave* is generated by atrial contraction and appears shortly after the P wave on an electrocardiogram. The *a* wave is followed by the *x descent,* which reflects a decrease in right atrial pressure caused by atrial relaxation. The *c* wave is sometimes visible as a secondary peak following the *a* wave and is caused by bowing of the tricuspid valve into the atrium during early right ventricular systole. As atrial diastolic filling proceeds, the *v wave* is created and it is generated soon after the T wave on an electrocardiogram. When ventricular systole ends and the ventricle relaxes, atrial pressure exceeds ventricular pressure, the tricuspid valve opens, and blood flows from the right atrium into the ventricle. Atrial emptying leads to a decrease in atrial pressure, thus producing the *y descent.* The *a* wave is usually larger than or similar in size to the *v* wave.[36]

Determining the CVP from the normal waveform

During continuous CVP measurement, the monitor displays a single pressure reading that represents an average pressure measurement over time. The mean CVP is often sufficient for clinical assessment in patients lacking significant primary cardiovascular or respiratory disease. However, changes in respiratory pattern, cardiac arrhythmias, and diseases that alter filling, emptying, or compliance of the right heart can lead to an inaccurate estimation of ventricular end-diastolic pressure (preload), resulting in errors in clinical interpretation. When any of these problems are evident, it is important to determine the CVP directly from the printed venous pressure tracing to ensure accuracy. The CVP and ECG waveforms are viewed simultaneously to determine the location of the *a* wave, which begins in the PR interval on the ECG. This should be distinguished from the *c* wave, which is found in the RT interval, and the *v* wave, which appears after the T wave.[37] Once the *a* wave is identified, determine the pressure at the top of the *a* wave and bottom of the *x* descent and calculate the mean to determine the CVP[36]:

$$CVP\ estimate = (a\ wave\ peak + x\ descent\ base)/2 \quad (11.2)$$

The reason the mean of the *a* wave is used to estimate the CVP is because it peaks at ventricular end-diastole. Immediately after end-diastole, the tricuspid valve closes with the onset of ventricular systole, an event that follows the appearance of the QRS wave on the electrocardiogram. Therefore an alternative method of determining the CVP is to locate the R wave[37] or the end of the QRS complex[36] on the ECG. A perpendicular line is drawn at this point extending down toward the CVP waveform and where they intersect represents the true CVP.

Abnormal CVP waveform

Waveform analysis provides a method of obtaining an accurate estimate of preload in the presence of cardiovascular or respiratory disease. It can also provide important supplementary information about cardiovascular function to help diagnose or confirm the presence of certain abnormalities. Several of these situations are described in the following subsections.

Respiratory changes

Venous return varies with respiratory phase and respiratory muscle activity. During inspiration, there is a decrease in pleural pressure generated by expansion of

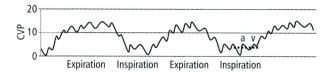

Figure 11.4 Baseline fluctuation in CVP waveform seen during forced expiration. The CVP should be estimated by calculating the mean of the *a* wave during early expiration (dashed line). The *a* wave and *v* wave are labeled.

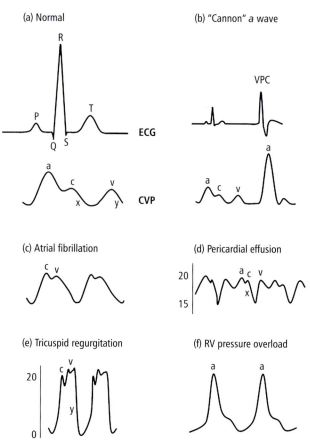

Figure 11.5 Illustration demonstrating (a) normal and (b–f) abnormal CVP waveforms. (b) Large "cannon" *a* waves are produced by simultaneous contraction of the right atrium and right ventricle and they can intermittently appear with certain arrhythmias, including second- and third-degree AV block, and some ventricular arrhythmias such as the ventricular premature complex (VPC) shown here. (c) Atrial fibrillation produces a prominent *c* wave. (d) Cardiac tamponade arising from pericardial effusion causes the CVP waveform to become flattened and there is a prominent *x* descent and small or absent *y* descent. (e) A broad and tall *c–v* wave is characteristic of tricuspid regurgitation. (f) Right ventricular (RV) pressure overload arising from pulmonary hypertension or pulmonic stenosis produces large, prominent *a* waves.

the chest wall and caudal movement of the diaphragm.[38] This decrease in transmural pressure is transmitted across the wall of the vena cava and causes a small decrease in CVP, which returns to baseline following passive, unforced expiration. For this reason, in the spontaneously breathing, relaxed patient, the CVP reading (the mean of the *a* wave) should be measured at the end of the expiratory phase to best correspond to right ventricular end-diastolic pressure.[1,6,38]

However, when there is increased expiratory effort, which may be seen patients that are vocalizing or dyspneic, CVP will be overestimated with this method. In that situation, CVP is best obtained during early expiration prior to the onset of active abdominal muscle contraction.[6] Again, the mean of the *a* wave is used but it is necessary to evaluate the printed CVP waveform to determine the most accurate place to obtain this measurement (see Fig. 11.4). Similarly, positive-pressure ventilation may also raise the displayed mean CVP. The waveform should be examined and CVP measured from a time point corresponding to end-expiration.

Arrhythmias

Certain cardiac rhythm disturbances, such as atrial fibrillation and junctional and ventricular arrhythmias, can lead to a lack of atrial contraction and therefore loss of the *a* wave on a CVP tracing. During atrial fibrillation, there is also a prominent *c* wave resulting from overfilling of the right atrium, which is unable to generate normal contractions (see Fig. 11.5c).[37] The most accurate CVP estimate will be obtained by viewing the CVP tracing and ECG simultaneously and selecting the pressure that is present toward the end of the QRS complex, which best represents ventricular end-diastole.[26]

Ventricular premature contractions (seen as ventricular premature complexes [VPCs] on an ECG), atrial fibrillation, atrial premature contractions (seen as atrial premature complexes [APCs] on an ECG), and second- or third-degree atrioventricular (AV) node block can intermittently produce large (cannon) *a* waves due to AV dissociation, where there is a transient increase in atrial

pressure caused by contraction of the atrium against a closed tricuspid valve during ventricular systole (see Fig. 11.5b).[39] When one of these arrhythmias is present, the CVP should be estimated from the normal *a* waves visible on the waveform tracing.[38]

Pericardial effusion with cardiac tamponade

Increased pericardial fluid pressure inhibits diastolic filling of the heart. This results in an increase in the mean CVP and flattening of the CVP waveform due to greater equalization of the pressures within the atria and ventricles. A prominent *x* descent is seen due to a rapid reduction in atrial pressure during ventricular systole, and the *y* descent is small or absent (see Fig. 11.5d).[38]

Tricuspid regurgitation

Tricuspid valvular disease results in obliteration of the *x* descent during ventricular systole by a large wave created by the backward flow of blood through the incompetent valve.[38,39] This wave is composed of the merging of the *c* wave and *v* wave. Both may be clearly visible when there is mild insufficiency, but they combine to form a broad wave with a single peak when severe insufficiency is present (see Fig. 11.5e).[39]

Pulmonic stenosis and pulmonary hypertension

Conditions such as pulmonic stenosis and pulmonary hypertension can result in large *a* waves as the right atrium contracts against the elevated right ventricular pressure (see Fig. 11.5f).[39]

Alternative techniques for assessing vascular volume

The gold standard of fluid therapy decision-making would be to assess appropriateness based on its effect on cardiac output. Unfortunately, the technical challenges associated with cardiac output measurement preclude its frequent use in veterinary medicine (see Chapter 12, Cardiac Output Monitoring, for more information regarding cardiac output assessment). Due to its simpler measurement technique and clinical utility, CVP measurement has become a commonly used hemodynamic monitoring tool in veterinary critical care. However, it does not reliably correlate with cardiac output. Therefore, CVP should always be interpreted in conjunction with other clinical and biochemical markers of intravascular volume status as well as with the knowledge of the animal's cardiac and renal function.

In the critical patient, the importance of performing serial, systematic physical examinations cannot be overemphasized, as these examinations may allow the clinician to detect early changes supportive of low circulating blood volume. Compensatory cardiovascular and renal changes in response to hypovolemia result in centralization of blood volume, renal sodium and water retention, and peripheral vasoconstriction. Initially, few clinical changes will be apparent when homeostatic mechanisms are sufficient to restore tissue perfusion. However, as the volume deficit worsens, these changes typically manifest as the development of mental obtundation, pale mucous membranes, delayed capillary refill time, tachycardia,

poor pulse strength, and cool extremities. When physical findings are equivocal, blood lactate concentration can provide a quantitative measure of the severity of impaired tissue perfusion and anaerobic metabolism. As shock worsens, arterial blood pressure will fall, and oliguria or anuria will develop. A high urine specific gravity will also be seen unless a concurrent disorder is present that is impairing renal concentrating ability. See Chapter 15, Monitoring Tissue Perfusion: Clinicopathologic Aids and Advanced Techniques, for more information about many of these other indices of perfusion.

In the absence of hypoalbuminemia or cardiac dysfunction, clinical signs suggestive of excessive intravascular blood volume include peripheral edema, chemosis, pleural or peritoneal effusion, serous nasal discharge, and in some cases, development of a new heart murmur or an increase in murmur intensity. Urine output is typically high and urine specific gravity low. If pulmonary edema is present, pulmonary crackles and respiratory difficulty may be evident. These findings, particularly when combined with rising CVP measurements, provide convincing evidence of volume overload.

Conclusion

In summary, the measurement of CVP is a useful adjunctive hemodynamic monitoring tool in critically ill patients and it is readily performed in any patient that has a central venous catheter. Trends, rather than isolated values, should be followed. A severely low or falling CVP suggests hypovolemia. A severely elevated or rising CVP can be seen with hypervolemia as well as with increased venous tone, reduced cardiac compliance, diminished cardiac function, or increased intrathoracic or intra-abdominal pressures. In conjunction with other clinical markers of cardiovascular function, CVP can serve as a valuable guide in the assessment and treatment of problems related to intravascular volume status and right-sided heart function.

References

1. Magder S. How to use central venous pressure measurements. Curr Opin Crit Care 2005;11:264–270.
2. Aldrich J, Haskins S. Monitoring the critically ill patient. In: Bonagura JD, Kirk RW, editors. Current Veterinary Therapy. Vol XII. Philadelphia: WB Saunders; 1995:98–105.
3. Day TK, Bateman S. Shock syndromes. In: DiBartola SP, editor. Fluid, Electrolyte and Acid–Base Disorders in Small Animal Practice. 3rd ed. St. Louis, MO: Saunders Elsevier; 2006:540–564.
4. Mathews KA. Monitoring fluid therapy and complications of fluid therapy. In: DiBartola SP, editor. Fluid, Electrolyte and Acid–Base Disorders in Small Animal Practice. 3rd ed. St. Louis, MO: Saunders Elsevier; 2006:377–391.

5. Waddell LS, Brown AJ. Hemodynamic monitoring. In: Silverstein DC, Hopper K, editors. Small Animal Critical Care Medicine. St. Louis, MO: Saunders; 2009:859–871.

6. Magder S. Central venous pressure: a useful but not so simple measurement. Crit Care Med 2006;34:2224–2227.

7. Gelman S. Venous function and central venous pressure. Anesthesiology 2008;108(4):735–747.

8. Qureshi AS, Shapiro RS, Leatherman JW. Use of bladder pressure to correct for the effect of expiratory muscle activity on central venous pressure. Intensive Care Med 2007;33:1907–1912.

9. Bolte AC, Dekker GA, van Eyck J, van Schijndel RS, van Geijn HP. Lack of agreement between central venous pressure and pulmonary capillary wedge pressure in preeclampsia. Hypertens Pregnancy 2000;19:261–271.

10. Monnet E. Cardiovascular monitoring. In: Wingfield WE, Raffe MR, editors. The Veterinary ICU Book. Jackson, WY: Teton NewMedia; 2002:266–280.

11. DiBartola SP, Bateman SW. Fluid therapy. In: DiBartola SP, editor. Fluid, Electrolyte and Acid–Base Disorders in Small Animal Practice. 3rd ed. St. Louis, MO: Saunders Elsevier; 2006: 48–54.

12. Ware WA. Cardiac tamponade and pericardiocentesis. In: Silverstein DC, Hopper K, editors. Small Animal Critical Care Medicine. St. Louis, MO: Saunders; 2009:180–183.

13. Walsh JT, Hildick-Smith DJR, Newell SA, Lowe MD, Satchithanada DK, Shapiro LM. Comparison of central venous and inferior vena cava pressures. Am J Cardiol 2000;85:518–520.

14. Magder S, Bafaqeeh F. The clinical role of central venous pressure measurements. J Intensive Care Med 2007;22:44–51.

15. Tkachenko BI, Evlakhov VI, Poyasov IZ. Relationship between venous return and right-atrial pressure. Bull Exp Biol Med 2001;131:421–423.

16. Radlinsky MG, Koenig A. Central venous access to the cranial vena cava via the omobrachial vein in the dog. J Vet Emerg Crit Care 2008;18(6):659–662.

17. Berg RA, Lloyd TR, Donnerstein RL. Accuracy of central venous pressure monitoring in the intraabdominal inferior vena cava: a canine study. J Pediatr 1992;120(1):67–71.

18. Machon RG, Raffe MR, Robinson EP. Central venous pressure measurements in the caudal vena cava of sedated cats. J Vet Emerg Crit Care 2007;5(2):121–129.

19. Anter AM, Bondok RS. Peripheral venous pressure is an alternative to central venous pressure in paediatric surgery patients. Acta Anaesthesiol Scand 2004;48:1101–1104.

20. Tugrul M, Camci E, Pembeci K, Al-Darsani A, Telci L. Relationship between peripheral and central venous pressures in different patient positions, catheter sizes, and insertion sites. J Cardiothorac Vasc Anesth 2004;18:446–450.

21. Chow RS, Kass PH, Haskins SC. Evaluation of peripheral and central venous pressure in awake dogs and cats. Am J Vet Res 2006;67(12):1987–1991.

22. Lakhal K, Ferrandiere M, Lagarrigue F, Mercier C, Fusciardi J, Laffon M. Influence of infusion flow rates on central venous pressure measurements through multi-lumen central venous catheters in intensive care. Intensive Care Med 2006;32(3): 460–463.

23. Magder S. Invasive intravascular hemodynamic monitoring: technical issues. Crit Care Clin 2007;23:401–414.

24. Gordon VL, Welch JP, Carley D, Teplick R, Newbower RS. Zero stability of disposable and reusable pressure transducers. Med Instrum 1987;21:87–91.

25. Fessler HE, Shade D. Measurement of vascular pressure. In: Tobin MJ, editor. Principles and Practice of Intensive Care Monitoring. New York: McGraw-Hill; 1998:91–106.

26. Hertzler LW. Technical considerations in obtaining hemodynamic waveform values. In: Ahrens TS, Taylor LA, editors. Hemodynamic Waveform Analysis. Philadelphia: WB Saunders; 1992:209–256.

27. Marik PE, Baram M, Vahid B. Does central venous pressure predict fluid responsiveness? Chest 2008;134:172–178.

28. Boulpaep EL. Arteries and veins. In: Boron WF, Boulpaep EL, editors. Medical Physiology. Philadelphia: Elsevier; 2005: 447–462.

29. Kuntscher MV, Germann G, Hartmann B. Correlations between cardiac output, stroke volume, central venous pressure, intra-abdominal pressure and total circulating blood volume in resuscitation of major burns. Resuscitation 2006;70:37–43.

30. Muller L, Louart G, Bengler C, Fabbro-Peray P, Carr J, Ripart J, de La Coussaye J, Lefrant J. The intrathoracic blood volume index as an indicator of fluid responsiveness in critically ill patients with acute circulatory failure: a comparison with central venous pressure. Anesth Analg 2008;107:607–613.

31. Lorsomradee S, Lorsomradee S, Cromheecke S, et al. Inferior vena cava diameter and central venous pressure correlation during cardiac surgery. J Cardiothorac Vasc Anesth 2007;21(4): 492–496.

32. Oliveira RH, Azevedo LC, Park M, Schettino GP. Influence of ventilator settings on static and functional haemodynamic parameters during experimental hypovolaemia. Eur J Anesthesiol 2009;26:66–72.

33. Hansen BD. Technical aspects of fluid therapy. In: DiBartola SP, editor. Fluid, Electrolyte and Acid–Base Disorders in Small Animal Practice. 3rd ed. St. Louis, MO: Saunders Elsevier; 2009: 344–376.

34. Barbeito A, Mark JB. Arterial and central venous pressure monitoring. Anesthesiology Clin 2006;24(4):717–735.

35. Greenway CV, Lister GE. Capacitance effects and blood reservoir function in the splanchnic vascular bed during non-hypotensive haemorrhage and blood volume expansion in anaesthetized cats. J Physiol 1974;237:279–294.

36. Ahrens TS, Taylor LA. Normal pulmonary capillary wedge and central venous pressure waveforms. In: Ahrens TS, Taylor LA, editors. Hemodynamic Waveform Analysis. Philadelphia: WB Saunders; 1992:23–52.

37. Shroeder RA, Barbeito A, Bar-Yosef S, Mark JB. Cardiovascular monitoring. In: Miller RD, editor. Miller's Anesthesia. 7th ed. Philadelphia: Churchill Livingstone Elsevier; 2009:1267–1386.

38. Mark JB. Getting the most from a CVP catheter. In: 52nd Annual Refresher Course Lectures, Clinical Updates and Basic Science Reviews. American Society of Anesthesiologists Annual Meeting; 2001 Oct 13–17; New Orleans, LA. American Society of Anesthesiologists. 2001:231.

39. Applefield MM. The jugular venous pressure and pulse contour. In: Walker HK, Hall WD, Hurst JW, editors. Clinical Methods: The History, Physical, and Laboratory Examinations. 3rd ed. Boston: Butterworth Publishers; 1990:107–111.

12

Cardiac output monitoring

Steve C. Haskins

Indications for cardiac output measurement

Evaluation of the cardiovascular status of critically ill patients is broadly divided into those parameters that relate to venous return to the heart and those that relate to forward flow from the heart. Parameters that evaluate venous return (preload; end-diastolic ventricular filling) include ease of jugular vein distention and central venous pressure, postcava diameter (radiography), and end-diastolic ventricular diameter (ultrasonography). Parameters that evaluate forward flow can be broadly divided as follows: (1) those that relate to cardiac output, such as heart rate, stroke volume, pulse quality, and cardiac output; (2) arterial blood pressure; (3) those that relate to arteriolar vasomotor tone, such as mucous membrane color and capillary refill time; and (4) those that relate to tissue perfusion, such as appendage temperature, urine output, gastric carbon dioxide tension, oxygen extraction ratio, venous oxygen tension, and metabolic acid–base balance (including blood lactate concentration).

There are various levels of knowledge involved in the evaluation of the cardiovascular status. Clinicians typically start with the collection of historical data and the physical examination of mental status, hydration status, ease of jugular vein distention, heart rate, pulse quality, mucous membrane color, capillary refill time (CRT), and appendage temperature. In many cases, based on the findings of this examination, a strong case can be made for hypovolemia, low cardiac output, or poor tissue perfusion and a therapy plan can be formulated. If the patient responds to therapy, no additional cardiovascular information is necessary. In other cases, the informa-

tion derived from the initial history and physical examination is insufficient to comfortably define patient status, or the patient's response to the initial therapy is insufficient to restore clearly delineable normal-range cardiovascular values. Subsequent therapeutic decisions require additional information. A second level of cardiovascular information is gained by measuring parameters such as central venous pressure (CVP), postcava diameter, end-diastolic left ventricular diameter, arterial blood pressure (ABP), and parameters of metabolic acid–base balance; there are chapters in this textbook describing these techniques. Many times this additional information helps clarify the patient's cardiovascular status and facilitates subsequent therapeutic decisions. A few residual patients either still cannot be defined or do not respond to therapy; in such cases, additional information is required. It is at this point that flow information such as cardiac output and oxygen delivery might be helpful. Cardiac output can be measured many ways but the common clinically applicable techniques involve indicator dilution.

Indicator dilution techniques

Indicator dilution techniques basically involve the injection of a known volume of fluid (V_1) with a known concentration of indicator (C_1) into an unknown larger volume (V_2) and then measuring the concentration of the indicator in the larger volume of fluid (C_2). The unknown volume (V_2) is then calculated by the following formula:

$$C_1 \times V_1 = C_2 \times V_2 \tag{12.1}$$

Advanced Monitoring and Procedures for Small Animal Emergency and Critical Care, First Edition. Edited by Jamie M. Burkitt Creedon, Harold Davis.
© 2012 John Wiley & Sons, Inc. Published 2012 by John Wiley & Sons, Inc.

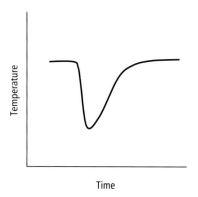

Figure 12.1 Temperature–time curve of a thermodilution cardiac output measurement. (Tracing can be displayed in either an upward or a downward direction.)

In a moving fluid such as the cardiovascular system, C_2 is calculated as the average change in indicator concentration over time.

Any indicator can be used as long as it can be measured with a rapidly responding sensor. In thermodilution, the indicator is temperature. A small volume of fluid (V_1) at a known temperature (T_1) is injected into the cranial vena cava or right atrium. This injected fluid flows and mixes with the blood through at least two heart valves. The change in temperature as the blood–fluid mix flows past a rapid-acting thermistor in the pulmonary artery or a peripheral artery is measured (see Fig. 12.1). The average change in temperature (T_2) is integrated from the change in temperature over time. The unknown volume of blood (V_2, the cardiac output) flowing along with the injected fluid is then calculated by the Stewart–Hamilton formula:

$$\text{Cardiac output} = V_1 \times (T_b - T_i) \times (\text{computation constant})$$
$$\div \, [\text{integrated area of the measured}$$
$$\text{temperature change over time} \, (T_2)]$$
$$(12.2)$$

where V_1 is the volume of the injectate, T_b is baseline blood temperature, and T_i is the temperature of the injectate. The computation constant is calculated from the density and specific heat of the injectate compared with the density and specific heat of blood, and the change in temperature of the injected fluid as it traverses the catheter. The computation constant is provided by the equipment manufacturer. The computer calculates cardiac output in milliliters or liters per minute, and this value must then be indexed to body size either as kilograms of body weight or square meters of body surface area.

Thermodilution has been demonstrated to be accurate and repeatable in *in vitro* models[1–4] and when compared *in vivo* with dye dilution,[5] electromagnetic flowmetry,[6] and transit-time flowmetry.[7]

Transpulmonary thermodilution cardiac output measurements, with the thermistor placed in a peripheral artery (thus avoiding the use of the balloon-tipped thermodilution catheter), have been reported to accurately reflect traditional thermodilution cardiac output measurements made with the pulmonary artery catheter.[8–12] Using the transpulmonary thermodiluation method, extravascular lung water (pulmonary edema) can also be estimated.

Cardiac output can also be measured continuously with specialized thermodilution catheters that incorporate a thermal filament near the proximal port of the catheter that is positioned in the cranial vena cava or right atrium. The thermal filament cycles on and off. The change in temperature of the heated blood is sensed by the downstream thermistor in the pulmonary artery. Values for cardiac output, ejection fraction, end-diastolic volume, end-systolic volume, and stroke volume are generated as an average for the last 5–10 minutes. This methodology has been reported to compare well with intermittent thermodilution cardiac output measurements,[13–16] although low-range cardiac outputs may be overestimated while high-range cardiac outputs may be underestimated.[17]

Thermodilution cardiac output measurements are the standard of practice for clinical measurements of cardiac output in people. Balloon-tipped thermodilution catheters are, however, expensive, variably difficult to place, and are invasive. Measurements are subject to significant intermeasurement variation and therefore repeated measures, to obtain an average, are necessary and take time. Many studies compare the cardiac output estimates of a particular methodology with thermodilution; variance and bias are usually blamed on the compared methodology without regard to the inherent variability of thermodilution. This approach elevates thermodilution to "gold standard" status and unfairly biases against the tested methodology.

While thermodilution catheters permit the measurement or calculation of a large number of important cardiovascular parameters, their use has a variable record with regard to improved patient survival.[18–24] Although one might expect that increased monitoring should provide the means for improved patient care and, therefore, survival, there is no overwhelming evidence for this. The lack of demonstrable statistically significant survival benefit does not, however, prove that the thermodilution catheter is a useless monitoring tool. Thermodilution catheters were used ubiquitously in human critical care and without regard for selecting patients who might truly be benefited. Of course, ultimate survival depends upon the effectiveness of the management of the underlying disease process, irrespective of the tools used to monitor the patient.

Lithium and indocyanine green (ICG) indicators are also used to measure cardiac output. The measurement is made by injecting a known amount of indicator into a central vein and withdrawing blood at a constant rate from an arterial catheter, past a lithium sensor or densitometer, respectively. Newer methods of ICG cardiac output use a transcutaneous finger photosensor[25] or ICG fluorescence[26] rather than an *ex vivo* cuvette densitometer. With the lithium indicator, cardiac output is calculated from the lithium dose and the area under the lithium concentration-versus-time curve:

$$\text{Cardiac output} = [\text{lithium dose (mM)}] \times 60$$
$$\div [\text{integrated area under the}$$
$$\text{concentration} - \text{time curve} \quad (12.3)$$
$$(\text{mM/sec}) \times (1\text{-PCV})]$$

where PCV stands for packed cell volume. Lithium dilution has been reported to compare well with thermodilution in dogs,[27] cats,[28] and foals.[29] One limitation to lithium and dye dilution techniques is the number of measurements that can be performed before background indicator concentrations start to interfere with subsequent measurements.

Balloon-tipped thermodilution catheter

Balloon-tipped catheters are available as two-lumen catheters for measuring pulmonary artery pressure and pulmonary artery occlusion pressure; as four-lumen catheters for measuring CVP, pulmonary artery pressure, and cardiac output (see Fig. 12.2); and as five- and six-lumen catheters for measuring CVP, pulmonary artery pressure, and cardiac output, for placement of pacing electrodes, and for continuous reflectance oximetry. Catheters are available in lengths of 80 (for pediatrics) or 110 (for adults) cm and in diameters of 4, 5, 6, 7, 7.5, or 8.5 Fr, depending upon the number of lumens and intended use. The cost of these catheters varies between about $80 for the simpler versions to $200 (in 2010) for the more comprehensive catheters. The 4-Fr catheter is the smallest diameter four-lumen catheter with thermodilution capabilities and can be used in cats and small dogs (1–3 kg). The 7-Fr four-lumen catheter can be used in dogs over 10 kg; 5- and 6-Fr catheters are suitable for dogs between 3 and 10 kg. Thermodilution cardiac output catheters are available from Arrow International (www.arrowintl.com) or Edwards Lifesciences (www.edwards.com). Cardiac output computers are available from many companies that market patient monitoring equipment (Baxter, Abbott, USCI, Siemens, Hewlett-Packard, Marquette, Space Labs, Spectramed, PPG, Elecath, Kontron, Lyons, Kone, Mennen, and Nihon Koden).

Insertion of the balloon-tipped thermodilution catheter and complications

Introduction of the catheter and repositioning of it after placement are facilitated by the use of an appropriate-sized introducer catheter, which incorporates a plastic cover sheath to protect the thermodilution catheter from contamination during the initial insertion as well as during subsequent repositioning.

The cardiac output computer and pressure monitor are turned on and readied. A bag of heparinized saline in a pressure bag is readied for the intrafusor. Introducer

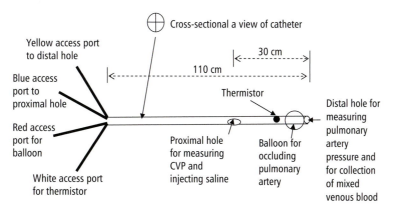

Figure 12.2 Schematic of a four-lumen, thermodilution, balloon-tipped catheter.

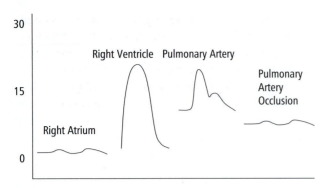

Figure 12.3 Schematic of representative pressure waveforms while introducing the balloon-tipped catheter into the pulmonary artery.

catheter kits and thermodilution catheter kits are opened. Catheters can be placed via the jugular vein or the saphenous or femoral vein. Introducer wires, introducer catheters, and thermodilution catheters are long and floppy, and are easily contaminated. Aseptic introduction must be assured. An area of at least 5-cm (2-inch) radius around the intended venipuncture site is clipped and aseptically prepared. Large sterile drapes are used to extend the sterile field.

First insert the introducer catheter and suture it in place. Next, the proximal port line of the thermodilution catheter is filled with sterile, heparinized saline and capped. The distal port line is flushed with heparinized saline and attached to a pressure transducer and a physiologic monitor for pressure measurements that will be used to identify the location of the catheter during its introduction. As the catheter is advanced toward the right atrium, a typical CVP tracing should be displayed on the monitor (see Fig. 12.3). Initially, angle the natural curvature of the catheter toward the sternum and the right ventricle. Marks on the catheter at 10-centimeter intervals identify how much of the catheter has been inserted. Typically the tip of the catheter will reach the right ventricle when it has been inserted to 25–40 cm, depending on the size of the patient. When the catheter enters the right ventricle the tracing will change to a typical ventricular pressure waveform (see Fig. 12.3). If the catheter has been introduced as far as 50 cm and has not entered the right ventricle, it has either coiled in the right atrium or passed into the caudal vena cava. The catheter should be withdrawn to 20 cm and reinserted. There is little directional control over the tip of the catheter and so, on subsequent reintroductions, the catheter should be rotated in one direction or another and readvanced until it ultimately ("accidentally") falls into the right ventricle. If the catheter end-hole butts up

against a vessel or chamber wall, there will be a sudden cessation of pressure waveform on the monitor. If the line is attached to a high-pressure, low-volume, constant-infusion device (to prevent clotting within the catheter between measurements), the pressure tracing will increase rapidly to the top of the screen. Withdraw the catheter slightly, rotate it, and advance it again.

If the catheter fails to enter the right ventricle after repeated rotating (first one way then the other) and readvancing, try advancing the catheter with the balloon inflated; try shifting the position of the animal, insofar as possible. If all else fails and patience is at an end, use fluoroscopy to guide the introduction of the catheter.

Once the tip of the catheter is in the right ventricle, the balloon is inflated (1 mL) and further advanced until it enters the pulmonary artery (see Fig. 12.3). Once in the pulmonary artery, with the balloon still inflated, the catheter is further advanced until it occludes a branch of the pulmonary artery, at which time the pressure tracing will change to a typical occlusion pressure (see Fig. 12.3). Deflation of the balloon allows the measurement of pulmonary artery pressure; reinflation of the balloon allows the measurement of pulmonary artery occlusion pressure. During subsequent inflations of the balloon, always monitor the pressure tracing. When the catheter is first introduced, there is usually a big loop of catheter in the right ventricle. Over time, between measurements, the catheter will migrate further into smaller branches of the pulmonary artery. Full inflation of the balloon at this time could rupture these smaller pulmonary vessels. If less than full balloon inflation occludes the vessels (as indicated by the appearance of a typical occlusion pressure waveform on the monitor), the balloon should be deflated and the catheter should be withdrawn a short distance until it requires the full 1-mL inflation to occlude the vessel. The balloon should be inflated only for the measurement of occlusion pressure and then should be deflated; it should not remain inflated for an extended duration because continuous inflation will cause vessel damage. Step-by-step instructions for pulmonary arterial catheterization are available in Protocol 12.1.

Once the catheter is ideally positioned so that all measurements (central venous, pulmonary artery, and occlusion pressure) can be obtained, it should be secured to the patient and bandaged aseptically and occlusively.

Sepsis is a major hazard of these catheters. They are long and floppy and are easily contaminated during placement if one is not careful. Once placed, they are "busy" catheters in that they are frequently used throughout the day to make measurements and procure blood

Protocol 12.1 Insertion of the balloon-tipped thermodilution catheter

Items Required
- Appropriate-sized thermodilution catheter set
- Appropriate-sized introducer set with catheter guard sheath
- Pressure transducer
- Noncompliant fluid tubing, if desired
- Patient monitor with integrated cardiac output computer and associated power cord, thermistor cable, and transducer cable
- Hair clippers and surgical scrub solutions
- Surgical cap, mask, and sterile gloves
- Sterile surgical drapes
- Basic surgical set and skin-suitable suture such as 3–0 to 2–0 nylon
- Sterile syringes with needles
- Three-way stopcocks
- Heparinized saline
- Bag of 0.9% NaCl heparinized to 1 U/mL
- Standard fluid administration set
- Pressure bag
- At least one assistant

Procedure
1. Collect necessary supplies.
2. Turn on the cardiac output computer and patient monitor. Input any necessary information into the computer (volume and temperature of injectate).
3. Spike the heparinized saline bag with the standard fluid administration set and insert into a pressure bag. Make sure the administration set is clamped and capped.
4. Attach electrocardiograph(ECG).
5. Clip and prepare with antiseptic solutions a wide area of skin over the intended vessel puncture site.
6. Perform a surgical aseptic hand scrub. Don cap, mask, sterile gown, and sterile gloves.
7. Drape off introduction site to create a large sterile field.
8. Open introducer and catheter sets. Fill proximal port line with heparinized saline; clamp and cap this line.
9. Attach distal catheter port to pressure transducer via a three-way stopcock and flush the system with heparinized saline. If any fluid line is inserted between the patient and the transducer, it must be noncompliant tubing.
10. Attach continuous flush line to the transducer and pressurize the bag to ≥200 mm Hg.
11. Zero the pressure transducer. Zeroing information can be found in Protocol 8.2.
12. Insert the introducer catheter per manufacturer's recommendations and suture in place.
13. Insert the thermodilution catheter through the introducer catheter to about 20 cm and verify that the pressure tracing reflects a central venous pressure waveform.
14. Advance the catheter with the natural curve of the catheter aimed toward the sternum of the animal; watch for a typical ventricular waveform.
15. If the catheter advances to the 50-cm mark without entering the right ventricle, withdraw it to the 20-cm mark and start again.
16. It may help to twist the catheter, a little or a lot, in either direction, to change the chance that it might enter the right ventricle.
17. If the pressure tracing becomes damped, flush the distal port with the transducer's fast flush device; if the pressure tracing abruptly ceases followed by a rapid, linear increase, the end-hole has butted up against a vessel or heart chamber wall and should be withdrawn slightly and then reinserted.
18. It may help to change the position of the animal.
19. Once the catheter tip has entered the right ventricle, inflate the balloon with 1 mL of air and advance it further until the pressure waveform indicates that the catheter tip has entered the pulmonary artery.
20. With the balloon inflated, advance the catheter until the pressure tracing reflects occlusion of a branch of the pulmonary artery; deflate the balloon and verify a good pulmonary artery tracing.
21. Bandage the catheter and introducer set aseptically and occlusively.

samples. Everything that is done with and around these catheters must be accomplished with the utmost care and asepsis. Thus, the operator should perform hand hygiene and don clean gloves each time the catheter, its ports, or its sheath is handled. See Chapter 54, Minimizing Nosocomial Infection, for more information.

Physical contact of these catheters against the endocardium, especially during introduction, is occasionally associated with arrhythmias. Simply stop or withdraw the catheter slightly and then recommence the procedure once the arrhythmia has abated. Persistent arrhythmia problems could be treated with an antiarrhythmic such as lidocaine.

Catheter-associated clot emboli may occur but there is not much one can do to prevent it. It is not typical to administer anticoagulants to patients with these catheters any more than it is for any other catheter. Heparin-coated catheters are now available that may decrease this problem. Air emboli may occur if air is inadvertently injected into the catheter or into the balloon port if the balloon has ruptured.

Pulmonary vessel trauma and rupture has been reported in people due to leaving the balloon inflated or by fully inflating the balloon after the catheter has migrated.[30] Additional rarely reported complications include pneumothorax, hemothorax, and knotting of the catheter (in the right ventricle) during removal.

Thermodilution cardiac output measurement

To measure pressure, a pressure transducer and physiologic monitor are required; to measure cardiac output, a compatible cardiac output computer is required; to measure venous blood oxygen saturation, a compatible oximeter is required; and to pace the heart, a suitable catheter-tipped pacemaker and control unit are required.

To make a cardiac output measurement, the thermistor connection is attached to the cardiac output computer. Some systems incorporate an injectate-measuring thermistor at the injection port. The computer will calculate a compensated value for the change in temperature of the injectate as it traverses the catheter. Otherwise the temperature of the injectate (room temperature or iced) will need to be measured and entered into the computer. Usually room-temperature fluid is used. Ice water temperature fluid may be necessary for signal detection when smaller volumes of fluid are used in larger patients. Injectate volume must be entered into the computer. Usually a small volume of fluid (3–5 to 10 mL; smaller volumes for smaller patients) of a crystalloid fluid such as saline is used. After recording all of the measured pressures, the operator must indicate to the computer that an injection is about to be made; the computer will indicate when it is ready for injection to begin. The designated volume of fluid is injected into the cranial vena cava or right atrium. The operator should try to make the injection at the end of exhalation and as fast as possible. The computer will measure the change in temperature as the fluid–blood mixture passes by the thermistor in the pulmonary artery and will then calculate the average change in temperature and cardiac output. Typically make three to five measurements, discard outliers, and average the rest to obtain a representative cardiac output value. Please see Protocol 12.2 for step-by-step instructions for performing pressure and cardiac output measurements.

Lithium cardiac output measurement

A central venous and an arterial catheter are placed. The lithium sensor is attached via a three-way stopcock to the arterial catheter and to the cardiac output computer. Arterial blood will be withdrawn past this sensor at a constant rate of 4 mL/min and into a collection container. Hemoglobin and sodium concentration are premeasured and entered into the computer. A sensor constant and the intended lithium dose are also entered into the computer. The dose of lithium is 0.005–0.008 mM/kg and is generally injected as a 0.015–0.15 mM/mL solution; a change in blood lithium concentration of 0.2–0.8 mM/L is recommended to obtain a good signal for cardiac output calculation. The calculated dose of lithium is placed into an extension set attached to the jugular catheter. The pump for withdrawal of arterial blood and the cardiac output computer are started. The dose of lithium is flushed into the anterior vena cava after 5–10 seconds (the computer needs a little time to establish a baseline; larger animals may require the longer delays). The sensor measures the change in lithium concentration over time and the computer calculates cardiac output. The measurement should be repeated at least once, outliers excluded, and the remaining values averaged. Please see Protocol 12.3 for detailed instructions.

Other measurements and calculations

The units of the raw cardiac output measurements are milliliters (or liters) per minute and must be indexed to the size of the patient. The size of the patient can be expressed as either kilograms of body weight or square meters (m^2) of surface area (see Table 12.1).

The measurements that can be obtained from the thermodilution catheter are central venous pressure, pulmonary artery pressure, pulmonary artery occlusion pressure, and cardiac output. In addition, mixed venous

Protocol 12.2 Thermodilution cardiac output measurement

Items Required
- Patient with indwelling pulmonary arterial catheter
- Cardiac output computer-equipped patient monitor with associated thermistor and pressure-transducer cables; power cord
- Injectate with known temperature—room temperature (measured) or iced fluid (0°C [32°F])

Procedure: Pressure Measurements
1. Perform hand hygiene and don clean examination gloves.
2. Inflate balloon while observing pressure tracing. It should take the entire 1-mL balloon volume.
3. If an occluded pressure waveform appears with less than the full 1 mL, deflate the balloon and withdraw the catheter a couple centimeters, and try again.
4. If the full 1-mL balloon inflation fails to occlude the vessel, leave the balloon inflated and advance the catheter until the vessel occludes.
5. Deflate the balloon after the occlusion pressure measurement has been made. Record the occlusion pressure.
6. Record the central venous pressure and arterial blood pressure.

Procedure: Cardiac Output Measurement
1. Perform hand hygiene and don clean examination gloves.
2. Make sure that the cardiac output computer knows the volume and temperature of the injectate (temperature is either measured or it must be input by the operator). Enter the computation constant if necessary. Make sure that the thermistor cable is attached to the computer.
3. Push the button on the cardiac output computer to tell it that you want to make a measurement; the computer will tell you when it is ready for you to inject.
4. At the end of a breath, rapidly inject a volume of injectate into the proximal port (patient weight less than 3 kg, use 3 mL; 3–25 kg, 5 mL; >25 kg, 10 mL).
5. Record the measurement.
6. Repeat measurement 3–5 times; discard outliers; average the remaining values.
7. Index to body size.

Protocol 12.3 Lithium cardiac output measurement

Items Required
- A lithium sensor and cardiac output computer
- Preplaced jugular venous and arterial catheters
- Three-way stopcock
- A roller pump and scavenge bag to withdraw blood at 4 mL/min

Procedure
1. Collect necessary supplies.
2. Perform hand hygiene and don clean examination gloves.
3. Premeasure hemoglobin and sodium concentration and enter into computer. Input sensor constant and intended lithium dose (0.005–0.008 mM/kg).
4. Attach lithium sensor, extension set, roller pump, and scavenge bag to the arterial catheter via the side-port of a three-way stopcock.
5. Measure and record central venous and arterial blood pressure.
6. Charge the extension set on the jugular catheter with the dose of lithium (0.005–0.010 mM/kg).
7. Start the roller pump and blood withdrawal at 4 mL/min and push the button to tell the computer that you are ready to make a measurement.
8. After 5–10 seconds, depending on the size of the animal (<5 kg, 5 seconds; 5–30 kg, 6–7 seconds; >30 kg, 8–10 seconds), rapidly inject the lithium at the end of a breath.
9. Repeat the measurement at least once and average similar values.
10. Index to body size.

blood samples can be obtained from the distal port of this catheter for pH and blood gas analysis. If a separate arterial catheter is placed, arterial blood pressure and arterial blood samples (for pH and blood gas analysis) can be obtained. In addition to cardiac output, measurements that can be obtained during lithium cardiac output measurements include central venous pressure and blood sampling, and arterial blood pressure and blood sampling (for pH and blood gas analysis).

Once cardiac output is measured, heart rate is measured separately and stroke volume can be calculated. When arterial and pulmonary pressure and cardiac output are measured, systemic arterial and pulmonary vascular resistance and left and right heart work indices can be calculated. When hemoglobin concentration and PO_2 are known, oxygen content can be calculated. When cardiac output and oxygen content are known, oxygen delivery can be calculated. When cardiac output and arterial and mixed-venous oxygen content are known, the oxygen consumption and extraction and the venous admixture can be calculated. Table 12.2 contains standard calculations.

Table 12.1 Body Weight to Surface Area Conversion Table*

Weight		Surface Area	Weight		Surface Area
Kilograms	Pounds	(sq meter)	Kilograms	Pounds	(sq meter)
0.5	1.1	0.06	26	57.2	0.89
1	2.2	0.10	27	59.4	0.91
2	4.4	0.16	28	61.6	0.93
3	6.6	0.21	29	63.8	0.95
4	8.8	0.25	30	66	0.98
5	11	0.29	31	68.2	1.00
6	13.2	0.33	32	70.4	1.02
7	15.4	0.37	33	72.6	1.04
8	17.6	0.40	34	74.8	1.06
9	19.8	0.44	35	77	1.08
10	22	0.47	36	79.2	1.10
11	24.2	0.50	37	81.4	1.12
12	26.4	0.53	38	83.6	1.14
13	28.6	0.56	39	85.8	1.16
14	30.8	0.59	40	88	1.18
15	33	0.61	41	90.2	1.20
16	35.2	0.64	42	92.4	1.22
17	37.4	0.67	43	94.6	1.24
18	39.6	0.69	44	96.8	1.26
19	41.8	0.72	45	99	1.28
20	44	0.74	46	101.2	1.30
21	46.2	0.77	47	103.4	1.32
22	48.4	0.79	48	105.6	1.34
23	50.6	0.82	49	107.8	1.36
24	52.8	0.84	50	110	1.38
25	55	0.86			

Source: Hand MS, Thatcher CD, Remillard RL, et al., Body surface area of dogs. In: *Small Animal Clinical Nutrition*. 4th ed. Topeka: Mark Morris Institute; 2000:1009.
*$(10.1 \times kg^{0.67})/100$.

Other methods of estimating cardiac output

Thermodilution cardiac output measurement is the standard against which other methodologies are often compared in the clinical measurement of cardiac output. Electromagnetic flowmetry is the gold standard for experimental blood flow measurement. Flow probes can be surgically placed around a suitably size-matched vessel of interest or flow catheters can be introduced into a large vessel. The application of a magnetic field perpendicular to the blood flow induces an electrical potential proportional to the blood flow velocity that can be easily and accurately calculated. Flow is calculated from flow velocity and conduit diameter. Other methods of measuring cardiac output have been recently reviewed.[31,32]

The Fick Method

The *Fick* principle assumes that flow is proportional to the rate of uptake of an indicator gas, and the difference between the concentration of the indicator gas entering and exiting the organ being studied:

$$Flow = (\text{indicator gas uptake}) \div [(\text{gas conc. in}) - (\text{gas conc. out})] \qquad (12.4)$$

Various marker gases have been used: oxygen, carbon dioxide, acetylene, and nitrous oxide. If any two parameters in this equation are known, the third can be calculated. When cardiac output is measured, for instance, arterial and venous oxygen content are calculated (from PO_2 and hemoglobin measurements; see Table 12.2), and oxygen consumption (VO_2) is calculated (flow times arterial–venous O_2 content). The venous blood sample used for these calculations must come from a central vein (pulmonary artery best; vena cava acceptable); cephalic or saphenous venous blood oxygen measurements will not do for this calculation. By the Fick equation, cardiac output can be calculated from oxygen consumption (calculated as the difference between inspired tidal volume and oxygen concentration and expired tidal volume and oxygen concentration) divided by arterial–venous O_2 content. Fick cardiac output estimates compared well with thermodilution cardiac output measurements in cats at low ($r = 0.89$) and normal ($r = 0.69$) cardiac outputs, but overestimated high ($r = 0.75$) cardiac outputs.[33] Fick cardiac output estimates compared well with dye-dilution cardiac output measurements in anesthetized dogs[34] and pigs.[13]

Arterial–venous oxygen content, oxygen extraction, venous oxygen, arterial–venous oxygen saturation

Oxygen consumption is usually not measured in clinical veterinary medicine so the whole Fick equation (Eq. 12.4) usually cannot be used. However, assuming that oxygen consumption has not changed too much (although it can easily halve [hypothermia; general anesthesia] or double [increased muscular activity] in common clinical situations), the arterial–venous oxygen content difference alone can be used to estimate the adequacy of tissue perfusion (directly related to cardiac output *if the animal is not vasoconstricted*). When oxygen delivery decreases, and oxygen uptake continues at its previous level, a greater proportion of oxygen is removed from the blood (oxygen extraction). This will

Table 12.2 Standard Formulas for Calculated Variables

Parameter	Formula
Body surface area	$(10.1 \times kg^{0.67})/100$
Alveolar PO_2 (room air)	[(barometric pressure-50) $\times$ 0.21]-($PaCO_2$/RQ), where 50 is the saturated water vapor pressure at 38.5°C, 0.21 is the fractional inspired oxygen, and RQ = 0.9
Arterial, mixed venous, and capillary oxyhemoglobin saturation	$([38{,}848/(202 \times PO_2 + 1.17 \times PO_2^2 + PO_2^3)] + 1)^{-1} \times 100$*
Arterial, mixed-venous, and pulmonary capillary oxygen content	$(1.34 \times Hb \times SO_2) + (0.003 \times PO_2)$, where 1.34 is 100% saturated hemoglobin oxygen content, SO_2 is hemoglobin saturation, PO_2 is partial pressure of oxygen in arterial, mixed venous, or capillary blood
Cardiac index	Cardiac output per square meter BSA or kilogram of body weight
Stroke volume index	CI/heart rate
Systemic vascular resistance index	(ABP-CVP) $\times$ 79.92/CI m^2 or (ABP-CVP)/CI kg
Pulmonary vascular resistance index	(PAP-PAOP) $\times$ 79.92/CI m^2 or (PAP-PAOP)/CI kg
Left and right cardiac work index	CI $\times$ ABPm $\times$ 0.0144 CI $\times$ PAPm $\times$ 0.0144
Left and right ventricular stroke work	SVI $\times$ ABPm $\times$ 0.0144 SVI $\times$ PAPm $\times$ 0.0144
Oxygen delivery	$CaO_2 \times$ (CI m^2 $\times$ 10) or (CI kg/100)
Oxygen consumption	$(CaO_2$-$CmvO_2) \times$ (CI m^2 $\times$ 10) or (CI kg/100)
Oxygen extraction	VO_2/DO_2 or CaO_2-$CmvO_2$/CaO_2
Venous admixture	$(CcO_2$-$CaO_2)/(CcO_2$-$CmvO_2)$
Arterial and venous blood carbon dioxide content	$(2.226 \times 0.0299 \times PCO_2 \times (1 + 10^{(pH-6.085)})) \times (1-((0.0289 \times Hb)/((3.352-(0.456 \times (SO_2/100))) \times (8.142$-$pH))))$**
Carbon dioxide production	$(CaCO_2$-$CmvCO_2) \times$ CI $\times$ 10

*Reeves RB, et al., Oxygen affinity and Bohr coefficients of dog blood. *J Appl Physiol* 1982;53:87–95.
**Douglas AR, et al., Calculation of whole blood CO_2 content *J Appl Physiol* 1988;65:473–477.

result in a decrease in venous oxygen and a greater difference between arterial and venous oxygen content. Arterial–venous oxygen content was reported to be 3.6 ± 1.2 mL/dL in normal dogs, increasing to 7.0 ± 1.9 mL/dL in moderately hypovolemic dogs.[35] In this same report, oxygen extraction increased from $21 \pm 6\%$ to $42 \pm 10\%$. Oxygen extraction is calculated by the following formula:

$$\text{Oxygen extraction} = (\text{Cont}_{\text{Art}} O_2 - \text{Cont}_{\text{Ven}} O_2)/ \quad \text{Cont}_{\text{Art}} O_2 \quad (12.5)$$

Central venous oxygen (partial pressure [PO_2] or saturation [SO_2]) alone (without calculating oxygen content) can also be used in this same context. Normal central venous PO_2 and SO_2 were reported to be 49 ± 6 and 78 ± 6, respectively, in normal dogs and decreased to 35 ± 5 and 56 ± 9 in moderate hypovolemia.[35] In another canine acute hemorrhage model,[36] PvO_2 decreased from 46 to 34 mm Hg. Venous PO_2 was reported to be significantly correlated with cardiac output in cats; however, there was notable variability.[33] In a cohort of critically ill humans, dobutamine augmentation of cardiac output, decreased oxygen extraction from 48% to 36% and increased mixed-venous oxygen saturation from 49% to 61%.[37] Other studies reported weak correlations between venous oxygen saturation and cardiac output in human intensive-care-unit patients[38] and in a piglet hemorrhagic shock model.[39]

Carbon dioxide–based Fick

The Fick principle and formula can also be used with carbon dioxide production:

$$\text{Flow} = (\text{carbon dioxide production})/(\text{CvCO}_2 - \text{CaCO}_2) \quad (12.6)$$

A commercial, noninvasive method for measuring cardiac output in intubated patients is available (NICO$_2$, Novametrix Medical Systems, Wallingford, CT). The method involves the transient partial rebreathing of carbon dioxide (for 50 seconds every 3 minutes). Cardiac output is calculated from end-tidal carbon dioxide concentrations during normal and CO$_2$ rebreathing episodes. End-tidal CO$_2$ (measured) and carbon dioxide solubility are used to calculate arterial CO$_2$ concentration. Inspired oxygen and arterial oxygenation are used to calculate a shunt fraction, which is used to correct for the shunted portion of cardiac output.[40,41] This method of analysis has been shown

to compare favorably with normal-range thermodilution cardiac output measurements (but overestimated cardiac output at low-range cardiac outputs and underestimated high-range cardiac outputs).[17] The NICO$_2$ system compared well with ultrasound transit time flowmetry and thermodilution during and after cardiopulmonary bypass,[7] and with lithium cardiac output measurements, across a spectrum of low to high cardiac outputs, in anesthetized dogs.[41] The NICO$_2$ system is noninvasive, easy to use, and provides near-continuous measurements.

Venous–arterial PCO$_2$

Carbon dioxide production is not measured in clinical veterinary practice and so the whole Fick equation (Eq. 12.6) cannot be used. However, assuming that carbon dioxide production has not changed too much (although it can easily halve [hypothermia; general anesthesia] or double [increased muscular activity] in common clinical situations), the venous–arterial PCO$_2$ difference alone can be used to estimate the adequacy of tissue perfusion (directly related to cardiac output *if the animal is not vasoconstricted*). When blood flow decreases, and carbon dioxide production continues at its previous level, an increase in venous carbon dioxide results in a greater difference between arterial and venous PCO$_2$. Venous–arterial PCO$_2$ was reported to be 4.2 ± 1.5 in normal dogs, increasing to 10.7 ± 3.9 in moderately hypovolemic dogs.[35] In a canine acute hemorrhage model, venous–arterial PCO$_2$ increased from 5.2 to 12.9 mm Hg.[36] Venous–arterial PCO$_2$ was 4.9 in critically ill people with normal cardiac output measurements and was 7.4 in patients with low cardiac output.[42] Venous–arterial PCO$_2$ decreased from 9 to 5 mm Hg with dobutamine augmentation of cardiac output.[37]

Pulse contour methods

The area under the pulse pressure waveform bears some correlation to stroke volume. The pulse pressure waveform can be qualitatively characterized by digital palpation of an arterial vessel; a tall, wide pulse is likely associated with a large stroke volume while a short, narrow pulse is likely associated with a small stroke volume. The pulse pressure waveform can also be measured by indirect sphygmomanometry or by direct arterial measurement.

Pulse contour methodologies calculate stroke volume from measured pulse pressure waveforms using algorithms that consider arterial impedance, compliance, and resistance. At a given arterial compliance there is a directional relationship between the change in the area under the pulse pressure waveform and the change in volume (stroke volume). Unfortunately, arterial compliance is not measured and so cardiac output must be periodically and independently verified. Once this measured cardiac output is fed into the computer, it back-calculates correction factors that will be used in future pulse-contour assessments (until it is again recalibrated). There are several commercial devices that continuously measure and assess the pulse pressure waveform.

The PiCCO$_2$ system (Pulsion Medical Systems, Irving, TX) requires a central venous and an arterial catheter. The PiCCO$_2$ system uses transpulmonary thermodilution to intermittently measure cardiac output (saline is injected into a jugular catheter and the change in temperature is measured by a thermistor in a special arterial catheter). The PiCCO$_2$ system also estimates cardiac filling volume, intrathoracic blood volume, and extravascular lung water. The PiCCO$_2$ system compared very well with thermodilution cardiac output measurements in critical human patients.[9,10,12,43–45] and in a piglet hemorrhagic shock model.[39]

The LiDCO Plus system (LiDCO Ltd Cambridge, UK) uses a pulse power analysis algorithm (PulseCO) that mathematically calculates changes in stroke volume; independent lithium indicator dilution cardiac output measurements are needed to calibrate the system. There is good agreement with thermodilution cardiac output measurements but large variability. Accuracy falls off with time and periodic recalibration (by remeasuring cardiac output) as often as every 1–2 hours may be necessary.[12] The PulseCO system has been reported to compare well with thermodilution and lithium cardiac output measurements (but overestimated cardiac output at low-range cardiac outputs and underestimated high-range cardiac outputs).[17,32,46,47] Early canine studies of pulse contour cardiac output estimates reported good correlation and accuracy compared with implanted electromagnetic flowmeter measurements[48,49] and thermodilution cardiac output measurements.[50] Several subsequent canine studies, however, have reported a high variability and poor correlation between pulse contour cardiac output estimates and lithium calibration cardiac output measurements.[51–53]

The MostCare™ device (Vytech Health, Padova, Italy) uses the pressure recording analytical method (PRAM), via perturbation theory, to estimate cardiac output just from the analysis of the pressure wave profile (requires only an arterial catheter). The PRAM algorithm characterizes the elastic properties of the arterial system from the analysis of the pulse pressure profile. The PRAM system also provides a parameter called cardiac cycle efficiency, which is an index of heart–vascular response coupling (+1 = best; −1 = worst). Cardiac cycle efficiency is a ratio between myocardial work and energy consumed, and represents an index of heart stress. PRAM compares very well with thermodilution cardiac output in people,[54] and with electromagnetic flowmetry and thermodilution cardiac output measurements in pigs across a wide range of cardiac outputs.[55]

The Portapres system (Finapress Medical Systems, Amsterdam, The Netherlands) is an ambulatory blood pressure monitoring unit that measures heart rate and blood pressure, calculates stroke volume and cardiac output, and calculates vascular resistance, compliance, and impedance. The technology compares well with thermodilution cardiac output in critically ill humans as a clinically acceptable trend monitor, but the substantial variation of measurements leads to a significant percentage of inaccurate measurements.[56,57]

The Flo Trac sensor and Vigileo monitor system (Edwards Lifesciences, Irvine, CA) utilizes user-entered anthropomorphic data (sex, age, weight, height, and surface area) to assign a value to compliance and vascular tone independent of external cardiac output measurements and system recalibration. For use in veterinary medicine, either the algorithms would need to be changed or false information would have to be entered to enable correct surface-area calculations. Flo Trac compared well with thermodilution cardiac output measurements.[32,45] The sensor can be used with any arterial catheter and no external calibration is required.

Transthoracic impedance

The transthoracic impedance method uses four paired electrodes to measure changes in transthoracic impedance during the cardiac cycle and then calculates an estimate of stroke volume. Over a cardiac cycle, the only intrathoracic fluid volume that changes is intrathoracic blood volume. The magnitude and rate of change reflects myocardial contractility. Baseline impedance is affected by other fluid accumulation diseases such as hydrothorax and pulmonary edema. A meta-analysis of thoracic impedance technology concluded that the technique may only be sufficiently accurate as a trend monitor.[58] There are several commercial devices that measure and assess the thoracic impedance.

The BioZ ICG system (Cardiodynamics, San Diego, CA, subsidiary of Sonosite, Bothel, WA) evaluates heart rate, blood pressure, cardiac output, systemic vascular resistance, systolic time ratio (an index of myocardial contractility), and thoracic fluid content. Studies generally report moderate correlation with thermodilution cardiac output measurements[59,60] or between thoracic fluid content and the amount of fluid removed by hemodialysis.[61]

Electrical cardiometry (Icon and Aesculon [Cardiotronic, Inc. La Jolla, CA]) utilizes electrical velocimetry (changes in thoracic conductivity caused by the alignment of red blood cells) to calculate heart rate, stroke volume, cardiac output, systolic time ratio, an index of contractility, and thoracic fluid index. Electrical velocimetry estimates of cardiac output compared favorably with transpulmonary thermodilution cardiac output measurements in piglets.[11]

The RheoCardioMonitor (ACMA, Ltd, Singapore) assesses cardiac output and compared well to thermodilution cardiac output measurements in pigs[62] and people.[63]

The Niccomo instrument (Medis, Ilmenau, Germany) measures heart rate and blood pressure and utilizes a physiological adaptive signal analysis (PASA) algorithm to calculate stroke volume, cardiac output, systemic vascular resistance, thoracic fluid content, left cardiac work index, several indices of contractility, and systolic time intervals. The company also produces computer-based impedance cardiography interfaces, using the same technology as the Niccomo that can run on any personal computer (Cardioscreen 1000 and 2000). The PASA-algorithm-derived cardiac output correlated well with thermodilution in people[64]; other studies reported only modest correlation between impedance-estimated cardiac output and transthoracic Doppler cardiography[65] and thermodilution cardiac output.[56]

Whole-body impedance estimates of cardiac output correlated well with thermodilution cardiac output measurements in one study[66] but not in another.[67]

Doppler ultrasound

Standard echocardiography, operated by experienced individuals, can be used to measure aortic or pulmonary valve diameter and the velocity–time integral, from which stroke volume can be calculated. Accurate assessment of the diameter of the outflow tract is difficult, and measurements are intermittent and not a readily viable option for critical care settings. Echocardiographic estimated cardiac output did not correlate well with thermodilution cardiac output measurements in cats.[33] In a hemorrhage model in dogs, the pulmonic valve, compared with the aortic valve, and proximal and distal aorta, was the site that generated the most repeatable Doppler measurements,[36] but none of the echocardiographic cardiac output determinations compared very well with thermodilution.

The ultrasound cardiac output monitor (USCOM, Uscom Ltd, Sydney, Australia) uses continuous-wave Doppler and anthropomorphic aortic and pulmonary valve data to calculate stroke volume. There are no reports of its use in dogs and cats.

Doppler probes can also be placed into the esophagus and positioned so as to face the descending thoracic aorta (Hemosonic 100, Arrow International, Reading, PA; Dynemo 3000, Sometec, Paris). The ultrasound transducer is positioned as close as possible to the direction of blood flow (corrections are made to the measurement to compensate for the angle between the direction of the ultrasound beam and that of the blood flow). The phase shift in the reflected ultrasound waves as they are carried downstream by the flowing blood is used to calculate blood flow velocity. Flow velocity and time are used to calculate stroke distance, and stroke distance times cross-sectional area of the aorta (measured or anthropomorphically determined) is used to calculate stroke volume. A major assumption of this technique is that a constant proportion of the cardiac output flows through the descending aorta (the remainder going through the brachiocephalic and coronary arteries). Unfortunately this is variable; hypovolemia decreases and vasodilation increases the proportion of the cardiac output entering the descending aorta. Although some reports suggest good correlation with thermodilution cardiac output,[44,68–70] other reports suggest a variable correlation.[71] Use of the technique has been reported in anesthetized dogs, but cardiac output values were not reported.[72] Transesophageal probes are large, anesthesia is required to introduce them, and they cannot be fixed in place for continuous measurements.

Other methods

Velocity encoded phase contrast magnetic resonance imaging is a very accurate technique for measuring flow in large vessels.[73] Nuclear scintigraphy can also be used to evaluate cardiac output.[74] The equipment is very expensive, requires considerable training to operate, and the measurements are intermittent. These techniques do not lend themselves to use in the intensive care unit.

Interpreting measurements

There is a large amount of cardiopulmonary function information that can be derived when cardiac output is measured (see Fig. 12.4 and Table 12.3). This allows for broader characterization of patient status and may improve survival opportunities for some patients. Since forward flow is dependent upon venous return, it is

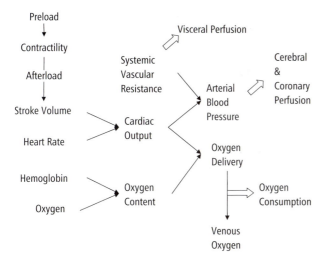

Figure 12.4 Integrated cardiopulmonary function: preload determines diastolic filling of the heart; contractility is the strength of load-independent contraction of the ventricles; afterload is the pressure against which the heart must contract to generate a stroke volume; stroke volume and heart rate determine cardiac output; hemoglobin concentration and the amount of oxygen loaded onto it determine oxygen content; cardiac output and systemic vascular resistance determine arterial blood pressure; arterial blood pressure is primarily important as a determinant of cerebral and coronary perfusion; systemic vascular resistance is primarily important as a determinant of visceral tissue perfusion; cardiac output and oxygen content determine oxygen delivery; oxygen delivery minus oxygen consumption determine venous oxygen.

appropriate to first evaluate preload parameters. Central venous pressure represents preload pressure to the right heart (0–10 mm Hg); pulmonary artery occlusion pressure represents preload pressure to the left heart (2–12 mm Hg). Low pressures suggest that there is room for additional blood volume augmentation if other parameters corroborate hypovolemia. High pressures may represent hypervolemia or heart failure, and suggest that additional volume loading may be unwarranted. Preload pressure has a variable relationship to preload volume, depending upon ventricular compliance. High preload pressure does not necessarily define high preload but it always necessitates a conservative fluid plan.

Next evaluate arterial blood pressure. Low mean arterial blood pressure (<60 mm Hg) could be caused by hypovolemia (check preload parameters), poor cardiac output (measure cardiac output; check for cardiac disease), or vasodilation (calculate systemic vascular resistance; check clinical vasomotor tone signs). High mean systemic arterial pressure (>140 mm Hg) is usually attributable to high vasomotor tone (iatrogenic hyper-

volemia is possible; high cardiac output and arteriosclerosis are unlikely).

Next evaluate cardiac output. Low cardiac output could be caused by the following: hypovolemia (check the preload parameters); cardiac disease (atrioventricular [AV] insufficiency, aortic stenosis, fibrosis, pericardial tamponade); poor contractility (if not measured, then presumed if preload parameters are high and forward flow parameters are low, in the absence of anatomic cardiac disease). Low cardiac output should be treated if it is associated with hypotension or evidence of poor tissue perfusion.

Next evaluate systemic vascular resistance. Low vascular resistance (vasodilation) may be associated with hypotension, in which case, it should be treated by administering a vasoconstrictor. Low vascular resistance associated with acceptable blood pressure does not need to be treated. High vascular resistance (vasoconstriction) may be associated with poor tissue perfusion. If associated with high blood pressure, the situation may benefit from judicious vasodilator therapy. However, if associated with marginal blood pressure, the condition should not be specifically treated because it is probably compensation for hypovolemia or marginal cardiac output, and vasodilator administration will probably cause hypotension.

Next evaluate oxygen content, delivery, consumption, and extraction. Low oxygen content is most likely caused by anemia. Low oxygen delivery may be caused by low oxygen content or low cardiac output. Low oxygen consumption may be caused by low oxygen delivery or impaired metabolism. High oxygen extraction is usually indicative of low oxygen delivery; low oxygen extraction may be caused by impaired cellular metabolism or peripheral arterial–venous shunting. Venous oxygen is low when oxygen extraction is high, and vice-versa; the assessments are the same.

Conclusion

Determination of cardiac output and systemic oxygen delivery can be helpful in patients with perfusion status that is poorly defined by other methods or that do not respond to therapy. Cardiac output can be measured many ways but the common clinically applicable techniques involve indicator dilution, usually either thermodilution with the balloon-tipped pulmonary arterial catheter or lithium dilution. Though it is unclear whether use of this advanced monitoring improves outcome, certainly outcome can only be improved if the technique is performed properly, the results interpreted correctly, and the appropriate therapy instituted.

Table 12.3 Cardiopulmonary Values in Normal Dogs[75]

Parameter	Units	Baseline $n = 97$ Mean ± SD	95% Confidence Interval
BW	kg	20.5 ± 6.9	
BSA	m²	0.74 ± 0.17	
Temp	°C	38.4 ± 0.6	38.3–38.5
pHa	Units	7.381 ± 0.025	7.376–7.387
$PaCO_2$	mm Hg	40.2 ± 3.4	39.5–41.0
HCO_3a	mEq/L	23.1 ± 2.0	22.7–23.5
BDa	mEq/L	−2.1 ± 2.3	−1.7 to −2.6
pHmv	Units	7.362 ± 0.027	7.356–7.367
$PmvCO_2$	mm Hg	44.1 ± 3.8	43.3–44.9
HCO_3mv	mEq/L	24.2 ± 2.1	23.7–24.6
BDmv	mEq/L	−1.9 ± 2.3	−1.4 to −2.3
a–mv pH	Units	0.020 ± 0.012	0.018–0.022
a–mv PCO_2	mm Hg	−3.9 ± 1.6	−3.6 to −4.2
a–mv HCO_3	mEq/L	−1.1 ± 0.7	−0.9 to −1.2
a–mv BD	mEq/L	0.2 ± 0.7	0.1–0.4
PaO_2	mm Hg	99.5 ± 6.8	98.1–100.8
SaO_2	%	96.3 ± 0.9	96.1–96.5
Hb	g/dL	13.6 ± 1.8	13.3–14.0
CaO_2	mL/dL	17.8 ± 2.3	17.4–18.3
$PmvO_2$	mm Hg	49.3 ± 5.8	48.2–50.5
$SmvO_2$	%	77.1 ± 5.5	75.6–78.2
$CmvO_2$	mL/dL	14.2 ± 2.2	13.8–14.7
Ca–vO_2	mL/dL	3.6 ± 1.0	3.4–3.8
PAO_2	mm Hg	105.8 ± 3.7	105.1–106.9
A–aPO_2	mm Hg	5.5 ± 6.9	3.6–7.4
ScO_2	%	96.9 ± 0.5	96.8–97.0
CcO_2	mL/dL	18.0 ± 2.3	17.5–18.5
Ven admix	%	3.6 ± 4.1	2.8–4.4
$CaCO_2$	mL/dL	45.8 ± 4.3	44.9–46.6
$CmvCO_2$	mL/dL	48.5 ± 4.4	47.6–49.4
Ca–vCO_2	mL/dL	2.7 ± 1.4	2.5–3.0
CVP	cm H_2O	3.1 ± 4.1	2.3–4.0
PAOP	mm Hg	5.5 ± 2.9	4.8–6.2
HR	Beats/min	87 ± 22	83.0–91.8

Table 12.3 (*Continued*)

Parameter	Units	Baseline n = 97 Mean ± SD	95% Confidence Interval
ABPm	mm Hg	103 ± 15	99.9–106.0
PAPm	mm Hg	14.0 ± 3.2	13.4–14.7
CO	mL/min	3360 ± 1356	3086–3633
CI	L/min/m^2	4.42 ± 1.24	4.17–4.67
	mL/min/kg	165 ± 43	156–174
SVI	mL/beat/m^2	51.9 ± 13.5	49.2–54.7
	mL/beat/kg	1.93 ± 0.46	1.84–2.02
SVRI	dyne·sec·cm^{-5}/m^2	1931 ± 572	1815–2045
	mm Hg/mL/min/kg	0.641 ± 0.173	0.606–0.676
PVRI	dyne·sec·cm^{-5}/m^2	196 ± 78	179–210
	mm Hg/mL/min/kg	0.065 ± 0.026	0.060–0.070
LCWI	kg·min/m^2	6.6 ± 2.3	6.2–7.1
	mm Hg/mL/min/kg	17,045 ± 5393	15,957–18,132
LVSWI	g·min/m^2	76.7 ± 24.5	71.7–81.6
	mm Hg/mL/min/kg	199 ± 54	188–210
LVRPP	Beats/min mm Hg	9057 ± 2937	8465–9649
RCWI	kg·min/m^2	0.91 ± 0.41	0.83–0.99
	mm Hg/mL/min/kg	2353 ± 981	2156–2551
RVSWI	g·min/m^2	10.4 ± 3.9	9.6–11.2
	mm Hg/mL/min/kg	27.1 ± 9.1	25.2–28.9
RVRPP	Beats/min mm Hg	1247 ± 510	1144–1350
DO$_2$	mL/min/m^2	790 ± 259	737–842
	mL/min/kg	29.5 ± 8.8	27.7–31.3
VO$_2$	mL/min/m^2	164 ± 71	148–181
	mL/min/kg	6.0 ± 2.6	5.5–6.5
O$_2$ extrac	%	20.5 ± 5.7	19.4–21.7
VCO$_2$	mL/min/m^2	128 ± 46	114–136

Source: Haskins SC, Pascoe PJ, Ilkiw JE, Fudge M, Hopper K, Aldrich J. Reference cardiopulmonary values in normal dogs. *Comparative Medicine* 2005;55:158–163.

BW, body weight; BSA, body surface area; a, arterial; mv, mixed venous; A, alveolar; c, capillary; a–v, arterial–mixed venous; m, mean; A–a, alveolar–arterial; PCO$_2$, partial pressure of carbon dioxide; HCO$_3$, bicarbonate; BD, base deficit; PO$_2$, partial pressure of oxygen; SO$_2$, hemoglobin saturation with oxygen; Hb, hemoglobin; C, content; O$_2$, oxygen; CO$_2$, carbon dioxide; ven admix, venous admixture; HR, heart rate; ABPm, mean arterial blood pressure; CVP, central venous pressure; PAPm, mean pulmonary arterial blood pressure; PAOP, pulmonary artery occlusion pressure; CO, cardiac output; CI, cardiac index; SVI, stroke volume index; SVRI, systemic vascular resistance index; PVRI, pulmonary vascular resistance index; LCWI, left cardiac work index; LVSWI, left ventricular stroke work index; RCWI, right cardiac work index; RVSWI, right ventricular stroke work index; LVRPP, left ventricular rate pressure product; RVRPP, right ventricular rate pressure product; DO$_2$, oxygen delivery; VO$_2$, oxygen consumption; O$_2$ extrac, oxygen extraction; VCO$_2$, carbon dioxide production.

References

1. Powner DJ, Snyder JV. In vitro comparison of six commercially available thermodilution cardiac output systems. Med Instrum 1978;12:122–127.

2. Bilfinger TV, Lin CY, Anagnostopoulos CE. In vitro determination of accuracy of cardiac output measurements by thermal dilution. J Surg Res 1982;33:409–414.

3. Dyson DH, McDonell WN, Horne JA. Accuracy of thermodilution measurement of cardiac output in low flows applicable to feline and small canine patients. Can J Comp Med 1984;48:425–427.

4. Norris SL, King EG, Grace M, Weir B. Thermodilution cardiac output—an in vitro model of low flow states. Crit Care Med 1986;14:57–59.

5. Sorensen MB, Bille-Brahe NE, Engell HC. Cardiac output measurement by thermal dilution: reproducibility and comparison with the dye-dilution technique. Ann Surg 1976;183:67–72.

6. Pelletier C. Cardiac output measurement by thermodilution. Can J Surg 1979;22:347–350.

7. Botero M, Kirby D, Lobato EB, Staples ED, Gravenstein N. Measurement of cardiac output before and after cardiopulmonary bypass: comparison among aortic transit-time ultrasound, thermodilution and noninvasive partial CO_2 rebreathing. J Cardiothorac Vasc Anaesth 2004;18:563–572.

8. Sakka SG, Reinahrt K, Meier-Hellman A. Comparison of pulmonary artery and arterial thermodilution cardiac output in critically ill patients. Intensive Care Med 1999;25:843–846.

9. Geodje O, Hoeke K, Lichtwarck-Aschoff M, Faltchauser A, Lamm P, Reichart B. Continuous cardiac output by femoral arterial thermodilution calibrated pulse contour analysis: comparison with pulmonary arterial thermodilution. Crit Care Med 1999;27:2407–2412.

10. Della Rocca G, Costa MG, Coccia C, Pompei L, DiMarco P, Vilardi V, Pietropaoli P. Cardiac output monitoring: aortic transpulmonary thermodilution and pulse contour analysis agree with standard thermodilution methods in patients undergoing lung transplantation. Can J Anaesth 2003;50:707–711.

11. Osthaus WA, Huber D, Beck C, Winterhalter M, Boethig D, Wessel A, Sumpelmann R. Comparison of electrical velocimetry and transpulmonary thermodilution for measuring cardiac output in piglets. Paediatr Anaesth 2007;17:749–755.

12. Hamzaoui O, Monnet X, Richard C, Osman D, Chemia D, Teboul JL. Effects of changes in vascular tone on the agreement between pulse contour and transpulmonary thermodilution cardiac outpt measurements within an up to 6-hour calibration-free period. Crit Care Med 2008;36:434–440.

13. Thrush D, Downs JB, Smith RA. Continuous thermodilution cardiac output agreement with Fick and bolus thermodilution methods. J Cardiothorac Vasc Anesth 1995;9:399–404.

14. Watt RC, Loeb RG, Orr J. Comparison of a new non-invasive cardiac output technique with invasive bolus and continuous thermodilution. Anesthesiology 1998;89:A536.

15. Zollner C, Polasek J, Kilger E, Pichler B, Jaenicke U, Briegel J, Vetter H, Haller M. Evaluation of a new continuous thermodilution cardiac output monitor in cardiac surgical patients: a prospective criterion standard study. Crit Care Med 1999;27:293–298.

16. O'Malley P, Smith B, Hamlin R, Nickel J, Nakayama T, MacVicar M, Mann B. A comparison of bolus versus continuous cardiac output in an experimental model of heart failure. Crit Care Med 2000;28:1985–1990.

17. Kothari N, Amaria T, Hegde A, Mandke A, Mandke NV. Measurement of cardiac output; comparison of four different methods. Ind J Thorac Cardiovasc Surg 2003;19:163–168.

18. Shoemaker WC, Appel PL, Kram HB, Waxman K, Lee TS. Prospective trial of supranormal values of survivors as therapeutic goals in high risk surgical patients. Chest 1988;94:1176–1186.

19. Ivanov R, Allen J, Calvin JE. The incidence of major morbidity in critically ill patients managed with pulmonary artery catheters: a meta-analysis. Crit Care Med 2000;28:615–619.

20. Binanay C, Califf RM, Hasselblad V, et al. Evaluation study of congestive heart failure and pulmonary artery catheterization effectiveness: the ESCAPE trial. JAMA 2005;294:1625–1633.

21. Hall JB. Searching for evidence to support pulmonary artery catheter use in critically ill patients. JAMA 2005;294(13):1693–1694.

22. Pinsky MR, Vincent JL. Let us use the pulmonary artery catheter correctly and only when we need it. Crit Care Med 2005;33:1119–1122.

23. Harvey S, Stevens K, Harrison D, Young D, Brampton W, McCabe C. An evaluation of the clinical and cost-effectiveness of pulmonary artery catheters in patient management in intensive care: a systematic review and randomised controlled trial. Health Technol Assess 2006;10: iii–iv, ix–xi, 1–133.

24. Friese RS, Shafi S, Gentilello LM. Pulmonary artery catheter use is associated with reduced mortality in severely injured patients: a National Trauma Data Bank analysis of 53,312 patients. Crit Care Med 2006;34:1597–1601.

25. Hori T, Yamamoto C, Yagi S, Lida T, Taniguchi K, Hasegawa T, Yamakado K, Hori Y, Takeda K, Maruyama K, Uemoto S. Assessment of cardiac output in liver transplantation recipients. Heptobiliary Pancreat Dis Int 2008;4:362–366.

26. Maarek HM, Holschneider DP, Harimoto J, Yang J, Scremin OU, Rubinstein EH. Measurement of cardiac output with indocyanine green transcutaneous fluorescence dilution technique. Anesthesiology 2004;100:1476–1483.

27. Mason DJ, O'Grady M, Woods P, McDonell W. Assessment of lithium dilution cardiac output as a technique for measurement of cardiac output in dogs. Am J Vet Res 2001;62:1255–1261.

28. Bealieu KE, Kerr CL, McDonell WN. Evaluation of a lithium cardiac output technique as a method for measurement of cardiac output in anesthetized cats. Am J Vet Res 2005;66:1639–1645.

29. Corley KTT, Donaldson LL, Furr MO. Comparison of lithium dilution and thermodilution cardiac output measurements in anaesthetised neonatal foals. Equine Vet J 2002;34:598–601.

30. Kelso LA. Complications associated with pulmonary artery catheterization. New Horizons 1997;6:259–263.

31. Mathews L, Singh KRK. Cardiac output monitoring. Ann Cardiac Anaesth 2008;11:56–68.

32. deWaal EEC, Kalkman CJ, Rex S, Buhre W. Validation of a new arterial pulse contour–based cardiac output device. Crit Care Med 2007;35:1904–1909.

33. Dyson DH, Allen DG, McDonell WN. Evaluation of three methods for cardiac output determination in cats. Am J Vet Res 1985;46:2546–2552.

34. Noe FE, Whitty AJ, Davies KR. Simultaneous computer-calculated carbon dioxide and oxygen direct Fick and dye dilution measurements of cardiac output in dogs. Acta Anaesthesiol Scand 1981;25:12–16.

35. Haskins SC, Pascoe PJ, Ilkiw JE, Fudge M, Hopper K, Aldrich J. The effect of moderate hypovolemia on cardiopulmonary function in dogs. J Vet Emerg Crit Care 2005;15:100–109.

36. Day TK, Boyle CR, Holland M. Lack of agreement between thermodilution and echocardiographic determination of cardiac output during normovolemia and acute hemorrhage in clinically healthy, anesthetized dogs. J Vet Emerg Crit Care 2007;17: 22–31.

37. Teboul JL, Mercat A, Lenique F, Berton C, Richard C. Value of the venous–arterial PCO$_2$ gradient to reflect the oxygen supply to demand in humans: effects of dobutamine. Crit Care Med 1998;26:979–980.

38. Mahutte CK, Jaffe MB, Sasse SA, Chen PA, Berry RB, Sassoon CSH. Relationship of thermodilution cardiac output to metabolic measurements and mixed venous oxygen saturation. Chest 1993;104:1236–1242.

39. Piehl MD, Manning JE, McCurdy SL, Rhue TS, Kocis KC, Cairns CB, Cairns BA. Pulse contour cardiac output analysis in a piglet model of severe hemorrhagic shock. Crit Care Med 2008; 36:1189–1195.

40. Guzzi L, Jaffe MB, Orr JA. Clinical evaluation of a new noninvasive method of cardiac output measurement: preliminary results in CABG patients. Anesthesiology 1998;89:A543

41. Gunkel CI, Valverde A, Morey TE, Hernandez J, Robertson SA. Comparison of non-invasive cardiac output measurement by partial carbon dioxide rebreathing with the lithium dilution method in anesthetized dogs. J Vet Emerg Crit Care 2004; 14:187–195.

42. Durkin R, Gergits MA, Reed JF, Fitzgibbons J. The relationship between the arteriovenous carbon dioxide gradient and cardiac index. J Crit Care 1993;8:217–221.

43. Godje O, Hoke K, Goetz AE, Felbinger TW, Reuter DA, Reichart B, Friedle R, Hannekum A, Pfeiffer UJ. Reliability of a new algorithm for continuous cardiac output determination by pulse-contour analysis during hemodynamic instability. Crit Care Med 2002;30:52–58.

44. Bein B, Worthmann F, Tonner PH, Paris A, Steinfath M, Hedderich J, et al. Comparison of esophageal Doppler, pulse contour analysis and real-time pulmonary artery thermodilution for the continuous measurement of cardiac output. J Cardiothorac Vasc Anaesth 2004;18:185–189.

45. Chakravarthy M, Patil TA, Jayaprakash K, Kalligudd P, Prabhakumar D, Jawali V. Comparison of simultaneous estimation of cardiac output by four techniques in patients undergoing off-pump coronary artery bypass surgery—a prospective observational study. Ann Card Anaesth 2007;10:121–126.

46. Pittman J, Bar-Yosef S, SumPing J, Sherwood M, Mark J. Continuous cardiac output monitoring with pulse contour analysis: a comparison with lithium indicator dilution cardiac output measurement. Crit Care Med 2005;33:2015–2021.

47. Linton NW, Linton RA. Estimation of changes in cardiac output from the arterial blood pressure waveform in the upper limb. Br J Anaesth 2001;86:486–496.

48. Cibulski AA, Lehan PH, Raju S, Keister TL, Bennet KR, Hellems HK. Pulmonary arterial pressure method for estimating the ventricular stroke volume. Am Heart J 1974;88:338–342.

49. Bourgeois MJ, Gilbert BK, Bernuth G, Wood EH. Continuous determination of beat-to-beat stroke volume from aortic pressure pulses in the dog. Circ Res 1976;39:15–24.

50. English JB, Hodges MR, Sentker K, Johansen R, Stanley TH. Comparison of aortic pulse-wave contour analysis and thermodilution methods of measuring cardiac output during anesthesia in the dog. Anesthesiology 1980;52:56–61.

51. Chen HC, Sinclair MD, Dyson DH, et al. Comparison of arterial pressure waveform analysis with the lithium dilution technique to monitor cardiac output in anesthetized dogs. Am J Vet Res 2005;66:1430–1436.

52. Cooper ES, Muir WW. Continuous cardiac output monitoring via arterial pressure waveform analysis following severe hemorrhagic shock in dogs. Crit Care Med 2007;35:1724–1729.

53. Duffy AL, Butler AL, Radecki SV, Campbell VL. Comparison of continuous arterial pressure waveform analysis with the lithium dilution technique to monitor cardiac output in conscious dogs with systemic inflammatory response synsdrome. Am J Vet Res 2009;70:1365–1373.

54. Romano SM, Pistolesi M. Assessment of cardiac output from systemic arterial pressure in humans. Crit Care Med 2002; 30:1834–1841.

55. Scolletta S, Romano SM, Biagioli B, Capannini G, Giomarelli P. Pressure recording analytical method (PRAM) for measurement of cardiac output during various haemodynamic states. Br J Anaesth 2005;95:159–165.

56. Hirschl MM, Kittler H, Woisetschlager C, Siostrzonek P, Staudinger T, Kofler J, Oschatz E, Bur A, Gwechenberger M, Laggner AN. Simultaneous comparison of thoracic bioimpedance and arterial pulse waveform–derived cardiac output with thermodilution measurement. Crit Care Med 2000;28:1798–1802.

57. Jellema WT, Wesseling KH, Groeneveid ABJ, Stoutenbeek CP, Thijs LG, van Lieshout JJ. Continuous cardiac output in septic shock by simulating a model of the aortic input impedance. Anesthesiology 1999;90:1317–1328.

58. Raaijmakers E, Faes TJC, Scholten RJPM, Goovaerts HG, Heethaar RM. A meta-analysis of three decades of validating thoracic impedance cardiography. Crit Care Med 1999;27: 1203–1213.

59. Albert NM, Hail MD, Li J, Young JB. Equivalence of the bioimpedance and thermodilution methods in measuring cardiac output in hospitalized patients with advanced, decompensated chronic heart failure. Am J Crit Care 2004;13: 469–479.

60. Kamath SA, Drazner MH, Tasissa G, Rogers JG, Stevenson LW, Yancy CW. Correlation of impedance cardiography with invasive hemodynamic measurements in patients with advanced heart failure: the bioimpedance cardiography (BIG) substudy of the ESCAPE trial. Am Heart J 2009;158:217–223.

61. Wynne JL, Ovadie LO, Akride CM, Sheppard SW, Vogel RL, Van De Water JM. Impedance cardiography: a potential monitor for hemodialysis. J Surg Res 2006;133:55–60.

62. Haryadi DG, Westenskow DR, Critchley LAH, Schookin SI, Zubenko VG, Beliaev KR, Morozov AA. Evaluation of a new advanced thoracic bioimpedance device for estimation of cardiac output. J Clin Monitoring Computing 1999;15:131–138.

63. Barin E, Haryadi DG, Schookin SI, Westenskow DR, Zubenko VG, Beliaev KR, Morozov AA. Evaluation of a thoracic bioimpedance cardiac output monitor during cardiac catheterization. Crit Care Med 2000;28:698–702.

64. Sherhag A, Kaden JJ, Kentschke E, Sueselbeck T, Borggrefe M. Comparison of impedance cardiography and thermodilution-derived measurements of stroke volume and cardiac output at rest and during exercise testing. Cardiovasc Drugs Therapy 2005;19:141–147.

65. Fellahi JL, Caille V, Charron C, Deschamps-Berger PH, Viellard-Baron A. Noninvasive assessment of cardiac index in healthy volunteers: a comparison between thoracic impedance cardiogaphy and Doppler echocardiography. Anesth Analg 2009;108: 1553–1559.

BISHOP BURTON COLLEGE

66. Koobi T, Kaukinen S, Turjanmaa VMH. Cardiac output can be reliably measured noninvasively after coronary artery bypass grafting operation. Crit Care Med 1999;27:2206–2211.

67. Imhoff M, Lehner JH, Lohlein D. Noninvasive whole-body electrical bioimpedance cardiac output and invasive thermodilution cardiac output in high-risk surgical patients. Crit Care Med 2000;28:2812–2818.

68. Cariou A, Monchi M, Joly LM, Bellenfant F, Claessens YE, Thebert D, Brunet F, Dhainaut JF. Noninvasive cardiac output monitoring by aortic blood flow determination: evaluation of the Sometec Dynemo-3000 system. Crit Care Med 1998;26:2066–2072.

69. Perrino AC Jr, Harris SN, Luther MA. Intraoperative determination of cardiac output using multiplane transesophageal echocardiography: a comparison to thermodilution. Anesthesiology 1998;89:350–357.

70. Tibby SM, Hatherill M, Murdoch IA. Use of transesophageal Doppler ultrasonography in ventilated pediatric patients: derivation of cardiac output. Crit Care Med 2000;28:2045–2050.

71. Estagnasie P, Djedaini K, Mier L, Coste F, Dreyfuss D. Measurement of cardiac output by transesophageal echocardiography in mechanically ventilated patients. Comparison with thermodilution. Intensive Care Med 1997;23:753–759.

72. Wall PL, Rudison MM, Lazic T, Reidesel DH. Transesophageal monitoring of aortic blood flow during nonemergent canine surgeries. J Vet Emerg Crit Care 2002;12:1–8.

73. Arheden H, Stahlberg F. Blood flow measurements. In: Roos A de, Higgins CB, eds. MRI and CT of the Cardiovascular System. 2nd ed. Philadelphia: Lippincott ,Williams & Wilkins; 2006:71–90.

74. Kupinski MA, Hoppin JW, Krasnow J, Dahlberg S, Leppo JA, King MA, Barrett CE. Comparing cardiac ejection fraction estimation algorithms without a gold standard. Acad Radiol 2006;13:329–337.

75. Haskins SC, Pascoe PJ, Ilkiw JE, Fudge M, Hopper K, Aldrich J. Reference cardiopulmonary values in normal dogs. Comparative Medicine 2005;55:158–163.

13

Bedside echocardiography

Romain Pariaut

Bedside transthoracic echocardiography is a powerful tool for rapid assessment of the cardiovascular system. It provides information that cannot be obtained from physical examination and radiography alone. Moreover, echocardiography is noninvasive, displays a dynamic, live image of cardiac structures, and, in contrast to radiography, it does not expose personnel and patient to ionizing radiation. However, bedside echocardiography has some obvious limitations. First, it demands technical skills in order to acquire good-quality images and experience to accurately interpret echocardiographic findings. Second, acquisition of high-quality images in an intensive care unit or an emergency room is often difficult because of space constraints, difficult positioning of patients, and poor lighting. Therefore, it is important to know these limitations and not overinterpret or rely too heavily on suboptimal echocardiographic images. Finally, bedside echocardiography should not replace a thorough physical examination or delay life-saving procedures.

Principles of echocardiography

Transthoracic echocardiography uses the physical principle of ultrasound wave reflection from tissue interfaces. The reflected waves are received by the transducer and processed by the echocardiograph, which displays a grayscale dynamic two-dimensional image of the heart. Ultrasound waves transmit poorly through gas; therefore lungs markedly interfere with cardiac imaging. Similarly, bones are obstacles to the propagation of ultrasound waves and prevent visualization of deeper structures. In dogs and cats, the heart can usually be imaged from one left and one right acoustic window along the sternal border, between the ribs, at the level of the pulmonary cardiac notch (fourth to fifth intercostal space). In this region of the thorax, the heart is in direct contact with the chest wall, without intervening lungs.[1]

The frequency of the ultrasound waves (always above 20,000 Hertz [Hz]) determines the resolution of the image and the depth of tissues that can be visualized. High-frequency transducers (around 10 megahertz [MHz]) increase the resolution of the image but only penetrate a few centimeters of tissue. They are used for cats and small dogs. Lower frequency transducers can image tissues 20–30 cm deep with a diminished resolution. Typically, transducers with a frequency of 5–8 MHz are used for medium-size dogs, and transducers with a frequency of 3–5 MHz are selected for large and giant-breed dogs. The transducer with the highest frequency that penetrates deep enough to provide an image of the entire heart should be selected.

In the two-dimensional (2D) mode, the echocardiograph displays a plane of the heart in real time. By moving the transducer, the operator can obtain anatomical views of the heart from various levels and angles. Echocardiographic views and measurements have been standardized.[2]

M-mode echocardiography was mainly used before two-dimensional echocardiography was developed. It provides a one-dimensional view of the heart that is displayed over time. Interpretation of M-mode images is much less intuitive than two-dimensional images. Because image resolution is much higher than in two-dimensional mode and more than one cardiac cycle can be displayed on a single frame, M-mode echocardiography is still

Advanced Monitoring and Procedures for Small Animal Emergency and Critical Care, First Edition. Edited by Jamie M. Burkitt Creedon, Harold Davis.
© 2012 John Wiley & Sons, Inc. Published 2012 by John Wiley & Sons, Inc.

used to measure left ventricular internal diameter and wall thicknesses over the cardiac cycle. In the emergency setting, M-mode echocardiography is usually not required, as the objective of the examination is primarily to obtain an overview of the cardiac structure and function. Additionally, all the measurements acquired from an M-mode image can also be obtained from a two-dimensional still image.

Doppler echocardiography is used to evaluate blood flow direction and velocity. It is based on the detection of a change in frequency of the ultrasound waves that are reflected after they hit red blood cells moving away from or toward the transducer. Accurate assessment of blood flow can only be obtained if the flow is nearly parallel to the ultrasound beam (Doppler angle of 0°). Accuracy of blood flow velocity measurements is markedly decreased when the Doppler angle is above 20°.[3] Typically, no signal can be detected if blood flow is perpendicular to the ultrasound beam. Doppler echocardiography can be divided into color mode and spectral mode. Color Doppler is the most useful tool for bedside echocardiography.

Color mode is the most recent development of the Doppler technique. It color-codes blood flow direction and velocity on a two-dimensional image. By convention, blood flowing toward the transducer is color-coded in red, and blood flow moving away from the transducer is color-coded in blue. Brighter colors indicate higher velocity flow. Blood turbulence is displayed in green or as a mosaic of colors, which makes color Doppler very useful for the assessment of valvular stenosis and insufficiency and vascular shunts. Doppler settings are adjusted to show a predetermined range of blood flow velocities. The preselected color map and range of velocities (velocity scale) are usually displayed on the top right of the monitor screen. For the purpose of bedside echocardiography, the scale is usually set to record the widest range of velocities.

Instrumentation

Many different models of echocardiographs are currently available. Each echocardiograph can usually be customized to the needs of the operator. However, every echocardiographic system should include the following important features. First, two or three transducers covering a range of frequencies are recommended to obtain adequate images in animals of various sizes. Phased-array transducers are specifically designed for echocardiography. They have a small contact surface, so they can easily be manipulated between the ribs. Linear transducers are not adapted for echocardiography. Second, color flow Doppler should be available, as

it allows rapid interrogation of large areas to assess abnormal blood flow. Third, a port to connect electrocardiograph (ECG) cables must be available on the echocardiograph. This allows continuous display of an electrocardiographic tracing on the monitor screen during the examination.

There is also the option to choose between a portable echocardiograph and a standard system. A portable, battery-powered machine is more convenient for use in a busy and crowded emergency room or intensive care unit. Traditional machines are heavy and can be cumbersome; maneuvering them to the patient's side is time-consuming and may cause damage to valuable equipment and personnel in the process. However, only one transducer can usually be connected to portable machines at one time, and with their small keyboards, many buttons often serve dual or triple function.

Echocardiographic examination

Transthoracic images of the heart can be obtained where lung tissue is not interposed between the heart and the chest wall. There is one window on the right side along the sternal border (parasternal), and one window on the left side along the sternal border in the region of the fourth to sixth intercostal space.

Patient positioning and preparation

To decrease lung interference, echocardiograms are usually performed with the patient in lateral recumbency on a "cutout" table that allows transducer manipulation from beneath the animal (see Fig. 13.1). One or two assistants restrain the patient in left or right lateral

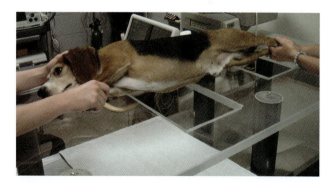

Figure 13.1 Patient positioning and "cutout" tabletop. The patient is restrained in right lateral recumbency. The thoracic limbs are pulled forward. The tabletop is made of Plexiglas and sits on a regular exam table. It is 56″ long and 25″ wide. Usually, one large cutout (15″ × 8″) is adequate. A pad can be made to cover the tabletop.

recumbency. Sedation is usually not needed. Dogs and cats can also be examined in standing position. If the patient is recumbent and cannot be repositioned or removed from its cage, the operator should try to slide the transducer underneath the patient's chest. If necessary, the ultrasound probe can be placed on the nondependent chest wall of a laterally recumbent animal, but with significant decrease in image quality. Air artifact is also a common limitation in dyspneic animals. Decrease in image quality may prevent accurate interpretation of the echocardiographic findings. However, in such situations, it is still usually possible to assess systolic function of the left ventricle and estimate the size of the cardiac chambers.

Good quality images can usually be obtained without hair clipping. A generous amount of ultrasonographic coupling gel is applied to create an air-free space between the skin and the transducer. The author never clips dogs or cats in his practice.

Transducer manipulation

Views from the right parasternal acoustic window are usually obtained first. They provide information on cardiac chamber size, valve structure, and left ventricular function. From the right-sided views, the direction of blood flow circulating from atrium to ventricle and then from ventricle to the circulatory system is almost perpendicular to the ultrasound beam and therefore cannot be reliably assessed with Doppler. Apical views from the left parasternal window provide more accurate assessment of blow flow. However, in the emergency setting, assessment of blood flow by Doppler is usually not critical. Indeed, turbulent blow flow caused by valve insufficiency or stenosis typically creates a heart murmur that can be identified on physical examination. Findings from the echocardiographic examination, combined with those from a thorough physical examination, will usually give a diagnosis.

The ultrasound beam fans out of the transducer in a plane, whose orientation is indicated by an index mark on the probe (see Fig. 13.3 in the later subsection Right Parasternal Short-Axis Views). This index mark is a plastic ridge on the transducer itself, so the operator holding the probe is aware of its position without having to look at it. By convention, the side of the transducer with the index mark corresponds to the right-hand side of the display.

Right parasternal long-axis views

These views are obtained from the right acoustic window. The right acoustic window is located by placing the transducer on the right ventral thorax at the level of the palpable precordial impulse. The precordial impulse is caused by ventricular contraction, usually at the level of the fifth or sixth intercostal space, and can be felt by placing a hand on the animal's chest.

In the long-axis view, the transducer should be aligned with the long axis of the heart. The image is oriented with the base of the heart to the right side of the screen, with the reference mark symbol on the top right side of the image and the reference index of the transducer pointing toward the heart base (i.e., oriented toward the patient's head in most cases). In deep-chested dogs, the heart is positioned vertically within the chest; therefore, in such cases the long axis of the heart is almost perpendicular to the spine. In most dogs and cats, the long axis of the heart is along a line that connects the xyphoid process to the caudal border of the scapula, creating a 45-degree angle with the spine. From this position, a simultaneous view of all four cardiac chambers, and a left ventricular outflow view that includes the ascending aorta, can be obtained (see Fig. 13.2). Anatomically, the aorta has a central position within the heart, which offers a reference point in order to determine how the transducer should be moved to image various portions of the heart. Left and right atria are on the right side of the midline plane. Therefore, if the animal is in right lateral recumbency, the atria will be closer to the table and will be visualized by decreasing the angle between the probe and the horizontal plane, represented by the "cutout" table or the patient's sagittal plane. If the transducer is tilted more vertically and slightly rotated clockwise, the ultrasound beam will intersect the aorta in a longitudinal plane. From this window, the right ventricle and atrium are seen at the top of the monitor image.

Right parasternal short-axis views

Right parasternal short-axis views are obtained with the animal and the probe in the same basic position as for the right parasternal long-axis view, and are acquired by rotating the probe 90° counterclockwise. The probe's reference mark is now oriented toward the elbow of the animal. The transducer is positioned to display the pulmonary artery to the right side of the screen when the base of the heart is in the image. Usually, the initial view obtained is at the level of the ventricular apex or the midventricular region (see Fig. 13.3). By moving the plane of the ultrasound beam from the apex to the base of the heart, the operator can examine various structures of the heart, displayed as successive two-dimensional planes. In small dogs and cats, the transducer is kept in its initial position and is tilted toward the head of the patient in order to image the base of the heart. When the transducer is positioned more perpendicular to

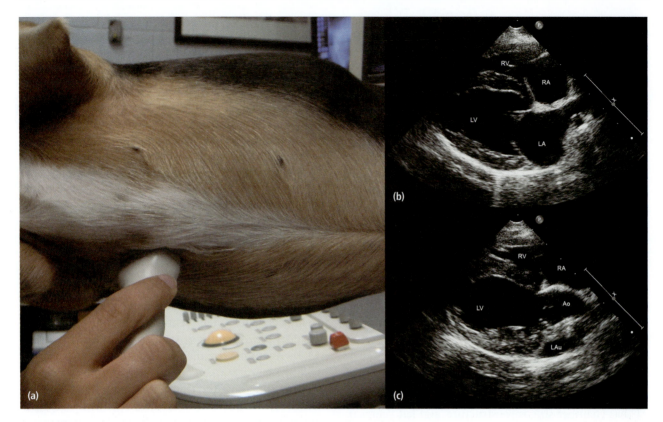

Figure 13.2 Two-dimensional long-axis views, right parasternal window. (a) Position of the transducer with the animal restrained in right lateral recumbency. See text for details. (b) Four-chamber view. Note the symbol on the top right side of the sector image, which corresponds to the reference mark on the transducer. (c) Left ventricular outflow tract view. LA, left atrium; Lau, left auricle; LV, left ventricle; RA, right atrium; RV, right ventricle; Ao, aorta.

the table, a view at the level of the left ventricular apex is obtained. In large dogs, the transducer is usually moved from its initial position one or two intercostal spaces cranially in order to obtain views of the base of the heart. The following views are usually obtained: apex level, papillary muscle level, mitral valve level, basal level. At the basal level, left atrium and auricle, right atrium, and aorta are imaged. By tilting the probe toward the head, the right ventricular outflow tract, pulmonic valve, and pulmonary arteries can be displayed (see Fig. 13.4).

Left apical views

Left-sided views are usually not essential to the evaluation of a patient in the emergency setting. Apical views should be obtained if the clinician is interested in assessing valve insufficiencies and stenotic areas by Doppler echocardiography. The animal is restrained in left lateral recumbency. If the patient is in standing position, its left side should face the operator. The transducer is placed at the level of the palpable precordial impulse, usually at the sixth intercostal space. On the left side, it corresponds to the apex of the left ventricle. If the animal is

in left lateral recumbency, the transducer is held almost parallel to the "cutout" table, oriented toward the left shoulder of the patient with the reference index down, facing the floor. With the transducer in this position, the heart is displayed upside down on the monitor, with the apex on top of the screen and the left cardiac chambers on the right side.

Echocardiographic assessment of cardiac anatomy and function

From the right parasternal acoustic window, the operator can subjectively evaluate the size of all cardiac chambers. The right atrium and the left atrium should be of similar size. The left atrial diameter is 1–1.5 times the diameter of the aorta at the level of the aortic cusps. Cardiovascular diseases may cause atrial enlargement. It is usually associated with increased circulating blood volume, as a result of primary cardiac disease, chronic anemia, or fluid overload. Atrial dilation is more severe if significant atrioventricular valve insufficiency is present. Left and right atria can also dilate in response to impaired diastolic function of the ventricles. Diastolic

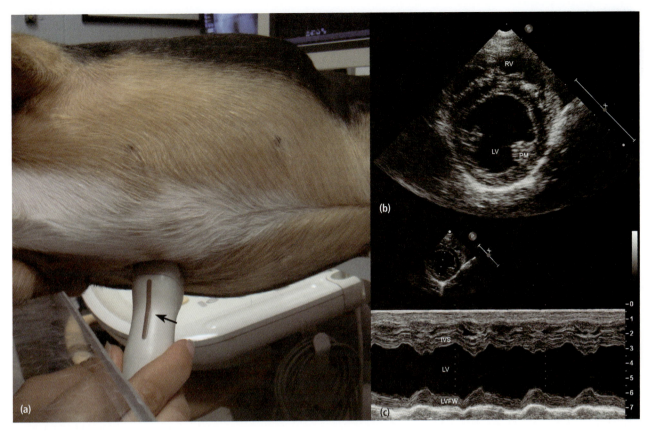

Figure 13.3 Short-axis views, right parasternal window. Note the position of the reference index (arrow). See text for details. (a) Position of the transducer with the animal in right lateral recumbency to visualize the left midventricular region. (b) Two-dimensional short-axis view at the level of the papillary muscles. (c) M-mode echocardiogram of the left ventricle at the level of the papillary muscles. The cursor is placed perpendicular to the interventricular septum and the left ventricular free wall on a live two-dimensional image. Four cardiac cycles are recorded on this M-mode image. The right ventricle is visualized at the top of the image as a thin echo-free (black) line. Then the M-mode shows the interventricular septum, the echolucent (black) left ventricle, and the left ventricular free wall. The pericardium is the bright white line just below the left ventricular free wall. The scale on the right side indicates the depth of the image in centimeters. LV, left ventricle; PM, papillary muscle; RV, right ventricle; IVS, interventricular septum; LVFW, left ventricular free wall.

dysfunction reflects abnormal relaxation or compliance of the ventricles, usually in response to concentric hypertrophy of the ventricular walls (e.g., with hypertension) or marked fibrotic replacement of normal cardiac tissue. Decreased ventricular filling in diastole results in progressive atrial dilation. Left atrial enlargement is directly correlated with the risk of pulmonary edema. Right atrial dilation is usually associated with increased systemic venous pressure, which may cause ascites and pleural effusion.

The right ventricular chamber is approximately one-third of the left ventricular internal diameter. The free wall of the right ventricle is equal to one-third or one-half the thickness of the left ventricular free wall.[4]

The interventricular septum and the left ventricular free wall are similar in thickness.

The mitral valve leaflets should be thin and should close on the plane of the mitral valve annulus in systole with no apparent bulging toward the left atrium.

The quality of left ventricular contraction can also be assessed from this view. The internal diameter of the left ventricle should decrease by 30%–40% in systole compared with diastole. For the experienced operator, a qualitative evaluation of ventricular contraction is usually sufficient to determine if cardiovascular abnormalities are present. This knowledge is only gained by frequently evaluating normal animals.

The two-dimensional right parasternal short-axis view at the level of the papillary muscles is used to take measurements of left ventricular size and function. Left ventricular systolic function is objectively described by the calculation of the fractional shortening (FS).

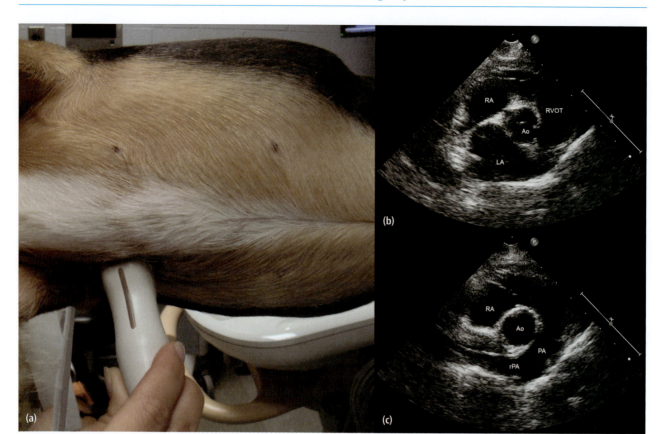

Figure 13.4 Short-axis views, right parasternal window. (a) Position of the transducer with the animal in right lateral recumbency to visualize the base of the heart. The probe is slightly tilted toward the head in order to image the right ventricular outflow tract and the main pulmonary artery. See text for details. (b) Two-dimensional short-axis view at the level of the left atrium. (c) Two-dimensional short-axis view at the level of the pulmonary arteries. LA, left atrium; Ao, aorta; RA, right atrium; RVOT, right ventricular outflow tract; PA, main pulmonary artery; rPA, right pulmonary artery.

Fractional shortening is based on the diameter of the left ventricle in diastole (LVIDd) and in systole (LVIDs) and is given as a percentage, calculated from the following formula:

$$\%FS = [(LVIDd - LVIDs)/LVIDd] \times 100 \qquad (13.1)$$

For example, a fractional shortening of 30% means that the left ventricular internal diameter is 30% smaller in systole than it is in diastole. In the author's echocardiography laboratory, normal dogs have a fractional shortening of 30%–45%, while FS is 40% on average in cats.

Left ventricular size comprises the measurements of the left ventricular internal diameter and wall thickness in end-diastole and end-systole. Ideally, an ECG is recorded and displayed on the monitor screen during the echocardiographic examination. It allows diastole to be accurately identified as the onset of the QRS complex

and systole as the peak of the T wave. Alternatively, measurements can be taken by visually recognizing left ventricular diastole and systole on the monitor screen. Diastole is measured on the still frame that displays the maximal left ventricular diameter; systole is measured at the minimal ventricular internal diameter. This method is less accurate than the previous one.

Measurements can also be obtained from an M-mode display of the left ventricle using the machine's caliper function to measure the left ventricular internal diameter in maximal left ventricular systole and diastole, and calculating %FS as above.

Measurements should be compared with published reference ranges in dogs and cats (see Tables 13.1 and 13.2). A qualitative visual assessment is usually applied to the right ventricle.

Cardiovascular diseases trigger concentric or eccentric hypertrophy of the ventricles. Thickening (concentric hypertrophy) of the ventricular walls results from

Table 13.1 Echocardiographic Values in Normal Dogs (Mean Values)

Weight (kg)	LVIDd (cm)	LVIDs (cm)	IVSd (cm)	LVFWd (cm)	LA (cm)	Ao (cm)
3	2.0	1.1	0.5	0.6	1.3	1.1
5	2.4	1.3	0.6	0.7	1.5	1.3
10	3.0	1.8	0.7	0.8	1.8	1.6
15	3.4	2.1	0.8	0.8	2.0	1.9
20	3.8	2.4	0.9	0.9	2.2	2.1
25	4.0	2.6	0.9	0.9	2.4	2.2
30	4.3	2.8	1.0	1.0	2.5	2.4
35	4.5	3.0	1.0	1.0	2.6	2.5
40	4.7	3.1	1.0	1.0	2.7	2.6
45	4.9	3.3	1.1	1.1	2.8	2.7
50	5.0	3.4	1.1	1.1	2.9	2.8
55	5.2	3.6	1.2	1.1	3.0	2.9
60	5.3	3.7	1.2	1.1	3.1	3.0
65	5.5	3.8	1.2	1.2	3.1	3.1

LVID, left ventricular internal diameter; IVS, interventricular septum; LVFW, left ventricular free wall; LA, left atrium; Ao, aorta; d, diastole; s, systole.
Adapted from: Kittleson MS, Kienle RD. *Small Animal Cardiovascular Medicine.* St. Louis: Mosby; 1998.

Table 13.2 Echocardiographic Values in Cats (Normal Range)

LVIDd (cm)	LVIDs (cm)	FS (%)	LVFWd (cm)	LVFWs (cm)
1.1–1.6	0.6–1.0	29–35	0.25–0.5	0.4–0.9

IVSd (cm)	IVSd (cm)	LA (cm)	Ao (cm)	LA/Ao
0.25–0.5	0.5–0.9	0.85–1.25	0.65–1.10	0.8–1.3

LVID, left ventricular internal diameter; FS, fractional shortening; LVFW, left ventricular free wall; IVS, interventricular septum; LA, left atrium; Ao, aorta; LA/Ao, left atrium–to–aorta ratio; d, diastole; s, systole.
Adapted from: Bonagura JD, O'Grady MR, Herring DS. Echocardiography: principles of interpretation. *Vet Clin North Am Small Anim Pract* 1985;15:1177.

increased resistance to ejection of blood into the vascular system. Signs of left ventricular hypertrophy indicate systemic hypertension, aortic stenosis and hypertrophic cardiomyopathy. Systemic hypertension occurs in dogs and cats. Subaortic stenosis is a cause of left ventricular concentric hypertrophy in large breed dogs. Dogs with severe subaortic stenosis have an increased risk of syncope and sudden death and may be presented on emergency after an episode of collapse. Physical examination will reveal a left basilar systolic murmur.[5] In cats, hyperthyroidism and hypertrophic cardiomyopathy cause left ventricular concentric hypertrophy. Hyperthyroidism is commonly associated with systemic hypertension.[6] In the case of feline hypertrophic cardiomyopathy, concentric hypertrophy is most likely a response to impaired myocardial contractility secondary to a mutation of genes coding for sarcomeric proteins. Echocardiographic diagnosis is based on a diastolic left ventricular free wall or interventricular septum thickness above 6 mm from a right parasternal short-axis view below the tip of the mitral valve leaflets. Hypertrophy at the base of the interventricular septum typically causes outflow tract obstruction and increased afterload, which further worsens concentric hypertrophy.[7] Right ventricular concentric hypertrophy results from pulmonic stenosis and pulmonary hypertension. Acquired right ventricular concentric hypertrophy usually indicates pulmonary hypertension, which may be secondary to various disease processes, including chronic respiratory disease, heartworm disease, left-sided heart failure, and pulmonary embolism.[4] The right ventricle's response to increased afterload is usually dilation in combination with wall thickening. Right ventricular dilation is more obvious if pulmonary hypertension is acute and severe, a condition known as cor pulmonale.[8] Valvular pulmonic stenosis is a common cause of right ventricular concentric hypertrophy. Pulmonic stenosis is more common in small-breed dogs and brachycephalic breeds, and is associated with a left basilar systolic murmur on auscultation. Concentric right ventricular hypertrophy secondary to congenital defects is typically characterized by severe concentric hypertrophy of the right ventricle with no or minimal dilation.[9] This difference in response of the right ventricle to congenital as opposed to acquired pressure overload can be appreciated during the echocardiographic examination.

Finally, the operator should be aware of the accuracy of measurements obtained from two-dimensional echocardiography. Studies have shown that, in dogs, coefficients of variation of echocardiographic parameters vary between 3% and 26% and on average between 10% and 15%.[10] The level of expertise of the operator and external factors that may impair optimal image acquisition may further decrease the accuracy of these measurements. Therefore, measurements should not be interpreted independently from the qualitative assessment of the cardiac structure and function, as well as the patient's history and physical examination findings.

Use of echocardiography for diagnosis of cardiovascular diseases

Echocardiographic evaluation of the patient with cardiac tamponade

Bedside echocardiography is an important tool to confirm a suspicion of cardiac tamponade. Pericardial effusion is the accumulation of fluid within the pericardial space, which can be acute or chronic. Acute cases result from hemorrhage within the pericardial space. Most commonly hemopericardium is associated with atrial hemangiosarcoma. Acute tamponade is characterized by the accumulation of a small amount of fluid within a noncompliant pericardial sac causing clinical signs of low cardiac output. Chronic tamponade results from the slow accumulation of a large volume of fluid, which slowly stretches the pericardium. Right intracardiac pressure rises until it causes right heart failure with ascites. Chronic tamponade may be associated with a cardiac tumor, but commonly the cause for tamponade is not found.[11] On echocardiogram, pericardial effusion appears as an echo-free (black) space around the ventricles. A small amount of effusion can be seen as a very small echo-free space in the left atrioventricular groove on a right parasternal long-axis view. The pericardium adheres to the large vessels at the heart base, which limits the accumulation of fluid in this region. The absence of fluid around the base of the heart can be used to differentiate pericardial effusion from pleural effusion, which accumulates homogeneously around the heart unless marked inflammation results in loculated effusion. Identification of the tip of the right auricle freely moving within the pericardial fluid in a right parasternal long-axis view, or the tip of the left auricle surrounded by fluid in a right parasternal short-axis view are also helpful signs to differentiate pericardial effusion from pleural effusion.[3]

A markedly dilated left auricle may mimic pericardial effusion in some echocardiographic views. In dogs and cats with severe left atrial dilation, the left auricle expands along the lateroposterior side of the left ventricle, creating an echo-free space off the lateral side of the left ventricle (see Fig. 13.5).

Echocardiographically, signs of cardiac tamponade include right atrial collapse during atrial diastole following atrial contraction, right ventricular collapse during ventricular diastole, and underfilling of the left side of the heart. Tamponade is best appreciated on a right parasternal long-axis view (see Fig. 13.6); its presence indicates that intrapericardial pressure is higher than right intracardiac chamber pressure.[3] Echocardiography is the best method with which to identify the cause of the effusion. It is important to thoroughly examine the area of the right atrium, right auricle, and right atrioventricular junction for an echogenic mass. An atrial mass is usually a hemangiosarcoma.[12] Pericardial fluid around the heart facilitates the detection of an atrial mass. It is the preference of the author to perform the echocardiogram before pericardiocentesis, if possible. The heart base should be examined for the presence of a mass. Most heart base masses are chemodectomas. On

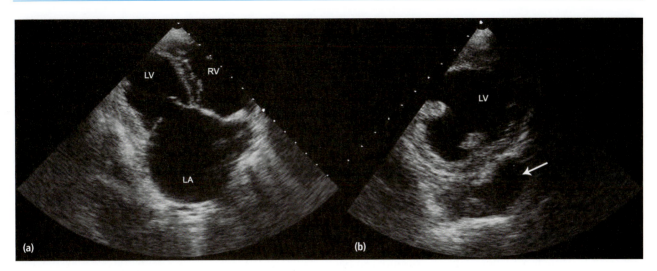

Figure 13.5 Severely enlarged left atrium mimicking pericardial effusion. (a) Two-dimensional four-chamber oblique view obtained from a right parasternal window in a deep-chested dog. The left atrium is markedly enlarged as a result of chronic mitral valve insufficiency. (b) Two-dimensional short-axis view at the level of the papillary muscles from a right parasternal window. The enlarged left auricle extends along the posterolateral side of the left ventricle (arrow). This can be mistakenly interpreted as pericardial effusion. LA, left atrium; LV, left ventricle; RV, right ventricle.

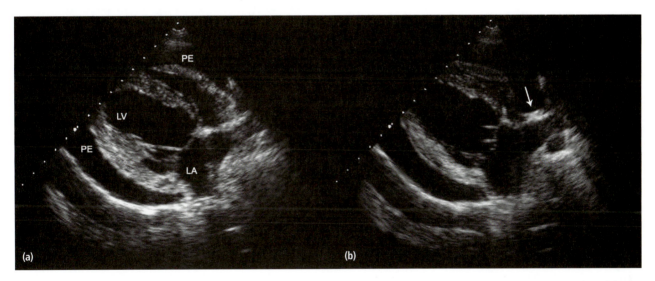

Figure 13.6 Cardiac tamponade in a dog. Two-dimensional long-axis four-chamber view from a right parasternal window. (a) Pericardial effusion is visualized as an echo-free space between the epicardium and the bright line that corresponds to the parietal pericardium. Pericardial effusion does not extend around the base of the heart. (b) Note the diastolic collapse of the right atrium (arrow) and the right ventricle. They are two sensitive findings for tamponade. LA, left atrium; LV, left ventricle; PE, pericardial effusion.

echocardiogram, chemodectomas are usually located at the base of the aorta, on top of the left atrium.[13]

Echocardiographic evaluation of the dog with chronic mitral valve disease

Chronic mitral valve disease, also known as mitral valve endocardiosis or myxomatous degenerative valve disease,

is the most common acquired cardiovascular disease in small dogs.[14] Moreover, this is the most common cause of left-sided congestive heart failure in dogs. Usually, management of dogs with pulmonary edema secondary to mitral valve disease does not require an echocardiographic examination. History, physical examination, and chest radiographs are sufficient to reach a diagnosis.

Flail leaflet from chordae tendineae rupture

Echocardiographic examination is indicated in dogs that do not rapidly respond to aggressive intravenous diuretic therapy and oxygen supplementation, or present with an acute worsening of a previously stable disease. Echocardiography may reveal chordae tendineae rupture as the cause for the severity of the clinical signs. Chordae tendineae rupture has been reported in up to 16% of a population of dogs with mitral valve disease.[15] Rupture of small, second-order chordae tendineae, which are attached to the midventricular surface of the leaflets, is usually of no clinical significance. However, the tips of the mitral valve cusps are anchored to papillary muscles by large, first-order chordae tendineae. Their disruption may lead to acute heart failure. Chordal rupture can be seen on echocardiography from the right parasternal long-axis view. A flail leaflet is identified by its chaotic motion with the tip of the valve extending beyond the mitral annular plane and pointing toward the left atrium in systole. The leaflet is then thrust into the left ventricle and toward the left ventricular outflow tract in diastole.[16] Moreover, thickened chordae tendineae that are ruptured from their attachment to the papillary muscles can be seen as bright hyperechoic filaments moving freely between the left ventricle and the left atrium. Rupture of chordae anchored to the anterior (septal) leaflet of the mitral valve is more common. Color Doppler reveals a large jet of mitral valve insufficiency.[15]

Left atrial rupture

Left atrial rupture is an uncommon complication of severe chronic mitral valve disease. It results from the chronic trauma to the endocardial surface of the left atrium by a high-velocity jet of mitral regurgitation. Left atrial rupture causes cardiac tamponade. Dogs are presented with signs of low cardiac output, extreme weakness, and collapse.[14] On echocardiogram, an atrial tear is not directly visible. Echocardiographic diagnosis is based on identification of signs of severe mitral valve disease: thickened mitral valve leaflets, severely dilated left atrium, color-flow Doppler indication of a large regurgitant jet. Pericardial effusion is present. Typically, a clot is seen in the pericardial space.[17]

Echocardiographic evaluation of the patient with dilated cardiomyopathy

Dilated cardiomyopathy may be the cause for congestive heart failure in dogs. It is rare in cats. Bedside echocardiography may help identify poor systolic function, which is an indication to use positive inotropic agents.[18] Echocardiography from the right parasternal acoustic window demonstrates both left ventricular dilation and systolic dysfunction. The degree of systolic dysfunction can be quantified by the calculation of fractional shortening. However, because of the variability of echocardiographic parameters, it is difficult to use fractional shortening to monitor response to inotropic agents.[19] Echocardiography can be used to decide if inotropes should be started, but clinical response determines if they should be continued. Color Doppler evaluation of the mitral valve frequently reveals mild to moderate regurgitation, which results from mitral valve annulus dilation. Pulmonary hypertension is a common complication of left heart disease, resulting from passive pulmonary venous congestion, active pulmonary arterial vasoconstriction, and vascular remodeling. Echocardiographic features of pulmonary hypertension include right ventricular dilation, right ventricular free wall thickening, and tricuspid valve insufficiency.

Echocardiographic evaluation of the patient with arrhythmogenic right ventricular cardiomyopathy

Arrhythmogenic right ventricular cardiomyopathy (ARVC) is most commonly identified in Boxer dogs. It is characterized by fibrofatty replacement of the right ventricular myocardium and severe ventricular arrhythmias. Dogs may be presented on emergency after an episode of collapse or with signs of cardiogenic shock due to rapid sustained ventricular tachycardia. Echocardiogram is frequently unremarkable in these dogs. Some will show signs of myocardial failure secondary to the expansion of the disease to the left side of the heart. It is important to know about cardiac function before using antiarrhythmics, as some of them have negative inotropic effects. Bedside echocardiography allows rapid assessment of ventricular function. Echocardiographic features of myocardial failure include left ventricular dilation in diastole and systole, and decrease in fractional shortening.[20] Isolated right ventricular enlargement, localized aneurysms, identified as an outpouching of the free wall of the right ventricle, and increased echogenicity of the myocardium reflecting adipose infiltration are reported echocardiographic findings in humans, but are usually not seen in dogs.[21] Arrhythmogenic right ventricular cardiomyopathy is also reported in cats. It is associated with ventricular arrhythmias, and most cats will have signs of congestive heart failure. Marked right ventricular and right atrial dilation, and tricuspid regurgitation are the main echocardiographic findings; these abnormalities are best seen from the right parasternal acoustic window.[22]

Echocardiographic evaluation of the cat with cardiomyopathy

Echocardiographic evaluation of the dyspneic cat

Decompensated myocardial disease is a common differential diagnosis in cats presented for respiratory distress. Dyspnea may result from pulmonary edema or pleural effusion. Cats with congestive heart failure should be treated with diuretics, thoracocentesis if indicated, and supplemental oxygen. Fluid therapy is contraindicated in these cats, even when presented with signs of shock.[23] Bedside echocardiography can be used to rapidly detect the presence of pleural effusion. The depth of the echocardiographic image should initially be increased to look for the accumulation of fluid around the heart and lung lobes. The depth is then decreased to focus on the heart itself. Cardiac disease should be suspected as the cause for the respiratory signs if marked atrial enlargement is present. Pleural effusion may occur in cats with isolated left atrial enlargement. Additionally, signs of myocardial disease, most commonly hypertrophic cardiomyopathy, may be present. Hypertrophic cardiomyopathy is diagnosed if the cat has an interventricular septum or left ventricular free wall thickness over 6 mm in diastole. Rapid diagnosis of advanced cardiac disease by bedside echocardiography may be critical to guide initial therapy.

Echocardiographic evaluation of the cat with pelvic limb paralysis

Acute pelvic limb paralysis in cats commonly results from arterial thromboembolism secondary to severe myocardial disease with left atrial dilation.[24] Physical examination findings including heart murmur or gallop, cold, painful pelvic limbs, and absent femoral pulses usually provide strong evidence of the disease. However, echocardiography may help confirm the diagnosis in some cases, and it provides additional information to adequately advise the owner and manage the patient. A right parasternal long-axis view will give information on the size of the left atrium, which is usually markedly dilated. A right parasternal short-axis at the level of the left atrium allows good visualization of the left auricle, where atrial thrombi are usually identified.[25]

Echocardiographic evaluation of the patient with infective endocarditis

Endocarditis is suspected in medium- to large-breed dogs with signs of acute ongoing infection and a new murmur or a change in intensity of a previously diagnosed murmur. Frequently endocarditis does not cause a cardiac murmur, and it is only diagnosed after an extensive workup that includes a full cardiology workup.[26] Bedside echocardiography can be used to identify large vegetative lesions. However, a veterinary cardiologist should always confirm such findings because it can be difficult to differentiate them from chronic degenerative valve changes. Vegetative lesions are most likely to be seen on the mitral valve. They less commonly develop on the aortic valve. A vegetation is typically an irregularly shaped, highly mobile mass attached to the free edge of a leaflet. The absence of mobility argues against the diagnosis of endocarditis. The lesion usually develops on the atrial side of the mitral valve and on the ventricular side of the aortic valve. The mass is usually homogeneous with echogenicity similar to that of the myocardium. Mitral valve endocarditis is commonly associated with mild to severe mitral regurgitation; aortic valve endocarditis, with aortic insufficiency. All echocardiographic windows should be used to increase the probability of detecting vegetations. Myxomatous mitral valve disease may mimic lesions of endocarditis.[3]

Echocardiographic evaluation of the patient with heartworm "caval syndrome"

The so-called heartworm caval syndrome is a complication of heartworm disease resulting from embolization of heartworms within the right cardiac chambers. Clinically, this is associated with shock, dyspnea, right-sided heart failure, and hemoglobinuria.

Echocardiographically, worms are easily seen trapped across the tricuspid valve, causing severe tricuspid regurgitation. Left ventricular chambers may appear smaller in size as a result of decreased forward blood flow through the pulmonary vessels. Signs of pulmonary hypertension, including concentric hypertrophy of the right ventricular free wall, enlargement of the right ventricle, and a flattened septum, may be present[27] (see Fig. 13.7).

Echocardiographic evaluation of volume status

Congestive heart failure may result from aggressive fluid therapy in dogs and cats with underlying cardiac disease. Bedside echocardiography may help estimate the risk for this complication. The operator should assess the size of the left atrium from the right parasternal long- and short-axis views. In dogs, it is unlikely that fluid therapy will lead to pulmonary edema if the left atrium is normal or mildly enlarged. At times, congestive heart failure arises in cats secondary to fluid therapy in the presence of a normal atrial size. The reason is that feline cardiomyopathy leads to poorly compliant ventricles and rapid elevation of

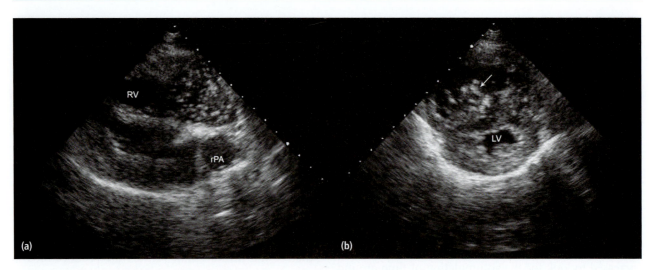

Figure 13.7 Caval syndrome in a dog. (a) Two-dimensional long-axis four-chamber view from a right parasternal window. Severely enlarged right atrium filled with heartworms that appear as two short parallel hyperechoic lines. Cross-section of a dilated right pulmonary artery is seen at the base of the heart, above the left atrium. (b) Two-dimensional short-axis view at the level of the left ventricular papillary muscles from a right parasternal window. Heartworms are visualized in the chamber of the right ventricle (arrow). Note the signs of severe pulmonary hypertension: concentric hypertrophy of the right ventricular free wall, dilated right ventricle, and flattened interventricular septum. Underfilling of the left ventricle is obvious as a result of decreased pulmonary venous flow caused by right ventricular failure. RV, right ventricle; rPA, right pulmonary artery; LV, left ventricle.

filling pressures with fluid overload. Thus, it may be difficult to identify cats at risk. With restrictive cardiomyopathy the heart may appear normal on echocardiogram. In the case of hypertrophic cardiomyopathy, interventricular septum and left ventricular thickening are sometimes the sole indicators of the disease. There is no simple way to rapidly assess diastolic dysfunction, which requires the use of advanced Doppler techniques.

Echocardiographic evaluation of the hypotensive patient

Regarding the management of a patient with hypotension, it is important to determine if hypotension results from decreased cardiac output, systemic vasodilation, or hypovolemia. On echocardiogram, a small left ventricular cavity with normal to increased systolic function indicates hypovolemia. In normovolemic patients, hypotension may result from low cardiac output. Bedside echocardiography can provide valuable information about cardiac contractility by measuring the fractional shortening, and help determine if inotropic drugs are indicated.[3]

Echocardiographic evaluation of the patient in cardiac arrest

Bedside echocardiography may be indicated during cardiopulmonary cerebral resuscitation (CPCR) to deter-
mine if mechanical cardiac activity is present. However, it should not interfere with CPCR. Pulseless electrical activity is characterized by cardiac electrical activity without a palpable pulse. However, weak cardiac contractions may not generate peripheral pulses. Echocardiography may help differentiate pseudopulseless electrical activity (cardiac contractions that do not generate a pulse) from pulseless electrical activity.[28]

Echocardiographic evaluation of the patient with pulmonary hypertension

Elevated pulmonary artery pressures characterize pulmonary hypertension. Echocardiographically, right ventricular changes in response to increased pressure include dilation of the right ventricle, flattening of the interventricular septum and paradoxical septal motion, and hypertrophy of right ventricular trabeculations and free wall. Acute pulmonary hypertension may result from pulmonary thromboembolism. However, the diagnosis is rarely confirmed by the detection of a thrombus in the main pulmonary artery or the origin of the left and right pulmonary arteries from a right parasternal short-axis view.[3]

Conclusion

In conclusion, bedside echocardiography can be used as a screening tool with minimal training. It can provide useful information when used in combination with physical examination in the emergency and critical care environment.

References

1. Evans HE. The respiratory system. In: HE Evans, ed. Miller's Anatomy of the Dog, 3rd ed. Philadelphia: Saunders; 1993:463–493.

2. Thomas WP, Gaber CE, Jacobs GJ, Kaplan PM, Lombard CW, Moise NS, Moses BL. Recommendations for standards in transthoracic two-dimensional echocardiography in the dog and cat. J Vet Intern Med 1993;7:247–252.

3. Feigenbaum H, Armstrong WF, Ryan T. Feigenbaum's Echocardiography, 6th ed. Philadelphia: Lippincott Williams & Williams; 2005.

4. Johnson L, Boon J, Orton EC. Clinical characteristics of 53 dogs with Doppler-derived evidence of pulmonary hypertension: 1992–1996. J Vet Intern Med 1999;13:440–447.

5. Freedom RM, Yoo SJ, Russell J, Perrin D, Williams WG. Thoughts about fixed subaortic stenosis in man and dog. Cardiol Young 2005;15:186–205.

6. Kienle RD, Bruyette D, Pion PD. Effects of thyroid hormone and thyroid dysfunction on the cardiovascular system. Vet Clin North Am Small Anim Pract 1994;24:495–507.

7. Baty CJ. Feline hypertrophic cardiomyopathy: an update. Vet Clin North Am Small Anim Pract 2004;34:1227–1234.

8. Yamashita H, Onodera S, Imamoto T, Obara A, Tanazawa S, Takashio T, Morimoto H, Inoue H. Functional and geometrical interference and interdependency between the right and left ventricle in cor pulmonale: an experimental study on simultaneous measurement of biventricular geometry of acute right ventricular pressure overload. Jpn Circ J 1989;53:1237–1244.

9. Shrope DP. Balloon valvuloplasty of valvular pulmonic stenosis in the dog. Clin Tech Small Anim Pract 2005;3:182–195.

10. Chetboul V, Tidholm A, Nicolle A, Sampedrano CC, Gouni V, Pouchelon JL, Lefebvre HP, Concordet D. Effects of animal position and number of repeated measurements on selected two-dimensional and M-mode echocardiographic variables in healthy dogs. J Am Vet Med Assoc 2005;227:743–747.

11. Shaw SP, Rush JE. Canine pericardial effusion: diagnosis, treatment, and prognosis. Compend Contin Educ Vet 2007;29:405–411.

12. Gidlewski J, Petrie JP. Pericardiocentesis and principles of echocardiographic imaging in the patient with cardiac neoplasia. Clin Tech Small Anim Pract 2003;18:131–134.

13. Aupperle H, Marz I, Ellenberger C, Buschatz S, Reischauer A, Shoon HA. Primary and secondary heart tumours in dogs and cats. J Comp Pathol 2007;136:18–36.

14. Rush JE. Chronic valvular disease in dogs. In: JD Bonagura, DC Twedt, eds. Kirk's Current Veterinary Therapy XIV. St Louis: Saunders; 2009:780–786.

15. Serres F, Chetboul V, Tissier R, Sampedrano CC, Gouni V, Nicolle AP, Pouchelon JL. Chordae tendineae rupture in dogs with degenerative mitral valve disease: prevalence, survival, and prognostic factors (114 cases, 2001–2006). J Vet Intern 2007;21:258–264.

16. Jacobs GJ, Calvert CA, Mahaffey MB, Hall DG. Echocardiographic detection of flail left atrioventricular valve cusp from ruptured chordae tendineae in 4 dogs. J Vet Intern Med 1995;9:341–346.

17. Prosek R, Sisson DD, Oyama MA. What is your diagnosis? Pericardial effusion with a clot in the pericardial space likely caused by left atrial rupture secondary to mitral regurgitation. J Am Vet Med Assoc 2003;222:441–442.

18. O'Grady MR, O'Sullivan ML. Dilated cardiomyopathy: an update. Vet Clin North Am Small Anim Pract 2004;34:1187–1207.

19. Galrinho A, Soares RM, Branco LM, Timoteo A, Feliciano J, Santana A, Ferreira R, Quininha J. Usefulness of low-dose dobutamine echocardiography in idiopathic dilated cardiomyopathy. Rev Prot Cardiol 2005;24:1491–1501.

20. Meurs KM. Boxer dog cardiomyopathy: an update. Vet Clin North Am Small Anim Pract 2004;34:1235–1244.

21. Basso C, Fox PR, Meurs KM, Towbin JA, Spier AW, Calabrese F, Maron BJ, Thiene G. Arrhythmogenic right ventricular cardiomyopathy causing sudden cardiac death in boxer dogs: a new animal model of human disease. Circulation 2004;109:1180–1185.

22. Fox PR, Maron BJ, Basso C, Liu SK, Thiene G. Spontaneously occurring arrhythmogenic right ventricular cardiomyopathy in the domestic cat: a new animal model similar to the human disease. Circulation 2002;102:1863–1870.

23. Rush JE. Therapy of feline hypertrophic cardiomyopathy. Vet Clin North Am Small Anim Pract 1998;28:1459–1479.

24. Smith SA, Tobias AH, Jacob KA, Fine DM, Grumbles PL. Arterial thromboembolism in cats: acute crisis in 127 cases (1992–2001) and long–term management with low-dose aspirin in 24 cases. J Vet Intern Med 2003;17:73–83.

25. Schober KE, Maerz I. Doppler echocardiographic assessment of left atrial appendage flow velocities in normal cats. J Vet Cardiol 2005;7:15–25.

26. Peddle GD, Drobatz KJ, Harvey CE, Adams A, Sleeper MM. Association of periodontal disease, oral procedures, and other clinical findings with bacterial endocarditis in dogs. J Am Vet Med Assoc 2009;234:100–107.

27. Hoch H, Strickland K. Canine and feline dirofilariasis: prophylaxis, treatment, and complications of treatment. Compend Contin Educ Vet 2008;30:146–151.

28. Tang A, Euerle B. Emergency department ultrasound and echocardiography. Emerg Med Clin North Am 2005;23:1179–1194.

14

Pericardiocentesis

Meredith L. Daly

In health, the fibrous pericardium has many important functions. It prevents excessive movement of the heart within the thoracic cavity, helps to minimize friction between the moving heart and the surrounding organs, protects the heart from extension of malignancy and infection from surrounding tissues, prevents excessive dilation of the heart, and aids in the regulation of ventricular coupling.[1] A small volume of fluid is normally present in the pericardial sac. The term pericardial effusion refers to an abnormal or excessive accumulation of fluid in the pericardial space. Pericardial effusion is the most common pericardial disease in dogs and cats.

Pathophysiology of cardiac tamponade

A small volume of fluid (0.25 ± 0.15 mL/kg) normally exists in the pericardial space.[1] Cardiac tamponade results from impaired ventricular filling secondary to increased intrapericardial pressure from *excess* fluid accumulation. Increased intrapericardial pressure secondary to fluid accumulation depends on several factors, the most important of which include the volume of fluid, the rate of fluid accumulation, and the distensibility of the fibrous pericardium. For example, in patients suffering acute pericardial fluid accumulation, a very small volume of fluid (50–100 mL in the dog) in the pericardial space may lead to a critical increase in intrapericardial pressure and resultant cardiac tamponade. However, if this fluid accumulates at a slower rate, parietal pericardial compliance will increase over time. This allows the pericardial sac to accommodate a significantly larger volume of fluid before intrapericardial pressure increases enough to result in cardiac tamponade. Therefore it stands to reason that a large volume of pericardial effusion is most commonly the result of a more chronic underlying disease process.

When intrapericardial pressure equilibrates with right atrial (typically 4–8 mm Hg) and right ventricular diastolic pressures, right-sided cardiac filling is impaired leading to cardiac tamponade. Further increases in pericardial fluid accumulation lead to concomitant increases in intrapericardial, right atrial, and right ventricular diastolic pressures. With excessive fluid accumulation, the intrapericardial pressure may rise to a level that exceeds the filling pressures of the left atrium and ventricle, leading to severe reductions in diastolic filling. Consequently, these patients suffer a marked reduction in stroke volume, and a resultant decrease in cardiac output. Neurohormonal compensatory mechanisms are activated, leading to an increase in heart rate, cardiac contractility, and systemic vascular resistance in an effort to improve effective circulating volume. However, as intrapericardial pressure continues to increase, these mechanisms are no longer able to compensate, and the result is a severe reduction in cardiac output and systemic arterial blood pressure. In patients with acute cardiac tamponade, signs consistent with low-output cardiac failure such as tachycardia, hypotension, and collapse dominate their clinical picture. However, in patients with more chronic elevations in intracardiac pressures, signs of right heart failure such as ascites and jugular venous distension are more common.[1]

Advanced Monitoring and Procedures for Small Animal Emergency and Critical Care, First Edition. Edited by Jamie M. Burkitt Creedon, Harold Davis.
© 2012 John Wiley & Sons, Inc. Published 2012 by John Wiley & Sons, Inc.

Clinical signs associated with pericardial effusion

The clinical presentation of patients suffering from acute and chronic pericardial effusion differs substantially.[1] Syncope or collapse is fairly common in patients presenting with acute cardiac tamponade, and is reported in up to 50% of canine patients with echocardiographic evidence of effusion.[2] Physical examination findings in patients suffering from acute disease are consistent with cardiogenic shock. Therefore, patients frequently exhibit most or all of the following in addition to the dull heart sounds classic for pericardial effusion: tachycardia, tachypnea, decreased arterial pulse pressure, jugular venous distension, and pulsus paradoxus. In health, systemic arterial blood pressure varies with the respiratory cycle, decreasing slightly during inspiration, and increasing with expiration. In patients with pericardial effusion, this variation may be more marked as a result of alterations in ventricular filling pressures secondary to pericardial fluid accumulation. This phenomenon is termed **pulsus paradoxus** and is characterized by an inspiratory decrease in systolic arterial blood pressure greater than 10 mm Hg.

In patients with more chronic fluid accumulation, the client complaint is often vague and nonspecific. Commonly reported findings include weight loss, inappetance, weakness, exercise intolerance, tachypnea, cough, and abdominal distension. Patients display signs of right-sided congestive heart failure such as dull lung sounds, hepatomegaly, ascites, and jugular venous distension. In addition, these patients may also exhibit physical examination findings consistent with acute decompensation, including decreased pulse quality, tachypnea, tachycardia, and pulsus paradoxus.

Pericardial effusion is usually secondary to congestive heart failure in feline patients. Therefore, cats with pericardial effusion often have abnormal cardiothoracic auscultatory findings including heart murmurs, gallop rhythms, and abnormal lung sounds.[3]

Diagnosis of pericardial effusion

There is no anamnestic detail or physical examination finding that is pathognomonic for pericardial effusion. The presence of multiple historical and physical examination abnormalities suggestive of pericardial fluid accumulation should prompt the clinician to perform additional testing to confirm a diagnosis of pericardial effusion. When the clinician suspects pericardial effusion, he or she may order thoracic radiography, electrocardiography, and/or echocardiography to aid in confirmation. Pericardial fluid analysis is often performed after pericardiocentesis and is occasionally helpful in determining etiology. Other less commonly utilized diagnostics include nonselective venous angiography, pneumopericardiography, transesophageal echocardiography, computed tomography, and magnetic resonance imaging.

Radiography

Thoracic radiography will reveal cardiac enlargement in up to 87% of dogs and 95% of cats that can range from mild to severe depending on the volume of fluid accumulation, with larger volumes typically indicating chronicity.[2,3] The cardiac silhouette is often globoid in appearance with loss of the normal cardiac contours. Pulmonary vascular markings may be diminished as a result of decreased cardiac output. Metastatic pulmonary disease may be present in patients with pericardial effusion secondary to neoplasia. Abnormal lung patterns have been seen in up to 60% of feline patients, likely due to the high frequency of congestive heart failure as an underlying cause for feline pericardial effusion.[3] In patients with cardiac tamponade, radiographs may reveal caudal vena caval distension, hepatomegaly, or pleural effusion. There may be evidence of tracheal deviation dorsally with tumors located at the heart base. Thoracic radiographs can also be normal in patients with acute cardiac tamponade; therefore radiography should be used in conjunction with additional diagnostic testing and thorough physical examination for the diagnosis of pericardial effusion.

Electrocardiography

Sinus tachycardia is the most common electrocardiographic rhythm in canine patients with pericardial effusion. Atrial or ventricular tachyarrhythmias have also been documented in both dogs and cats; however, in many patients the electrocardiogram is normal. Low-amplitude QRS complexes and ST segment elevation are seen quite commonly.[2,4] From 6% to 64% of canine patients exhibit evidence of **electrical alternans** on routine electrocardiography (see Fig. 14.1).[4,5] This is typically seen in patients with large-volume effusions and is thus rare in the feline patient. Electrical alternans results from shifting of the heart's electrical axis in relation to the electrocardiograph leads as the heart oscillates within the fluid-filled pericardial space. The shifting relationship between the heart's electrical axis and the electrocardiograph leads results in phasic variations in QRS or T-wave amplitude on the electrocardiogram (ECG). Because the ECG is often normal in patients with pericardial effusion, it is not considered a sensitive diagnostic test.

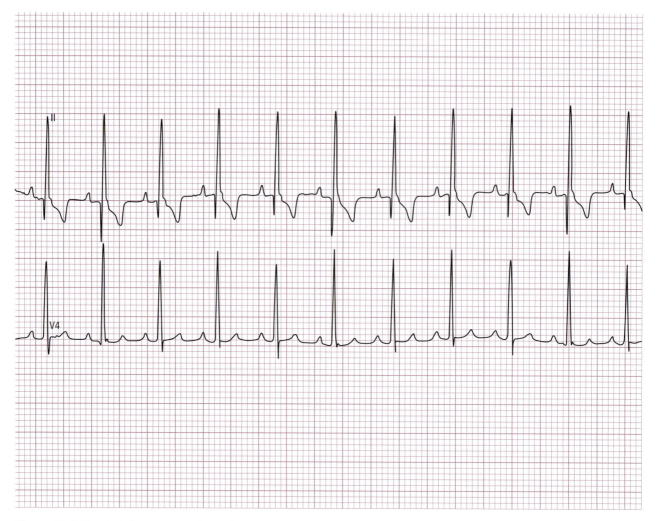

Figure 14.1 Electrical alternans in a dog with pericardial effusion. Note the change in R-wave amplitude from one complex to the next such that every other complex is similar. Also note that electrical alternans may be visualized quite easily in one lead and more difficult to see in another.

Echocardiography

Echocardiography is the noninvasive reference standard for the diagnosis of pericardial effusion in humans and animals; it has eclipsed thoracic radiography and electrocardiography as the most sensitive and specific diagnostic test available in routine clinical practice. Effusion is identified as an echo-free or hypoechoic space between the epicardium and the pericardium (see Fig. 14.2). Echocardiography can identify even very small volumes of fluid accumulation and can also be used to identify cardiac tamponade, cardiac mass lesions, severe valvular endocardiosis leading to left atrial rupture, diminished left or right ventricular internal diameter, ventricular wall thickening, paradoxical interventricular septal motion, or pleural effusion that may accompany pericardial effusion. Because it can identify the underlying

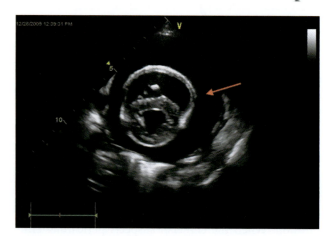

Figure 14.2 Pericardial effusion in a dog identified as an echo-free space (see arrow) between the epicardium and the pericardium. (Courtesy Boileau JS.)

etiology for the effusion in some patients, echocardiography can also be useful in determining long-term prognosis. See Chapter 13, Bedside Echocardiography, for more information about obtaining adequate echocardiographic images.

Pericardial fluid analysis

The diagnostic yield of pericardial fluid analysis in canine patients is generally low; nevertheless it can be useful for the diagnosis of suppurative, mycotic, transudative, and modified transudative effusions. Depending on gross characteristics or cytological findings, fluid samples may be submitted for bacterial or fungal culture and sensitivity to determine appropriate antimicrobial therapy. However, most pericardial effusions in the dog are bloody or blood-tinged. The overlap of cell counts between serosanguinous and hemorrhagic effusions makes the differentiation between these fluid types problematic. In addition, cells from cardiac neoplasias in the dog do not reliably exfoliate into the pericardial space, limiting the clinician's ability to accurately diagnose neoplasia via fluid cytology. The discrimination between neoplastic and reactive mesothelial cells is also challenging, making a diagnosis of mesothelioma difficult. Despite these limitations, pericardial fluid analysis should be performed routinely, as it provides crucial information in some cases. In feline patients cytological analysis tends to be more rewarding, as the underlying etiologies of pericardial effusion in this species are quite different from those in the dog (see Table 14.1).

Pericardiocentesis

Diagnostic pericardiocentesis is indicated in any patient with pericardial effusion. Therapeutic pericardiocentesis is essential for the stabilization of patients suffering from cardiac tamponade and for definitive therapy in patients with infectious pericarditis. If a patient is hemodynamically unstable, fluid therapy prior to or during the pericardiocentesis procedure is indicated. Baseline blood work including a packed cell volume, serum total protein concentration, and coagulation profile (prothrombin time, activated partial thromboplastin time) is recommended prior to performing the procedure, if the patient's clinical condition persists.

Pericardiocentesis can be performed with the patient in sternal, left lateral, or right lateral recumbency. The author prefers left lateral recumbency, as the cardiac notch is larger on the right side, which minimizes the risk of lung injury. In addition, placing patients in left lateral recumbency decreases the chance of inadvertent laceration of the coronary vessels. A potential disadvan-

Table 14.1 Pericardial diseases in the dog (D) and cat (C)

Congenital pericardial disease
Peritoneal pericardial diaphragmatic hernia[a]
Partial or complete pericardial agenesis
Pericardial cysts (D)

Acquired pericardial disease and pericardial effusion
Idiopathic pericardial effusion (D)[a]
Neoplasia[a]
Congestive heart failure (C more than D)[a]
Feline infectious peritonitis (C)[a]
Septic effusion
 Bacterial
 Fungal
 Viral
 Protozoal
Exudative effusion
Transudative or modified transudative effusion
Chylous effusion (D)
Coagulopathy
Left atrial rupture (D)
Systemic disease
 Uremia
 Hypoalbuminemia
 Sepsis
Trauma
Pneumopericardium (D)
Iatrogenic hemorrhage
Hyperthyroidism (C)

Note: diseases occur in both dog and cat unless otherwise noted.
[a]Common.

tage of pericardiocentesis performed from the right side of the thorax is aspiration of deoxygenated blood directly from the right ventricle, which appears grossly similar to the classic "port-wine"-colored hemorrhagic effusion seen most commonly in dogs. Some clinicians may prefer pericardiocentesis be performed from the left side for this reason, as blood obtained by inadvertent left ventricular puncture is oxygenated, and thus grossly distinguishable from hemorrhagic pericardial effusion. Comparing the packed cell volume of the sample with that obtained from peripheral blood can readily make the distinction between blood and effusion. These values will differ significantly in most patients, with the exception of those suffering from acute hemorrhage in the absence of preexisting fluid accumulation. Additionally, pericardial effusion will not clot, so depositing some fluid into an empty red-top tube at the beginning of pericardiocentesis and observing for clot formation can help distinguish effusion from fresh ventricular blood.

Lastly, pericardiocentesis may also be performed from the right side with the patient in sternal recumbency, as this position may be more favorable in the hemodynamically unstable patient.

The optimum site for catheter insertion must be determined. Ideally, echocardiography is used to identify the site with the largest volume fluid accumulation between the thoracic wall and the heart. However, if this imaging modality is not available, blind pericardiocentesis can be performed at the right fourth or fifth intercostal space just below the costochondral junction where the precordial pulse is most readily palpable.

The area between the right third and eighth intercostal spaces from the costochondral junction to the sternum should be clipped and cleaned with aseptic surgical scrub technique. Hand hygiene should be performed and sterile gloves should be donned for the duration of the procedure. An electrocardiogram should be attached to the patient and monitored continuously throughout the procedure to facilitate detection of dysrhythmias generated by inadvertent contact with or puncture of the myocardium. Arterial blood pressure should be monitored at regular intervals throughout the procedure using either invasive or noninvasive monitoring tools.

A local anesthetic block of 2% lidocaine should be administered at the intended site of catheter insertion and associated underlying intercostal musculature and pleura to minimize patient discomfort. Pericardiocentesis can be performed in many canine patients simply with the aid of local anesthesia; however, the addition of chemical restraint will be needed in almost all feline patients. The combination of an opioid and a benzodiazepine provides excellent sedation while minimizing cardiovascular instability seen with many other sedative combinations. Alternatively, etomidate administered in combination with other sedatives may also be considered.

Several different catheter types can be used. The author prefers a 14- to 16-gauge 5.5-inch over-the-needle catheter for canine patients. Additional side-holes may be cut near the tip of the catheter with a scalpel to facilitate drainage, with care taken to smooth sharp edges at the periphery of these holes (see Fig. 14.3). Smaller catheter sizes will be needed for small-breed dogs and cats. The author prefers a 22-gauge 1- to 1.5-inch needle or butterfly catheter attached to a 12- to 20-mL syringe for these smaller patients.

A stab incision should be made with a number-11 scalpel blade through the skin at the site of catheter insertion. The catheter should be inserted perpendicular to the skin on the cranial aspect of the rib with care taken to avoid the intercostal vessels. The catheter should

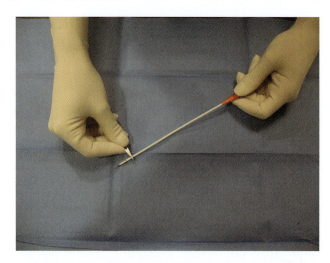

Figure 14.3 Correct method for cutting additional side holes in pericardial catheter to facilitate drainage.

be slowly advanced in 1-cm increments until fluid is seen in the catheter hub. As the needle is advanced, pale yellow or serosanguinous pleural effusion may be obtained, particularly in patients with chronic pericardial effusion; however, this should not be confused with pericardial effusion, which is typically deep red and hemorrhagic in character in dogs. Upon entering the pericardial space, the catheter should be advanced an additional 1–1.5 cm and then fed off the tip of the stylet. The stylet should subsequently be removed and the catheter attached to extension tubing, a three-way stopcock, and a 12- to 60-cc syringe (depending on patient size). Subtle scratching of the tip may be noted as the catheter enters the pericardial space; however, once within the pericardial space, scratching felt at the tip of the catheter is likely due to the catheter contacting the epicardial surface. As this has the potential to induce ventricular arrhythmias, the catheter should be slightly retracted, and the ECG should be carefully monitored.

After a small amount of fluid is retrieved, steps should be taken to differentiate between intracardiac and intrapericardial fluid (see Box 14.1). Pericardial effusion does not clot unless the hemorrhage is very recent, and the packed cell volume of pericardial effusion will often differ significantly from that of peripheral blood. Lastly, the supernatant in a spun sample of pericardial effusion is often xanthochromic, or yellow in color, due to the presence of by-products of hemoglobin breakdown resulting from previous hemorrhage. Once it has been determined that the retrieved fluid is from the pericardial space, as much fluid as possible should be retrieved from the patient's pericardium (in the absence of active hemorrhage) and quantified. Reduction of the effusion

Box 14.1 Methods to differentiate pericardial effusion from blood retrieved by inadvertent cardiac aspiration

Evaluate sample for clotting

Place sample in red-top tube and observe for 3 minutes:

- Pericardial effusion will rarely clot.
- Blood aspirated from heart will clot readily.

Evaluate packed cell volume (PCV) of sample

Place sample in microhematocrit tube and compare with sample of peripheral blood placed in microhematocrit tube:

- PCV of pericardial effusion will differ from that of peripheral blood.
- PCV of blood aspirated from heart will match that of peripheral blood.

Evaluate sample supernatant

Place red-top tube containing sample in centrifuge for 5 minutes at 3400 rpm and evaluate supernatant:

- Supernatant of pericardial effusion may be yellowish due to breakdown products of previous hemorrhage.
- Supernatant of blood aspirated from heart will be clear to slightly cloudy (serum).

and resolution of tamponade should be confirmed by echocardiography. See Protocol 14.1 for step-by-step instructions.

Postpericardiocentesis monitoring

Patients should be closely monitored for evidence of hemodynamic instability resulting from reaccumulation of pericardial fluid, ongoing hemorrhage, or ventricular arrhythmias. In patients with active hemorrhage, fluid can leak from the pericardial space into the pleural cavity, resulting in life-threatening hemorrhage. Ventricular arrhythmias following pericardiocentesis can range from mild to severe, the latter of which may necessitate treatment with antiarrhythmic medications. The author recommends inpatient monitoring for at least 24 hours following pericardiocentesis with serial evaluation of heart rate, respiratory rate, and blood pressure, frequent thoracic auscultation for dull heart or lung sounds consistent with fluid accumulation, and serial evaluation of urine output and mentation, both of which may change as a result of altered perfusion. Intensive monitoring of these physical examination findings coupled

with continuous electrocardiography and intermittent echocardiography will facilitate prompt recognition of complications such as hemorrhage or dysrhythmias.

Complications of pericardiocentesis

Pericardiocentesis is a relatively safe procedure if it is performed as recommended and appropriate precautions are taken to minimize the risk of complications. Relative contraindications to pericardiocentesis include coagulopathy, active hemorrhage due to atrial rupture or actively bleeding neoplasia, and small-volume effusions in the absence of tamponade. Commonly recognized complications of pericardiocentesis include inadvertent ventricular puncture, ventricular or supraventricular arrhythmias, cardiac or coronary artery laceration, exsanguination, tumor rupture, or dissemination of neoplasia or infectious agents into the thoracic cavity (see Table 14.2).[6] Ventricular puncture occurs when the catheter is advanced too far into the pericardial space. Once in the wall of the ventricle, the catheter will move with each ventricular systole, and ventricular arrhythmias may be evident on the surface ECG. If cardiac puncture occurs, the catheter should be incrementally withdrawn from the ventricular wall. This is often not a serious complication if recognized and corrected promptly. However, failure to recognize ventricular puncture may result in removal of large amounts of blood from the ventricle and possible exsanguination. In addition, manipulation of the catheter while it is within the ventricular wall may result in cardiac laceration and rupture with catastrophic hemorrhage. Monitoring the patient as recommended with electrocardiography will facilitate early detection of dysrhythmias generated by cardiac puncture. Utilization of echocardiography and blood pressure monitoring, as well as monitoring retrieved fluid for clotting and packed cell volume as directed previously, will facilitate the prompt recognition of hemorrhage. Early intervention is critical in these patients; however, most patients

Table 14.2 Complications of pericardiocentesis

Ventricular puncture
Dysrhythmias
Coronary artery laceration
Cardiac laceration
Exsanguination
Tumor rupture
Dissemination of neoplasia
Dissemination of infection

Protocol 14.1 Pericardiocentesis

Items Required
- Clippers with clean blade
- Surgical antiseptics for preparation
- 14- to 22-gauge over-the-needle catheter
- Scalpel blade #11
- Three-way stopcock
- Fluid extension tubing
- 12- to 60-cc syringe
- Bowl for collecting expelled effusion
- Sterile tubes
  - Red-top to monitor for clotting, for culture as needed
  - Lavender-top for cytology
- Sterile gloves
- 2% lidocaine for local anesthetic block (not to exceed safe dosage)
- Lidocaine 2 mg/kg intravenously, for possible ventricular arrhythmias
- Electrocardiograph
- Noninvasive blood pressure monitor
- Portable ultrasound if available
- Chemical restraint as needed
- Oxygen supplementation as needed
- Two or more assistants

Procedure
1. Collect necessary supplies.
2. Obtain baseline peripheral blood samples.
3. Aseptically attach syringe and extension tubing to three-way stopcock such that catheter will attach to extension tubing, leaving one stopcock port open for fluid expulsion into collection bowl.
4. Place patient in preferred recumbency.
5. Determine optimum site for pericardiocentesis with ultrasound or by palpation.
6. Clip and aseptically prepare pericardiocentesis site.
7. Connect patient to electrocardiograph and blood pressure monitor.
8. Administer local block of 2% lidocaine through the subcutaneous tissues and intercostal musculature.
9. Administer chemical restraint if needed.
10. Perform hand hygiene and don sterile gloves.
11. Make a stab incision through the skin with scalpel blade.
12. Incrementally advance catheter–stylet pair through the skin, subcutaneous tissues, and intercostal musculature until pericardial fluid is seen in the hub of the catheter.
13. Advance catheter and stylet additional 1 cm, then feed catheter off stylet.
14. Remove stylet and attach catheter hub to available three-way stopcock port. Aspirate fluid.
15. Aseptically place fluid samples in red- and lavender-top tubes. Examine aspirated fluid for evidence of clotting; determine packed cell volume and serum total protein concentration (PCV/TP) of fluid and compare with peripheral blood to confirm appropriate catheter placement in pericardial space.
16. Deposit remaining fluid into collection bowl. Quantitate volume of retrieved fluid and store samples in refrigerator prior to submission for cytologic analysis.
17. Once all fluid is removed, withdraw catheter from pericardial space.
18. Verify reduction of the effusion via echocardiography if possible.

with active hemorrhage due to coronary artery laceration or cardiac rupture will not survive.

Summary

Pericardiocentesis is a relatively safe procedure that can be life-saving for patients with cardiac tamponade. Pericardial effusion is most readily diagnosed with thoracic ultrasound, which can also be helpful to guide pericardiocentesis. Fluid samples should be used to ensure pericardial effusion is being collected rather than ventricular blood, and for additional diagnostic testing. Monitoring perfusion parameters and the patient's ECG is crucial during and following the procedure.

References

1. Sisson DK, Thomas WP. Chapter 29: Pericardial disease and cardiac tumors. In: Fox PR, Sisson DK, Moise NS, eds. Textbook of Canine and Feline Cardiology: Principles and Clinical Practice. 2nd ed. St Louis: WB Saunders; 1999:679–701.

2. Stafford JM, Martin M, Binns S, Day MJ. A retrospective study of clinical findings, treatment and outcome in 143 dogs with pericardial effusion. J Small Anim Pract 2004;45:546–552.

3. Hall DJ, Shofer FJ, Meier CK, Sleeper MM. Pericardial effusion in cats: a retrospective study of clinical findings and outcome in 146 Cats. J Vet Intern Med 2007;21:1002–1007.

4. Berg RJ, Wingfield W. Pericardial effusion in the dog: a review of 42 cases. J Am Anim Hosp Assoc 1984;20:721–730.

5. Bonagura JD. Electrical alternans associated with pericardial effusion in the dog. J Am Vet Med Assoc 1981;178:574–579.

6. Kittleson MD. Chapter 25: Pericardial disease and cardiac neoplasia. In Kittleson MD, Kienle RD, eds. Small Animal Cardiovascular Medicine. 1st ed. St Louis: Mosby; 1998;413–431.

15

Monitoring tissue perfusion: clinicopathologic aids and advanced techniques

Brian C. Young

Optimal tissue perfusion with complete restoration of cumulative oxygen debt, resolution of acidosis, and resumption of aerobic metabolism in all tissues, are ultimate goals of shock resuscitation and lead to improved outcomes and decreased morbidity in critically ill patients.[1] Under-resuscitation causes prolonged oxygen deprivation and may lead to cellular and organ dysfunction, and ultimately patient demise. Over-resuscitation can lead to abdominal compartment syndrome (ACS), dilutional coagulopathy, volume-overload pulmonary edema, exacerbation of cerebral edema, and acute respiratory distress syndrome (ARDS). Methods to assess global and regional tissue perfusion and microcirculatory function are therefore being investigated as guides for precise, successful hemodynamic resuscitation and cardiovascular optimization without iatrogenic complication.

Monitoring perfusion always begins with an initial physical examination of the patient at presentation (primary survey) and continues with serial examinations thereafter. Triage and the primary patient survey are discussed elsewhere (see Chapter 1, Triage, and Chapter 2, The Small Animal Emergency Room) but several important details regarding evaluation of perfusion deserve repeat mention. Several physical examination parameters give information about global and regional perfusion. Vitally important parts of the assessment include mentation, mucous membrane color and quality, capillary refill time (CRT), heart rate (HR), distal pulse quality, and subjective distal extremity temperature. If not contraindicated (i.e., suspected cardiogenic shock), fluid resuscitation is immediately initiated in the poorly perfused patient while the physical

examination is completed. Further diagnostics, such as arterial blood pressure measurement, pulse oximetry (SpO_2), venous and arterial blood gases (VBG/ABG), electrolytes, blood glucose, packed cell volume, total protein, and lactate, are then pursued. A hemodynamically unstable patient is typically resuscitated to normalization of physical examination parameters, mean arterial pressure (MAP), and potentially, urine output (UOP).[2]

Pathophysiology of microcirculatory dysfunction

Several research groups have demonstrated microcirculatory hypoperfusion despite successful resuscitation to traditional perfusion parameters (HR, MAP, and UOP) in animal models and up to 85% of severely injured human patients.[3–8] Untreated compensatory shock and occult shock (ongoing tissue hypoperfusion despite normal vital signs) are associated with increased morbidity, increased mortality, and multiple organ dysfunction syndrome (MODS) in critically ill humans.[9–11] Theoretical pathogeneses for occult hypoperfusion-related MODS include direct damage from ischemia, subsequent reperfusion injury, instigation of overwhelming systemic inflammatory response syndrome (SIRS) and/or compensatory anti-inflammatory response syndrome (CARS), and development of irreversible cellular dysfunction. Global ischemia activates endothelial adhesion molecules, platelet activating factor (PAF), and the coagulation system in addition to breaking down endothelial glycocalyx[12] and increasing vascular permeability.[13]

Advanced Monitoring and Procedures for Small Animal Emergency and Critical Care, First Edition. Edited by Jamie M. Burkitt Creedon, Harold Davis.
© 2012 John Wiley & Sons, Inc. Published 2012 by John Wiley & Sons, Inc.

Additionally, prolonged hypoxia can interrupt ATP-dependent processes such as active electrolyte pumping, with subsequent cessation of cellular metabolism. This may lead to cell swelling, apoptosis, or necrosis. Research laboratories, emergency departments, operating suites, and intensive care units have begun to develop and utilize tools to elucidate the condition of the microcirculation in an attempt to identify occult shock and restore or maintain optimal tissue perfusion. This chapter introduces these techniques and discusses their clinical applications.

The literature consists of numerous experimental studies and an increasing number of human clinical trials that have significantly broadened our understanding of the pathophysiologies of several common disease states. These include septic shock, hemorrhagic shock, polytrauma, injury related to return of spontaneous circulation (ROSC) after cardiopulmonary cerebral resuscitation (CPCR), and anesthesia-induced hypotension. The microcirculation is a dynamic regulator of nutritional delivery to and waste removal from organs through cellular membranes, interstitial fluid, and blood constituents. The microcirculation is adversely affected in many disease states (see Table 15.1 for relevant veterinary diseases). Several factors lead to alterations in tissue oxygen supply and utilization at the cellular level. A typical response to overwhelming inflammation involves increased leukocyte adhesion to the endothelium and release of cytokines and reactive oxygen species (ROS). This increases chemotaxis, endothelial damage, and vascular permeability. Vascular tone is adversely affected by SIRS and severe sepsis. Abnormalities of vasomotor function affect both arteries and veins. During SIRS, venous capacitance vessels, which normally contain 75% of the total circulating volume (the unstressed portion), may fail to constrict in response to sympathetic signaling. This venous vasodilation and the resultant pooling of blood in the venous circulation may lead to decreases in preload and cardiac output (CO). Protein-rich fluid exudation from the vascular space simultaneously decreases effective circulating volume and increases interstitial edema, creating additional barriers to nutrient diffusion.

An appropriate physiologic response to shock harnesses the sympathetic nervous system, causing adrenal release of catecholamines. Initially, β-adrenergic stimulation enhances chronotropy, inotropy, CO, and oxygen delivery (DO_2). Alpha-adrenergic receptors facilitate vasoconstriction and centralization of blood flow to the brain, heart, and lungs at the expense of other capillary beds (hepatosplanchnic and musculocutaneous). This potent insult to regional perfusion may persist despite normalization of systemic hemodynamics.[14,15]

Table 15.1 Diseases affecting the microcirculation

Systemic inflammatory response syndrome (SIRS)[46,182–184]
Acute necrotizing pancreatitis
Polytrauma[185]
Hemorrhagic shock
Hypovolemic shock
Heat-induced illness
Immune-mediated diseases: hemolytic anemia, thrombocytopenia, polyarthropathy
Steroid-responsive meningitis
Hemorrhagic gastroenteritis (HGE)
Uroperitoneum
Disseminated neoplasia
Envenomation
Gastric ulceration
Acute respiratory distress syndrome
Feline hepatic lipidosis
Abdominal compartment syndrome

Severe sepsis[182,183,186–189]
Bacterial peritonitis
Pyothorax
Pneumonia
Pyometra
Bacterial prostatitis
Urosepsis
Gastrointestinal translocation
Soft-tissue infection
Parvovirus
Endocarditis
Bloodstream infection
Bacterial meningoencephalitis
Hepatic abscessation

Ischemia-reperfusion injury[190]
Gastric dilatation–volvulus
Aortic thromboembolism
Pulmonary thromboembolism
Pulmonary reexpansion injury
Post–cardiopulmonary cerebral resuscitation
Any state of hypoperfusion

Anaphylaxis[191–193]
Vaccine reaction
Insect sting
Envenomation
Antivenin
Drug reaction
Transfusion reaction (acute hemolytic, transfusion-related lung injury)

In addition to heterogeneous diversion of blood via shunted venules (distributive hypoxia), the microcirculation suffers several other insults, which affects its environment.[10,16–18] These include tumor necrosis factor (TNF-α), endothelial swelling, alterations in nitric oxide

concentration >2 mmol/L at 6 hours into treatment was associated with significantly increased mortality.

Technology available to measure blood lactate concentration

Blood lactate measurements are readily accessible in veterinary medicine using blood gas machines (NOVA, Stat Profile Critical Care Xpress, NOVA Biomedical Corporation, Waltham, MA; Rapidlab, Bayer Diagnostics, East Walpole, MA), handheld monitors (istat, istat Corporation, East Windsor, NJ), and several recently introduced point-of-care instruments.[42,56,57]

Blood lactate concentration can be measured via enzymatic colorimetry or enzymatic amperometry. Enzymatic colorimetry utilizes spectrophotometry to measure NADH produced from lactate dehydrogenase-catalyzed oxidation of L-lactate by NAD^+. The NADH levels indicate the amount of lactate present in the sample. This technology is most often found in blood chemistry analyzers. In contrast to the relatively slow process of spectrophotometry, enzymatic amperometry reads results from small amounts of whole blood samples within 2 minutes. Enzymatic amperometry detects hydrogen peroxide produced by the lactate oxidase-catalyzed conversion of lactate to pyruvate, proportional to the lactate level of the sample.[58] Hydrogen peroxide is detected as an anodic current by a sensor, which translates the measurement into a lactate value. Bench-top blood gas analyzers often include lactate monitoring capabilities and require only a small amount of heparinized whole blood.

Recently, several handheld lactate monitors have been evaluated for use in dogs and cats. Point-of-care lactate monitors have greatly improved the accessibility and affordability of measuring blood lactate in clinical veterinary patients. Compared with serum chemistry analyzers, bench-top blood gas machines (NOVA and Rapidlab, above) and point-of-care monitors (such as istat, above; Accusport, Sports Resource Group, Inc. London, UK; Lactate Pro, Arkray Inc, Kyoto, Japan; Lactate Scout, Sens Lab GmbH, Leipzig, Germany; and Accutrend, Roche Diagnostics, Basel, Switzerland) require a very small amount of blood and provide results within seconds to minutes. Careful review of recent literature provides important information regarding the accuracies of newer point-of-care monitor use in canine and feline clinical patients.[42,56–59]

Performing blood lactate concentration measurement

Sample acquisition should be taken into consideration when evaluating lactate concentration in veterinary patients. Ideally, blood samples for bench-top analyzers should be acquired using blood gas syringes prefilled with lyophilized heparin to avoid dilutional effects of liquid heparin.[60] Cats can have marked, transient spikes in blood lactate in stressful situations,[61] such as restraint for venipuncture. Also, blood lactate concentration is expected to increase any time the anaerobic threshold has been breached, which will occur with excessive struggling, seizuring, and physical exertion. Serial blood lactate measurements taken from indwelling sampling catheters may avoid stressing the patient and adversely affecting interpretation of results. Prolonged venous stasis may increase regional blood lactate concentrations and should be avoided when acquiring a peripheral venous sample. Although blood lactate from peripheral samples in dogs were statistically higher than concurrent jugular venous and femoral arterial samples, all values were reasonably close to one another and the differences were not clinically significant.[41] The study concluded <2.5 mmol/L is the normal blood lactate concentration in dogs.

There is no documented benefit to monitoring arterial as opposed to venous blood lactate levels.[24]

It has been recommended that heparinized, whole blood samples be run as soon as possible and within 30 minutes, as lactate increases over time even if the sample is stored on ice.[43] Separation of plasma or serum from erythrocytes is recommended when samples cannot be immediately analyzed.[43] To arrest glycolytic enzymes, plasma and serum samples can be stored in sodium fluoride, on ice, for later colorimetric analysis. With adequate cardiovascular function, blood lactate has a half-life of 60 minutes in humans.[62] See Box 15.1 for detailed procedures for blood lactate concentration measurement.

Acid–base monitoring

Tissue hypoperfusion and ensuing metabolic acidosis can be assessed using pH, bicarbonate (HCO_3), base deficit (BD), and lactate. Hydrogen ions are produced both from lactate formation and the rapid breakdown of high- and intermediate-energy phosphates. It has recently (2007) been shown in a canine hemorrhagic shock model that, in addition to lactate, several unmeasured anions (citrate, fumarate, and α-ketoglutarate) contribute to metabolic acidosis during tissue oxygen debt.[63] These unmeasured ions are intermediates of the Krebs cycle and may be evidence of mitochondrial dysfunction. Other potential causes of metabolic acidosis include an increased strong ion gap (SIG), which has been independently shown to predict mortality in people when it is the major cause of metabolic acidosis.[39]

Box 15.1 Guidelines for blood lactate concentration measurement

Guidelines are appropriate for bench-top blood gas analyzers and for point-of-care lactate monitors:
1. Minimize stress and begin with a relatively calm patient, if possible.
2. Use a blood gas syringe with lyophilized heparin to decrease dilutional errors. (Some point-of-care monitors may require unheparinized blood.)
3. The sample may be acquired from direct arterial or venous puncture or from an indwelling catheter (free-flowing, stress-free samples are ideal).
4. Run the sample measurement as soon as possible. If the sample cannot be run within several minutes, it should be put on ice. There is a significant, artifactual increase in lactate within 30–60 minutes of time delay.
5. It is reasonable to monitor trends in abnormal blood lactate levels in critically ill clinical patients over the course of several hours (serial samples every 4–6 hours).

Collecting a sample for later testing:
1. Collect blood in a syringe and centrifuge the sample (after clot formation if no anticoagulant is used).
2. Separate the plasma or serum from the erythrocytes.
3. Refrigerate the serum or plasma in sodium fluoride (if available) to prevent further lactate production.

Shedding of heparan sulfate from damaged endothelial cells may also cause metabolic acidosis in a canine hemorrhagic shock model.[63] Normalization of lactate does not necessarily equate to adequate resuscitation, especially when the patient displays a persistent metabolic acidosis. Therefore, metabolic acidosis of unknown origin in critically ill patients, with or without hyperlactatemia, is a significant finding that warrants further monitoring and potentially additional resuscitative efforts. Blood collection for interpretation of acid–base status is discussed in Chapter 47, Blood Sample Collection and Handling (see also Chapter 50, Acid–Base Evaluation).

Monitoring the arterial or venous BD has long been recognized as a marker of cellular function. The BD is the amount of base in millimoles needed to titrate 1 L of arterial whole blood to a pH of 7.4, with fully saturated hemoglobin, at 37°C, and a $PaCO_2$ of 40 mm Hg. A high BD correlates with type A hyperlactatemia, and suggests continued O_2 debt and cellular dysfunction. It is well accepted as a predictor of hemodynamic changes, increased length of hospital stay,

transfusion requirements, MODS, and mortality in human patients.[64–67] Initial BD, in combination with lactate, is a sensitive screening tool for illness severity and outcome prediction.[49,51] A preliminary retrospective study of canine trauma patients reported admission BD to be a predictor of mortality and requirement for red blood cell transfusion.[68]

Although significant time and effort have been dedicated to evaluating BD,[51,67,69] it is considered by many to be a poor indicator of shock reversal and is not currently recommended as a definitive resuscitation endpoint.[70,71] However, the availability of BD on any blood gas analysis makes it an inexpensive and readily available marker of perfusion, useful for initial evaluation of shock.[64,69] As with other dynamic patient variables, noting trends in serial BD measurements may reveal occult hypoperfusion in hospitalized patients with normal vital parameters. Two separate research groups have demonstrated profound differences in MODS and mortality (50%–68% versus 4.5%–9%) in critically ill humans who did not correct BD or lactate after 24 hours of treatment.[51,67] Kincaid[67] also correlated persistently increased BD with decreased VO_2 in human trauma patients, suggesting an uncoupling of oxygen delivery and consumption. Similar to lactate, pH, HCO_3, and BD are only indirect measures of global tissue perfusion and may engender a false sense of security in patients with ongoing regional hypoperfusion.

Oxygen-derived variables
Oxygen extraction ratio

Oxygen delivery (DO_2), consumption (VO_2), and extraction ratio (O_2ER) have been investigated using the pulmonary artery catheter (PAC) to elucidate patient response to shock in animal models and clinical human patients.[72–75] In normal physiologic equilibrium, tissues are provided with far more oxygen than necessary for normal metabolic activity (*supply independence*), but at some point ("**critical DO_2**"; usually at O_2ER of 70%), decreased DO_2 leads to anaerobic metabolism, lactate production, and decreased VO_2 (*supply dependence*). Shoemaker et al.[76,77] observed supranormal cardiac index (CI), DO_2, and VO_2 in human polytrauma survivors requiring general anesthesia and surgical intervention. Initial prospective, randomized clinical data suggested a decrease in mortality when patients were resuscitated to a goal-directed, supranormal CI and DO_2 with fluid therapy and pharmacologic intervention using inotropes and vasopressors.[78,79] However, these promising results have not been duplicated despite extensive efforts[80,81] and the interventions may be harmful.[82–84] One major line of criticism of this line of research is that the patients may not have received resuscitation efforts early enough in their disease processes to confer significant outcome benefits. Also, it is important to recognize DO_2 and O_2ER, as indicators of global oxygen transport, may not detect ongoing deficits in individual organs. Kincaid et al.[67] showed a lack of outcome prediction and great interpatient variability in serial VO_2 measurements in human trauma patients, questioning the validity of VO_2 as a resuscitation endpoint.

Other clinical investigators have focused their efforts on the O_2ER, which additionally requires arterial and pulmonary artery catheters. Increasing oxygen extraction is an important compensatory physiologic mechanism to maintain VO_2 in states of suboptimal DO_2. The O_2ER is representative of the cumulative oxygen debt to be corrected with reperfusion and metabolism of toxic metabolites, both requiring the adequate function of many organ systems. The O_2ER (VO_2/DO_2) is calculated as

$$VO_2/DO_2 = (CaO_2 - CmvO_2)/CaO_2 \qquad (15.1)$$

using samples taken simultaneously from both a peripheral artery and the pulmonary artery to determine arterial (CaO_2) and mixed venous ($CmvO_2$) oxygen content. See Box 15.2 for VO_2 and DO_2 calculation formulae, which require pulmonary arterial catheterization (PAC) and cardiac output monitoring. Protocol 15.1 describes the steps taken to calculate the O_2ER.

The need for a PAC and lack of clear consensus regarding interpretation of results limit the use of DO_2,

VO_2, and O_2ER in veterinary patients. Recent studies and reviews have challenged the cost versus benefit of PAC use in critically ill humans.[85–88] However, the concept of oxygen-derived variables can be applied to interrogation of patient status using venous oximetry.

Venous oximetry

Values that have gained renewed research interest are mixed ($SmvO_2$) and central venous ($ScvO_2$) oxygen saturations, which can be measured continuously via specialized fiberoptic catheters attached to reflectance oximetry, or serially with a co-oximeter (NOVA, Rapidlab as above). After fully oxygen-saturated hemoglobin (bound within erythrocytes) leaves the left ventricle, it travels to tissue capillaries, where oxygen diffuses from the hemoglobin to the surrounding interstitium, with 25%–30% of the oxygen leaving the hemoglobin molecule under homeostatic conditions. The normal resultant $ScvO_2$ and $SmvO_2$ are >70% and >65%, respectively. Increasing oxygen extraction from the hemoglobin is a compensatory mechanism to maintain tissue oxygenation during states of decreased DO_2. An increased O_2ER has been shown to significantly correlate with increased morbidity and mortality among the human intensive care patient population.[89–91] Other possible causes of low $ScvO_2$ include hyperthyroidism, seizure disorders, and pyrexia.

Rivers et al.[1] revolutionized clinical shock resuscitation practice by introducing a resuscitation protocol associated with an absolute risk reduction in mortality of 16% for humans with severe sepsis or septic shock. Strict, protocol-driven shock resuscitation [see Fig. 15.1, which outlines early goal-directed therapy (EGDT)] to specific CVP, MAP, UOP, and $ScvO_2$ endpoints, improved survival at all time points, improved illness severity scores, decreased the incidence of MODS, and improved coagulation parameters (prothrombin time, fibrin-split products, and D-dimer concentration). The control group was resuscitated to standard CVP, MAP, and UOP endpoints, without a specific protocol and without taking $ScvO_2$ into consideration. In the treatment group, a specific protocol was used, in which a $ScvO_2$ >70% was attained via MAP and CVP optimization, red blood cell transfusion and/or dobutamine infusion, as indicated by patient hematocrit (HCT) and CI. Early goal-directed therapy emphasizes the benefits of aggressively intervening as early as possible (within 6 hours of presentation) to prevent development of MODS and death. The standard-therapy patient group received larger volumes of fluids, blood products, and vasopressors throughout hospitalization, which have all been individually correlated with worsened outcomes.[92,93]

Box 15.2 Useful formulae to calculate oxygen extraction ratio

$DO_2 = [\text{blood flow (CO)}] \times CaO_2$

$VO_2 = [\text{blood flow (CO)}] \times (CaO_2 - CmvO_2)$

$O_2ER = \dfrac{(CaO_2 - CmvO_2)}{CaO_2} = \dfrac{VO_2}{DO_2} = \dfrac{(SaO_2 - SmvO_2)}{SmvO_2}$

$CaO_2 = (1.34 \times Hb \times SaO_2) + (0.003 \times PaO_2)$

CaO_2, arterial oxygen content; $CmvO_2$, mixed venous oxygen content; CO, cardiac output; DO_2, oxygen delivery; Hb, hemoglobin concentration; O_2ER, oxygen extraction ratio; SaO_2, saturation of Hb with O_2 in arterial blood; $SmvO_2$, saturation of Hb with O_2 in mixed venous blood; VO_2, oxygen consumption. All values must be checked for unit agreement before computation.

Protocol 15.1 How to calculate an oxygen extraction ratio (O_2ER)[199]

Items Required
- Patient with indwelling pulmonary arterial catheter (PAC) and peripheral arterial access (catheter or direct puncture)
- Examination gloves
- Supplies to aseptically prepare catheter port(s)
- Blood gas syringes—2
- Aseptically prepared 6-mL blood scavenging syringe filled with 1 mL heparinized 0.9% NaCl (two of these syringes if peripheral arterial sample will be from a catheter)
- Pressure bandage if performing direct arteriopuncture

Procedure
1. Obtain arterial and mixed venous blood samples, both using the following technique:
   a. Prepare supplies to collect an arterial blood gas sample (arteriopuncture or via arterial catheter) and mixed venous blood gas sample (via PAC).
   b. Perform hand hygiene and don clean examination gloves.
   c. Open a blood gas syringe filled with lyophilized heparin and expel air.
   d. Suspend pressure monitoring in preparation for sample collection from a three-way stopcock.
   e. The stopcock is turned off to the pressure transducer.
   f. Collect all samples anaerobically using aseptic technique.
   g. Slowly and gently remove (scavenge) a 3- to 6-mL presample of blood into heparinized saline solution that can be returned to the patient through a venous catheter.
   h. The stopcock is turned off to the patient to change syringes.
   i. Once the sample is slowly and gently obtained, excess air must be removed from the collection syringe immediately and the sample taken to the laboratory for blood gas measurement.
   j. Return scavenged blood via a venous catheter port.
   k. The catheter is then flushed and pressure monitoring can continue.
   l. Measure blood gases on both peripheral and pulmonary arterial samples as soon as possible.
2. Calculate $O_2ER = (CaO_2 - CmvO_2)/CaO_2$:
   a. $CaO_2 = (1.34 \times Hb \times SaO_2) + (0.003 \times PaO_2)$ (see Note)
   b. $CmvO_2 = (1.34 \times Hb \times SmvO_2) + (0.003 \times PmvO_2)$ (see Note)
   Note: Some suggest disregarding dissolved oxygen as it only slightly increases oxygen content

CaO_2, arterial oxygen content; $CmvO_2$, mixed venous oxygen content; Hb, hemoglobin concentration; O_2ER, oxygen extraction ratio; PAC, pulmonary arterial catheter; SaO_2, saturation of Hb with O_2 in arterial blood; $SmvO_2$, saturation of Hb with O_2 in mixed venous blood. All values must be checked for unit agreement before computation.

In addition to being a sensitive and specific indicator of global tissue perfusion, $ScvO_2$ is easy to measure clinically, requiring only a central venous catheter, a co-oximeter or a specialized blood gas machine with a co-oximetry function, proper sampling technique, and education. The measured saturation (not calculated from the PvO_2) is the proven strategy shown to effectively guide resuscitation in critically ill patients.[94] Partial pressure of oxygen may not accurately reflect $ScvO_2$, since the oxyhemoglobin dissociation curve can be altered in critical illness due to changes in pH, temperature, CO_2, and 2,3-DPG. There is debate as to the accuracy of $ScvO_2$ as an estimate of $SmvO_2$ and contradictory conclusions exist.[95–98] In critically ill patients, $ScvO_2$ is greater than $SmvO_2$, likely due to preferential maintenance of cerebral perfusion, compared with splanchnic

circulation, and $ScvO_2$ may lag behind changes in $SmvO_2$.[99] An experimental canine study showed a difference between the two variables, but changes paralleled each other.[100] Although $ScvO_2$ may vary in its correlation with $SmvO_2$, it has been independently validated as a resuscitation endpoint.

Furthermore, both veterinary and human patients with normal traditional perfusion parameters can remain in shock at a cellular level, as evidenced by $ScvO_2$,[101,102] which correlates with morbidity and mortality in humans.[11] Indeed, changes in $SmvO_2$ and $ScvO_2$ often precede abnormalities in HR and MAP, and thus represent a harbinger of patient deterioration. The Rivers group[99] concluded that $ScvO_2$ is an effective and practical resuscitation endpoint that should be targeted by optimizing MAP, CVP, HCT, and CI. In fact,

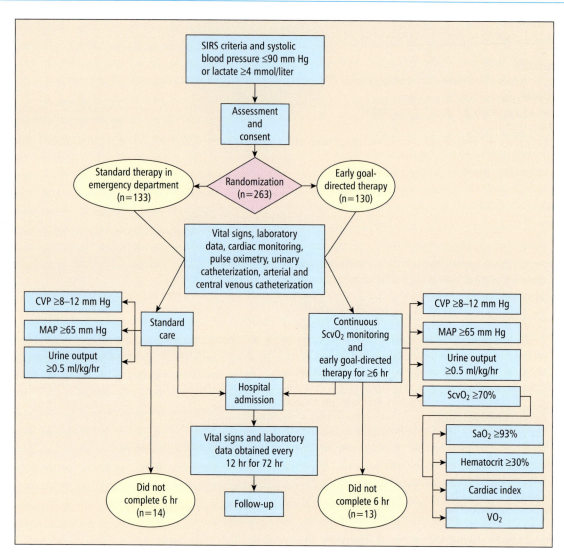

Figure 15.1 Study algorithm for early goal-directed therapy. CVP denotes central venous pressure; MAP, mean arterial pressure; and ScvO₂, central venous oxygen saturation. (Used with permission from Rivers et al. Early goal-directed therapy in the treatment of severe sepsis and septic shock. *New Eng J Med* 2001;345:1368–1377 © 2001 Massachusetts Medical Society. All rights reserved.)

the Surviving Sepsis Campaign (SSC) has recently endorsed ScvO₂ as an endpoint in its resuscitation bundle.[2] This specific intervention bundle has not been formally investigated in veterinary medicine but remains an excellent subject for future research. There are several recent trials confirming EGDT as an effective resuscitation bundle in human patient populations.[91,103–108]

Several other clinical uses have been suggested for ScvO₂. Changes in ScvO₂ may be more useful than MAP in determining the effectiveness of a fluid challenge.[109] Central venous oxygen saturation can also signal clinically silent blood loss and guide transfusion therapy in trauma patients,[110] as well as indicate the relative success of CPCR.[111] A ScvO₂ >72% was seen with return of spontaneous circulation.

Limitation to ScvO₂—cytopathic hypoxia

A controversy surrounding the use of ScvO₂ as a resuscitation endpoint for septic shock is that it may not be an accurate assessment of perfusion in patients with cytopathic hypoxia. In septic conditions, a normal or increased ScvO₂ or SmvO₂ may reflect a decrease in VO₂ secondary to microcirculatory and mitochondrial distress syndrome (MMDS), despite adequate or increased DO₂. MMDS is characterized by increased circulating inflammatory mediators, ROS, lipid peroxidation, DNA damage, loss of blood flow autoregulation, unresponsive hypotension, decreased systemic vascular resistance (SVR), normal to increased CO, increased gastric CO₂, increased blood lactate, acid–base abnormalities, and O₂ debt. MMDS is likely a combination of microcirculatory dysfunction–flow heterogeneity, and mitochondrial dysfunction regardless of oxygen availability.

As a result, humans in septic shock can have a normal $ScvO_2$, despite severe regional tissue dysoxia, due to microcirculatory shunting and/or a decreased O_2ER.[90,112] Yet a swine septic shock model showed an increased O_2ER throughout the hyperdynamic and hypodynamic phases of sepsis.[113]

Nicotinamide adenine dinucleotide

Nicotinamide adenine dinucleotide (NADH is the reduced form) is a major reducing agent, along with flavin adenine dinucleotide (FADH), needed to accept electrons from the oxidizing oxygen molecules along the assembly line of aerobic metabolism. Oxidation of NADH to NAD^+ represents the first step in the electron transport chain that drives oxidative phosphorylation (ATP production) in the inner mitochondrial compartment.

Defects in cellular oxygen utilization have been demonstrated to occur late in septic shock, after the resuscitation period,[114] which may explain the utility of $ScvO_2$ in EGDT. The poly(ADP-ribose) polymerase (PARP-1) enzyme, when activated by free radical peroxynitrite ($ONOO^-$), catalyzes the cleavage of NAD^+ into ADP-ribose and nicotinamide, leading to NADH depletion, thus halting aerobic respiration.[115,116] PARP-1 has also been implicated in the pathogenesis of LPS-induced vascular contractile dysfunction in rodents[117] and apoptosis.[118] This enzyme has therefore been identified as a possible target for pharmacologic intervention in septic shock.

As oxygen availability becomes decreased, more NADH remains in the reduced form. NADH has been shown to decrease in states of hyperoxia or increased tissue activation and is increased respectively with anesthesia, hypoxia, ischemia, and death.[119] Organ levels of NADH fluorescence (450 nm) can be measured via spectroscopic fluorometry to document regional oxygen availability in laboratory animals.[120] However, recent experimental work shows normal NADH levels throughout the hyperdynamic phase of sepsis, with subsequent decreased levels observed during septic shock.[113] The research concludes that decreased NADH appears to be a major factor in ATP depletion in advanced severe sepsis. It is unclear whether this is due to decreased NADH production, NO-related enzyme dysfunction,[121] or accelerated consumption through pyruvate metabolism to lactate.[113]

More useful clinical information can be obtained by simultaneously measuring NADH fluorescence and O_2 supply to the tissues (hemoglobin dynamics). Some multiparametric monitoring systems (MMS) can simultaneously measure microcirculatory tissue blood flow using a laser Doppler flowmetry approach (LDF), in addition to NADH fluorescence, tissue oxyhemoglobin-to-deoxyhemoglobin ratio, and tissue reflectance.[119,122]

Regional perfusion monitoring

Peripheral tissue gases

Notably, evaluation of tissue oxygenation has been introduced using subcutaneous or skeletal muscle monitoring. Monitoring transcutaneous oxygenation provides a noninvasive to minimally invasive measurement of regional tissue perfusion with a timescale for microcirculatory changes in shock and resuscitation closer to that of the gastrointestinal tract.[123] Transcutanous oxygenation suffers during shock, with both tissue O_2 and tissue CO_2 correlating less with well with PaO_2 and $PaCO_2$ during shock and initial resuscitation. Subcutaneous and skeletal tissues remain acidotic relative to the arterial pH during early resuscitation.

Transcutaneous partial pressure O_2 ($PtcO_2$) and partial pressure CO_2 ($PtcCO_2$) can be monitored with minimally invasive microprobes or noninvasive gel electrode pads, which are easily applied to clean skin and provide continuous data.[124,125] As the sensors warm with skin contact, the monitored segment of stratum corneum changes from a gel to a sol state, allowing transcutaneous gas diffusion. There is an initial 20-minute calibration period after probe placement, and probes are moved every 4 hours to prevent burns.[124] A different sensor has been described that noninvasively measures continuous $PtcCO_2$ and SpO_2 on the earlobe.[126]

Transcutaneous monitoring has been common practice in lieu of ABG monitoring in human neonatal critical care for decades. Data from human clinical studies shows a correlation between $PtcO_2$ and neurologic outcome.[127] Low $PtcO_2$ and high $PtcCO_2$ were significantly correlated with organ failure and death in human emergency department patients. All patients with a $PtcCO_2$ >60 mm Hg for >30 minutes died.[124] In the same study, $PtcO_2$ and $PtcCO_2$ were shown to be more sensitive indicators of occult hypoperfusion compared with changes in MAP or SpO_2 during the initial 3 hours of resuscitation.

Logistical dilemmas with this technology that impede the accuracy of monitoring include tissue edema, tissue trauma, and regional changes in thermoregulation that are commonly present in critically ill patients. Also, the measured $PtcO_2$ is representative of only a very limited area of cells, capillaries, and larger blood vessels. It will not accurately detect hidden hypoxic regions because of the heterogeneity of regional perfusion.

An experimental canine study group demonstrated good correlations with DO_2 and $ScvO_2$ measuring muscle PO_2 (PmO_2) via invasive microprobe fluoroscopy.[128] The same probe measured PmO_2, muscle PCO_2 ($PmCO_2$), and muscle pH (pHm). The group was able to show a decrease in PmO_2 before development of systemic hypotension, thus providing a sensitive method of detecting compensated shock. The return to baseline PmO_2 after resuscitation was comparable with oxygen delivery variables. However, the $PmCO_2$ and pHm lag behind resuscitation efforts by up to 4 hours. This research provides additional clear evidence of occult regional hypoperfusion despite resuscitation to traditional endpoints.

Near-infrared spectroscopy

Near-infrared spectroscopy (NIRS)[129] uses principles of light transmission and absorption to determine tissue oxygen saturation (StO_2); mitochondrial oxygen consumption via cytochrome a,a_3; PO_2; PCO_2; and pH. NIRS has been used to examine cerebral and muscle oxygenation after hypoxic injury[130] and was found to decrease in proportion to blood loss in human volunteers.[131] McKinley et al.[132] found correlations in human trauma patients between StO_2 and DO_2, BD, and lactate. Hall et al.[133] published a canine reference range for monitoring StO_2 using a portable NIRS device in healthy dogs. The most reliable measurements were obtained with a probe placed on the skin over the sartorius muscle.

Since skin and skeletal muscle tissues are relatively resistant to hypoxia-related damage, they may not be the ideal regional circulatory beds to monitor in critically ill patients. Furthermore, the subcutaneous tissue and skeletal muscle $PtcO_2$ and $PtcCO_2$ return to baseline levels before intestinal tissue, which is a potential drawback of this method since splanchnic hypoperfusion correlates with increased MODS and mortality. Skeletal muscle pH, which lags behind changes in O_2 and CO_2, has been suggested to correlate best with blood loss and incomplete resuscitation.[134] An ideal resuscitation endpoint would represent return of normal homeostasis to all regional capillary networks.

Monitoring gastrointestinal tract perfusion

The gastrointestinal tract suffers disproportionately early in shock states and is one of the last organ systems to be reperfused during resuscitation.[135,136] The countercurrent vascular flow of intestinal villi makes the mucosa exquisitely susceptible to hypoxia. There is also solid evidence of sepsis-related splanchnic dysfunction, including intestinal epithelial breakdown, gastric mucosal erosion and hemorrhage, ileus, local immunodysfunction, disruptions of enteric microflora populations, and bacterial translocation. Occult splanchnic hypoperfusion may insidiously cause patient deterioration and MODS. Low intramucosal pH (pHi) in a canine model correlated with increased mortality.[137] It is therefore logical to develop techniques to quantify gastrointestinal mucosal perfusion as a specific marker of continued shock. Sublingual capnometry ($PslCO_2$) and pHi are two monitoring techniques that have been well described in human medicine but have failed to enter standard clinical practice.[138,139]

Gastric tonometry

Tissue CO_2 reflects accumulation of waste products from metabolism of high-energy phosphate species during hypoxia, as well as intracellular buffering of hydrogen ions from anaerobic glycolysis. Tissue beds may experience changes in both metabolism and blood flow. Gastric intramucosal acidosis is attractive clinically as a functional monitoring parameter. In contrast to blood lactate, tissue CO_2 accumulation is rapidly cleared upon shock reversal. Gastric tonometry measures the gastric mucosal interstitial fluid via a specialized nasogastric (NG) tube. A thin bubble at the end of the NG tube is filled with saline and allowed to equilibrate with the gastric mucosa for 1 hour. The subsequent saline pCO_2 is measured and translated to the approximate pHi via a modified Henderson–Hasselbalch equation utilizing a simultaneous arterial HCO_3.

The pHi correlates with local tissue perfusion[137] and may predict subsequent deterioration of global hemodynamic status.[140–144] Friedman et al.[145] found improved mortality prediction in humans with severe sepsis by evaluating pHi and lactate together, at presentation and 24 hours later. Unfortunately, prospective, randomized, controlled goal-directed trials in critically ill humans using pHi as a resuscitation endpoint have been unable to show any morbidity or mortality benefit.[146,147]

Some potential drawbacks of pHi that contribute to inconsistent measurements in clinical practice include the need for concurrent arterial sampling, debate regarding concurrent acid blocking pharmacologic agents, and interference with implementation of enteral nutrition. In addition, the pHi calculation is dependent on arterial HCO_3, which may be vastly different from gastric tissue HCO_3. Further criticisms of pHi as an ideal resuscitation endpoint include the added expense of specialized NG tubes and the significant lag time from test initiation to results. However, pHi is argued to be more sensitive than

$ScvO_2$ since it can detect tissue perfusion deficits independent of a concurrent change in $ScvO_2$.[148,149] Puyana et al.[150] have shown pHi to lag behind shock-related changes in small-intestinal tissue in an experimental porcine hemorrhagic shock model.

Sublingual microcirculation

More recently, sublingual tissue has become a target for local tissue monitoring. Sublingual tissue is developmentally derived from splanchnic tissue, is exquisitely sensitive to changes in DO_2, and provides information similar to gastric mucosal tonometry. Techniques described for use in this anatomic area include tonometry[151,152] and orthogonal polarization spectral (OPS) imaging.

Sublingual tonometry provides a less invasive, more practical way to access microcirculatory status than gastric techniques. It is also faster and less cumbersome to perform than pHi and can be used without a concurrent ABG. A sublingual tonometer is a handheld instrument that can be used cage-side. Sublingual tonometry has been found to correlate significantly with gastric PCO_2, CI, and blood lactate in all types of shock,[111,142] and to accurately represent microcirculatory changes in septic humans.[153] Porcine hemorrhagic shock research models show excellent correlation between buccal/$PslCO_2$ and MAP, CO, tissue perfusion, and mortality.[154,155] Marik et al.[139] have focused research on serial differences between $PslCO_2$ and $PaCO_2$ (CO_2 gap) during the first 8 hours of shock resuscitation in critically ill humans. Baseline CO_2 gap was a better predictor of survival than the change in lactate or SvO_2. This group and Weil et al.[142] did find $PslCO_2$ to be a significant indirect outcome predictor, by multivariate analysis. In critically ill patients, $PslCO_2$ has been shown to normalize before lactate, which has a significant lag time to normalization after resuscitation.[139,142]

The sublingual microcirculation can also be measured via laser Doppler flow (LDF) technology.[156] Monochromatic laser light (820 nm) penetrates the skin and is reflected by moving cells. The scattered light is transmitted to the laser Doppler photodiode, where it is amplified, analyzed, and transformed to an analog signal. Using changes in reflected wavelength, LDF can yield information regarding the relative velocity and number of erythrocytes in a region of superficial microcirculation.

Direct visualization of superficial cutaneous and organ capillary beds is an area of investigation that has relatively recently been reviewed and a clinical consensus of useful quantitative variables reported.[157] Experimental studies have evaluated the microcirculation in endotoxemia and peritonitis animal models (including a canine study[158]) using intravital microscopy to show heterogeneous regional perfusion, low capillary density, and impaired flow velocity.[4,159,160] Two newer examples of this microcirculatory imaging technology include OPS imaging[161] and its further development, sidestream dark field (SDF).[162] Sidestream dark field employs the addition of stroboscopic light-emitting diodes on a videomicroscope.[163] The light-emitting diodes help prevent surface reflections to improve image quality.

Microcirculatory imaging utilizes handheld video microscopy to directly visualize sublingual capillary density and microcirculatory blood flow (velocity and heterogeneity). This technology is based on the principle that green polarized light illuminates tissue to a depth of 3 mm. The scattered light is then absorbed by hemoglobin in the superficial vasculature. Optical filtration eliminates reflected superficial light and produces a high-contrast image of the microcirculation. Although the vessels are not visible, red blood cells appear dark and their movement through the microcirculation can be observed. The image can then be quantitatively analyzed, yielding objective data regarding microvascular perfusion and flow. Reports from the human clinical literature typically describe evaluating the sublingual tissue with OPS imaging.[7] Specific parameters reported have included total vessel density (TVD), perfused vessel density (PVD), proportion of perfused vessels (PPV), functional capillary density (FCD), microvascular flow index (MFI), flow velocity score, and flow heterogeneity index.[164,165]

Sakr et al.[8] and Trzeciak et al.[165] used OPS imaging to demonstrate significant microcirculatory impairment in human sepsis nonsurvivors. Sakr et al.[8] showed an association between circulatory impairment and subsequent development of MODS and death. Additionally, Trzeciak et al.[165] demonstrated markedly impaired early (within 6 hours) microcirculatory parameters using OPS imaging in human septic shock EGDT patients who progressed to develop hypotension, increased vasopressor requirements, lower SvO_2, and death. Lack of microcirculatory blood flow over time was consistent with decreased survival in critically ill human patients.[7]

As a functional monitoring parameter, OPS imaging has been used to assess the microcirculatory response to dobutamine in human septic shock patients.[166] Continuous infusions of dobutamine led to increased sublingual capillary perfusion and decreased regional blood lactate levels. Genzel-Boroviczeny et al.[167] showed an increased FCD of the skin of anemic preterm human infants receiving blood transfusions.

An important challenge of monitoring buccal sublingual tissue in veterinary medicine is the logistics of safely and reliably measuring this anatomic location in the conscious patient. This technology could prove useful in veterinary patients with decreased levels of consciousness, anesthetized patients, and those requiring mechanical ventilation. Investigation has begun in clinical canine patients. A veterinary study concluded that the canine microcirculation could be evaluated objectively in healthy dogs under general anesthesia.[168] The study reported the need for patient immobility and nonpigmented mucous membranes in order to obtain optimal images. Specifically, the imaging was performed at the mucogingival junction, above the maxillary canine tooth.

Clinical application of advanced perfusion monitoring techniques in veterinary medicine

Noninvasive hemodynamic monitoring will continue to improve and change the practice of critical care medicine. Downstream parameters more accurately reflect cellular well being. However, there is unlikely to be a single parameter that will be able to solely guide resuscitation and maintain optimal microcirculatory perfusion. In fact, experts recommend interpreting any monitoring variable, such as $ScvO_2$, in the context of HR, MAP, CVP, lactate concentration, and UOP.[169,170] As with routine serial complete blood counts and biochemical screens in critically ill patients, routine evaluation of all available perfusion monitoring parameters (global and regional) provides the most information to evaluate overall patient status and detect changes in condition. Moreover, downward trends in regional or global perfusion parameters serve as early markers of patient deterioration.

It has been recommended to aggressively treat shock as soon as possible to attain the best patient morbidity and mortality outcomes.[94] For example, human septic shock patients whose EGDT endpoints could not be stabilized were sedated and intubated for mechanical ventilation to decrease VO_2.[1] Mounting evidence supports expedient resuscitation as the only way to effectively treat microcirculatory failure and prevent irreversible cellular damage or organ failure.

Taking scientific evidence into consideration,[171] shock resuscitation recommendations can be suggested for veterinary patients. Generally accepted upstream resuscitation endpoints include achieving normal HR, MAP >70 mm Hg, and PaO_2 >80 mm Hg. The value of CVP in resuscitation of dogs and cats in shock has not been determined. Resuscitation efforts should also be guided by serial physical examination findings such as mentation, mucous membrane color, CRT, distal pulse quality, and subjective extremity temperature. Evaluation of distal extremity temperature in human surgical ICU patients is documented to predict CI, $SmvO_2$, and lactate concentration.[172]

Critical care medicine will continue to incorporate functional hemodynamic monitoring to assess resuscitation efforts and therapeutic trials.[173] Functional hemodynamic monitoring principles apply to fluid resuscitation in shock (monitoring changes in lactate and $SmvO_2$); predicting fluid challenges in hemodynamically unstable patients (arterial pulse pressure variation and CVP trends); and assessing the effects of inotropic–vasopressor therapy. It has also been suggested that functional hemodynamic monitoring may be used to guide pharmacologic vasodilation aimed at recruiting weak microcirculatory units and increasing blood flow.[7,174,175] For example, prostacyclin can improve pHi and DO_2 in critically ill humans.[176,177] In a canine model of endotoxemia, Zhang et al.[178] were able to show improvements in CI and cranial mesenteric blood flow after administering SIN-1, a NO donor. Accordingly, complete inhibition of NOS resulted in increased mortality in a randomized, controlled, multicenter, clinical human trial, suggesting a protective role of NO, likely related to maintenance of microcirculatory flow via vasodilation.[179]

In human critical care medicine, the concept of the treatment bundle[180] is becoming a standard of care for complex disease states such as severe sepsis, septic shock, ventilator-associated pneumonia, and acute respiratory distress syndrome (ARDS). A treatment bundle consists of several evidence-based treatment recommendations combined into a protocol to improve patient outcome. Perfusion markers are becoming incorporated into sepsis resuscitation and management bundles[2] as a logical way to ensure microcirculatory and organ function and to improve patient survival.[181]

Summary

Tissue hypoperfusion can persist undetected by traditional perfusion parameters (heart rate, blood pressure, urine output), and occult hypoperfusion increases morbidity and mortality. Several markers of global and regional perfusion exist in current research, including blood lactate concentration, gastric tonometry, sublingual capnometry, the NADH:NAD ratio, orthogonal polarization spectral (OPS) imaging, oxygen-derived variables, and near-infrared spectroscopy (NIRS). Evaluation of multiple parameters can aid in optimizing hemodynamic resuscitation, tissue perfusion, and patient outcome.

References

1. Rivers E, Nguyen B, Havstad S, et al. Early goal-directed therapy in the treatment of severe sepsis and septic shock. N Engl J Med 2001 Nov 8;345(19):1368–1377.
2. Dellinger RP, Levy MM, Carlet JM, et al. Surviving Sepsis Campaign: international guidelines for management of severe sepsis and septic shock: 2008. Crit Care Med 2008 Jan;36(1):296–327.
3. Wo CC, Shoemaker WC, Appel PL, et al. Unreliability of blood pressure and heart rate to evaluate cardiac output in emergency resuscitation and critical illness. Crit Care Med 1993 Feb;21(2):218–223.
4. Lam C, Tyml K, Martin C, et al. Microvascular perfusion is impaired in a rat model of normotensive sepsis. J Clin Invest 1994 Nov;94(5):2077–2083.
5. Scalea TM, Maltz S, Yelon J, et al. Resuscitation of multiple trauma and head injury: role of crystalloid fluids and inotropes. Crit Care Med 1994 Oct;22(10):1610–1615.
6. Rady MY, Rivers EP, Nowak RM. Resuscitation of the critically ill in the ED: responses of blood pressure, heart rate, shock index, central venous oxygen saturation, and lactate. Am J Emerg Med 1996 Mar;14(2):218–225.
7. De Backer D, Creteur J, Preiser JC, et al. Microvascular blood flow is altered in patients with sepsis. Am J Respir Crit Care Med 2002 Jul 1;166(1):98–104.
8. Sakr Y, Dubois MJ, De Backer D, et al. Persistent microcirculatory alterations are associated with organ failure and death in patients with septic shock. Crit Care Med 2004 Sep;32(9):1825–1831.
9. Beal AL, Cerra FB. Multiple organ failure syndrome in the 1990s. Systemic inflammatory response and organ dysfunction. JAMA 1994 Jan 19;271(3):226–233.
10. Ince C, Sinaasappel M. Microcirculatory oxygenation and shunting in sepsis and shock. Crit Care Med 1999 Jul;27(7):1369–1377.
11. Blow O, Magliore L, Claridge JA, et al. The golden hour and the silver day: detection and correction of occult hypoperfusion within 24 hours improves outcome from major trauma. J Trauma 1999 Nov;47(5):964–969.
12. Rehm M, Bruegger D, Christ F, et al. Shedding of the endothelial glycocalyx in patients undergoing major vascular surgery with global and regional ischemia. Circulation 2007 Oct 23;116(17):1896–1906.
13. Karimova A, Pinsky DJ. The endothelial response to oxygen deprivation: biology and clinical implications. Intensive Care Med 2001 Jan;27(1):19–31.
14. Edouard AR, Degremont AC, Duranteau J, et al. Heterogeneous regional vascular responses to simulated transient hypovolemia in man. Intensive Care Med 1994 Jul;20(6):414–420.
15. Riddez L, Hahn RG, Brismar B, et al. Central and regional hemodynamics during acute hypovolemia and volume substitution in volunteers. Crit Care Med 1997 Apr;25(4):635–640.
16. Machiedo GW, Zaets SB, Berezina TL, et al. Trauma-hemorrhagic shock–induced red blood cell damage leads to decreased microcirculatory blood flow. Crit Care Med 2009 Mar;37(3):1000–1010.
17. Bateman RM, Sharpe MD, Ellis CG. Bench-to-bedside review: microvascular dysfunction in sepsis—hemodynamics, oxygen transport, and nitric oxide. Crit Care 2003 Oct;7(5):359–373.
18. Aird WC. The role of the endothelium in severe sepsis and multiple organ dysfunction syndrome. Blood 2003 May 15;101(10):3765–3777.
19. Reffelmann T, Kloner RA. The "no-reflow" phenomenon: basic science and clinical correlates. Heart 2002 Feb;87(2):162–168.
20. Brooks GA. Intra- and extra-cellular lactate shuttles. Med Sci Sports Exerc 2000 Apr;32(4):790–799.
21. Allen S, Hold JL. Lactate: physiology and clinical utility. J Vet Emerg Crit Care 2008;18(2):123–132.
22. Pang DS, Boysen S. Lactate in veterinary critical care: pathophysiology and management. J Am Anim Hosp Assoc 2007 Sep–Oct;43(5):270–279.
23. Karagiannis MH RA, Kerl ME, Mann FA. Lacate measurement as an indicator of perfusion. Compendium Vet CE 2006(April):287–298.
24. Vernon C, Letourneau JL. Lactic acidosis: recognition, kinetics, and associated prognosis. Crit Care Clin 2010 Apr;26(2):255–283.
25. Lagutchik MS OG, Wingfield WE, Hackett TB. Lactate kinetics in veterinary critical care: a review. J Vet Emerg Crit Care (San Antonio) 1996;6(2):81–95.
26. Levy B, Sadoune LO, Gelot AM, et al. Evolution of lactate/pyruvate and arterial ketone body ratios in the early course of catecholamine-treated septic shock. Crit Care Med 2000 Jan;28(1):114–119.
27. Suistomaa M, Ruokonen E, Kari A, et al. Time-pattern of lactate and lactate to pyruvate ratio in the first 24 hours of intensive care emergency admissions. Shock 2000 Jul;14(1):8–12.
28. Gore DC, Jahoor F, Hibbert JM, et al. Lactic acidosis during sepsis is related to increased pyruvate production, not deficits in tissue oxygen availability. Ann Surg 1996 Jul;224(1):97–102.
29. Gutierrez G, Wulf ME. Lactic acidosis in sepsis: a commentary. Intensive Care Med 1996 Jan;22(1):6–16.
30. Chrusch C, Bands C, Bose D, et al. Impaired hepatic extraction and increased splanchnic production contribute to lactic acidosis in canine sepsis. Am J Respir Crit Care Med 2000 Feb;161(2 Pt 1):517–526.
31. Levy B. Lactate and shock state: the metabolic view. Curr Opin Crit Care 2006 Aug;12(4):315–321.
32. Trzeciak S, Dellinger RP, Chansky ME, et al. Serum lactate as a predictor of mortality in patients with infection. Intensive Care Med 2007 Jun;33(6):970–977.
33. De Backer D, Creteur J, Zhang H, et al. Lactate production by the lungs in acute lung injury. Am J Respir Crit Care Med 1997 Oct;156(4 Pt 1):1099–1104.
34. Mizock BA. Hyperlactatemia in acute liver failure: decreased clearance versus increased production. Crit Care Med 2001 Nov;29(11):2225–2226.
35. Schurr A, Payne RS, Miller JJ, et al. Brain lactate is an obligatory aerobic energy substrate for functional recovery after hypoxia: further in vitro validation. J Neurochem 1997 Jul;69(1):423–426.
36. Revelly JP, Tappy L, Martinez A, et al. Lactate and glucose metabolism in severe sepsis and cardiogenic shock. Crit Care Med 2005 Oct;33(10):2235–2240.
37. Bakker J, Gris P, Coffernils M, et al. Serial blood lactate levels can predict the development of multiple organ failure following septic shock. Am J Surg 1996 Feb;171(2):221–226.
38. Husain FA, Martin MJ, Mullenix PS, et al. Serum lactate and base deficit as predictors of mortality and morbidity. Am J Surg 2003 May;185(5):485–491.
39. Gunnerson KJ, Saul M, He S, et al. Lactate versus non-lactate metabolic acidosis: a retrospective outcome evaluation of critically ill patients. Crit Care 2006 Feb;10(1):R22.
40. Mikkelsen ME, Miltiades AN, Gaieski DF, et al. Serum lactate is associated with mortality in severe sepsis independent of

organ failure and shock. Crit Care Med 2009 May;37(5):1670–1677.

41. Hughes D, Rozanski ER, Shofer FS, et al. Effect of sampling site, repeated sampling, pH, and PCO$_2$ on plasma lactate concentration in healthy dogs. Am J Vet Res 1999 Apr;60(4):521–524.

42. Acierno MJ, Johnson ME, Eddleman LA, et al. Measuring statistical agreement between four point of care (POC) lactate meters and a laboratory blood analyzer in cats. J Feline Med Surg 2008 Apr;10(2):110–114.

43. Christopher MM, O'Neill S. Effect of specimen collection and storage on blood glucose and lactate concentrations in healthy, hyperthyroid and diabetic cats. Vet Clin Pathol 2000;29(1):22–28.

44. McMichael M, Lees GE, Hennessey J, et al. Serial plasma lactate concentrations in 68 puppies aged 4–80 days. J Vet Emerg Crit Care 2005;15(1):17–21.

45. Lagutchik M, Olgilvie GK, Hackett TB. Increased lactate concentrations in ill and injured dogs. J Vet Emerg Crit Care 1998;8(2):117–127.

46. Holahan ML, Brown AJ, Drobatz KJ. The association of blood lactate concentration with outcome in dogs with idiopathic immune-mediated hemolytic anemia: 173 cases (2003–2006). J Vet Emerg Crit Care (San Antonio) 2010 Aug;20(4):413–420.

47. Butler A, Campbell VL, Wagner AE. Lithium dilution cardiac output and oxygen delivery in conscious dogs with systemic inflammatory response syndrome. J Vet Emerg Crit Care 2008;18(3):246–257.

48. de Papp E, Drobatz KJ, Hughes D. Plasma lactate concentration as a predictor of gastric necrosis and survival among dogs with gastric dilatation–volvulus: 102 cases (1995–1998). J Am Vet Med Assoc 1999 Jul 1;215(1):49–52.

49. Dunham CM, Siegel JH, Weireter L, et al. Oxygen debt and metabolic acidemia as quantitative predictors of mortality and the severity of the ischemic insult in hemorrhagic shock. Crit Care Med 1991 Feb;19(2):231–243.

50. Abramson D, Scalea TM, Hitchcock R, et al. Lactate clearance and survival following injury. J Trauma 1993 Oct;35(4):584–588; discussion 8–9.

51. Smith I, Kumar P, Molloy S, et al. Base excess and lactate as prognostic indicators for patients admitted to intensive care. Intensive Care Med 2001 Jan;27(1):74–83.

52. Nguyen HB, Rivers EP, Knoblich BP, et al. Early lactate clearance is associated with improved outcome in severe sepsis and septic shock. Crit Care Med 2004 Aug;32(8):1637–1642.

53. Jones AE, Shapiro NI, Trzeciak S, et al. Lactate clearance vs central venous oxygen saturation as goals of early sepsis therapy: a randomized clinical trial. JAMA 2010 Feb 24;303(8):739–746.

54. Nel M, Lobetti RG, Keller N, et al. Prognostic value of blood lactate, blood glucose, and hematocrit in canine babesiosis. J Vet Intern Med 2004 Jul–Aug;18(4):471–476.

55. Stevenson CK, Kidney BA, Duke T, et al. Serial blood lactate concentrations in systemically ill dogs. Vet Clin Pathol 2007 Sep;36(3):234–239.

56. Acierno MJ, Mitchell MA. Evaluation of four point-of-care meters for rapid determination of blood lactate concentrations in dogs. J Am Vet Med Assoc 2007 May 1;230(9):1315–1318.

57. Ferasin L, Dodkin SJ, Amodio A, et al. Evaluation of a portable lactate analyzer (Lactate Scout) in dogs. Vet Clin Pathol 2007 Mar;36(1):36–39.

58. Stevenson CK, Kidney BA, Duke T, et al. Evaluation of the Accu-trend for lactate measurement in dogs. Vet Clin Pathol 2007 Sep;36(3):261–266.

59. Thorneloe C, Bedard C, Boysen S. Evaluation of a hand-held lactate analyzer in dogs. Can Vet J 2007 Mar;48(3):283–288.

60. Hopper K, Rezende ML, Haskins SC. Assessment of the effect of dilution of blood samples with sodium heparin on blood gas, electrolyte, and lactate measurements in dogs. Am J Vet Res 2005 Apr;66(4):656–660.

61. Rand JS, Kinnaird E, Baglioni A, et al. Acute stress hyperglycemia in cats is associated with struggling and increased concentrations of lactate and norepinephrine. J Vet Intern Med 2002 Mar–Apr;16(2):123–132.

62. Vincent JL, Dufaye P, Berre J, et al. Serial lactate determinations during circulatory shock. Crit Care Med 1983 Jun;11(6):449–451.

63. Bruegger D, Kemming GI, Jacob M, et al. Causes of metabolic acidosis in canine hemorrhagic shock: role of unmeasured ions. Crit Care 2007;11(6):R130.

64. Davis JW, Shackford SR, Holbrook TL. Base deficit as a sensitive indicator of compensated shock and tissue oxygen utilization. Surg Gynecol Obstet 1991 Dec;173(6):473–476.

65. Davis JW, Parks SN, Kaups KL, et al. Admission base deficit predicts transfusion requirements and risk of complications. J Trauma 1996 Nov;41(5):769–774.

66. Davis JW, Kaups KL. Base deficit in the elderly: a marker of severe injury and death. J Trauma 1998 Nov;45(5):873–877.

67. Kincaid EH, Miller PR, Meredith JW, et al. Elevated arterial base deficit in trauma patients: a marker of impaired oxygen utilization. J Am Coll Surg 1998 Oct;187(4):384–392.

68. Stillion J. Admission base excess as a predictor of mortality and blood transfusion requirement in dogs and cats with blunt trauma. J Vet Emerg Crit Care 2010;20(S1):A13.

69. Shah NS, Kelly E, Billiar TR, et al. Utility of clinical parameters of tissue oxygenation in a quantitative model of irreversible hemorrhagic shock. Shock 1998 Nov;10(5):343–346.

70. Englehart MS, Schreiber MA. Measurement of acid–base resuscitation endpoints: lactate, base deficit, bicarbonate or what? Curr Opin Crit Care 2006 Dec;12(6):569–574.

71. Marik PE, Baram M. Noninvasive hemodynamic monitoring in the intensive care unit. Crit Care Clin 2007 Jul;23(3):383–400.

72. Heyland DK, Cook DJ, King D, et al. Maximizing oxygen delivery in critically ill patients: a methodologic appraisal of the evidence. Crit Care Med 1996 Mar;24(3):517–524.

73. McKinley BA, Valdivia A, Moore FA. Goal-oriented shock resuscitation for major torso trauma: what are we learning? Curr Opin Crit Care 2003 Aug;9(4):292–299.

74. Velmahos GC, Demetriades D, Shoemaker WC, et al. Endpoints of resuscitation of critically injured patients: normal or supranormal? A prospective randomized trial. Ann Surg 2000 Sep;232(3):409–418.

75. Rixen D, Siegel JH. Bench-to-bedside review: oxygen debt and its metabolic correlates as quantifiers of the severity of hemorrhagic and post-traumatic shock. Crit Care 2005 Oct 5;9(5):441–453.

76. Shoemaker WC, Appel PL, Kram HB, et al. Prospective trial of supranormal values of survivors as therapeutic goals in high-risk surgical patients. Chest 1988 Dec;94(6):1176–1186.

77. Shoemaker WC, Wo CC, Thangathurai D, et al. Hemodynamic patterns of survivors and nonsurvivors during high risk elective surgical operations. World J Surg 1999 Dec;23(12):1264–1270; discussion 70–71.

78. Boyd O, Grounds RM, Bennett ED. A randomized clinical trial of the effect of deliberate perioperative increase of oxygen delivery on mortality in high-risk surgical patients. JAMA 1993 Dec 8;270(22):2699–2707.

79. Bishop MH, Shoemaker WC, Appel PL, et al. Prospective, randomized trial of survivor values of cardiac index, oxygen delivery, and oxygen consumption as resuscitation endpoints in severe trauma. J Trauma 1995 May;38(5):780–787.

80. Yu M, Levy MM, Smith P, et al. Effect of maximizing oxygen delivery on morbidity and mortality rates in critically ill patients: a prospective, randomized, controlled study. Crit Care Med 1993 Jun;21(6):830–838.

81. Gattinoni L, Brazzi L, Pelosi P, et al. A trial of goal-oriented hemodynamic therapy in critically ill patients. SvO$_2$ Collaborative Group. N Engl J Med 1995 Oct 19;333(16):1025–1032.

82. Hayes MA, Timmins AC, Yau EH, et al. Elevation of systemic oxygen delivery in the treatment of critically ill patients. N Engl J Med 1994 Jun 16;330(24):1717–1722.

83. Kremzar B, Spec-Marn A, Kompan L, et al. Normal values of SvO$_2$ as therapeutic goal in patients with multiple injuries. Intensive Care Med 1997 Jan;23(1):65–70.

84. McKinley BA, Kozar RA, Cocanour CS, et al. Normal versus supranormal oxygen delivery goals in shock resuscitation: the response is the same. J Trauma 2002 Nov;53(5):825–832.

85. Robin E, Costecalde M, Lebuffe G, et al. Clinical relevance of data from the pulmonary artery catheter. Crit Care 2006;10 Suppl 3:S3.

86. Connors AF Jr, Speroff T, Dawson NV, et al. The effectiveness of right heart catheterization in the initial care of critically ill patients. SUPPORT Investigators. JAMA 1996 Sep 18;276(11):889–897.

87. Shah MR, Hasselblad V, Stevenson LW, et al. Impact of the pulmonary artery catheter in critically ill patients: meta-analysis of randomized clinical trials. JAMA 2005 Oct 5;294(13):1664–1670.

88. Hadian M, Pinsky MR. Evidence-based review of the use of the pulmonary artery catheter: impact data and complications. Crit Care 2006;10 Suppl 3:S8.

89. Edwards JD. Oxygen transport in cardiogenic and septic shock. Crit Care Med 1991 May;19(5):658–663.

90. Krafft P, Steltzer H, Hiesmayr M, et al. Mixed venous oxygen saturation in critically ill septic shock patients. The role of defined events. Chest 1993 Mar;103(3):900–906.

91. Polonen P, Ruokonen E, Hippelainen M, et al. A prospective, randomized study of goal-oriented hemodynamic therapy in cardiac surgical patients. Anesth Analg 2000 May;90(5):1052–1059.

92. Wiedemann HP, Wheeler AP, Bernard GR, et al. Comparison of two fluid-management strategies in acute lung injury. N Engl J Med 2006 Jun 15;354(24):2564–2575.

93. Hebert PC, Wells G, Blajchman MA, et al. A multicenter, randomized, controlled clinical trial of transfusion requirements in critical care. Transfusion Requirements in Critical Care Investigators, Canadian Critical Care Trials Group. N Engl J Med 1999 Feb 11;340(6):409–417.

94. Rivers EP, Ahrens T. Improving outcomes for severe sepsis and septic shock: tools for early identification of at-risk patients and treatment protocol implementation. Crit Care Clin 2008 Jul;24(3 Suppl):S1–S47.

95. Tahvanainen J, Meretoja O, Nikki P. Can central venous blood replace mixed venous blood samples? Crit Care Med 1982 Nov;10(11):758–761.

96. Berridge JC. Influence of cardiac output on the correlation between mixed venous and central venous oxygen saturation. Br J Anaesth 1992 Oct;69(4):409–410.

97. Martin C, Auffray JP, Badetti C, et al. Monitoring of central venous oxygen saturation versus mixed venous oxygen saturation in critically ill patients. Intensive Care Med 1992;18(2):101–104.

98. Herrera A, Pajuelo A, Morano MJ, et al. [Comparison of oxygen saturations in mixed venous and central blood during thoracic anesthesia with selective single-lung ventilation]. Rev Esp Anestesiol Reanim 1993 Nov–Dec;40(6):349–353.

99. Rivers EP, Ander DS, Powell D. Central venous oxygen saturation monitoring in the critically ill patient. Curr Opin Crit Care 2001 Jun;7(3):204–211.

100. Reinhart K, Rudolph T, Bredle DL, et al. Comparison of central-venous to mixed-venous oxygen saturation during changes in oxygen supply/demand. Chest 1989 Jun;95(6):1216–1221.

101. Rady MY, Rivers EP, Martin GB, et al. Continuous central venous oximetry and shock index in the emergency department: use in the evaluation of clinical shock. Am J Emerg Med 1992 Nov;10(6):538–541.

102. Young B, Prittie JE, Fox PR, Barton LJ. Evaluation of post-resuscitation global perfusion parameters in dogs presenting in shock. J Vet Emerg Crit Care 2007;17:S12 (abst).

103. Pearse R, Dawson D, Fawcett J, et al. Early goal-directed therapy after major surgery reduces complications and duration of hospital stay. A randomised, controlled trial [ISRCTN38797445]. Crit Care 2005;9(6):R687–R693.

104. Jakob SM. Multicenter study on peri-postoperative central venous oxygen saturation in high-risk surgical patients. Crit Care 2006;10:R158.

105. Otero RM, Nguyen HB, Huang DT, et al. Early goal-directed therapy in severe sepsis and septic shock revisited: concepts, controversies, and contemporary findings. Chest 2006 Nov;130(5):1579–1595.

106. Donati A, Loggi S, Preiser JC, et al. Goal-directed intraoperative therapy reduces morbidity and length of hospital stay in high-risk surgical patients. Chest 2007 Dec;132(6):1817–1824.

107. Jones AE, Focht A, Horton JM, et al. Prospective external validation of the clinical effectiveness of an emergency department–based early goal-directed therapy protocol for severe sepsis and septic shock. Chest 2007 Aug;132(2):425–432.

108. Huang DT, Clermont G, Dremsizov TT, et al. Implementation of early goal-directed therapy for severe sepsis and septic shock: a decision analysis. Crit Care Med 2007 Sep;35(9):2090–2100.

109. Magder S, Bafaqeeh F. The clinical role of central venous pressure measurements. J Intensive Care Med 2007 Jan–Feb;22(1):44–51.

110. Scalea TM, Hartnett RW, Duncan AO, et al. Central venous oxygen saturation: a useful clinical tool in trauma patients. J Trauma 1990 Dec;30(12):1539–1543.

111. Nakagawa Y, Weil MH, Tang W, et al. Sublingual capnometry for diagnosis and quantitation of circulatory shock. Am J Respir Crit Care Med 1998 Jun;157(6 Pt 1):1838–1843.

112. Vincent JL, Gerlach H. Fluid resuscitation in severe sepsis and septic shock: an evidence-based review. Crit Care Med 2004 Nov;32(11 Suppl):S451–S454.

113. Hart DW, Gore DC, Rinehart AJ, et al. Sepsis-induced failure of hepatic energy metabolism. J Surg Res 2003 Nov;115(1):139–147.

114. Simonson SG, Welty-Wolf K, Huang YT, et al. Altered mitochondrial redox responses in gram negative septic shock in primates. Circ Shock 1994 May;43(1):34–43.

115. Lautier D, Lagueux J, Thibodeau J, et al. Molecular and biochemical features of poly (ADP-ribose) metabolism. Mol Cell Biochem 1993 May 26;122(2):171–193.

116. D'Amours D, Desnoyers S, D'Silva I, et al. Poly(ADP-ribosyl) ation reactions in the regulation of nuclear functions. Biochem J 1999 Sep 1;342(Pt 2):249–268.

117. Szabo A, Salzman AL, Szabo C. Poly (ADP-ribose) synthetase activation mediates pulmonary microvascular and intestinal mucosal dysfunction in endotoxin shock. Life Sci 1998; 63(23):2133–2139.

118. Simbulan-Rosenthal CM, Rosenthal DS, Iyer S, et al. Involvement of PARP and poly(ADP-ribosyl)ation in the early stages of apoptosis and DNA replication. Mol Cell Biochem 1999 Mar;193(1–2):137–148.

119. Mayevsky A, Chance B. Oxidation–reduction states of NADH in vivo: from animals to clinical use. Mitochondrion 2007 Sep; 7(5):330–339.

120. Kraut A, Barbiro-Michaely E, Mayevsky A. Differential effects of norepinephrine on brain and other less vital organs detected by a multisite multiparametric monitoring system. Med Sci Monit 2004 Jul;10(7):BR215–20.

121. Brealey D, Brand M, Hargreaves I, et al. Association between mitochondrial dysfunction and severity and outcome of septic shock. Lancet 2002 Jul 20;360(9328):219–223.

122. Mayevsky A, Manor T, Pevzner E, et al. Tissue spectroscope: a novel in vivo approach to real time monitoring of tissue vitality. J Biomed Opt 2004 Sep–Oct;9(5):1028–1045.

123. Clavijo-Alvarez JA, Sims CA, Pinsky MR, et al. Monitoring skeletal muscle and subcutaneous tissue acid–base status and oxygenation during hemorrhagic shock and resuscitation. Shock 2005 Sep;24(3):270–275.

124. Tatevossian RG, Wo CC, Velmahos GC, et al. Transcutaneous oxygen and CO_2 as early warning of tissue hypoxia and hemodynamic shock in critically ill emergency patients. Crit Care Med 2000 Jul;28(7):2248–2253.

125. Boekstegers P, Weidenhofer S, Kapsner T. Skeletal muscle partial pressure of oxygen in patients with sepsis. Crit Care Med 1994;22:640–650.

126. Bendjelid K, Schutz N, Stotz M, et al. Transcutaneous PCO_2 monitoring in critically ill adults: clinical evaluation of a new sensor. Crit Care Med 2005 Oct;33(10):2203–2206.

127. Valadka AB, Gopinath SP, Contant CF, et al. Relationship of brain tissue PO_2 to outcome after severe head injury. Crit Care Med 1998 Sep;26(9):1576–1581.

128. McKinley BA, Parmley CL, Butler BD. Skeletal muscle PO_2, PCO_2, and pH in hemorrhage, shock, and resuscitation in dogs. J Trauma 1998 Jan;44(1):119–127.

129. Guery BP, Mangalaboyi J, Menager P, et al. Redox status of cytochrome a,a3: a noninvasive indicator of dysoxia in regional hypoxic or ischemic hypoxia. Crit Care Med 1999 Mar;27(3): 576–582.

130. Taylor JH, Mulier KE, Myers DE, et al. Use of near-infrared spectroscopy in early determination of irreversible hemorrhagic shock. J Trauma 2005 Jun;58(6):1119–1125.

131. Torella F, Cowley RD, Thorniley MS, et al. Regional tissue oxygenation during hemorrhage: can near infrared spectroscopy be used to monitor blood loss? Shock 2002 Nov;18(5): 440–444.

132. McKinley BA, Marvin RG, Cocanour CS, et al. Tissue hemoglobin O_2 saturation during resuscitation of traumatic shock monitored using near infrared spectrometry. J Trauma 2000 Apr;48(4):637–642.

133. Hall K, Powell LL, Beilman GJ. Measurement of tissue oxygen saturation levels using portable near-infrared spectroscopy in clinically healthy dogs. J Vet Emerg Crit Care 2008;18(6): 594–600.

134. Sims C, Seigne P, Menconi M, et al. Skeletal muscle acidosis correlates with the severity of blood volume loss during shock and resuscitation. J Trauma 2001 Dec;51(6):1137–1145; discussion 45–46.

135. Takala J. Splanchnic perfusion in shock. Intensive Care Med 1994 Jul;20(6):403–404.

136. Mythen MG, Webb AR. The role of gut mucosal hypoperfusion in the pathogenesis of post-operative organ dysfunction. Intensive Care Med 1994;20(3):203–209.

137. Grum CM, Fiddian-Green RG, Pittenger GL, et al. Adequacy of tissue oxygenation in intact dog intestine. J Appl Physiol 1984 Apr;56(4):1065–1069.

138. Tang W, Weil MH, Sun S, et al. Gastric intramural PCO_2 as monitor of perfusion failure during hemorrhagic and anaphylactic shock. J Appl Physiol 1994 Feb;76(2):572–577.

139. Marik PE, Bankov A. Sublingual capnometry versus traditional markers of tissue oxygenation in critically ill patients. Crit Care Med 2003 Mar;31(3):818–822.

140. Gutierrez G, Palizas F, Doglio G, et al. Gastric intramucosal pH as a therapeutic index of tissue oxygenation in critically ill patients. Lancet 1992 Jan 25;339(8787):195–199.

141. Rackow EC, O'Neil P, Astiz ME, et al. Sublingual capnometry and indexes of tissue perfusion in patients with circulatory failure. Chest 2001 Nov;120(5):1633–1638.

142. Weil MH, Nakagawa Y, Tang W, et al. Sublingual capnometry: a new noninvasive measurement for diagnosis and quantitation of severity of circulatory shock. Crit Care Med 1999 Jul;27(7):1225–1229.

143. Marik PE, Iglesias J, Maini B. Gastric intramucosal pH changes after volume replacement with hydroxyethyl starch or crystalloid in patients undergoing elective abdominal aortic aneurysm repair. J Crit Care 1997 Jun;12(2):51–55.

144. Kolkman JJ, Otte JA, Groeneveld AB. Gastrointestinal luminal PCO_2 tonometry: an update on physiology, methodology and clinical applications. Br J Anaesth 2000 Jan;84(1):74–86.

145. Friedman G, Berlot G, Kahn RJ, et al. Combined measurements of blood lactate concentrations and gastric intramucosal pH in patients with severe sepsis. Crit Care Med 1995 Jul;23(7): 1184–1193.

146. Gomersall CD, Joynt GM, Freebairn RC, et al. Resuscitation of critically ill patients based on the results of gastric tonometry: a prospective, randomized, controlled trial. Crit Care Med 2000 Mar;28(3):607–614.

147. Palizas F, Dubin A, Regueira T, et al. Gastric tonometry versus cardiac index as resuscitation goals in septic shock: a multicenter, randomized, controlled trial. Crit Care 2009; 13(2):R44.

148. Silva E, De Backer D, Creteur J, et al. Effects of fluid challenge on gastric mucosal PCO_2 in septic patients. Intensive Care Med 2004 Mar;30(3):423–429.

149. Boerma EC, Mathura KR, van der Voort PH, et al. Quantifying bedside-derived imaging of microcirculatory abnormalities in septic patients: a prospective validation study. Crit Care 2005;9(6):R601–R606.

150. Puyana JC, Soller BR, Zhang S, et al. Continuous measurement of gut pH with near-infrared spectroscopy during hemorrhagic shock. J Trauma 1999 Jan;46(1):9–15.

151. Marik PE. Sublingual capnometry: a non-invasive measure of microcirculatory dysfunction and tissue hypoxia. Physiol Meas 2006 Jul;27(7):R37–R47.

152. Boswell SA, Scalea TM. Sublingual capnometry: an alternative to gastric tonometry for the management of shock resuscitation. AACN Clin Issues 2003 May;14(2):176–184.

153. Creteur J, De Backer D, Sakr Y, et al. Sublingual capnometry tracks microcirculatory changes in septic patients. Intensive Care Med 2006 Apr;32(4):516–523.

154. Pellis T, Weil MH, Tang W, et al. Increases in both buccal and sublingual partial pressure of carbon dioxide reflect decreases of tissue blood flows in a porcine model during hemorrhagic shock. J Trauma 2005 Apr;58(4):817–824.

155. Cammarata GA, Weil MH, Fries M, et al. Buccal capnometry to guide management of massive blood loss. J Appl Physiol 2006 Jan;100(1):304–306.

156. Maier S, Holz-Holzl C, Pajk W, et al. Microcirculatory parameters after isotonic and hypertonic colloidal fluid resuscitation in acute hemorrhagic shock. J Trauma 2009 Feb;66(2):337–345.

157. Awan ZA, Wester T, Kvernebo K. Human microvascular imaging: a review of skin and tongue videomicroscopy techniques and analysing variables. Clin Physiol Funct Imaging 2010 Mar;30(2):79–88.

158. Drazenovic R, Samsel RW, Wylam ME, et al. Regulation of perfused capillary density in canine intestinal mucosa during endotoxemia. J Appl Physiol 1992 Jan;72(1):259–265.

159. Farquhar I, Martin CM, Lam C, et al. Decreased capillary density in vivo in bowel mucosa of rats with normotensive sepsis. J Surg Res 1996 Feb 15;61(1):190–196.

160. Fries M, Weil MH, Sun S, et al. Increases in tissue PcO$_2$ during circulatory shock reflect selective decreases in capillary blood flow. Crit Care Med 2006 Feb;34(2):446–452.

161. Groner W, Winkelman JW, Harris AG, et al. Orthogonal polarization spectral imaging: a new method for study of the microcirculation. Nat Med 1999 Oct;5(10):1209–1212.

162. Ince C. The microcirculation is the motor of sepsis. Crit Care 2005;9 Suppl 4:S13–S19.

163. Goedhart PT, Khalilzada M, Bezemer R, et al. Sidestream dark field (SDF) imaging: a novel stroboscopic LED ring-based imaging modality for clinical assessment of the microcirculation. Opt Express 2007 Nov 12;15(23):15101–15114.

164. De Backer D, Hollenberg S, Boerma C, et al. How to evaluate the microcirculation: report of a round table conference. Crit Care 2007;11(5):R101.

165. Trzeciak S, Dellinger RP, Parrillo JE, et al. Early microcirculatory perfusion derangements in patients with severe sepsis and septic shock: relationship to hemodynamics, oxygen transport, and survival. Ann Emerg Med 2007 Jan;49(1):88–98, e1–e2.

166. De Backer D, Creteur J, Dubois MJ, et al. The effects of dobutamine on microcirculatory alterations in patients with septic shock are independent of its systemic effects. Crit Care Med 2006 Feb;34(2):403–408.

167. Genzel-Boroviczeny O, Christ F, Glas V. Blood transfusion increases functional capillary density in the skin of anemic preterm infants. Pediatr Res 2004 Nov;56(5):751–755.

168. Silverstein DC, Pruett-Saratan A 2nd, Drobatz KJ. Measurements of microvascular perfusion in healthy anesthetized dogs using orthogonal polarization spectral imaging. J Vet Emerg Crit Care (San Antonio) 2009 Dec;19(6):579–587.

169. Reinhart K, Bloos F. The value of venous oximetry. Curr Opin Crit Care 2005 Jun;11(3):259–263.

170. Pinsky MR, Payen D. Functional hemodynamic monitoring. Crit Care 2005;9(6):566–572.

171. Tisherman SA, Barie P, Bokhari F, et al. Clinical practice guideline: endpoints of resuscitation. J Trauma 2004 Oct;57(4):898–912.

172. Kaplan LJ, McPartland K, Santora TA, et al. Start with a subjective assessment of skin temperature to identify hypoperfusion in intensive care unit patients. J Trauma 2001 Apr;50(4):620–627; discussion 7–8.

173. Hadian M, Pinsky MR. Functional hemodynamic monitoring. Curr Opin Crit Care 2007 Jun;13(3):318–323.

174. Spronk PE, Ince C, Gardien MJ, et al. Nitroglycerin in septic shock after intravascular volume resuscitation. Lancet 2002 Nov 2;360(9343):1395–1396.

175. Pinsky MR. Hemodynamic evaluation and monitoring in the ICU. Chest 2007 Dec;132(6):2020–2029.

176. Bihari D, Smithies M, Gimson A, et al. The effects of vasodilation with prostacyclin on oxygen delivery and uptake in critically ill patients. N Engl J Med 1987 Aug 13;317(7):397–403.

177. Radermacher P, Buhl R, Santak B, et al. The effects of prostacyclin on gastric intramucosal pH in patients with septic shock. Intensive Care Med 1995 May;21(5):414–421.

178. Zhang H, Rogiers P, Friedman G, et al. Effects of nitric oxide donor SIN-1 on oxygen availability and regional blood flow during endotoxic shock. Arch Surg 1996 Jul;131(7):767–774.

179. Grover R, Lopez A, Lorente JA. Multicenter, randomized, placebo controlled, double-blind study of the nitric oxide synthase inhibitor 546C88: effect on survival in patients with septic shock. Crit Care Med 1999;27(Suppl):A33 (abs).

180. Levy MM, Pronovost PJ, Dellinger RP, et al. Sepsis change bundles: converting guidelines into meaningful change in behavior and clinical outcome. Crit Care Med 2004 Nov;32(11 Suppl):S595–S597.

181. Nguyen HB, Corbett SW, Steele R, et al. Implementation of a bundle of quality indicators for the early management of severe sepsis and septic shock is associated with decreased mortality. Crit Care Med 2007 Apr;35(4):1105–1112.

182. Gebhardt C, Hirschberger J, Rau S, et al. Use of C-reactive protein to predict outcome in dogs with systemic inflammatory response syndrome or sepsis. J Vet Emerg Crit Care (San Antonio) 2009 Oct;19(5):450–458.

183. Rau S, Kohn B, Richter C, et al. Plasma interleukin-6 response is predictive for severity and mortality in canine systemic inflammatory response syndrome and sepsis. Vet Clin Pathol 2007 Sep;36(3):253–260.

184. DeClue AE CL. Acute respiratory distress syndrome in dogs and cats: a review of clinical findings and pathophysiology. J Vet Emerg Crit Care 2007;17(4):340–347.

185. Durkan S, de Laforcade A, Rozanski E, Rush JE. Suspected relative adrenal insufficiency in a critically ill cat. J Vet Emerg Crit Care 2007;17(2):197–201.

186. Greiner M, Wolf G, Hartmann K. A retrospective study of the clinical presentation of 140 dogs and 39 cats with bacteraemia. J Small Anim Pract 2008 Aug;49(8):378–383.

187. Costello MF, Drobatz KJ, Aronson LR, et al. Underlying cause, pathophysiologic abnormalities, and response to treatment in cats with septic peritonitis: 51 cases (1990–2001). J Am Vet Med Assoc 2004 Sep 15;225(6):897–902.

188. Brady CA, Otto CM, Van Winkle TJ, et al. Severe sepsis in cats: 29 cases (1986–1998). J Am Vet Med Assoc 2000 Aug 15;217(4):531–535.

189. Kenney EM, Rozanski EA, Rush JE, et al. Association between outcome and organ system dysfunction in dogs with sepsis: 114 cases (2003–2007). J Am Vet Med Assoc 2010 Jan 1;236(1):83–87.

190. McMichael M MR. Ischemia-reperfusion injury pathophysiology, part I. J Vet Emerg Crit Care 2004;14(4):231–241.

191. Fitzgerald KT, Flood AA. Hymenoptera stings. Clin Tech Small Anim Pract 2006 Nov;21(4):194–204.

192. Litster A, Atkins C, Atwell R. Acute death in heartworm-infected cats: unraveling the puzzle. Vet Parasitol 2008 Dec 10;158(3): 196–203.

193. Berdoulay P SM, Starr J. Serum sickness in a dog associated with antivenin therapy for snake bite caused by *Crotalus adamaneus*. J Vet Emerg Crit Care 2005;15(3):206–212.

194. Arieff AI, Graf H. Pathophysiology of type A hypoxic lactic acidosis in dogs. Am J Physiol 1987 Sep;253(3 Pt 1):E271–E276.

195. Arieff AI, Park R, Leach WJ, et al. Pathophysiology of experimental lactic acidosis in dogs. Am J Physiol 1980 Aug;239(2): F135–F142.

196. Vail DM, Ogilvie GK, Fettman MJ, et al. Exacerbation of hyper-lactatemia by infusion of lactated Ringer's solution in dogs with lymphoma. J Vet Intern Med 1990 Sep–Oct;4(5):228–232.

197. Burkitt JM, Haskins SC, Aldrich J, et al. Effects of oral administration of a commercial activated charcoal suspension on serum osmolality and lactate concentration in the dog. J Vet Intern Med 2005 Sep–Oct;19(5):683–686.

198. Boysen SR, Bozzetti M, Rose L, et al. Effects of prednisone on blood lactate concentrations in healthy dogs. J Vet Intern Med 2009 Sep–Oct;23(5):1123–1125.

199. T Preuss DL-MW. Blood sampling from a pulmonary artery catheter. In: Lynn-McHale DJ, Wiegnad KC, eds. AACN Procedure Manual for Critical Care. St. Louis: Elsevier Saunders; 2005: 476–481.

16

Cardiopulmonary cerebral resuscitation

Sean D. Smarick

Cardiopulmonary arrest (CPA) is the sudden cessation of spontaneous and effective circulation and ventilation. It is the common pathway to death from any disease process. Cardiopulmonary cerebral resuscitation (CPCR) is the treatment to establish effective perfusion to the heart and brain with the ultimate goal of returning the patient to a normal life.[1,2] The entire veterinary healthcare team is crucial in the preparation for and execution of CPCR in veterinary medicine.

Preparing for a cardiopulmonary arrest

Every veterinary practice from a vaccination clinic to a multispecialty referral hospital should have systems in place to address a CPA. Appropriate equipment and drugs must be available, and staff members at all levels must be adequately trained to fulfill their roles during an arrest event.[2,3]

Equipment and drugs required

Equipment and drugs used in CPCR should be readily available. A tackle box with CPCR supplies kept in a consistent place, usually near the surgery suites or treatment area, is the minimum recommended for nonemergency practices. Emergency practices usually designate a central area for all CPCR supplies, often with a multi-drawer resuscitation (or "crash") cart, oxygen, and suction readily available.[2,3]

Resuscitation boxes and carts are available from medical suppliers; however, tackle boxes and tool carts can provide alternatives (see Fig. 16.1). Some practices maintain mechanical means to seal the crash box or cart to ensure its integrity, whereas others incorporate CPCR supplies with those used in intravenous (IV) access, treatments, or anesthetic inductions to maintain familiarity and maximize efficiency of space and resources.

A checklist is necessary to ensure the crash cart or box and other related equipment are adequately stocked and in working order. The checklist and any necessary restocking should be performed as personnel begin and end shifts, and after each resuscitation. Using an A–I mnemonic (A, airway; B, breathing; C, circulation; D, drugs; E, electrocardiograph [ECG]; F, fibrillation; G, gauge; H, hypothermia; I, intensive care) first proposed by Peter Safar in 1961,[4] the organization of the resuscitation area and equipment can be accomplished. A basic checklist can be found in Table 16.1. Stocking considerations for individual practices are addressed next.

Airway—items required to secure the airway

Once a CPA has been recognized, securing an airway is the first priority. Laryngoscopes, cuffed endotracheal tubes (and a syringe for inflating the cuff), and a suction system are minimally needed. Lidocaine in an atomizer or syringe is often needed for cats with laryngospasm, even in CPA situations. The suction system may range from a bulb syringe to a central suction outlet with a collection bottle, tubing, and Yankauer tip. A tracheostomy pack (see Chapter 24, Temporary Tracheostomy) may also be a consideration.[2,3,5]

Breathing—items needed to provide positive-pressure ventilation

Positive-pressure ventilation is generally performed during in-hospital CPCR; it can be provided by an adult

Advanced Monitoring and Procedures for Small Animal Emergency and Critical Care, First Edition. Edited by Jamie M. Burkitt Creedon, Harold Davis.
© 2012 John Wiley & Sons, Inc. Published 2012 by John Wiley & Sons, Inc.

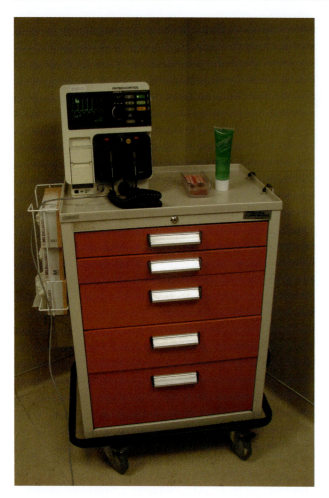

Figure 16.1 "Crash" or resuscitation cart. Equipment and drugs used in CPCR should be kept together in a readily available, standard place. They can be easily stored in a tool chest or a purpose-specific box.

Table 16.1 Basic CPCR supplies

Airway
  Endotracheal tubes
  Laryngoscope(s) with blades
  Muzzle gauze or tubing to secure ET tubes
  Cuff inflation syringe(s)
  Suction device
  Lidocaine 2% solution in an atomizer or syringe

Breathing
  Bag–valve (adult, pediatric, neonatal) and/or Bain's
    nonrebreathing circuit
  Oxygen source

Circulation
  IV and IO access supplies
  IV fluids and administration sets

Drugs
  Emergency drugs
    Atropine
    Epinephrine +/− vasopressin
    Sodium bicarbonate
  +/−Anesthetic reversals
    Naloxone
    Yohimbine/atipamezole
    Flumazenil
  Syringes and needles
  Red-rubber or polypropylene catheter
  Sterile water for injection

ECG
  ECG with leads attached
  Electrode gel

Fibrillation treatment
  Defibrillator
  Electrode gel

CPCR, cardiopulmonary cerebral resuscitation; ECG, electrocardiograph; ET, endotracheal; IO, intraosseous; IV, intravenous.

or pediatric bag–valve–mask (without the mask), a Bain's nonrebreathing circuit, or an anesthetic machine connected to an oxygen source. The source of oxygen can be centralized, with outlets and flow meters in strategic areas, or it can be portable or fixed compressed-oxygen cylinders such as E, M, or H tanks connected directly to the anesthetic machine or via a regulator and flow meter to the Bain's circuit or bag–valve setup.

Circulation—items used during cardiac compressions to enhance blood circulation

No specialized equipment is needed to provide closed-chest (CC) compressions; however, there are devices available such as pneumatic pistons or banded backboards that can perform compressions.[5] Open-chest (OC) compressions require an emergent thoracotomy, so the minimal requirements are sterile gloves, a scalpel, a pair of mayo scissors, self-retaining retractors (abdom-

inal or rib spreaders), and a Rommel tourniquet. See Chapter 17, Open-Chest Cardiopulmonary Cerebral Resuscitation, for more information.

Inspiratory impedance threshold valves are experimental in veterinary patients but have shown significant promise in the human literature and are recommended in people.[5] These devices enhance circulation by helping ensure adequate venous return to the heart during CPCR.

Intravenous fluids are warranted when hypovolemia may be a contributing cause to CPA. At minimum, vascular access supplies (see below) and isotonic crystalloids must be stocked; consideration should be given to synthetic colloids.[1,2,6,7]

Drugs used during cardiopulmonary cerebral resuscitation

Injectable atropine, epinephrine, and sodium bicarbonate are the basic drugs every crash box or cart should have. Anesthetic reversals such as naloxone, yohimbine/atipamezole, and flumazenil are recommended if narcotics, alpha-2 agonists, and valium, respectively, are used in the practice. Injectable vasopressin and calcium along with amiodarone, lidocaine, magnesium, and other antiarrhythmics are drugs used in people and may play a role in veterinary CPAs. A drug chart based on patient weight or a dosing sheet generated for each individual patient (see example in Fig. 16.2) should be available.[1,2,6,7]

To administer drugs (including IV fluids) beyond oxygen, vascular access is ideally obtained through cephalic intravenous catheter placement, via jugular venous cut-down and catheterization (scalpel, hemostats, suture, and scissors), or by intraosseous (commercial, spinal, or hypodermic) needle placement into the proximal humerus or trochanteric fossa of the femur. Alternatively, percutaneous, facilitated, or cut-down peripheral intravenous catheterization can be attempted. Until vascular access is obtained, naloxone, atropine, vasopressin, epinephrine, and lidocaine (referred to by the acronym NAVEL) can be administered by a red-rubber or polypropylene catheter placed through the endotracheal tube into the bronchi with appropriate-sized syringes and sterile water for injection.[2,5–7]

Electrocardiograph—required during cardiopulmonary cerebral resuscitation

An electrocardiograph (ECG) is recommended for all but the most basic of practices, as a significant proportion of electrical cardiac rhythms in a CPA warrant specialized treatment, namely, ventricular fibrillation. An ECG is stored in the resuscitation area or on the crash cart. Electrode gel is needed to obtain a diagnostic ECG, while *isopropyl alcohol is strictly avoided* due to the explosion hazard in the presence of an electric defibrillator.[2,5,6]

Fibrillation treatment—often required during cardiopulmonary cerebral resuscitation

The only consistently effective treatment for ventricular fibrillation is electrical defibrillation; therefore, having a defibrillator on the crash cart or in the treatment or anesthetic area is recommended. The unit should remain connected to an electrical outlet to keep the internal battery charged. With newer biphasic defibrillators gaining popularity, there are numerous refurbished monophasic units available that also include an ECG. Electrode gel is required as a coupling substance between the paddles and the patient; as mentioned previously, isopropyl alcohol and other chemicals are strictly avoided because they can create an explosion hazard. (See Chapter 18, Defibrillation, for more information.)

Gauge the efficacy—equipment used to gauge the efficacy of cardiopulmonary cerebral resuscitation

Short of the return of spontaneous circulation (ROSC), it is difficult to gauge the effectiveness of resuscitation efforts without equipment. Equipment to help assess the effectiveness of CPCR includes an end-tidal carbon dioxide monitor (capnometer) or a direct blood pressure monitor connected to an arterial catheter.[1,5] These items therefore warrant consideration when creating a practice's resuscitation area.

Hypothermia

As hypothermia postresuscitation is thought to result in better neurological outcomes and, conversely, hyperthermia is thought to result in worse outcomes, a tympanic membrane, esophageal, or rectal thermometer is recommended to ensure the patient does not become hyperthermic and to monitor passive or active cooling efforts.[5]

Intensive care

Immediate and prolonged critical care of the reanimated patient is crucial to avoid rearrest and to maximize the potential for a good (neurological) outcome.

Maintaining adequate blood pressure, oxygenation, and ventilation is paramount. Monitoring blood pressure directly with a transducer system or indirectly with a Doppler or oscillometric monitor allows titration of pressors such as norepinephrine, dopamine, or vasopressin. Dysrhythmias, which are often encountered after ROSC, can compromise perfusion and further tax the myocardium, so continuous ECG monitoring is warranted along with the appropriate antiarrhythmic use. Oxygen supplementation may be needed to maintain normoxia, monitored by arterial blood gas analysis or pulse oximetry. Normocapnea, assessed by arterial or central venous blood gas analysis or capnometry (measuring end-tidal PCO_2 [$PetCO_2$]), is maintained as needed with positive-pressure ventilation. A critical care ventilator is ideal in this situation; however, anesthetic ventilators and "hand bagging" (manual inflation using a bag–valve, Bain's circuit, or anesthetic machine and circle system) may be adequate.

Arrest Information

Date		Time	

Patient Name	
Last name	
Patient #	
Weight (kg)	**kg**

Time

	Time
CPA	
*ROSC	

Airway

ET Tube Size		Intubation Time	

Code Outcome	
*ROSC (See above)	Unsuccessful
	Successful/Euthanasia

Breathing

Ventilaton			
Baines	Bag Valve	Vent	Other_____

O2 Rate (200ml/kg)		L/min	BPM (8-15 BPM)	

Circulation

Compression Type	Closed chest (100BPM)	Open chest	I A C

IV Site	Cephalic ga in	Jugular ga in	Saphenous ga in	IO ga in	**Time**

IV Fluid

Start Time	Fluid			Volume	Finish Time
	LRS	0.9% NaCl	Other_____	ml	
	LRS	0.9% NaCl	Other_____	ml	
	LRS	0.9% NaCl	Other_____	ml	

Drugs

* Doses in this chart are reflected in ml and are for IV admin Doses

Medication/Conc	Time			
Atropine 0.54mg/ml				
Epinephrine 1mg/ml				
Vasopressin 20u/ml				
Na Bicarb 1mEq/ml				

Med/Dose	3kg	5 kg	7kg	10kg	15kg	20kg	25kg	30kg	40kg	50kg
Atropine 0.02mg/kg	0.1	0.2	0.25	0.37	0.55	0.75	0.93	1.1	1.5	1.85
Epinephrine 0.02mg/kg	0.06	0.1	0.14	0.2	0.3	0.4	0.5	0.6	0.8	1
Vasopressin 0.4u/kg	0.06	0.1	0.14	0.2	0.3	0.4	0.5	0.6	0.8	1
Na Bicarb 1mEq/kg	3	5	7	10	15	20	25	30	40	50

* Doses in chart should include volume and route

* For IT admin Dose= epi x10, atr x2, vaso x2

EKG

Initial Rhythm	Asystole	PEA	Sinus Bradycardia	V Fib	Other _____
Time	Asystole	PEA	Sinus Bradycardia	V Fib	Other _____
Time	Asystole	PEA	Sinus Bradycardia	V Fib	Other _____
Time	Asystole	PEA	Sinus Bradycardia	V Fib	Other _____

Fibrillation

Time	Charge (J)	Type	
		external	Internal
		external	Internal
		external	Internal
		external	Internal

Gauge

	Time				
Time					
ETCO2					
Diastolic BP					

Figure 16.2 Example of a form used to guide and record treatments performed during CPCR. A drug chart based on patient weight or a dosing sheet generated for each individual patient should be available.

Lastly, as every organ system will have suffered some degree of ischemia and secondary reperfusion injury, multiple organ dysfunction syndrome should be anticipated and addressed as needed with appropriate monitoring and treatment beyond the scope of this chapter.[1,2,5–7]

By running through the A–I mnemonic, the veterinary team member can establish drug and equipment checklists appropriate for each clinic or hospital. Having the right drugs and equipment in stock and in working order is crucial to being prepared to perform CPCR; however, the skills to work as a team and to use the drugs and equipment properly are equally important.

Staff training in preparation for cardiopulmonary arrest

Staff members should understand their roles on the team during CPCR and should be trained appropriately. From initial hire orientation, the individual team member can become familiar with the CPCR systems in place. Having a new technician participate in completing the checklist and subsequent stocking may help develop familiarity with the location of the practice's drugs and equipment. A CPCR training program includes both didactic instruction and hands-on skill development. Participating in human basic cardiac life support courses provides applicable overlap and the added benefit of being prepared (and legally protected) to address a client's, coworker's, or loved one's CPA. Without regular training, skills diminish.[5] Thus, drills using commercial pet resuscitation mannequins or even simply a toy stuffed animal give the team the opportunity to maintain its resuscitation skills.

Notifying the staff of cardiopulmonary arrest

The veterinary care team must be alerted when a CPA occurs. Therefore, each practice should have in place a system that notifies the team that a CPA has occurred. Notification can be in the form of an overhead page or an internal audible alarm. Either or both should be predetermined and universally recognized by the hospital team. Once a CPA is suspected, the system is activated and the resuscitation team reports immediately to the predetermined resuscitation area or the location where the CPA has taken place.

Initiating cardiopulmonary cerebral resuscitation

Early recognition of a CPA and institution of resuscitative efforts are paramount to a successful outcome. The decision to initiate CPCR will often fall on the veterinary technician caring for a pet in the intensive care unit (ICU), in the surgical suite area, or during triage. Depending on the individual state board rules, standing orders should be developed by the veterinarians in the practice so veterinary technicians can initiate CPCR and lead the effort until a veterinarian is available to direct the resuscitation.

The veterinary technician should be vigilant in monitoring anesthetized patients and those that are critically ill for signs of impending arrest, and should be proficient in triage to recognize patients presenting to the practice with immediately life-threatening signs. The best treatment for CPA is not CPCR but rather prevention of the CPA in the first place.[1,2,5–7]

Once a CPA is suspected, the resuscitation team is assembled and CPCR is instituted unless a do not attempt resuscitation (DNAR) order is in place. The care givers should be aware of the desires of the pet owner regarding advance resuscitative directives (i.e., "code status") of hospitalized pets. Code status should be communicated in patient rounds and should appear in a predetermined, consistent, and standardized fashion in the patient's record, treatment orders, cage card, or ID collar.[2,5]

Recognizing cardiopulmonary arrest

Patients that collapse, lose consciousness, or have absent spontaneous respirations (i.e., no chest movement) have signs that suggest CPA. *All patients undergoing CPA experience these signs*, but not all patients with these signs are necessarily dying. No auscultable apex heartbeat and absence of femoral pulses confirm a CPA.[2,3] Less obvious signs that distinguish the patient at high risk of CPA include significant changes or obvious abnormalities in the following: mentation; respiratory rate and effort; heart rate and pulse quality; mucous membrane color; or capillary refill time.

In the anesthetized or critically ill patient, monitoring equipment provides useful information in a nonresponsive, perhaps not spontaneously breathing patient. Esophageal stethoscopes, Doppler blood pressure flow detectors, and multiparameter monitors that measure and report direct vascular pressures, pulse oximetry, $PetCO_2$, and ECG are invaluable in the recognition of an impending arrest.

The esophageal stethoscope is a cost-effective tool that can alert the anesthetist to real-time changes in the apex beat's rate, rhythm, or intensity; a Doppler blood pressure flow detector does the same for peripheral pulses and allows for the determination of systolic blood pressure. Precipitously decreasing heart rates, pulse intensity, severe tachyarrhythmias or bradyarrhythmias, or hypotension can all lead to a CPA. An ECG provides more detailed information regarding the heart's rate and rhythm and is a valuable tool for rhythm evaluation. Pulse oximetry has technical challenges but any changes in the waveform or oxygen saturation should be investigated rather than assumed to be a false alarm. Precipitously decreasing $PetCO_2$ values or a decreasing, stair-stepping capnogram can signal an impending CPA (see Chapter 26, Capnography). While not every alarm or abnormality signals an impending arrest, the integration of available information into an accurate clinical picture can help prevent CPA or give the care-giving team some warning that CPCR will be required soon.

Assembling the team to perform cardiopulmonary cerebral resuscitation

With an impending or confirmed CPA, the team in the hospital responsible for performing CPCR is notified with the predetermined and universally understood page or signal. The team may include nontraditional caregivers such as receptionists and kennel or maintenance personnel, who can be invaluable by assisting in the resuscitation or record keeping. As stated previously, these individuals should not only be acquainted with their roles prior to being called upon, but also have ample practice and be proficient in the tasks they are being asked to carry out.

Depending on the degree of training and effective teamwork, the ideal number on a resuscitation team varies. Ideally the veterinarian would have no other task than directing the CPCR; however, staffing numbers in veterinary hospitals may make this unrealistic. On the team there could be a person for each position: ventilator, chest compressor, abdominal compressor, vascular access, drug administrator, and recorder. The author would recommend three people as the minimum number of team members; however, there is no evidence to suggest an ideal number.

Performing cardiopulmonary cerebral resuscitation

Each member of the resuscitation team plays a key role in executing CPCR. The role each member plays can span the entire A–I paradigm. Many of the skills and much of the knowledge are general nursing skills and not specific to CPCR, such as endotracheal intubation; however, there are caveats to those basic skills and specific ones to resuscitation that cumulate into effective CPCR.

Pursuing an "ABC" (airway–breathing–circulation) approach is still considered to be the first priority in

veterinary medicine. The majority of veterinary arrests are not due to primary cardiac disease amenable to defibrillation as is the case in humans, in whom a "C(D)AB" approach has been generally adopted. Veterinary patients with a compromised airway or hypoxemia as inciting cause would suffer in the human paradigm, and therefore, intubation and oxygen supplementation are recommended in dogs and cats.[2,3,5]

Securing the airway

The airway should be established with a cuffed endotracheal tube (see Chapter 23, Tracheal Intubation); extending the neck (in the absence of suspected cervical injuries) and pulling the tongue forward may open a closed airway and allow for spontaneous breathing. Suction any material from the caudal pharyngeal or laryngeal area. The endotracheal tube must be secured to ensure the airway remains patent and to minimize tracheal trauma.[2,3]

A Heimlich maneuver can be used in an attempt to dislodge an upper airway foreign body, performed by a quick inward and cranial force between the umbilicus and xyphoid generated by the fingers in small patients or palm of the hand or fist in larger ones. Alternatively, an external chest compression may have the same effect in generating enough intrathoracic pressure to force the object free. See Chapters 23, Tracheal Intubation, and 24, Temporary Tracheostomy, for information regarding rapid airway access and tracheostomy.

While the endotracheal tube is in place, any time the patient is moved, and intermittently during the resuscitation, tube placement should be confirmed. This is accomplished by (bilateral) thoracic and stomach auscultation to ensure breath sounds and not bubbling are heard; by visualization of the tube traveling through the arytenoids; by direct palpation of tissue (larynx) around the tube 360°; or by capnometry with measurement of some carbon dioxide.[2,3]

Breathing—providing positive-pressure ventilation during cardiopulmonary cerebral resuscitation

Positive-pressure ventilation (PPV) should be performed at a rate of approximately 8 breaths per minute. The chest should visibly rise, and peak inspiratory pressures should not exceed 15–20 cm H_2O. Increased rates are acceptable in hypoxemic or hypoventilated patients; however, as PPV has negative effects on coronary perfusion pressure, cardiac output, and survival, a conservative approach should be taken to maintain adequate oxygenation.[2,3,5]

Once the endotracheal tube is in place, it is connected to a bag–valve or an anesthetic circuit with bag reservoir. The bag is squeezed to provide a breath and is then allowed to recoil completely to avoid positive end-expiratory pressure (PEEP); expiration occurs passively and should occur without resistance.[5] When using an anesthetic machine, before attaching the system to the patient's endotracheal tube, the circuit must be flushed of any anesthetic gas by depressing the oxygen flush valve and squeezing the reservoir bag into an open pop-off valve. The expiratory pop-off valve is then closed to generate a good breath using the reservoir bag, then opened again to avoid excessive gas accumulation in the bag and high pressure in the airways. The opening and closing of the pop-off valve must be repeated to generate breaths. When using a Bain's nonrebreathing circuit, the tip of the reservoir bag must be occluded as with the pop-off valve.

Oxygen flow is required to provide a volume of gas in the reservoir bag. Even the standard "semiclosed" anesthetic circuit, when used as described above, requires relatively high fresh gas flow rates to fill the reservoir bag such that fresh gas is available for each breath. Bain's and other nonrebreathing circuits generally require fresh gas flows twice the minute volume (200–250 mL/kg/min) to avoid rebreathing. Bag–valves can be used with just room air but connecting them to oxygen at high flows provides near 100% oxygen (the specific flow rate is dependent on the manufacturer and model).

The acupuncture GV 26 site has been reported to increase respiratory rates in CPAs and is stimulated by placing a ~25-gauge needle into the nasal philtrum.[8]

Circulation—circulating blood during cardiopulmonary cerebral resuscitation

Once the diagnosis of pulselessness is established, circulation must be maintained until the underlying cause of the CPA is addressed. The primary goal of this assisted circulation is to support the heart and brain. To this end, external chest compressions are initiated immediately. Circulatory (IV or IO) access is also attempted at this time.[2,3,5,6]

Closed chest (CC) CPCR is theorized to propel blood forward by the cardiac pump and the thoracic pump models. The **cardiac pump theory** states that blood circulates during chest compressions due to direct compression of the ventricles with intact atrioventricular valves preventing retrograde flow. The **thoracic pump theory** states that blood circulates during external chest compressions because compression increases intrathoracic pressure, which results in a pressure gradient from the thin-walled, valved veins to the thick-walled arteries;

release of compression leads to venous refilling. Both theories are probably at work but the cardiac pump has been reported to predominate in animals <15 kg. In small animals, hand placement is over the heart (5–6th intercostal space) in lateral recumbency or circumferentially around the thorax. In larger animals, the hands are best placed over the widest portion of the thorax in lateral recumbency or over the caudal sternum in dorsal recumbency (be careful to avoid the xyphoid).[2,3]

Compressions are performed at a rate of at least 100 compressions per minute, decreasing the thoracic diameter by approximately one third, and maintaining a ratio ("**duty ratio**") of 1:1 for compression and relaxation. During the noncompression phase, all pressure should be released from the thorax to allow for venous return to the right heart. Ideally chest compressions are not interrupted for interventions such as IV access and intubation, as interruption significantly affects coronary perfusion pressure and chances of ROSC.[2]

If CC-CPCR is not effective, a number of alternatives can be employed. Changing compressors, placement of hands, varying the rate, and varying compression depth may offer some benefit. Due to studies showing no benefit over standard CPCR, simultaneous ventilation–compression CPCR and the application of MAST trousers is not recommended. In people, **interposed abdominal compressions**, which are performed midway between the umbilicus and xyphoid to generate a pressure of 100 mm Hg, are recommended if the personnel are available.[2,3,5,7] If the patient's size and conformation are amenable, a person can place one hand on the chest and one hand on the belly; interposed abdominal compressions are then accomplished by alternating compressions between the left and right arm.

In veterinary and human medicine, debate continues regarding the use and timing of open chest (OC) compressions. If there is a chest wall defect or loss of compliance, penetrating thoracic trauma, cardiac tamponade, or pleural space disease, an emergency thoracotomy is recommended. If CC compressions have not resulted in ROSC within 5 minutes, OC compressions can be considered. It is not recommend to wait >5 minutes into the resuscitative efforts to start OC-CPCR, as beyond that time, any benefit may be lost. See Chapter 17, Open-Chest Cardiopulmonary Cerebral Resuscitation, for a discussion of OC-CPCR.

Drugs—for cardiopulmonary cerebral resuscitation

The administration of some drugs may warrant ECG evaluation (see below); however, others are immediately or empirically indicated.

Preoperative or sedative drugs or ones used as part of a balanced or total intravenous anesthetic must be immediately reversed during an anesthetic arrest. For example, naloxone should be administered when a narcotic has been used and a CPA has occurred. If there is a known underlying or contributing cause to an arrest, then drugs to address that cause should be immediately given. For example, when a hyperkalemic patient arrests, sodium bicarbonate should be administered.[2,5,6]

Compressions alone are unlikely to provide enough circulation to the heart to enable its return to function. A vasopressor is warranted in CPA to help increase coronary perfusion pressures to a level associated with ROSC, no matter the initial ECG rhythm. Currently, epinephrine is still considered the first-line vasopressor and is administered at a dose of 0.01–0.02 mg/kg, repeated every 3–5 minutes. "High-dose" (0.1–0.2 mg/kg) epinephrine has not been shown to be superior (except in intratracheal administration) over "low-dose" (0.01–0.02 mg/kg) epinephrine. For endotracheal administration, a higher dose is used to ensure high enough blood concentrations that α effects predominate.[2,5,6]

Vasopressin is an alternative to epinephrine in CPCR, and it may be used in dogs once at 0.2–0.8 U/kg as an alternative to epinephrine, either initially or in place of the second dose; no feline studies have been performed.[9] A successful clinical resuscitation with vasopressin in the dog has been reported.[10]

In people, the change in the ABC paradigm to a C(D) AB is generally driven by the majority of patients having ventricular fibrillation. About the same percentage of dogs and cats have a rhythm in which the anticholinergic is warranted as have ventricular fibrillation. Using this rationale, atropine can justifiably be given empirically at a dose of 0.02–0.04 mg/kg IV/IO every 3–5 minutes (maximum, three times); dose should be doubled if given intratracheally.[2,5,6]

The administration of drugs is ideally given by the central intravenous route followed by the intraosseous, (cranial) peripheral intravenous, and lastly the intratracheal route. In dogs receiving CC-CPCR, the time to reach half the peak drug concentration from the cephalic vein averaged over a minute longer than when given centrally.[2,5,6] This timing must be weighed against the ease of gaining access. Proficiency in jugular venous cutdowns and the placement of intraosseous needles is valuable for cardiopulmonary cerebral resuscitation scenarios and for shock resuscitation.

Intratracheal (IT) administration can be used for naloxone, atropine, vasopressin, epinephrine, and lidocaine (NAVEL, as mentioned earlier). For IT administration, drug doses should be at least doubled (and in the case of epinephrine, the "high dose" used); suspended in 5–10 mL of sterile water for injection (preferable) or 0.9% NaCl; injected via long red-rubber or polypropylene catheter to the level of the carina; and followed with two breaths. Peripherally injected drugs should be followed by a 5- to 20-mL bolus of IV fluids with elevation of the extremity.[2,5,6]

Intravenous fluid administration is warranted in cases of hypovolemia but has been associated with worse outcomes in euvolemic arrests.[2,5,6]

In cases of pre-existing severe metabolic acidosis, hyperkalemia, after prolonged (>10 minutes) CPA, and in some intoxications, buffer therapy is suggested. Currently sodium bicarbonate is the only recommended buffer; it is administered empirically at 1 mEq/kg slow IV, repeated every 5 minutes.[2,5,6]

Electrocardiography in cardiopulmonary cerebral resuscitation

The significant ECG rhythms of CPA in veterinary patients as described by Rush and Wingfield in 1992 were pulseless electrical activity (PEA; also formerly known as EMD—electromechanical dissociation; 23.3%), asystole (22.8%), ventricular fibrillation (VF; 19.8%), and sinus bradycardia (19%).[11]

The protocols for treating the bradyarrhythmias (PEA, asytole, sinus bradycardia) are similar. However, because the treatment for bradyarrhythmia and the treatment for VF are different, the ECG becomes invaluable in distinguishing these two arrest-rhythm patient populations. It is important to remember that the CPA patient's ECG rhythm can change many times through the CPCR effort. As an example, patients may initially have VF, or may start out in asystole and go on to develop VF after a period of CPCR.[2,5,6]

Fibrillation treatment

The definitive treatment for ventricular fibrillation is electrical defibrillation. Antiarrhythmics have a very limited role during VF. Due to recent studies in people, amiodarone has replaced lidocaine (now Class Indeterminate) as the drug for shock-resistant VF. The suggested veterinary dose is 5 mg/kg IV. Bretylium is no longer recommended as it is no longer available. In known hypomagnesemic states or torsades de pointes, magnesium sulfate (30 mg/kg diluted in D5W and given IV push) is a recommendation in people.[2,5,6]

Caregiver safety is paramount during defibrillation and is ensured by not using isopropyl alcohol for electrode conductivity (either for defibrillator or ECG electrode contact), observing for caregiver contact, and announcing the impending delivery of the shock ("I'm clear, you're clear, we're all clear!").[7] If the initial shock is unsuccessful, pharmacologic interventions are instituted and CPCR is resumed for 2 minutes to reoxygenate the myocardium. Research continues to investigate the ideal timing of shocks and compressions.[2,5] Continued, minimally interrupted CC or OC compressions before and after defibrillation shocks are important in the success of ROSC. For a more detailed discussion of defibrillation see Chapter 18, Defibrillation.

Gauging the effectiveness of cardiopulmonary cerebral resuscitation

Evaluation of how each step of the resuscitation and the effort as a whole are being executed is crucial for a successful resuscitation.[2,3,5–7] Additionally, the attending veterinarian must consider what (potentially reversible) conditions contributed to the CPA, and treat accordingly.

The resuscitation team leader along with the members should revisit "A" through "E": Assess the airway is still intact, the ventilation (breathing) rate is appropriate, the circulation is maximized (e.g., the compressor is not fatiguing), if another round or different drugs are to be administered, and what the ECG is now reading.

The ultimate reinforcement of a job well done is ROSC; this may not come despite ideal execution. Pulse checks and pupil size do not offer any gauge to the effectiveness of CPCR. If the patient has an indwelling arterial line, obtaining diastolic pressures >30 mm Hg are associated with ROSC.[5,11] End-tidal expired carbon dioxide can be used as a marker of CPCR effectiveness. Carbon dioxide in the breath requires the delivery of oxygen from the lungs to tissues and the return of carbon dioxide to the lungs that is subsequently ventilated to the detector. End-tidal expired carbon dioxide tensions exceeding 15–20 mm Hg have been correlated to ROSC and survival in veterinary and human studies.[1] When using $PetCO_2$ to monitor the efficacy of CPCR, one must remember that alterations in breathing rate will affect $PetCO_2$, that the administration of bicarbonate will increase $PetCO_2$, and that pressor administration will cause the $PetCO_2$ to drop. A dramatic rise is associated with ROSC as the increased concentrations of carbon dioxide are washed out from the venous system.[2,5]

If the search for reversible causes has been unrewarding, CPCR is being provided according to plan, diastolic pressures are >30 mm Hg, and $PetCO_2$>1–20 mm Hg, then there is little more to do than continue on until the veterinarian believes the efforts are futile (usually not greater than 20 minutes).[2,5,12] However, if ROSC is achieved, CPCR continues into prolonged life support.

Hypothermia following return of spontaneous circulation

Upon ROSC, hypothermia should be considered because improved clinical outcomes have been demonstrated experimentally in dogs and clinically in people. Induction of mild hypothermia at 32–34°C for 12–24 hours after ROSC has improved neurological outcome in both experimental dogs and clinically treated humans. Cooling can be accomplished by surface ice packs or cooling blankets, sedation and neuromuscular blockade, and 30 mL/kg IV fluids at 4°C.[5]

Intensive care following return of spontaneous circulation

Intensive care is needed to address the complex pathology in the postresuscitation phase following ROSC. Each organ system should be aggressively monitored and supported. Factors known to be important in the recovery of postarrest patients include maintenance of normocapnea, normoxia, and adequate systemic blood pressure.

Maintenance of normocapnea monitored with capnometry and blood gases is important because hypercapnea causes cerebral vasodilation and can increase intracranial pressure, something that is already a concern in the postarrest state. Hypocapnea can conversely lead to damaging cerebral vasoconstriction and hypoxia. Oxygen supplementation should be titrated with pulse oximetry and arterial blood gases to avoid hypoxemia and excessive hyperoxia, as high PaO_2 is thought to increase reactive oxygen species and result in worse neurologic outcomes.

Maintaining MAP>100 mm Hg is recommended to maintain blood flow to the brain. Arrhythmia control is warranted if a dysrhythmia is affecting perfusion. Constant-rate infusions (CRIs) of inotropes, pressors, and antiarrhythmics are usually required to maintain adequate blood pressure post-ROSC. The veterinary technician should anticipate close blood pressure and ECG monitoring, and the administration of multiple CRIs with syringe or infusion pumps.

As for any patient with global ischemia and reperfusion, SIRS, MODS, or DIC, the care giver is faced with vigilant monitoring of and comprehensive care for every organ system to effect a successful outcome in providing CPCR.[2,5,12]

Acknowledgments

The author wishes to thank Corey Korinko and Amanda Cole for their assistance with this chapter.

References

1. Hofmeister EH, Brainard BM, Egger CM, et al. Prognostic indicators for dogs and cats for cardiopulmonary arrest treated for cardiopulmonary cerebral resuscitation at a university teaching hospital. J Am Vet Med Assoc 2009;235:50–57.
2. Plunkett SJ, McMichael M. Cardiopulmonary resuscitation in small animal medicine: an update. JVIM 2008;22:9–25.
3. Cole SG, Otto CM, Hughes D. Cardiopulmonary cerebral resuscitation in small animals—a clinical review (Part I). J Vet Emerg Crit Care 2003;12:261–267.
4. Safar P. On the history of modern resuscitation. Crit Care Med 1996;24(2):S4.
5. 2005 American Heart Association guidelines for cardiopulmonary resuscitation and emergency care. Circulation 2005;112(suppl IV).
6. Cole SG, Otto CM, Hughes D. Cardiopulmonary cerebral resuscitation in small animals—a clinical review. (Part II). J Vet Emerg Crit Care 2003;13:13–23.
7. Guidelines 2000 for cardiopulmonary resuscitation and emergency care. Circulation 2000;102(suppl I).
8. Janssens L, Altman S, Rogers PA. Respiratory and cardiac arrest under general anaesthesia: treatment by acupuncture of the nasal philtrum. Vet Rec 1979;105(12):273–276.
9. Scroggin RD, Quandt J. The use of vasopressin for treating vasodilatory shock and cardiopulmonary arrest. J Vet Emerg Crit Care 2009;19(2):145–157.
10. Schmittinger CA, Astner S, Astner L, et al. Cardiopulmonary resuscitation with vasopressin in a dog. Vet Anaesth Analg 2005 Mar;32(2):112–114.
11. Rush JE, Wingfield WE. Recognition and frequency of dysrhythmias during cardiopulmonary arrest. J Am Vet Med Assoc 1992 Jun 15;200(12):1932–1937.
12. Waldrop JE, Rozanski EA, Swanke ED, et al. Causes of cardiopulmonary arrest, resuscitation management, and functional outcome in dogs and cats surviving cardiopulmonary arrest. J Vet Emerg Crit Care 2004;14(1):22–29.

Additional resources

Complete 2010 American Heart Association Guidelines for cardiopulmonary resuscitation and emergency cardiovascular care science. Circulation 2010 Nov 2;122(18_suppl_3): S640–S946. Available at: http://circ.ahajournals.org/content/122/18_suppl_3.toc.

17

Open-chest cardiopulmonary cerebral resuscitation

Janelle R. Wierenga

Cardiopulmonary arrest (CPA) is the single pathway to death from any underlying disease and is common in small animal emergency and critical care medicine. Some underlying disease conditions are treatable in the acute CPA setting if they can be identified. Other disease conditions are not treatable or not identifiable in the acute setting, making resuscitation efforts from CPA difficult. Immediate cardiopulmonary cerebral resuscitation (CPCR) is indicated in sudden cardiac arrest. Delay in initiation of cardiac compressions in CPCR has been shown to result in decreased return of spontaneous circulation (ROSC). In human studies evaluating delay of CPCR in CPA due to ventricular fibrillation (VF), every minute of untreated VF decreases survival by 7%–10%.[1] Even with immediate CPCR the success of resuscitation to ROSC and survival to discharge is low in veterinary medicine at only 5%–10%.[2–4] Survival rates depend on the underlying disease condition, the inciting cause of the arrest, and the resuscitation efforts and timing.

Indications for open-chest cardiopulmonary cerebral resuscitation

"Open-chest" or "internal" CPCR through an emergency thoracotomy was the standard of care for CPA in the early 20th century.[5] Now, closed-chest CPCR is generally instituted first unless specific situations or disease conditions exist that may be indications for immediate open-chest CPCR.[5,6] A full discussion of closed-chest CPCR can be found in Chapter 16, Cardiopulmonary Cerebral Resuscitation.

Any condition that prevents healthcare workers from achieving adequate perfusion to the lungs, heart, and brain through closed-chest CPCR is a potential indication for internal CPCR with direct cardiac massage. The 2010 American Heart Association Guidelines for Cardiopulmonary Resuscitation and Emergency Cardiovascular Care state that open-chest CPCR is recommended or may be considered for specific indications. The Guidelines recommend open-chest CPCR in the case of intraoperative arrest during a laparotomy or thoracotomy procedure, or in the case of CPA shortly following a cardiothoracic surgery (Class IIa, Level of Evidence C), and state that it may be useful in some cases of CPA secondary to penetrating trauma (Class IIb, Level of Evidence C).[7]

After closed-chest CPCR has been chosen as the first method of CPCR, there is controversy regarding whether and when one should abandon closed-chest efforts and proceed to open-chest CPCR. Some literature recommends initiating open-chest CPCR if there is no response to external chest compressions within 2–5 minutes,[6,8–11] while others allow 5–10 minutes of closed-chest CPCR.[5,12–15] There is a consensus, however, that if the healthcare team is going to perform open-chest CPCR, it should be initiated relatively early in the resuscitation effort. When instituted after 20 minutes of closed-chest compressions, internal cardiac massage is ineffective in achieving ROSC.[5,16,17] It has been suggested that inadequate forward blood flow during closed-chest efforts is more likely to occur in animals over 20 kg, in which the thoracic pump method probably predominates (see Chapter 16, Cardiopulmonary Cerebral Resuscitation).[5,16] Situations in which open-chest CPCR may be indicated are listed in Box 17.1.

Advanced Monitoring and Procedures for Small Animal Emergency and Critical Care, First Edition. Edited by Jamie M. Burkitt Creedon, Harold Davis.
© 2012 John Wiley & Sons, Inc. Published 2012 by John Wiley & Sons, Inc.

Box 17.1 Possible indications for open-chest CPCR

- Failure of closed-chest CPCR efforts
- Pericardial effusion
- Pleural space disease
  - Pneumothorax
  - Moderate or marked pleural effusion
  - Diaphragmatic hernia
- Thoracic-wall trauma
  - Rib fractures
  - Flail chest
  - Penetrating injuries through thoracic wall and into thoracic cavity

---

Box 17.2 Equipment in surgical pack for open-chest CPCR

- Scalpel handle
- Mayo and Metzenbaum scissors
- Hemostats
- Needle holder
- Sharp and blunt suture scissors
- Tissue forceps
- Sterile gauze
- Sterile drape
- Finochietto rib retractors

Rationale

Coronary blood flows from the proximal aorta into the myocardium via the coronary arteries during diastole; blood returning from the myocardium drains into the right atrium. Thus, coronary perfusion pressure (CoPP) is equal to the difference between diastolic aortic pressure (DAoP) and right atrial pressure (RAP):

$$CoPP = DAoP - RAP \quad (17.1)$$

Research in animal models and in humans with CPA has shown that adequate CoPP is associated with successful resuscitation and ROSC. A CoPP greater than or equal to 15 mm Hg during CPCR has been associated with increased ROSC and survival to discharge.[1] Clinical studies in humans demonstrate an increase in CoPP and increased ROSC with internal cardiac massage compared with external chest compressions.[18,19] Internal cardiac massage has been shown to produce coronary perfusion pressures 3 times greater than external chest compressions.[20] Studies have shown significant increase in cardiac output, arterial blood pressure, forward blood flow, CoPP, and cerebral perfusion pressure with internal cardiac massage, and an increase in ROSC and improvement in neurological outcome in canine models of cardiopulmonary arrest.[21–25] Nevertheless, the 2010 American Heart Association Guidelines for Cardiopulmonary Resuscitation and Emergency Cardiovascular Care state that there is insufficient evidence of benefit or harm to recommend the routine use of open-chest CPCR in people, except in the specific situations mentioned above.[7]

There are additional potential benefits of open-chest CPCR. Unlike external chest compressions, open-chest CPCR allows direct visualization of the heart and assessment of ventricular filling. The healthcare worker can directly evaluate for ventricular fibrillation, asystole, or an atonic heart muscle during internal cardiac massage, which can help direct therapy when appropriate treatment is unclear during closed-chest efforts. Open-chest CPCR also allows for the occlusion of the descending aorta, which maximizes cardiac output to the most crucial organs—the heart, brain, and lungs. Descending aortic compression is also useful in critical hemorrhage into the abdomen by decreasing further blood loss.

Performing open-chest cardiopulmonary cerebral resuscitation

Equipment and preparedness

The equipment for open-chest CPCR should be ready and immediately available in a crash cart (see Fig. 16.1). Emergency thoracotomy equipment should be readily accessible in the crash cart, preferably contained within a single sterilized surgery pack to improve the ease and speed of obtaining all necessary equipment. The sterile surgical pack equipment is listed in Box 17.2 and shown in Figure 17.1. A sterile #10 scalpel blade should be easy to obtain along with sterile gloves, clippers, aseptic scrub, and isopropyl alcohol. Devices for clamping the descending aorta should also be aseptically prepared, such as Rumel tourniquet, Penrose drain, umbilical tape, or vascular clamps (see Fig. 17.2). A device with similar function to a Rumel tourniquet can be created using a red-rubber catheter, umbilical tape, and hemostats. A 12- to 18-Fr red-rubber catheter is cut to 3–4 cm in length at the tapered end of the catheter. The umbilical tape is passed around the descending aorta with both ends of the tape facing outward (Fig. 17.3a). A mosquito hemostat is fed through the red-rubber catheter and used to grasp and thread the umbilical tape through the red-rubber catheter (Fig. 17.3b). The red-rubber tube is then moved toward the vessel and the vessel is compressed (Fig. 17.3c). The umbilical tape is held in place around the compressed vessel by placing the hemostats perpendicularly on the umbilical tape next to the red rubber on the side further from the vessel, as shown in Figure 17.3d.

Performing an emergency thoracotomy

The patient should be placed in right lateral recumbency to prepare for a left lateral thoracotomy at the left sixth intercostal space as shown in Figure 17.4. Throughout, external chest compressions should continue as is possible. The region is prepared quickly with minimal fur clipping at the fourth through sixth intercostal spaces and minimal cleaning with a surgical scrub. Sterile gloves are worn and the skin is incised along the cranial aspect of the left sixth rib extending from the dorsal aspect of the scapula to 3–5 cm dorsal to the sternum. Rapid transection of the latissimus dorsi, serratus ventralis, scalenous, and pectoral muscles will be

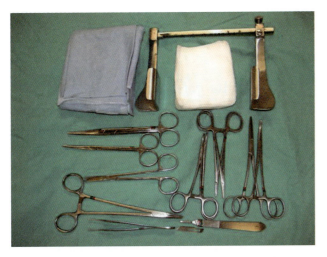

Figure 17.1 Surgical pack for emergency thoracotomy for open-chest CPCR.

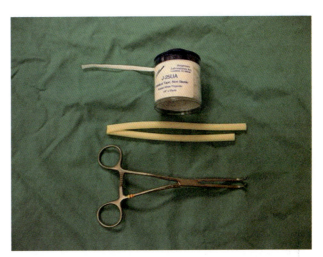

Figure 17.2 Penrose drain, umbilical tape, and vascular clamps for clamping the descending aorta.

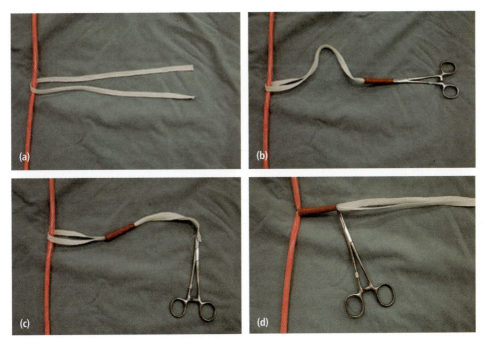

Figure 17.3 Red-rubber catheter, umbilical tape, and hemostats that can be made (a–c) into a tourniquet for compression or clamping (d) of the descending aorta.

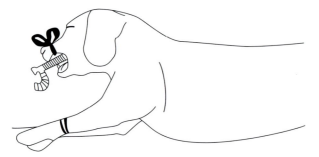

Figure 17.4 Placement of patient and location of incision for emergency thoracotomy in order to perform internal cardiac massage. Patient is placed in right lateral recumbency for a left lateral thoracotomy at the left sixth intercostal space. The skin is incised along the cranial aspect of the left sixth rib extending from the dorsal aspect of the scapula to 3–5 cm dorsal to the sternum. Reprinted from Arlene Coulson and Noreen Lewis, *An Atlas of Interpretative Radiographic Anatomy of the Dog and Cat*, 2nd edition, Blackwell Publishing, 2008 (figure 407, page 282).

necessary to reach the external and internal intercostal muscles. The external and internal intercostal muscles are incised along the cranial aspect of the rib with either a scalpel blade or Metzenbaum scissors to the level of the pleura. Care should be taken to avoid lacerating the lateral thoracic vessels that run alongside the sternum or the intercostal vessels that run along the caudal aspect of each rib. It is also recommended not to penetrate the pleural space with the scalpel blade or scissors due to the potential for trauma to the lung parenchyma, heart muscle, or coronary vessels; this can be very difficult in the emergent setting. Manual ventilation of the patient should cease briefly while the pleura is bluntly penetrated with hemostats and the pleural entry extended dorsally and ventrally. Finochietto rib retractors are placed between the ribs to provide intrathoracic exposure with enough space to insert the hand for internal cardiac massage. A pericardiectomy should be performed if there is pericardial disease such as effusion or restrictive pericarditis. The pericardium is grasped with tissue forceps and an incision is made with Metzenbaum scissors ventral to the phrenic nerve through the pericardium and extended ventrally. Pericardotomy or partial pericardectomy should be adequate in the case of effusion. Direct manual cardiac massage is then initiated. When CPA occurs in intraoperative situations, cardiac massage can be performed directly via a thoracotomy or by incising through the diaphragm in a laparotomy procedure.

Complications associated with emergency thoracotomy include laceration of vessels such as the lateral thoracic vessels along the sternum, intercostal vessels, or coronary vessels; laceration of the lung parenchyma, leading to leakage of air from the lungs and the potential need for suture closure or a partial or complete lung lobectomy; laceration of the heart muscle, leading to profound hemorrhage; penetration into a cardiac chamber, leading to exsanguination; or rib fractures secondary to overzealous retraction with the rib retractor.[5,16] The complication rate associated with the procedure has been documented to be low in humans even with the invasive nature of open-chest CPCR and the need to enter the thoracic cavity rapidly. In humans less than 2% of the open-chest CPCR patients have iatrogenic cardiac trauma or injury associated with the thoracotomy.[26,27]

Performing internal cardiac massage

Direct compression of the heart has been shown to triple the coronary perfusion pressure compared with external chest compressions.[20] The heart can be massaged in a single hand, between two hands, or between a hand and the internal body wall. Studies have shown that two-handed cardiac massage can be more beneficial than providing cardiac massage with one hand, though this will be limited by patient size, heart size, patient conformation, the entry site into the thoracic cavity, and the availability of appropriate instruments such as rib retractors.[6,28] The heart can be palmed if it is small enough, squeezed between two hands, or pressed up against the inside of the thoracic cavity to compress the chambers (see Fig. 17.5). Cardiac compression rates should be greater than 100 beats per minute according to the 2010 American Heart Association Guidelines for Cardiopulmonary Resuscitation and Emergency Cardiovascular Care.[29] Compression rates of greater than or equal to 120 beats per minute have been associated with increased coronary perfusion pressures and up to 150 beats per minute with increased pressures and perfusion to vital organs in dogs.[30] To allow for adequate refilling of the heart, realistic compression rates for internal cardiac massage of 120–140 compressions per minute are recommended.[5,16]

As stated previously, sterile gloves should be used to decrease contamination of the thoracic cavity during the emergency thoracotomy and internal cardiac massage. The compressor should be changed at least every 2–5 minutes (with minimal interruption to compression) to avoid decreased coronary perfusion that could occur with hand fatigue. Each compressor should wear sterile gloves for internal cardiac massage.[1,17] Hand placement is important, as inadvertent penetration of the heart muscle with fingers can occur, leading to catastrophic hemorrhage (see Fig. 17.5d). It is recommended to cup

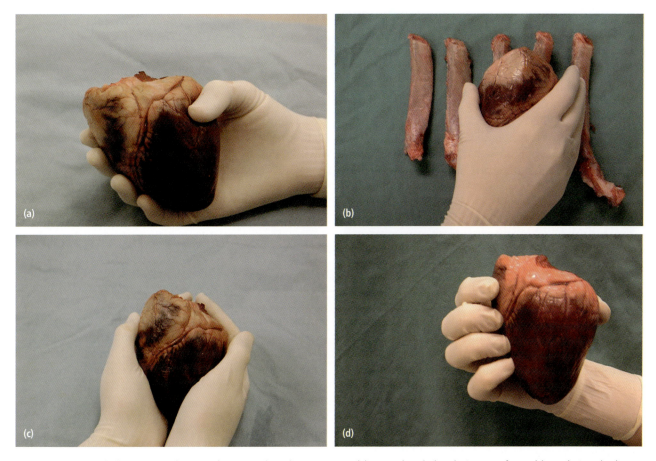

Figure 17.5 Hand placement techniques for internal cardiac massage: (a) a one-handed technique performed by palming the heart; (b) a one-handed technique performed by compressing the heart against the rib cage; (c) a two-handed technique for internal cardiac compression; (d) shows how inadvertent penetration of the heart muscle can occur if the fingers point inward toward the heart during internal cardiac massage.

the hand around the heart using either the one-handed or two-handed technique for internal cardiac massage.

The heart should be evaluated visually and by gentle palpation for adequate filling, atonic musculature, and ventricular fibrillation during open-chest CPCR. The heart is directly accessible for defibrillation if indicated. In small animals, asystole or pulseless electrical activity (PEA) was the most common arrest rhythm identified, though in one study ventricular fibrillation was almost as common as PEA and asystole.[31–35] Defibrillation in open-chest CPCR can be performed with internal defibrillator paddles wrapped in sterile saline-soaked gauze sponges and placed on either side of the heart. The energy recommended for defibrillation in open-chest CPCR is approximately 1/10th of the energy used with external defibrillation, using 0.5–1 Joules per kilogram of body weight.[5,16,36] It is recommended to perform internal cardiac massage immediately after defibrillation for 1–3 minutes before performing further defibrilla-

tion.[1] It is recommended to use the least amount of energy needed to defibrillate the critical mass of the heart.[20] Ventricular fibrillation is more difficult to convert if the patient has been in ventricular fibrillation for longer than 5 minutes or is refractory to increasing doses of energy in defibrillation.[5,16,20] See Chapter 18, Defibrillation, for more information.

Augmentation techniques

Emergency thoracotomy for internal cardiac massage increases the possibility of the return of spontaneous circulation by improving CoPP. Augmentation techniques that can be used during open-chest CPCR help increase CoPP and therefore may improve the chances of ROSC and survival. Compression of the descending aorta can increase CoPP and cerebral perfusion pressure by directing the cardiac output to the cranial half of the body. Descending aortic compression can also help prevent hemorrhage occurring distal to the site of aortic occlusion. The aorta can be compressed using a Rumel tourniquet, red-rubber tube, Penrose drain, or umbilical tape that is passed around the major vessel (see Figs. 17.2 and 17.3). Digital compression of the descending aorta can be performed, as an alternative to a tourniquet, by compressing the vessel dorsally against the ventral aspect of the vertebral bodies.[6] Aortic compression should be gradually removed over 10–15 minutes to help minimize ischemia-reperfusion injury and cardiovascular collapse.[10]

Postresuscitation care

Emergency thoracotomy for open-chest CPCR is invasive, traumatic to the tissues, and is a clean to clean-contaminated procedure that involves specific postresuscitation care. The pleural space should be flushed with sterile saline to dilute possible contaminants that may have entered the thoracic cavity during the procedure. Intrathoracic samples should be taken for anaerobic and aerobic cultures after lavage, prior to closing the thoracotomy.[5,16] Closure of the thoracotomy should be performed aseptically, usually involving consultation with or closure by an experienced surgeon.[36] Nonabsorbable monofilament suture or wire is passed around the adjacent ribs with care to avoid the intercostal vessels on the caudal aspect of the ribs. This can be done by passing the needle backward or using hemostats to bluntly pass the sutures around the ribs. The sutures are tightened with a square knot closure with a minimum of four throws. After the closure around the ribs, the tissue is sealed and there is no longer communication with the pleural space. Sometimes no fur clipping or surgical scrub is possible prior to thoracotomy; in such cases, fur probably should not be clipped even once the thorax is closed, to prevent excessive intrathoracic fur contamination. A thoracostomy tube can be placed prior to closure or thoracocentesis can be performed after closure to evacuate the air from the pleural space from the thoracotomy. Information on thoracostomy tube placement and thoracocentesis is available in Chapter 30, Pleural Space Drainage.

Due to the need to enter the thoracic cavity quickly, minimal preparation is done prior to emergency thoracotomy. Despite this, infection rates postresuscitation for open-chest CPCR patients are low, reportedly less than 10% in humans.[6,26,27] Appropriate-spectrum intravenous antibiotics should be instituted after ROSC and should be continued during hospitalization. The antibiotics may need to be administered after discharge as indicated by length of hospitalization and actual contamination during the thoracotomy. It is also important

to remember that the patient successfully resuscitated after an open-chest CPCR effort has not usually received anesthesia or analgesia, unless the arrest occurred intra-operatively. Therefore, it is important to administer analgesics to these patients at safe doses once spontaneous circulation has been established. Analgesics should be administered at doses that do not cause cardiovascular or respiratory depression but control pain associated with the procedure.

Postresuscitation monitoring and care are similar to those patients resuscitated with external CPCR. The cardiovascular system should be evaluated frequently to continuously by monitoring blood pressure and an electrocardiogram, and by serially evaluating the patient's perfusion parameters such as mucous membrane color, heart or pulse rate, pulse quality, and capillary refill time. The respiratory system should be monitored with pulse oximetry or arterial blood gases for hypoxemia, end-tidal capnography for hypercapnia secondary to hypoventilation, respiratory rate and effort evaluation, and frequent auscultation of the thorax for decreased lung sounds associated with a persistent or worsening pneumothorax or pleural effusion. Monitoring of the neurologic system is recommended with serial neurological examinations, pupil size and symmetry, pupillary light reflex, palpebral response, and changes in mentation to evaluate for injury to the brain secondary to compromised perfusion.

The blood glucose, electrolytes, and acid–base status should be monitored for alterations in metabolic status. The patient should also be monitored for organ dysfunction or injury such as insult to the kidneys resulting in renal failure; insult to the gastrointestinal tract resulting in hematemesis, hematochezia, or melena; or injury to the liver leading to liver enzyme elevation.

Summary

In summary, open-chest CPCR may be indicated in specific disease conditions such as those associated with pericardial diseases, pleural space diseases, and thoracic wall injury. Open-chest CPCR may be indicated when external chest compressions do not result in adequate forward flow of blood. Open-chest CPCR has been shown to result in increased coronary and cerebral perfusion pressures, and consequently increased ROSC and survival in patients. The procedure to enter the thoracic cavity is performed quickly in order to minimize the time that forward blood flow is compromised. Emergency thoracotomy can lead to traumatic complications such as vessel and intrathoracic organ laceration along with infection, though reported complication rates are low. Specific care is taken to decrease the incidence of infection. Postresuscitative care and monitoring is similar to any patient that has a sudden cardiac arrest, with monitoring of all organ systems and intensive monitoring of the cardiovascular, respiratory, and neurologic systems.

References

1. ECC Committee, Subcommittees, and Task Force of the American Heart Association. 2005 American Heart Association guidelines for cardiopulmonary resuscitation and emergency cardiovascular care. Circulation 2005;112(Suppl):IV1–IV203.

2. Kass KH, Haskins SC. Survival following cardiopulmonary resuscitation in dogs and cats. JVECC 1992;2(2):57–65.

3. Wingfield WE, Van Pelt DR. Respiratory and cardiopulmonary arrest in dogs and cats: 265 cases (1986–91). JAVMA 1992; 200(12):1993–1996.

4. Waldrop JE, Rozanski EA, Swanke ED, O'Toole TE, Rush JE. Causes of cardiopulmonary arrest, resuscitation management, and functional outcome in dogs and cats surviving cardiopulmonary arrest. JVECC 2004;14(1):22–29.

5. Haldane S, Marks SL. Cardiopulmonary cerebral resuscitation: techniques (part 1). Comp Cont Ed Pract Vet 2004;26:780–789.

6. Cole SG, Otto CM, Hughes D. Cardiopulmonary cerebral resuscitation in small animals—a clinical practice review (part I). JVECC 2002;12(4):261–267.

7. Cave DM, Gazmuri RJ, Otto CW, et al. Part 7: CPR techniques and devices: 2010 American Heart Association Guidelines for cardiopulmonary resuscitation and emergency cardiovascular care. Circulation 2010;122(Suppl 3):S720–S728.

8. Evans AT. New thoughts on cardiopulmonary resuscitation. Vet Clin North Am Small Anim Pract 1999;29:819–829.

9. Kruse-Elliot KT. Cardiopulmonary resuscitation: strategies for maximizing success. Vet Med 2001;16(1):51–58.

10. Barton L, Crowe DT. Open chest cardiopulmonary resuscitation. In: Bonagura JD, ed. Kirk's Current Veterinary Therapy XIII. Philadelphia: W.B. Saunders; 2000:147–149.

11. Burkett DE. Cardiopulmonary cerebral resuscitation: an update. In: Proceedings, International Veterinary Emergency Critical Care Society VI. 1998;104–108.

12. Pottle A, Bullock I, Thomas J, Scott L. Survival to discharge following open chest cardiac compression (OCCC). A 4-year retrospective audit in a cardiothoracic specialist centre: Royal Brompton and Harefield NHS Trust, United Kingdom. Resuscitation 2002;52:269–272.

13. Hackett TB. Cardiopulmonary cerebral resuscitation. Vet Clin North Am Small Anim Pract 2001;31:1253–1264.

14. Marks SL. Cardiopulmonary resuscitation and oxygen therapy. Vet Clin North Am Small Anim Pract 1999;29:959–969, vii.

15. Wingfield WE. Cardiopulmonary arrest. In: Wingfield WE, Raffe MR, eds. The Veterinary ICU Book. Jackson, WY: Teton NewMedia; 2002.

16. Haldane S, Marks SL. Cardiopulmonary cerebral resuscitation: emergency drugs and postresuscitative care (part 2). Comp Cont Ed Pract Vet 2004;26:791–799.

17. ECC Committee, Subcommittees, and Task Force of the American Heart Association. 2000 American Heart Association guidelines for cardiopulmonary resuscitation and emergency cardiovascular care. Circulation 2000;102(Suppl):I1–I384.

18. Takino M, Okada T. The optimum timing of resuscitative thoracotomy for non-traumatic out-of-hospital cardiac arrest. Resuscitation 1993;26(1):69–74.

19. Boczar ME, Howard MA, Rivers EP, Martin GB, Horst AM, Lewandowski C, Tomlanovich MC, Nowak RM. A technique revisited: hemodynamic comparison of closed- and open-chest cardiac massage during human cardiopulmonary resuscitation. Crit Care Med 1995;23:498–503.

20. Callaway CW. Chapter 50: Cardiopulmonary–cerebral resuscitation. In: Shoemaker, Ayres, Grenvik, and Holbrook, eds. Textbook of Critical Care Medicine. 3rd ed. Philadelphia: W.B. Saunders; 1995:311–324.

21. Kern KB, Sanders AB, Badylak SF, Janas W, Carter AB, Tacker WA, Ewy GA. Long-term survival with open-chest cardiac massage after ineffective closed-chest compression in a canine preparation. Circulation 1987;75(2):498–503.

22. Luce JM, Ross BK, O'Quin RJ, Culver BH, Sivarajan M, Amory DW, Niskanon RA, Alferness CA, Kirk WL, Pierson LB, Butler J. Regional blood flow during cardiopulmonary resuscitation in dogs using simultaneous and nonsimultaneous compression and ventilation. Circulation 1983;67:258–265.

23. Kern KB, Sanders AB, Janas W, Nelson JR, Badylak SF, Babbs CF, Tacker WA, Ewy GA. Limitations of open-chest cardiac massage after prolonged, untreated cardiac arrest in dogs. Ann Emerg Med 1991;20(7):761–767.

24. DeBehnke DJ, Angelos MG, Leasure JE. Comparison of standard external CPR, open-chest CPR, and cardiopulmonary bypass in a canine myocardial infarct model. Ann Emerg Med 1991;20(7):754–760.

25. Arai T, Dote K, Tsukahara I, Nitta K, Nagaro T. Cerebral blood flow during conventional, new, and open-chest cardiopulmonary resuscitation in dogs. Resuscitation 1984;12(2):147–151.

26. Anthi A, Tzelpis GE, Alivizatos P, Michalis A, Palatianos GM, Geroulanos S. Unexpected cardiac arrest after cardiac surgery: incidence, predisposing causes, and outcome of open chest cardiopulmonary resuscitation. Chest 1998;113(1):15–19.

27. Bircher N, Safar P. Manual open-chest cardiopulmonary resuscitation. Ann Emerg Med 1984;13(9):770–773.

28. Barnett WM, Alifimoff JK, Paris PM, Stewart RD, Safar P. Comparison of open-chest cardiac massage techniques in dogs. Ann Emerg Med 1986;15(4):408–411.

29. Neumar RW, Otto CW, Link MS, et al. Part 8: Adult advanced cardiovascular life support: 2010 American Heart Association Guidelines for cardiopulmonary resuscitation and emergency cardiovascular care. Circulation 2010;122(Suppl 3):S729–S767.

30. Halperin HR, Tsitlik JE, Guerci AD, Mellits ED, Shi AY, Chandra N, Weisfeldt ML. Determinants of blood flow to vital organs during cardiopulmonary resuscitation in dogs. Circulation 1986;73(3):539–550.

31. Soo LH, Gray D, Young T, Hoff N, Skene A, Hampton JR. Resuscitation from out-of-hospital cardiac arrest: is survival dependent on who is available at the scene? Heart 1999;81:47–52.

32. Stiell IG, Wells GA, DeMaio VJ, Spaite DW, Field BJ, Munkley DP, Lyver MB, Luinstra LG, Ward R. Modifiable factors associated with improved cardiac arrest survival in a multicenter basic life support/defibrillation system: OPALS Study Phase I Results. Ann Emerg Med 1999;33(1):44–50.

33. Varon J, Marik PE, Fromm RE. Cardiopulmonary resuscitation. A review for clinicians. Resuscitation 1998;36(2):133–145.

34. Zoch TW, Desbiens NA, DeStefano F, Stueland DT, Layde PM. Short- and long-term survival after cardiopulmonary resuscitation. Arch Intern Med 2000;160:1969–1973.

35. Cole SG, Otto CM, Hughes D. Cardiopulmonary cerebral resuscitation in small animals—a clinical practice review (part II). JVECC 2003;13(1):13–23.

36. Hachimi-Idrissi S, Leeman J, Hubloue T, Huyghens L, Corne L. Open chest cardiopulmonary resuscitation in out-of-hospital cardiac arrest. Resuscitation 1997;35(2):151–156.

Additional resources

Complete 2010 American Heart Association Guidelines for cardiopulmonary resuscitation and emergency cardiovascular care science. Circulation 2010 Nov 2;122(18_Suppl_3): S829–S861.

18

Defibrillation

Matthew S. Mellema, Craig Cornell, and Casey J. Kohen

Fibrillation may be defined as a form of cardiac arrhythmia marked by fine irregular contractions of the cardiac muscle due to rapid repetitive excitation of myocardial fibers without coordinated contraction of the affected chambers. Fibrillation reflects unsynchronized, random, and continuously changing electrical activity in the myocardium. Fibrillation is typically further categorized by defining the chambers of the heart affected by this arrhythmia (e.g., atrial fibrillation or ventricular fibrillation). This additional level of categorization is essential as fibrillation of the atria and the ventricle have very different effects on cardiac output and often have vastly different underlying causes.

Atrial fibrillation results in the loss of coordinated atrial contraction (the "atrial kick"), which reduces ventricular filling during diastole. This reduction can be as significant as 25% of diastolic filling in some settings. Reductions in diastolic filling (all else being equal) will result in a decrease in cardiac preload and subsequently smaller stroke volumes (Starling's law of the heart). Patients often tolerate reductions in preload of this magnitude as long as there is adequate time for passive filling of the ventricles. However, in some instances of atrial fibrillation the ventricular rate may also be quite rapid (e.g., greater than 160 beats per minute[bpm] in a dog) if the atrioventricular (AV) node conduction is such that a large number of the atrial depolarizations are conducted to the ventricles. Atrial fibrillation in which the ventricular rate is also rapid can lead to more marked reductions in cardiac output due to inadequate time for passive diastolic filling of the ventricles. Atrial fibrillation also results in more stagnant flow of blood in the atria, which promotes intravascular coagulation and thromboembolic sequelae.

The prothrombotic consequences of atrial fibrillation are generally considered more crucial to address early in human patients than in small animal patients. At present, there is a notable lack of evidence in veterinary medicine regarding the risk-to-benefit ratio of prophylactic anticoagulation in patients with atrial fibrillation.

Atrial fibrillation is often the result of atrial distension secondary to structural cardiac disease (e.g., AV valve insufficiencies, primary myocardial dysfunction); however, atrial fibrillation can also occur in the absence of structural heart disease (lone atrial fibrillation), particularly in large and giant breed dogs. Dogs in atrial fibrillation may present in congestive heart failure or due to signs of decreased forward flow such as weakness, lethargy, or exercise intolerance. Atrial fibrillation in cats is most often associated with myocardial disease such as hypertrophic cardiomyopathy. Atrial fibrillation may be managed medically or through cardioversion (see the next section, Defibrillation and Cardioversion, and the later section, Cardioversion) depending on whether structural heart disease is present or absent. An additional consideration is whether the patient has acutely developed atrial fibrillation or whether the arrhythmia is long-standing. Management of chronic atrial fibrillation is more often approached via rate control rather than rhythm control due to the less-favorable outcomes achieved with cardioversion in these cases.[1,2]

Ventricular fibrillation is far more acutely life-threatening than atrial fibrillation. While atrial fibrillation leads to a loss of atrial contraction, animals can survive without effective atrial contraction if ventricular rates are not excessively high as well. However,

Advanced Monitoring and Procedures for Small Animal Emergency and Critical Care, First Edition. Edited by Jamie M. Burkitt Creedon, Harold Davis.
© 2012 John Wiley & Sons, Inc. Published 2012 by John Wiley & Sons, Inc.

ventricular fibrillation results in ineffective ventricular contraction, which is incompatible with life for all but the shortest periods of time. Ventricular fibrillation results in cardiac arrest and is a life-ending event unless immediately addressed. While atrial fibrillation is often the result of structural heart disease in dogs and cats, ventricular fibrillation has been associated with a wide range of extra-cardiac causes, including shock, hypoxemia, electrolyte and acid–base disorders, electrical shock, excessive sympathetic tone (or sympathomimetic agents), hypothermia, and drug reactions. Structural heart disease or damage can also lead to ventricular fibrillation; examples include aortic stenosis, primary myocardial disease, and secondary myocardial disease (e.g., contusion, myocarditis, myocardial infarction).[3–7] Heritable causes of ventricular fibrillation must also be considered. A congenital disease in a group of German Shepherds has been described in which related dogs are predisposed to sudden death due to ventricular arrhythmias including fibrillation.[7]

Ventricular fibrillation results in cardiac output dropping to zero or near-zero values. Patients will rapidly lose consciousness and pulses will be absent. This is important to keep in mind when simultaneously evaluating the patient and the electrocardiogram (ECG). If the ECG appears to indicate ventricular fibrillation yet the patient is conscious and has pulses, then ECG artifacts due to such processes as muscle tremors or shivering should be investigated. Conversely, the identification of ventricular fibrillation in an unconscious patient with no palpable pulses should prompt the immediate initiation of CPCR unless such resuscitation has been previously identified as inappropriate for this specific patient (see Chapter 16, Cardiopulmonary Cerebral Resuscitation). Cardiac compressions should be started while the equipment for defibrillation is prepared.

Defibrillation and cardioversion

Defibrillation is a process by which the entire myocardium is depolarized simultaneously. Fibrillation rhythms are dependent on re-entry pathways being sustained, and the goal of defibrillation is to disrupt the aberrant conduction occurring via these pathways and thus terminate the fibrillatory rhythm. In theory, defibrillation may be achieved via electrical, mechanical (e.g., precordial thump), or chemical means. However, the success of chemical and mechanical defibrillation is generally regarded as so unlikely that they are very rarely recommended (and recommended only when electrical defibrillation is unavailable).[8,9] For the remainder of this chapter the term defibrillation will refer only to the application of electric current to the myocardium and not to chemical defibrillation.

Defibrillation is achieved via the delivery of electric current to the myocardium and, as such, success is partially dependent on how much of the current applied to the patient reaches the myocardium. The current is delivered via the paddles of a defibrillator. Paddles may be applied either externally, to the thorax, or internally, to the pericardium or epicardium. Impedance to current flow is dependent on some factors that the clinician controls and some that he or she does not control. Those factors that the caregiver can influence include paddle size, quality of the contact between tissue and paddle, and how much air is in the chest (e.g., choosing to deliver the energy at end-exhalation rather than end-inhalation is recommended). Factors outside of the caregiver's control include the absolute amount of air and tissue in the chest as well as the chest width. At present, defibrillation is achieved via the delivery of *direct* current rather than *alternating* current (although the application may be bidirectional—see below). Although direct current (DC) may be utilized in portions of an energy grid for energy transmission, it is converted to alternating current (AC) before reaching the end user in most parts of the world. AC defibrillators have been developed and were once thought to be superior to DC models, but the superiority of DC defibrillation has since been established.[10] However, despite the former usage of AC defibrillators (and what television programs might lead one to believe), shocking a patient with a *spliced electrical cord plugged into a wall socket* is unlikely to accomplish anything other than harming the patient.[10]

Cardioversion involves the use of defibrillator equipment to convert rhythms *other* than ventricular fibrillation. Generally this is done in an attempt to convert an arrhythmia to a sinus rhythm. Although in the vast majority of patients arrhythmias are addressed via the administration of antiarrhythmic drugs, electrical cardioversion may be attempted in refractory cases. The mechanism is the same as was described previously for defibrillation: the disruption of conduction via aberrant re-entry pathways. Cardioversion is typically reserved for supraventricular or ventricular tachyarrhythmias that are severe enough that pulses are not palpable, the patient is symptomatic, and pharmacologic approaches have failed. Historically, cardioversion has been viewed as an intervention of last resort, but is increasingly being viewed as a viable early alternative to antiarrhythmic drug therapy for acute rhythm control.

Equipment

It is strongly recommended by the authors that defibrillators be kept in the same area as a "crash cart" (see Fig. 16.1) or other area where CPCR supplies are stored. Defibrillator equipment should be routinely tested and maintained as per the manufacturer's instructions. All personnel who might be called upon to assist in cardiopulmonary cerebral resuscitation (CPCR) or cardioversion should be instructed in the operation of the equipment and where supplies and accessories for the equipment are stored. Accessories and supplies may include coupling gel, adhesive patches, pediatric external paddles, and a variety of sizes of internal paddles. A minor surgical pack and rib retractors should also be stored in the same area for times when internal defibrillation is to be attempted.

Until the late 1980s all defibrillators used monophasic waveforms in the delivery of defibrillatory energy. Monophasic defibrillators deliver a single pulse of positive current. The current is unidirectional, traveling from one paddle to the other (hopefully across the myocardium on its way). Biphasic defibrillators initially deliver a similar (but not identical) positive current that is then followed by a negative current in the opposite direction. The application of biphasic current, when successful, allows for depolarization of the myocardium with the application of lower total energy and thus less risk of myocardial damage. Defibrillators manufactured after 1990 began using biphasic waveforms and currently all major manufacturers use this waveform. The actual waveform and the way energy is delivered vary among manufacturers. ZOLL (Chelmsford, MA) uses a proprietary rectilinear biphasic waveform, while other manufacturers (e.g., Physio-Control, Inc.) use truncated exponential biphasic waveforms.

The ZOLL rectilinear biphasic waveform was developed specifically for *external* defibrillation. It takes into account high and/or varied thoracic impedance levels due to patient or technique factors (e.g., reduced current flow caused by large lung volume, large chest size, and/or poor electrode-to-chest contact). The rectilinear waveform maintains a stable shape in response to impedance, and the constant current in the first phase reduces potentially harmful peak currents.[11]

The truncated exponential biphasic (TEB) waveform was developed for *internal* use in implantable cardioverter-defibrillators (ICDs), where impedance is generally low relative to external methods. If a TEB waveform is utilized in an external defibrillation–cardioversion attempt, then thoracic impedance may alter the waveform's shape. Research has shown that, as the biphasic waveform's shape changes, its efficacy varies.[12] In contrast, the ZOLL rectilinear waveform remains stable in shape, and current delivery dynamics are similar for patients over a wide range of impedances. This reduces the potentially adverse effect of patient impedance on successful defibrillation.[11]

Another recent development in defibrillators is the degree to which the device can make decisions regarding the diagnosis and treatment of the arrhythmia. Automated external defibrillators (AEDs), are designed to assist individuals with minimal training perform CPR, defibrillation, and cardioversion in people. Currently there is no evidence regarding the effectiveness of AEDs in veterinary medicine. Failure of the diagnostic algorithm used in an implantable defibrillator used to treat ventricular tachycardia in a Boxer dog should raise concern about the risk of using AEDs designed for human patients in veterinary medicine.[13] Recommended dosage ranges are listed in Table 18.1.

Safety issues

The application of electrical current to a patient can be done safely even in the hectic environment of CPCR if specific procedural steps are taken. Attempting defibrillation without having taken such steps runs the risk of significant adverse events occurring such as the following: accidental delivery of current to clinic personnel; burning the patient; or igniting the patient's hair coat. These hazards may be particularly relevant to the veterinary clinical setting wherein the patients often have thick, matted hair coats and may be receiving oxygen via unsealed facemasks. These factors may increase the risk of ignition compared with human patients receiving similar care. The accidental delivery of current to clinic personnel can result in painful shocks, burns, and arrhythmias in the person accidentally dosed. To avoid such a scenario, safety measures such as ensuring that the patient is on a nonconducting surface, that no one is touching the patient, that contact gel does not extend beyond the surface of the pads, and that a warning shout such as "Clear!" is given (*and given with sufficient time for personnel* **to actually get clear** *if they are not*), and that the operator visually verifies that personnel, including himself or herself, are clear. The accidental burning of the patient is most likely to occur when contact is poor and arcing of electrical current occurs, or when isopropyl alcohol is used for contact rather than gel. Contact gel intended for defibrillation pads is preferred over other types of gels and pastes. These gels not only enhance contact between the pads and patient skin, they can prevent arcing and reduce impedance. Gel should

Table 18.1 Recommended energy doses for defibrillation or synchronized cardioversion using monophasic or biphasic equipment

Body Wt (kg)	External—Defibrillation				External—**Refractory** VF		External—Synchronized Cardioversion				Internal—Defibrillation	
	Monophasic		Biphasic		Monophasic	Biphasic	Monophasic		Biphasic		Monophasic *or* Biphasic	
	Lower Dose	Higher Dose	Lower Dose	Higher Dose	Maximum Dose	Maximum Dose	Lower Dose	Higher Dose	Lower Dose	Higher Dose	Lower Dose	Higher Dose
2.5	5	12.5	5	12.5	25	25	1.25	10	1.25	10	0.5	1.25
5	10	25	10	25	50	50	2.5	20	2.5	20	1	2.5
10	20	50	20	50	100	100	5	40	5	40	2	5
15	30	75	30	75	150	150	7.5	60	7.5	60	3	7.5
20	40	100	40	100	200	200	10	80	10	80	4	10
30	60	150	60	150	300	200	15	120	15	120	6	15
40	80	200	80	200	300	200	20	160	20	160	8	20
50	100	250	100	200	300	200	25	200	25	200	10	25
60	120	300	120	200	300	200	30	240	30	200	12	30

VF, ventricular fibrillation.

be applied to the pad surface liberally while ensuring that an excessive amount has not been applied such that it extends beyond the pad itself. The application of excessive coupling gel can lead to tracts of gel extending toward (or reaching) the hands of the person holding the paddles. Coupling gel is not applied to the pads of internal defibrillator paddles. Instead, they are wrapped in one or two layers of saline-soaked gauze sponges (4 × 4-inch) prior to application to the pericardium or epicardium (depending on whether the pericardium has been opened).

While small- to medium-sized dogs may be placed in dorsal recumbency for defibrillation, this position may prove unsafe in some larger patients. Stabilizing a large dog in dorsal recumbency using only the defibrillator pads may place the person holding the pads in such a position that they are at risk of touching the patient or the table during the delivery of current. Further, other personnel may reflexively reach out to try to stabilize a patient that is tipping over while the energy is being applied. For such large patients it is advised that a posterior plate or adhesive pads (see Fig. 18.1) be used to enhance patient and personnel safety. Lastly, patients should always be placed on a nonconducting surface rather than directly on a metal examination table prior to defibrillation.

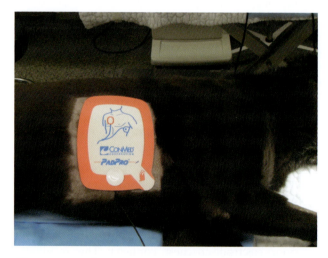

Figure 18.1 Adhesive ECG/external-pacing/defibrillator pads in place on the thorax of an adult dog. Shaving the area prior to placement will reduce thoracic impedance and decrease energy requirements relative to placement on an unshaved site.

Indications for use

The predominant indication for defibrillation is for the treatment of ventricular fibrillation or ventricular flutter. In one retrospective study of in-hospital cardiac arrest in dogs and cats, defibrillation was indicated in 28% of dogs and 16% of cats.[14] Ventricular flutter is an unstable rapid ventricular tachyarrhythmia that often converts to ventricular fibrillation in a short time. It should be noted that many patients may develop ventricular fibrillation during a resuscitation attempt even when it is not initially present. Induced ventricular fibrillation may spontaneously resolve in young, healthy animals in a research laboratory setting, but in clinical patients, time should **never** be wasted waiting to see if ventricular fibrillation is going to resolve on its own.[15] Immediate action is indicated and required. Survival rates decrease by 7%–10% for each minute the ventricles fibrillate and thus survival approaches zero percent after 10–12 minutes of ventricular fibrillation.[16–20]

The indication for defibrillation is less clear for the other predominant arrest rhythms seen in small animal practice: asystole and pulseless electrical activity. Although there is no indication to apply defibrillatory currents to an asystolic myocardium, it likely does little harm in this setting and occasionally it may turn out that what appeared to be asystole was, in fact, *fine ventricular fibrillation*. Fine ventricular fibrillation is a form wherein the undulations of the baseline are minimal and thus it may appear similar to asystole at times.[21]

Procedure and technique

Defibrillation is nearly always done concurrently with CPCR and needs to be properly integrated into the overall resuscitation attempt. If closed-chest CPCR is being performed, then typically external defibrillation will be the means initially employed. If ventricular fibrillation cannot be converted with external defibrillation, then internal defibrillation may be more successful and could be attempted. If internal cardiac massage is being attempted, then internal defibrillation is likely to be the first mode attempted although external defibrillation can still be performed even if the chest is open.[22–24]

Defibrillation should be performed as soon as possible once ventricular fibrillation is identified. Chest compressions and the "A-B-Cs" (i.e., airway, breathing, circulation) of CPCR should be performed while the machine is being readied and charged. Defibrillation can be achieved in *most* patients without shaving; however, in the authors' experience, dogs with thick matted hair coats often cannot be defibrillated without prior shaving. There is evidence from human patients that even the chest hair of male humans is sufficient to significantly increase thoracic impedance and impair current delivery during defibrillation attempts.[25] Standard adult paddles are used for medium- and large-sized dogs (>13.5 kg); pediatric paddles (see Fig. 18.2) can be used for cats and small dogs. It is better to have paddles too large than too

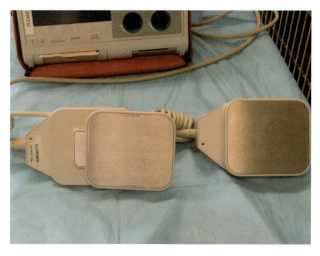

Figure 18.2 Adult and pediatric paddles from a biphasic defibrillator. Some models may have separate pediatric paddles that must be plugged into the base. In the model shown, the pediatric paddles are located beneath the larger paddles (which have been partially removed on the paddle shown to the left).

small, generally. An experimental study using a dog model of ventricular fibrillation has demonstrated that defibrillation is somewhat more effective when larger paddles (12.8-cm diameter) are used rather than smaller paddles (8-cm diameter) in dogs ranging from ~30 to 70 pounds body weight (BW).[26] After gel has been applied to the pad surface of the paddles they should be held as firmly as possible against each side of the chest wall directly over the area of the heart. If possible, compressing the thorax between the paddles and discharging the energy while the lungs are deflated is advised. The optimal force for the application of the paddles to the thorax has been shown to range from 8 to 12 kg force; however, it has been shown that as few as 14% of humans performing defibrillation are able to generate this much force, nor is force application readily measurable in the clinical setting.[27] As so few human operators are able to generate the optimal force required, the authors advise applying the paddles with as much force as can be sustained for the duration of the defibrillation attempt. Modern defibrillators are often designed to use multipurpose adhesive electrodes. These electrodes can be used for diagnosis, defibrillation, and pacing. It is unlikely that these electrodes will function properly unless the patient's skin is clean, dry, and free from hair.

Defibrillating the patient with a permanent pacemaker in place bears special mention. If the patient has a pacemaker, the electrodes for the defibrillator **should not** be placed over or close to the pacing generator to minimize the risk of damage during defibrillation.[28]

Protocol 18.1 External defibrillation

Items Required
- Defibrillator
- Coupling gel
- Clippers, as needed for excessive fur

Procedure
1. Analyze the electrocardiogram (ECG) and confirm ventricular fibrillation is present.
2. Collect necessary supplies.
3. Ensure that rubbing alcohol or other flammable solvents are not present on the thorax (dilute with water and dry rapidly if needed).
4. Calculate energy dosage and set defibrillator to this dosage.
5. Apply coupling gel to the pad surface of the paddles.
6. Charge paddles.
7. Interrupt chest compressions and apply paddles to each side of the chest with as much pressure as can be sustained.
8. Temporarily suspend positive-pressure ventilation if it is being provided.
9. Announce to those present that energy is about to be delivered ("Clear!") and visually verify that all personnel (including oneself) are clear.
10. Deliver the energy by discharging the paddles.
11. Evaluate ECG rapidly (<1 sec) while compressor is getting ready to begin again.
12. Restart CPCR, including compressions and positive-pressure ventilation.
13. In approximately 2 minutes, re-evaluate ECG again and restart at step 1 if ventricular fibrillation is still present.

Note: In patients with thick, matted hair coats it may be necessary to rapidly clip the coat over the thorax in order to successfully and safely deliver the energy dose.

Protocol 18.2 Internal defibrillation

Items Required
- Defibrillator with internal paddles
- Saline-soaked sterile gauze
- Patient undergoing open-chest CPCR

Procedure
1. Analyze the ECG and confirm ventricular fibrillation is present.
2. Direct access to the thoracic cavity may be achieved by one of several means, depending on the setting:
   a. Lateral thoracotomy: If emergency access to the thoracic cavity is needed solely for the purpose of open chest cardiopulmonary cerebral resuscitation (CPCR), then a lateral thoracotomy is the preferred approach.
   b. Median sternotomy: This approach is generally reserved for intraoperative CPCR when a median sternotomy has already been performed prior to the arrest.
   c. Transdiaphragmatic approach: If open-chest CPCR is to be attempted when the abdomen is already open (e.g., an arrest during a laparotomy), then the thorax may be entered via an incision in the diaphragm.
3. Collect necessary supplies.
4. Calculate energy dosage and set defibrillator to this dosage (see Table 18.1).
5. Plug internal paddles into defibrillator base per manufacturer's instructions.
6. Cover each paddle with one to two layers of 4 × 4-inch gauze.
7. Moisten each gauze wrapping with sterile 0.9% saline.
8. Charge paddles.
9. Interrupt cardiac massage and apply paddles to the heart with one paddle over the region of the right atrium and one over the area of the left ventricle. Apply gentle, but firm, pressure.
10. Positive pressure ventilation may be briefly suspended if necessary to properly place paddles.
11. Announce to those present that energy is about to be delivered ("Clear!") and visually verify that all personnel (including oneself) are clear.
12. Deliver the energy by discharging the paddles.
13. Evaluate ECG rapidly (<1 sec) while the person performing cardiac massage is getting ready to begin again.
14. Restart CPCR, including cardiac massage and positive-pressure ventilation.
15. In approximately 2 minutes, re-evaluate ECG again and restart at step 1 if ventricular fibrillation is still present. Steps 2 and 4–6 are generally only applicable to the first attempt.

The recommended sequence of events in external and internal defibrillation is described in Protocols 18.1 and 18.2, respectively. For internal defibrillation, the protocol is similar in most regards to that for external defibrillation. However, as noted previously, saline-soaked gauze is substituted for gel or paste. Also, the internal paddles (see Fig 18.3) are concave and intended to cradle the heart between them. Firm but not excessive contact should be maintained between the internal paddles and the cardiac structures.

As described previously and in Table 18.1, energy dosage is based on body weight in kilograms and differs for monophasic versus biphasic as well as for internal versus external (see Energy Dose Selection below, for a more detailed discussion of dose determination). It is

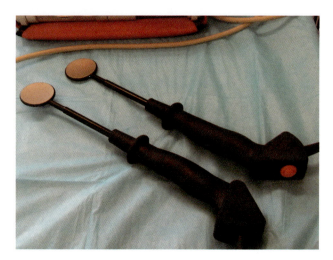

Figure 18.3 Internal paddles are concave with elongated handles to remove the operator's hands from where the current will be discharged. One paddle should be placed over the right atrium and one over the left ventricle.

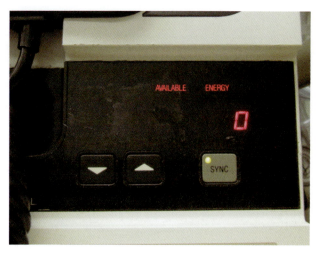

Figure 18.4 A close-up view of a monophasic defibrillator. In this view the synchronization button is shown lit. This synchronized mode is employed when cardioversion is attempted.

essential to recall that dosages for internal defibrillation are approximately one-tenth those needed for external defibrillation. Regardless of the initial energy dosage used, it is generally advised that on subsequent attempts the energy delivered be increased by 50%–100% after an unsuccessful defibrillation attempt. It should also be noted that the practice of delivering multiple shocks in rapid succession is no longer recommended by the American Heart Association.[28]

Cardioversion

Cardioversion involves the use of defibrillator equipment to convert rhythms other than ventricular fibrillation. The major differences between cardioversion and defibrillation involve the setting (e.g., performed outside of the emergency room or intensive care unit), circumstances (e.g., nonventricular fibrillatory rhythm), and the timing (e.g., scheduled procedure) of the process. Cardioversion for lone atrial fibrillation is generally a scheduled procedure done under general anesthesia or at least with significant pre-emptive analgesic administration. This type of cardioversion is not typically regarded as an emergency procedure and will not be covered further herein.

However, cardioversion may be performed in the acute setting to address supraventricular (SVT) or ventricular (VT) tachyarrhythmias that are life threatening, severe, and/or refractory to pharmacological treatment. As these patients may not necessarily be unconscious, it is advised that they receive analgesics or be anesthetized

prior to attempting cardioversion (which is painful). A major difference between cardioversion in these circumstances as compared to defibrillation as discussed above is the timing of the energy delivery. Ventricular fibrillation is a chaotic rhythm and timing the delivery to a specific phase of the cardiac cycle is not applicable or possible. However, in the treatment of rapid VT or SVT, the issue of timing becomes relevant. The application of electrical current to the myocardium during the repolarization process (during the T wave on an ECG) can lead to ventricular fibrillation. The period around the peak of the T-wave on an ECG is a time at which the myocardium is particularly prone to fibrillating. As such many modern defibrillators come with a synchronization option that can be turned on to help avoid delivering the energy during this most vulnerable period. The synchronization setting will prompt the equipment to deliver the energy during the R or S wave of the QRS complex and avoid the more vulnerable period associated with the T wave. If cardioversion of a refractory VT or SVT is to be attempted using a defibrillator, then it is strongly advised that one use equipment in which the synchronization feature is available *and* switched on (see Fig 18.4). As a rule, defibrillators should always be used in synchronized mode unless ventricular fibrillation is the arrhythmia being treated. However, it must be noted that achieving synchronization is not always possible even with the best equipment. In this case, the American Heart Association guidelines recommend the administration of a high-energy unsynchronized shock.[28] When electrical cardioversion is being attempted, the initial energy setting may be selected at approximately half of

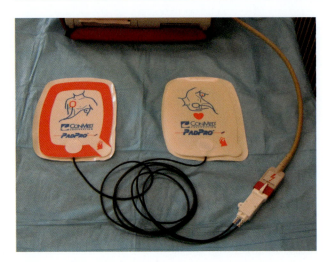

Figure 18.5 Adhesive ECG/external-pacing/defibrillator pads can be placed in advance if a patient is at increased risk of developing ventricular fibrillation or requires external cardiac pacing. These same pad types are shown in place on a patient in Figure 18.1.

the calculated dosage for defibrillation in the same sized patient. The protocol for delivering the energy is similar to the protocol described above for defibrillation except that time should be taken to ensure that the synchronization mode is working properly. Many modern defibrillators will give a visual indication of what complexes are being recognized as QRS complexes. Additionally, as cardioversion is often attempted in a less acute setting than defibrillation it may be possible to take measures such as clipping the hair coat off of the thoracic cage and applying adhesive pads rather than using handheld paddles (as an additional safety measure to reduce risk of shocking personnel). These adhesive pads (see Figure 18.5) can also be left on during the initial monitoring period in case fibrillation occurs or cardioversion is again required.

Energy dose selection

Selecting the proper energy dose (see also Table 18.1) is important to successfully terminate the arrhythmia while avoiding injury to the patient. One of the most important determinants of the proper dose is body size. Smaller animals can be defibrillated with smaller amounts of energy than larger animals. There is a strong correlation between body size and the energy required for defibrillation, but the relationship appears to be nonlinear. Geddes found that external defibrillation using a monophasic damped sine wave required $0.73 \times BW^{1.52}$ joules.[29,30] The nonlinear relationship between size and dose means that smaller animals would be expected to

be defibrillated using fewer joules per kilogram than larger animals. The amplitude, duration, and polarity of electrical current delivered to the heart also affect the dose required. Defibrillators using biphasic waveforms require less energy to defibrillate than monophasic waveforms. Lee found that dogs required 30% less energy for defibrillation using a biphasic waveform than a monophasic waveform.[31] The probability of successful defibrillation increases as the energy dose increases, but the risk of injury also increases. Babbs found that the median effective dose for monophasic defibrillation in dogs weighing an average of 14 kg was 1.5 J/kg. The median dose required to cause injury was 30 J/kg and the median lethal dose was 470 J/kg.[32] Although the difference between the median effective dose and the median dose causing injury seems very large there is an overlap between the dose some patients may require for defibrillation and a dose that will injure some patients. Examination of the dose–response curves published by Babbs shows that the overlap occurs at about 10 J/kg in dogs.[32] Although patients can be defibrillated at a lower energy using biphasic waveforms, using a biphasic defibrillator at energy levels recommended for monophasic defibrillators does not appear to increase the risk of injury to the patient.[33]

The evidence from animal studies showing that smaller patients require less energy per kilogram than larger patients and that doses greater than 10 J/kg are likely to cause injury seem to be reflected in the 2010 American Heart Association (AHA) guidelines.[33] For monophasic defibrillation the recommended dose for adults is about 5 J/kg (360 J for a 70-kg adult) while the dose for smaller children was 2–4 J/kg. For biphasic defibrillation in adults the AHA recommends using the manufacturer's dose. If the manufacturer's dose is unknown, 200 J is recommended. The 2010 AHA guidelines for pediatric defibrillation state that the optimal first-attempt energy dose for biphasic defibrillation is unknown. The current recommendation is to use a dose of 2–4 J/kg for monophasic or biphasic pediatric defibrillation. For refractory ventricular fibrillation subsequent doses should be at least 4 J/kg. Higher doses for refractory ventricular fibrillation may be considered but the maximum dose should not exceed 10 J/kg or the adult maximum dose.

Cardioversion of supraventricular tachycardia is often successful at low doses of 0.5–1 J/kg, although higher doses may be required. Cardioversion of atrial fibrillation and ventricular tachycardia generally requires higher energy levels, starting at about 50% of the maximum defibrillation dose and sometimes increasing in a stepwise manner up to the maximum defibrillation dose.

The dose required for defibrillation when the electrodes are placed directly on the heart (internal defibrillation) is much lower than the dose required for transthoracic (external) defibrillation. Geddes[30] found that $(84 \times 10^{-6}) \times$ (heart weight in grams)$^{1.95}$=(average joules required for defibrillation). Van Fleet found that a wide safety margin exists between the dose required for defibrillation compared with the dose required to produce injury or death.[34] Doses for internal defibrillation in adult humans are well established in the range 5–20 J. There is little published information regarding internal defibrillation in human pediatric patients. The doses traditionally used in veterinary medicine are 10% of the dose used for external defibrillation (0.2–0.5 J/kg).[35]

Drug and defibrillator interactions

Although the amount of time a patient remains in fibrillation is the most important determinant of successful defibrillation, certain medications can contribute to the ease or difficulty of converting a fibrillatory rhythm. The defibrillation threshold determines the level of energy needed to depolarize enough myocytes to terminate the fibrillation. This threshold can be altered by certain medications commonly used in emergency patients.[36] An increase in this threshold requires increased energy settings for successful defibrillation. Medications that have been shown to increase defibrillation threshold include amiodarone, lidocaine, and mexiletine (see Table 18.2). Unfortunately, these medications are used commonly in the emergency setting to treat ventricular tachyarrhythmias. Despite concurrent use of these medications, defibrillation should still be attempted as soon as possible. Procainamide has been shown to have little effect on defibrillation threshold. Medications that

decrease the defibrillation threshold include sotalol and beta-blockers. In studies that investigated the effects of medications on defibrillation threshold, the effects were more pronounced with monophasic waveform defibrillators than the more modern biphasic defibrillators. This suggests that the contributions of concurrent medications on successful defibrillation may be less clinically important if using a biphasic defibrillator.

Patient care in the postcardioversion or postdefibrillation period

The care for post-cardioversion patients will be dependent on the severity of illness present prior to cardioversion. If the patient was in congestive heart failure prior to cardioversion, then continued care for this syndrome will likely be required. If the patient was predominantly exhibiting signs of forward failure, these may abate postcardioversion; however, significant morbidity secondary to reperfusion injury may necessitate ongoing care for some time. Continued monitoring of perfusion parameters and cardiac rhythm are indicated until the patient is deemed stable. Many patients undergoing emergency *defibrillation* will require extensive monitoring and care following a return to spontaneous circulation. Standard postresuscitation protocols should be followed and are covered elsewhere in this text. In addition, care may be required for surface wounds as a result of the defibrillator use.

Table 18.2 Common cardiac drug effects on defibrillation threshold

Increase (more energy required for defibrillation)
- Amiodarone
- Lidocaine
- Mexilitine

Little Effect (no major alteration in energy required)
- Procainamide

Decrease (less energy required for defibrillation)
- Sotalol
- Beta-adrenergic blockers

References

1. Klein, A.L., R.D. Murray, and R.A. Grimm. Role of transesophageal echocardiography-guided cardioversion of patients with atrial fibrillation. J Am Coll Cardiol 2001;**37**(3):691–704.
2. Arya, A., et al. First time and repeat cardioversion of atrial tachyarrhythmias—a comparison of outcomes. Int J Clin Pract 2010;**64**(8):1062–1068.
3. Kienle, R.D., W.P. Thomas, and P.D. Pion. The natural clinical history of canine congenital subaortic stenosis. J Vet Intern Med 1994;**8**(6):423–431.
4. Basso, C., et al. Arrhythmogenic right ventricular cardiomyopathy causing sudden cardiac death in boxer dogs: a new animal model of human disease. Circulation 2004;**109**(9):1180–1185.
5. Calvert, C.A., et al. Clinical and pathologic findings in Doberman pinschers with occult cardiomyopathy that died suddenly or developed congestive heart failure: 54 cases (1984–1991). J Am Vet Med Assoc 1997;**210**(4):505–511.
6. Hamlin, R.L. Animal models of ventricular arrhythmias. Pharmacol Ther 2007;**113**(2):276–295.
7. Gelzer, A.R., N.S. Moise, and M.L. Koller. Defibrillation of German shepherds with inherited ventricular arrhythmias and sudden death. J Vet Cardiol 2005;**7**(2):97–107.
8. Madias, C., et al. Precordial thump for cardiac arrest is effective for asystole but not for ventricular fibrillation. Heart Rhythm 2009;**6**(10):1495–1500.

9. Stoner, J., et al. Amiodarone and bretylium in the treatment of hypothermic ventricular fibrillation in a canine model. Acad Emerg Med 2003;**10**(3):187–191.

10. Lown, B. Electrical reversion of cardiac arrhythmias. Br Heart J 1967;**29**(4):469–489.

11. Amato-Vealey, E. and P.A. Colonies. Demystifying biphasic defibrillation. Nursing 2005;**35**(8 Suppl E D):6–11; quiz 12.

12. Kerber, R.E., et al. Energy, current, and success in defibrillation and cardioversion: clinical studies using an automated impedance-based method of energy adjustment. Circulation 1988;**77**(5):1038–1046.

13. Nelson, O.L., et al. The use of an implantable cardioverter defibrillator in a Boxer Dog to control clinical signs of arrhythmogenic right ventricular cardiomyopathy. J Vet Intern Med 2006;**20**(5):1232–1237.

14. Kass, P.H. and S.C. Haskins. Survival following cardiopulmonary resuscitation in dogs and cats. J Vet Emerg Crit Care 1992;**2**(2):57–65.

15. Jalife, J. Ventricular fibrillation: mechanisms of initiation and maintenance. Annu Rev Physiol 2000;**62**:25–50.

16. Herlitz, J., et al. Rhythm changes during resuscitation from ventricular fibrillation in relation to delay until defibrillation, number of shocks delivered and survival. Resuscitation 1997;**34**(1):17–22.

17. Ladwig, K.H., et al. Effects of early defibrillation by ambulance personnel on short- and long-term outcome of cardiac arrest survival: the Munich experiment. Chest 1997;**112**(6):1584–1591.

18. Mosesso, V.N., Jr., et al. Use of automated external defibrillators by police officers for treatment of out-of-hospital cardiac arrest. Ann Emerg Med 1998;**32**(2):200–207.

19. Nichol, G., et al. A cumulative meta-analysis of the effectiveness of defibrillator-capable emergency medical services for victims of out-of-hospital cardiac arrest. Ann Emerg Med 1999;**34**(4 Pt 1):517–525.

20. Yakaitis, R.W., et al. Influence of time and therapy on ventricular defibrillation in dogs. Crit Care Med 1980;**8**(3):157–163.

21. Lightfoot, C.B., et al. Physician interpretation and quantitative measures of electrocardiographic ventricular fibrillation waveform. Prehosp Emerg Care 2001;**5**(2):147–154.

22. Knaggs, A.L., et al. Automated external defibrillation in cardiac surgery. Resuscitation 2002;**55**(3):341–345.

23. Braimbridge, M.V., et al. External DC defibrillation during open heart surgery. Thorax 1971;**26**(4):455–456.

24. Rastelli, G.C., et al. Experimental study and clinical appraisal of external defibrillation with the thorax open. J Thorac Cardiovasc Surg 1968;**55**(1):116–122.

25. Sado, D.M., et al. Comparison of the effects of removal of chest hair with not doing so before external defibrillation on transthoracic impedance. Am J Cardiol 2004;**93**(1):98–100.

26. Thomas, E.D., et al. Effectiveness of direct current defibrillation: role of paddle electrode size. Am Heart J 1977;**93**(4):463–467.

27. Deakin, C.D., et al. Determining the optimal paddle force for external defibrillation. Am J Cardiol 2002;**90**(7):812–813.

28. Link, M.S., et al. Part 6: electrical therapies: automated external defibrillators, defibrillation, cardioversion, and pacing: 2010 American Heart Association Guidelines for Cardiopulmonary Resuscitation and Emergency Cardiovascular Care. Circulation 2010;**122**(18 Suppl 3):S706–S719.

29. Geddes, L.A., et al. Electrical dose for ventricular defibrillation of large and small animals using precordial electrodes. J Clin Invest 1974;**53**(1):310–319.

30. Geddes, L.A., et al. The electrical dose for ventricular defibrillation with electrodes applied directly to the heart. J Thorac Cardiovasc Surg 1974;**68**(4):593–602.

31. Lee, S.G., H.S. Moon, and C. Hyun. The efficacy and safety of external biphasic defibrillation in toy breed dogs. J Vet Emerg Crit Care 2008;**18**(4):362–369.

32. Babbs, C.F., et al. Therapeutic indices for transchest defibrillator shocks: effective, damaging, and lethal electrical doses. Am Heart J 1980;**99**(6):734–738.

33. Link, M.S., et al. Part 6: Electrical therapies: automated external defibrillators, defibrillation, cardioversion, and pacing; 2010 American Heart Association Guidelines for cardiopulmonary resuscitation and emergency cardiovascular care. Circulation 2010;**122**(18 Suppl 3):S706–S719.

34. Van Vleet, J.F., et al. Effect of shock strength on survival and acute cardiac damage induced by open-thorax defibrillation of dogs. Am J Vet Res 1978;**39**(6):981–987.

35. Plunkett, S.J. and M. McMichael. Cardiopulmonary resuscitation in small animal medicine: an update. J Vet Intern Med 2008;**22**(1):9–25.

36. Dopp, A.L., J.M. Miller, and J.E. Tisdale. Effect of drugs on defibrillation capacity. Drugs 2008;**68**(5):607–630.

Additional resources

Complete 2010 American Heart Association Guidelines for cardiopulmonary resuscitation and emergency cardiovascular care science. Circulation **2010** Nov 2;**122**(18_suppl_3): S829–S861.

19

Temporary cardiac pacing

Craig Cornell

Cardiac pacemakers maintain cardiac function in patients whose hearts have slowed or stopped beating. Artificial pacemakers were developed by people who observed the tragic and premature deaths of patients whose hearts were capable of contraction, but lacked the stimulus to initiate a heartbeat. Techniques for artificially stimulating a heartbeat have been known for hundreds of years. Luigi Galvani used electricity to stimulate muscular contraction in the eighteenth century[1] and William Harvey used his finger to pace the heart of a dove in the seventeenth century.[2] It was not until the twentieth century that devices were developed that could stimulate or "pace" the heart in a reliable manner, and it is only in the last 40 or 50 years that artificial pacemakers have been practical. Transcutaneous cardiac pacing was one of the first types of temporary pacing to be used clinically. Although it was first used in the 1950s,[3] it only became truly practical in the early 1980s after the design was improved to reduce the associated discomfort associated with its use to a more tolerable level.[4] Transvenous, epicardial, percutaneous transmyocardial, and transesophageal pacing techniques were subsequently developed. Because dogs were used as research subjects, development of techniques for pacing the canine heart usually preceded the techniques' introduction in people. The first clinical use of an implantable pacemaker in a dog occured relatively early in the history of artificial pacing, in 1967. With the aid of the pacemaker that dog lived to the age of 16.[5]

Permanent and temporary pacing techniques are used in different ways. Permanent implantable pacemakers are used for long-term therapy of bradyarrhythmias. Temporary pacemakers are used for emergency treatment of bradyarrhythmias and as a prophylactic measure in patients that are at risk of developing a serious bradyarrhythmia. Temporary pacing can also maintain a normal heart rhythm until the patient recovers from a reversable cause of a bradyarrhythmia or until a permanent pacemaker is implanted. In general, temporary pacing techniques are used only for a few hours to a few days.

An artificial electrical pacing system consists of two major components: a generator and an electrode. The generator controls the frequency and strength of the electrical stimulus, and in some cases senses the intrinsic electrical activity of the patient's heart. In dual-chamber pacing, in which separate electrical signals are sent to the atria and the ventricles, the generator also controls the delay between the atrial and ventricular stimuli. The electrode delivers the electrical stimulus to the heart.

Indications for temporary pacing

Temporary pacing is the therapy of choice for emergency treatment of hemodynamically unstable patients with any of the dysrhythmias listed in Table 19.1. Temporary pacing is useful as a prophylactic measure for support of asymptomatic bradyarrhythmic patients that require anesthesia. Anesthesia has been observed, in both human and veterinary medicine, to exacerbate profoundly the severity of bradyarrythmias in some individuals, and patients are sometimes referred for specialist care after an anesthesia-exacerbated bradyarrhythmia prevented completion of a surgical procedure. Since implantation of a permanent pacemaker usually requires general anesthesia, temporary pacing is useful during implantation to maintain a normal heart rate until the permanent pacemaker is functional.

Advanced Monitoring and Procedures for Small Animal Emergency and Critical Care, First Edition. Edited by Jamie M. Burkitt Creedon, Harold Davis.
© 2012 John Wiley & Sons, Inc. Published 2012 by John Wiley & Sons, Inc.

Table 19.1 Dysrhythmias for which temporary pacing is the therapy of choice for emergency treatment of hemodynamically unstable patients

Third-degree AV block
Second-degree AV block
Persistent atrial standstill
Sick sinus syndrome
Sinus arrest
Sinus bradycardia that does not respond to drug therapy
Asystole

Some patients with bradyarrhythmias also have concomitant tachyarrhythmias. In this situation the clinician is faced with a dilemma, as many antiarrhythmic drugs used to treat tachyarrhythmias can increase the severity of the bradyarrhythmia. Prophylactic temporary pacing can prevent life-threatening bradycardia during antiarrhythmic therapy on a short-term basis or during implantation of a permanent pacemaker when long-term antiarrhythmic therapy will be required to control a tachyarrhythmia.

Patients with right or left bundle branch block can develop complete bundle branch block (and subsequent life-threatening bradyarrhythmia) during a procedure that has the potential to damage the functional bundle branch. A good example of this would be a patient with left bundle branch block who also requires catheterization of the right ventricle or pulmonary artery for balloon valvuloplasty to treat pulmonic stenosis. The right bundle branch is smaller and more prone to injury than the left, and patients requiring right heart catheterization frequently develop right bundle branch block. Temporary pacing may also be indicated in patients about to undergo a procedure that risks damage to the sinus node, atrioventricular (AV) node, or bundle of His.

A note on terminology

Anyone reviewing the literature on temporary pacing will discover that the terms used to describe different types of pacing are varied and often confusing. Transthoracic pacing, for example, has been used to describe three different techniques: electrodes placed on the skin of the chest, electrodes passed through the chest wall and sutured to the epicardium, and electrodes inserted through the chest wall and ventricular wall and contacting the endocardium. Temporary transvenous pacing is sometimes referred to as temporary endocardial pacing. Transcutaneous pacing is sometimes known as external pacing, noninvasive pacing, or transthoracic pacing. Temporary epicardial pacing has also been called trans-

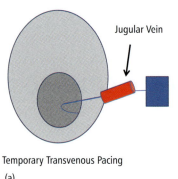

Temporary Transvenous Pacing

(a)

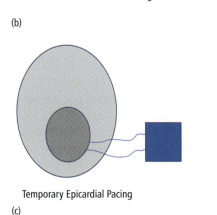

Transcutaneous Pacing

(b)

Temporary Epicardial Pacing

(c)

Figure 19.1 Schematics depicting different methods of temporary cardiac pacing: (a) temporary transvenous pacing; (b) transcutaneous pacing; (c) temporary epicardial pacing.

thoracic pacing. Thump pacing, percussion pacing, fist pacing, and manual external pacing have all been used by different authors to describe pacing accomplished by striking the chest wall or heart. Transesophageal pacing is often called transesophageal atrial pacing (TAP). The technique of using a needle to insert a pacing lead into the ventricular chamber has been called transthoracic pacing, transmyocardial pacing, and percutaneous transthoracic pacing.

In this review, temporary pacing techniques are defined as follows: Placing a pacing electrode into the right ventricle by way of a vein is **temporary transvenous pacing** (see Fig. 19.1a). Pacing using adhesive electrodes placed on the skin on the chest is **transcutaneous pacing** (see Fig. 19.1b). **Transesophageal pacing** uses an electrode inserted in the esophagus. Striking the precordium with the fist is **thump pacing**. A pacing electrode inserted percutaneously into the right or left ventricle is **transthoracic pacing. Temporary epicardial pacing** uses detachable electrodes attached to the epicardium and passed through the chest wall during a thoracotomy (see Fig. 19.1c).

Types of temporary pacing

The ideal temporary pacing system would possess the following characteristics: it would be able to be applied quickly, it would be minimally invasive, it would have a low risk of causing serious injury to the patient, and it would not cause discomfort while it is being used. While several different types of temporary pacing are available to the clinician, no single technique meets all of these requirements (see Table 19.2). Transvenous and transcutaneous pacing are the most commonly used techniques. Other pacing techniques are used much less frequently, often in specific situations such as after thoracotomy has been performed for cardiac surgery.

Temporary transvenous pacing

Temporary transvenous pacing is one of the most reliable and frequently used types of temporary pacing. The technique is relatively safe and reliable and it is practically the only technique that allows both electrode insertion and pacing in a conscious patient. It is also one of a few techniques that can be used to pace patients for a day or more. With appropriate catheters and pacing generators, transvenous AV sequential pacing or ventricular (such as VDD) pacing can be accomplished.

Insertion of a transvenous temporary pacing lead can be performed without general anesthesia. The patient should be prepared for the procedure by administering appropriate sedative drugs if indicated. Continuous monitoring of ECG, pulse, and blood pressure is useful to detect hypotension or severe bradycardia.

Several factors should be considered when selecting the site for inserting the pacing lead. Although vascular anomalies are uncommon (in the author's experience about 1% or 2% of patients), they can complicate insertion of the pacing lead.[6] One of the most frequently encountered anomalies is a persistent left cranial vena cava. This anomaly makes it very difficult to insert the pacing lead into the ventricle via the left jugular vein. If the temporary pacemaker is to be used to support the patient during permanent pacemaker implantation, it may be useful to save the right jugular vein for the permanent pacing lead. The right jugular vein is usually easier to use if the person inserting the permanent lead is right handed, and the right jugular vein is less likely to be associated with a vascular anomaly such as persistent left cranial vena cava. The right or left lateral saphenous veins often can be used for insertion of a temporary pacing lead. The saphenous vein may be too small to

Table 19.2 Characteristics of different modes of temporary cardiac pacing

	Transvenous	Transcutaneous	Transesophageal	Thump	Transthoracic	Epicardial
Anesthesia required for lead placement	Usually only local anesthesia needed	No	Yes	No leads needed	Technique should not be used if conscious	Yes
Anesthesia required when pacing	No	Yes	Yes	Usually yes	No	No
Atrial pacing	Yes	No	Yes	No	No	Yes
Ventricular pacing	Yes	Yes	Usually no	Yes	Yes	Yes
Dual chamber pacing	Yes, with multiple or special electrodes	No	No	No	No	Yes, with multiple electrodes
Easy to start in an emergency	No	Yes, although the need to clip hair delays pacing	Yes	Yes	Yes	No

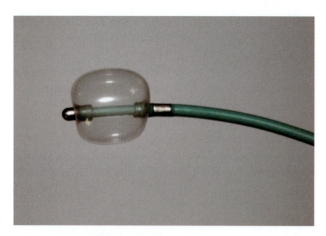

Figure 19.2 Some transvenous pacing catheters have a balloon at the tip. When inflated, blood flow helps direct the catheter appropriately by pulling the balloon across the tricuspid valve into the right ventricular apex.

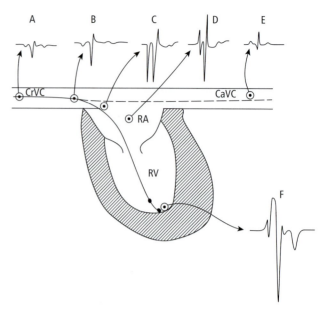

Figure 19.3 An ECG can be used to determine the location of the pacing lead by observing the polarity and amplitude of the P waves and QRS complexes. Note that as the pacing lead reaches the right ventricular apex the P wave appears large and positive, and ventricular depolarization appears as a large negative complex.

accommodate an introducer for a 4-Fr temporary pacing lead in dogs weighing less than 10 or 15 kg. In some very large dogs a 110-cm pacing lead may be unable to reach the right ventricle from a saphenous vein. Bulmer[7] described a technique for inserting an introducer in the femoral vein. Once the insertion site has been selected the fur should be clipped and the skin aseptically prepared. The patient should be protected from electrical hazards to avoid microshock.

A percutaneous introducer sheath with a hemostasis valve or a special over-the-needle catheter with or without a hemostatsis valve is used for venous access. Obviously, it is important to be sure that the catheter or introducer can accommodate the pacing lead. The introducer sheath is inserted using the Seldinger technique and secured. The pacing lead is then inserted through the introducer.

Prior to inserting the pacing lead, one should inspect and test the equipment. For instance, some transvenous pacing catheters have a balloon at the tip (see Fig. 19.2). When inflated, blood flow helps direct the catheter appropriately by pulling the balloon across the tricuspid valve into the right ventricular apex. Balloon integrity should be tested prior to catheter insertion. The easiest, most reliable way to insert a transvenous pacing lead is by using fluoroscopy to direct the lead. It is possible to use other methods to determine the location of the pacing lead. An ECG recorded from the catheter tip can be used to determine the loction of the pacing lead by observing the polarity and amplitude of the P waves and QRS complexes (see Fig. 19.3). Bing[8] described the technique in man, and Moïse described the technique in

dogs.[9] Baird[10] described a technique in which the pacing generator is turned on while the lead is inserted. The stimulus from the pacing lead causes muscular contractions to show the location of the electrode. Observation of the ECG, using standard limb leads, will show when the atrium or ventricle is being paced. Echocardiography has also been used to assist in determining the location of the pacing lead.[11–13] See Protocol 19.1 for detailed instructions on temporary transvenous pacemaker placement.

Transcutaneous pacing

Transcutaneous pacing is particularly well suited for emergency use and for prophylactic use in situations where there is a risk of developing bradyarrhythmias. Transcutaneous pacing was one of the first pacing techniques developed, having first been used in 1952.[3] It was not until improvements in electrode design and pulse duration were introduced in the 1980s that the use of transcutaneous pacing became widespread. Many modern defibrillators designed for emergency use now also include a transcutaneous pacing function.

The procedure for pacing is relatively simple. Once adhesive electrodes are applied to the appropriate

Protocol 19.1 Placement of a temporary transvenous pacemaker

Items Required
- Fluoroscope or electrocardiogram [ECG] to determine location of the electrode
- 2% lidocaine solution in syringe with needle
- Percutaneous introducer kit, or a suitable intravenous (IV) catheter and an access port
- Temporary pacing lead
- Pacing generator with fresh batteries
- Sterile scalpel, scissors, needle driver, thumb forceps
- Suture
- Sterile surgical drapes
- Sterile sponges
- Sterile gloves
- Bandage material
- Assistants
- Patient monitoring equipment (ECG, blood pressure monitor)

Procedure: Introducer placement
1. Collect necessary supplies.
2. Select insertion site, position patient appropriately, and place monitoring equipment.
3. Clip fur at least 5 cm (2 inches) in all directions from planned insertion site and aseptically prepare the skin. Inject local anesthetic agent (<0.5 mL 2% lidocaine) subcutaneously around the point of insertion.
4. Perform hand hygiene, don sterile gloves, and drape the sterile insertion field.
5. Use a scalpel blade to cut a small hole completely through the skin.
6. Insert an intravenous catheter into the vein. This catheter must be large enough to allow a guide wire to pass through it.
7. Pass the guide wire through the intravenous catheter and into the vein. Remove the intravenous catheter while keeping the guide wire in the vein.
8. Insert the tapered dilator into the sheath and pass the dilator and sheath over the guide wire.
9. Dilate the vein and insert the introducer: Push the dilator and sheath over the guide wire through the hole in the skin, through the wall of the vein, and into the lumen of the vein. Remove the dilator and guide wire from the introducer sheath, leaving the introducer in the vein.
10. Suture the introducer to the skin. Check to see that there is no leakage from the port of the hemostasis valve on the introducer.
11. Cover the opening on the hemostasis valve to maintain sterility.

Procedure: Pacing lead placement through introducer
1. If the electrode catheter does not have a bend in the tip, form one to facilitate passage into the right atrium. Most catheters are packaged to produce this bend, but the bend may be lost if the catheter has been resterilized.
2. Lead introduction:
    a. If the introducer is in the jugular vein, insert the lead through the access port, jugular vein, cranial vena cava, right atrium, tricuspid valve, and right ventricle until it contacts the right ventricular endocardium.
    b. If the introducer is in the lateral saphenous vein, insert the lead through the access port, saphenous vein, femoral vein, caudal vena cava, right atrium, tricuspid valve, and right ventricle until it contacts the right ventricular wall. Sometimes resistance is encountered as the lead reaches the inguinal region. Abduction of the leg usually allows the lead to pass.
3. For bipolar leads, connect the negative terminal of the generator to the distal electrode on the lead and the positive terminal of the generator to the proximal electrode of the lead.
4. Set the rate on the generator and increase the strength of the stimulus until it captures the ventricle (produces a ventricular complex on the ECG and a palpable pulse).
5. Adjust the sensitivity to recognize intrinsic beats. Avoid setting the pacemaker so that it senses T waves, P waves, shivering, or other artifacts that may inhibit pacing.
6. Secure the lead to the access port.
7. Protect the access port with a bandage.

ECG, electrocardiogram; IV, intravenous.

location on the shaved skin of the thorax, pacing can begin. Proper application of the electrodes is important for successful pacing. The size of the electrode, how well it is in contact with the patient's skin, its location on the patient, and the electrode's polarity are important factors that influence the ability to capture the heart. Figure 19.4 shows an example of electrode patches used for transcutaneous pacing.

Transcutaneous pacing electrode location

Several studies regarding electrode size and placement have been published.[14–17] Geddes et al.[14] mapped the thoraces of 18 dogs and determined that the positive elec-

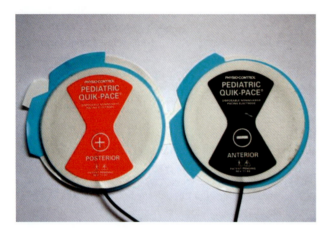

Figure 19.4 Transcutaneous pacing electrode patches.

trode on the right side of the chest was not critical but a distinct window for optimal pacing corresponded with placement of the negative electrode over the apex beat on the left side of the chest (see Fig. 19.5). It should be noted that this window coincides with the optimum window for defibrillation,[18] so pacing electrodes may prevent optimal placement of defibrillation electrodes. DeFrancesco et al.[16] found that the optimal location for electrode placement was directly over the precordial impulses on the left and right hemithoraces. The negative electrode was placed on the left side near the sternum and the positive electrode was placed on the right side more dorsally. Lee et al.[15] tested several different electrode configurations and found that the most effective position was with the electrode centered on the costochondral junction of the sixth rib on the right and left hemithoraces. Unfortunately the authors did not indicate the polarity of the electrodes. The studies performed by Geddes, DeFrancesco, and Lee all seem to be describing the same location for the optimal placement of the electrode on the left side of the thorax. Perhaps because placement of the right electrode is less critical, the three studies found similar but slightly different optimal locations for the electrode on the right side. DeFrancesco used the right precordial impulse, Lee used the costochondral junction on the sixth rib, and Geddes found that for most but not all dogs the right electrode should be more cranial than the left. Falk et al.[19] tested the pacing threshold in humans for three electrode configurations: (1) the negative electrode placed in the

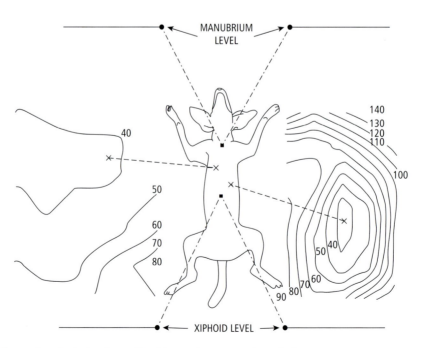

Figure 19.5 Map of the canine chest showing optimal transcutaneous pacing window.

left parasternal location and the positive electrode placed in the lower right scapular border; (2) the negative electrode placed in the left parasternal location and the positive electrode placed in the lower left scapular border; and (3) the negative electrode placed at the apex and the positive electrode placed in the right parasternal region. Falk found little difference in the pacing threshold using either of these electrode configurations, but he found that electrode polarity is critical and that reversing the polarity can result in extremely high capture thresholds or result in failure to capture. Most manufacturers seem to use electrode configurations similar to those used by Falk. Manufacturers use diagrams to indicate how the electrodes should be placed on a human patient. In many cases they do not indicate the polarity of the electrode. Normally, the electrode that would be placed in the left parasternal or left anteriolateral (apex) position on a human should be placed on the dog's left side over the apex. The electrode placed in the right parasternal or the posterior position in a human should be placed on the dog's right side.

Transcutaneous pacing electrode size

Optimal electrode size appears to be weakly correlated to body size.[14] DeFrancesco et al.[16] used adult pacing electrodes. Lee[15] found that for beagles the optimal electrode size was 4×5 cm (20 cm^2). Geddes[14] found that there was little advantage in using electrodes greater than 5 cm in diameter in dogs. Both ZOLL Medical and Physio Control recommend using pediatric electrodes for patients less than 15 kg.

Other transcutaneous electrode considerations

To function properly the electrodes must make good contact with the skin. The skin should be clean and free from hair so that the adhesive on the electrode patches adhere well. DeFrancesco et al. recommended using ECG paste and an elastic bandage to hold the electrode in place. Multifunction electrode patches may be advantageous in dogs if there is a significant likelihood that defibrillation will be required, because the optimal pacing and defibrillation windows on the dog are nearly identical.[18]

Performing transcutaneous cardiac pacing

All of the steps required to prepare for pacing can be performed with the patient awake, but before any electrical stimulus can be applied the patient must be anesthetized. Conscious animal patients will not tolerate transcutaneous pacing because of pain. The need to shave the thorax in animals probably increases the dis-

comfort associated with transcutaneous pacing. People report that minor skin nicks or cuts greatly increase discomfort.

Electrocardiographic electrodes must be attached to the pacing electrodes so that the patient's intrinsic QRS complexes can be sensed by the pacemaker. It may be necessary to try different leads in order to sense the QRS complexes properly. Asynchronous pacing, in which the pacemaker does not stop in response to the patient's own heartbeats, may be used with little risk to the patient[20,21] if the pacemaker is being inhibited by artifacts or does not sense the QRS complexes.

Pacing is initiated by selecting the desired heart rate and increasing the strength of the stimulus until the ventricle is captured. The pacemaker will also cause contraction of the muscles in the chest, which will cause the patient to move. The stimulus can also lighten the plane of anesthesia. See Protocol 19.2 for detailed instructions on transcutaneous cardiac pacing.

Protocol 19.2 Transcutaneous cardiac pacing

Items Required
- Transcutaneous pacing generator
- Pacing electrode patches
- Clippers
- ECG electrodes

Procedure
1. Prepare to monitor the ECG, pulse, and blood pressure.
2. Collect necessary supplies.
3. Select adult or pediatric electrode patches based on body size, remembering that if the patch is not designed for defibrillation, it may interfere with defibrillation.
4. Clip fur from planned electrode site. Avoid abrading or cutting skin.
5. Place the electrode on the right hemithorax directly over the precordial impulse. Place the electrode on the left hemithorax directly over the precordial impulse.
6. Inspect the electrode to be sure there is complete contact with the skin.
7. Turn on the machine.
8. Connect the ECG electrodes. A good ECG tracing is required for demand pacing. The QRS complex should stand out in relation to the T and P waves.
9. Anesthetize the patient if not already unconscious.
10. Determine if the pacemaker is sensing intrinsic beats for demand pacing. Set the desired pacing rate.
11. Adjust the output of pacing generator until the ventricle is captured (ventricular complexes appear on the ECG and pulses are produced).

Temporary epicardial pacing

Temporary epicardial pacing is a specialized technique that is generally used in patients recovering from cardiac surgery. Temporary epicardial pacing allows more flexibility in where the electrode(s) can be located and the mode of pacing than any other temporary pacing technique. The electrodes used for temporary epicardial pacing are thin and resemble wire suture. They have needles on both ends; one end of each electrode is attached to the heart, while the other end passes through the chest wall and skin and is connected to a pacing generator. The surgeon usually decides where the electrodes will be placed. Since several electrodes (etc.) may be used, it is important to identify the function of each lead. The pacemaker is operated by inserting the electrode into the appropriate connector on the generator. The pacing leads should be secured to the patient's body so that the leads will not be pulled out if the patient moves or the generator is dropped. When pacing is no longer needed the electrode is designed to be removed by gently pulling on it. A 2007 review[22,23] provides a more detailed description of the technique.

Thump pacing

Mechanical force applied to the heart or precordium has a long history of being used to treat bradyarrhythmias. Anyone working in the operating room during thoracic or cardiac surgery has probably had an experience similar to that of Paul M. Zoll, a major figure in the history of pacing and defibrillation. During heart surgery on wounded soldiers during World War II, Zoll observed that the heart was sensitive to manipulation and that even a light touch could stimulate a heartbeat.[24] This observation inspired Zoll to develop artificial pacemakers, including a mechanical pacemaker[25] that was used in dogs and over 100 people.[4] Nevertheless, the technique of "thump" or "fist" pacing, which use a series of thumps to the precordium to maintain a physiological heart rate, is still not well known. Several authors have described it as an almost forgotten technique.[26,27]

It is important to recognize that the use of precordial thumps for the treatment of bradyarrythmias is much safer and more effective than the use of a thump for treating tachyarrhythmias. The American Heart Association's 2005 cardiopulmonary resuscitation (CPR) guidelines only mention the use of a single precordial thump as a technique for termination of ventricular tachycardia or ventricular fibrillation, not for bradyarrhythmias. The American Heart Association found only limited evidence regarding the effectiveness of a precordial thump in treating tachyarrhythmias and made no recommendation for or against its use.[28] Since the 2005 guidelines were published other studies have been published that suggest that a single precordial thump is ineffective in converting ventricular tachyarrhythmias.[29,30] Reexamination of evidence that supports thump pacing has led to the inclusion into newer resuscitation guidelines of thump or fist pacing for emergency treatment of bradycardia caused by complete AV block when electrical pacing is not available.[26,31] Based on the Consensus on Science and Treatment Recommendations of the International Liaison Committee on Resuscitation, the European Resuscitation Council (in 2005) incorporated percussion pacing into its advanced life support guidelines.[31]

Fist pacing requires less effort than chest compression, and hemodynamically fist pacing is just as effective as transcutaneous or transvenous pacing.[32] The force required to stimulate a heartbeat with fist pacing is much less than that required to produce an adequate pulse using chest compression. This makes thump pacing easier, less tiring to perform, and less likely to cause injury than chest compression. The 2005 American Heart Association CPR guidelines recommend a 1.5- to 2-inch depression of the sternum for effective chest compression, which requires a force of 100–125 pounds. This amount of force frequently causes rib fractures in human patients and is extremely tiring for the individuals performing CPR.[33–35] Zeh[36] found that the required mechanical energy for fist pacing in people is approximated by allowing the ulnar side of the fist to fall from a height of 20–30 cm above the chest. Zoll[25] examined the technique in dogs and humans and found that

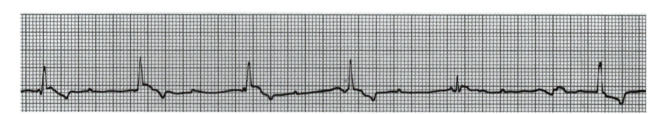

Figure 19.6 Every QRS complex on this ECG tracing was initiated by a thump delivered to the chest. Each QRS produced a pulse wave that could be seen on a direct arterial pressure monitor.

the force required to stimulate a heartbeat was 0.04–0.7 joules in dogs and 0.04–1.5 joules in people. The human subjects were able to tolerate the stimuli at this level and complained of severe discomfort only when the stimuli was increased to 2–3 joules. If the thorax is open and the heart has been exposed, a light flick of the finger is usually all that is needed to stimulate a beat.

The author was able to use thump pacing to maintain normal heart rate and blood pressure in a large dog for 10 minutes while a temporary transvenous pacing lead was inserted. In the ECG shown in Figure 19.6, every QRS complex was initiated by a thump delivered to the chest. Each QRS produced a pulse wave that could be seen on a direct arterial pressure monitor. The heart rate dropped precipitously whenever thump pacing was stopped.

Transesophageal pacing

Transesophageal pacing has not been widely used or extensively studied in clinical veterinary medicine, but the technique has been used successfully in dogs in research, and a device, promoted for use in veterinary medicine, was on the market in the 1980s (Stat-Pace II Model V, Seecor Inc. Fort Worth, TX). Transesophageal pacing is minimally invasive and can be initiated quickly in an emergency. The transesophageal method paces the atria, but unfortunately, it does not reliably pace the ventricles. Therefore, if the bradyarrhythmia is due to AV block or complete bundle branch block another type of pacing should be used. Two recent reports[37,38] on the use of transesophageal pacing in dogs found that it was impossible to capture the ventricle with any electrode position or stimulus strength, but it was possible to capture the atrium.

Protocol 19.3 Transesophageal cardiac pacing

Items Required
- Transesophageal pacing generator
- Transesophageal pacing lead
- Electrocardiograph

Procedure
1. Collect necessary supplies.
2. Anesthetize the patient.
3. Attach the ECG to the pacing electrode catheter.
4. Insert the pacing electrode catheter into the esophagus until it reaches a point close to the atrium. It is assumed that the electrodes are closest to the atrium when the ECG shows maximum amplitude of the P wave.
5. Set the desired pacing rate.
6. Adjust the output of the pacing generator until the atrium is captured (complexes appear on the ECG and pulses are produced).

Transesophageal pacing is indicated when drug therapy is not effective in treating sinus bradycadia, sinus block, or sinus arrest, particularly during anesthesia. These bradyarrhythmias are often caused by sick sinus syndrome, or by the use of cholinergic or beta-blocking drugs. Generators used for transesophageal pacing typically do not have a sensing function and only operate in asynchronous mode (they provide electrical stimulation regardless of the patient's intrinsic cardiac electrical activity). Transesophageal pacing can cause movement by stimulating muscular contraction. See Protocol 19.3 for instructions on transesophageal cardiac pacing.

Transthoracic pacing

Until the 1980s it was difficult and time consuming to begin and maintain pacing in an emergency. Transvenous pacing was theoretically possible but it is difficult to establish venous access and to guide a pacing lead into the ventricle during CPR. Fluoroscopy is unlikely to be available and flow-directed catheters or ECG guidance is useless if the patient is in asystole. It probably occured to someone that if intracardiac injection of drugs was possible, it might also be possible to insert a pacing electrode into the ventricle through the needle. The use of percutaneously inserted pacing electrodes dates back to at least 1958. Although the risk of injury associated with transthoracic pacing is significant, it could be started much more quickly in an emergency than transvenous pacing, and if the alternative is death, great risks may be justified.

Gessman[39] demonstrated the use of the technique experimentally in 24 dogs using a subxiphoid and parasternal approach. Although no acute deaths occured, examination after euthanasia showed significant complications, including hemothorax, hemopericardium without tamponade, and laceration of a coronary vein. By 1981 the Electro-Catheter Corporation reported that 40,000 transmyocardial pacing kits were in use in more than 1000 hospitals[40]; 1981 was also the year that Zoll introduced an improved transcutaneous pacemaker. The reliability and comfort of noninvasive transcutaneous pacing techniques began to improve in the 1980s and quickly supplanted transthoracic pacing. Today transthoracic pacing is largely obsolete, and the equipment needed to perform the technique is difficult to obtain. However, it is possible to improvise an introducer and electrode. Roberts[40] described a method to make a pacing electrode using a 20-gauge spinal needle and 4-0 stainless steel suture wire. The electrode kit manufactured by Electro-Catheter Corp contained a blunt-tipped, 18-gauge, 6-inch cannula with a trocar-tipped obturator, a 34-cm × 0.97-mm "J" tipped bipolar pacing electrode,

Protocol 19.4 Transthoracic (transmyocardial) cardiac pacing

Items Required
- Transmyocardial pacing kit or equivalent improvised equipment
- Pacing generator
- Electrocardiograph
- Sterile gloves

Procedure
1. Transmyocardial pacing is generally only performed in extreme life-threatening situations, when the patient is unconscious.
2. Collect necessary supplies.
3. Ideally the area where the needle will be inserted should be clipped and aseptically scrubbed.
4. Perform hand hygiene and don sterile gloves.
5. Insert the needle percutaneously into either the left or right ventricular chamber. Use ultrasound guidance, or insert blindly in the fifth intercostal space.
6. Remove the obturator from the needle and insert the curved end of the pacing lead.
7. Once the curved portion of the pacing lead is inside the ventricle the needle is withdrawn, leaving the pacing lead in place.
8. Use the adapter to connect the lead to the generator. The distal portion of the lead should be connected to the negative pole of the pacing generator.
9. Set the desired pacing rate on the generator.
10. Adjust the output of the pacing generator until the ventricle is captured (ventricular complexes appear on the ECG and pulses are produced).
11. Determine if the pacemaker is sensing intrinsic beats for demand pacing.

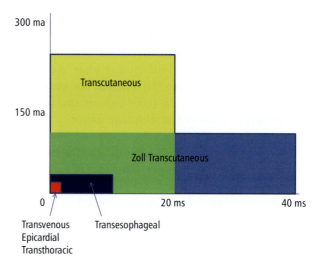

Figure 19.7 Graphic representation of strength and duration of pacing impulses provided by different types of pacemakers.

pacing when they occur. Some pacemakers are able to pace both the atrium and the ventricle, while some pace only one or the other. Dual chamber pacing may improve hemodynamic function compared with ventricular pacing. Temporary pacing generators that are designed for electrodes that directly contact the endocardium or epicardium can be used for transvenous, epicardial, or transmyocardial pacing. Transesophageal and transcutaneous pacing require much stronger stimuli to capture the heart; both the amplitude and the duration of the output pulse are much larger than that required for electrodes that directly contact the heart (see Fig. 19.7). Generators designed for transesophageal or transcutaneous pacing should not be used for any other type of pacing. Some pacemakers allow more sophisticated functions than the basic ones described below.

Output pulse

Output is the strength of the stimulus (output pulse) delivered to the heart. Output is usually measured in milliamperes (mA) but some manufacturers measure output in volts. The amplitude of the stimulus required varies with the type of pacing (see Fig. 19.7). Transcutaneous pacing requires the strongest stimulus and transvenous or epicardial pacing requires the lowest amplitude. The ability to capture the ventricle is a function of duration of the stimulus as well as its amplitude. Longer duration stimuli can achieve capture at a lower output than shorter stimuli. Similar to their pulse amplitude requirements, transcutaneous pacing uses the longest duration pulse and transvenous pacing uses the shortest duration pulse. The output required for capture is also affected by the area of the pacing electrode, its location in relation to the heart, drug therapy, and serum electrolyte concentrations.

and an adapter that is used to connect the electrode to a pacing generator. With the obturator in place, the cannula is inserted into the right ventricle. The obturator is removed and the pacing electrode is inserted. A plastic sleeve that can be used to straighten the "J" tip of the electrode to facilitate insertion is included in the kit. The "J" tip is designed to help keep the electrode in the ventricle. Once the electrode tip is inside the ventricle the cannula is removed and the electrode can be connected to the pacing generator. Transthoracic pacing should only be considered in extreme life-threatening situations, when safer options have failed or are unavailable. See Protocol 19.4 for instructions on transthoracic pacing.

Pacing generators and their operation

Pacing generators provide the electrical stimulus that initiates a heartbeat. The generator may also have the ability to sense the patient's own intrinsic heartbeats and pause

In some cases the stimulus can be detected if it produces a pacing "spike" on the ECG. **Pacing spikes** vary in amplitude depending on the lead selected on the ECG and the amplitude of the stimulus. The pacemaker will indicate (usually by illuminating a light on the display) when a stimulus is being delivered. **Capture** means that the stimulus provided by the pacemaker has resulted in depolarization of the heart. Electrical capture is evidenced by a wide QRS complex if the pacing lead is in or on a ventricle. Mechanical capture occurs when the stimulus produces a pulse as well as myocardial depolarization. Evidence of a pacing spike that does not result in myocardial depolarization is known as failure to capture. Output settings are determined by increasing the amplitude until capture is just achieved and then increasing the strength 1.5–3 times the threshold. Excessive output settings increase the discomfort associated with transcutaneous or transesophageal pacing and can also result in increased risk of movement caused by skeletal muscle contraction, pacing the diaphragm, and causing burns of the skin or esophagus.

Sensitivity

The pacing generators currently available for transvenous or transcutaneous pacing have the ability to detect electrical activity that originates in the the heart (intrinsic beats) and pause artificial pacing when intrinsic depolarizations occur. The transesophageal pacing generators currently available only operate in asynchronous mode (they do not sense intrinsic electrical activity). The sensitivity function is important because a stimulus delivered during certain phases of the heartbeat can cause ventricular fibrillation, although the risk of this occurring due to pacing appears to be extremely low. The pacemaker detects intrinsic beats by using the pacing lead, or standard limb leads in the case of transcutaneous pacemakers, to measure the amplitude of the QRS complex. The sensitivity control sets the minimum amplitude that is assumed to identify an intrinsic QRS complex. If, for example, the sensitivity control is set for 4 mV, signals that are detected with an amplitude of more than 4 mV are assumed to be intrinsic beats and will cause the pacemaker to pause. When the pacemaker senses an intrinsic beat it is displayed to the operator. The indicator is usually a light on generators used for transvenous pacing, or an indicator mark inserted over the QRS complex on the ECG display on transcutaneous pacing generators. The failure to detect intrinsic beats is called **undersensing**. There are other sources of electrical signals in the body and the environment that can be detected by the pacemaker. P and T waves are the most common. Muscular contractions produced by shivering or trembling are common sources of myopotentials in the body. Electrocautery units, clippers, and the electric

motors in surgery tables are examples of equipment found in hospitals that can produce signals that may be detected by the pacemaker. Since the pacemaker senses only these signals' amplitudes and is blind to their origins, if these signals exceed the pacemaker's sensitivity setting they will prevent pacing. This is known as **oversensing**, which could result in periods of ventricular asystole. The objective in adjusting the sensitivity setting is to exceed the amplitude of P waves, T waves, or noise in the environment but not exceed the amplitude of the intrinsic QRS. This may not be possible in every case and if the source of the interference cannot be eliminated, the only other option would be to switch the pacemaker to asynchronous mode where the pacemaker will not pause regardless of the amplitude of the detected signal.

A–V delay

Transvenous and temporary epicardial pacing techniques can be used to pace the atrium as well as the ventricle. During dual chamber pacing there must be a delay after the atrial stimulus to allow the atrial contraction to be completed before delivering the ventricular stimulus—this pause is called the **A–V delay**. This duplicates the delay that normally occurs between atrial and ventricular contraction in the animal, and that is normally represented on the ECG as the P-R interval. In some patients A–V synchrony can augment stroke volume 25%. Ideally, the A–V delay should be adjusted to optimize hemodynamic function by monitoring changes in stroke volume or cardiac output in near-real time with the velocity–time integral (VTI), contour analysis of the pressure waveform, change in pulse pressure, or continuous mixed venous oxygen saturation. If this is not possible, a delay of 120 ms may be used.[7]

Rate

The rate setting determines the interval between output stimuli; therefore, it determines the heart rate. Typically a heart rate between 60 and 100 beats per minute is used in dogs (with smaller dogs receiving the higher rate) and 100 beats per minute in cats. Rapid pacing should be avoided because it can lead to heart failure over time.

Nursing care of the patient undergoing temporary pacing

The nursing care required for patients with temporary pacemakers depends on the type of pacing being performed. Patients being paced by invasive pacing techniques such as transvenous, temporary epicardial, or transthoracic pacing will need to have a dressing applied where the pacing catheter or wires enter the body. Whenever the wires or catheters are covered with bandages it is possible to damage or sever them when the bandage is being removed. It is easy to dislodge the electrodes used for invasive pacing, so the cables and generator must be secured to the patient in a way that avoids tension if the patient moves or the generator is dropped. The use of a vest with pockets for the generator helps secure the generator to the patient. Patients with invasive temporary pacemakers have a direct, low-resistance electrical pathway to the heart, which theoretically puts them at increased risk of ventricular fibrillation or other dysrhythmia with only very small electrical shock impulses. In this situation, the small electrical impulse is called a **microshock;** special care is required to prevent it. Death due to electrical shock is uncommon and almost completely preventable. Staff who care for patients with invasive pacemakers should be aware of sources of microshock and how to avoid microshock in patients. Faulty electrical equipment, current leakage, and static electricity are all potential sources of electrical current that could cause microshock.[41] Many modern medical devices use symbols to indicate when they may be safely used (see Fig. 19.8).

Box 19.1 Procedures used to prevent microshock[41–44]

- Identify electrically sensitive patients. Some institutions post a warning sign on the patient's cage.
- Never use damaged or poorly maintained electrical equipment. Avoid using extention cords.
- Wear rubber gloves whenever the leads or terminals of the pacemaker must be touched.
- Pacing leads should always be insulated whenever they are not connected to a pacing generator. They should never be allowed to touch electrically conductive or wet surfaces.
- Water, urine, and other fluids can conduct electricity. Keep the patient and pacing equipment as dry as possible.
- Electrically powered devices that come into contact with patients, such as clippers, fans, and warming devices, can be dangerous.
- Touching a grounded metal object before touching a patient, and touching the patient away from the leads or pacemaker first, reduces the risk of microshock from static electricity.
- Certain modern electrical devices designed to be in contact with a patient will be labeled to show whether they are safe to use in electrically sensitive patients and patients who may require defibrillation. See Figure 19.8.

Electrocution hazard

Class B Designed to prevent macroshock

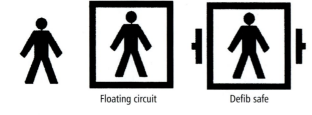

Floating circuit   Defib safe

Class C Designed to prevent microshock

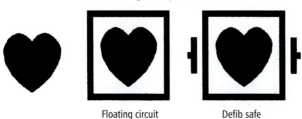

Floating circuit   Defib safe

Figure 19.8 Symbols related to electrical safety. Some pieces of medical equipment bear symbols to indicate their safety for use around patients with pacemakers.

Class B equipment is designed to prevent injury if the equipment is attached to the patient's skin. Class C equipment is designed to be safe when equipment breaches the skin, such as pacing leads, and CVP and PA catheters.[42] See Box 19.1 for procedures used to prevent microshock in patients with pacemakers.

Monitoring the patient with a temporary pacemaker

One of the most important parameters to monitor is the patient's pulse. Every impulse produced by the generator should produce a pulse, and every intrinsic beat should produce a pulse and be sensed by the pacing generator. Palpation of the apical impulse is ideal because there is minimal delay between mechanical capture and a palpable impulse. Auscultation of heart sounds, Doppler pulse detection, pulse oximetry, or direct arterial pressure waveform monitoring are also useful monitoring techniques. Although the pacing generator will indicate when an impulse has been delivered and when an intrinsic beat appears to have occurred, an ECG is required to determine if the generator is sensing correctly and that the output impulse is capturing the ventricle (or atrium). It is important to realize that pacing spikes can look similar to QRS complexes and may be interpreted as such by an ECG monitor, and that electrical capture (electrical activity) does not always mean that mechanical capture (cardiac contraction) has occurred.

The objective of pacing is to maintain adequate blood pressure and cardiac output, so it is important to monitor these functions. Cardiac output is rarely measured, but level of consciousness, body temperature, the temperature of the extremities, urine production, and blood lactate concentration can be used to monitor perfusion.

Troubleshooting

Failure to capture

The pacing indicator shows that the pacemaker has produced a stimulus. The ECG may show a pacing spike, but the stimulus does not produce a ventricular complex or a contraction (no palpable pulse). See Table 19.3 for recommendations on troubleshooting capture failure.

Undersensing

Undersensing is the pacemaker's failure to detect intrinsic beats. The pacemaker does not recognize and is not pausing when intrinsic beats occur. The ECG may show

a pacing spike in the QRS or T wave. See Table 19.4 for troubleshooting tips for undersensing.

Oversensing

Oversensing is used to describe the situation in which the pacemaker interprets other (nonventricular) sources of electrical signal as a ventricular depolarization and therefore fails to deliver an output impulse. During oversensing, the pacing generator indicates that the patient has produced a heartbeat. If the pacemaker is in demand mode, pacing will pause. The ECG will not show a QRS complex at the time the generator sensed a beat. Instead a P wave, T wave, muscle tremor, panting, electrocautery, or some other form of electrical interference may be visible on the ECG. See Table 19.5 for methods of troubleshooting oversensing.

Table 19.3 Troubleshooting failure to capture

Transvenous electrode is not in contact with the heart.	Reposition the electrode.
Transcutaneous electrode is not in contact with the skin.	Use a bandage to hold electrode against the skin. Be sure skin has been properly prepared and use a new electrode.
Polarity of the electrode is reversed.	Check to see if polarity is correct. If the polarity was reversed, change the electrodes or connections to the correct configuration. It may be possible to capture the heart by increasing the output of the generator.
Connections are loose.	Inspect and tighten connections.
Battery has failed.	Replace the battery.
Output is inadequate.	Increase the stimulus.
The heart cannot respond to stimulus.	Patient is not viable, electrolyte abnormality, drug overdose.
The ECG shows a QRS is produced by pacemaker but this does not produce a pulse.	Increase the output of the pacemaker and if this does not produce a pulse, treat as if the patient has pulseless electrical activity (PEA).

Table 19.4 Troubleshooting undersensing

Sensitivity control is set too high.	Lower sensitivity setting.
Transvenous electrode is not in contact with the heart.	Reposition the electrode.
Poor-quality ECG or improper lead selection for transcutaneous pacing.	Remove sources of interference, be sure ECG electrodes are making good contact with the patient, and select a lead that produces large QRS complexes.
Pacemaker is set for asynchronous pacing.	Check setting.

Table 19.5 Troubleshooting oversensing

Electrical interference is present.	Identify and eliminate the source of the interference.
Sensitivity setting is too low.	Raise the sensitivity setting.
Low-amplitude QRS complex is lost in noise in the lead selected for transcutaneous pacing.	Select a better lead for sensing.
P waves or T waves are larger than QRS in lead selected for transcutaneous pacing.	Select a better lead for sensing.
Generator appears to be sensing P waves in transvenous pacing.	The pacing lead may not be in the apex of the right ventricle. Reposition the electrode.

Summary and manufacturer information

Temporary cardiac pacing can be a life-saving measure for patients with or at risk of severe bradyarrhythmia from multiple causes. There are many different methods by which temporary pacing can be applied, some of which are simple and relatively noninvasive considering the benefit. Temporary pacing has relatively few complications, most of which can be remedied with basic care and troubleshooting procedures.

Manufacturer information

Manufacturers of temporary pacing generators that can be used for transvenous, epicardial, or transthoracic pacing

- Galix Biomedical Instrumentation, Miami Beach, FL; www.galix-gbi.com
- Medtronic, Minneapolis, MN; www.medtronic.com
- Oscor, Palm Harbor, FL; www.oscor.com
- Osypka Medical, Inc., La Jolla, CA; www.osypkamed.com/en/
- Pace Medical, Waltham, MA; www.pacemedicalinc.com
- St Jude Medical, St. Paul, MN; www.sjm.com

Manufacturers of temporary pacing generators that can be used for transcutaneous pacing

- Phillips Healthcare, www.healthcare.philips.com
- Physio Control, Redmond, WA; www.physio-control.com
- Zoll Medical, Chelmsford, MA; www.zoll.com

Manufacturers of temporary pacing generators that can be used for transesophageal pacing

- Cardiocommand, Tampa, FK; www.cardiocommand.com
- FIAB Medical Devices, Florence, Italy; www.fiab.it

References

1. Galvani L. Commentary on the Effect of Electricity on Muscular Motion. 1791.
2. Harvey W. On the Motion of the Heart and Blood in Animals. 1628.
3. Zoll PM. Resuscitation of the heart in ventricular standstill by external electric stimulation. N Engl J Med 1952;247:768–771.
4. Zoll PM, Zoll RH, Belgard AH. External noninvasive electric stimulation of the heart. Crit Care Med 1981;9:393–394.
5. Buchanan JW. First pacemaker in a dog: a historical note. J Vet Intern Med 2003;17:713–714.
6. Cunningham SM, Rush JE. Transvenous pacemaker placement in a dog with atrioventricular block and persistent left cranial vena cava. J Vet Cardiol 2007;9:129–134.
7. Bulmer BJ. VDD pacing in dogs: when, why and how to perform single-lead atrial synchronous, ventricular inhibited (VDD) pacing. J Vet Cardiol 2006;8:25–39.
8. Bing OH, McDowell JW, Hantman J, Messer JV. Pacemaker placement by electrocardiographic monitoring. N Engl J Med 1972;287:651.
9. Moïse NSS, Charles E. In: Short CE, ed. Principles & Practice of Veterinary Anesthesia. Baltimore: Williams & Wilkins; 1987:204.
10. Baird CL. Transvenous pacemaking—a bedside technique. Br Heart J 1971;33:191–192.
11. Aguilera PA, Durham BA, Riley DA. Emergency transvenous cardiac pacing placement using ultrasound guidance. Ann Emerg Med 2000;36:224–227.
12. Macedo W Jr, Sturmann K, Kim JM, Kang J. Ultrasonographic guidance of transvenous pacemaker insertion in the emergency department: a report of three cases. J Emerg Med 1999; 17:491–496.
13. Nanda NC, Barold SS. Usefulness of echocardiography in cardiac pacing. Pacing Clin Electrophysiol 1982;5:222–237.
14. Geddes LA, Voorhees WD 3rd, Babbs CF, Sisken R, DeFord J. Precordial pacing windows. Pacing Clin Electrophysiol 1984;7:806–812.
15. Lee S, Nam SJ, Hyun C. The optimal size and placement of transdermal electrodes are critical for the efficacy of a transcutaneous pacemaker in dogs. Vet J 2010;183:196–200.
16. DeFrancesco TC, Hansen BD, Atkins CE, Sidley JA, Keene BW. Noninvasive transthoracic temporary cardiac pacing in dogs. J Vet Intern Med 2003;17:663–667.
17. Noomanová N, Perego M, Perini A, Santilli RA. Use of transcutaneous external pacing during transvenous pacemaker implantation in dogs. Veterinary Record 2010;167:241–244.
18. Geddes LA, Grubbs SS, Wilcox PG, Tacker WA Jr. The thoracic windows for electrical ventricular defibrillation current. Am Heart J 1977;94:67–72.
19. Falk RH, Ngai ST. External cardiac pacing: influence of electrode placement on pacing threshold. Crit Care Med 1986;14: 931–932.
20. Voorhees WD 3rd, Foster KS, Geddes LA, Babbs CF. Safety factor for precordial pacing: minimum current thresholds for pacing and for ventricular fibrillation by vulnerable-period stimulation. Pacing Clin Electrophysiol 1984;7:356–360.
21. Nowak B. [Is asynchronous ventricular pacemaker stimulation dangerous? Results of an international survey]. Dtsch Med Wochenschr 2005;130:997–1001.
22. Reade MC. Temporary epicardial pacing after cardiac surgery: a practical review. Part 2: selection of epicardial pacing modes and troubleshooting. Anaesthesia 2007;62:364–373.
23. Reade MC. Temporary epicardial pacing after cardiac surgery: a practical review. Part 1: general considerations in the management of epicardial pacing. Anaesthesia 2007;62:264–271.
24. Jeffrey K. Cardiac pacing and electrophysiology at millennium's end: historical notes and observations. Pacing Clin Electrophysiol 1999;22:1713–1717.
25. Zoll PM, Belgard AH, Weintraub MJ, Frank HA. External mechanical cardiac stimulation. N Engl J Med 1976;294: 1274–1275.
26. Eich C, Bleckmann A, Schwarz SK. Percussion pacing—an almost forgotten procedure for haemodynamically unstable bradycardias? A report of three case studies and review of the literature. Br J Anaesth 2007;98:429–433.

27. Iseri LT, Allen BJ, Baron K, Brodsky MA. Fist pacing, a forgotten procedure in bradyasystolic cardiac arrest. Am Heart J 1987;113:1545–1550.

28. 2005 American Heart Association Guidelines for Cardiopulmonary Resuscitation and Emergency Cardiovascular Care. Part 7.2: Management of cardiac arrest. Circulation 2005;112:IV-58–66.

29. Haman L, Parizek P, Vojacek J. Precordial thump efficacy in termination of induced ventricular arrhythmias. Resuscitation 2009;80:14–16.

30. Amir O, Schliamser JE, Nemer S, Arie M. Ineffectiveness of precordial thump for cardioversion of malignant ventricular tachyarrhythmias. Pacing Clin Electrophysiol 2007;30:153–156.

31. Nolan JP, Deakin CD, Soar J, Bottiger BW, Smith G. European Resuscitation Council guidelines for resuscitation 2005. Section 4. Adult advanced life support. Resuscitation 2005;67(Suppl 1): S39–S86.

32. Chan L, Reid C, Taylor B. Effect of three emergency pacing modalities on cardiac output in cardiac arrest due to ventricular asystole. Resuscitation 2002;52:117–119.

33. Hoke RS, Chamberlain D. Skeletal chest injuries secondary to cardiopulmonary resuscitation. Resuscitation 2004;63:327–338.

34. Lederer W, Mair D, Rabl W, Baubin M. Frequency of rib and sternum fractures associated with out-of-hospital cardiopulmonary resuscitation is underestimated by conventional chest X-ray. Resuscitation 2004;60:157–162.

35. Geddes LA, Boland MK, Taleyarkhan PR, Vitter J. Chest compression force of trained and untrained CPR rescuers. Cardiovasc Eng 2007;7:47–50.

36. Zeh E, Rahner E. [The manual extrathoracal stimulation of the heart. Technique and effect of the precordial thump (author's transl)]. Z Kardiol 1978;67:299–304.

37. Schmidt M, Estrada A, Vangilder J, Maisenbacher H, Prosek R. Safety and feasibility of transesophageal pacing in a dog. J Am Anim Hosp Assoc 2008;44:19–24.

38. Sanders RA, Green HW 3rd, Hogan DF, Trafney D, Batra AS. Efficacy of transesophageal and transgastric cardiac pacing in the dog. J Vet Cardiol 2010;12:49–52.

39. Gessman LJ, Wertheimer JH, Davison J, Watson J, Weintraub W. A new device and method for rapid emergency pacing: clinical use in 10 patients. Pacing Clin Electrophysiol 1982;5:929–933.

40. Roberts JR, Greenberg MI. Emergency transthoracic pacemaker. Ann Emerg Med 1981;10:600–612.

41. Hull CJ. Electrocution hazards in the operating theatre. Br J Anaesth 1978;50:647–657.

42. Graham S. Electrical safety in the operating theatre. Curr Anaesth Crit Care 2004;15:350–354.

43. Baas LS, Beery TA, Hickey CS. Care and safety of pacemaker electrodes in intensive care and telemetry nursing units. Am J Crit Care 1997;6:302–311.

44. Ward CS. Electrical safety in the theatre. Curr Anaesth Crit Care 1992;3:42–47.

SECTION III

Respiratory

SECTION

20

Oxygen therapy

Jennifer Boyle

Respiratory distress is one of the more frequently seen emergency presentations in veterinary medicine. Signs of respiratory distress include tachypnea (increased respiratory rate), increased respiratory effort, open-mouth breathing, nostril flaring, lip movement with respiration, and cyanosis (blue color to the mucous membranes). Oxygen therapy is warranted initially in all patients with signs of respiratory distress.

Indications for oxygen supplementation

Oxygen makes up 20.9% of the earth's atmosphere. Animals' cells require oxygen for basic metabolism and the creation of energy. Without oxygen, the cells and thus the body will die.

Oxygen enters the body through the pulmonary alveoli, becomes dissolved in plasma, binds to hemoglobin, and is carried to tissues by the cardiovascular system. When the airway becomes compromised or the lungs are not functioning properly, this process may be interrupted, leading to **hypoxemia** (deficient oxygenation of the blood, defined here as a partial pressure of oxygen in the arterial blood [PaO_2] <80 mm Hg). Most patients with hypoxemia have evidence of respiratory distress on physical examination. General causes of hypoxemia include hypoventilation, low inspired oxygen, ventilation/perfusion (V/Q) mismatch, diffusion barrier impairment, and right-to-left extrapulmonary blood shunting.[1] All of these conditions are likely to respond at least somewhat to oxygen therapy, except for right-to-left shunting. Additional conditions in which oxygen therapy may be beneficial include sepsis, hyperthermia, anemia, shock, pulmonary hypertension, seizures, and head trauma.[2]

For any patient in distress (respiratory or otherwise), oxygen supplementation should be provided immediately while assessing for a patent airway. If an upper airway obstruction is suspected, immediate invasive action such as endotracheal intubation or tracheostomy may be indicated to secure an airway and prevent respiratory arrest (see Chapters 23 and 24 for more detailed information). Regardless of the underlying cause of distress, oxygen should be supplemented while the patient is fully examined and appropriate definitive or supportive therapy is performed.

Oxygen sources

Oxygen can be supplied in many different ways. For instance, a clinic may have centralized in-house oxygen or rely solely on portable oxygen tanks; a central source may have wall- or ceiling-mounted outlets (see Fig. 20.1); or tanks may supply oxygen cages (see Fig. 20.2) or be attached to an anesthetic machine. Please see Box 20.1 for details.

Methods of oxygen administration

It is important to provide the optimal oxygen support while minimizing stress. There are multiple methods of oxygen supplementation, including noninvasive, moderately invasive, and invasive techniques.

Noninvasive techniques
Flow-by oxygen supplementation

Flow-by oxygen supplementation is the easiest method of oxygen administration, but it most often results in

Advanced Monitoring and Procedures for Small Animal Emergency and Critical Care, First Edition. Edited by Jamie M. Burkitt Creedon, Harold Davis.
© 2012 John Wiley & Sons, Inc. Published 2012 by John Wiley & Sons, Inc.

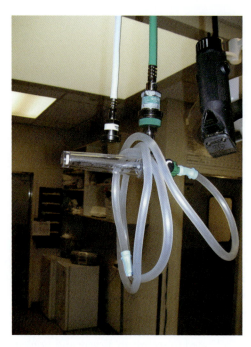

Figure 20.1 Ceiling-mounted central oxygen supply with flowmeter.

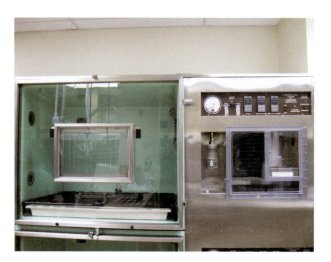

Figure 20.2 Commercial oxygen cage.

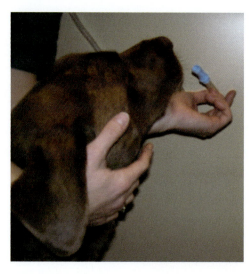

Figure 20.3 Administration of oxygen using the flow-by technique.

> **Box 20.1** Oxygen sources
>
> - Individual oxygen tanks with regulator (flowmeter)
> - Anesthetic machine: The anesthetic circuit can be bypassed by attaching a "Y" connector to the oxygen supply before it enters the circle.
> - Wall- or ceiling-mounted central source
> - Oxygen cage

> **Box 20.2** Equipment required for flow-by oxygen administration
>
> - Oxygen source with regulator (flowmeter)
>   - Individual oxygen tank
>   - Wall- or ceiling-mounted central source
>   - Anesthetic machine
> - Oxygen tubing or hose

relatively modest oxygen supplementation compared with other methods. The technique involves placing a flowing oxygen source very close (2–4 cm)[1] to the patient's nose or to the patient's mouth if the animal is open-mouth breathing (see Fig. 20.3). Although flow-by oxygen supplementation is generally less stressful to the patient than the placement of a face mask, even at a very high oxygen flow rate (3–15 L/min),[3] flow-by typically does not provide the concentration of oxygen required to improve oxygenation. Inspired oxygen (FiO_2) of between 29.5% and 48% has been measured at an oxygen flow rate of 2 L/min,[1] but true FiO_2 ultimately

depends not only on the flow rate but also on the patient's resistance to having the oxygen held up to its face and the distance of the oxygen source from the airway opening. Equipment required for flow-by oxygen administration is listed in Box 20.2.

There are three main advantages of the flow-by method: it is easy and immediate, it requires minimal equipment, and it is generally well tolerated. The disadvantages are the relatively low achievable FiO_2 and that it requires constant manual application (personnel required to hold the apparatus) in the mobile patient.

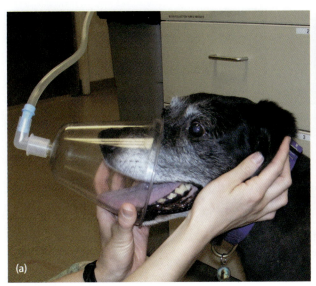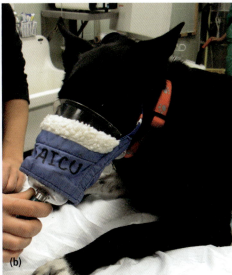

Figure 20.4 (a) Administration of oxygen using a loose-fitting facemask. (b) Use of a loose nylon muzzle to secure an oxygen mask to a dog's face.

Face mask

Face masks are easy to use and effective at quickly delivering oxygen; however, face masks are typically only used short term because they require constant manual application (see Fig. 20.4). The mask can be connected via tubing to the oxygen source, and if used for long periods of time (postanesthesia recovery or in immobile patients), the oxygen should be humidified. Masks can deliver high inspired oxygen concentrations; for instance, 50%–60% oxygen can be achieved with an oxygen flow rate of 8–12 L/min.[4] The patient's face and nose should fill the mask as much as possible to reduce the amount of dead space in the mask. However, care should be taken to avoid pressing the nose and mouth against the wall of the mask, which could occlude gas flow and patient ventilation.

Some animals do not tolerate face mask application well due to the degree of respiratory distress, hyperthermia, or demeanor. Forced application of a tight-fitting face mask often defeats the purpose of oxygen therapy because patient struggling increases both stress and oxygen consumption. To reduce patient struggling and increase patient compliance, the mask's diaphragm (rubber portion of the face mask) can be removed. This may decrease the efficiency of oxygen delivery, but as previously stated, the patient's comfort is a major factor in oxygen therapy efficacy. Another option is to place an oversized nylon muzzle over the face mask and secure the whole apparatus to the patient (see Fig. 20.4). This allows the patient to move its head freely while still receiving oxygen supplementation. Again, patients

> **Box 20.3** Equipment required for face mask oxygen administration
>
> **Equipment/supplies required for mask:**
> - Oxygen source with regulator (flowmeter)
>   - Individual oxygen tank
>   - Wall- or ceiling-mounted central source
>   - Anesthetic machine
> - Oxygen tubing or hose
> - Appropriate size mask
> - Nylon muzzle, oversized (optional)

should be carefully monitored to ensure that airflow is not restricted and that the patient appears comfortable. Box 20.3 includes a list of equipment required for face mask oxygen administration.

There are three main advantages of the face mask oxygen delivery system: it is easy and effective, requires minimal equipment, and can achieve high FiO₂. The disadvantages are that it may not be well tolerated and it requires manual application.

Oxygen bag (oxygen hood)

This technique combines the flow-by and face mask methods. It works well for obtunded patients because high concentrations of oxygen can be provided (75%–95%)[5] while all parts of the animal caudal to the head are exposed, allowing procedures to be performed. A very high oxygen flow rate must be used to avoid

Protocol 20.1 Oxygen bag (hood) setup and application

Items Required
- Oxygen source with regulator (flowmeter)
  - Individual oxygen tank
  - Wall- or ceiling-mounted central source
  - Anesthetic machine
- Oxygen tubing or hose
- Clear plastic bag large enough not to collapse during inhalation

Procedure
1. Collect necessary supplies.
2. Place clear plastic bag over the patient's head.
3. Place the oxygen tubing inside the bag, 2–4 cm from the patient's nose. The bag should remain open along the animal's neck to allow gas to escape.

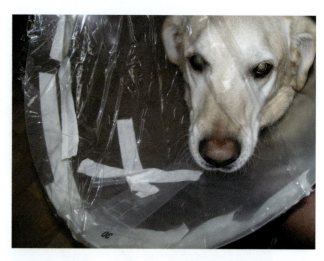

Figure 20.5 Oxygen collar (oxygen tent) method using E-collar. Note the oxygen supply tubing secured to the dependent aspect of the collar. Note also the opening in the plastic wrap in the upper right-hand portion of the image, to allow ventilation.

collapse of the bag (5–8 L/min).[6] This technique tends to be better tolerated than the oxygen mask. Care must be taken with this method because condensation can develop inside the plastic cover, the animal can overheat, and carbon dioxide can build up. The plastic should cover only about two-thirds of the hood, leaving an opening for heat, carbon dioxide, and condensation to vent. See Protocol 20.1 for oxygen bag setup and application.

There are several advantages to the oxygen hood delivery method: it's easy and effective, noninvasive, requires minimal equipment, can achieve high FiO_2, and is useful for obtunded patients. Disadvantages are that it may not be well tolerated, requires manual application in alert patients, a very high flow rate is needed, and there is risk of overheating and carbon dioxide accumulation in the bag if it is inadequately ventilated.

Oxygen collar (oxygen tent)

An alternative to the face mask or oxygen hood is the oxygen tent. An oversized Elizabethan collar (E-collar) is placed on the patient. An oxygen hose is run alongside the neck, into the caudal aspect of the E-collar, and secured to the E-collar with tape or staples ventral to the patient's mandible (see Fig. 20.5). Clear plastic wrap is then placed over the forward edge of the E-collar, leaving an opening to allow for carbon dioxide to escape. Oxygen concentrations of up to 80% generally can be achieved.[4] Flow rates of approximately 1 L/10 kg body weight usually provide an adequate inspired oxygen concentration. Patients generally tolerate the oxygen collar technique quite well, and they do not often require close attendance for its application. Oxygen tents should be used cautiously with large panting dogs because the tent

Protocol 20.2 Oxygen collar (oxygen tent) setup and application

Items Required
- Oxygen source with regulator (flowmeter)
  - Individual oxygen tank
  - Wall- or ceiling-mounted central source
  - Anesthetic machine
- Oxygen tubing or hose
- E-collar oversized for the patient and equipment to secure the collar on the animal
- Clear plastic wrap
- Adhesive tape

Procedure
1. Collect necessary supplies.
2. Place the E-collar on the patient and secure routinely.
3. Run the oxygen tubing alongside the neck, into the caudal aspect of the E-collar, and secure to the E-collar with tape or staples ventral to the patient's mandible.
4. Place clear plastic wrap over the forward edge of the E-collar, leaving a dorsal opening adequate for gas, moisture, and carbon dioxide escape. Tape the plastic wrap in place.
5. Set oxygen flow rate at approximately 1 L/10 kg body weight.

can become rapidly overheated and overhumidified. See Protocol 20.2 for details.

The advantages to the oxygen collar technique are that it's generally well tolerated, effective, minimally invasive, requires minimal equipment, can achieve high FiO_2, and does not require constant manual application.

Disadvantages are that it requires high oxygen flow rates, there is risk of overheating, and carbon dioxide and condensation can accumulate.

Oxygen cage

An oxygen cage is a good option for patients that are in severe respiratory distress or likely to decompensate rapidly if manually restrained. There is minimal stress involved and the patient can receive the benefit of oxygen supplementation while being visually evaluated. A commercial oxygen cage environment's oxygen concentration, temperature, and humidity can be adjusted and monitored. The oxygen cage is a good option for longer term use because it does not require manual application of the oxygen but allows complete patient observation. Commercially available oxygen cages have integrated venting systems that prevent carbon dioxide accumulation. Oxygen therapy in a cage allows the patient to position itself comfortably (see Fig. 20.2).

Unfortunately, oxygen cages are relatively expensive to operate, and by their nature they limit technician and clinician access to the patient. It takes time for the cage to fill with oxygen, and each time the cage door is opened, the oxygen concentration in the cage drops toward or to room air concentration. When performing time-consuming patient treatments, a facemask may be required to supplement oxygen while the door is open. Most oxygen cages are too small to adequately accommodate large dogs without significant overheating, but they work well for small dogs and cats. Even with temperature control, large or panting dogs can quickly overheat. Portable fans and cooling packs can be used to lower the temperature in the cage without opening the door.

If a commercially made oxygen cage is not available, a neonatal or veterinary incubator can be used for small patients (see Fig. 20.6). Even pet carriers can be modified by covering some of the holes and providing an oxygen source. Elevated temperatures and increased carbon dioxide levels may be a problem with this technique. Oxygen cages and incubators usually have a venting system that allows for the evacuation of carbon dioxide and may have a filter that scavenges excess gas from the environment, whereas pet carriers and other forms of containers rely on fresh oxygen flow to flush out the carbon dioxide in the box. The atmosphere is about 0.038% or 380 ppm carbon dioxide. Exhaled gas contains as much as 4% carbon dioxide, or about 100 times the amount normally inhaled.[7]

There are several advantages to the oxygen cage: it is well tolerated, creates minimal stress, is noninvasive, can achieve high FiO_2, and it is a controlled environment.

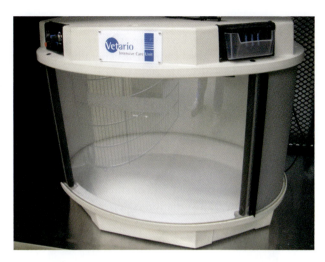

Figure 20.6 A veterinary incubator that can be used as an oxygen supplementation cage for very small patients.

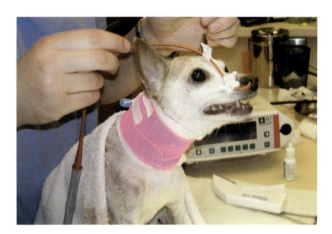

Figure 20.7 Red rubber catheter being used for nasal insufflation in a dog.

The disadvantages are that it is expensive, allows limited access to patient, has a risk of overheating, and that hands-on manipulations of the animal interfere with oxygen supplementation.

Moderatively invasive techniques

Nasal oxygen insufflation catheters

Nasal insufflation is an effective method for oxygen administration. Nasal oxygen insufflation uses supplies readily available in most clinics, is inexpensive, and is relatively well tolerated. It allows for excellent access to the patient without compromising oxygen provision. In this technique, a red rubber catheter or infant feeding tube is placed into the nasal cavity and secured externally to the patient (see Fig. 20.7). The red rubber catheter or feeding tube is then attached to an oxygen source.

Nasal oxygen insufflation is a great option for dogs that are too large for or may become overheated in an oxygen cage. Although the nasal catheter is generally well tolerated once in place, it is advisable to fit the patient with an E-collar to avoid patient removal. An FiO_2 between 40% and 65% can be achieved with flow rates of 50–100 mL/kg/min.[3,8,9] In panting or open-mouth breathing patients, the FiO_2 is decreased.

Placement of bilateral nasal catheters allows for higher oxygen flow, although some patients do not tolerate having both nares blocked. Use of smaller catheters may help when bilateral insufflation is performed. FiO_2 with bilateral catheters can be 60% with a flow rate of 100 mL/kg and up to 80% at 200 mL/kg. Therefore, use of bilateral nasal oxygen catheters can produce a adequate FiO_2 to cause oxygen toxicity (cell damage from high concentrations of oxygen) if administered long term (>24 hours).[5,10]

High oxygen flow rates can cause trauma to the nasopharyngeal mucosa. To help prevent mucosal drying, the oxygen should be humidified, although for short-term oxygen supplementation <24 hours, nonhumidified oxygen may not cause problems (see later section for information about humidification). Other complications of nasal catheters include gastric distension, nasal discharge, and epistaxis. Nasal insufflation is contraindicated in patients with nasal masses, rhinitis, nasal fractures, or epistaxis. See Protocol 20.3 and Figures 20.8 through 20.11 for detailed instructions on placement of nasal oxygen insufflation catheters.[1,4,5,6]

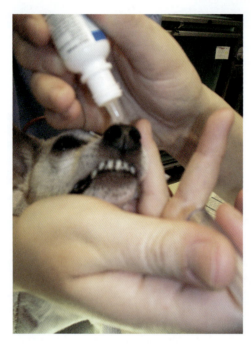

Figure 20.8 Administering proparacaine drops intranasally prior to nasal catheter placement aids in placement.

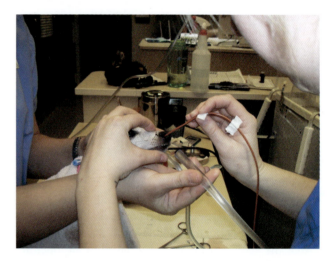

Figure 20.10 Insertion of a nasal catheter.

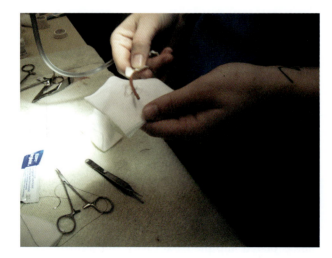

Figure 20.9 Applying lubricant gel to catheter helps ease catheter passage and enhance patient comfort.

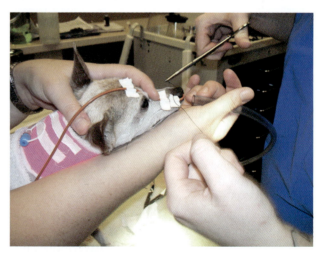

Figure 20.11 Suturing nasal catheter in place using nylon suture and adhesive tape "butterflies" on the red rubber catheter.

Protocol 20.3 Nasal oxygen insufflation catheter: placement and use

Items Required
- Oxygen source with regulator (flowmeter)
  - Individual oxygen tank
  - Wall- or ceiling-mounted central source
  - Anesthetic machine
- Red rubber urinary catheter or infant feeding tube:
  - For small patients: 3.5–5F tubes
  - For medium-size dogs: 5–8F tubes
  - For larger dogs: 8–10F tubes
- Lubricating jelly
- Proparacaine ophthalmic drops or 2% lidocaine
- ½–1-inch adhesive medical tape
- Nonabsorbable suture material and suturing instruments, or skin staple gun
- Bubble humidifier
- Intravenous extension set (if needed)
- Christmas tree adapter (if needed)
- E-collar
- Assistant

Procedure
1. Collect necessary supplies, selecting appropriate size tube. Although no precise guidelines exist, the nares diameter should be estimated and a smaller catheter placed. See previous recommendations.
2. Premeasure the tube to the medial or lateral canthus of the eye and mark the tube. Measuring to the medial canthus will place the tube tip in the nasal passage; measuring to the lateral canthus will place its tip in the nasopharynx. Patients may more readily tolerate insufflation into the nasopharynx.
3. The assistant should restrain the patient from behind and point the patient's nose toward the ceiling.
4. Apply a few drops of topical 2% lidocaine or proparacaine ophthalmic drops in the nose to desensitize the nasal mucosa. Do not exceed 1 mg/kg lidocaine in cats or 2 mg/kg lidocaine in dogs. Allow the topical anesthetic time to take effect prior to inserting the catheter.
5. Apply a small amount of lubricating jelly or lidocaine gel on the outside of the tube to ease passage of the tube.
6. In the cat, insert the catheter in a ventral-medial direction. In the dog, initially insert the catheter in a dorsal-medial direction, then ventromedially. Insert the catheter a little at a time, releasing the catheter between each advancement to avoid accidental displacement if the patient moves. Advance only to the premarked level (see step 2).
7. Once in place, the tube can be sutured to the side of the patient's muzzle (or as close to the nasal planum as possible) and then either sutured or stapled on the side of the face, up the bridge of the nose, or to the forehead. Adhesive tape "butterflies" can be made around the catheter to serve as anchoring points for the suture or staples.
8. An adapter may be required to secure the catheter to the oxygen tubing.
9. Place E-collar.

Nasal catheters have several advantages. They are inexpensive, minimal equipment is required, they allow excellent patient accessibility, and the technique can achieve moderate to high FiO₂ with low oxygen flow rates. Some disadvantages are that they are not always well tolerated, are moderately invasive, and placement can be stressful.

Nasal prongs

Nasal prongs are intended for human use but can be used for larger dogs as well (EMT Medical Company, Direct Home Medical Supply; multiple other suppliers online). The prongs are placed in the patient's nostrils and secured behind the dog's ears. The prongs' tubing can be taped or sutured in place, and it may be helpful to build a tape "bridge" between the right and left portions of the tubing across the top of the dog's muzzle. Nasal prongs are easier to place than a nasal catheter; however, they generally require higher flow rates than nasal catheters and their tips are always situated in the nasal passages, so they may be less comfortable. As with nasal catheters, oxygen should be humidified if it is going to be administered long term. See Protocol 20.4 for detailed instructions on nasal prong placement.

Protocol 20.4 Nasal prongs: application

Items Required
- Oxygen source with regulator (flowmeter)
  ○ Individual oxygen tank
  ○ Wall- or ceiling-mounted central source
  ○ Anesthetic machine
- Nasal prongs set
- ½–1-inch medical adhesive tape
- Nonabsorbable suture material and suturing instruments, or skin staple gun
- Bubble humidifier
- Christmas tree adapter (if needed)
- E-collar

Procedure
1. Collect necessary supplies.
2. Place nasal prongs in each nostril. Run the length of the tubing behind the patient's ears and secure with integrated tab, as applicable.
3. Create an adhesive tape "butterfly" tab on the side of each nasal prong and secure the nasal prongs near the skin beside the patient's nose using suture or staples.
4. A "tape bridge" can also be used to help keep the prongs in place. (Run the tape over the bridge of the nose, either adhesive side toward fur or with two adhesive sides stuck together.)
5. Attach tubing to oxygen source (use Christmas tree adapter if needed).
6. Place E-collar.

Some advantages to nasal prongs are that they are relatively noninvasive, require minimal specialized equipment, and provide excellent patient accessibility. Some disadvantages are they may not be well tolerated. Higher flow rates are required for prongs but they provide lower FiO_2 than nasal catheter.

Nasotracheal catheter

Nasotracheal oxygen administration is a very useful in the patient with upper airway disease such as laryngeal dysfunction or collapsing trachea. A catheter is placed into the trachea via the nares. The FiO_2 achieved is generally as high as with nasal insufflation; however, the flow rate should be 50% of the nasal rates and oxygen should always be humidified.[5] See Protocol 20.5 for detailed instructions on nasotracheal catheter placement.[1,5]

The advantages to nasotracheal catheters are they are inexpensive, require minimal equipment, provide excellent patient accessibility, and can achieve high FiO_2 with a very low flow rate. The disadvantages are that they may

not be well tolerated, it is moderately invasive, and placement can be stressful.

Transtracheal catheters

Transtracheal catheters are useful for administering oxygen to patients with upper airway obstructions or when passage of a tube through the nasal cavity is contraindicated. This technique involves the percutaneous placement of a sterile catheter into the tracheal lumen using aseptic technique. Transtracheal oxygen supplementation is typically performed short term. In an emergency situation, a hypodermic needle attached to a fluid extension set can be used to administer intratracheal oxygen. This technique allows for the use of lower flow rates and less patient discomfort than with nasal catheters. Transtracheal oxygen administration has also been shown to increase PaO_2 more than nasal insufflation.[4] An FiO_2 of 60% to 80% can be achieved with an oxygen flow rate of 1–2 L/min.[4] Oxygen used with this technique should be humidified. See Protocol 20.6 for detailed instructions on transtracheal catheter placement.[5,6]

The advantages of transtracheal catheters are they provide excellent patient accessibility, can achieve high FiO_2 with very low flow rate, and are generally well tolerated. Some disadvantages are they are moderately invasive to invasive, the placement is stressful, and they require constant monitoring.

Invasive techniques

Endotracheal intubation

In patients with severe respiratory distress or marked upper airway obstruction, it may be necessary to secure an airway by intubating with an endotracheal tube. The cuff should be inflated after intubation to provide protection to the airway. Unless the patient is severely obtunded or unconscious, anesthesia will be required because alert patients do not tolerate endotracheal intubation. Detailed instructions for endotracheal intubation can be found in Chapter 23, Tracheal Intubation, Protocol 23.1 (canine), and Protocol 23.2 (feline).

The major advantages of endotracheal intubation in the respiratory distress patient are the abilities to deliver 100% oxygen, to control the airway, and to provide manual or mechanical ventilation if needed. Intubated patients must be closely monitored at all times to prevent accidental or patient removal of the tube. This method requires the use of an oxygen source with a breathing circuit attached. Whenever the patient is repositioned, the endotracheal tube should be disconnected from breathing circuit and reconnected once the patient is in

Protocol 20.5 Nasotracheal catheter placement

Items Required
- Oxygen source with regulator (flowmeter)
  - Individual oxygen tank
  - Wall- or ceiling-mounted central source
  - Anesthetic machine
- Red rubber urinary catheter or infant feeding tube
  - For small patients: 3.5–5F tubes
  - For medium-size dogs: 5–8F tubes
  - For larger dogs: 8–10F tubes
- Lubricating jelly
- Proparacaine ophthalmic drops or 2% lidocaine
- ½–1-inch medical adhesive tape
- Suture material and suturing instruments, or skin staple gun
- Bubble humidifier
- Intravenous extension set (if needed)
- Christmas tree adapter (if needed)
- E-collar
- Assistant

Procedure
1. Collect necessary supplies, selecting appropriate-size tube. Although no precise guidelines exist, the nares diameter should be estimated and a smaller catheter placed. See preceding recommendations.
2. Premeasure the tube to the fifth intercostal space and mark with indelible marker. This length should place the tube's tip just cranial to the tracheal bifurcation.
3. With the patient in sternal recumbency, point the patient's nose toward the ceiling.
4. Apply a few drops of topical 2% lidocaine or proparacaine ophthalmic drops in the nose to desensitize the nasal mucosa. Do not exceed a total dose of 1 mg/kg lidocaine in cats or 2 mg/kg lidocaine in dogs. Allow the topical anesthetic time to take effect prior to inserting the catheter.
5. Apply a small amount of lubricating jelly or lidocaine gel on the outside of the tube to facilitate passage of the tube.
6. In the cat, insert the catheter in a ventral-medial direction. In the dog, initially insert the catheter in a dorsal-medial direction, then ventromedially. Insert the catheter a little at a time, releasing the catheter between each advancement to avoid accidental displacement if the patient moves.
7. Once the catheter is in the mid-nasopharynx, the patient's head should be held in an extended position (rostral and dorsal) to ease tube passage into the trachea.
8. The patient may cough during the insertion, in which case lidocaine can be infused via the tube to desensitize the larynx, minding the total dosing maximum from step 4.
9. Advance the tube to the level premarked in step 2.
10. Once in place, the tube can be sutured to the side of the patient's muzzle (or as close to the nasal planum as possible) and then either sutured or stapled on the side of the face, up the bridge of the nose, or to the forehead. Adhesive tape "butterflies" can be made around the catheter to serve as anchoring points for the suture or staples.
11. An adapter may be needed to attach the catheter to the oxygen tubing.
12. Place E-collar.

its new position to prevent the tube twisting in and thus traumatizing the trachea.

Administering oxygen by way of endotracheal intubation allows maximum control of oxygen supplementation, allows for positive pressure ventilation, requires low oxygen flow rates, minimizes patient emotional stress due to anesthesia, and is inexpensive. The major disadvantages to endotracheal intubation are the requirement for general anesthesia in conscious patients and the need for intensive monitoring while the tube is in place.

Tracheostomy tube placement

A tracheostomy may be required to bypass an upper airway obstruction. This technique requires general anesthesia unless the patient is already unconscious. Commercial tracheostomy tubes are commonly used, but regular oral endotracheal tubes can be used if

Protocol 20.6 Transtracheal catheter placement for oxygen supplementation

Items Required
- Oxygen source with regulator (flowmeter)
  - Individual oxygen tank
  - Wall- or ceiling-mounted central source
  - Anesthetic machine
- Bubble humidifier
- Clippers with clean blade
- Surgical aseptic preparation supplies
- Sterile gloves
- 2% lidocaine in a syringe fitted with a 22-gauge or smaller needle
- A large bore over-the-needle or through-the-needle central venous catheter or commercial tracheal catheter
- Adapter from 3.5 mm or smaller endotracheal tube or Christmas tree adapter
- ½–1-inch medical adhesive tape
- Suture material and suturing instruments, or skin staple gun

Procedure
1. Collect necessary supplies.
2. Clip fur from and aseptically prepare an area with a radius at least 5 cm from the proposed insertion point. The catheter should be inserted on the ventral midline of the trachea, two to three tracheal rings below the cricoid cartilage.
3. Administer 2% lidocaine subcutaneously to the area to allow for catheter insertion. Do not exceed a total dose of 1 mg/kg lidocaine in cats or 2 mg/kg lidocaine in dogs. Allow the topical anesthetic time to take effect prior to inserting the catheter.
4. Perform hand hygiene and don sterile gloves.
5. Using aseptic technique, insert the catheter on the trachea's ventral midline, two to three tracheal rings below the cricoid cartilage, and direct caudally such that the tip of the catheter lies at the carina.
6. Secure the catheter hub to the neck. Adhesive tape "butterflies" can be made around the catheter hub to serve as anchoring points for the suture or staples.
7. Place a light dressing around the patient's neck.
8. Connect to a humidified oxygen source with appropriate adapter from preceding equipment list.

tracheostomy tubes are not available. The cuff should not be inflated unless the patient is receiving positive pressure ventilation. Additionally, the tube should not be sutured in place. Ideally, aseptic technique is used, but in an emergency, the site can be clipped and swabbed with 70% alcohol. This method requires use of an oxygen source with a breathing circuit. As with endotracheal intubation, this technique requires close monitoring to prevent the patient from dislodging the tube.

E-collars should not be placed because they can lie across the insertion site and potentially obstruct the tube. Details about temporary tracheostomies are found in Chapter 24, Temporary Tracheostomy, and Protocol 24.1.

The advantages of the tracheostomy tube are the same as those for the endotracheal tube; additionally, tracheostomy tubes are tolerated in awake patients. The disadvantages are that placement usually requires general anesthesia, and frequent care is necessary to prevent obstruction of tube with respiratory secretions. Chapter 25 contains details on management of artificial airways such as temporary tracheostomy tubes.

General care of patients receiving oxygen therapy

Patients requiring oxygen therapy should be monitored closely. It is important to monitor temperature, pulse rate and quality, respiratory rate and effort, mucous membrane color, and capillary refill time. Blood gas analysis or pulse oximetry are important to track progress and response to therapy in patients that require respiratory support.[2] See Chapters 21 and 22 for more information on oximetry and blood gas analysis, respectively.

Because pure oxygen gas contains no moisture, supplemental oxygen therapy can dry the airways. During longer term oxygen therapy, this airway drying can lead to increased viscosity of mucosal secretions and damage to respiratory epithelium, both of which increase the risk of infection. Although there are no specific guidelines as to what constitutes long term, patients that require oxygen therapy for more than a few hours probably benefit from humidification. See Chapter 25, Artificial Airway Management, for details regarding airway humidification recommendations during longer term oxygen administration.

When weaning patients from supplemental oxygen, it is advisable to taper over a 24- to 48-hour period, so that the patient's response can be observed and monitored.[2]

Complications of oxygen therapy

Oxygen toxicity

Patients exposed to high levels of FiO_2 (>50%) can experience oxygen toxicity in <24 hours. Although 40%–50% oxygen can be administered long term without risk,[1,11] administration of 100% oxygen for >12 hours or 80%–90% for >18 hours can lead to signs of oxygen toxicity.[2] Most of the described methods of oxygen supplementation, with the exception of the oxygen cage, do not allow for precise control of FiO_2 below 100%. Oxygen toxicity is sometimes difficult to recognize because the clinical signs can look like those seen with other causes of lung disease. Fortunately, it is reversible if caught early enough and oxygen supplementation is discontinued. If oxygen therapy cannot realistically be discontinued or significantly reduced due to persistent hypoxemia, mechanical ventilation will be required, which may allow the FiO_2 to be reduced. See Chapter 27, Mechanical Ventilation, for more information about indications for and performance of mechanical ventilation.

Absorption atelectasis

When airway obstruction is present, alveolar gases eventually diffuse completely into the blood, causing alveolar collapse. Normally the gas in the alveolus contains a significant amount of nitrogen from atmospheric air. Nitrogen does not diffuse well into the blood from the alveolus, so absorption atelectasis is usually a very slow process. However, when high concentrations of oxygen are introduced, oxygen gas replaces some or most of the nitrogen, and absorption atelectasis is hastened.[1]

Hypoventilation

Carbon dioxide in the blood is the stimulus for ventilation in the normal animal. However, for patients with chronic pulmonary disease, hypoxemia can become the stimulus for respiratory drive. In such cases, oxygen supplementation can lead to severe hypoventilation by inhibiting the respiratory drive.[1] Therefore, monitoring of PCO_2 or end-tidal carbon dioxide ($ETCO_2$) should be considered.

Catheter "whip"

High oxygen flow rates can cause an oxygen insufflation catheter to "whip" within the nasal or tracheal cavity, causing trauma.[6]

Other complications

Prolonged oxygen therapy has also been associated with suppression of erythropoiesis, pulmonary vasodilatation, and systemic arteriolar vasoconstriction.[1]

Summary

Both invasive and noninvasive techniques for providing oxygen therapy were discussed. The technique chosen depends on the patient's degree of respiratory distress. The goal is to increase FiO_2 using the lowest effective flow rates and the least amount of stress to the patient. Ideally, one should start with the least invasive technique appropriate for the patient's condition. If no improvement is seen or the patient's condition worsens, more invasive techniques may be required. The patient's condition should be monitored and reevaluated at frequent intervals so that adjustments can be made to maximize the effect of oxygen therapy.

References

1. Tseng LW, Drobatz KJ. Oxygen supplementation and humidification. In: King LG, ed. Textbook of Respiratory Disease in Dogs and Cats. St. Louis, MO: Saunders; 2004:205–213.
2. Marks SL. Oxygen Supplementation (Notes), Baton Rouge, LA.
3. Rozanski E. Common procedures in respiratory medicine. In: Proceedings of the Central Veterinary Conference East; 2008.
4. Powell LL. (in collaboration with Roberto Novo, DVM, MS, DACVS). Respiratory emergencies. Harris County Veterinary Medical Association Speaker Notes, 2005–2008.
5. Devey JJ. The respiratory distress patient—approach and applied oxygen therapy. In: Proceedings of the Second Annual VetsNow Emergency Critical Care Congress; 2005.
6. Davis HH. Oxygen therapy—chasing the blues away. In: Proceedings of the American Animal Hospital Association Conference; 2008.
7. Universal and Industrial Gases, Inc. Available at: www.uigi.com/carbondioxide.html.
8. Mann FA, Wagner-Mann C, Allert A, et al. Comparison of intranasal and intratracheal oxygen administration in healthy awake dogs. Am J Vet Res 1992;53(5):856–860.
9. Drobatz KJ. Emergency management of respiratory distress. In: Proceedings of the District of Columbia Academy of Veterinary Medicine; 2004.
10. Dunphy ED, Mann FA, Dodam JR, et al. Comparison of unilateral versus bilateral nasal catheters for oxygen administration in dogs. J Vet Emerg Crit Care 2002;12(4):245–251.
11. Drobatz KJ. Approach to the emergency patient. In: Proceedings of the District of Columbia Academy of Veterinary Medicine; 2004.

BISHOP BURTON COLLEGE

21

Pulse oximetry and CO-oximetry

Devon A. Ayres

The vast majority of oxygen in the bloodstream is carried on hemoglobin. Hemoglobin molecules of different morphology (i.e., deoxyhemoglobin, oxyhemoglobin) have different light absorption characteristics. Oximetry is the use of light to quantify the percentage of blood hemoglobin that is present as oxyhemoglobin (is bound to oxygen), and its laboratory use dates back to the 1930s. Oximetry can be used to measure the adequacy of hemoglobin oxygenation in a patient's blood. The earliest patient bedside oximeters were developed in the 1960s but did not receive common use because they often overheated skin and were uncomfortable. The pulse oximetric method used today was invented by Takuo Aoyagi in 1972 and was integrated into commercial monitors for use in humans in the early 1980s.[1]

Until pulse oximeters were introduced in the 1980s, there was no way to continuously monitor a patient's arterial hemoglobin oxygen saturation. The pulse oximeter uses a ratio of near-infrared and red wavelengths of light to determine the percentage of hemoglobin present as oxyhemoglobin, and it allows for continuous evaluation of a patient's blood oxygenation. Because of its continuous nature and the ease of use, pulse oximetry greatly reduced the incidence of lethal hypoxemia during anesthetic events and became a standard piece of monitoring equipment in human medicine during the 1980s. Until pulse oximetry was available, the only way to measure a patient's arterial oxygenation was to analyze blood *ex vivo*, which required time, expertise, expensive equipment, and did not allow for continuous monitoring.

A CO-oximeter is a benchtop analyzer that uses multiple wavelengths of light to recognize and quantify multiple hemoglobin species, including oxyhemoglobin, deoxyhemoglobin, carboxyhemoglobin (bound to carbon monoxide), and methemoglobin (denatured). CO-oximeter manufacturers use a number of proprietary algorithms to correct and calculate hemoglobin values.

Pulse oximetry and to some extent CO-oximetry have become firmly entrenched in the monitoring of anesthetized, acutely ill, and critically ill patients. This chapter focuses on the principles of oximetry and how to best use the technology to improve patient care.

Hemoglobin forms

Erythrocytes (red blood cells) are the primary oxygen transport system in the mammalian body. They contain hemoglobin, a protein (globin) with rings of ferrous iron (heme) that can bind, or become "saturated" with, oxygen. When oxygen is bound to the heme group, the hemoglobin is called **oxyhemoglobin** and transports oxygen through the arterial bloodstream to tissues. Oxyhemoglobin is bright red, which gives arterial blood its distinctive color. **Deoxyhemoglobin** (also known as reduced hemoglobin) is hemoglobin without oxygen bound to it, with intact heme groups available for oxygen binding. Deoxyhemoglobin is darker in color than oxyhemoglobin, which imparts venous blood with its darker color. Oxyhemoglobin and deoxyhemoglobin constitute 97%–98% of a normal mammal's total hemoglobin content, and they are together known as **functional hemoglobin** (see later).[2]

Hemoglobins that are incapable of binding oxygen, known as **dyshemoglobins**, include methemoglobin,

Advanced Monitoring and Procedures for Small Animal Emergency and Critical Care, First Edition. Edited by Jamie M. Burkitt Creedon, Harold Davis.
© 2012 John Wiley & Sons, Inc. Published 2012 by John Wiley & Sons, Inc.

carboxyhemoglobin, and sulfhemoglobin. **Methemoglobin** occurs naturally and develops when the iron of the heme group is oxidized from the ferrous form to the ferric form. There are multiple enzymes that can convert methemoglobin back to deoxyhemoglobin, but when these pathways are no longer functional, the hemoglobin remains in the methemoglobin state. **Carboxyhemoglobin** is created when hemoglobin binds to carbon monoxide rather than to oxygen. Unfortunately, hemoglobin's affinity for carbon monoxide is >200 times its affinity for oxygen, which means that hemoglobin binding to carbon monoxide is very difficult to reverse. Carbon monoxide binding to hemoglobin prevents oxygen binding and carriage, which is why carbon monoxide toxicity can be fatal. **Sulfhemoglobin** is a very rare form of dyshemoglobin that is formed when hemoglobin reacts with sulfide in the presence of oxygen. This process occurs during the degeneration pathway of hemoglobin and in the formation of Heinz bodies.[3] A method of hemoglobin saturation measurement that takes into account the abnormal hemoglobin fractions such as carboxyhemoglobin and methemoglobin is said to report **fractional hemoglobin** saturation, discussed in more detail later.

Functional and fractional hemoglobin saturations

Hemoglobin is considered functional if it can bind, carry, and unbind oxygen. Oxyhemoglobin and deoxyhemoglobin are therefore together known as the functional hemoglobin species. The percentage of total functional hemoglobin that is oxygenated is called **functional hemoglobin saturation** (functional SO_2) and is calculated using this equation:

$$\text{Functional } SO_2 = [(HbO_2)/(HbO_2 + HHb)] \times 100 \tag{21.1}$$

where HbO_2 is oxyhemoglobin and HHb is deoxyhemoglobin. Standard pulse oximeters measure and report functional hemoglobin saturation; they do not take into account the abnormal hemoglobin species.[4]

Fractional hemoglobin saturation (fractional SO_2) refers to the ratio of oxyhemoglobin to all hemoglobin species present, including methemoglobin and carboxyhemoglobin. Fractional SO_2 is calculated as a percentage using this equation:

$$\text{Fractional } SO_2 = [(HbO_2)/(HbO_2 + HHb + COHb + MetHb)] \times 100 \tag{21.2}$$

where COHb is carboxyhemoglobin and MetHb is methemoglobin.

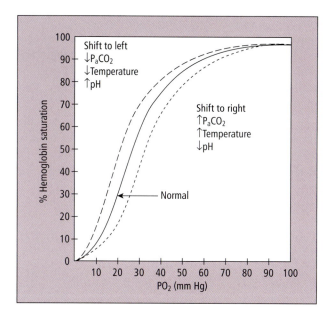

Figure 21.1 Oxyhemoglobin equilibrium curve. Note the sigmoidal relationship between partial pressure of oxygen and hemoglobin saturation with oxygen. Within the normal range of PaO_2 (on room air at sea level), hemoglobin saturation remains above 90% but drops precipitously below a PO_2 of 60 mm Hg. If the PO_2 were taken to infinity, the curve would be completely flat at a hemoglobin saturation (SO_2) of 100%. PCO_2, partial pressure of carbon dioxide in the blood; PO_2, partial pressure of oxygen in the blood.

Modern CO-oximeters and pulse CO-oximeters can measure the presence of all these hemoglobin species, so they can report fractional SO_2, although many can also be programmed to report functional SO_2 if the operator prefers. When a CO-oximeter is also capable of measuring sulfhemoglobin, that species is also included in the calculation used by that machine to report fractional SO_2.

Both functional and fractional SO_2 can provide valuable information about a patient's status. One must consider the information provided by both methods prior to selecting whether either or both values will be obtained. Functional hemoglobin saturation gives a good idea of lung function as reflected by the partial pressure of oxygen in arterial blood (PaO_2; see Fig. 21.1) in patients breathing room air. The relationship between functional SO_2 and PO_2 is relatively reliable, such that if one knows the SO_2, the PO_2 can be back-calculated. PaO_2 as estimated by pulse oximetry is one of the most common methods for quickly assessing lung function in patients with respiratory signs.

However, if abnormal amounts of dyshemoglobin are present, only fractional hemoglobin saturation accurately reflects the blood oxygen content and thus the dyshemoglobinemia's impact on the patient. Because functional hemoglobin saturation considers only the percentage of normal hemoglobin species that is oxygen bound, it ignores conditions such as methemoglobinemia or carboxyhemoglobinemia but would still be superior at reflecting the patient's lung function. Take the following example:

A canine patient breathing room air at sea level has increased respiratory rate and effort, and has a total of 16 g of hemoglobin per deciliter of arterial blood. Of that hemoglobin, 13 g are oxyhemoglobin, 0.5 g are deoxyhemoglobin, 2.4 g are methemoglobin, and 0.1 g is carboxyhemoglobin.

$$Functional\ SaO_2 = [(13\ g/dL)/(13\ g/dL + 0.5\ g/dL)] \times 100$$
$$= 96\%$$

$$Fractional\ SaO_2 = [(13\ g/dL)/(13\ g/dL + 0.5\ g/dL$$
$$+ 2.4\ g/dL + 0.1\ g/dL)] \times 100 = 81\%$$

The functional arterial blood hemoglobin saturation of 96% indicates that the patient has a PaO_2 within the expected range and therefore makes lung dysfunction unlikely as the source of the dog's respiratory distress. The fractional SaO_2 reveals that only 81% of the dog's total arterial hemoglobin is saturated with oxygen, which suggests that the 2.4 g/dL of methemoglobin may be the source of its distress. Although the lungs are able to oxygenate the blood, the dysfunctional methemoglobin molecules make fewer of the dog's total hemoglobin molecules available for oxygen carriage to tissues; this can result in tissue hypoxia and respiratory signs.

Types of oximeters: What they measure and report

Oximetry is the use of light to quantify the percentage of blood hemoglobin that is present as oxyhemoglobin. **Pulse oximetry,** which yields an "SpO_2" measurement, specifically refers to the noninvasive measurement of functional hemoglobin in arterial blood using a bedside monitoring device that can detect an arterial pulse. Thus *standard pulse oximeters report functional hemoglobin saturation.* **CO-oximetry,** which (when performed on arterial blood) yields an "SaO_2" measurement, generally measures the presence of functional hemoglobins (oxy- and deoxy-) in addition to the presence of dyshemoglobins (usually carboxy- and met-). Therefore, CO-oximetry can report the fractional hemoglobin saturation, or the percentage of all hemoglobin in the body (not just the functional molecules) that is present as oxyhemoglobin. In an animal with a dyshemoglobinemia such as carbon monoxide toxicity, the fractional hemoglobin saturation will be lower than the functional hemoglobin saturation (see previous example using methemoglobinemia). **Pulse CO-oximeters,** which combine the technology of a CO-oximeter and the bedside continuous nature of the pulse oximeter, are being used in humans as a noninvasive test for carbon monoxide toxicity and methemoglobin-inducing drug overdoses. Pulse CO-oximeters are not yet in routine use in veterinary medicine.

Pulse oximetry

The science behind a pulse oximeter

Understanding how a pulse oximeter functions can be of great value to the operator. Comprehending how the monitor works will allow the operator to recognize the limitations of the device and troubleshoot problems with readings.

A pulse oximeter estimates oxyhemoglobin percentage by using two wavelengths of light: red at 660 nm and infrared at 940 nm.[5] The machine emits these wavelengths of light from its probe's light-emitting diode (LED) into the patient's tissue bed. This emitted light reaches a receiver in the probe either by reflecting off the tissue or by through transmission to the receiving end of a probe, depending on the probe's style. A photo detector measures the received signal and sends the information to a signal-processing unit.

As this light is introduced into the tissue, each type of hemoglobin absorbs a different wavelength of light. The oximeter uses the differential light absorption characteristics of deoxyhemoglobin and oxyhemoglobin to calculate the arterial blood's functional hemoglobin saturation. The correlation of light absorption patterns and SpO_2 are based on human studies and experimentation, but it has been demonstrated that these calculations are accurate in veterinary patients.[6]

Surrounding tissues such as bone, fat, and venous blood also absorb light, so to target arterial hemoglobin in its measurements, the pulse oximeter considers only pulsatile (arterial) wavelength absorption in the calculations. Thus pulse oximeters function best when placed over tissue with good arterial (pulsatile) blood flow. Pulse oximetry measurements should only be trusted if the monitor displays the patient's correct pulse rate because light from other sources can reach and affect the probe's receiver.

Dysfunctional hemoglobin species also absorb some light at these wavelengths, and thus they can falsely elevate or depress readings if they are present in large amounts. For example, methemoglobin absorbs light at 660 nm *and* 940 nm, which shifts the reported "oxyhemoglobin" value toward 80%–85%, whereas carboxyhemoglobin can falsely elevate the SpO_2 because it absorbs

940 nm light like oxyhemoglobin.[5] Put simply, the presence of methemoglobin usually causes falsely depressed SpO_2 values, and carboxyhemoglobin usually causes falsely elevated SpO_2 values.

Equipment available

Many pulse oximeters are commercially available, both from human and veterinary medical supply companies. Models are available from Nellcor, Masimo, Cardell, Apexx, Respironics, and numerous other companies. Reviewing different brands and models is beyond the scope of this chapter; however, certain general guidelines should be followed. When selecting a pulse oximeter, many factors must be taken into account. Ease of use, probes available, battery life, and cost are just a few of the factors that must be considered before purchase. The newest models may or may not provide more accurate information. A study done at the University of Pennsylvania demonstrated that one older instrument provided more accurate SpO_2 values.[7] Therefore, it is recommended that any model of pulse oximeter be used within a facility prior to its purchase (most manufacturers and distributors allow for trial periods). Pulse oximeters that are independent units, as opposed to those that are part of multiparameter monitors, may be of greater use. These monitors are typically smaller with a longer battery life, allowing for more convenient cage-side monitoring.

Waveform display option

Many pulse oximeters are available with a waveform screen display option that reports the quality of the pulse being measured by the oximeter. The waveform screen displays a graphic interpretation of the peripheral pulse wave, which is called a photoplethysmograph (PPG). The PPG is generated using the pulse oximeter's 660 nm light wave to create an "image" of the pulse,[8] and the PPG's amplitude directly corresponds to pulse quality at the site. The PPG should have sinusoidal form with a small second shoulder on the wave.[9]

Sensor options

Many pulse oximeters have more than one sensor available. Although the lingual clip is the most common, some models include a reflectance/rectal sensor or an esophageal sensor. In the author's experience, a clip-style sensor is the most versatile and easiest to place. However, the models with rectal sensors can be of great use. Although these sensors may be difficult to use when inserted per rectum (feces often obscure the LED), they may be used to acquire readings from the tail.

Other equipment options

Other parameters to consider are whether or not alarms are preset for maximum and minimum acceptable values, cost of replacement probes and batteries, cost of replacement chargers, service contracts, and warranties.

Care and storage of pulse oximeters

When not in use, pulse oximeters should be stored on their chargers. The probe wire should be carefully looped either next to or around the monitor but not wound so tightly as to cause damage to the internal wires. As with any electronic device, care should be taken to avoid exposing the monitor to water, chemicals, and direct sunlight.

Probes should be cleaned in between each use following manufacturer's instructions. Most probes can be cleaned with mild soap and water; others tolerate cleaning with isopropyl alcohol or chlorhexidine. However, some diodes will be damaged by the use of chemicals.

Indications for pulse oximetry

Due to the relative ease of performing pulse oximetry, it is used often as a first test to assess a patient's oxygenation status. Compared with arterial blood gas measurements, pulse oximetry is noninvasive because it does not require vascular puncture or the removal of blood. It can be performed cage side, during anesthetic procedures, and when obtaining an arterial blood sample may be difficult. Pulse oximetry also allows for continuous monitoring, which is invaluable under potentially changeable conditions like general anesthesia and critical illness.

Although continuous pulse oximetry is vital to the safety of anesthetized patients, one must understand the relationship between PO_2 and SO_2 (see Fig. 21.1) to properly interpret an SpO_2 value in a patient receiving supplemental oxygen. FiO_2 is the fraction of oxygen in inspired gas. When a patient is breathing 100% oxygen (FiO_2 1.0), the patient's PaO_2 should be >500 mm Hg. Considering the relationship between PO_2 and SO_2 described in Fig. 21.1, note that the PaO_2 must drop well below 500 mm Hg (in fact, below 100 mm Hg) to change the SpO_2. Therefore, a patient can have a severe lung problem with inadequate oxygenating ability and still have an unchanged SpO_2 when receiving oxygen supplementation (as in general anesthetic procedures).

Patients who have changes in their respiratory pattern (increase in rate or effort) should have their SpO_2 checked. The acquisition of an accurate normal SpO_2 value is an easy way to rule out hypoxemia as the cause of a patient's respiratory distress.

It must be stressed that pulse oximetry does not assess ventilation. Ventilation determines and is indirectly determined by the partial pressure of carbon dioxide in the blood (PCO_2). Blood or end-tidal PCO_2 should be monitored in critically ill and anesthetized patients (see Chapters 22, Blood Gas Analysis, and 26, Capnography, for more information).

Performing pulse oximetry

Obtaining an accurate reading depends on many factors. Readings that are questionable cause delays in appropriate treatment. Before attempting to obtain a reading, make sure that the probe is clean and undamaged. If the model being used has different settings, use the setting that corresponds most accurately to the patient's heart rate. For example, pulse oximeters designed for human patients often have neonatal, pediatric, and adult settings. Use the neonatal setting for patients with higher heart rates and the adult setting for patients with lower heart rates; the setting used should reflect the pulse rate, not the size or weight of the patient.

Site selection

The next step is to select an appropriate site for a reading. Mucous membranes typically provide the most accurate readings (see Fig. 21.2a). Potential sites for use are listed in Table 21.1. The most common site used in anesthetized animals is the tongue, although this is not often well tolerated by conscious patients. The pinna may be the most accessible site but often gives erroneous results.[10] Occasionally inguinal skin folds can be used. The site selected should be warm, well perfused, and clean. If the patient is markedly hypovolemic or hypothermic, the site chosen should be as close to a central vessel as possible (tongue, lips) to provide the most accurate results.[10]

Artifactually low readings may be obtained from areas with poor arterial perfusion. Clipping fur from the site and cleaning it may help reduce interference. Pigmented tissue may give falsely low readings or no reading at all. The probe site should be moistened frequently with water or lubricant to help improve accuracy and to protect the underlying tissue because the clip can restrict local blood flow and the continuous light emission can burn if left in one place too long. If a continuous reading is necessary, the site should be checked often for damage and the probe rotated to a new spot at least every few hours. If the clip compresses the tissue to such an extent that blood is driven from the capillary space, falsely low readings may occur.

Reflectance probes may also be used on the tail base. By clipping the ventral aspect of the base of the tail, a large artery can be accessed for monitoring. Placing the probe against the skin and securing it in place with tape or flexible bandaging material can provide accurate readings. If this method is used, the patient should have the site monitored hourly for cleanliness and tissue damage that can occur from overly tight or wet bandages, or probe burns.

Obtaining a measurement

Once the probe has been attached to the site it may take several seconds for a pulse reading to be obtained. It is imperative that the pulse rate acquired by the pulse oximeter match the patient's actual pulse rate. If the pulse oximeter reads an incorrect number, the reading should not be trusted and another reading must be taken. Increased respiratory rate or effort and panting can register as a pulse rate and give incorrect values. See Protocol 21.1 for specific steps to acquire an SpO_2 reading.

Once it has been determined that the pulse rate displayed is accurate and the PPG shows a strong waveform, the SpO_2 can be determined. It should be noted that individual readings are of less value than multiple readings over a period of time. Patient trends should be closely monitored. Figure 21.2 shows different sites and PPG waveforms that may be seen during pulse oximetry measurements.

Factors interfering with pulse oximetry measurement

Some patients may present a challenge when attempting to obtain a SpO_2 reading due to physical problems. Jaundice can cause interference with red and infrared light. It also may be more difficult to obtain a pulse wave on obese animals or animals with significant edema. Patients suffering from peripheral vasoconstriction, vascular disease, or low cardiac output may not have enough blood flow to arteriolar beds to obtain an accurate SpO_2 value.[10,11] Patients with SpO_2 readings below 94% ideally should have arterial blood gas values obtained because pulse oximetry becomes less reliable at values below the normal range; many studies have demonstrated that pulse oximetry is inaccurate at saturation values below 80%.[11,12] Methylene blue has also been reported to interfere with pulse oximeter readings.[13] See Table 21.2[14,15] for a list of factors affecting the ability to obtain an accurate pulse oximeter reading.

It can be a significant challenge to obtain an SpO_2 reading from a cat. Not only are cats often more resistant to handling than dogs, they are more easily stressed and have fewer accessible sites for monitoring. Unfortunately, feline patients also present a challenge

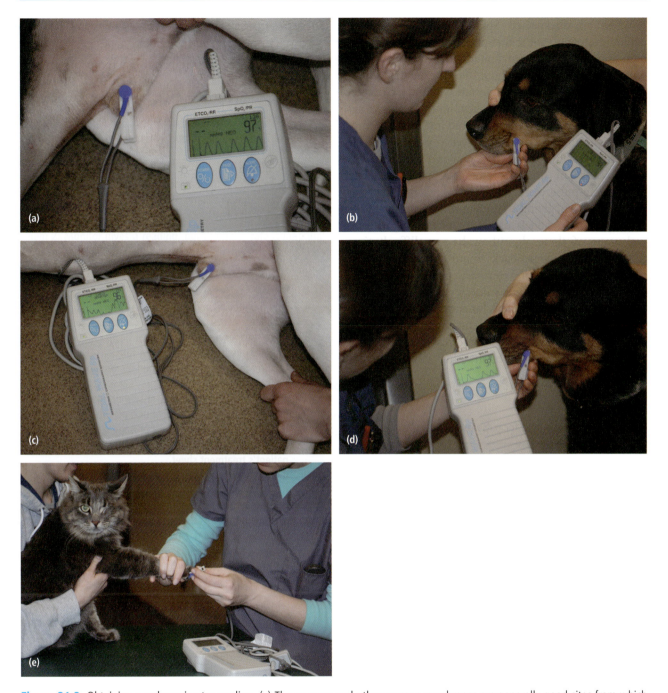

Figure 21.2 Obtaining a pulse oximetry reading. (a) The prepuce and other mucous membranes are generally good sites from which to measure SpO$_2$. (b) Obtaining a pulse oximetry reading on a dog's lip. (c) A pulse oximetry reading with a poor PPG waveform. This pulse oximetry reading should not be used; another site should be selected or blood gas analysis performed if necessary. (d) A high-quality pulse oximetry reading in a dog. Note the strong waveform and the small second shoulder (dicrotic notch) on the PPG, both marks of a high-quality graph. (e) Obtaining a reading on a cat's digits.

for obtaining samples for arterial blood gas analysis. Feline patients generally tolerate pulse oximeter clip placement on their digits more readily than on their lips.[10]

Patients with abnormal or unrepeatable SpO$_2$ values should have CO-oximetry or blood gas analysis per-formed to clarify the findings. When pulse oximetry is used as a guide to tailor or wean respiratory support, as is common in ventilator patients or those being weaned from supplemental oxygen, the patient's clinical signs must be considered in addition to the SpO$_2$ reading because the SpO$_2$ reading can be incorrect.

are low due to local oxygen consumption, the low local PO_2 leads to oxygen disassociating from the hemoglobin and moving down its concentration gradient into the cell for metabolism.

The PaO_2 is 80–110 mm Hg in a normal animal breathing room air at sea level. The relationship between PO_2 and SO_2 (as depicted in Fig. 21.1) is *not linear*. Above a PO_2 of ~100 mm Hg, huge changes in PO_2 (to 550 mm Hg, for instance, as is expected at an FiO_2 of 1.0) make almost no change in the SO_2 because hemoglobin is nearly 100% saturated already. Conversely, below a PO_2 of approximately 60 mm Hg, small decreases in PO_2 lead to enormous drops in SO_2 and therefore in the amount of oxygen that can be carried on hemoglobin to the tissues. Thus although 90% is considered a good "grade," it is absolutely *not* a good SpO_2: it signifies clinically relevant hypoxemia because the patient's PaO_2 is likely ≤70 mm Hg at an SpO_2 of 90%. Another thing to consider is that when a patient is receiving supplemental oxygen, any SpO_2 below 98%–100% may indicate a problem. For instance, a patient on 100% oxygen with an SpO_2 of 90% is physiologically safe but has compromised lung function that may become immediately and life-threateningly apparent once oxygen support has been removed.

CO-oximetry

The science behind a CO-oximeter

CO-oximeters are benchtop analyzers that measure hemoglobin oxygen saturation in a blood sample rather than through tissue. A CO-oximeter uses between four and eight different wavelengths of light, most between 475 nm and 600 nm, to measure the fractions of all relevant species of hemoglobin; values typically reported include total hemoglobin (tHb), oxyhemoglobin (O_2Hb), deoxyhemoglobin (HHb), methemoglobin (MetHb), and carboxyhemoglobin (COHb). Most CO-oximeters do not recognize sulfhemoglobin. If sulfhemoglobinemia is suspected due to applicable toxin ingestion, care should be taken when interpreting values provided by CO-oximetry. Sulfhemoglobinemia can cause a falsely elevated result for methemoglobin and a falsely decreased result for carboxyhemoglobin.[17]

To determine the total hemoglobin concentration (tHb) in a blood sample, CO-oximeters use **conductimetry** to estimate the sample's hematocrit (HCT). Whole blood conducts an electrical current due to the electrolytes in plasma,[4] but erythrocytes, leukocytes, and platelets do not. Alterations in conductivity of the blood then correlate to approximate cell counts, such that diminished electrical conductivity indicates an increase in the

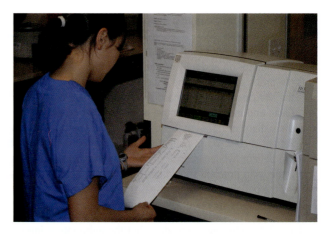

Figure 21.3 Output from a multiparameter benchtop analyzer including a CO-oximeter.

ratio of nonconductive cells to conductive plasma (a higher HCT). Leukocytes and platelets do not have enough mass to affect conductimetry significantly,[18] so the CO-oximeter estimates the HCT based on the electricity transmitted through the sample. The CO-oximeter then uses a standard calculation to determine the tHb from the HCT.

Once the CO-oximeter has determined tHb, the percentages of tHb that are oxy-, de-, carboxy-, and methemoglobins can be calculated. The CO-oximeter directly measures each of the species' concentrations via spectrometric means as just described and then reports them in percentages of tHb. For example, carboxyhemoglobin percentage would be calculated as:

$$COHb, \% = (COHb/tHb) \times 100$$

Many CO-oximeters are combined with basic analyzers that also provide blood gas values, metabolites, and electrolytes. Some also report calculated values such as the alveolar-arterial oxygen gradient (A-a; see Chapter 22), bicarbonate concentration, and base deficit, which makes these machines good all-purpose analyzers for an intensive care setting or emergency department (see Fig. 21.3).

Equipment available

Many CO-oximeters are available from human biomechanical companies, although no company currently advertises a veterinary model. Human CO-oximeters may or may not yield accurate results in dogs and cats because species-specific algorithms are needed. Some models allow the operator to manually enter which species' blood is being introduced. The CO-oximeter generally aspirates blood through a small probe and gives results rapidly on small sample sizes.

Maintenance of a CO-oximeter

Maintenance for most multivalue large CO-oximeters includes replacing a number of consumables at manufacturer-designated times in addition to replacing consumables when an error in calibration or quality control is detected. One highlight of the unit is the ability to preset the machine for automatic quality controls and calibrations. Some models automatically lock out any functions that do not pass quality control. Although this may lead to frustration among staff, it is essential to prevent errors in clinical judgment based on inaccurate readings.

Indications for CO-oximetry

Patients that will benefit from CO-oximetry include those that have known or suspected exposure to drugs that cause hemoglobin conversion to methemoglobin (see Box 21.1)[19–21] or those that have been exposed to carbon monoxide (as in smoke inhalation). Patients with high levels of carboxyhemoglobin can have normal SpO$_2$ values because pulse oximeters cannot differentiate carboxyhemoglobin from oxyhemoglobin. Patients in which carbon monoxide exposure is suspected should have CO-oximetry performed because "classic" bright red mucous membranes are not always seen.[22] Patients with brown or muddy mucous membranes, and those with unexplained respiratory distress, warrant CO-oximetry evaluation for methemoglobinemia.

Box 21.1 Substances known to cause methemoglobinemia[19–21]

Medications
- Azo dye (urinary antiseptic)
- Hydroxycarbamide (hydroxyurea)
- Local anesthetics
  - Benzocaine
  - Lidocaine
- Methimazole and propylthiouracil
- Methylene blue
- Metoclopramide
- Nitroglycerin, nitroprusside
- Sulfa antibiotics

Environmental toxins and human medications
- Acetaminophen
- Antimalarials
- Burning wood and plastic
- Naphthalene (mothballs)

Dyshemoglobinemias

Methemoglobinemia

Normal methemoglobin values in the canine and feline are less than 1%.[23] Values between 10% and 20% cause skin discoloration, usually most noticeable in the mucous membranes. Values above 20% yield clinical signs such as anxiety and dyspnea with exertion, and values between 30% and 50% cause fatigue, confusion, dizziness, and tachypnea. Values between 50% and 70% can lead to coma, seizures, and arrhythmias. Values above 70% are generally lethal.[24]

Carboxyhemoglobinemia (carbon monoxide toxicity)

Normal carboxyhemoglobin values in canine and feline patients are less than 1%. Although increases in methemoglobin percentages lead to consistent clinical signs, increases in carboxyhemoglobin values can cause a variety of signs at different degrees of elevation in individual animals. Most commonly, carboxyhemoglobin at 10%–20% causes nausea.[2] Values between 20% and 30% often cause dizziness and generalized weakness. If greater than 30% of hemoglobin is converted to carboxyhemoglobin, dyspnea during exercise and confusion occur. Once carboxyhemoglobin comprises 40% to 50% of an animal's total hemoglobin, the patient is likely to present with significant neurologic signs such as syncope, seizures, and severe obtundation.[2] Percentages of carboxyhemoglobin greater than 60% can cause hypotension, coma, respiratory failure, and death. Although household carbon monoxide poisoning is now rare due to improved home heating systems, CO-oximetry should be used to rule out carboxyhemoglobinemia in cases in which it is a differential.

Performing CO-oximetry

CO-oximetry is minimally invasive because it requires a small blood sample; arterial blood is required if arterial oxygen content information is desired, but venous blood is adequate to diagnose dyshemoglobinemia. Samples should be drawn from an artery or central vein whenever possible, and patient size and disposition should be considered when choosing a sampling site. Potential sampling sites include the dorsal pedal artery, the femoral artery, the jugular vein, and sublingual veins. More peripheral veins such as the cephalic and saphenous veins can be used but may not render accurate values in hypoperfused patients. Samples obtained from the tongue, usually from patients under anesthesia, are considered venous samples, but some studies have shown that these values are very close to arterial values in the normal patient.[25] If the sample is being taken from a catheter, follow all appropriate scavenging techniques to ensure that the sample is not tainted with saline flush or intravenous fluids (see Chapter 47, Blood Sample Collection and Handling, for appropriate sampling techniques from indwelling catheters).

Benchtop CO-oximeters require anticoagulated samples, usually with sodium heparin or lithium heparin. Follow the unit manufacturer's guidelines when choosing an appropriate anticoagulant, although typically ethylenediaminetetraacetic acid (EDTA), citrate, oxalate, and sodium fluoride are not recommended.

Once the sample has been drawn it should be analyzed immediately, although sometimes immediate analysis is impossible. Although it has been established that ice-water storage for blood gas analysis samples is best,[26] follow all manufacturer guidelines concerning sample storage for CO-oximetry because often the manufacturer recommends samples be stored at room temperature. Once a blood sample has been obtained, it is imperative that it is well mixed and is not exposed to room air, which can falsely increase pH and oxygenation. Samples should be handled carefully to avoid hemolysis that could result in a falsely low HCT value.

Factors affecting CO-oximetry measurements

Several problems may arise while obtaining CO-oximetry measurements. Arterial samples must be used when one wishes to evaluate lung function or estimate PaO_2; venous samples will not suffice in such cases. Inadequate sample mixing, incorrect anticoagulant use, clot formation, air exposure, air bubbles, or prolonged hold time prior to analysis can all cause erroneous results. Some drugs such as hydroxocobalamin and cyanocobalamin (antidotes for cyanide poisoning) can cause interference because of their dark red color.[27,28]

Blood products and CO-oximetry

Bovine hemoglobin-based oxygen carriers such as Oxyhemoglobin (OPK Biotech, Cambridge, MA) do not interfere with CO-oximetry. Hemoglobin-based oxygen carriers, also known as Hb-200, carry oxygen differently than endogenous hemoglobin molecules, and therefore they have a different oxyhemoglobin equilibrium curve. This does not appear to affect CO-oximetry values, although it may affect CO_2 values: a 10% difference was found in calculated versus actual values.[29]

Other biologic products can lead to inaccurate CO-oximetry results. Patients that have received human albumin transfusions can have inaccuracies due to changes in electrolyte concentrations in the plasma.[18] It has also been shown that hyperbilirubinemia can cause falsely elevated COHb levels as measured by CO-oximetry.[30] There are mixed opinions on whether fetal hemoglobin can interfere with carboxyhemoglobin readings,[31,32] but dogs, cats, and horses are born with 100% adult hemoglobin, which eliminates this concern in the species of interest.

The future of oximetry

Recently the Masimo Corporation (Irvine, CA) announced the world's first bedside pulse CO-oximeter using wavelengths of light absorbed by carboxyhemoglobin and methemoglobin. Pulse CO-oximetry was marketed to human emergency departments for use as a point-of-care monitor for carbon monoxide toxicities. Multiple studies have been performed to evaluate the accuracy of the pulse CO-oximeter in humans and have yielded mixed results.[33,34] These contradictory data suggest that more information needs to be gathered prior to relying solely on pulse CO-oximetry for diagnoses and assessments of hemoglobin function. Until pulse CO-oximetry becomes more reliable and veterinary studies are performed, obtaining intermittent CO-oximetry values obtained from a laboratory analyzer will have to suffice.

Summary

Both pulse oximetry and CO-oximetry have their places in veterinary medicine. It is essential to understand the limitations of both and when one modality would be preferred over the other. Appreciating the strengths and weaknesses of these monitors as diagnostic tools will lead to improved patient care and expedite diagnosis and treatment.

Acknowledgment

The author wishes to thank Dr. Monica Clare for her assistance in preparation of this chapter.

References

1. Severinghaus JW, Astrup PB. History of blood gas analysis: VI. Oximetry. J Clin Monit 1986;2(4):270–288.
2. Turgeon ML. Normal erythrocyte lifecycle and physiology. In (eds?) Clinical Hematology: Theory and Procedures. Hagerstown, MD: Lippincott Williams & Wilkins; 2004:82–83.
3. Blood DC, Studdert VP. In: (eds? same as authors?) Saunders Comprehensive Veterinary Dictionary. 2nd ed. Bath, UK: The Bath Press; 1999:1095.
4. Toben B. Pitfalls in the measurement and interpretation of hemoglobin, oxyhemoglobin saturation, and oxygen content in point-of-care devices. RT Decision Makers Respir Care 2008;21(1):1–5.

5. Haskins SC. Interpretation of blood gas measurements. In: King L, ed. Textbook of Respiratory Disease in Dogs and Cats. St. Louis, MO: Saunders; 2004:187–193.

6. Grosenbaugh D, Alben J, Muir W. Absorbance spectra of interspecies hemoglobins in the visible and near-infrared regions. J Vet Emerg Crit Care 1997;7(1):36–42.

7. Burns PM, Driessen B, Boston R, et al. Accuracy of a third (*Dolphin Voyager*) versus first generation pulse oximeter (Nellcor N-180) in predicting arterial oxygen saturation and pulse rate in the anesthetized dog. Vet Anaesth Analg 2006;33:281–295.

8. Srinivas K, Gopal Reddy L, Srinivas R. Estimation of heart rate variability from peripheral pulse wave using PPG sensor. Proc Int Fed Med Biol Eng 2007;325–328.

9. Hlimonenko I, Meigas K, Vahisalu R. Waveform analysis of peripheral pulse wave detected in the fingertip with photoplethysmograph. Measure Sci Rev 2003;3(2):49–52.

10. Hendricks JC, King LG. Practicality, usefulness, and limits of pulse oximetry in critical small animal patients. J Vet Emerg Crit Care 2003;l3(1):5–12.

11. Fairman NB. Evaluation of pulse oximetry as a continuous monitoring technique in critically ill dogs in the small animal intensive care unit. J Vet Emerg Crit Care 1992;2(2):50–56.

12. Sendak MJ, Harris AP, Donham RT. Accuracy of pulse oximetry during arterial oxyhemoglobin desaturation in dogs. Anesthesiology 1988;68:111–114.

13. Sidi A, Paulus DA, Rush W, et al. Methylene blue and indocyanine green artificially lower pulse oximetry readings of oxygen saturation. J Clin Monit 1987;3(4):249–256.

14. Raffe MR. Oximetry and capnography. In: Wingfield WE, Raffe MR, eds. The Veterinary ICU Book. Jackson Hole, WY: Teton NewMedia; 2002:86–95.

15. Mathews KA. Assessment & measurement of oxygenation and ventilation. In: Mathews KA, ed. Veterinary Emergency Care Manual. Guelph, Ontario, Canada: LifeLearn; 2006:580–581.

16. Ford MD, Delaney KA, Ling LJ, et al. In: eds. Clinical Toxicology. Philadelphia, PA: WB Saunders; 2001.

17. Demedts P, Wauters A, Watelle M, et al. Pitfalls in discriminating sulfhemoglobin from methemoglobin. Clin Chem 1997;43(6):1098–1099.

18. Nova Biomedical Operator's Manual, Nova Biomedical, Copyright 2001, Waltham, MA.

19. Boothe DM. Adverse reactions to therapeutic drugs in the CCU patient. In: Wingfield WE, Raffe MR, eds. The Veterinary ICU Book. Jackson Hole, WY: Teton NewMedia; 2002:1070–1071.

20. Aepfelbacher F, Breen P, Manning W. Methemoglobinemia and topical pharyngeal anesthesia. N Eng J Med 2003;348(1):85–86.

21. Harvey JW, Sameck JH, Burgar FJ. Benzocaine-Induced methemoglobinemia in dogs. J Am Vet Med Assoc 1979;175(11):1171–1175.

22. Berent AC, Todd J, Sergeeff J, et al. Carbon monoxide toxicity: a case series. J Vet Emerg Crit Care 2005;15(2):128–135.

23. Wray JD. Methaemoglobinaemia caused by hydroxycarbamide (hydroxyurea) ingestion in a dog. J Sm Anim Sci 2008;49:211–215.

24. Harvey JW. Methemoglobinemia and Heinz body hemolytic anemia. In: Kirk RW, Bonagura J, eds. Current Veterinary Therapy XII. Philadelphia, PA: WB Saunders; 1994.

25. Wagner AE, Muir WW, Bednarski RM. A comparison of arterial and lingual venous blood gases in anesthetized dogs. J Vet Emerg Crit Care 1991;1(1):14–18.

26. Rezende ML, Haskins SC, Hopper K. The effects of ice-water storage on blood gas and acid-base measurements. J Vet Emerg Crit Care 2007;17(1):67–71.

27. Jones K. Hydroxocobalamin (Cyanokit): A new antidote for cyanide toxicity. Adv Emerg Nurs J 2008;30(2):112–121.

28. Pamidi P, DeAbreu M, Kim D, et al. Hydroxocobalamin and cyanocobalamin interference on co-oximetry based hemoglobin measurements. Int J Clin Chem 2009;401(1–2):63–67.

29. Lurie F, Driessen B, Jahr JS, et al. Validity of arterial and mixed venous oxygen saturation measurements in a canine hemorrhage model after resuscitation with varying concentrations of hemoglobin-based oxygen carrier. Anesth Analg 2003;96:46–50.

30. Lampert R, Brandt L. The effect of hyperbilirubinemia on the measurement of oxygenated hemoglobin (O_2Hb), carboxyhemoglobin (COHb) and methemoglobin (MetHb) using multiwave oximeter in mixed venous blood. Anesth Analg 1993;42(10):702–709.

31. Vreman HJ, Stevenson DK. Carboxyhemoglobin determined in neonatal blood with a CO-oximeter unaffected by fetal oxyhemoglobin. Clin Chem 1994;40(8):1522–1527.

32. Lynch PLM, Bruns DE, Boyd JC, et al. Chiron 800 System CO-oximeter module overestimates methemoglobin concentrations in neonatal samples containing fetal hemoglobin. Clin Chem 1998;44:1569–1570.

33. Coulange M, Barthelemy A, Hug F, et al. Reliability of the new pulse CO-oximeter in victims of carbon monoxide poisoning. Undersea Hyperbaric Med 2008;35(2):107–111.

34. Nagano T, Iseki K, Niki T, et al. Experience in employing pulse CO-oximetry. Masui 2008;57(5):621–623.

22

Blood gas analysis

Sarah Gray and Lisa L. Powell

Abnormalities in oxygenation and ventilation

Hypoxemia is defined as a partial pressure of oxygen in the artery (PaO_2) of less than 80 mm Hg. In general, there are five causes of hypoxemia: hypoventilation, decreased inspired oxygen content, ventilation/perfusion (V/Q) mismatch, intrapulmonary shunt, and diffusion impairment. Hypoventilation (increased partial pressure of carbon dioxide [$PaCO_2$] in the blood) can be caused by primary central nervous system (CNS) suppression of ventilation, the administration of medications that suppress ventilation (opioids, anesthetic agents), neuromuscular disease affecting ventilation (tick paralysis, botulism), upper airway obstruction, pleural space disease, chest wall injury (flail chest, pain), and respiratory muscle fatigue. Decreased inspired oxygen content is associated with higher altitudes or from anesthetic machine errors. General etiologies are listed in Box 22.1.

V/Q mismatch and intrapulmonary shunting (V/Q mismatch taken to an extreme) are the most common causes of hypoxemia. **V/Q mismatch** occurs due to decreased ventilation to normally perfused lungs and results in a low V/Q ratio. This type of hypoxemia can be caused by narrowed airways as with asthma or chronic bronchial disease. The narrowing is either secondary to bronchospasm or increased mucus secretions, limiting oxygen entry into the alveolus. **Intrapulmonary shunting** is an extreme "low V/Q" state—a "zero V/Q state"—that occurs when collapsed alveoli or alveoli filled with nongas substance are perfused but (due to the collapse or nongas substance) are not ventilated at all (zero ven-

tilation). Diseases like aspiration pneumonia and pulmonary edema commonly cause intrapulmonary shunting. Shunts can also occur due to abnormal blood flow, as with right-to-left shunting of blood due to cardiac abnormalities (extrapulmonary shunts: patent ductus arteriosus and septal defects), although these are less common than lung disease. **Diffusion impairment** results in incomplete arterialization of the pulmonary capillary blood due to thickening of the gas exchange layer in the alveoli. Under normal conditions the equilibration of oxygen occurs rapidly, but with a thickened gas exchange layer more time is needed, resulting in

---

Box 22.1 Causes of hypoxemia and causes of hypoventilation

Causes of hypoxemia
- Hypoventilation
- Decreased inspired oxygen content
- Ventilation/ perfusion (V/Q) mismatch
- Intrapulmonary shunt
- Diffusion impairment

Causes of hypoventilation
- Central nervous system disease
- Medications (opioids, anesthetic agents)
- Neuromuscular disease
- Upper airway obstruction
- Pleural space disease (severe)
- Chest wall injury
- Respiratory muscle fatigue

Advanced Monitoring and Procedures for Small Animal Emergency and Critical Care, First Edition. Edited by Jamie M. Burkitt Creedon, Harold Davis.
© 2012 John Wiley & Sons, Inc. Published 2012 by John Wiley & Sons, Inc.

hypoxemia. Diffusion impairment is believed to be an uncommon cause of hypoxemia in small animals.

When evaluating a patient's oxygenation and ventilation status, the gold standard is to obtain an arterial blood sample for direct analysis of the partial pressures of these gases in the blood: **blood gas analysis**. Blood gases—the analyzers available, results, and interpretation—are the topics of this chapter.

Blood gas analyzers

The types of analyzers available for use include benchtop and portable models. Dedicated blood gas benchtop analyzers are generally only used in academic facilities and large institutions due to their maintenance requirements and expense. Benchtop analyzers use a polarographic oxygen electrode and the Severinghaus carbon dioxide (CO_2) electrode to analyze the level of gas in the blood sample. The amount of CO_2 in the sample is evaluated based on comparison to a known amount of CO_2, which is supplied by conventional gas tanks. This severely limits the portability of the benchtop analyzers.

Portable (or "bedside") blood gas analyzers accurately measure oxygen and CO_2 using a small foil-wrapped cartridge containing a pH electrode, a polarographic oxygen (O_2) electrode, and a CO_2 electrode. When the cartridge is sealed, the CO_2 equilibrates with bicarbonate within the cartridge. Upon removal of the foil package, the gas surrounding the CO_2 is the known partial pressure of CO_2 in the ambient air, and the electrode calibrates to this pressure upon insertion into the machine.

There are many advantages to the use of portable blood gas analyzers. These machines are usually less expensive than the benchtop devices, can analyze full blood gases on a very small blood sample, and are portable. The availability of bedside analyzers has enhanced the care of critically ill veterinary patients, allowing for more frequent monitoring, diagnosis of ventilation and oxygenation problems, and the ability to guide therapy and prognosis of patients with significant respiratory disease.[1]

Sample analysis

To be clinically useful, the arterial blood sample has to provide an accurate reflection of the patient's status. This requires appropriate blood sampling and handling. Please see Chapter 5, Arterial Puncture and Catheter Placement, and Chapter 47, Blood Sample Collection and Handling, for more information.

The basic method of determining the gas content in the blood involves obtaining an arterial blood sample and inserting it into the blood gas analyzer within a short period of time.

The blood gas analyzer measures the pH, the PO_2, and the PCO_2 of the sample, and the bicarbonate concentration and base deficit are calculated. The pH is measured using a pH-sensitive membrane. The pH is determined by measuring the voltage difference across this membrane.

The PCO_2 measurement is made by measuring the hydrogen ion difference between two solutions after allowing a chemical reaction that results in hydrogen ion production:

$$CO_2 + H_2O \rightarrow H_2CO_3 \rightarrow H^+ + HCO_3^-. \qquad (22.1)$$

Resultant hydrogen ion production is determined using a pH-sensitive membrane similar to that used for the pH measurement. The hydrogen ion production is directly proportional to the PCO_2 of the blood sample.

The PO_2 is measured using a Clark electrode, which uses oxidation and reduction reactions involving the oxygen in the sample to quantify the partial pressure of oxygen present. The change in current as a result of the oxidation-reduction reactions is proportional to the PO_2 of the blood gas sample. Once pH, PCO_2, and PO_2 are measured, a microprocessor then calculates the bicarbonate, base deficit, and temperature-corrected gas values (see later).[2]

Temperature correction

Blood gas analysis is performed at 37°C, which may or may not reflect patient body temperature and thus *in vivo* blood gas values. When the patient's temperature is entered into the blood gas analyzer, the machine can calculate the blood gas results accurate for the individual patient. However, changes in temperature alter gas solubility (Charles law) and alter hemoglobin's affinity for oxygen. Taken together with the fact that the metabolic, vascular, and respiratory effects of hyper- and hypothermia are not fully understood, temperature correction of blood gases remains controversial.[3]

Blood gas sampling

The most commonly sampled arterial sites are the dorsal pedal (dorsal metatarsal) and femoral arteries. Less commonly sampled sites are the brachial, radial, auricular, and lingual arteries. Sampling is generally done using palpation and knowledge of anatomy. The dorsal pedal artery can be palpated over the dorsomedial aspect of the metatarsal; the femoral can be palpated on the medial aspect of the thigh. A single sample can be drawn using a needle and heparinized syringe, or a catheter can be placed for blood gas sampling and for direct blood pressure monitoring. The type of material used in catheters can affect handling of the catheter with placement but also the likelihood of causing thrombophlebitis.[4] Monitoring for evidence of thrombosis is important, especially in the peripherally placed anatomic sites because this my compromise blood flow to distal tissues. Refer to Chapter 5, Arterial Puncture and Catheter Placement, for more information.

Sample handling

To ensure accuracy of blood gas results, knowledge of appropriate sample handling is important. Exposure of the sample to room air and delayed analysis will alter the measurements. Air bubbles in the sample syringe should be expelled immediately. Due to gas diffusion, exposure to room air will cause a drop in the sample $PaCO_2$ (PCO_2 of room air is approximately zero) and change in the sample PaO_2 (PO_2 of room air is approximately 150 mm Hg at sea level). Analysis delay will also alter the accuracy of the blood gas results. Blood cells remain metabolically active for some time *ex vivo*, and cellular effects can alter the accuracy of the blood gas results when delayed samples are not chilled. If sample analysis must be delayed, the sample should be stored anaerobically in an ice water bath at $4°C$; this allows up to a 6-hour delay in analysis without significantly affecting results.[5,6]

Blood gas analysis requires whole blood samples, and as such anticoagulants must be used to allow testing. Dilutional errors can affect sample results. Heparin is commonly used as an anticoagulant during blood sampling. Studies have shown that dilution of the sample with liquid heparin lowers the $PaCO_2$, affects the measure of oxygen, and also can affect electrolytes, lactate, and bicarbonate results. A <10% dilution with heparin minimizes effects on the analytes; this dilution can be achieved with the **evacuated syringe method** using a 3-cc syringe and 22-gauge needle. Liquid sodium heparin (1000 U/mL) 0.5 mL is drawn into the syringe, and then the plunger is drawn to the 3-cc mark to allow the heparin to coat the entire syringe. Then the contents of the syringe are removed by drawing back to the 3-cc mark and expelling all the air and any heparin forcibly. This air/heparin expel procedure is repeated three times, and the syringe is filled with at least 1 cc of blood, which represents a 3.9% dilution.[7] See Chapter 5, Arterial Puncture and Catheter Placement, for further details about this technique.

Evaluating arterial blood gas results

Normal arterial blood gas values for dogs and cats are listed in Box 22.2.[8]

> **Box 22.2** Normal arterial blood gas values for dogs and cats
>
> **Dog[8] (at sea level)**
> - PaO_2: 92 mm Hg (80–105)
> - $PaCO_2$: 37 mm Hg (32–43)
> - SaO_2: more than 95%
>
> **Cat[8] (at sea level)**
> - PaO_2: 105 mm Hg (95–115)
> - $PaCO_2$: 31 mm Hg (26–36)
> - SaO_2: more than 95%

Assessment of the partial pressure of carbon dioxide

The partial pressure of carbon dioxide (PCO_2) is the amount of CO_2 dissolved in the blood and is determined by the balance between production in the tissues and elimination from the body.

PCO_2 is primarily a measure of ventilation because when CO_2 production increases, increases in respiratory rate and/or tidal volume (ie, minute ventilation) will normalize the PCO_2 in a healthy animal. Alterations in $PaCO_2$ are usually associated with neurologic or neuromuscular disease, medications, or pathology of the airway, pleural space, or chest wall.

Control of ventilation is primarily driven by the medulla. Increased PCO_2 diffuses into the cerebrospinal fluid and lowers the pH, which stimulates chemoreceptors and leads to increased ventilation. Hypoxemia can also trigger central chemoreceptors to increase ventilation when the PaO_2 is less than 60 mm Hg. The carotid bodies and aortic bodies are peripheral chemoreceptors that can stimulate ventilation secondary to decreased PaO_2, increased $PaCO_2$, or a drop in pH.[9]

Although this chapter focuses on arterial blood gas analysis, note that PCO_2 (unlike PO_2) is quite similar in the venous blood as in the arterial blood. Therefore venous blood can and is used to evaluate PCO_2, with normal values expected to be only a few millimeters of mercury higher than in arterial samples. The same is not true for evaluation of PO_2, which must be performed on arterial blood to provide information about the lung's ability to oxygenate the blood; venous PO_2 cannot provide such information.

Elevated PCO₂ (hypercapnia)

By definition respiratory acidosis or hypercapnia is an increase in the partial pressure of carbon dioxide ($PaCO_2$ >43 mm Hg in the dog, >36 mm Hg in the cat). This most commonly occurs due to decreased alveolar ventilation, which can occur for several reasons. CNS dysfunction, as with anesthetics, traumatic brain injury, neoplasia, infections, or cerebral edema, can affect CNS control of ventilation. Cervical diseases affecting the spinal cord, such as intervertebral disk disease, neoplasia, infection, or inflammation, can also lead to hypoventilation due to effects on the upper and lower (phrenic nerve) motor neurons responsible for diaphragmatic innervation. Peripherally mediated neuromuscular disease such as tetanus, botulism, and tick paralysis can also lead to a respiratory acidosis due to hypoventilation. Diseases of the pleural space, such as severe pleural effusion or pneumothorax, or diaphragmatic hernia can also result in hypoventilation. Obstructive diseases of the upper and lower airway alter airway resistance and lead to hypercapnia. Tracheal collapse, an upper airway mass, or a foreign body can lead to upper airway obstruction and hypercapnia. Lower airway diseases such as asthma or bronchitis can also cause hypercapnia. Respiratory acidosis will result when there is increased CO_2 production in the tissues without the appropriate compensation in ventilation, as in heat stroke and malignant hyperthermia; however, such situations are much less common than inadequate CO_2 elimination as the cause for hypercapnia.

Depending on the cause, interventions may vary significantly, so the primary goal is to determine the underlying cause and attempt to fix it (i.e., reverse respiratory depressant medications, decrease anesthetic depth, relieve pleural space disorders). A $PaCO_2$ greater than 60 mm Hg is a significant problem and warrants immediate correction of the underlying problem.

Decreased PCO₂ (hypocapnia)

Respiratory alkalosis, or hypocapnia, is a decrease in the partial pressure of carbon dioxide ($PaCO_2$ <32 mm Hg in the dog, <26 mm Hg in the cat). This commonly occurs secondary to lung disease, which stimulates pulmonary afferents to drive ventilation, or poor oxygenation, which triggers both central and peripheral chemoreceptors and increases ventilation. Poor oxygenation can be caused by primary lung disease (leading to low PaO_2 or hypoxemia) or from disease states that affect the ability to transport or use oxygen. Examples of disease processes that lead to poor tissue oxygenation not associated with pulmonary disease include anemia, decreased cardiac output (shock, poor cardiac contractility), and mitochondrial dysfunction (as with sepsis or cyanide toxicity). Also animals with metabolic acidosis have a compensatory respiratory alkalosis (from hyperventilation → low $PaCO_2$) in an attempt to normalize the pH. See Chapter 50, Acid-Base Evaluation,

for more information about acid-base status. A drop in the $PaCO_2$ below 25 mm Hg can result in compromised cerebral blood flow and should be addressed immediately.[10]

Assessment of the partial pressure of oxygen in arterial blood (PaO₂)

Oxygen is carried in the blood in only two forms. One form is the portion of gas dissolved in the blood and measured as a partial pressure (PO_2). This represents only 2%–3% of the total arterial blood oxygen content.[11] The other form is the oxygen bound to hemoglobin in the red blood cells. In arterial blood gas analysis, the PaO_2 is measured to evaluate the lung's ability to oxygenate blood, often called simply "lung function." The diffusion of oxygen into the pulmonary capillaries occurs via diffusion down a concentration gradient. Alveolar partial pressure of oxygen (PAO_2) is higher than the partial pressure of oxygen in the pulmonary capillary as it leaves the pulmonary arteriole and approaches the alveolus. At the alveolar-pulmonary capillary junction, oxygen passively diffuses across the alveolar membrane into the pulmonary capillaries. The rate of diffusion is driven by Fick's law, which states that the diffusion of a gas across a membrane is directly proportional to the area of the tissue membrane and the pressure gradient, and inversely proportional to the thickness of the membrane.[12] Clinically, this means that diffusion will be altered if the surface area for gas exchange is decreased or if the respiratory membrane is thickened (which is uncommon in small animals). Decreased surface area for gas exchange occurs secondary to airway constriction (low V/Q) or lung unit collapse or consolidation (no V/Q: intrapulmonary shunting). PaO_2 is essentially a measure of how many perfused lung units are ventilated adequately to allow oxygen to diffuse into the pulmonary capillary as it heads to the left heart for systemic circulation. Hence PaO_2 is used as a primary measure of pulmonary function.

A PaO_2 less than 80 mm Hg is considered hypoxemia, and oxygen supplementation should be considered. A PaO_2 less than 60 mm Hg is considered severe hypoxemia, and immediate intervention is necessary.

Pulmonary function assessment using arterial blood gas data

Once arterial blood gas values are attained, further analysis may be helpful to determine the severity of the pulmonary dysfunction and to rule out hypoventilation as the cause of hypoxemia. A summary of these analyses is available in Box 22.3.

Box 22.3 Pulmonary function assessment using arterial blood gas data

Alveolar-arterial oxygen gradient

- A-a gradient $= PAO_2 - PaO_2$
  $$= [FiO_2(P_b - P_{H20}) - PaCO_2/RQ] - PaO_2$$

  - Normal ≤ 15 mm Hg at FiO_2 0.21 (room air), normal ≤ 150 mm Hg at FiO_2 1.0 (100% oxygen); values in excess of 15 mm Hg on room air indicate pulmonary dysfunction
  - Use: At any P_b, at any $PaCO_2$
  - Reliable only at room air or 100% oxygen

The "120" rule
- $PaCO_2 + PaO_2 \geq 120$: adequate lung function
- $PaCO_2 + PaO_2 < 120$: abnormal lung function
  - Use: Only at sea level on room air

PaO_2/FiO_2
- $PaO_2/FiO_2 = $ "P:F ratio"
  - Normal ≥ 500 mm Hg; mild pulmonary dysfunction 300–500 mm Hg; moderate pulmonary dysfunction consistent with ALI 200–300 mm Hg; severe pulmonary dysfunction consistent with ARDS <200 mm Hg
  - Use: At any FiO_2
  - Expected values apply only to sea level; extrapolated, reliable values would be available at other P_b

$FiO_2 \times 5$ rule
- Normal $PaO_2 \geq (FiO_2, \%) \times 5$
  - Use: At any FiO_2
  - Expected value of $PaO_2 \geq 5 \times FiO_2$ applies only to sea level; extrapolated, reliable values would be available at other P_b

Total arterial oxygen content
- $CaO_2 = (SaO_2 \times Hgb \times 1.34) + (0.003 \times PaO_2)$
  - Normal in dogs: 16.9–18.0 mL/dL
  - Relevant at all P_b, PCO_2, and FiO_2

Alveolar to arterial gradient (A-a gradient)

After gas exchange occurs, the oxygen content in the pulmonary capillary is normally the same as the oxygen content in the alveolus (PaO_2 ~105 mm Hg at sea level on room air) because diffusion is complete. Oxygenated pulmonary capillary blood then flows to the left heart for systemic circulation. However, a small amount of blood (from bronchial and Thebesian circulations) normally returns to the left heart deoxygenated; this small amount of deoxygenated blood mixes with the arterialized blood returning from the pulmonary capillaries, which drops the PaO_2 below the PAO_2. The normal difference between PAO_2 and PaO_2 (the "**A-a gradient**" or "A-a difference") should be less than 15 mm Hg and is generally considered "physiologic shunting." However, when an increased amount of blood enters the left atrium without being oxygenated (for instance, because it perfused lung units that were not well ventilated due to a low V/Q or no V/Q scenario), the excessive deoxygenated blood further dilutes the properly arterialized blood coming from functional lung units. This situation is commonly referred to as **venous admixture** or intrapulmonary **shunting.** To determine whether there is increased pulmonary shunting, the A-a gradient can be calculated; increased gradients are associated with underlying pathology and help direct diagnostics and intervention.

$$\text{A-a gradient} = PAO_2 - PaO_2$$
$$= [FiO_2(P_b - P_{H20}) - PaCO_2/RQ] - PaO_2$$

$$(22.2)$$

Where the FiO_2 is the fraction of inspired oxygen (0.21 or 21% on room air), P_b is the barometric pressure (~760 mm Hg at sea level), and P_{H20} is the vapor pressure of water. P_{H2O} does vary with temperature, but generally 47 mm Hg is used because this is the vapor pressure of water at 37°C (human body temperature). The $PaCO_2$ is measured from the arterial blood gas sample, and RQ is the respiratory quotient, which is approximately 0.8. This assessment also works when the patient is receiving 100% oxygen, in which case the expected gradient is less than 150 mm Hg. For fractional inspired oxygen levels between room air and pure oxygen, the expected gradient has not been established and must be extrapolated.[5]

The "120" rule

Because the PCO_2 affects PAO_2 (see expanded Equation 22.2), when an animal is at sea level breathing room air, one can estimate what PaO_2 to expect when one knows the $PaCO_2$ by using **the "120" rule.** When an animal is breathing *room air at sea level*, the sum of $PaCO_2$ and PaO_2 is generally 120 to 160 mm Hg. When the sum of $PaCO_2$ and PaO_2 is less than 120, pulmonary dysfunction is present.[5] The major inherent limitation to this method is the requirement for room air, sea level conditions. The major advantage is its ease of use.

$$PaCO_2 + PaO_2 \geq 120: \text{adequate lung function}$$
$$PaCO_2 + PaO_2 < 120: \text{abnormal lung function}$$

$$(22.3)$$

PaO$_2$/FiO$_2$ ("the P:F ratio")

Equation 22.3 can be used to evaluate pulmonary function at any FiO$_2$, which provides an advantage over the A-a gradient and the 120 rule. The value is acquired simply by dividing the PaO$_2$ by the FiO$_2$:

$$PaO_2/FiO_2 = \text{"P:F ratio"} \quad (22.4)$$

where the FiO$_2$ is expressed as a decimal. With normal pulmonary function, the **P:F ratio** should exceed 500 mm Hg. The P:F ratio can be used to approximate the severity of pulmonary dysfunction; values between 300 and 500 mm Hg are associated with mild dysfunction, between 300 and 200 mm Hg are considered to have moderate dysfunction, and less than 200 mm Hg are considered to have severe pulmonary dysfunction. This calculated ratio, along with several other criteria such as acute onset of respiratory distress, bilateral dorsocaudal pulmonary infiltrates, absence of fluid overload or congestive heart failure (pulmonary artery occlusion pressure <18 mm Hg; see Chapter 12), and an appropriate underlying disease process, is also used to identify patients with acute lung injury (ALI) and acute respiratory distress syndrome (ARDS).[13] Values less than 500 mm Hg indicate there is compromised pulmonary function and definitive intervention and diagnostics are indicated. The advantage of this method is that it is simple, quick, and can be used at any FiO$_2$. The main disadvantage is the method's disregard for the effect of ventilation (PCO$_2$), although this is only really an issue when making the calculation on room air.

FiO$_2$ × 5

Another way to approximate the expected PaO$_2$ is to multiply the FiO$_2$ (as a percentage) by 5. With normal pulmonary function the PaO$_2$ would be approximately 100 mm Hg, which is about 5 times the FiO$_2$. This can then be extrapolated out to estimate what the PaO$_2$ should be with normal pulmonary function. Values attained that are lower than this indicate dysfunction.[5] Advantages and disadvantages are identical to those described for the P:F ratio.

Calculation of the total oxygen content

As stated earlier, O$_2$ is carried in the blood two ways: dissolved in plasma and attached to hemoglobin. Total blood O$_2$ content can be calculated easily using the blood gas analyzer results. For arterial blood,

$$CaO_2 = (SaO_2 \times Hgb \times 1.34) + (0.003 \times PaO_2) \quad (22.5)$$

where CaO$_2$ is the total arterial blood oxygen content, SaO$_2$ is the saturation of hemoglobin with oxygen expressed as a decimal (see later), and 1.34 and 0.003 are constants. Normal O$_2$ content in dogs is reported to be 16.9 − 18.0 mL/dL,[14] although an idealized canine value is closer to 20 mL/dL. Note that red blood cell mass has a far more profound effect on total blood oxygen content than does PO$_2$ within the survivable range.

Venous samples

Although arterial samples are preferable for assessment of both oxygenation and ventilation, a venous sample can also help evaluate the respiratory system.

Venous PCO$_2$ (PvCO$_2$)

There is an expected arterial-venous gradient for PCO$_2$. Venous blood contains CO$_2$ from the metabolically active tissue bed(s) upstream from where the sample was acquired, and as such, it generally has a PCO$_2$ approximately 5 mm Hg higher than arterial blood. CO$_2$ produced in the tissues is carried in several forms by the blood to the lungs for removal. The dissolved PCO$_2$ represents approximately 10% of the total CO$_2$.[5] Most of the CO$_2$ is buffered within the red blood cell and then transported as bicarbonate to the lungs where this process is reversed to facilitate removal of CO$_2$ by the lungs. The disadvantage of venous samples is that in certain disease states, the **arterial-to-venous PCO$_2$ gradient** may increase. Such disease states include anemia, where there is a decrease in the ability to buffer the CO$_2$. Venous stasis will also increase the gradient. As a general guide, a PvCO$_2$ less than 48 mm Hg indicates hypoventilation assuming no concurrent perfusion compromise.

Venous PO$_2$ (PvO$_2$)

The PvO$_2$ can be used to determine the **oxygen extraction ratio (OER)**, a ratio that sheds some light on the adequacy of oxygen delivery in comparison with the patient's oxygen consumption. Traditionally, calculation of the OER requires a mixed venous sample collected from the distal port of a pulmonary arterial catheter; however, blood from a central venous line (a catheter with a distal port near the right atrium) is probably adequate for most purposes. See Chapter 15, Monitoring Tissue Perfusion: Clinicopathologic Aids and Advanced Techniques, for more information regarding the oxygen extraction ratio. Normal PvO$_2$ values range from 40 to 50 mm Hg. As a general rule, when PvO$_2$ is less than 30 mm Hg, this may be an indication of decreased oxygen delivery, and diagnostics to determine the cause should be considered if the patient's clinical condition supports this finding.

Saturation of hemoglobin with oxygen

Blood gas analyzers often report the saturation of oxygen (SO_2). This value represents the amount of oxygen bound to the hemoglobin molecule and is reported as a percentage of hemoglobin saturation with oxygen. Blood in which all hemoglobin oxygen sites are bound with oxygen is 100% saturated; blood in which 75% of hemoglobin oxygen sites are bound with oxygen is 75% saturated. The arterial hemoglobin oxygen saturation (SaO_2) is calculated from the pO_2, pH, and bicarbonate values; it assumes normal conditions for the calculation.[5] The oxyhemoglobin equilibrium curve shows the relationship between the PaO_2 and the SaO_2 graphically; it is a sigmoid curve where initially there is rapid binding of oxygen and the hemoglobin molecule. Pulse oximetry is a noninvasive method of estimating the PaO_2 using the oxyhemoglobin dissociation curve. See Chapter 22, Pulse Oximetry and CO-oximetry, for more information about the oxyhemoglobin equilibrium curve and these monitoring tools.

Summary

Blood gas analysis allows detailed assessment of a patient's respiratory function. Arterial blood gases provide the opportunity to monitor a patient's pulmonary function in response to time and therapy, particularly when simple tools like the A-a gradient and the P:F ratio are used. Arterial and venous blood gases can be used to inform the clinician and technician about the patient's ventilatory adequacy. Venous oxygen tension can be used as a marker of adequacy of tissue perfusion. Blood gas analysis is readily available and relatively inexpensive with the use of bedside monitoring equipment.

References

1. Wahr JA, Tremper KK, Hallock L, Smith K. Accuracy and precision of a new, portable, handheld blood gas analyzer, the IRMA®. J Clin Monit 1996; 2(4):317–324.

2. Shapiro BA. Blood gas analyzers. In: Shapiro BA, Peruzzi WT, Templin R, eds. Clinical Application of Blood Gases. 5th ed. St. Louis, MO: Mosby; 1994:313–321.

3. Shapiro BA. Temperature correction of blood gas values. In: Shapiro BA, Peruzzi WT, Templin R, eds. Clinical Application of Blood Gases. 5th ed. St. Louis, MO: Mosby, 1994:227–233.

4. Waddell L. Advanced vascular access. In: Proceedings of Western Veterinary Conference; 2004.

5. Haskins SC. Interpretation of blood gas measurements. In: King LG, ed. Textbook of Respiratory Disease in Dogs and Cats. St. Louis, MO: Saunders; 2004:181–193.

6. Shapiro BA. Obtaining blood gas samples. In: Shapiro BA, Peruzzi WT, Templin R, eds. Clinical Application of Blood Gases. 5th ed. St. Louis, MO: Mosby; 1994:301–312.

7. Hopper K, Rezende ML, Haskins SC. Assessment of the effect of dilution of blood samples with sodium heparin on blood gas, electrolyte, and lactate measurements in dogs. Am J Vet Res 2005;66(4):656–660.

8. DiBartola SP. Introduction to acid-base disorders. In: DiBartola SP, ed. Fluid, Electrolyte, and Acid-Base Disorders in Small Animal Practice. 3rd ed. St. Louis. MO: Saunders; 2006: 229–251.

9. Campbell VL, Perkowski SZ. Hypoventilation. In: King LG, ed. Textbook of Respiratory Disease in Dogs and Cats. St. Louis, MO: Saunders; 2004:53–61.

10. Johnson RA, de Morais HA. Respiratory acid-base disorders. In: DiBartola SP, ed. Fluid, Electrolyte, and Acid-Base Disorders in Small Animal Practice. 3rd ed. St. Louis. MO: Saunders, 2006:283–296.

11. Pierce LNB. Practical physiology of the pulmonary system. In: Pierce LNB, ed. Management of the Mechanically Ventilated Patient. 2nd ed. St. Louis. MO: Saunders; 2007:26–60.

12. West JB. Diffusion, how gas gets across the blood-gas barrier. In: West JB, ed. Respiratory Physiology: The Essentials. 8th ed. Baltimore, MD: Lippincott Williams & Wilkins; 2008:25–34.

13. Wilkins PA, Otto CM, Baumgardner JE, et al. Acute lung injury and acute respiratory distress syndromes in veterinary medicine: consensus definitions: The Dorothy Russell Havemeyer Working Group on ALI and ARDS in veterinary medicine. J Vet Emerg Crit Care 2007;17(4):333–339.

14. Haskins SC, Pascoe PJ, Ilkiw JE, et al. The effect of moderate hypovolemia on cardiopulmonary function in dogs. J Vet Emerg Crit Care 2005;15(2):100–109.

23

Tracheal intubation

Jeni Dohner and Rebecca S. Syring

The ability to establish an airway through tracheal intubation, as well as maintain patency once accomplished, is a vital skill that all veterinarians and veterinary technicians should master. An understanding of airway anatomy and the differences in conformation between cats and dogs will help one choose an appropriate intubation technique when airway access is required (see Fig. 23.1).

One should be comfortable with the different types of endotracheal (ET) tubes, as well as ancillary materials that may be needed to perform ET intubation. If initial attempts to gain airway access result in failure, one should also be knowledgeable of advanced techniques that can be used to quickly secure an airway.

Because of the often chaotic and unpredictable nature of emergency situations, it is recommended that you have a space set aside in your practice that has all of the supplies needed for rapid intubation readily accessible. This may be the same space that is set aside for cardiopulmonary cerebral resuscitation (CPCR). This designated space should be inventoried and restocked regularly, depending on the frequency of use, to assure that all supplies are present and in proper working order. Having such a space set aside will facilitate a rapid response and hopefully minimize stress in a crisis situation.

Indications for intubation

There are many reasons for tracheal intubation in dogs and cats (see Table 23.1). In many instances, this may be a routine intubation for general anesthesia and surgery. However, in an emergency and critical care setting, intubation may be required in unstable animals to facilitate

treatment of that animal. Therefore, a rapid response time is critical, and communication between team members is vital during intubation, particularly when CPCR is needed (see Chapter 16, Cardiopulmonary Cerebral Resuscitation). The same can be said when emergent intubation is required for upper airway obstruction as occurs with foreign bodies, soft tissue swelling due to anaphylaxis or trauma, tumors, laryngeal paralysis, brachycephalic airway syndrome, and tracheal collapse. In some cases an ET tube cannot be passed due to the obstruction, requiring alternative intubation techniques, such as retrograde intubation (discussed later in this chapter) or tracheostomy tube placement, discussed in detail in Chapter 24, Temporary Tracheostomy.

Animals with decreased levels of consciousness may require tracheal intubation to maintain a functional and protected airway. The primary purpose of intubation in these animals is to provide a protected airway from oral and gastric secretions that could be aspirated, resulting in respiratory distress and/or pneumonia. Any animal with a decreased or absent gag reflex, which can be easily checked by gently stimulating the back of the tongue or soft palate with a cotton swab or tongue depressor, should be considered a candidate for ET intubation. A decreased gag response may be seen in animals that have been sedated with propofol or barbiturates.

Another reason that animals with decreased levels of consciousness may require ET intubation is if they are not ventilating appropriately. Severe head trauma or other intracranial diseases resulting in increased intracranial pressure (i.e., brain tumors, meningitis) may result in stuporous to comatose states. These animals may exhibit insufficient ventilation, resulting in carbon dioxide (CO_2) retention, which can further increase

Advanced Monitoring and Procedures for Small Animal Emergency and Critical Care, First Edition. Edited by Jamie M. Burkitt Creedon, Harold Davis.
© 2012 John Wiley & Sons, Inc. Published 2012 by John Wiley & Sons, Inc.

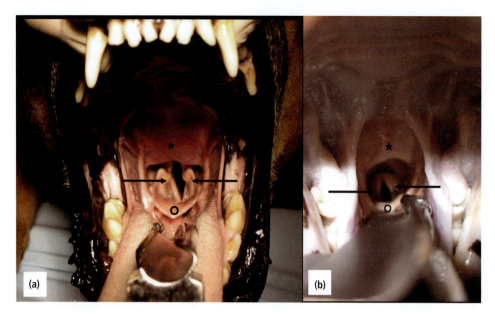

Figure 23.1 Anatomy of the oropharynx of the (a) dog and (b) cat. A laryngoscope is placing pressure on the base of the tongue to expose the larynx and surrounding anatomy. The arrows are pointing to the arytenoids (vocal folds). The asterisk indicates the soft palate. The O indicates the epiglottis.

Table 23.1 Indications for tracheal intubation

Cardiopulmonary cerebral resuscitation
Upper airway obstruction
  Foreign body
  Soft tissue swelling
  Trauma
  Laryngeal paralysis
  Masses
  Tracheal collapse
Decreased levels of consciousness
  Sedation
  Head trauma
  Intracranial disease
Decreased ability to ventilate
  Lower motor disease (flaccid/ascending paralysis)
    Tick paralysis
    Polyradiculoneuritis (coonhound paralysis)
    Botulism
    Myasthenia gravis
  Phrenic nerve damage
    Cervical lesions
  Head trauma
  Hypokalemia
Mechanical ventilation
General anesthesia
Endotracheal wash

intracranial pressure. Intubation and positive pressure ventilation may be required to rid the body of excess CO_2.

Animals with muscular weakness may not be able to ventilate adequately, resulting in hypercarbia, respiratory acidosis, and ultimately hypoxemia. Muscular weakness may occur due to neurologic dysfunction as the result of cervical injuries (resulting in injury to the phrenic nerve that controls the diaphragm or other respiratory interneurons that control the intercostal muscles) or lower motor neuron disease causing flaccid paralysis (i.e., myasthenia gravis, Coonhound paralysis, polyradiculoneuritis, or botulism). Severe hypokalemia is another important reason for marked muscular weakness. Care should be taken to monitor for appropriate diaphragmatic movement (diaphragm moving caudally and causing expansion of the abdomen during inhalation) and chest wall expansion in these patients because respiratory muscle fatigue can occur. With worsening respiratory muscle weakness, hypoventilation, resulting in hypercapnia and respiratory acidosis, may occur and require intubation and mechanical ventilation (see Chapter 27, Mechanical Ventilation). Animals with megaesophagus, which can be seen in some animals with generalized flaccid paralysis, may require airway protection from regurgitation.

The animal with a condition that causes severe hypoxia (PaO_2 <60 mm Hg) in the face of oxygen supplementation may require intubation and mechanical ventilation. In any animal requiring intubation for

Table 23.2 Materials needed for endotracheal intubation

Canine
  Three different-size ET tubes, cuffs previously checked if applicable
    One of estimated size
    One each of size smaller and larger
  Laryngoscope
  Sterile aqueous lubricant
  Gauze squares for grasping the tongue
  Length of muzzle gauze for tying in ET tube
  Appropriate-size air syringe
    3–5 mL: small dog/5–10 mL: large dog
  Atraumatic clamp if using rubber tube
  Cotton-tipped applicators
  Oxygen, mask

Feline
  Three different-size ET tubes, cuffs previously checked if applicable
    One of estimated size
    One each of size smaller and larger
  Laryngoscope, curved blade if available
  Sterile aqueous lubricant
  Gauze squares for grasping the tongue
  Length of muzzle gauze for tying in ET tube
  Appropriate-size air syringe
    3 mL usually sufficient
  Atraumatic clamp if using red rubber ET tube
  2% lidocaine to prevent laryngospasm
  Stylet
  Cotton-tipped applicators
  Oxygen, mask

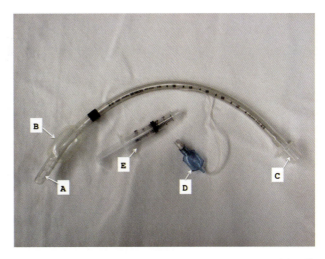

Figure 23.2 Anatomy of an ET tube. (A) Murphy eye; (B) cuff; (C) adapter; (D) pilot balloon; (E) cuff inflation syringe.

mechanical ventilation, sterile technique is extremely important when placing the ET tube because bacterial contamination can increase the risk of pneumonia and sepsis. Sterile ET tube placement requires the use of sterile gloves, a clean laryngoscope, and a sterile ET tube. Placement of a sterile ET tube is also important for diagnostic airway washes.

Equipment needed for intubation

Intubation of dogs and cats requires equipment beyond the ET tube itself and varies slightly by species (see Table 23.2).

ET tubes

Cuffed ET tubes

The cuff on the ET tube is used for two purposes: to prevent gas leaks around the tube and to reduce risk of aspiration of gastric and oral secretions (see Fig. 23.2). Prevention of gas leaks is necessary when using inhaled anesthetic agents to reduce environmental contamination and to facilitate positive pressure ventilation without loss of tidal volume. To prevent gas leakage out of the airways or fluid entrance around the ET tube, the cuff must be inflated to a degree that exerts some degree of pressure against the wall of the trachea. The cuff should be inflated to the lowest pressure that achieves the goals just described, to a pressure no greater than 25 cm H_2O, to reduce the risk for injury to the tracheal wall. Excessive cuff pressure can result in tracheitis, necrosis of the tracheal mucosa, damage to the cartilaginous rings resulting in tracheal dilation, and tearing of tracheal membranes.

There are two main types of cuffs on ET tubes: high-pressure, low-volume cuffs made of a thicker material that conforms to the outside of the ET tube when deflated (see Figs. 23.3a and b) and low-pressure, high-volume cuffs made of a thinner, more compliant material that remains raised with ridges of excess material when deflated (see Fig. 23.3c). Low-pressure, high-volume cuffs are preferred when possible because they generate less pressure for a given volume of inflation, resulting in less tracheal trauma.

Intracuff pressure, which approximates the pressure the cuff exerts on the tracheal wall, can be measured with a sphygmomanometer attached to the pilot balloon to ensure it does not exceed 25 cm H_2O. In the absence of the ability to measure intracuff pressure, either the minimal occlusive volume technique or the minimal leak technique should be used to inflate the cuff.

With the minimal occlusive volume technique, air should be injected into the cuff while ausculting over the trachea while delivering a breath until no leak can be

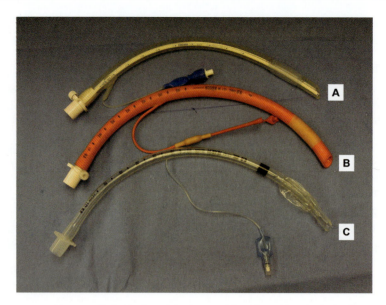

Figure 23.3 Three different types of large cuffed ET tubes. (A) silicone; (B) rubber; (C) polyvinyl chloride (PVC). Note the differences in the cuff between (A) and (B) (low volume, high pressure) and (C) (high volume, low pressure). Note that the silicone tube has been curved for the purposes of this image with a length of suture; silicone ET tubes are straight.

detected. At this point, a small amount of air should be removed from the cuff until a small leak can be heard (e.g., 0.5 cc of air). Small amounts of air should then be gradually instilled until the leak can no longer be heard. This technique minimizes the risk for aspiration but may result in a greater degree of tracheal injury than when using the minimal leak technique.

With the minimal leak technique, air should be injected into the cuff while ausculting over the trachea during breath delivery until no leak is noted. At this point air is removed from the cuff in 0.1-cc increments until a very small leak can be detected. This technique results in less injury to the tracheal wall but may increase the risk for aspiration of secretions and can only be performed with ET tubes that have a spring-locked pilot balloon.

Murphy-type tubes are the most commonly used cuffed ET tubes (see Figs. 23.2 and 23.3). This type of tube has a beveled tip with an eye hole ("Murphy eye") in the wall opposite the bevel to ensure airflow if the end hole is occluded against the tracheal wall. These tubes can be composed of silicone (Fig. 23.3a), rubber (Fig. 23.3b), or polyvinyl chloride (Fig. 23.3c). Each of these materials possesses different physical properties, which should be considered when choosing an ET tube for the small animal patient.

Polyvinyl chloride (PVC) and silicone ET tubes possess many similar attributes: they are made of a clear to semiopaque material that allow visualization of airflow and material within the tube. These tubes are less irritating to the airways than red rubber tubes. PVC tubes have a preformed curve, whereas silicone tubes are straight (the authors curved the ET tube pictured in Fig. 23.3 with a piece of purple suture to fit it in the image; without the suture, it is straight). Both types of tubes are more flexible than red rubber tubes, with silicone tubes the most flexible. A stylet may be needed with smaller silicone tubes to prevent them from bending during intubation. PVC tubes are labeled as single-use tubes, but they can be cleaned with typical antiseptic solutions and reused. The biggest advantage of PVC tubes is that they possess the low-pressure, high-volume cuffs that may be the least damaging to the trachea. Both types of tubes have self-sealing, spring-loaded pilot balloons, making it easier to ensure that the volume of air instilled into the cuff is retained.

Rubber ET tubes are affordable but have several properties that may make them less desirable for routine use. The tube is prone to drying out and cracking with repeated use, resulting in air leaks. Their opaque nature makes it difficult to assess air movement within the tube because accumulation of condensation cannot be noted and the cleanliness of the interior surface cannot be easily assessed. The rubber is more likely to retain agents used for cleaning and therefore may cause more tracheal irritation. Rubber tubes have high-pressure, low-volume cuffs that are associated with greater injury to the tracheal wall. Lastly, rubber ET tubes do not have a spring-loaded pilot balloon; therefore, an atraumatic clamp (Europlas Flowclamp Hemostat, Pollack International

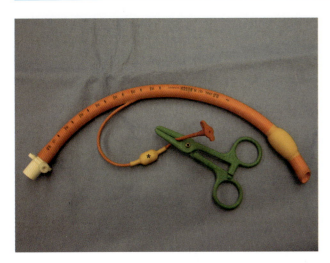

Figure 23.4 Because the pilot balloon (asterisk) on a rubber tube is not spring loaded, an atraumatic clamp should be applied to the cuff tubing to prevent accidental deflation of the cuff.

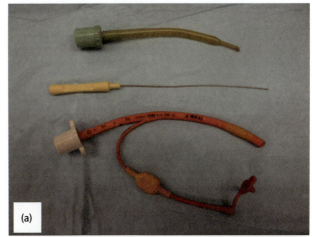

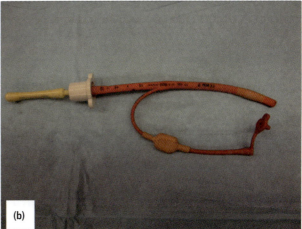

Figure 23.5 (a) Options for intubation of smaller animals such as cats and pediatric patients: an uncuffed Cole ET tube (top) and a smaller cuffed ET tube and metal stylet. (b) The metal stylet inserted into the smaller cuffed ET tube, with care that the tip of the stylet does not protrude from the end of the tube. The stylet provides support to the more flexible tube to facilitate intubation.

Ltd, Rosh Ha'ayin, Israel) must be applied to the cuff tubing to prevent cuff deflation while the patient is intubated (see Fig. 23.4).

Uncuffed ET tubes

It is difficult to find ET tubes smaller than 3.0 mm that are cuffed. When smaller animals such as cats, pediatric animals, or exotic pets require intubation, an uncuffed ET tube may need to be used. Cole ET tubes are designed with a wide portion proximally and a narrow portion distally; the area where the tube narrows is called the shoulder of the tube. These tubes are designed so the narrow portion of the tube is inserted into the larynx and trachea and the shoulder portion of the tube is situated at the level of the arytenoids to form a seal to minimize the risk for aspiration (see Fig. 23.5a). When using uncuffed tubes, it is important to use the largest tube that can be fit into the trachea without causing injury; this helps create the best seal for providing positive pressure breaths during anesthesia, limit air/gas leaks, and minimize the risk for aspiration.

Laryngoscope with illumination

The use of a handheld laryngoscope during routine intubation dramatically increases airway visualization and facilitates timely and accurate intubation in both cats and dogs. Laryngoscope lights should be routinely checked and repaired to ensure that the light bulb is in working order when needed for emergent situations. A variety of blades are available to attach to the handle of the laryngoscope. Short curved blades work best in cats,

whereas the straight blades, which are available in varying lengths, work best for most dogs (see Fig. 23.6).

Stylets

With smaller or extremely flexible ET tubes, placement of a stiff stylet into the interior of the tube during intubation may aid in tube placement. This is particularly true in cats with laryngospasm. Care should be taken to ensure that the tip of the stylet does not protrude beyond the tip of the ET tube to minimize injury to the larynx and trachea (see Fig. 23.5b).

Lidocaine (2%)

Topical lidocaine can be applied to the arytenoids prior to intubation to minimize laryngospasm and facilitate

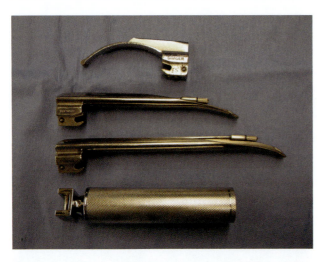

Figure 23.6 Illuminated laryngoscope. The top blade, a pediatric curved blade, is most useful in cats. The straight Miller blades (middle and bottom) are most useful for dogs.

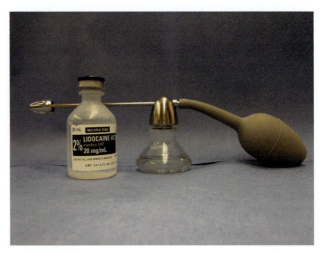

Figure 23.7 An atomizer used to distill lidocaine onto the arytenoids to facilitate intubation.

intubation. In addition, it can reduce the amount of premedication and induction agent needed to establish an airway. Lidocaine can be placed into a needleless syringe, or an atomizer (see Fig. 23.7) can be used to deliver it to the perilaryngeal tissues. Cats are more sensitive to the toxic effects of lidocaine; therefore, care should be taken to ensure that the dose administered is safe. In most cats, a dose of 0.5 mL of less of 2% lidocaine should be sufficient to provide local anesthesia without causing toxicity.

Securing the ET tube

Once the ET tube is properly inserted into the airway, securing the tube in place is of utmost importance to limit airway trauma and reduce the risk for inadvertent extubation. Cloth muzzle gauze (Kendall Curity Bandage Roll, Tyco Healthcare, Mansfield, MA) should be tied around the ET tube caudal to the adapter but rostral to the pilot balloon tube tubing and positioned at the level just behind the canine teeth and then secured to the upper or lower jaw or behind the ears. Alternatively, a section of intravenous (IV) fluid tubing can be used rather than muzzle gauze. One advantage of IV fluid tubing is that it can be washed and reused between patients, limiting waste. However, fluid tubing provides a less secure grip on the ET tube and can be a source for bacterial contamination.

Intubation techniques

As mentioned previously, preparation is critical in successful ET intubation in emergency situations. All supplies that may be needed should be accessible and ET

tubes of all sizes should be readily available for daily use. ET tubes should be regularly checked for cracking, and cuffs should be inflated to find potential leaks or weaknesses in the material.

Choosing appropriate ET tube size

ET width

Selecting an appropriate-size ET tube is important to facilitate rapid intubation, minimize tracheal trauma, and ensure that the airway is appropriately protected. If too large a tube is used, it may cause trauma to the airway and result in swelling and rupture. If too small a tube is used, it will result in leaks around the cuff and protection of the airway will be compromised. Overinflating the cuff to compensate for an undersized ET tube can result in tracheal necrosis and rupture.[1] In addition, increased airway resistance may be seen when the ET tube is too small.

Various techniques can be used to aid in choosing an appropriate-size ET tube. Unfortunately, these techniques are not routinely reliable and may not be applicable to certain breeds. Time and experience with intubation of many different sizes and breeds is often needed before one is able confidently to select the correct ET size. Initially, you will simply need to look at the animal and make an estimate on tube size. You should have readily available to you an ET tube that is both one size larger and one size smaller than the tube you initially chose in case visual inspection reveals a narrower or wider airway opening than initially expected.

One method of selecting an ET tube is by correlating body weight to tracheal size.[2-4] Although these size

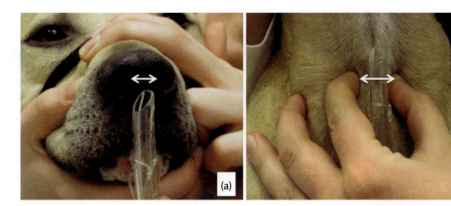

Figure 23.8 Techniques for estimating ET tube size. (a) The width of the nasal septum is measured and used as a guide for selection of ET tube size. (b) The extrathoracic trachea is palpated and used as a guide for selection of ET tube size.

charts may be used as a general guideline, this may not prove accurate in certain animals, such as brachycephalic breeds and those animals with abnormal body condition score (those that are excessively thin or overweight).[2]

Another method for selecting ET tube size is by evaluating the width of the nasal septum. The ET tube should be held up to the narrowest point between the nares (see Fig. 23.8a). The ET tube with an outer diameter that best matches the width of the nasal septum should be used. However, a recent study found that this technique was only effective 21% of the time, and there was no actual correlation between internal or external diameter of the tube and nasal septum width in dogs.[2]

Palpation of the width of the extrathoracic trachea just above the thoracic inlet can also be used to estimate ET tube size (see Fig. 23.8b). This technique was found to be more effective than nasal septum measurement, successful 46% of the time, but it still had a wide margin of error.[2] Palpation of the trachea can be difficult in brachycephalic breeds and in obese pets.

ET tube length

The ET tube length is just as important as its width. Fortunately, this measurement is much easier to perform. When placed, the adapter, to which external tubing for oxygen delivery and ventilatory support is attached, should be positioned just cranial to the incisor teeth while the distal portion of the tube should end at the level of the thoracic inlet. This can be easily measured by holding an ET tube up to the patient's neck and estimating distance prior to intubation. This length of tubing is important because excessively long ET tubes contribute to mechanical dead space and increase the work of breathing. A long tube may also divert at the tracheal bifurcation into a bronchus, resulting in venti-

lating only a portion of the lungs (single bronchus or "one-lung" intubation). If the tube is measured to be too long, it can easily be cut to the appropriate length. Remove the adapter at the rostral end, cut to size, and reattach the adapter to the tube.

Intubating dogs

The dog should ideally be in sternal recumbency, although lateral recumbency can be used if needed in large dogs. If the dog is breathing spontaneously, preoxygenation is ideal. Emergency situations in which the animal is agonal, still has jaw tone, or is struggling may require some sedation. Drugs that can be reversed such as benzodiazepines should be considered. Short-acting agents such as propofol or thiopental may also be utilized for rapid intubation. If performing general anesthesia, premedication and induction agents are used. Neuromuscular blocking agents may also be used in certain situations where traditional sedation protocols are not feasible.

An assistant should open the mouth by placing one hand just behind the maxillary canine teeth with the thumb and index finger (thumb and middle finger in large dogs) (see Fig. 23.9a). The other hand should grasp the distal portion of the tongue using a dry gauze square. The tongue should be pulled out over the lower incisors and ventral, thus opening the oral cavity for easier visualization. The head should be pulled rostrally and dorsally, which straightens the neck and facilitates full view of the pharynx and larynx (see Fig. 23.9b).

At this time the person intubating should place the laryngoscope blade into the oral cavity. The tongue should be depressed just rostral to, but not touching, the base of the epiglottis. The epiglottis, which normally sits covering the laryngeal opening, should flip ventrally to reveal the arytenoids (vocal cords) (see Fig. 23.9c). At

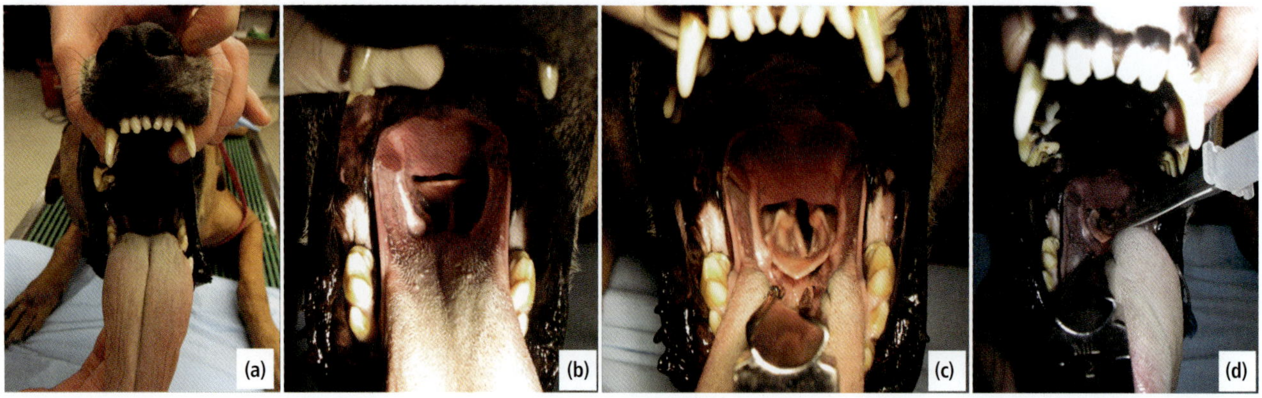

Figure 23.9 A diagram of the intubation sequence of a dog. (a) The dog is placed in sternal recumbency and the upper jaw should be grasped behind the canine teeth while the tongue is pulled rostrally between the canine teeth while the lower jaw is opened. (b) View of the caudal oropharynx when the mouth is properly opened for intubation. Note that the epiglottis is elevated, obscuring view of the glottis and arytenoids. (c) The laryngoscope is inserted into the mouth and the tip is used to place pressure on the base of the tongue. Care should be taken to avoid touching the epiglottis with the laryngoscope blade to minimize airway trauma. When properly positioned, a good view of the glottis and arytenoids is achieved. (d) Following intubation, direct visualization of the ET tube between the arytenoids is the most accurate way to ensure proper intubation.

times the epiglottis is caught behind the soft palate and the laryngoscope can be used to gently release it. Care should be taken not to apply pressure to the epiglottis because edema can result.

If not done previously, the appropriate-size ET tube is selected, and sterile aqueous lubricant is applied to the distal end. Care should be taken not to occlude the Murphy eye (if applicable). The ET tube should be advanced over the epiglottis without contact and through the vocal cords (see Fig. 23.9d). The ET tube should be oriented with the bevel to the right of the person inserting the tube (in tubes with Murphy eyes, the Murphy eye would be to the left). In this orientation, the curve of the ET tube follows the curve of the trachea.

The adapter should ideally remain just cranial to the incisors on midline with the nasal septum to avoid the tube being inadvertently chewed and inhaled by the patient. The tube should be secured with a length of muzzle gauze or similar material. The gauze is first tied around the ET tube near the junction of the adapter. In large dogs it should be secured around the muzzle behind the canines. In small dogs the gauze can be secured around the head behind the ears.

With an appropriate size syringe, air should be injected into the pilot balloon to inflate the cuff to a maximum of 20 to 25 cm H_2O. If the ability to measure pressure is unavailable, use the smallest amount needed to maintain a slight leak (see previous section). This will ensure that the tracheal mucosa is minimally compromised. Red rubber ET tubes do not have a spring-locked pilot balloon to occlude the cuff. Thus the pilot balloon

tubing should be occluded using an atraumatic clamp so that the cuff will not deflate when removing the air syringe (see Fig. 23.4).

While the ET tube is being tied in and the cuff inflated, a manual resuscitator can be connected to the adapter to provide breaths. If general anesthesia is being performed, the breathing system would than be connected to the patient. See Protocol 23.1 for concise step-by-step instructions on intubating dogs.

Intubating cats

As with dogs, cats should ideally be in sternal recumbency. This should be easier to perform because their smaller size facilitates easier handling. If the cat is breathing spontaneously, preoxygenation is ideal. Emergency situations where the animal is agonal, still has jaw tone, or is struggling may require sedation. Drugs that can be reversed such as benzodiazepines should be considered. Short-acting agents such as propofol or thiopental may also be utilized for fast intubation. If performing general anesthesia, premedication and induction agents are used. Neuromuscular blocking agents may also be used in certain situations where traditional sedation protocols are not feasible.

An assistant should open the mouth by placing one hand just behind the maxillary canine teeth with the thumb and index finger. The other hand should grasp the distal portion of the tongue using a dry gauze square. The tongue should be pulled rostrally over the lower incisors and ventral, thus opening the oral cavity for easier visualization. The head should be pulled rostrally

Protocol 23.1 Endotracheal intubation in a dog

Items Required
- Three different-size endotracheal tubes
  - Cuffs previously checked if applicable
    - One of estimated size
    - One each of size smaller and larger
- Laryngoscope
- Sterile aqueous lubricant
- Gauze squares for grasping the tongue
- Length of muzzle gauze for tying in ET tube
- Appropriate size air syringe
  - 3–5 mL: small dog/5–10 mL: large dog
- Atraumatic clamp if using rubber tube
- Cotton-tipped applicators
- Oxygen, mask
- Assistant (usually required in an emergency)

Procedure
1. Collect necessary supplies.
2. For conscious animals, heavy sedation to light anesthesia will be required.
3. Position the dog in sternal recumbency (lateral recumbency can be used if needed in large dogs).
4. Provide preoxygenation if possible.
5. Assistant: Open the mouth by using thumb and one finger of the dominant hand to grasp behind the maxillary canine teeth and the nondominant hand to grasp the distal portion of the tongue using a dry gauze square. Pull the tongue out over the lower incisors and ventral, opening the oral cavity widely. Pull the head rostrally and dorsally, to facilitate intubator's full view of the pharynx and larynx.
6. Intubator: Place the laryngoscope blade into the oral cavity. Depress the tongue just rostral to, but not touching, the base of the epiglottis. The epiglottis should flip ventrally to reveal the arytenoids.
7. Select the appropriate-size ET tube and apply sterile aqueous lubricant to the distal end, avoiding the Murphy eye.
8. Advance the ET tube over the epiglottis without contact and through the arytenoids. Orient the ET tube with the bevel to the right of the person inserting the tube (in tubes with Murphy eyes, the Murphy eye would be to the left).
9. The adapter should remain just cranial to the incisors on midline. Secure the tube with a length of muzzle gauze or similar material. First tie the gauze around the ET tube near the junction of the adapter. In large dogs it should be secured around the muzzle behind the canines. In small dogs the gauze can be secured around the head behind the ears.
10. With an appropriate-size syringe, inject air into the pilot balloon to inflate the cuff to a maximum of 20 to 25 cm H_2O. If the ability to measure pressure is unavailable, use the smallest amount needed to maintain a slight leak when breaths are manually delivered.
    a. If using a red rubber ET tube, occlude the pilot balloon tubing with an atraumatic clamp.
11. While the ET tube is being secured and the cuff inflated, a manual resuscitator can be connected to the adapter to provide breaths. If general anesthesia is being performed, the breathing system would than be connected to the patient.

and dorsally, which straightens the neck and facilitates full view of the pharynx and larynx.

At this time the person intubating the cat should place the laryngoscope blade into the oral cavity. The tongue should be depressed rostral to, but not touching, the base of the epiglottis. If available, short curved laryngoscope blades tend to work better in cats. The epiglottis, which normally sits covering the laryngeal opening, should flip down to reveal the arytenoids (vocal cords). Extreme care should be taken when intubating a cat because they are more prone to laryngeal edema and inflammation than dogs.

Cats are also prone to laryngospasm, which can result in upper airway obstruction and make intubation virtually impossible. If this is the case, 2% lidocaine can be used to paralyze the vocal cords to facilitate intubation. One drop applied to each vocal cord with a needleless tuberculin syringe should be sufficient. The vocal cords should not be touched by the syringe. An atomizer may also be used if available to spray each vocal cord. Usually, 30 seconds to a minute is needed for the 2% lidocaine to take effect. Because of the risk of laryngospasm and difficult intubation in cats, preoxygenation is suggested to avoid hypoxemia secondary to hypoventilation.

If not done previously, the appropriate-size ET tube is selected and sterile aqueous lubricant is applied to the distal end. Care should be taken not to occlude the Murphy eye (if applicable). The ET tube sizes used in cats are smaller, so they tend to be more flaccid. A stylet may be used to stiffen the ET tube and allow easier passage through the vocal cords. Care must be taken to ensure that the end of the stylet does not protrude past the end of the ET tube because airway puncture or laceration could result. The ET tube should be advanced over the epiglottis without contact and through the vocal cords. The ET tube should be oriented with the bevel to the right of the person inserting the tube (in tubes with Murphy eyes, they would be to the left). In this orientation, the curve of the ET tube follows the curve of the trachea.

The adapter should ideally stay just cranial to the incisors on midline with the nasal septum to avoid the tube being inadvertently chewed by the patient. The tube should be tied in with a length of muzzle gauze or similar material. The gauze is first tied around the ET tube at the adapter and can be secured around the head behind the ears.

With a 3-cc syringe, air should be injected into the pilot balloon to inflate the cuff to a maximum of 20 to 25 cm H_2O. If the ability to measure pressure is unavailable, use the smallest amount needed to maintain a slight leak (see previous section). This will ensure that the tracheal mucosa is minimally compromised. Red rubber ET tubes do not have a spring-locked pilot balloon to occlude the cuff. The pilot balloon tubing will need to be occluded using an atraumatic clamp so that the cuff will not deflate when removing the air syringe (see Fig. 23.4).

While the ET tube is being tied in and the cuff inflated, a manual resuscitator can be connected to the adapter to provide breaths. In general anesthesia the breathing system would be connected to the patient. See Protocol 23.2 for concise step-by-step instructions for intubating cats.

Intubation of difficult airways

Difficult intubation should be expected and planned for in animals with oropharyngeal trauma, upper airway obstruction, and brachycephalic airway syndrome. In most situations, difficult intubations can be remedied by providing a deeper level of sedation with injectable anesthetic agents, optimizing patient positioning, using a laryngoscope, and illuminating the oral cavity. If excessive secretions are present in the oropharynx, it should be cleared away with gauze, cotton-tipped applicators, or suction to improve airway visualization. A closed-tip suction catheter or red rubber catheter can be attached to a vacuum source via tubing (see Chapter 25, Artificial Airway Management).

If intubation cannot be accomplished using these methods, intubation with a smaller size ET tube than expected should be attempted to gain control of the airway. Once an adequate plane of anesthesia has been achieved, the tube can be replaced with a larger tube if a leak is present.

If the ET tube is not stiff enough, as happens with smaller size and silicone tubes, a stylet can be placed into the tube to make the tube less flimsy. This is particularly helpful when attempting to bypass masses in the oral cavity, which may cause the tip of the tube to deviate away from the larynx. Care should be taken to ensure that the tip of the stylet does not extend beyond the tip of the tube to prevent injury to the airway.

A "guidewire," such as a 5F or 8F polyurethane or red rubber catheter can be used to facilitate difficult intubations. The catheter can be inserted into the airway and then the ET tube fed over the catheter into the airway. The catheter is then removed once an airway has been established.

Retrograde intubation is another technique that can be used to facilitate ET intubation when standard techniques are not successful. Similar to the technique used for transtracheal washing, a long through-the-needle catheter is inserted into the airway either between two tracheal rings or through the cricothyroid ligament. Unlike during transtracheal washing, the catheter bevel should be directed up when inserted into the airway. Once in, the hub of the needle is lowered (so that the tip of the needle and catheter point toward the head), the needle removed from the airway, and the catheter is fed in an oral direction up through the larynx. This catheter with or without internal guidewire is then used as a guidewire, over which to pass and guide the ET tube into the airway, and then removed.

Jet ventilation with a long large-bore catheter (i.e., 14- to 16-gauge, 9- to 13-inch IV catheter) can be utilized as a means to maintain oxygen saturation and CO_2 elimination when intubation cannot be achieved (see Chapter 29, High-Frequency Ventilation). This technique is primarily used during bronchoscopy when an ET tube cannot be used because the bronchoscope is too large to pass through the it. The catheter is inserted orotracheally alongside the bronchoscope.

Alternatively, transtracheal oxygen delivery and jet ventilation can be used as an emergency procedure when orotracheal intubation cannot be achieved. With transtracheal jet ventilation, a 16-gauge catheter (Venocath-16, Venisystems, Abbott Ireland, Sligo, Ireland) is inserted percutaneously into the trachea through the cricothy-

Protocol 23.2 Endotracheal intubation in a cat

Items Required
- Three different-size endotracheal tubes, cuffs
  - Previously checked if applicable
    - One of estimated size
    - One each of size smaller and larger
- Laryngoscope, curved blade if available
- Sterile aqueous lubricant
- Gauze squares for grasping the tongue
- Length of muzzle gauze for tying in ET tube
- Appropriate-size air syringe
  - 3 mL usually sufficient
- Atraumatic clamp if using red rubber ET tube
- 2% lidocaine to prevent laryngospasm, in either needleless 1-mL syringe or in an atomizer
- Stylet
- Cotton-tipped applicators
- Oxygen, mask
- Assistant (usually required in an emergency)

Procedure
1. Collect necessary supplies.
2. For conscious animals, heavy sedation to light anesthesia will be required.
3. Position the cat in sternal recumbency.
4. Provide preoxygenation if possible: more important than in most dogs due to potential for laryngospasm.
5. Assistant: Open the mouth by using thumb and one finger of the dominant hand to grasp behind the maxillary canine teeth and the nondominant hand to grasp the distal portion of the tongue using a dry gauze square. Pull the tongue out over the lower incisors and ventral, opening the oral cavity widely. Pull the head rostrally and dorsally, to facilitate intubator's full view of the pharynx and larynx.
6. Intubator: Place the (ideally curved) laryngoscope blade into the oral cavity. Depress the tongue just rostral to, but not touching, the base of the epiglottis. The epiglottis should flip ventrally to reveal the arytenoids.
7. If the cat has laryngospasm, apply 2% lidocaine to the vocal cords: either one drop applied to each vocal cord with a needleless tuberculin syringe or sprayed using an atomizer. Do not contact the arytenoids. Usually, 30 to 60 seconds are required for the lidocaine to take effect.
8. Select the appropriate-size ET tube and apply sterile aqueous lubricant to the distal end, avoiding the Murphy eye. If the tube is very flaccid, a stylet may be used to stiffen the ET tube. The stylet must not protrude past the end of the ET tube.
9. Advance the ET tube over the epiglottis without contact and through the arytenoids. Extreme care should be taken when intubating a cat because they are more prone to laryngeal edema and inflammation than dogs. Orient the ET tube with the bevel to the right of the person inserting the tube (in tubes with Murphy eyes, the Murphy eye would be to the left).
10. The adapter should remain just cranial to the incisors on midline. Secure the tube with a length of muzzle gauze or similar material. First tie the gauze around the ET tube near the junction of the adapter, and then tie the gauze around the head behind the ears.
11. With a 3-cc syringe, inject air into the pilot balloon to inflate the cuff to a maximum of 20 to 25 cm H_2O. If the ability to measure pressure is unavailable, use the smallest amount needed to maintain a slight leak when breaths are manually delivered.
    a. If using a red rubber ET tube, occlude the pilot balloon tubing with an atraumatic clamp.
12. While the ET tube is being secured and the cuff inflated, a manual resuscitator can be connected to the adapter to provide breaths. If general anesthesia is being performed, the breathing system would than be connected to the patient.

roid ligament or between two tracheal rings and directed distally. It is important to secure this catheter adequately to the outside of the neck with sutures to prevent catheter migration, which could result in marked subcutaneous emphysema. The catheter can be connected to the anesthesia machine via an adapter (i.e., connect a 1-cc syringe to the catheter, and then cut off the end and attach that to noncompliant oxygen tubing). The flush valve on the anesthesia machine is used to provide breaths to the animal.[5]

Rarely, an emergency tracheostomy may be required to secure an airway in cats and dogs. In most instances, however, airway access can be obtained via the one of the techniques described here, and a tracheostomy can be performed, if needed, in a controlled manner (see Chapter 24, Temporary Tracheostomy).

Techniques to confirm tracheal intubation

Accidental intubation of the esophagus is a common occurrence due to close proximity of the esophagus to the trachea. Confirmation of correct placement into the trachea should be performed after insertion. Visual confirmation of the ET tube passing between the vocal cords is the only definitive way of confirming correct placement. Various other methods can be used to ensure proper placement is maintained, but these techniques may not be as reliable as direct visualization:

1. The animal may cough when the ET tube is advanced into the trachea. This usually only occurs if the animal is not heavily sedated.
2. Condensation may be seen through a clear tube on exhalation signifying air movement.
3. Palpation of the ventral cervical region should reveal one rigid structure. The presence of two rigid tubular structures indicates that the ET tube is in the esophagus.
4. Auscultation of the lungs while a breath is given to listen for lung sounds.
5. The chest wall should expand while a breath is being given. The abdomen should be not become distended to the same extent as the chest.
6. Capnometry can be used to detect the PCO_2 of the gas expelled from the tube. If the ET tube is in the esophagus, no CO_2 should be detected. If the tube is correctly placed in the trachea, CO_2 should be measurable and a waveform should be associated with breathing. It is important to note that this technique will not be useful to confirm intubation in animals with cardiac arrest due to the absence of circulation and therefore lack of CO_2 return to the lungs.

If at any time the parameters just listed raise the question of proper placement, direct visualization should be performed.

Risks and complications of tracheal intubation

Although placement of an ET tube has many benefits to the patient, complications can occur if proper technique is not utilized. One must weigh the benefits and risks before intubating a patient.

Cats appear to be at greater risk for complications associated with tracheal intubation.[6–8] Cats are prone to laryngospasm, which can make tracheal intubation difficult. Laryngospasm can be minimized by applying 2% lidocaine to the arytenoids before intubation and avoiding contact with the epiglottis and arytenoids while passing the ET tube. Airway trauma is also more likely to occur in cats. Excessive force during intubation and overinflation of the cuff may happen inadvertently due to their small size.

Dogs, particularly brachycephalic breeds, can have elongated soft palates that entrap the epiglottis. Brachycephalic breeds also have redundant oral tissue and hypoplastic tracheas, making intubation more difficult, which can result in pharyngeal and laryngeal edema. Dogs are also susceptible to vagal stimulation during intubation, which can cause bradycardia and dysrhythmias.

Choosing the appropriate size and length of ET tube (see previous section) can make the difference between a successful intubation and multiple failed attempts that cause trauma to the pharynx and larynx. Forceful intubation and excessive pressure exerted by the laryngoscope blade can result in edema of the epiglottis and vocal cords. This could lead to an upper airway obstruction and the need for alternative techniques (such as tracheostomy) to establish and maintain a patent airway. Forceful intubation could also result in unintentional tearing of an arytenoid.[8]

Overinflation of the cuff can cause tracheal trauma. When repositioning an intubated animal, the ET tube should be disconnected from the anesthetic circuit to prevent excessive traction on the trachea. Excessive traction and torsion on the ET tube can result in tracheal necrosis and/or rupture. This is particularly important during anesthesia for dental procedures, where excessive manipulation of the oral cavity may occur during cleaning and extractions.

When prolonged cuff inflation is needed, as during mechanical ventilation and lengthy general anesthesia, it is recommended that the cuff be deflated, repositioned, and reinflated periodically (at least daily). This will ensure adequate blood flow to all areas of the trachea. There can be complications associated with this, including inadvertent aspiration of oral and gastric secretions or movement of the tube into the esophagus. Care must be taken during repositioning of the ET tube.

Increased pressure from the inflated cuff and decreased blood flow to the trachea can result in tracheal necrosis, rupture, and stenosis. This is more commonly seen in cats than dogs.[6,7] Tracheal necrosis can lead to tears in the tracheal wall. This causes subcutaneous emphysema and pneumomediastinum. Increasing mediastinal pressures can result in a pneumothorax, pneumoretroperitoneum, and even pneumoperitoneum. Most cases of tracheal rupture do not require surgery but can take several weeks before the leak seals and subcutaneous emphysema reabsorbs.[6,7] Medical management in the form of oxygen supplementation, alleviating excessive subcutaneous emphysema with needle aspiration, and analgesics for discomfort is usually sufficient while the tracheal tear seals on its own. If the leak is persistent or severe, surgical repair of the tear may be required. Scar tissue that forms as the tracheal mucosa heals may result in tracheal stenosis at the site of injury. Depending on the severity, it may cause respiratory problems in the future that require surgery.

Extubation

Animals should only be extubated after confirmation that the gag reflex has been reestablished and their airway can be protected. The oral cavity should be assessed for excessive secretions prior to extubation. Excessive oral secretions may occur with salivation, hemorrhage or regurgitation, and they could be aspirated when the animal is extubated. Any secretions should be suctioned or swabbed from the oral cavity before removing the ET tube.

The cuff should be fully deflated prior to extubation, except in cases where the airway may be compromised. Leaving a small amount of air in the cuff while extubating may be beneficial in animals with megaesophagus and in brachycephalic breeds. In some of these cases, it may be best to wait until the animal is actively coughing and trying to chew the tube. It is important to keep the ET tube on midline with the nasal septum so that shearing does not occur.

Once extubated, the animal should be closely monitored for complications that may warrant reintubation. The head should be kept elevated to avoid aspiration from regurgitation, and flow-by oxygen should be administered. Respiration and oxygenation should be monitored until the animal is fully awake.

Summary

ET intubation is an essential skill for all veterinarians and veterinary technicians. It is a lifesaving measure in patients with cardiopulmonary arrest and those in severe respiratory distress, and it is required during most general anesthetic procedures. Proper equipment and technique help minimize trauma and complications associated with intubation, and special techniques exist to help facilitate difficult intubation. Veterinarians and veterinary technicians should practice these skills frequently to be prepared in case of an emergency.

References

1. Alderson B, Senior AHA, Dugdale JM. Tracheal necrosis following tracheal intubation in a dog. J Small Anim Pract 2006;47(12): 754–756.

2. Lish J, Ko JC, Payton ME. Evaluation of two methods of endotracheal tube selection in dogs. J Am Anim Hosp Assoc 2008; 44:236–242.

3. Waddell KW, Ponder CA. In: Carroll GL, ed. Small Animal Anesthesia and Analgesia. Ames, IA: Blackwell; 2008:260–265.

4. McKelvey D, Hollingshead KW. Veterinary Anesthesia and Analgesia. 3rd ed. St. Louis, MO: Mosby; 2003:66–74, 166–170.

5. Haskins SC, Orima H, Yamamoto Y, et al. Clinical tolerance and bronchoscopic changes associated with transtracheal high-frequency jet ventilation in dogs and cats. J Vet Emerg Crit Care 1992;2:6–10.

6. Hardie EM, Spodnick GJ, Gilson SD, et al. Tracheal rupture in cats: 16 cases (1983–1998). J Vet Med Assoc 1999;214(4):508–512.

7. Mitchell SL, McCarthy R, Rudloff E, Pernell RT. Tracheal rupture associated with intubation in cats: 20 cases (1996–1998). J Vet Med Assoc 2002;216(10):1592–1595.

8. Hofmeister EH, Trim CM, Kley S, Cornell K. Traumatic endotracheal intubation in the cat. Vet Anaest Analg 2007;34(3): 213–216.

24

Temporary tracheostomy

F.A. (Tony) Mann and Mary M. Flanders

Indications

The primary indication for temporary tracheostomy tube placement is to relieve life-threatening upper airway obstruction due to trauma, foreign body, laryngeal paralysis, or neoplasia. Other indications include facilitating removal of lower airway secretions when there is compromised cough reflex, allowing manual or mechanical ventilation when orotracheal intubation is not practical, reducing airway resistance in patients where increased intracranial pressure is a concern, and permitting inhalant anesthesia during certain intraoral surgical procedures.

Equipment

Most commercially available tracheostomy tubes are made of plastic or silicone. The most versatile tubes contain an inflatable cuff and inner cannula as well as the standard obturator and tube tie (see Figs. 24.1 and 24.2). Some tube sizes are too small to contain a cuff and inner cannula, so many small dogs and cats do not benefit from those two accessories. The cuff is only needed when positive pressure ventilation is necessary, such as with patients requiring general anesthesia or ventilator therapy. In fact, the cuff may be disadvantageous in management of airway obstruction in awake patients because of the possibility of secretions accumulating around the deflated cuff. High-volume, low-pressure cuffs are preferred for patients requiring ventilation, and when these cuffs are deflated there is significant surface area of the wrinkled cuff to harbor accumulations of secretions. The inner cannula is helpful for tube hygiene and maintenance because the cannula may be easily removed and replaced. Without the inner cannula, there is more emphasis on tracheal suctioning, and more frequent tube changes may be necessary. Single-lumen tubes must be removed and replaced with a new tube or reinserted into the stoma site after each cleaning.

When an appropriate commercial tracheostomy tube is not available, a tracheostomy tube may be fashioned from a standard endotracheal tube (see Fig. 24.3). Choose an endotracheal tube that is approximately one size smaller than you would choose for orotracheal intubation. Remove the endotracheal tube connector and bisect the tube along its length until the uncut portion of the tube is the necessary tracheostomy tube length. If the need to inflate the cuff is anticipated, the cuts can be carefully made to preserve the inflation channel. The two halves of the bisected portion of the tube may be used as a flange to which the ties can be attached. Reattach the endotracheal tube connector at the flange-tube junction. The flange may be shortened to a convenient length prior to attaching the ties. One disadvantage of this modified tube when the inflation channel is preserved is that the natural curve of the tube is about 90 degrees rotated; however, no untoward patient consequences with this deviation have yet to be reported.

The size of tracheostomy tube is important to a successful procedure and good outcome. Ideally, the tracheostomy tube should be a half to a third of the tracheal diameter to minimize iatrogenic tracheal trauma and decrease the incidence of postintubation stenosis. Also, an appropriate-size tube that allows some airflow around it may prevent respiratory arrest should tube occlusion

Advanced Monitoring and Procedures for Small Animal Emergency and Critical Care, First Edition. Edited by Jamie M. Burkitt Creedon, Harold Davis.
© 2012 John Wiley & Sons, Inc. Published 2012 by John Wiley & Sons, Inc.

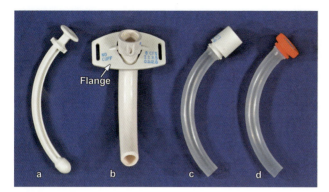

Figure 24.1 Commercially available uncuffed tracheostomy tube with disassembled components: (a) obturator, which is inserted into the tracheostomy tube immediately before placement and removed as soon as the tube is in the trachea; (b) tracheostomy tube, which is secured with umbilical tapes attached to eyelets in the flange and tied behind the neck; (c) inner cannula, which is placed in the tracheostomy tube and replaced at regular intervals, and (d) closed-end cannula, which can be used to temporarily occlude the tracheostomy tube to see if the patient can breathe around the tube.

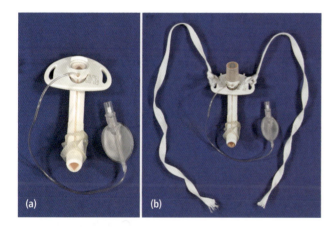

Figure 24.2 Commercially available cuffed tracheostomy tube (a) without inner cannula and (b) with inner cannula locked in place and umbilical tapes tied to eyelets in the flange. Note: The cuff would only be inflated when positive-pressure ventilation is necessary; a deflated cuff increases the surface area on which secretions could accumulate thereby complicating tracheostomy hygiene.

occur. However, a tube that is too small may cause resistance to airflow if the patient must breathe entirely through the tube with no airflow around it. Tube size should allow air passage both around and through the tube for uncuffed tubes and for tubes with deflated cuffs. Available tracheostomy tube sizes that may be applied to dogs and cats range from 00 to 10. Sizes 00 to 5.5 are

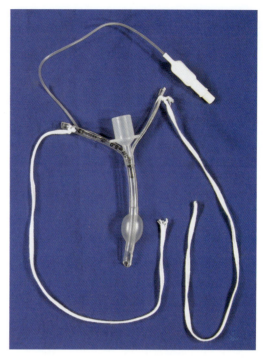

Figure 24.3 Tracheostomy tube fashioned from a standard endotracheal tube. Note: The inflation channel can be preserved if the cuff is needed. Preserving the inflation channel results in a curve to the tube that is rotated about 90 degrees to the desired curve.

neonatal/pediatric sizes and are too small to be available with inner cannulas, whereas sizes 6.0 or larger may come with removable inner cannulas. Tracheostomy tube sizes are equivalent to endotracheal tube sizes but can be misleading because they do not necessarily correlate to the millimeter diameters of the tubes. For example, a size 6.0 tracheostomy tube may have an inner diameter of 6.4 mm, but an outer diameter of 10.8 mm. Therefore, one should always check the inner and outer diameter dimensions typically located on the tube flange to choose the tube that will best fit the trachea in question. The largest possible inner diameter is always desired, but the outer diameter will determine if the tube will appropriately fit in the trachea.

Tube length should extend six to seven tracheal rings down from the placement site. Ideal tube length may not be achieved in all veterinary patients because of the limits of what is commercially available, but tailor-made tubes fashioned from endotracheal tubes can be used when the length of commercially available tubes is too far from appropriate.

Other equipment needed for tracheostomy tube placement includes an endotracheal tube for orotracheal intubation, standard anesthetic supplies, clippers,

> **Box 24.1.** Minimally suggested surgical instruments required for tracheostomy
>
> - Two towel forceps
> - Scalpel handle to accommodate a number 10 or 15 blade
> - Thumb forceps (Adson-Brown or DeBakey tissue forceps)
> - Metzenbaum scissors
> - Needle holders
> - Two mosquito hemostatic forceps
> - Suture scissors.
> - Ideally, self-retaining retractors, such as Gelpi perineal retractors (preferably two) or a Weitlaner retractor

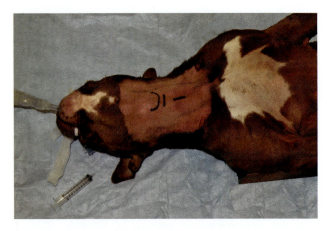

Figure 24.4 Positioning and preparation for tracheostomy tube placement. The dog is in dorsal recumbence with the thoracic limbs pulled caudally. The airway is captured with an endotracheal tube attached to anesthetic tubing. The curved mark on the skin represents the area of the caudal aspect of the thyroid cartilage, the straight mark immediately caudal to the curved mark represents the cricoid cartilage, and the midline straight mark indicates the proposed skin incision. Note the widely clipped and prepared surgical field. The syringe is present as a reminder that the endotracheal tube needs to be deflated and the endotracheal tube removed as the tracheostomy tube is inserted.

prepping scrub and solution, barrier drape, sterile surgical gloves, sterile gauze, surgical instruments, suture material, and, if not supplied with the tracheostomy tube, umbilical tape for securing the tube after it is in place. The minimally suggested surgical instruments, which may be packaged together in a tracheostomy pack, are two towel forceps, a scalpel handle to accommodate a number 10 or number 15 scalpel blade, thumb forceps (Adson-Brown or DeBakey tissue forceps), Metzenbaum scissors, needle holders, two mosquito hemostatic forceps, and suture scissors. It is also handy to have some self-retaining retractors, such as a Gelpi perineal retractor (preferably two) or a Weitlaner retractor, which may be included in the tracheostomy pack or wrapped separately. Suction capability and an oxygen source should be readily available during the procedure (see Text Box 24.1).

Positioning and aseptic preparation

The emergent "slash" tracheostomy should be a rare occurrence; there is usually time to capture the airway with an endotracheal tube and prepare the patient for a controlled surgical approach (see Chapter 23, Tracheal Intubation). Once intubated and in an appropriate plane of general anesthesia, the patient is placed in dorsal recumbence (see Fig. 24.4). The neck is extended and the thoracic limbs are pulled caudally and secured to the table with ties or tape. A positioning aid, such as a thoracic positioning trough, may be used to keep the patient from leaning to one side.

An area large enough for a ventral midline skin incision made longitudinally from the cricoid cartilage to the fourth or fifth tracheal ring is clipped and prepared; this area should extend sufficiently far laterally to create an area on each side wide enough to allow easy skin cleaning and tube maintenance. In most cases, a sufficient surgical field can be achieved by clipping the ventral neck from the angle of the mandibles to the manubrium and laterally past the level of the jugular veins (see Fig. 24.4). For longhaired dogs and cats, overhanging fur should be trimmed. Breeds with excessive skin folds may require skin to be deflected dorsally and taped or temporarily tacked with sutures to prevent the skin folds from contaminating or occluding the tracheostomy area when the animal is no longer in dorsal recumbence.

After clipping and vacuuming, a rolled towel may be placed underneath (dorsal to) the neck to stabilize the neck and prevent the surgical site from sinking away during surgical manipulations, and a standard aseptic surgical skin preparation is performed.

Procedure

The prepared surgical site is isolated with a barrier drape secured with two towel forceps (see Fig. 24.5). A single drape fenestrated over the proposed skin incision is usually sufficient, but quarter draping may be performed if desired. Quarter draping requires at least four towel forceps. Make a ventral midline cervical skin incision just caudal to the larynx for a distance of approximately 3 to 4 cm, depending on the size of the patient (see Fig. 24.5a). Apply a self-retaining retractor to hold open the

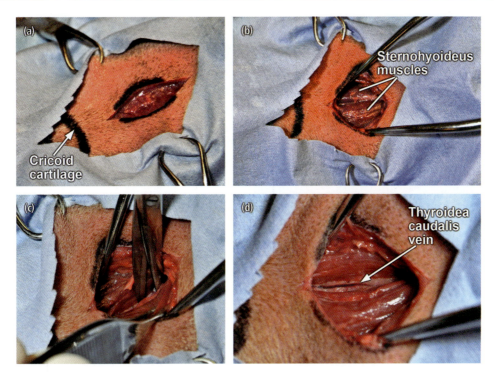

Figure 24.5 Surgical approach to the trachea for tracheostomy tube placement. Cranial is to the left in all frames. (a) The skin incision is made immediately caudal to the cricoid cartilage over approximately the first through fourth tracheal rings. (b) The skin edges are retracted with a Gelpi retractor to facilitate identification of the sternohyoideus muscles and their midline division. (c) Metzenbaum scissors are used to bluntly separate the sternohyoideus muscles on the midline. (d) The thyroidea caudalis vein located on the midline on the dorsal aspect of the sternohyoideus muscles is avoided to minimize hemorrhage.

skin edges and clear just enough subcutaneous tissue to identify the midline division of the sternohyoideus muscles (see Fig. 24.5b). Using Metzenbaum scissors, bluntly separate the sternohyoideus muscles on the midline (see Fig. 24.5c), taking care to avoid the thyroidea caudalis vein on the midline between these two muscles (see Fig. 24.5d). Retract the thyroidea caudalis vein to one side along with one of the sternohyoideus muscles (see Fig. 24.6a). Reposition the self-retaining retractors on the sternohyoideus muscles to expose the trachea and clear the loose fascia off the ventral trachea at the proposed tracheotomy site (see Fig. 24.6b). Application of a second self-retaining retractor at a right angle to the original retractor to retract the skin in a craniocaudal direction enhances exposure of the tracheal rings and interannular ligaments (see Fig. 24.6c).

Using a scalpel blade, incise the interannular ligament between the second and third tracheal rings (see Fig. 24.7). This tracheal location is chosen because the area of the second through fourth tracheal rings is the preferred stomal site for permanent tracheostomy should it be required at a later time. Do not incise the interannular ligament beyond 50% of the tracheal circumfer-

ence. Place stay sutures (3-0 or 2-0 nylon for cats/small dogs or medium/large dogs, respectively) around the second and third tracheal rings, knot the sutures to create large suture loops, and tag the suture strands with mosquito hemostatic forceps (see Fig. 24.8). Use the stay sutures to manipulate the interannular opening while the endotracheal tube is removed and the tracheostomy tube is inserted (see Fig. 24.9). During the postoperative course, the stay sutures can be used for manipulation during reinsertion of a tube that has been inadvertently dislodged or requires changing; therefore, it is recommended they not be removed intraoperatively. The tracheostomy tube is inserted with the obturator in place (see Fig. 24.9b), but the obturator is quickly removed and replaced with an inner cannula as soon as the tracheostomy tube is positioned in the trachea (see Fig. 24.10). Secure the tracheostomy tube by attaching umbilical tape to the flange eyelets and tying the tapes behind the neck (see Fig. 24.11). Ties are secured firmly behind the animal's neck, leaving enough room for two fingers to be placed between the neck and ties. There should be no need to suture the tracheostomy wound, unless the incision was made too large. In that case, a

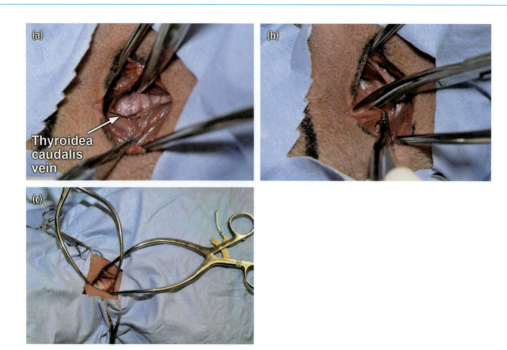

Figure 24.6 Isolating the trachea prior to tracheotomy for tracheostomy tube placement. Cranial is to the left in all frames. (a) The thyroidea caudalis vein is retracted laterally with one of the sternohyoideus muscles, the right sternohyoideus muscle in this case. (b) The Gelpi retractor is repositioned to retract the sternohyoideus muscles, and the loose fascia covering the ventral surface of the trachea is incised with Metzenbaum scissors. (c) A second Gelpi retractor is placed for craniocaudal retraction of skin and loose fascia, exposing the tracheal rings.

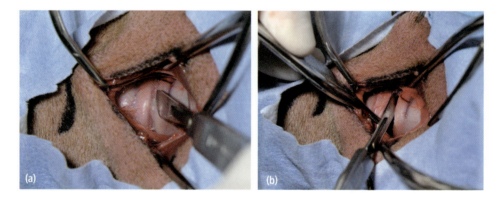

Figure 24.7 Incising the interannular ligament for tracheostomy tube placement. Cranial is to the left in both frames. (a) The interannular ligament between the second and third tracheal rings is isolated. (b) After the initial interannular incision, the scalpel blade is turned upward to extend the incision, taking care to not damage the underlying endotracheal tube or its cuff. The tracheotomy is limited to 50% or less of the tracheal circumference.

few interrupted sutures may be placed in the subcutaneous tissue and/or skin to decrease the size of the wound; however, care should be taken not to make the wound too small because the wound is contaminated and must be able to drain. See Protocol 24.1 for concise step-by-step instructions.

Once the surgical procedure is completed, the area is gently cleaned. Medical tape tabs may be applied to the two stay sutures, one bearing the word "UP" and the other the word "DOWN," to clearly indicate which way one should hold the stay sutures in the event of a tube dislodgement emergency. We prefer to leave the incision area uncovered for easy observation of swelling, bleeding, accumulated secretions, and tube position, and for prompt intervention as needed. If a bandage is applied, wait until the animal is awake and standing or in ventral

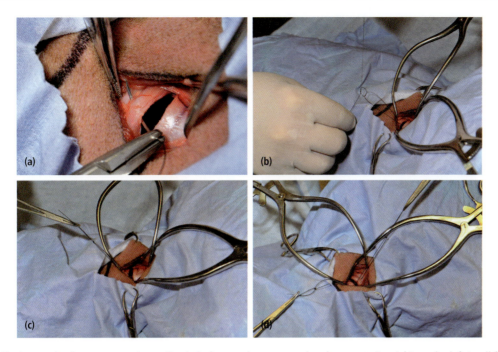

Figure 24.8 Placing tracheal stay sutures immediately before tracheostomy tube placement. Cranial is to the left in all frames. (a) The suture needle is placed around the second tracheal ring, the ring just cranial to the tracheotomy. (b) The suture is knotted such that a long loop will be retained. (c) The free ends of the stay suture are tagged temporarily with a mosquito hemostatic forceps. (d) A second identical stay suture is placed around the third tracheal ring, the ring just caudal to the tracheotomy.

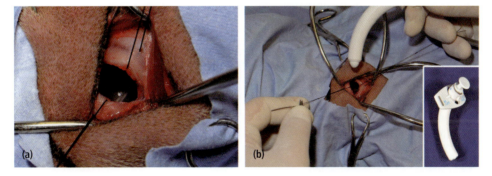

Figure 24.9 Preparing to insert a tracheostomy tube. Cranial is to the left in both frames. (a) The cranial and caudal stay sutures are retracted to pull open the tracheotomy. Note the endotracheal tube within the tracheal lumen. The cuff will now be deflated and the endotracheal tube removed as the tracheostomy tube is inserted. (b) The obturator is inserted into the tracheostomy tube immediately before placing the tube into the trachea. The purpose of the obturator is to keep blood and other secretions from being scraped into the tracheostomy tube lumen during placement.

recumbence. A bandage applied to the neck in a recumbent patient could change position when the patient recovers and becomes more active. The altered bandage position could cause patient discomfort or interfere with tube positioning. The bandage must be changed at least once daily to observe for tube site complications. Simply peeking under the bandage is insufficient.

Contraindications

There is no absolute contraindication for placing a tracheostomy tube when upper airway obstruction is causing respiratory distress. However, endotracheal intubation is always the preferred method of capturing an airway in an animal with airway distress. Once the

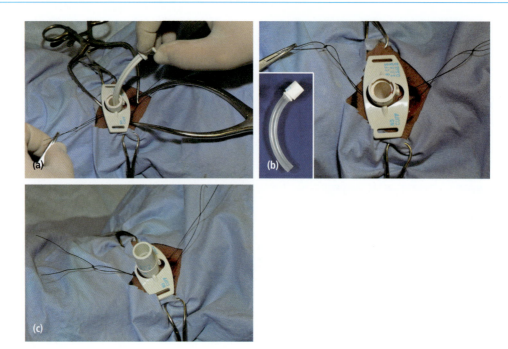

Figure 24.10 Insertion of a tracheostomy tube. Cranial is to the left in all frames. (a) The obturator is removed as soon as the tracheostomy tube is in place. (b) After removing the obturator, the inner cannula (inset) is placed into the tracheostomy tube. (c) The inner cannula has been inserted into the tracheostomy tube and locked in place. The hemostatic forceps are removed from the stay sutures and the stay sutures are left in place.

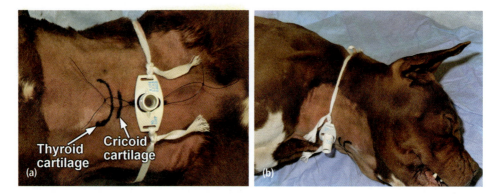

Figure 24.11 Completed tracheostomy tube placement. (a) Umbilical tapes are tied to the eyelets in the tracheostomy tube flange. The knotted stay sutures are left in place. The stay sutures are used to facilitate replacement of the tracheostomy tube in the case of inadvertent or planned removal. (b) The umbilical tapes are tied on the back of the neck.

airway is controlled, tracheostomy may be performed under controlled conditions. The quick "slash" tracheostomy is rarely needed but may be necessary if endotracheal intubation is not possible.

Relative contraindications for tracheostomy tube placement include uncorrected coagulopathy, symptomatic thrombocytopenia, unstable cervical spine, increased intracranial pressure, presence of a cervical mass that would interfere with the surgical approach,

and recent cervical surgery. If tube tracheostomy is indicated in patients with any of these conditions, the condition is brought under control or preparations are undertaken to deal with the consequences prior to placement of the tracheostomy tube. Plasma may be given to coagulopathic patients, and meticulous hemostasis should be exercised during surgical placement to avoid excessive blood loss in patients with coagulopathy and thrombocytopenia. Careful positioning and cautious

Protocol 24.1. Temporary tracheostomy tube placement

Items Required
- Appropriate type and size tracheostomy tube
  - Alternatively, standard endotracheal (ET) tube fashioned into tracheostomy tube, one size smaller than for ET intubation
- Appropriate-size ET tube for ET intubation, with cuff syringe
- Clippers with clean blade
- Surgical scrub supplies
- Barrier drapes
- Sterile surgical gloves
- Sterile gauze
- Surgical instruments (see Text Box 24.1)
- Suture material
- Umbilical tape
- Assistant
- Suction capability
- Oxygen/standard anesthetic supplies and equipment

Procedure
1. Collect necessary supplies.
2. Anesthetize and orotracheally intubate the patient with a cuffed ET tube.
3. Position the animal in dorsal recumbence with a towel rolled under the neck. Clip and aseptically prepare a large surgical field on the ventral cervical surface.
4. Perform hand hygiene, and don cap, mask, and sterile gloves.
5. Isolate the prepared surgical site with a barrier drape.
6. Make a ventral midline cervical skin incision just caudal to the larynx for a distance of approximately 3 to 4 cm.
7. Apply a self-retaining retractor to hold open the skin edges and clear just enough subcutaneous tissue to identify the midline division of the sternohyoideus muscles.
8. Using Metzenbaum scissors, bluntly separate the sternohyoideus muscles on the midline, taking care to avoid the thyroidea caudalis vein on the midline between these two muscles. Retract the thyroidea caudalis vein to one side along with one of the sternohyoideus muscles.
9. Reposition the self-retaining retractors on the sternohyoideus muscles to expose the trachea and clear the loose fascia away at the proposed tracheotomy site. Application of a second self-retaining retractor at a right angle to the original retractor to retract the skin in a craniocaudal direction enhances exposure.
10. Using a scalpel blade, incise the interannular ligament between the second and third tracheal rings. Do not incise the interannular ligament beyond 50% of the tracheal circumference.
11. Place stay sutures around the second and third tracheal rings, knot the sutures to create large suture loops, and tag the suture strands with mosquito hemostatic forceps.
12. Use the stay sutures to manipulate the interannular opening while the orotracheal tube is removed. Insert the tracheostomy tube with the obturator in place, and then quickly remove the obturator and replace it with an inner cannula.
13. Leave the stay sutures in place for postoperative nursing care manipulations.
14. Secure the tracheostomy tube by attaching umbilical tape to the flange eyelets and tying the tapes behind the neck.
15. Do not suture the tracheostomy wound unless the incision was made too large. In that case, place a few interrupted sutures in the subcutaneous tissue and/or skin to decrease the size of the wound, taking care not to make the wound too small.
16. Once the surgical procedure is completed, the area is gently cleaned and left uncovered for easy observation.

manipulation must be performed in patients at risk for cervical and intracranial neurologic complications. The consequences of invading a cervical mass or previous surgical site in the neck must be weighed against the need for tracheostomy tube placement. Tracheostomy tube placement may be lifesaving in the face of relative contraindications, as long as proper preparations and precautions are used.

Possible complications during the procedure

Intraoperative complications with tracheostomy tube placement can be avoided by diligent attention to surgical technique. Hemorrhage can be minimized with meticulous attention to hemostasis and avoidance of inadvertent vessel damage. The thyroidea caudalis vein (see Fig. 24.5d) is a single midline vein on the dorsal aspect of the sternohyoideus muscles that can be avoided by careful separation of these muscles, but care must also be taken not to tear or puncture the vessel with self-retaining retractors. Recurrent laryngeal nerve damage can be prevented by limiting the clearing of peritracheal fascia to the ventral aspect of the trachea over the intended interannular ligament and associated tracheal rings. Incising an interannular ligament that is too close to the larynx or too far caudal can be avoided by precise attention to the regional anatomy. Inadvertent puncture of the endotracheal tube cuff during interannular ligament incision or puncturing the cuff during stay suture placement can be avoided by palpation of the inflated cuff and close communication with the anesthetist to deflate and reposition the endotracheal tube and cuff before making the tracheal incision and placing sutures.

Tracheostomy tube maintenance

Patient management and monitoring begin immediately after the procedure to minimize the risk of airway obstruction from dislodgment or occlusion of the tube. Regular care may be scheduled every 2 to 3 hours but may be needed as often as every 15 minutes if a patient's condition warrants. The objectives of regular management are to prevent buildup of secretions that may block the tube, provide aseptic wound care, and humidify inspired air. Frequent observation is the best way to gauge the need for increased tube care. Abnormal respiratory pattern, coughing, or pawing at the tube or face should signal the need to check for occlusions and increase the frequency of tube care. Additional information about tracheostomy tube care can be found in Chapter 25, Artificial Airway Management.

Airway humidification

Regular maintenance consists of humidifying inspired air by instilling 0.5 to 3 mL of sterile isotonic saline into the tube hourly (small patients, 0.5 mL; large dogs, up to 3 mL). Aseptic instillation is achieved by cleansing the external portions of the tracheostomy tube and surrounding skin with 0.05% chlorhexidine solution, aspirating sterile saline for injection into a sterile syringe, removing the hypodermic needle used to aspirate the saline, and quickly injecting the saline into the tracheostomy tube without coming in contact with surroundings. Alternatively, the airway can be humidified with a humidity exchange filter (also called a **heat moisture exchanger** or "artificial nose") if the tube is attached to a rebreathing circuit, or a nebulizer can be used. Humidity exchange filters (Gibeck Humid Vent 1) are dispos-

able devices that interface between the tracheostomy tube and breathing circuit of a ventilator or anesthetic machine and trap exhaled moisture, which then humidifies the inhaled gas. Aerosol therapy (nebulization) can be used as a means of airway humidification. Nebulization with sterile isotonic saline can be used in sessions of 10 to 15 minutes every 4 to 6 hours. Sterile water can be nebulized if humidification is the sole purpose, but saline is better for loosening thick airway secretions to facilitate their removal. Nebulization produces particles small enough to oversaturate the lungs if used excessively.

Tracheostomy site hygiene

The tracheostomy site and surrounding skin should be examined frequently, at least whenever the tube is cleaned. Good wound care decreases the medium for bacterial growth and increases patient comfort. Prior to tending to the tracheostomy wound, the caregiver should disinfect hands and don gloves. Sterile gloves are preferred, but clean examination gloves suffice when sterile gloves are not practical. Skin surrounding the incision, especially under the flange of the tube, should be gently cleansed with sterile cotton-tipped applicators or gauze sponges soaked in dilute (0.05%) chlorhexidine solution. Begin at the wound edges and work away from the incision. Squeeze excess solution from the cleaning materials before the skin is cleaned. Keep antiseptic soaps and antibacterial ointments away from the incision and wound area because they can irritate exposed tracheal mucosa. Address an increase in exudate from the incision promptly to prevent abscess formation and skin maceration. If gauze pads or fenestrated tracheostomy sponges are used, apply fresh ones after each wound care session. The area of cleaned skin must be completely dry before new sponges are placed. Gauze pads should never be trimmed or cut because fibers could embed in secretions from the surgical incision or be inhaled into the airway. Fold sponges in a triangle pattern and place them on each side of the site under the flange and ties. Triangular folding allows the long base of the triangle to contact the wound, leaving a pointed apex more externally located for ease of grasping during dressing changes. Special fenestrated sponges are placed above the tube, with the side panels extending down under the flange and ties. Wound areas can also be maintained without pad materials to allow easier visualization of the tissue around the tube and incision area.

Tube tie inspection

The wound maintenance session is an excellent time to inspect the ties. Ties should be checked regularly for security. Tapes tied with a double bow will hold firmly but can be easily loosened. Ties secured with a knot may be difficult to remove, and thus scissors should be hanging on the cage or readily available near the patient. A tube that is untied even briefly is in danger of being pulled or coughed out. If not secured, a tube can be expelled in an instant with unexpected force. Ties that are too tight will cause discomfort, whereas ties that are too loose will allow the tube to slide freely within the trachea and can cause mucosal damage. When changing soiled ties, secure the clean ties before removing the old ones.

Tracheostomy tube suctioning

Regular suctioning of the tracheostomy tube helps prevent accumulation of secretions that may cause occlusions. Because of the possibility of tracheal mucosal irritation and the gagging or bradycardia that can be caused by vagal stimulation of this area, suctioning the trachea without a tube in place must be done with great care. Patients should be preoxygenated for several breaths from an oxygen source held at the tracheostomy tube opening. Using aseptic technique, a small sterile suction catheter made of pliable tubing with side fenestrations is then introduced. Suctioning is not begun until the suction catheter is in place; intermittent light suction is then applied as the catheter is withdrawn with a circular motion. Most suction catheters are controlled by a thumb port to allow adjustment of the amount of suction. The entire suctioning procedure should be completed in less than 15 seconds. The patient is allowed a few moments to "catch its breath," supplemental oxygen is again held near the tracheostomy tube opening, and suctioning is repeated if necessary. If power-driven suction is unavailable, a handheld suction unit (available at automotive stores) fits medical suction tubing and can be used for patient care. Because the action of suctioning can initiate gagging or vomiting, patients should not be suctioned immediately after eating. Stop suctioning immediately if respiratory or cardiac changes or excessive patient discomfort occur.

Tracheostomy tube cleaning

For double-lumen tubes, the inner cannula is removed as often as the patient's condition warrants but at least every 4 to 6 hours. The inner cannula is removed and immediately replaced with a second sterile inner cannula, making sure that the locking mechanism is secured in place. When copious secretions are noted, it may be necessary to instill saline into the outer lumen tube and suction that tube before placing the new inner cannula. The removed cannula is placed in a soak solution of 0.05% chlorhexidine for cleaning. Alternately, a cleansing soak bath of 50:50 0.9% NaCl and 3% H_2O_2 may be used. When debris and secretions are present, the inner surface may be cleaned with sterile applicators, pipe cleaners, brushes, or gauze passed through the tube. The cannula is then placed in the chlorhexidine solution until the next tube change is due. When the inner cannula is next changed, the sanitized cannula is removed from the antiseptic solution and thoroughly rinsed with sterile water or saline before being reused.

If a single-lumen tube is used, it is preferable to replace the tube with a fresh one. However, if frequent tube changes are needed, less damage and irritation to the tissue occurs if saline is instilled and suction applied while the tube remains in place. The frequency of suctioning varies according to each patient. Patients with conditions that produce excessive secretions may need frequent suctioning or more frequent humidification than those with minimal secretions. Patients with conditions that produce moderate secretions may be suctioned every 4 to 6 hours. Cats seem to need more frequent maintenance than dogs because they have a tendency to produce thick mucus, especially on the second and third day after tube placement. Blockage of the tube by secretions is the most common life-threatening occurrence in tracheostomy patients.

Facilitation of respiratory secretion removal

Postural drainage and *coupage* (percussion) after nebulization can help to mobilize secretions in dependent bronchial areas and stimulate coughing to clear them. To perform this technique, the patient should be positioned in ventral or lateral recumbence and the chest rapidly, gently slapped repeatedly with a cupped hand. The technique should be performed on both sides of the chest. With the animal in sternal position, coupage may be done on both sides of the chest simultaneously, working from the rear toward the head and from the lower portion of the chest upward. Great care must be taken so that the tracheostomy tube does not become dislodged during postural drainage and coupage. If coupage results in coughing, tube placement should be checked when the coughing subsides. Coughing may not be obvious in patients with tracheostomy tubes but may still be productive, and therefore any coughing that is accomplished contributes to mobilization of secretions. As such, additional suctioning should be performed after this treatment. Increasing amounts or changes in consistency of secretions can be a warning of greater risk of tracheal occlusion and warrant more frequent suctioning, increased humidification frequency, or nebulization, coupage, and postural drainage. If an occlusion is suspected, it is preferable to remove the inner cannula or replace the tube. Attempts to force a suction catheter tip down the tube or to clear the tube by running any form of stylet through it will force material into the patient's airway.

Replacement of tracheostomy tubes

We recommend that tracheostomy tubes (both single and double lumen) be replaced at least as frequently as every 24 hours. All materials should be prepared and available, and an assistant should restrain the patient. The importance of placing stay or traction sutures during the tracheostomy procedure cannot be overemphasized because of their usefulness in making tube changes safer and easier. Tabs attached to the stay sutures labeled "UP" and "DOWN" facilitate tube exchange. These sutures are used to part the tracheal lumen opening, the ties on the tube are loosened, and the tube is removed. The new tube is then placed, ensuring that it actually enters the trachea and not the subcutaneous tissue, and new neck ties are secured. This procedure should be done as quickly as possible after preoxygenation, and oxygen should remain available in case the patient becomes distressed. A mask and eye protection are recommended for the caregiver when the patient's condition produces excessive secretions to keep expelled secretions out of the caregiver's face during inspection of the incision and tube care.

General patient observations

When respiratory distress is relieved, patients often relax and are able to rest. Many dogs and most cats assume a position with the head down or neck bent that will seem to block the free flow of air to and from the tracheostomy tube; however, the flexed neck rarely causes a problem. The rate and character of respiration should be closely observed rather than constantly waking, disturbing, or repositioning the patient. Any change in breathing pattern, such as dyspnea, tachypnea, or hyperpnea, warrants intervention.

Environmental considerations and patient hygiene

Cages must be kept clean and free from materials that could be inhaled, such as lint from bedding and excess hair shed by the patient. Fur inevitably accumulates in the cage and creates a hazard. For patients that seem to be at greater risk for aspiration of such debris, a gauze shield can be placed over the tube opening; human stoma shields might also be adapted for this purpose. Cats should be provided with long strips of cut paper for litter rather than clay or any material that could produce dust or small particles that could adhere to the incision or be inhaled. For cats that refuse to void except in their customary litter materials, the litter box should be offered regularly and then removed from the cage, especially because many hospitalized cats seem to prefer to sleep in their litter boxes. Tracheostomy patients require general hygiene care as with any hospitalized patient, but common sense dictates modification of certain nursing procedures. For example, tub bathing could result in aspiration of soap and water into the tracheostomy tube or the wound around the tube.

Attention to hydration status

Close monitoring of hydration is important in tracheostomy patients. Normally inhaled air is heated and humidified by the nasopharynx and tracheobronchial tree so that alveolar air is 100% humidified at body temperature and contains four to six times the water vapor content of room air. Inspired air that bypasses the upper airways increases humidification requirements and desiccates the respiratory mucosa, resulting in viscous secretions, impaired mucociliary transport, inflammation, small airway collapse, decreased functional residual capacity, reduced pulmonary compliance, and increased risk of infection. A compensatory increase in vaporization by respiratory mucosa results in cooling of the liquid surface and patient heat loss. Animals on diuretic therapy and small hypermetabolic patients need to be encouraged to drink or be given continuous parenteral or enteral fluid support. Patients should be weighed daily because weight loss or gain can aid in the evaluation of patient hydration. Most patients capable of food and water intake seem to have little trouble eating and drinking with a tracheostomy tube in place. However, it is still good nursing practice to observe animals while they are eating and drinking. Food and water bowls may need to be adjusted to avoid possible aspirations, especially in short-necked or brachycephalic animals. If problems are noted with bowls or the acts of eating and drinking, food and water should be kept out of the cage and offered intermittently while the patient is supervised.

Tracheostomy tube removal

The longer a tracheostomy tube must remain in place, the more likely intubation complications and stenosis become. The tube should be removed as soon as assisted ventilation is no longer needed, the patient can move a normal volume of air around or without the tube, or the condition that required the procedure is resolved. When a patient is to be weaned from the tube, replace the existing tube with a tube of the next smaller size and closely observe the patient for 10 to 15 minutes for signs of dyspnea. If no distress is noted, then a smaller diameter tube is placed at the next scheduled maintenance session. If a patient shows signs of respiratory distress, the tube that was just removed (i.e., the larger tube) is replaced and tube removal attempted again in 12 to 24 hours. If breathing is adequate with the smaller tube in place, this tube is occluded with a cap or occlusion cannula and the patient is observed for 30 minutes. If no dyspnea is noted, the tube is removed. If a patient already has the smallest available tube in place, then weaning must be attempted by complete removal of the tube and close observation of the patient for 15 minutes. If distress occurs, the tube must be immediately replaced. Tracheostomy wounds are allowed to heal by second intention. The area is cleaned daily of any drainage with sterile saline. Patients with temporary tracheostomy tubes require 24-hour observation and are almost never released to home care. Patients with tracheostomy wounds in the process of healing may be returned to an owner's care with strict instructions that the animal must not be bathed, cannot be allowed to swim, cannot wear collars or neck leads, and should be returned for reexamination and further directions.

Summary

Temporary tracheostomy tube placement is a skill all emergency and intensive care veterinarians should master. A well-prepared technical staff with a good nursing plan in place makes care of patients with temporary tracheostomies less stressful for all concerned and helps to ensure a satisfactory outcome for patients and the medical team.

25

Artificial airway management

Lila K. Sierra and Lesley G. King

An artificial airway (AA) is any tubelike device inserted into the trachea to provide an unobstructed pathway to the lower airways. AAs may be used to bypass an airway obstruction, protect the airway, allow maintenance of airway hygiene, or permit mechanical ventilation. Management of an AA involves maintaining and monitoring its patency while decreasing the risk of complications.

Normal airway defense mechanisms

The nose and pharynx serve as the first line of defense for the respiratory tract. In normal animals, the nasal turbinates warm and humidify inspired air, allow thermoregulation, and filter large inhaled particles. Smaller particles that pass farther down the airway become trapped by the second line of defense, the **mucociliary escalator**. Made up of mucus-producing goblet cells and ciliated epithelium, the sticky cilia of the escalator line the airway from the trachea to the bronchioles and continually beat cranially, causing the mucus to ascend toward the pharynx. In addition, the cough reflex, integral to airway defense, expels material that would otherwise remain in the airways. Bypassing any of these natural defenses can result in serious impairment of airway clearance and long-term respiratory damage. When you take into account the complexity of the respiratory system and all of the potential complications that an AA can pose, the need for intensive nursing management becomes clear.

Nursing the artificial airway is both a science and an art

The *science* of AA management is the compensation for functions of the bypassed natural defenses while maintaining a clear airway. Because AAs circumvent normal airway humidification, systemic hydration, humidification, and nebulization are all important. The *art* of AA management lies in the anticipation of, preparation for, and appropriate action in the face of any complication that may arise. Experience lends a hand in this arena. As time goes on, technicians sometimes develop a sixth sense regarding the idiosyncrasies of AAs.

Even the most stable and well-fitted AA poses a constant high risk to the patient's life. Although the properly-placed AA should provide an improved breathing conduit, obstructions, dislodgements, and other complications can happen in an instant and are immediately life threatening. Therefore, anticipation of worst case scenarios is a vital tool when dealing with a patient with an AA. Possible complications of AAs and approaches to their prevention and management are discussed in detail later.

It is vital to prepare for AA-related emergencies. One can mentally play out different scenarios to list the equipment that could be required. For example, an uncooperative patient who has just removed its tracheostomy tube might require sedation to safely replace it, so having sedatives ready at hand might be useful. Another patient might develop an obstruction distal to the AA, in which case having easy access to suction can minimize reaction time. When a patient with an AA first enters the unit, items that may be required can be neatly

Advanced Monitoring and Procedures for Small Animal Emergency and Critical Care, First Edition. Edited by Jamie M. Burkitt Creedon, Harold Davis.
© 2012 John Wiley & Sons, Inc. Published 2012 by John Wiley & Sons, Inc.

Table 25.1 Extended-term endotracheal tube station

- Endotracheal tubes
  - Have extra tubes available for quick, convenient reintubation
  - Have a few smaller sized tubes available for difficult airways
- Laryngoscope with functioning light source
- Sterile gloves
  - Several pairs of varying sizes should be available to accommodate all of the staff
- Lidocaine spray
  - For laryngeal spasm (cats)
- Sterile aqueous lubricant
- Gauze squares
  - For extracting the tongue or swabbing out the mouth
- Endotracheal tube ties
  - Muzzle gauze or IV extension tubing
- Air syringe or Posey Cufflator Manometer
- Hemostats
  - Can be used to occlude the pilot balloon (red rubber ET tube) or hold gauze squares to swab out the back of the mouth
- Suction canister and vacuum system
- Suction tubing
- Suction catheters
  - Oral (e.g., Yankauer)
  - ET (e.g., Kendall Safe-T-Vac suction catheter)
- Bottle of sterile water for irrigation
  - Used for rinsing out suction catheters after use
  - Dedicate one bottle for oral suction and one for ET suction to avoid cross-contamination
- Oral hygiene rinse
- Glycerin
- Mouth prop
- Sedative or injectable anesthetic, predrawn to appropriate dose

Table 25.2 Temporary tracheostomy tube/permanent tracheostomy station

- Tracheostomy tubes
  - Having several backup tracheostomy tubes optimizes reaction time when replacement is necessary
  - Some inner cannulas can be purchased separately, depending on the manufacturer
  - Resterilize used tracheostomy tubes where applicable (metal trach tubes) for continued availability
- Air syringe and/or Posey Cufflator Manometer
  - For cuffed trach tubes
- Sterile gloves
  - Several pairs of varying sizes should be available to accommodate all of the staff
- Tracheostomy tube care kits
  - Most kits allow for several uses but need to be discarded if they become too dirty
  - If there is not a kit available, you can make your own using:
    - Sterile unfenestrated drape (to use as a sterile field)
    - Two sterile bowls (one for cleaning and one for rinsing)
    - Sterile gauze squares
    - Sterile cotton swabs
    - Sterile pipe cleaners or small brushes
- Bottle of hydrogen peroxide
  - Used to soak and remove secretions from tracheostomy tubes
- Bottle of sterile water or saline
  - Dedicated to that patient to avoid contamination
  - Used to rinse tracheostomy tubes
- Sterile gauze squares
- Sterile cotton swabs
- Tracheostomy tube ties
  - Umbilical tape or Velcro ties
- Suction canister and vacuum system
- Suction tubing
- Suction catheters (e.g., Kendall Safe-T-Vac suction catheter)

organized and made easily accessible near the patient in the event a crisis should arise. A list of suggested materials is provided in Tables 25.1 and 25.2.

Practice drills are an effective way to improve technical proficiency and promote teamwork. Implementation of the plan should prove unproblematic if every precaution has been meticulously anticipated and prepared for.

General considerations for airway management

It is difficult if not impossible to provide a prescriptive list for AA management because the type and frequency of care requires depends on many factors, such as the type of AA in place, the reason for its placement, and the type and severity of any pulmonary disease present. Some patients require sedation or general anesthesia; others often require none (such as those with temporary or permanent tracheostomies). Oxygen supplementation may or may not be required, and other injuries or diseases may be present that have an impact on nursing care of the airway. Serial thorough physical examinations assist in scheduling therapy for the patient. Although the basic overall measures for AA management are presented here, treatments should be tailored to the requirements of each individual.

Systemic hydration

Patients with AAs can lose a significant amount of water from the airway, causing dehydration of the airway mucus and potentially clinically important systemic water loss. Normal airway mucus contains a great deal of water, and local airway water loss increases airway mucus viscosity, making it very difficult for normal defense mechanisms to remove material from the airways. For patients with AAs in place, intravenous fluid therapy is highly recommended to ensure adequate hydration, which helps loosen respiratory secretions. Secretions that are more watery allow for easier airway clearance whether it is by coughing or suctioning. Humidification and nebulization should never be used as alternatives to systemic hydration.

Airway humidification

Humidification involves the saturation of inspired gases with water vapor (water in the gas phase). The amount of water vapor that can be carried in inspired gas depends on temperature: warmer gas carries more water. In the normal animal, the nasal turbinates warm the inspired air, and because the air flows over their large surface area, they concurrently saturate it with water vapor. AAs bypass the nasal turbinates, and those that are open to the environment (not connected to a rebreathing circuit) are thus susceptible to heat loss and desiccation. Direct exposure to cool, dry air increases inflammation, damage to epithelial cells, and sticky mucus production. The mucociliary escalator becomes compromised and is unable to remove the thickened secretions. Humidifying inspired gas helps alleviate these complications. In fact, all oxygen administered to spontaneously breathing AA patients and all inspired gases in ventilated patients should be humidified all of the time.

Types of humidifiers

Oxygen "bubblers" or **bubble humidifiers** are the easiest and most cost-efficient type of humidifier for AA patients that are breathing spontaneously (Airlife Bubbler Humidifier, Cardinal Health, McGaw Park, IL; see Fig. 25.1). Filled with sterile water, they can be connected to an oxygen flowmeter (Ohmeda Oxygen Flowmeter, Ohmeda Medical, Laurel, MD) that titrates the flow of oxygen as required. This is a simple way to humidify inspired gases: the oxygen flows from a tube at the bottom of the sterile water canister and bubbles to the surface before delivery to the patient. As the oxygen bubbles rise to the surface, they become saturated with water vapor.

Heat and moisture exchangers (HMEs) or **"artificial noses"** are a form of passive humidification (Portex Thermovent Heat and Moisture Exchangers, Smiths Medical, Keene, NH; see Fig. 25.2). Commonly used for ventilated patients, these disposable plastic filters attach

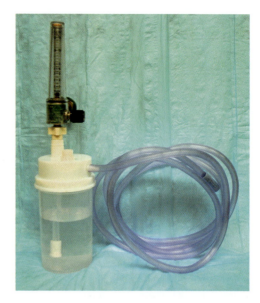

Figure 25.1 Bubble humidifier. All oxygen administered in the critical care unit should be humidified. Options for humidification include this Airlife Bubbler Humidifier with an Ohmeda Oxygen Flowmeter, attached to oxygen tubing for delivery to the patient.

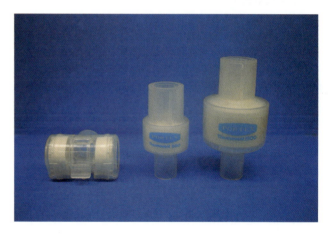

Figure 25.2 Heat and moisture exchangers (Portex Thermovent Heat and Moisture Exchangers, Smiths Medical, Keene, NH) or "artificial noses." These devices can provide an inexpensive and readily accessible way to humidify inspired gas.

directly to the AA and are designed to "recycle" the moisture and heat from exhaled air and to filter viruses and bacteria. Unfortunately, HMEs tend to become occluded with excess respiratory secretions, which can cause an obstruction. Therefore, careful consideration should be made when using these devices, and they should be avoided in patients producing large amounts of airway secretions. Artificial noses add some dead space and some resistance to airflow, so they are best avoided in

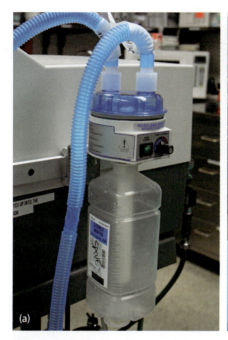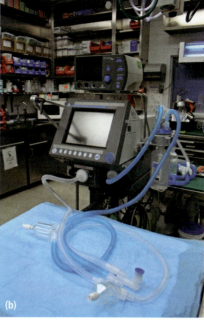

Figure 25.3 Theramist Nebulizer Heater and Wick (Pegasus Research Corp., Costa Mesa, CA). (a) Note the heating unit atop the water bottle, with the large white wick descending into the fluid. Adjust the thermostat carefully to provide optimal humidification without risk of thermal injury to the respiratory tract. (b) The nebulizer system incorporated into a ventilator circuit (note the two water traps—clear plastic cups with white drain outlets—located distally on the ventilator circuit to capture condensation).

spontaneously breathing patients with tracheostomy tubes.

Heated humidifiers (Thera-mist Nebulizer Heater, Pegasus Research Corp., Costa Mesa, CA) are more expensive but are very effective and are easy to use with mechanical ventilators (see Fig. 25.3). A disposable wick and sterile water container are connected to a heater and incorporated into the ventilator circuit. Because the inspired gases are warmed, a larger amount of water vapor can be delivered to the airway compared with passive humidifiers. The thermostat can be adjusted as needed to add more heat and moisture to the inspired gas. Warmed inspired gas may be used to increase the body temperature of hypothermic patients, although this method is not recommended as the sole source of warming because the risk for hyperthermia and thermal injury to the airways increases if the inspired air is warmer than 42°C/107.6°F.[1] The human medical literature suggests that humidifier thermostats should be set as close to a patient's normal body temperature with emphasis on monitoring airway temperatures continuously.[2] As the warmed gases saturated with water vapor gases go down the ventilator tubing to the patient, the temperature of the gas drops. When the inspired gas cools, it cannot carry as much water vapor, so water condenses and showers out as droplets in the tubing.

Drainable water traps should be added at the lowest point of the ventilator tubing, allowing removal of the water as it accumulates. If it is not removed, excess condensation can back up into the ventilator circuit causing resistance and creating a risk of aspiration.

Airway nebulization

Nebulizers deliver aerosolized droplets of sterile saline or water to the respiratory tract. Thus they differ from humidifiers because nebulized water is in the liquid phase rather than humidified water vapor in the gas phase. When inhaled, the droplets shower onto the respiratory mucosa to hydrate the tissues and moisten secretions, making them easier to expel. Droplet size has a profound impact on how deeply these aerosolized water droplets travel into the lungs. For example, droplets larger than 10 microns deposit in the upper airway and nasal turbinates. Any droplets smaller than 0.5 microns are too light and will be exhaled again rather than landing on the airway mucus. For the droplets to shower into the bronchial mucus, the ideal size is 3–8 microns.[3]

Because nebulization involves the creation of water or saline droplets, drugs can be dissolved in the solution. Drugs such as bronchodilators and corticosteroids can be delivered to the patient by inhalation. The advantage of this local drug delivery is decreased systemic drug absorption and side effects, and the potential for delivery of high concentrations of the drug directly to the target tissues. Because the efficacy of the medication depends on patient compliance and tolerance of the use of a mask, nebulized drugs are not as widely used in veterinary patients as they are in humans. Conversely, humidification cannot be used to deliver inhaled drugs because water is in the gaseous (not liquid) phase when gas is humidified.

Because nebulization is such an effective way to deliver large volumes of water to the airway, it is usually not administered continuously. The duration of nebulization sessions can be adjusted according to the patient's needs. Animals with normal lungs that have AAs in place may only require 15 minutes of nebulization therapy every 4–6 hours, provided there is an alternate humidification system in place between treatments. In contrast, some animals with AAs that have severe pneumonia might benefit from continuous nebulization. Potential complications of nebulization are discussed later.

Types of nebulizers

Pneumatic nebulizers, also called **jet nebulizers** or **atomizers**, use a compressed air or oxygen source by which a mist is created under pressure. Although they are a less expensive option, depending on the kind of compressor utilized, they can be bulky and noisy. In addition, droplet sizes and the amount of mist produced are unpredictable because they depend on the strength of the pressurized source. For hypoxic patients, disposable pneumatic nebulizers that attach to metered oxygen outlets are available (Airlife Nebulizer Cap & 0.45% NaCl Inhalation Solution, Cardinal Health McGaw Park, IL), allowing constant nebulization with the added advantage of concurrent oxygen support (see Fig. 25.4).

Ultrasonic nebulizers (ULTRA-NEB '99 by Devil Bliss Healthcare Worldwide, Somerset PA; see Fig. 25.5), in contrast, produce more uniform droplets using high-frequency vibrations from a transducer. Ultrasonic nebulizers deliver smaller droplets in higher volumes, allowing deeper penetration into the airways.

Many factors should be weighed when selecting a nebulizer for an intensive care unit (ICU). Considerations may include ease of use, noise, ability to integrate into an oxygen supplementation system, reusability and disinfection procedures, power and consistency in droplet production, and cost, among others. See Table 25.3 for a list of advantages and disadvantages of different nebulizer types.

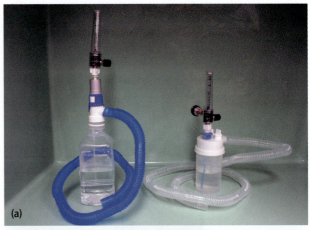

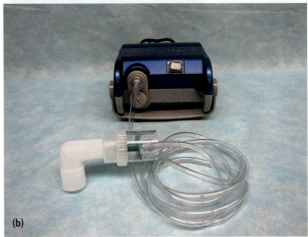

Figure 25.4 (a) Airlife Nebulizer Cap and 0.45% NaCl Inhalation Solution with Ohmeda Oxygen Flowmeter and corrugated plastic tubing. Either of these units can be titrated to deliver various concentrations of oxygen and humidification. (b) Compressor nebulizer without supplemental oxygen feature (Hudson RCL Opti-Neb Pro, Teleflex Medical, Research Triangle Park, NC).

Complications of nebulization

Nebulization offers many benefits for airway management, but as with any therapy, complications may ensue. Although complications are uncommon, they can include airway irritation, bronchospasm, overhydration, hyperthermia, and iatrogenic infection.

Inhaling aerosolized liquids, depending on their tonicity and content (i.e., antibiotics), may irritate the tissues of the upper and lower airways. Occasionally, nebulization can stimulate strong, forceful coughing and bronchoconstriction. Mucosa can become inflamed and swollen, further obstructing lower airways. In response to inflammation, increased secretion of thick mucus can exacerbate respiratory distress by occluding the narrowed bronchi. This domino effect can occur

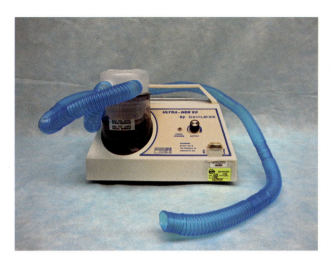

Figure 25.5 Ultrasonic nebulizer system (ULTRA-NEB '99 by Devil Bliss) delivers uniform droplets deep into the respiratory tract but does not have the added advantage of supplemental oxygen delivery.

Table 25.3 Comparison of pneumatic and ultrasonic nebulizers

Pneumatic nebulizers
- Pros
  - Inexpensive
  - Disposable; single use
  - Can deliver supplemental oxygen
- Cons
  - May not be portable; tend to be bulky
  - Noisy
  - Performance variable; may not aerosolize adequately
  - Require pressurized gas or oxygen source

Ultrasonic nebulizers
- Pros
  - Relatively quiet
  - Rapid delivery
  - Deliver smaller, uniform droplets
  - Newer designs smaller and portable
  - Intended for multiple use
- Cons
  - Expensive
  - Cannot deliver supplemental oxygen
  - Require power source or batteries
  - Contamination possible if not properly disinfected

suddenly and should be considered an emergency. In the event of bronchospasm (coughing and sudden dyspnea) during a nebulization session, nebulization should be discontinued immediately and supplemental oxygen provided. Bronchodilator therapy may be required if the patient fails to recover rapidly after removal of the nebulizer.

Systemic overhydration may develop as a result of continuous direct nebulization or nebulizing large volumes of a highly saturated mist. The body can absorb the water, causing an inadvertent water imbalance. Performing brief but frequent nebulization sessions (15 minutes every 4–6 hours) is usually sufficient to keep the airway moist without causing fluid overload. Patients requiring continuous nebulization should be monitored for hyponatremia or hypervolemia. Nebulization of saline rather than sterile water minimizes the risk of electrolyte imbalance as a result of absorption from the respiratory mucosa.

Humidifiers and nebulizers equipped with a heating element require frequent observation and adjustment. As mentioned earlier, excessive heating of inhaled gases can cause patient hyperthermia and thermal injury to the respiratory tract.

Contamination of the nebulizer unit is a common cause of iatrogenic respiratory infection. Nebulizer hoses left uncovered may contact the floor, become colonized with bacteria, and aerosolize microorganisms. Inadequate disinfection between patient uses can also promote contamination with microorganisms. A nebulizer should be dedicated to a single patient and measures taken to keep the system clean. Covering the end of the hose, by inserting it into a clean glove between uses, is usually adequate. Hoses should be changed any time they do not appear clean. Disposable systems are available and useful as a quick maintenance-free, single-use option.

Airway suctioning

Suctioning the AA is vital in maintaining airway patency. Respiratory secretions often collect distal to, around, and within the lumen of the AA, resulting in obstruction. If an AA is in place, the secretions are often copious and may be extremely thick and viscous, particularly if the airway becomes desiccated. Following humidification and nebulization, the loosened secretions may move in an orad direction, subsequently occluding the AA. In the normal airway, the cough reflex is a vital part of the clearance of secretions. Depending on the type of AA, the cough reflex may be partially impeded, if not obliterated (i.e., when the patient is anesthetized). Medical intervention is necessary to remove excess debris and avoid respiratory distress. The frequency of suctioning depends on the volume and quality of the secretions being produced, but it is often required no less frequently than every 4 hours.

Suction catheters

A variety of suction catheters are commercially available. The ideal catheter should be sterile, soft, flexible,

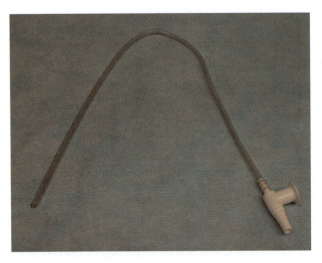

Figure 25.6 Kendall Safe-T-Vac Suction Catheter for airway suctioning. Note the "Murphy eye" feature at the tip of the catheter and proximal "thumb" port for manual suction control.

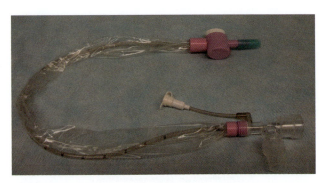

Figure 25.7 Kimberly-Clark Ballard Trach Care Closed Suction System can be incorporated into a ventilator circuit providing quick, easy access for AA suctioning without detaching the patient from the ventilator. The catheter is fed aseptically using the plastic encasement and suction controlled by the button located proximally.

have more than one distal opening (usually one side port and one end port) at the tip, and a proximal port for manual control of the suction (Kendall Safe-T-Vac Suction Catheter, TYCO Healthcare Group LP, Mansfield, MA; see Fig. 25.6) Suction catheters are available in a variety of sizes; those between 5 and 10F are suitable for most small animal patients. The largest gauge catheter possible should be selected, as long as it can be passed effortlessly through the AA without obstructing the tube. Larger diameter suction catheters may be necessary to evacuate thicker material from the airways. In emergent situations, if specialized suction catheters are unavailable, sterile red rubber catheters can be substituted. Red rubber catheters should not be routinely used because they lack a proximal port and therefore do not allow the operator to control the amount of suction applied to the airway.

Closed-system suction catheters are available for use in ventilator patients. The catheter is encased in a plastic bag that can be fitted into the ventilator circuit and advanced intermittently to apply suction without breaking sterility or opening the circuit (Kimberly-Clark Ballard Trach Care Closed Suction System, Ballard Medical Products Draper, UT; see Fig. 25.7).

The source of negative pressure for suction depends on the capability of the hospital. Larger hospitals may be equipped with central vacuum systems with suction outlets typically wall mounted; with the use of a regulator, the vacuum flow can be titrated (see Fig. 25.8a). Portable electric suction units can be purchased and set up similarly as an alternative (see Fig. 25.8b). Hospitals that use AAs beyond brief healthy anesthetic

procedures should be equipped with some type of suction device.

Procedures, risks, and complications of airway suctioning

Many risks are associated with suctioning. Nosocomial infection is one possible complication. With the obvious risk of introducing bacteria into the airway during this procedure, the use of sterile materials and aseptic technique is imperative.

Iatrogenic hypoxia can be minimized by preoxygenation of the patient prior to and between each pass of the suction catheter. High concentrations of oxygen are administered for a short period of time prior to the procedure. Ideally, to ensure optimal hemoglobin saturation, patients should be preoxygenated for 5–10 minutes before the intervention. Some ventilators are outfitted with a "100% Oxygen" button that flushes the ventilator circuit for up to 2 minutes; however, the ventilator settings can also temporarily be manually changed for the same effect. Patients not being mechanically ventilated can be given high oxygen flow rates through an Ambu bag or as "flow-by" oxygen directed in front of their AA opening (see Chapter 20, Oxygen Therapy). Monitoring with a pulse oximeter prior to, during, and after suctioning is strongly recommended (see Chapter 21, Pulse Oximetry and CO-Oximetry).

Suction passes should be brief, taking no longer than 5 seconds.[4] The catheter should extend just a couple centimeters past the end of the AA, but no further. Suctioning too deep into the airway can result in airway

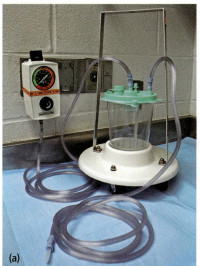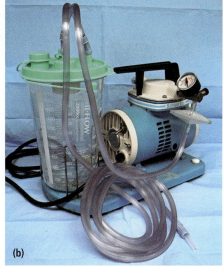

Figure 25.8 (a) Central vacuum system with wall-mounted suction regulator connected to a portable suction canister. The suction regulator can be metered for a variety of purposes (airway suctioning, continuous thoracic drainage, etc.). (b) Portable Suction System, Schuco-Vac 130 Suction Machine.

inflammation, airway collapse, bronchial spasm and coughing, lung collapse, activation of the vagal reflex, vomiting, or accidentally displacing the AA during coughing. If the amount of suction can be controlled, the vacuum device should be adjusted to provide a moderate, but not excessive, degree of negative pressure. The recommended range for suctioning should be between 80 and 120 mm Hg.[1] Extreme and prolonged negative pressure can exacerbate airway collapse and atelectasis as complications of the suction procedure.

Ideally, suction should only be applied once the catheter tip is at its target depth within the airway. Therefore, the catheter's proximal port should not be occluded as the catheter is advanced so as not to apply suction during advancement. Once the catheter has been advanced to the desired depth in the airway, suction is applied intermittently as the catheter is withdrawn, by tapping the thumb on the proximal port. In addition, increased removal of secretions can sometimes be attained if the catheter is twisted as it is slowly withdrawn from the airway. Observing the patient's respiratory pattern, listening at the AA opening, auscultation of the cervical trachea below the tube, auscultation of the lungs, and pulse oximetry are all useful ways to determine whether the obstruction has been removed or if further intervention is required. Between suction passes, it is best to allow the patient to recover with supplemental oxygen while you perform a quick physical evaluation to assess for distress before repeating the procedure.

The instillation of sterile saline directly into the AA remains controversial. Theoretically, the injection of small amounts of physiologic saline (2–3 mL at a time) into a dry airway might allow hydration of sticky exudates, thereby facilitating their removal. However, we believe that the saline probably flows quickly past mucus concretions into the lower airways and alveoli, rather than staying in the upper airway long enough to soak into the material. Additionally, instillation of saline under pressure may simply flush mucus plugs deeper into the airways, where they can occlude small bronchi. Although on rare occasions instillation of saline has been helpful, complications such as increased infection and further insult to the airway may outweigh the benefits.[4] In general, nebulization is a more effective way of moistening secretions. Therefore, saline instillation is usually limited to those patients who absolutely need it in a crisis or in which nebulization has not been effective. See Protocol 25.1 for detailed suctioning instructions.

Chest physiotherapy

Chest physiotherapy goes hand in hand with nebulization and should follow each nebulization session. Paralyzed, sedated, or recumbent patients, especially larger sized animals and those that are obese, often experience a certain degree of atelectasis. Alveolar collapse occurs because of lung compression by the animal's body weight and is most severe in the ventral lung. Thus the

Protocol 25.1 Artificial airway suctioning procedure (for endotracheal tubes, temporary tracheostomy tubes, permanent tracheostomy sites)

Items Required
- Suction source
  - Central vacuum system with a regulator
  - Portable suction compressor
- Suction tubing
- Suction catheters of appropriate size (largest possible that will easily glide into AA)
- Sterile gloves
- Sterile injectable saline and syringes (for flushing if required)
- Oxygen source
- Assistant(s)
- Predrawn sedation protocol in the event of anxiety or distress
- Pulse oximeter
- Electrocardiogram (ECG)

Procedure
1. Collect necessary supplies.
2. Instrument patient with ECG and pulse oximeter.
3. Preoxygenate patient for 5–10 minutes unless the situation is emergent (e.g., obstruction).
4. Set suction regulator between 80 and 120 mm Hg.
5. Perform hand hygiene and don sterile gloves.
6. Aseptically insert suction catheter, without applying suction, to the depth of the entrance of the airway (shallow suctioning), down the length of the tube (premeasured suctioning), or a few centimeters past the end of the artificial airway (deep suctioning).
7. Activate suction catheter by placing finger over the proximal port of the catheter, and tap the port as the catheter is withdrawn to apply rapid intermittent suction.
8. Swirl the catheter within the artificial airway lumen as the catheter is withdrawn to maximize secretion removal.
9. Apply suction no longer than 5 seconds and withdraw the catheter from the airway.
10. Reapply supplemental oxygen and monitor for hypoxia, arrhythmias, or patient discomfort. Allow the patient to recuperate completely before repeating the procedure.
11. Repeat the suctioning procedure one to three times, or as needed until secretions run clear and the patient is comfortable. Avoid oversuctioning, which will worsen inflammation and secretions.

simplest and most important form of chest physiotherapy is frequent repositioning of the patient to correct atelectasis. If the patient will tolerate sternal recumbency, this is often the best position for the lungs,[5] although this can vary in animals with respiratory disease. However, animals with hip or back pain may not accept sternal positioning. If possible, a reasonable compromise is to achieve sternal recumbency in the front limbs but allow lateral recumbency in the rear. Typically, the patient is changed from right lateral to left lateral recumbency every 2–4 hours.[5] The larger and more immobile the patient, the more frequently its position should be changed.

Encouraging coughing and clearance of loosened respiratory material is just as important as maintaining airway hydration. Coughing serves two functions: it helps to decrease atelectasis and it clears airway secretions. To cough, the animal must first take a maximal inspiration, which can help to decrease atelectasis. Following inspiration, the next stage of a cough is an initial buildup of airway pressure against a closed glottis. When the glottis is opened, the sudden release of pressure pushes material in an orad direction. In addition, airway smooth muscle contraction further milks material toward the pharynx. When an AA is in place, the animal cannot build up pressure in the airway at the beginning of the cough because the AA remains open even if the glottis is closed; therefore, coughing is less effective in patients with an AA in place. Some coughing efforts may occur, and in that case one walks a fine line in how much coughing should be permitted without causing the AA to obstruct or dislodge.

Coughing is stimulated by airway stretching, compression, or inflammation. Physical exercise encourages the patient to take breaths with increased tidal volumes, thereby stretching the airway and encouraging coughing as well as decreasing atelectasis. Thus walking patients after nebulization is another useful method of physiotherapy because it promotes increased tidal volumes and induces coughing. Gentle exercise cannot be overemphasized in the management of patients with pneumonia; clearance of airway infection is most challenging in paralyzed patients that cannot move around. In addition, if coupage (see later) is contraindicated, as in patients with thoracic wall injuries or coagulopathies, walking and exercise may be used as a substitute.

Coupage

Coupage creates vibrations within the chest that may help to mobilize exudates and stimulate coughing. Typically, nebulization is performed first, to make the secretions as liquid as possible. Then coupage is performed by gently but firmly tapping on the chest in rapid succession with a cupped hand. The force applied depends on the size of the patient; large dogs often tolerate the application of quite a lot of force to the chest wall, unless they are painful. Alternative methods may include the use of battery-operated vibrating massage devices available on the commercial market for use in people. Coupage should be applied to both sides of the thorax. Positioning of the patient during coupage may also assist with airway drainage. For example, a patient with right-sided lung disease may benefit from coupage applied to the right side of the chest while the patient is in left lateral recumbency. Some deep-chested dogs may be persuaded to roll onto their back for application of coupage, facilitating drainage from the most ventral lung lobes. Sedation or anesthesia may completely hinder the cough mechanism. In such cases, it may be appropriate to suction the airway after coupage.

Pharmacologic intervention

A variety of drugs may be administered to patients with AAs. Medications may include those used to treat the primary problem or its complications, and those used to manage the AA itself. For example, a postoperative brachycephalic dog with a tracheostomy tube might receive corticosteroids to treat soft palate and pharyngeal swelling, or antibiotics for aspiration pneumonia. A full description of all of the drugs that might be administered for treatment of all underlying problems is beyond the scope of this chapter. Instead, we focus on the medications that warrant special attention in the management of an AA.

General anesthesia

Dogs and cats with endotracheal tubes in place require general anesthesia to tolerate orotracheal intubation. A variety of drugs are used to maintain general anesthesia over a period of several hours to days. Typically, to maintain optimal cardiovascular and respiratory function, a combination of drugs is used. The drugs are often given as continuous intravenous infusions of injectable anesthetics, rather than as intermittent boluses or as inhalants. Careful monitoring is needed whenever patients are maintained under anesthesia for prolonged periods of time. Oxygen supplementation, ventilator support, fluid therapy, and pressors should be given as needed.

Sedatives and anxiolytics

Most dogs and cats with tracheostomy tubes are awake. Patients that are anxious or dysphoric may receive sedation, and those that are in pain may receive analgesics. It is important to remember that drug efficacy varies by individual, and there is often some trial and error involved in drug choices.

Animals with anxiety, excessive panting, and upper airway obstruction may benefit from administration of a sedative. Acepromazine is a commonly used tranquilizer suitable for many of these patients. The advantages of acepromazine include its relatively long duration of effect (hours); disadvantages include the risk of drug-induced vasodilation and hypotension. Therefore, although acepromazine is used commonly in this patient population, it is administered in low doses and repeated to effect (0.005–0.02 mg/kg IV, every 4–6 hours). Benzodiazepines such as diazepam and midazolam can also be used either as bolus doses (0.2–0.4 mg/kg IV) or as continuous IV infusions (0.05–0.3 mg/kg/hour). Benzodiazepines should be used cautiously because they can induce excitement in some dogs and cats.

Analgesics

Side effects of narcotic analgesics include suppression of coughing because of their centrally acting antitussive effects. Narcotics can also cause panting in dogs, which can be a problem with an AA. Panting against the AA's increased airway resistance can cause or exacerbate hyperthermia; panting can also cause rapid and complete occlusion of the AA with large mucus plugs.

Mucolytic drugs

Mucolytic agents such as N-acetylcysteine may be used as an adjunct to nebulization to facilitate the removal of respiratory secretions. N-acetylcysteine breaks disulfide bonds in the respiratory mucus, making it more watery and easier for the mucociliary escalator to move. N-acetylcysteine can be administered orally, intravenously, or by inhalation. Oral use may be limited by its bitter taste and the inadvisability of oral intake in some patients with AAs in place. When administered by inhalation in nebulization fluid, it can cause bronchospasm; therefore, caution is advisable when using this route. IV administration may be the safest option, although the drug must be diluted, filtered, and administered slowly.

Management of patients with endotracheal tubes

Endotracheal (ET) tubes are the most commonly used AA, and they are most familiar to veterinarians and veterinary technicians. ET tube placement is easier and quicker, less expensive, and less invasive than tracheostomy tube placement, although general anesthesia is required for insertion and maintenance.

Patients that are intubated for any length of time can develop adverse sequelae. Detailed and frequent nursing care is paramount not only to address the needs of the recumbent anesthetized patient but to prevent secondary complications. Although special attention to oral and airway hygiene can help minimize complications associated with ET intubation, the most reliable way to decrease intubation-associated morbidity is to extubate the animal as soon as possible.

Endotracheal tube qualities

Numerous varieties of ET tubes are commercially available, differing from each other with regard to physical composition, specialty, and reusability. Silicone tubes are soft, pliable, and made to withstand repeated sterilization. Polyvinylchloride (PVC) plastic tubes, in contrast, are packaged aseptically and designed for single use. Red rubber tubes can be sanitized and reused; however, over time, repeated use and cleaning degrades the integrity of the material. Figure 22.3 shows the three different types of ET tubes. Although Chapter 23, Tracheal Intubation, contains a more detailed discussion of ET tube attributes, it bears mentioning here that disposable sterile ET tubes should generally be used in patients that require AA management, namely in those undergoing longer term anesthesia or positive pressure ventilation.

Pressure from an inflated ET tube cuff on the tracheal mucosa can cause severe tracheal trauma, particularly if the cuff is overinflated or the tube is in place for a length of time. Low-pressure, high-volume cuffs have a wider surface area in contact with the trachea, which applies less pressure, resulting in a decreased incidence of tracheal mucosal ischemia and necrosis. However, the seal may not be as effective for airway protection from oropharyngeal secretions. High-pressure, low-volume cuffs are inflated with a smaller volume but apply more pressure over a small surface area. Although this makes for

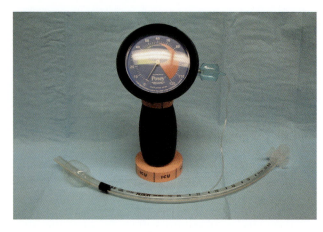

Figure 25.9 The Posey Cufflator Manometer is a useful tool to monitor ET tube cuff inflation pressure.

a better seal, it is more likely to cause tracheal mucosal ischemia, necrosis, or rupture if overinflated or if used for extended periods of time.

A manometer such as the Posey Cufflator TM (J.T. Posey Company. Arcadia, CA; see Fig. 25.9) can be used to monitor cuff inflation pressures to avoid overinflation and help prevent complications. Tracheal mucosa perfusion pressures range between 25 and 35 mm Hg, so maintaining a cuff pressure below 25 cm H_2O can minimize the risks of tracheal wall ischemia.

It is important to remember that although ET tube cuffs help decrease the aspiration of foreign materials, they do not provide complete protection. Even with appropriately inflated cuffs, fluid containing bacteria may seep down into the airways between the cuff and the tracheal mucosa. Careful selection of the proper tube size, continuous monitoring of cuff efficacy, and vigilant maintenance of the oral cavity (see later) are all equally important in avoiding aspiration pneumonia.

Oral hygiene

Animals intubated for prolonged periods of time develop a number of oral problems. The swallowing reflex is suppressed by anesthesia, which results in accumulation of oral secretions in the pharynx and caudal commissures of the lips. Gastrointestinal tract contents may be regurgitated from the esophagus into the pharynx. Furthermore, the pharynx rapidly becomes colonized with pathogenic gram-negative bacteria that can proliferate in accumulated secretions. Meticulous oral care is an important part of maintaining oral hygiene, thereby decreasing the risk of airway bacterial invasion during reintubation or accidental aspiration. It has been proven and widely documented in humans that one in four ICU infections are attributed to ventilator-associated

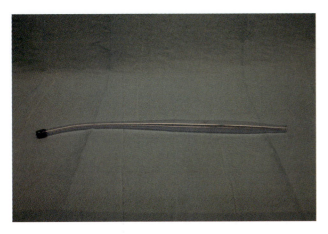

Figure 25.10 Kendall Argyle Yankauer Suction Tube. This stiff catheter allows ease of maneuverability when suctioning out the oral cavity. A thumb port, located proximally, provides suction control.

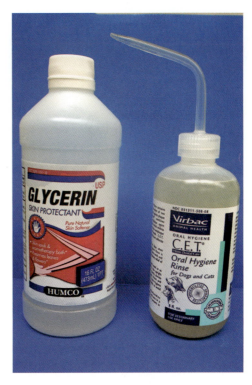

Figure 25.11 Glycerin Skin Protectant (left) and Virbac Animal Health C.E.T. Oral Hygiene Rinse (right). These items are used for oral care in patients with indwelling ET tubes.

pneumonia (VAP), that 90% of pneumonia cases in the human ICU are VAP, and that oral hygiene is now a standard of care to effectively reduce incidence of VAP in intubated patients.[6]

During ET intubation, routine oral care consists of inspection, suctioning, lavaging, moistening, and padding the delicate oral tissues. Stiff suction catheters, such as Yankauer tubes (Kendall Argyle Yankauer Suction Tube, TYCO Healthcare Group Mansfield, MA; see Fig. 25.10), can be easily maneuvered in and around the mouth and pharynx to gently remove excess secretions.

A commercial antibacterial oral rinse such as C.E.T. Oral Hygiene Rinse (Virbac Animal Health, Forth Worth, TX) should be used to cleanse the oral cavity. This mouth rinse contains chlorhexidine gluconate (0.12%), cetylpyridinium chloride (0.05%), and zinc. The rinse should be applied liberally inside the oral cavity using gauze sponges or a syringe, and then the excess is swabbed or suctioned away. One should be certain to clean around the teeth and remove all accumulated secretions in the back of the pharynx. Afterward, glycerin may be used as an emollient for lips and mucous membranes but should be diluted 1:1 with water as directed. (Humco Texarkana, TX; see Fig. 25.11) Oral care should be performed at least every 4 hours or more frequently if warranted by the nature or volume of secretions.[4]

Folded wads of gauze squares, soaked in the glycerin/ water solution, can be positioned in the mouth and around the tube to create a cushion to prevent pressure injury. The patient's tongue should be wrapped with soaked gauze sponges to prevent desiccation and swelling (see Fig. 25.12). It is also important periodically to

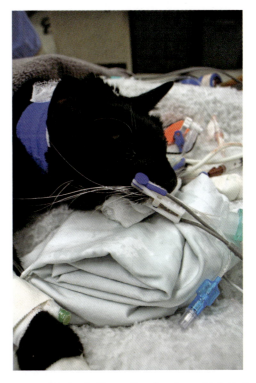

Figure 25.12 Mechanically ventilated patient with folded gauze squares (saturated with glycerin and water) padding the oral cavity. Repositioning the pulse oximeter probe regularly decreases tissue trauma.

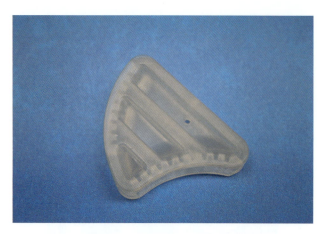

Figure 25.13 Dental wedge. Small grooves around the perimeter of the wedge hold the patient's teeth, which provides secure positioning of the mouth and helps prevent lip and tongue injury.

Table 25.4 Recommended schedule for ET tube care

- Auscult all portions of the patient airway and chest q2h
  - Auscultation may be done as frequently as necessary
- Evaluate ET tube q2–4h
  - Suction when necessary
  - Flush only when needed
- Oral care q4h
  - Flush, swab, and suction oropharyngeal cavity
  - Note and monitor tissues for swelling or ulceration
  - Replace gauze squares with freshly moistened ones (water and glycerin)
  - Readjust mouth prop
- Nebulize and coupage q2–4h
  - Continuous nebulization may be necessary for select cases
- Deflate and reposition tube q4–6h
  - Monitor cuff pressure if possible (e.g., Posey Cufflator manometer)
- Replace ET tube q24–48h or as needed
- Monitor comfort and sedation continuously

change the position of pulse oximeter probes placed in or on the mouth to prevent tissue injury.

Visual inspection of the oral cavity may reveal oropharyngeal ulceration, lingual swelling, or trauma to the lips. Treatment of these injuries associated with prolonged ET intubation involves keeping the tissues clean and avoidance of further pressure damage from the tube, gauze ties, pulse oximeter probe, or teeth. To avoid lip and tongue damage from teeth and the tube, a mouth prop or gag (Dental Wedge, Jorgensen Laboratories Inc., Loveland, CO) is helpful. The wedge is lined with ridges along each side for tooth positioning. It is designed for secure placement between the premolars and molars while allowing the mouth to remain comfortably open (see Fig. 25.13).

ET tube ties naturally accumulate material from the mouth, including bacteria. A nonporous material such as fluid extension tubing provides less surface area for bacteria and is easy to clean, so it can be a useful option to secure tubes. If muzzle gauze is used to secure the ET tube, it should be changed often because it provides a large surface area for bacteria and is impossible to clean.

Endotracheal tube care

ET tube care consists of evaluating tube patency, suctioning, flushing, repositioning, and replacing the tube when necessary. The tube should be evaluated no less often than every 2–4 hours and addressed as often as required by the patient. Table 25.4 provides a suggested schedule for ET tube maintenance and care.

To evaluate the patency of the ET tube, the upper and lower airways should be auscultated to help determine if there is an obstruction in the tube. When the tube itself is the source of a partial obstruction, the sounds are often loudest when the stethoscope is placed on the cervical area. Moist popping sounds usually indicate fluid or mucus buildup. Dry wheezing within the tube, similar to breathing through a straw, may be a sign of partial obstruction with thick or inspissated debris. In patients whose ET tubes are not connected to a breathing circuit, the naked ear may detect sounds emanating from the ET tube opening. Placing a hand or a teased-out cotton ball in close proximity to the tube's opening can also help gauge how much gas is successfully passing through with each exhalation.

Even patients with healthy lungs that are intubated for a period of time accumulate airway secretions; trauma to the tracheal mucosa from the tube itself results in increased secretions. Any material aspirated from the oropharynx causes additional inflammation. Bacterial infection may ensue due to compromise of pulmonary defense mechanisms, resulting in further inflammation and exudate production. The cough reflex has been intentionally eliminated by anesthesia, to allow ongoing intubation. Therefore, when secretions are auscultated in the ET tube, suctioning may be required to maintain a clear airway. Moistening the airway using humidification or nebulization, followed by coupage, may help further mobilize the secretions prior to suctioning. Because suctioning causes some trauma to the airway mucosa, it should be minimized and only applied as needed when auscultation suggests the presence of secretions in the AA.

Occasionally a patient continues to have a dry non-productive but still partially obstructed airway despite all efforts. As discussed earlier, there remains speculation whether instilling small aliquots of sterile saline into an airway helps or hinders management. With the risk of introducing bacteria into the lungs, causing further inflammation, and stimulating severe coughing, this decision should be made judiciously and saline infused sparingly in our opinion. If there is no alternative, then aliquots of 2–3 mL of sterile saline can be instilled into the ET tube, either by direct injection using a syringe or through a sterile catheter placed into the airway through the tube. Catheters used for this purpose can include red rubber urinary catheters or long through-the-needle IV catheters. The catheter is measured against a similar tube prior to insertion into the airway and should only be inserted slightly deeper than the length of the tube. Following instillation of saline, the suction catheter is passed into the airway and suctioning is performed as described perviously and in Protocol 25.1.

To minimize tracheal injury, the ET tube cuff should be deflated and the tube repositioned approximately every 4 hours.[4] When using a tube with a high-pressure, low-volume cuff, changing the position by just a centimeter allows normal circulation to return to the mucosa of the previous site. Care should be taken to avoid accidental extubation while repositioning the tube and to avoid advancing the tube too deeply into the airway, which could result in bronchial intubation. The cuff should be reinflated to no more than 25 cm H_2O pressure. If a manometer is not available, the cuff should be filled with an air syringe, just enough to prevent an audible air leak when the lungs are manually inflated (see Chapter 23, Tracheal Intubation, for more details).

ET tubes should be removed and replaced with a new sterile tube every 24–48 hours.[4] Patients with extensive accumulation of thick secretions in the lumen of the tube may need tube replacement much more frequently (as often as every few hours) if suctioning fails. Personnel should be prepared to change the tube at a moment's notice, and an area near the patient should be set up with all of the necessary equipment including replacement sterile tubes and laryngoscopes, to minimize response times (see Table 25.1).

Humidification and nebulization can be performed in several ways on intubated patients. Sedated intubated patients with intact respiratory drive may simply require an oxygen bubbler humidifier or a nebulizer system placed in front of the opening of the airway to provide optimal humidification. Chest physiotherapy is encouraged, although loosened material may need to be manually evacuated afterward using suction. Patients on a mechanical ventilator should have a heated humidifier incorporated into the breathing circuit, with the thermostat carefully adjusted to provide optimal humidity. Excessive heat can injure delicate airway tissues. Pooling of condensation increases ventilator circuit resistance, and water can potentially flow from the circuit into the patient's airway. Therefore, the humidifier should be set low, with the patient's temperature continuously monitored, and water traps (see Fig. 25.3b) should be placed at dependent points in the ventilator circuit and emptied as needed. Heat and moisture exchange devices or "artificial noses" can be inserted between the ET tube and the ventilator circuit. These devices trap heat and water vapor, and transfer them from the exhaled air to the inhaled air, thereby recycling them. There is a tendency for noses to become clogged with secretions, making them less desirable for cases with pneumonia or for long-term ventilation.

Management of patients with temporary tracheostomy tubes

A *tracheotomy* is the procedure of making an incision in the trachea, whereas a *tracheostomy* is the temporary or permanent opening established in the trachea during the tracheotomy procedure. The most common indication for temporary tracheostomy is circumvention of an upper airway obstruction. In addition, some long-term ventilator cases may also benefit from temporary tracheostomy because extended periods of endotracheal intubation can traumatize the oropharynx and larynx. Furthermore, temporary tracheostomies allow a much lighter plane of sedation in ventilated patients, allowing assessment of neurologic function and minimizing some adverse effects of prolonged anesthesia.

Tracheostomy tube placement requires general anesthesia and is a surgical procedure; see Chapter 24, Temporary Tracheostomy, for instructions on how to create a temporary tracheostomy. During the tracheotomy procedure, long stay sutures are positioned around the tracheal rings on each side of the stoma to allow manipulation of the rings during and after tracheostomy tube placement. Typically, the tracheostomy tube is not sutured directly to the skin of the neck because movement of the head and neck can pull the tube out of the airway if it is attached to the skin. Instead, umbilical twill tape or Velcro foam straps are fastened to each side of the tube's flange or neck plate and then tied behind the patients head, thus securing it in place (see Fig. 23.11). The skin incision is usually not closed with sutures. Instead, it is left open with the long tracheal ring stay sutures in place. If the tracheostomy tube needs to be replaced, the stay sutures allow quick removal and replacement of the tube. A moderate amount of

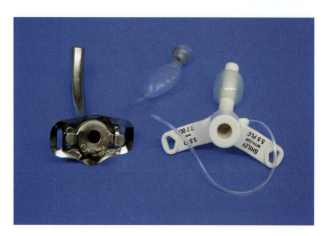

Figure 25.14 Two tracheostomy tube types. Jackson (metal) uncuffed tracheostomy tube on left. Shiley (PVC) cuffed tracheostomy tube on right.

discharge from the stoma site is common for the first few days. It should be cleaned from the skin several times daily, but care should be taken to avoid touching the tissues inside the incision.

Types of tracheostomy tube

A wide variety of tracheostomy tubes are available to suit veterinary needs (see Fig. 25.14 for two types). The clinician should take into consideration the likelihood of positive pressure ventilation, the patient's anatomy and disease process, and the length of time the tube is likely to remain in place when selecting a tube type. A basic review of tube selection is found in Chapter 24, Temporary Tracheostomy. The discussion here emphasizes tube choice based on length of intubation and maintenance.

Silicone tracheostomy tubes

Silicone tubes are soft and flexible, and they easily conform to the patient's airway. Both cuffed and cuffless versions are available. Their composition makes them less likely to accumulate bacteria and pulmonary secretions, therefore most are made without an inner cannula. This type of tube is useful for longer term tracheostomy when the volume of secretions has decreased. During the first few days after tracheostomy, most dogs and cats produce large amounts of airway secretions, and therefore the lack of an inner cannula can be a problem; thus a silicone tube may be a good choice as a replacement tube rather than as the initial tube placed after tracheotomy. An added advantage is the ability of silicone tubes to withstand multiple sterilizations.

Polyvinylchloride tracheostomy tubes

PVC tubes are single use and disposable, and they are the most frequently used in short-term veterinary ICU practice. The material is porous and more likely to accrue bacteria and mucosal debris, making it difficult to clean. Disinfectants are ill advised because they can absorb into the plastic and degrade the integrity of the tube. Larger tubes have a separate inner cannula, and separate disposable inner cannulas can be purchased to prolong the life of the outer cannula. Smaller sized tubes are not equipped with a removable inner cannula because it would excessively decrease the inner lumen diameter. Cuffed and uncuffed versions are available. Because of the availability of cuffed tubes with an inner cannula, this is the most commonly used tracheostomy tube for mechanically ventilated patients.

Metal tracheostomy tubes

Jackson tubes are made of stainless steel or silver and always cuffless. All sizes are available with inner cannulas, making them ideal for smaller patients. They can be easily cleaned and are autoclavable. Thus Jackson tubes can be reused for multiple patients over time, and they are therefore a cost-effective option. Because there is no bulky cuff, it may be possible to use a larger diameter tube than would be possible if a cuffed tube were used. They have grown less popular in humans due to their weight and tendency to irritate the tracheal mucosa. Although that is still a concern in veterinary patients, the practicality of their use for short-term management keeps them a popular choice.

Cuffed and uncuffed tracheostomy tubes

As with endotracheal tubes, tracheostomy tubes can be cuffed or cuffless. Cuffed tubes are valuable to protect the airway in patients at risk for aspiration or to provide a seal when mechanical ventilation is required; cuffless tubes should be used in others. The cuff is a soft balloon located at the distal end of the tube, which can be filled with air, sterile water, sterile saline, or foam (depending on the manufacturer's recommendations). The balloon can be deflated or inflated at a moment's notice should problems arise.

Cuff pressure must be monitored and readjusted frequently to avoid damaging the trachea. As discussed earlier, maintaining cuff pressure below 25 cm H_2O minimizes tracheal mucosal injury. High-volume, low-pressure cuffs generally minimize tracheal mucosal damage, although they are bulky during placement and may limit the size of tracheostomy tube that can be accommodated in the airway.

Smaller tracheas may not be able to accommodate bulky cuffed tubes; this is a particular problem in cats, pediatrics, and brachycephalic breeds. In these patients, very small-cuff tracheostomy tubes significant narrow the airway, which increases airway resistance. In such cases, a larger cuffless tracheostomy tube can be substituted without sacrificing internal diameter, as long as positive pressure ventilation is not required.

Stable tracheostomy cases may be less at jeopardy for aspiration once they are awake and have adequate cough and gag reflexes. In such instances, a cuffless or deflated tracheostomy cuff may be preferred, thereby minimizing tracheal damage while allowing the patient to breathe around the tube.

Impact of tracheostomy tube cannula type on airway management

Depending on the composition, size, and manufacturer, tracheostomy tubes may have single or double cannulas.

A double cannula tracheostomy tube comes equipped with a removable inner cannula, allowing it to be cleaned and replaced quickly. This is an ideal feature in cases producing large amounts of sticky respiratory secretions. Unlike single-cannula tubes, the patency of a double-cannula tracheostomy tube can generally be maintained for longer periods of time without tube replacement.

Tracheostomy tube attachment to a breathing circuit

When mechanical ventilation or anesthesia is expected, the proximal end of the tracheostomy tube needs to fit snugly into the breathing circuit. Most tubes, except for Jackson tubes, provide a 15-mm hub for this purpose. External adaptors are available to suit various size tracheostomy tubes; the adaptor fits between the tube's cannula and the breathing circuit (see Fig. 25.15).

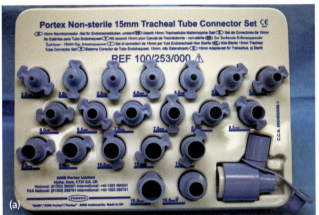
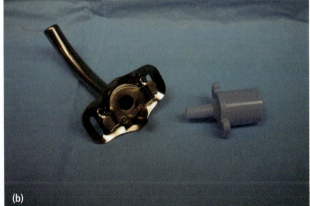
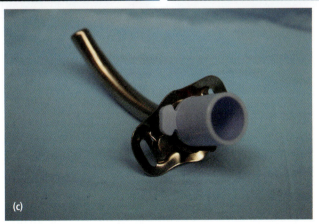

Figure 25.15 (a) Portex Non-sterile 15 mm Tracheal Tube Connector Set (SIMS Portex Limited, Kent, UK). These adaptors can be fitted into tracheostomy tubes lacking an appropriate hub to connect to breathing circuits. (b) Select an appropriately sized hub to fit into the inner cannula. (c) Jackson tracheostomy tube with 15-mm hub adapter.

Temporary tracheostomy tube care

Two people are usually required to provide basic tracheostomy tube care: one to position the patient and the other to perform the procedure. However, it is crucial that all the staff in the room remain on high alert in the event an emergency ensues because more hands may be needed. Manual restraint or mild sedation might be indicated for the awake or uncooperative patient. Deeper sedation or immediate induction of general anesthesia may be necessary for a patient in distress. A well-equipped tracheostomy supply station should be set up near the patient to decrease reaction time in a crisis. A list of suggested materials is provided in Table 25.2, and a recommended schedule for temporary tracheostomy tube care is found in Table 25.5.

Cannula maintenance and tube patency

Tracheostomy care begins with cannula maintenance. Although no strict guidelines exist, the inner cannula should be inspected and cleaned every 2–4 hours, or as often as the patient dictates it. Those with extremely productive secretions require vigilant monitoring and more frequent intervention to avoid tube obstruction episodes. Using aseptic technique, the inner cannula should be removed and visually inspected for debris.

Table 25.5 Recommended schedule for temporary tracheostomy tube care

- Auscult q2h
  - Auscultation may be done as frequently as necessary
- Evaluate tracheostomy tube q2–4h
  - Suction when necessary
  - Flush only when needed
- Cannula care q2–4h
  - May be continuous depending on productivity of secretions
  - Remove and clean cannula
  - Note consistency and character of secretions
- Stoma care q4–6h
  - Clean around stoma
  - Note character of the site (presence of discharge, presence of subcutaneous emphysema, etc.)
  - Evaluate for obstruction from neck skin folds or evaluate skin fold sutures, if applicable
- Nebulize and coupage q4–6h
  - Continuous nebulization may be necessary for select cases
- Deflate and/or monitor cuff pressure q4h
- Replace tracheostomy tube when necessary
- Monitor comfort and anxiety continuously
- House the patient in a central location that allows staff to see, hear, and access the patient quickly

The outer cannula can also be examined for any obvious material that can be swabbed out of the lumen with sterile cotton swabs. For patients receiving positive pressure ventilation, a new replacement cannula should be quickly inserted after removing the old one, thereby reducing the time the patient is disconnected from the ventilator circuit. The used inner cannula is placed in a sterile vessel filled with hydrogen peroxide. Soaking the tracheostomy tube in 3% hydrogen peroxide loosens the mucus and secretions that have adhered to it (see Chapter 24 for additional recommendations). Sterile pipe cleaners or small sterile brushes are then used to remove remaining debris (see Fig. 25.16). The inner cannula is rinsed thoroughly with sterile saline or water to remove any remaining hydrogen peroxide, which would cause tracheal irritation. The tube is carefully shaken or dried with sterile gauze squares. Finally, the inner cannula is replaced in the tracheostomy tube or saved in a sterile container for later use.

In addition to visual inspection of the tube during maintenance, a stethoscope should be used to auscult the upper and lower airways to detect diminished air movement, wheezing, or whistling sounds. The naked ear can also detect these sounds emanating from the entrance of the tube in spontaneously breathing patients. A reduction of airflow can be detected by placing a hand or teased-out cotton ball in front of the opening of the tube. If evidence of airway obstruction continues despite cleaning the inner cannula, there may be an obstruction at the distal end of the tracheostomy tube, in which case the entire tube may need to be removed and replaced.

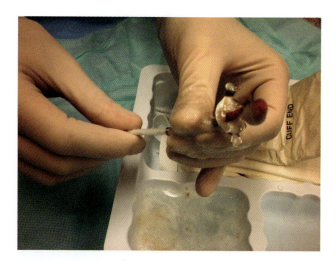

Figure 25.16 Tracheostomy tube care: cleaning the inner cannula. It is very common for peroxide to effervesce in the presence of blood, mucus, or other tissues adhered to the tracheostomy tube.

There is no set time to change out the entire tracheostomy tube, and this is typically done only when efforts to clear an obstruction have failed. Single-cannula tracheostomy tubes usually require more changes than those with an inner cannula. Flushing and suctioning the tube should be reserved for those with viscous secretions or debris, or patients with a decreased or absent cough reflex.

Stoma site care

The stoma of the tracheostomy site should be inspected approximately every 4 hours and monitored for inflammation, discharge, and pain; the operator should palpate around the stoma for evidence of subcutaneous emphysema. The consistency and origin of any discharge should be documented. Changes in the type of secretions within the lumen of the tracheostomy tube may indicate pneumonia, tissue necrosis, or hemorrhage, whereas changes in those from the stoma can indicate incisional infection. Using aseptic technique, the skin *around the stoma* should be cleaned using a 2% chlorhexidine scrub or half-strength hydrogen peroxide (3% strength diluted 1:1 with sterile water) on gauze squares to remove any debris. Sterile cotton swabs moistened with sterile water may be used to carefully clear material from the more delicate tissues of the stoma, but scrubs and ointments should not contact the wound. Soiled neck ties should be changed as needed to prevent them from becoming a source of infection.

Cuff maintenance

If there is an inflated cuff, the cuff pressure should be checked and adjusted if needed every 4 hours. A Posey Manometer can be used to check the pressure on high-volume, low-pressure cuffed tracheostomy tubes. Unlike ET tubes, it is not possible to adjust the position of a tracheostomy tube within the trachea to minimize pressure on one location of the tracheal mucosa. Instead, changing the amount of pressure in the cuff allows the tracheal mucosa to reperfuse. In patients that are completely awake and able to protect their airway, the cuff should be left deflated.

Airway humidification

The frequency of nebulization depends on the degree of desiccation of the airway and whether or not the patient has pneumonia. Ideally, nebulization should be continuous for patients with large amounts of exudative secretions or those with severe respiratory infections, and every 4–6 hours for more stable cases. This can be challenging, particularly in patients that are awake and mobile. If sitting with the patient in front of a nebulizer unit is not possible, an alternative solution is to place patients in a smaller open cage (with bars) with the nebulizer turned on "high." If the animal is asleep or sedated, it is useful to take advantage of that time to place the nebulizer hose in front of the AA opening. Nebulization during client visitation can be useful for patients that behave best for their owners. Most clients welcome the opportunity to help nurse their pets back to health and are happy to sit with them for a nebulizing session. Nebulization sessions are typically 15–30 minutes long.[1]

A word of caution: a tracheostomy patient should not be placed inside an enclosed cage (such as an oxygen cage) for nebulization unless absolutely necessary. Most of the time, early airway obstructions are easily audible to caregivers before they become severe enough that the patient starts to react physically. The incidence of obstruction increases during nebulization, and if the patient is left unattended, especially in a busy room or behind a glass panel, an early obstruction episode may be missed. If there is no alternative to placement inside the oxygen cage for nebulization, a member of the critical care team should be designated to stand vigil and monitor for any emergencies until the session is completed and the patient can be moved out of the cage. Patients with tracheostomy tubes in place should be housed in a central area to allow maximum visibility (and audibility) to all the staff.

Artificial noses (HMEs) should be avoided in tracheostomy patients because they can easily become occluded with respiratory secretions.

Hypoxic tracheostomy patients pose a significant challenge to the critical care team because of the need to deliver supplemental oxygen. A pneumatic nebulizer can be connected to an oxygen flowmeter, allowing oxygen supplementation during nebulization. Additionally, an oxygen delivery hose can be adapted into the nebulizer tubing to provide a higher fraction of inspired oxygen. If the patient is recumbent or sedated, the hoses can easily be positioned in front of the opening of the tracheostomy tube. Patients that are both hypoxic and mobile present a challenge. There may be no choice but to house these animals in an oxygen cage, but this presents considerable risk. As discussed earlier, oxygen cages muffle airway sounds that would otherwise be heard by the critical care personnel, including those sounds indicating early airway obstruction or respiratory distress. Extra precautions such as continuous pulse oximetry, stationing a team member in close proximity to the patient, and increasing peripheral vision around the room should be implemented to avoid emergent issues.

Physiotherapy

Chest physiotherapy such as coupage and gentle exercise should be encouraged after nebulization but under strict supervision. There is a fine line between adequate and excessive coughing in patients instrumented with a tracheostomy tube. Too little coughing produces inadequate airway clearance, whereas forceful coughing poses a risk of accidentally dislodging the tube. Antitussives such as butorphanol can be titrated to achieve the desired effect in animals that tend to cough.

Anxiolysis

Management of comfort and anxiety is extremely important to improving recovery time and decreasing complications as a result of stress. Not all patients react the same when it comes to dealing with a tracheostomy tube; some are incredibly stoic, whereas others may panic from the mere sensation of the tube. Adverse reactions might include severe coughing or attempts to scratch the tube out of place. If muscle activity leads to increased generation of heat, hyperthermia can develop quickly because of defective thermoregulation because the animal is unable to move air over the surface of the tongue during panting. Panting in these cases actually leads to the paradoxical situation of increasing body temperature because it involves the high work of breathing through the small tube aperture.

Some patients require pharmacologic intervention for anxiolysis. The goal is to maintain a plane of calm, comfort, and analgesia if needed, to allow the patient to continue with a normal daily routine. Most tracheostomy patients get used to living with tracheostomy tubes in place and will leave them alone, but a small subpopulation can be expected to encounter setbacks and require moderate to full sedation to tolerate the tube.

Special considerations for the patient with temporary tracheostomy

Table 25.6 lists the common complications seen in patients with temporary tracheostomy tubes.

Table 25.6 Complications of temporary tracheostomy tubes

- Airway obstruction
- Tube displacement
- Hemorrhage
- Infections (pneumonia or stoma infection)
- Subcutaneous emphysema
- Tracheal mucosal injury and necrosis

Animals with severe pneumonia that require a temporary tracheostomy tube can be among the most difficult and time consuming to manage. Copious amounts of secretions can accumulate inside the cannula, requiring almost continuous cleaning and/or changing. Hypoxic patients may need to be housed inside oxygen cages on higher oxygen concentrations or even require mechanical ventilation. These patients may require constant attendance due to the dynamics of their disease processes. Dedicating a trained technician for that patient facilitates constant patient monitoring and management while freeing up clinicians and the rest of the team members to handle other cases.

Head and neck conformation in brachycephalic breeds makes it difficult to manage their tracheostomy tubes. This creates a major challenge for the critical care team because brachycephalic dogs are also the most likely to require AAs. Because of the frequent incidence of tracheal hypoplasia, tracheostomy tubes may need to be significantly smaller than those used in other dogs of similar size. Smaller cuffed tubes should be avoided because the presence of the bulky cuff further decreases airflow. In these breeds, larger cuffless Jackson tracheostomy tubes may provide the greatest ease of placement, with the added benefit of a removable inner cannula. The shape of the tube should be scrutinized. An inappropriately shaped tracheostomy tube can curve too far in the tracheal lumen and become obstructed against the tracheal mucosa, or alternatively not curve enough and be easily displaced from the airway. A shortened ET tube may be placed through the stoma as a short-term option but is yet more difficult to maintain because of the lack of an inner cannula.

In some cases, the presence of a tracheostomy tube may not be enough to maintain a patent airway. In some breeds, especially pugs and bulldogs, the stoma can become obstructed by folds of fat or loose skin that can drape over the stoma, obstructing the airway from the outside. The problem may not be apparent during the initial placement of the tracheostomy tube because the animal is in dorsal recumbency. Once the animal is placed in sternal recumbency, it can be determined whether skin folds may need to be addressed. Skin folds can be temporarily sutured out of the way. Alternatively, strategically placed stay sutures can be placed on the skin folds on each side of the neck, umbilical tape can be threaded through the loops, and the skin can be gently pulled back and the tape tied behind the neck.

Most dogs and cats accept a tracheostomy tube without significant problem, but some have difficulty breathing while sleeping because of the position they assume while trying to sleep. These animals typically attempt to sleep in their usual recumbency but obstruct their tubes in the process and develop respiratory distress. Alternatively, they may try to sleep in a standing position because they are too frightened, uncomfortable, or anxious to lie down. A key role in nursing the temporary tracheostomy patient is rehabilitating the patient's habits to conform to its new airway. Take time to ease their anxiety and coax them to lie down in a position that allows them to rest without interfering with their breathing. Arrange bedding to fit the way the patient wants to lie down. An assortment of pillows, rolled towels, or folded sheets may be used to prop up the head, keeping the area in front of the tracheostomy tube free of obstruction. Gently holding the patient's head at an angle that allows maximum airway movement can also help calm it down. At times, pharmacologic intervention may be necessary to reduce their anxiety so they can be manipulated, but with time, patients may begin to pick up on the new habit and lay down on their own. It may take numerous tries to find the comfort zone for each patient. It is also crucial to remember that one major rule-out for anxiety and sleeping while standing up is respiratory distress, so one should evaluate the respiratory status of a tracheostomy patient that cannot get settled.

Management of patients with permanent tracheostomy (stoma)

A permanent tracheotomy is a salvage procedure performed to achieve long-term airway patency when all other options have been exhausted and the upper airway is irreversibly obstructed. A stoma (permanent opening) is surgically created in the ventral neck by suturing the tracheal mucosa to the skin, allowing free air passage without the use of a tracheostomy tube. During the first few days to weeks after formation of the stoma, there is usually considerable accumulation of mucus and secretions around the opening, and there is a high risk of occlusion, particularly in cats. Over time, the upper tracheal mucosa becomes epithelialized and the volume of secretions decreases considerably and eventually becomes negligible.

Permanent tracheostomy care

Table 25.7 shows a recommended schedule for care of the patient with permanent tracheostomy.

Stoma site care

Using the same guidelines as for temporary tracheostomy tubes, the stoma should be monitored every 4–6 hours for signs of obstruction, infection, or bleeding. The skin around the stoma should be aseptically cleaned

Table 25.7 Recommended schedule for permanent tracheostomy care

- Auscult q2h
  - Auscultation may be done as frequently as necessary
- Stoma care q4–6h
  - Clean around stoma
  - Note character of the site (presence of discharge, presence of subcutaneous emphysema, etc.)
  - Evaluate for obstruction by neck skin folds; evaluate skin fold sutures, if applicable
- Nebulize and coupage q4–6h
  - Continuous nebulization may be necessary for select cases
- Monitor comfort and anxiety q2–6h
- House the patient in a central location that allows staff to see, hear, and access the patient quickly

with either an antiseptic soap such as chlorhexidine (2%) mixed with water or half-strength hydrogen peroxide (3% strength diluted 1:1 with sterile water) as needed. As the tissues around the stoma start to heal and contract over the first few days, the opening of the stoma needs constant supervision because it can narrow to the point of airway obstruction and may require the emergent insertion of a tracheostomy tube. Occasionally, patients may need subsequent surgeries to expand the opening.

Airway care

The most common and life-threatening complication of permanent tracheostomy is airway obstruction. Dried mucus and secretions from within the trachea may lodge in the airway or at the entrance of the stoma, preventing airflow. Saline nebulization of the airway every 4–6 hours, or more often, helps moisten tissues and mucus, and it allows easier clearance of secretions. If the patient cannot expel material on its own, sterile cotton swabs moistened with sterile water may be used to carefully swab the interior of the stoma, taking extra care to not go in too far. As a final alternative, a small amount of sterile saline may be infused into the stoma to loosen debris and assist the patient in a more forceful, productive cough. Suctioning the interior of the stoma can lend some assistance but should be used cautiously because of the risk of mucosal trauma from the suction.

Special considerations for the patient with permanent tracheostomy

The animal should be closely supervised during initial attempts to eat and drink to avoid aspiration through

Table 25.8 Complications of permanent tracheostomies

- Obstruction of the airway
- Aspiration (pneumonia, foreign bodies, liquids)
- Tracheal necrosis
- Tracheal stenosis

the stoma. Bathing and obviously swimming are strongly discouraged for the rest of the patient's life. Potential complications of permanent tracheostomy are listed in Table 25.8, and Table 25.9 offers troubleshooting tips.

Table 25.9 Troubleshooting endotracheal tubes, temporary tracheostomy tubes, and permanent tracheostomies

Symptoms	Possible Causes	Course of Action
ET tube/trach tube/ stoma sounds: wet, gurgling, popping; dry/ raspy/whistling/ wheezing/"breathing through a straw"	Accumulated secretions +/− potential obstruction	• Increase nebulization/humidification to moisten secretions and induce productive coughing • Remove and clean inner cannula (trach tube) • Suction +/− flush if necessary (material or obstruction may be distal to tube or stoma) • Replace ET/trach tube if unable to remove obstruction
Mucus plugs	Dry airway	• Increase nebulizer frequency
Viscous secretions	Dehydration	• Evaluate systemic hydration • Increase inner cannula/stoma cleaning • Suction +/− flush if necessary (material or obstruction may be distal to tube or stoma) • Replace ET/trach tube if unable to remove obstruction
Tracheal secretions: Purulent	Infection	• Document and monitor for progression; submit aerobic cultures or cytology; treat accordingly
Hemorrhagic	Trauma from suctioning	• Reduce suction frequency • Meter suction between 80 and 120 mm Hg • Increase humidification and promote patient airway clearance
	Blood vessel injury from mucosal erosion	• Emergency intervention required if hemorrhage persists
Mucosa/tissue	Tracheal mucosal sloughing	• Decrease iatrogenic trauma (suctioning, cuff overinflation, etc.)
Inability to pass suction catheter	Catheter not able to pass curvature of trach tube cannula	• Suction without inner cannula (trach tube)
	Suction catheter too large	• Use smaller catheter
	Accumulated secretions within tube lumen	• Suction/flush/replace if necessary to loosen/remove secretions
Dislodged trach tube	Forceful cough, shaking, excessive pulling	• Consider pharmacologic intervention to soothe patient (antitussive/analgesic/anxiolytic/bronchodilator, etc.)
	Heavy trach tube (metal) Trach tube curvature inappropriate for patient anatomy	• Replace trach tube; make sure tube is appropriate for patient needs
	Loosened trach ties	• Resecure tube

Table 25.9 (*Continued*)

Symptoms	Possible Causes	Course of Action
Accidental extubation	Awake patient Repositioning ET tube too far proximally Deflated or damaged cuff Loose ET tube ties	Resedate/reanesthetize patient; replace ET tube; resecure tube
Labored breathing	ET tube or trach tube obstruction (proximally or distally) = mucus plug	• See course of action for mucus plugs
	Trach tube curvature inappropriate for tracheal anatomy = obstruction	• Replace trach tube with more appropriately shaped tube or short ET tube
	ET tube kinked	• Deflate and reposition ET tube
	Mainstem bronchus intubation (ET tube)	• Deflate and back out ET tube
	Bronchospasm	• Discontinue nebulization and administer oxygen; consider bronchodilators
	Pneumothorax, pneumomediastinum (ET tube)	• Check for barotrauma or tracheal tears; treat accordingly
	Tracheal stricturing (permanent trach stoma)	• Place trach tube (or ET tube through stoma)
	Airway interference +/− obstruction from skin folds (trach tube/stoma)	• Resect granulation tissue • Suture back skin folds
	Aspiration	• Check cuff for inflation/defects (ET and trach tube)
	Tube dislodgement	• Check for condensation backup in ventilator circuits • Evaluate trach patients for vomiting, regurgitation, or inadvertent aspiration through stoma
Stoma changes:	Trauma from manipulation	• Restrict iatrogenic trauma (cleaning/suctioning) and patient-induced manipulation (scratching/pawing/etc.); consider analgesics/anxiolytics
Bleeding	Blood vessel hemorrhage	• Emergency intervention may be required
Purulent discharge	Infection	• Treat accordingly
Subcutaneous emphysema	Air escape into incision (permanent trach)	• Document and monitor progression
	Tracheal tear (ET and trach tube)	• Treat accordingly
	Barotrauma	• Emergency intervention may be required if severe

References

1. Raffe MR. Respiratory care. In: Wingfield WE, Raffe MR, eds. The Veterinary ICU Book. Jackson Hole, WY: Teton NewMedia; 2002:147–165.

2. Branson RD, Campbell RS, Chatburn RL, et al. AARC clinical practice guidelines: humidification during mechanical ventilation. Respir Care 1992;37:887–890.

3. Hendricks JC. Airway hygiene. In: King LG, ed. Textbook of Respiratory Disease in Dogs and Cats. St. Louis, MO: Saunders; 2004:214-217.

4. Clare M. Care of the ventilator patient. In: Silverstein DC, Hopper K, eds. Small Animal Critical Care Medicine. St. Louis, MO: Saunders; 2009:912–916.

5. Davis HH. Nursing of the critically ill patient. In: Proceedings of the Atlantic Coast Veterinary Conference; 2001.

6. Pear SM, Ridley KJ. Infection Control Today—Oral Care Vital to V.A.P. Prevention; January 29, 2009; Infection Prevention—Comprehensive Oral Care: A critical component of VAP prevention; September 2008.

26

Capnography

Linda S. Barter

Terminology

A continuous plot of carbon dioxide (CO_2) in the respired gas versus time is called a **capnogram** and recorded by an instrument known as a **capnograph**. A **capnometer** detects the highest and lowest values for CO_2 in the respired gas and reports them as inspired and end-expired (also known as end-tidal) partial pressures or concentrations. The practices of measuring and recording CO_2 are called capnometry and capnography, respectively. Many monitors function as both capnometers and capnographs, displaying both numerical and graphical information about CO_2 in the respired gas. As with all monitoring tools, a capnogram is only a snapshot in time of one aspect of the patient's respiratory system function and should be evaluated in light of each patient's clinical condition.

Types of carbon dioxide analyzers

There are two types of CO_2 analyzers: mainstream and sidestream.

Mainstream

In **mainstream** analyzers, a sample cell or cuvette is inserted directly in the airway between the tracheal tube and the breathing circuit. An infrared sensor fits over the sample cell and emits light through windows in the sample cell (see Fig. 26.1). Light reaching the photodetector on the opposing side of the sensor measures PCO_2. Because the measurements are made directly in the airway, this technology eliminates the need for sampling tubes and scavenging but limits its use to the intu-

bated patient. The capnographic waveforms generated by mainstream analyzers are crisper than those from sidestream analyzers because they reflect real-time CO_2 measurements and suffer no deformity due to dispersion of gases in a sample line.

To prevent condensation on the sample cell windows, which can cause falsely high CO_2 readings, the mainstream sensor is heated. Thermal injury to the patient is possible; however, newer analyzers now have limited upper temperatures to avoid such problems. Disadvantages of mainstream analyzers are that they can be bulky and can have relatively large internal volume. This bulk puts traction on the endotracheal tube, which may increase the risk of inadvertent extubation, and their internal volume adds to apparatus dead space. These factors are more troublesome in smaller patients. The sensor unit in older models was fragile and easily broken; however, newer models are of simpler design and are lightweight, increasing their durability and suitability to daily use in veterinary practice. Many models use disposable sensor windows, available in standard and pediatric sizes (see Fig. 26.1), which can be changed between patients, to prevent contamination and minimize apparatus dead space.

Sidestream

In **sidestream** capnography the CO_2 measuring unit (monitor) is remote from the patient. A small pump within the monitor aspirates gas from the patient's airway through a long sampling tube. Ports onto which a sample line can be attached can be found on some endotracheal tube adaptors, some breathing circuit Y-pieces, or most commonly, lightweight connectors

Advanced Monitoring and Procedures for Small Animal Emergency and Critical Care, First Edition. Edited by Jamie M. Burkitt Creedon, Harold Davis.
© 2012 John Wiley & Sons, Inc. Published 2012 by John Wiley & Sons, Inc.

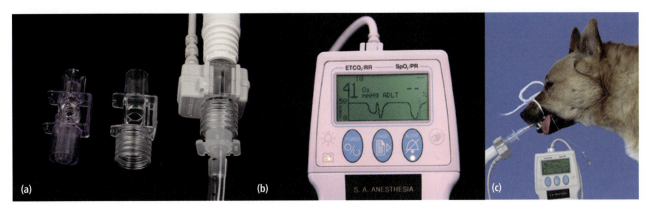

Figure 26.1 Mainstream capnography. (a) From left to right are micro cuvette, standard cuvette, and standard cuvette inside the infrared sensor connected between an endotracheal tube and the patient breathing circuit. (b) The display screen of a portable mainstream capnograph. (c) Mainstream capnograph in use on an anesthetized dog.

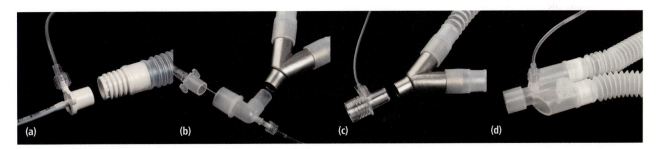

Figure 26.2 Different connection options for a sidestream capnograph gas sampling line. (a) Endotracheal tube adaptor with sample line adaptor. No additional apparatus dead space is added by attaching the capnograph in this way. (b) An elbow connector with adaptor port through which a small-bore catheter has been placed, which will be situated in the distal third of the endotracheal tube lumen to improve accuracy of sidestream gas sampling. (c) Short in-line connector between endotracheal tube and breathing circuit to which gas sampling line can be attached. (d) Some circuit Y-pieces have built-in sampling line connection ports.

designed to be inserted between the endotracheal tube or mask and the breathing circuit (see Fig. 26.2).

With sidestream capnography, gas analysis is delayed because it takes time for the gas to reach the monitor and some time to make the measurement (depending on the technology used). The effect of this delay is that capnographic waveforms generated by sidestream analyzers do not appear synchronously with each breath as is the case with mainstream capnography. Additionally, capnographic waveforms produced by sidestream monitors tend to be more rounded than those produced by mainstream devices in the same situations (see Fig. 26.3). The delay due to transit time depends on the length and diameter of the tubing and the rate at which gas is aspirated (this can vary from 50 to 250 mL/min depending on the monitor). As gas aspirated from the airway travels through the tubing to the monitor, the gas molecules can move around and start to mix (i.e., the CO_2-containing gas starts to mix with non-CO_2-containing gas). The faster the transit time between

the airway and the monitor, the less mixing will occur and the more representative will be the capnogram of actual changes in respiratory gas composition. Slow rates of aspiration, long sample lines, and large-bore sample lines result in capnogram waveforms with slurred up- and downstrokes (see section on capnographic interpretation).

Sidestream analyzers remove gas from the patient's breathing circuit. This must be accounted for when calculating fresh gas flow rates and also means that if patients are anesthetized with an inhaled anesthetic agent, then the gas must be appropriately scavenged or returned to the patient's breathing system. Gas may pass through conduits within the analyzer that cannot be cleaned or sterilized. This may pose an infectious disease risk to subsequent patients if analyzed gas is returned to the patient. The small-bore sample lines used by sidestream analyzers can easily become obstructed with moisture or aspirated secretions, and methods must be instituted to collect moisture, such as the use of Nafion

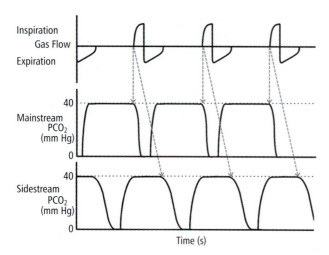

Figure 26.3 Comparison of capnograms obtained from mainstream and sidestream capnographs. The upper tracing depicts gas flow during the respiratory cycle, with gas flow above the line representing inspiration and gas flow below the line representing expiration. The middle tracing is a mainstream capnogram and the lower a sidestream capnogram recorded from the same patient at the same time. The dashed lines connecting the flow tracing with the capnograms illustrate the delay in registering changes in PCO_2 by capnography. The magnitude of this delay with a sidestream analyzer varies with the monitor settings and equipment (see text for details). A major difference between the two types of analyzers can be seen in the shape of the capnograms. Mainstream capnograms tend to record sharper changes in PCO_2, creating more vertical up-and-down strokes on the capnogram when compared with sidestream capnograms (see text for more details).

tubing (Nafion, E I du Pont de Nemours Company) or water traps.

Sidestream CO_2 analyzers may be single-purpose monitors or part of a larger monitoring unit with capabilities to analyze other respiratory gases as well as inhaled anesthetic agents. A unique advantage of sidestream capnographs is the ability to use them to monitor nonintubated patients. For example, expired gases may be sampled from the nasal cavity using nasal cannulas, or these monitors may be connected to feeding tube to obtain information to ensure correct placement (see indications section for more detail).

Equipment setup

In smaller patients mainstream CO_2 analyzers are technically superior to sidestream analyzers.[1,2] Due to their faster response time PCO_2 measurements are more reliable, especially when tidal volumes are small and respiratory rates are elevated. The main disadvantage of mainstream measurements is the addition of apparatus

dead space. This can lead to rebreathing of CO_2 and either elevation in $PaCO_2$ or increased work of breathing and altered ventilatory patterns to maintain a normal $PaCO_2$.[3] The size of the sampling cuvette relative to the tidal volume of the patient should be considered when choosing the type of analyzer to use on an individual (mainstream versus sidestream). Other considerations in making that decision would include whether there is any additional apparatus dead space as well as the length of time you intend to utilize the monitor. Routine mainstream capnography would not be recommended for long-term use in small patients.[3] It is always good to minimize apparatus dead space; however, small internal volume connectors or cuvettes also have a small internal diameter. As such a compromise is made to avoid unnecessary increases in airway resistance due to reduced airway diameter. It would be generally recommended not to use a connector with an internal diameter any smaller than that of the endotracheal tube placed in the patient.

Sidestream analyzers can be connected to the patient airway with the addition of minimal to no apparatus dead space (see Figure 26.2d). The cost of making this choice is reduced accuracy. A general figure for total minute ventilation is 200 mL/kg/min. Gas aspiration rates of the monitor must be considerably lower than total minute ventilation of the patient to prevent dilution of expired gas with fresh gas during sampling. If not, the capnograph waveform would be deformed and end-expired CO_2 underestimated. However, slow aspiration rates mean a long delay before gas is analyzed and distortion of the capnographic waveform. The sampling line should thus be as short as possible to minimize this delay time. Microstream aspiration technology with miniaturized sample chambers should be used if expired CO_2 is to be measured on spontaneously breathing small patients (<3–4 kg) for any length of time for improved accuracy and reduced deadspace.[4,5]

The closer to the alveolus that respiratory gas is sampled, the more faithfully the capnogram represents alveolar gas. However, a major problem with sampling from within the airways as is required with the sidestream technique is machine aspiration of secretions and water vapor. In intubated patients, sampling catheters placed within the lumen of the endotracheal tube reduce mucus aspiration (see Fig. 26.2b).

Physiology

Aerobic metabolism in tissues consumes oxygen, glucose, and other substrates and eventually produces energy, CO_2, and water. CO_2 produced in cells easily diffuses into the surrounding interstitial fluid raising local partial pressure of carbon dioxide (PCO_2). Arterial blood entering the tissues has a lower PCO_2 than the interstitial tissue and thus CO_2 diffuses from the interstitial fluid into blood. Venous blood leaves the tissues with a PCO_2 higher than that of arterial blood but equal to that of interstitial fluid. Venous blood carries the CO_2 produced by metabolism to the lungs to be removed from the body by ventilation. The process of ventilation replaces CO_2-rich gas from the alveoli with CO_2-free gas from the atmosphere or breathing circuit.

Alveolar partial pressure of CO_2 reflects a balance between CO_2 delivery to the alveoli by the cardiovascular system and its removal by ventilation. In the steady state, alveolar partial pressure of CO_2 is directly related to the metabolic production of CO_2 and inversely related to alveolar ventilation. CO_2 is highly diffusible such that in perfused alveoli, alveolar and arterial partial pressures of CO_2 are considered equivalent. Gas sampled at the end of expiration (end-expired or end-tidal gas) is representative of alveolar gas and is thus used as an estimate of arterial PCO_2.

Under the control of both the central and peripheral chemoreceptors, the body normally maintains arterial PCO_2 within a tight range by adjusting ventilation to the amount of CO_2 produced. Normal range for arterial PCO_2 is from 35 to 45 mm Hg, with some slight variations between species.[6,7]

Hyperventilation describes the situation where alveolar ventilation is in excess of metabolic CO_2 production resulting in alveolar (and thus arterial) PCO_2 levels below the normal range (hypocapnia). Low $PaCO_2$ values are associated with respiratory alkalosis and reduced cerebral blood flow. Hypoventilation describes the opposite situation where alveolar ventilation is insufficient to remove the metabolically produced CO_2 causing alveolar (and arterial) PCO_2 levels to rise above the normal range (hypercapnia). Most anesthetic and sedative drugs result in dose-dependent respiratory depression and respiratory acidosis. A $PaCO_2 > 60$ mm Hg is generally considered respiratory depression significant enough to warrant positive pressure ventilation in small animal patients.

Technology of carbon dioxide measurement

A number of techniques are available for measuring CO_2 including infrared absorption, Raman scattering, and mass spectrometry.

Infrared absorption

Infrared (IR) absorption is the most popular technique for CO_2 measurement. Monitors utilizing IR technology are typically the most compact and least expensive. IR absorption is the only technique used for CO_2 measurement in mainstream analyzers. Polyatomic gases like CO_2 have specific and unique absorption spectra of IR light. The amount of light absorbed in a specific spectrum is proportional to the concentration of the absorbing molecule. The concentration of gas can then be determined by comparing the measured light absorbance with that of a known standard. Infrared absorption can be used to measure any polyatomic gas (e.g., nitrous oxide and the halogenated anesthetic agents), which may be advantageous if purchasing a single monitor for use in anesthetized patients.

IR monitors have a short warmup period and a fast response time for CO_2 measurement, allowing them to measure inspired and expired concentrations. Water vapor absorbs infrared light and thus can spuriously increase measured CO_2. Water must therefore be removed from the expired gas by use of water traps or Nafion tubing (Nafion, E I du Pont de Nemours Company). There is some overlap between the absorption of nitrous oxide and CO_2. Most newer monitors that measure nitrous oxide in addition to CO_2 are able to correct for the effect of nitrous oxide on CO_2 readings.

Microstream capnographs are based on a modified approach to IR absorption. Molecular correlation spectroscopy is used to generate a narrow band of infrared light that precisely matches the absorption spectrum of CO_2 and eliminates interference with other gases. The high CO_2 specificity and sensitivity allows for a very short light path, and measurements can be made on a very small gas sample. In turn this allows the use of low sample rates (50 mL/min compared with typical rate of 150 mL/min for conventional IR analyzers) without compromising accuracy or response time. This reduces entry of moisture into the sample line and also reduces the competition for tidal volume that may compromise measurement accuracy in small patients or those with high respiratory rates.

Raman scatter

Raman scatter is a technique able to measure CO_2, oxygen, nitrogen, nitrous oxide, and halogenated anesthetic agents. Gas is sampled into an analyzing chamber where it is illuminated by a high-intensity monochromatic argon laser beam. When the laser beam hits molecules with interatomic bonds, a fraction of the energy is absorbed and reemitted at various wavelengths characteristic of the particular molecule that absorbed it. These monitors have a short warmup period, fast response time, require little maintenance, and are very accurate.

Mass spectrometry

Mass spectrometry is not commonly used for CO_2 measurement in clinical practice because these machines tend to be expensive and bulky. A unique feature of mass spectrometers is that a single unit can be used to measure gas concentration from up to 30 different locations. As such these are most commonly found in large hospitals. Gases are aspirated into a vacuum chamber where an electron beam ionizes and fragments the components of the sample. Ions are then accelerated through a magnetic field that separates them based on their mass-to-charge ratio. Individual detector plates allow for determination of the concentration of each component of the gas mixture. These analyzers typically measure only gases for which they have been preprogrammed to find. Adding the capability to measure new gases may require new hardware and/or software and may be costly. Because these units measure gases in concentrations (as opposed to infrared analyzers and Raman spectrometers that measure gases as partial pressures), they assume that the sum of the gases they can detect is 100%. If an unmeasured gas is present in significant concentrations, this may result in erroneously high measured CO_2 concentrations.

Indications for capnography/capnometry

Indications for performing capnography or capnometry are listed in Table 26.1.

Confirming correct endotracheal tube placement

Capnography or capnometry may be useful in to situations in which it is challenging to determine visually the correct endotracheal tube placement. Repeated upstrokes in the capnogram (repetitive increases in the PCO_2) suggest the presence of ventilation. It is theoretically possible to sample CO_2-containing gas from the stomach, but the values for end-expired partial pressure of CO_2 are likely to be much lower, reduce with time, and not fluctuate in a pattern consistent with respiration. Positioning of the endotracheal tube tip just inside the glottis may produce acceptable end-expired PCO_2 levels and a normal capnogram. Such tube placement risks easy dislodgement and inadequate airway protection. In low perfusion states (e.g., cardiac arrest, shock) verification of correct endotracheal tube placement by capnography is complicated by the presence of abnormally low end-expired PCO_2 and a dampened waveform because little CO_2 is being delivered to the lung for expiration.

Detection of apnea

If a patient becomes apneic, the capnograph or capnometer typically sounds an alarm when CO_2 stays at zero for a given period of time. Such monitoring is easily achieved if the patient is intubated. The sampling line of a sidestream analyzer can be attached to nasal prongs for the detection of apnea in nonintubated patients.

Monitoring ventilation

The gas exhaled at the end of expiration should be primarily alveolar gas, and thus end-expired PCO_2 is representative of alveolar PCO_2. Due to the high diffusivity of CO_2, alveolar and arterial PCO_2 equilibrate and end-expired PCO_2 is used to estimate arterial PCO_2. Capnography and capnometry can therefore be used to assess the adequacy of ventilation in spontaneous or mechanically ventilated patients.

Monitoring pulmonary perfusion

Large drops in cardiac output (hypovolemic shock or cardiac arrest) result in exponential drops in expired PCO_2. Therefore, very low or precipitously dropping PCO_2 should lead the operator to suspect cardiovascular collapse. Capnography may be useful in monitoring cardiopulmonary resuscitation efforts. End-expired PCO_2 has been used to predict the survivability from cardiac arrest. A successful outcome from cardiopulmonary resuscitation is more likely if expired PCO_2 levels are >10–15 mm Hg during resuscitation efforts.[8–10]

Correct nasogastric tube placements

Connection of a sidestream analyzer to gastric tubes may provide additional evidence for correct placement. Detection of any significant level of CO_2 should create suspicion of inaccurate placement.

Equipment problems

Capnography may be used to detect malfunctioning or incorrect assembly of breathing circuits, anesthetic machines, and ventilators. Problems such as malfunctioning

Table 26.1 Clinical indications for capnography

- Ensuring correct placement of endotracheal tube
- Detection of apnea
- Monitoring adequacy of ventilation
- Monitoring pulmonary perfusion during cardiopulmonary resuscitation
- Ensuring correct placement of nasogastric tube
- Detection of equipment problems

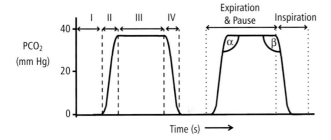

Figure 26.4 The normal capnogram. The capnogram can be divided into four phases, I through IV, and forms two angles, the alpha (α) and beta (β) angles. The phases of the respiratory cycle have been superimposed on the capnogram to the right side of the figure.

unidirectional valves, exhausted CO_2 absorbers, and inadequate fresh gas flows may be detected by alterations in the capnogram waveform (see next section).

Interpretation of the capnogram

The normal capnogram, seen in Figure 26.4, can be divided into four phases (I–IV).

Phase I

Phase I is the normally flat baseline segment of the capnogram. During the first part of this phase, inspiration is occurring. At the very end of this phase, the direction of gas flow reverses as expiration begins. During early expiration, expired gas comes from anatomic dead space. Anatomic dead space has not participated in gas exchange, and as such gas from these regions is identical in composition to inspired gas (normally CO_2 free).

Phase II

Phase II is the upstroke of the capnogram waveform. This corresponds to the period of expiration where CO_2-containing alveolar gas begins to be exhaled in a mixture with gas from anatomic dead space. As expiration proceeds the expired gas is composed of rapidly increasing proportions of alveolar gas. and the CO_2 levels quickly rise.

Phase III

Phase III is the plateau of the capnogram. During this phase PCO_2 is normally almost constant as alveolar gas, normally of nearly uniform composition, is expired. Expiration actually ends partway through this phase and is usually followed by a pause. During this pause PCO_2 typically remains constant on the capnogram even though no gas is flowing in or out of the patient. This

occurs because there is expired alveolar gas remaining stationary within the region of breathing circuit from which the gas is being sampled by the capnograph. This part of the plateau may be cut short by small tidal volumes, high fresh gas flow rates, and/or high gas sampling rates (see abnormal capnograms for more details). The angle between phases II and III of the capnogram is known as the alpha angle and is normally close to 100–110°.

Phase IV

Phase IV is the rapid downstroke on the capnogram corresponding to inspiration. During this phase fresh normally CO_2-free gas passes the sampling port as it is inspired into the lungs. The angle between phases III and IV is known as the beta angle and normally close to 90°.

Abnormal capnograms

Abnormal phase I

If the capnogram fails to return to baseline during inspiration, then the shape of the waveform should be considered. If the response time of the analyzer is slow, particularly in the face of high respiratory frequencies, then the capnogram may adopt a sine wave formation (see Fig. 26.5a). This is a relatively common capnographic waveform in cats. Such a waveform has no distinct alveolar plateau, and erroneous values for inspiration and expiration may result (falsely elevated baseline and underestimated peak expired CO_2, respectively).

If the capnogram fails to return to baseline during inspiration and is not the result of a slow response time (i.e., the shape of the waveform is relatively normal), then there must be CO_2 in the inspired gas. Common reasons for this include exhausted CO_2 absorber in a circle system, malfunctioning inspiratory valve in a circle system, or inadequate fresh gas flow in a nonrebreathing system (see Fig. 26.5b).

Periodic elevations in baseline can occur if external pressure is applied to the patient's chest during the inspiratory period. If this occurs, then gas is forced out of the lungs and a small rise in PCO_2 is registered on the capnogram during what would normally be the baseline period (see Fig. 26.5c).

Abnormal phase II

With sidestream capnographs, gas sampling rate affects the shape of the capnogram. Slow sampling rates decrease the slope of phase II, shorten the alveolar plateau, and decrease the slope of phase IV (see

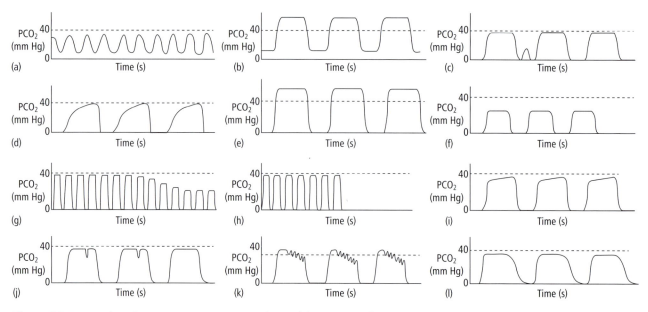

Figure 26.5 Examples of common capnogram waveforms. (a) Sine wave form common with sidestream analysis on small patient with high respiratory rate; (b) rebreathing of CO$_2$-containing gas; (c) expiratory effort between regular breaths; (d) bronchoconstriction/airway obstruction; (e) hypoventilation; (f) hyperventilation; (g) slow-speed capnogram suggesting reduced pulmonary blood flow; (h) slow-speed capnogram indicating accidental extubation, patient disconnection, or sudden apnea; (i) uneven alveolar emptying; (j) spontaneous inspiratory efforts during mechanical ventilation; (k) cardiogenic oscillations; (l) faulty inspiratory valve.

Fig. 26.3). This delayed equipment response time typically results in increases in both the alpha and beta angle of the capnogram. If the slope of phase II is decreased in the absence of delayed equipment response time, it suggests slow expiration. Such an abnormality is often also associated with a sloped alveolar plateau and increases in alpha angle but normal beta angle (see Fig. 26.5d). Important causes of slow expiration are patient conditions causing airway narrowing or external conditions such as a partially obstructed or kinked endotracheal tube.

Abnormal phase III

Normally, peak expiratory PCO$_2$ values are only a few mm Hg lower than PaCO$_2$. A normally shaped capnogram with an elevated alveolar plateau (see Fig. 26.5e) reflects hypoventilation. This is very common in anesthetized or sedated patients. If the patient is not receiving supplemental oxygen, hypoventilation is a common cause of hypoxemia.

A normally shaped capnogram with lower than normal alveolar plateau (see Fig. 26.5F) may reflect hyperventilation. In this instance end-expired and arterial PCO$_2$ levels are close in value. If the patient is being mechanically ventilated, ventilator settings should be evaluated. Other causes for lower than normal alveolar plateau include reduced CO$_2$ production (hypothermia)

or reduced delivery of CO$_2$ to the lungs (low cardiac output). Trends in peak expired CO$_2$ over time can be useful to demonstrate the effect of reduced pulmonary blood flow on the capnogram. Figure 26.6 displays tracings of a systemic arterial pressure waveform and corresponding capnogram recorded at slow paper speed. A period of hypotension can be seen to correspond to reduced alveolar plateau levels on the capnogram, which returned to previous levels when systemic pressure was restored.

The existence of alveolar dead space (ventilated but unperfused areas of the lung), such as would occur secondary to pulmonary thromboembolism, creates a situation in which peak expired PCO$_2$ levels are substantially lower than arterial PCO$_2$ measurements. Unperfused alveoli will not have participated in gas exchange and so contain gas identical in composition to inspired gas, which is normally CO$_2$ free. During expiration this gas mixes with the gas from perfused alveoli diluting the PCO$_2$ in the expired alveolar gas. When examining a capnogram recorded at slow paper speed, the alveolar plateaus of each wave are typically fairly uniform in a stable patient (see early part of Fig. 26.5g). Sudden reductions in pulmonary blood flow, such as occurs with pulmonary thromboembolism, typically result in exponential decreases in the peak alveolar plateau as long as ventilation continues (see progression of Fig. 26.5g) as

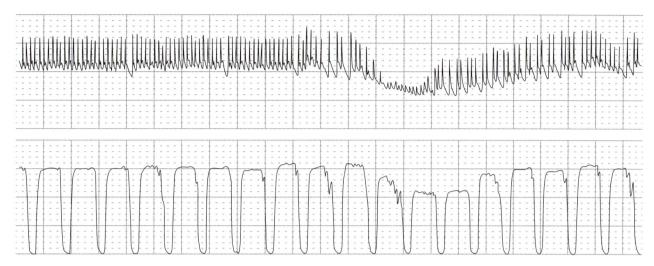

Figure 26.6 The effect of reduced pulmonary blood flow on the capnogram. The upper tracing is arterial blood pressure recorded from the dorsal pedal artery of an anesthetized dog. The lower tracing is a capnogram recorded concurrently from the same patient. Note that the period of hypotension results in a corresponding reduction in the height of the alveolar plateau on the capnogram.

opposed to an abrupt disappearance of the capnogram waveform as would occur with disconnect or accidental extubation of a patient (see Fig. 26.5h).

An abnormally low alveolar plateau could also be seen if a sidestream analyzer were to have a leak in the gas sampling line and constantly aspirate room air, thus diluting the exhaled gas and creating falsely low PCO_2 measurements.

Conditions causing uneven filling and emptying of alveoli (ventilation perfusion mismatch) result in a slanted plateau phase of the capnogram (and an increased alpha angle) (see Fig. 26.5i). If exhalation is particularly slow, then peak PCO_2 levels may not be reached before inhalation occurs, and as such end-expired PCO_2 values will be below alveolar and thus arterial PCO_2 values.

The normal alveolar plateau is roughly horizontal (see Fig. 26.4). Artifactual dips and bumps in the plateau phase may result from pushing on the thorax of an anesthetized patient causing gas to move out and into the lungs. In an animal being mechanically ventilated, spontaneous ventilatory efforts may be interspersed among mechanical breaths and cause dips or clefts in the alveolar plateau (see Fig. 26.5j). Reasons for these respiratory efforts should be investigated including insufficient anesthetic depth, inadequate mechanical ventilation, hypoxemia, inadequate analgesia, and hyperthermia.

Cardiogenic oscillations are undulations in the capnogram that are synchronous with cardiac contractions (see Fig. 26.5k). Contraction of the right ventricle and filling of the pulmonary vasculature expels a small volume of gas from the lungs with each beat. In combination with gas aspiration by a sidestream analyzer, oscillations in PCO_2 during the respiratory pause may become evident. This is a common and inconsequential finding in dogs.

Abnormal phase IV

Normally the capnogram returns briskly to baseline from the alveolar plateau, creating a beta angle of almost 90° as fresh gas is inspired thus replacing the CO_2-containing gas at the sampling site. If the slope of this phase is reduced (i.e., the beta angle is increased; see Fig. 26.5l), then either inspiration is occurring abnormally slowly (not common because it does not take much gas to replace the small volume of exhaled gas at the sampling site) or there is CO_2 in the inspired gas. This could occur with inadequate fresh gas flows on a nonrebreathing circuit or malfunctioning inspiratory valve on a circle system.

Protocol 26.1 describes a step-by-step approach to capnogram interpretation.

Summary

Capnography is a noninvasive method for continuous assessment of ventilation because $ETCO_2$ provides a very good estimate of PCO_2 in most cases. Gas sampling can be either mainstream or sidestream, each of which has advantages and disadvantages. Capnography is most accurate in intubated patients but can also be used in awake, nonintubated patients for continuous noninvasive PCO_2 monitoring. Finally, evaluation of

Protocol 26.1 Capnogram interpretation: a step-by-step guide

Procedure

1. Are there regular waves of CO_2 providing evidence of ventilation?
2. Does the baseline return to zero (normal) or is there evidence of rebreathing (elevated baseline)?
3. Is the upstroke steep (normal) or is there evidence of slow expiration (slanted upstroke)?
4. Is the alveolar plateau even (normal) or is there evidence of uneven alveolar emptying (slanted plateau) or interruption of the expiratory period by inspiratory efforts (clefts in plateau)?
5. Are end-expired PCO_2 values within an acceptable range, and are they consistent with the patient's respiratory parameters?
6. Is the downstroke steep (normal), or is there evidence of slow inspiration or rebreathing (slanted downstroke)?

capnographic waveforms can aid in the detection of patient or equipment abnormalities.

References

1. Badgwell JM, Heavner JE. End-tidal carbon dioxide pressure in neonates and infants measured by aspiration and flow-through capnography. J Clin Monit 1991;7:285–288.

2. Pascucci RC, Schena JA, Thompson JE. Comparison of a side-stream and mainstream capnometer in infants. Crit Care Med 1989;17:560–562.

3. Schmalisch G, Foitzik B, Wauer RR, et al. Effect of apparatus dead space on breathing parameters in newborns: "flow-through" versus conventional techniques. Eur Respir J 2001;17:108–114.

4. Kugelman A, Zeiger-Aginsky D, Bader D, et al. A novel method of distal end-tidal CO2 capnography in intubated infants: comparison with arterial CO2 and with proximal mainstream end-tidal CO2. Pediatrics 2008;122:e1219–1224.

5. Hagerty JJ, Kleinman ME, Zurakowski D, et al. Accuracy of a new low-flow sidestream capnography technology in newborns: a pilot study. J Perinatol 2002;22:219–225.

6. Middleton DJ, Ilkiw JE, Watson AD. Arterial and venous blood gas tensions in clinically healthy cats. Am J Vet Res 1981;42:1609–1611.

7. Haskins S. Monitoring the anesthetized patient In: Tranquilli WJ, Thurmon JC, Grimm KA, eds. Lumb & Jones' Veterinary Anesthesia & Analgesia. 4th ed. Ames, IA: Blackwell; 2007:533–558.

8. Sanders AB, Kern KB, Otto CW, et al. End-tidal carbon dioxide monitoring during cardiopulmonary resuscitation. A prognostic indicator for survival. JAMA 1989;262:1347–1351.

9. Trevino RP, Bisera J, Weil MH, et al. End-tidal CO2 as a guide to successful cardiopulmonary resuscitation: a preliminary report. Crit Care Med 1985;13:910–911.

10. Gudipati CV, Weil MH, Bisera J, et al. Expired carbon dioxide: a noninvasive monitor of cardiopulmonary resuscitation. Circulation 1988;77:234–239.

27

Mechanical ventilation

Kate Hopper

A mechanical ventilator is a machine that performs some or all of the work of breathing and is used to support respiratory function in patients with respiratory failure. The primary function of the lung is oxygenation of the arterial blood and removal of carbon dioxide from the venous blood. The ability of the lung to oxygenate the pulmonary capillary blood depends largely on the surface area available for gas exchange and the preservation of the delicate structure of the gas exchange barrier. In contrast, removal of carbon dioxide primarily depends on the movement of fresh gas into the alveoli, thereby flushing out carbon dioxide–rich gas on exhalation, a process known as ventilation. Patients with respiratory failure can generally be divided into one of two groups: those with oxygenation failure and those with ventilatory failure.

Indications for mechanical ventilation[1]

There are three main indications for mechanical ventilation. The first is severe hypoxemia despite oxygen therapy. Severe hypoxemia is indicated by cyanosis, a $PaO_2 < 60\,mm\,Hg$, or an $SpO_2 < 90\%$. Patients with severe hypoxemia have significant lung disease such as pneumonia, acute respiratory distress syndrome, pulmonary edema, or pulmonary contusions.

The second indication for mechanical ventilation is severe hypoventilation despite therapy. Severe hypoventilation is marked by a $PCO_2 > 60\,mm\,Hg$ (see Chapter 22 for a further discussion of blood gas analysis). The PCO_2 is controlled primarily by alveolar minute ventilation. This is the total amount of fresh gas that reaches the alveoli in a minute and is equal to the product of the respiratory rate and effective tidal volume. Consequently, causes of severe hypoventilation are diseases that impair the ability of patients to maintain an adequate respiratory rate and/or tidal volume. Such diseases include brain disease, cervical spinal cord disease, peripheral neuropathies, diseases of the neuromuscular junction, and myopathies. Not all patients that have severe hypoxemia or severe hypoventilation require mechanical ventilation, but these criteria help identify candidates for ventilation. An understanding of the primary disease process and other patient data will help determine the necessity of mechanical ventilation in individual patients.

The third indication for mechanical ventilation is excessive respiratory effort, even if the patient can maintain acceptable blood gas values. Determination of excessive respiratory effort is based on clinical judgment, and mechanical ventilation is indicated in these patients to avoid imminent exhaustion and subsequent arrest. These patients usually have lung disease.

Ventilator settings

The ventilator makes gas flow into the lungs by the generation of positive airway pressure in a manner similar to that achieved by squeezing the rebreathing bag on an anesthetic machine when "bagging" a patient. Every ventilator has a variable number of available settings that can be altered to change the nature of the breath delivered. Despite the apparent complexity of many ventilators, there are only a few key settings that are essential to understand to provide effective ventilation. When choosing ventilator settings, the operator must first

Advanced Monitoring and Procedures for Small Animal Emergency and Critical Care, First Edition. Edited by Jamie M. Burkitt Creedon, Harold Davis.
© 2012 John Wiley & Sons, Inc. Published 2012 by John Wiley & Sons, Inc.

choose a mode of ventilation and then select machine settings based on general guidelines (described later). These initial settings may be adjusted based on some understanding of the nature of the patient's respiratory disease. Following initiation of mechanical ventilation the ventilator settings are then titrated as necessary to achieve the blood gas goals desired.

Ventilator breath types[1,2]

The three main ventilator breath patterns commonly used in veterinary medicine are Assist/Control (A/C) ventilation, synchronized intermittent mandatory ventilation (SIMV), and continuous spontaneous ventilation. Some machines only have one breath pattern option, such as an anesthetic-type ventilator, whereas more modern intensive care unit ventilators may offer all three options.

The two primary breath patterns used to provide positive pressure ventilation are A/C and SIMV. In A/C ventilation, all the breaths delivered are completely generated by the machine (mandatory breaths). In this mode of ventilation, a minimum respiratory rate is set by the operator. If the trigger sensitivity is set appropriately, the patient can increase the respiratory rate, but all breaths delivered will be full ventilator (mandatory) breaths. The size of these ventilator breaths will depend on machine settings entered by the operator. Ventilator breaths can either be pressure- or volume-controlled breaths. In volume control ventilation, the operator presets the desired tidal volume, and the peak airway pressure generated depends on the size of the tidal volume chosen and the compliance (how stiff or stretchy the lung is) of the respiratory system. In pressure-controlled ventilation, the operator presets the desired peak airway pressure, and the tidal volume generated depends on the level of airway pressure chosen and the compliance of the respiratory system. A/C ventilation provides maximum support of the respiratory system and is used in patients with severe disease or patients with no respiratory drive (those making little or no attempts to breathe on their own).

In SIMV, the operator can set the number of full ventilator (mandatory) breaths delivered, and between these breaths the patient can breathe spontaneously as much or as little as it wishes. The machine tries to synchronize the ventilator breaths with the patient's own respiratory efforts. As this mode combines full ventilator breaths with spontaneous patient breaths, it is generally used for animals that need <100% assistance from the ventilator, such as neurologically abnormal animals with a less reliable respiratory drive or patients with lung disease that are improving and do not need as much support as A/C provides.

The two common options for provision of continuous spontaneous ventilation are continuous positive airway pressure (CPAP) and pressure support ventilation (PSV). In CPAP the ventilator delivers no breaths; all breaths are spontaneous breaths, meaning they are completely patient generated: the respiratory rate, inspiratory time, and tidal volume are all determined by the patient. Constant positive airway pressure provides just that: a constant level of positive airway pressure (the amount is preset by the operator) throughout the respiratory cycle. It decreases resistance to gas flow and increases respiratory system compliance, enhancing gas exchange and oxygenation. In addition the machine alarms if the animal does not generate adequate breaths or develops apnea, so it is a useful monitoring mode for weaning patients or for monitoring intubated patients.

As in CPAP, all PSV breaths are spontaneous breaths; the ventilator does not deliver any breaths. In PSV, the tidal volume generated by the patient is augmented by the machine. The amount of support provided during inspiration depends on how much pressure is selected by the operator. This mode reduces the effort required to maintain spontaneous breathing in patients with adequate respiratory drive and inadequate ventilatory strength. Pressure support ventilation can be used alone, in conjunction with CPAP, or to augment the spontaneous breaths during SIMV.

Tidal volume

The normal tidal volume reported for dogs and cats is in the range of 10–15 mL/kg. Lower tidal volumes (6–8 mL/kg) may be targeted in animals with severe lung disease. When using volume control ventilation, the operator presets the desired tidal volume. Because over-distension of the lung is extremely dangerous, it is recommended to start with no more than 10 mL/kg as a preset tidal volume; the tidal volume can always be increased if it is determined to be insufficient once the patient is connected to the machine. If pressure control ventilation is used, then the operator presets a desired peak airway pressure, and once the animal is connected to the machine the tidal volume achieved with the preset pressure is assessed. A tidal volume of around 10 mL/kg would be a very acceptable result.

Airway pressure

Patients with normal lungs such as anesthetic patients or patients with ventilatory failure should only require low peak airway pressures in the range of 8–15 cm H_2O, ideally not exceeding 20 cm H_2O. Animals with lung disease have stiff lungs and consequently require higher airway pressures to achieve the same tidal volume. Peak airway pressures as high as 30–35 cm H_2O may be required in animals with very severe lung disease. When using pressure control ventilation, the desired airway pressure is preset by the operator. Once the animal is connected to the machine, the tidal volume achieved with that airway pressure can be assessed. Alternatively, in volume control the tidal volume is preset, and the associated airway pressure must be assessed. Initially airway pressures of 10–15 cm H_2O should be targeted; higher airway pressures can be used if indicated by inadequate pulmonary function.

Trigger

Most modern ventilators allow the patient to trigger machine breaths, allowing ventilation to be better matched to the patient's efforts. The trigger, or sensitivity setting, on the ventilator determines what the machine will recognize as a patient's inspiratory effort. Appropriate trigger sensitivity is essential to ensure the ventilator recognizes genuine respiratory efforts made by the patient. This increases patient comfort and allows the patient to increase its own respiratory rate, if desired. The trigger variable can be too sensitive so that nonrespiratory efforts such as patient handling may initiate breaths, which should be avoided. An airway pressure drop of −2 cm H_2O or a gas flow change of 2 L/min are reasonable trigger sensitivity settings to start with; these settings can then be altered as necessary once the patient is connected to the machine.

Positive end expiratory pressure

Positive end expiratory pressure (PEEP) maintains pressure in the breathing circuit during exhalation so that the patient cannot exhale completely. This pressure holds the lung open and improves oxygenating efficiency of the lung and helps recruit collapsed alveoli. Additionally it may reduce ventilator-induced lung injury. A small amount of PEEP (~2 cm H_2O) is commonly set in all ventilator modes to reduce atelectasis. In patients with lung disease, much higher levels of PEEP may be required to improve oxygenating ability. In continuous spontaneous ventilation, CPAP is the equivalent of PEEP.

I : E ratio/respiratory rate

An operator-set respiratory rate is available on most if not all ventilators. A normal respiratory rate of 15–20 breaths with an inspiratory time of ~1 second is usually selected when the patient is initially established on the machine. This can then be changed as appropriate for the patient. The ratio of the duration of inspiration to exhalation (I : E ratio) may be preset by the operator or may be a default setting within the machine. Commonly an I : E ratio of 1:2 is utilized to ensure the patient has fully exhaled before the onset of the next breath. As respiratory rates are increased, the expiratory time is sacrificed to "squeeze" in the necessary number of breaths in 1 minute. High respiratory rates can lead to a situation known as breath stacking or intrinsic positive end expiratory pressure (intrinsic PEEP) because the animal is not able to fully exhale before the start of the next inspiration. To avoid this problem it is recommended to use an I : E ratio of 1:1 or higher. If a higher respiratory rate is required, a shorter inspiratory time will allow maintenance of an acceptable I : E ratio.

Guidelines for initial ventilator settings

As previously stated, the ideal ventilator settings for a given patient cannot be predicted. It is likely that animals with lung disease will need more aggressive settings than those with ventilatory failure. It is necessary to choose some initial settings prior to connecting the patient to the machine. First the type of ventilation must be selected: A/C, SIMV, or continuous spontaneous ventilation. If A/C or SIMV is chosen, it may be necessary to decide between volume control or pressure control ventilation. The more modern and advanced the ventilator, the more options you will have. The settings that need to be selected will depend on the type of ventilation chosen. In volume control the tidal volume is preset by the operator. Once the patient is connected to the machine, the operator will need to note the peak inspiratory pressure associated with this tidal volume and determine if it is acceptable or not. In pressure control ventilation, the airway pressure is preset by the operator, and once the patient is connected to the machine the operator will need to note the tidal volume and determine if it is acceptable or not.

The initial machine settings can be based on guidelines such as those shown in Table 27.1. These settings can then be altered as necessary once the patient is connected to the ventilator. It is best to have the ventilator turned on and confirm it is working appropriately before connecting the patient. When this is not possible, for example, beginning ventilation in the patient on an anesthetic machine, then it is best to start with quite low settings and increase them as required to avoid inadvertent overdistension of the lung. It is imperative to always have a method by which to perform manual ventilation close at hand at all times during PPV in case of equipment malfunction, power failure, or operator error.

Table 27.1 Suggested initial ventilator settings for patients with normal lungs

Ventilator Parameter	Initial Settings: Normal Lungs
Fraction of inspired oxygen	100%
Tidal volume (volume control)	5–15 mL/kg
Inspiratory pressure (pressure control)	8–15 cm H_2O
Respiratory rate	10–30 breaths/min
Positive end expiratory pressure	0–5 cm H_2O
Inspiratory time	~1 s
Inspiratory-to-expiratory ratio	1:2
Inspiratory trigger	−1 to −2 cm H_2O

Table 27.2 Suggested initial ventilator settings for patients with lung disease

Ventilator Parameter	Initial Settings: Lung Disease
Fraction of inspired oxygen	100%
Tidal volume (volume control)	5–10 mL/kg
Inspiratory pressure (pressure control)	10–20 cm H_2O
Respiratory rate	10–30 breaths/min
Positive end expiratory pressure	3–8 cm H_2O
Inspiratory time	~1 s
Inspiratory-to-expiratory ratio	1:2
Inspiratory trigger	−1 to −2 cm H_2O

Lung disease

When setting the ventilator up for a patient with lung disease, it is to be predicted that the pressure settings will need to be more aggressive than those guidelines provided in Table 27.1. This is because pulmonary parenchymal disease reduces the compliance of the lung (makes the lung more stiff). This means that higher pressures will be needed to achieve the same tidal volume. It is now recognized that excessive distension of the lung is a major cause of ventilator-induced lung injury.[2] For this reason it is recommended to minimize the tidal volume when ventilating patients with significant lung disease. In very severe lung disease such as the acute respiratory distress syndrome, it may be necessary to target a tidal volume as low as 6 mL/kg, whereas in more moderate lung disease tidal volumes no greater than 10 mL/kg may be best.[3] Table 27.2 provides some suggested initial ventilator settings for patients with lung disease.

Initial stabilization on the ventilator

When the patient is first connected to the machine, an FiO_2 of 100% is advised as a safety measure. Hopefully the FiO_2 can be reduced once the stability of the patient is verified. When ventilating patients with lung disease, it can be beneficial to keep them in sternal recumbency for the initial stabilization period. These animals almost always oxygenate better in sternal compared with lateral recumbency. After connection, the patient's chest is observed for appropriate movement. If there is insufficient or excessive chest inflation, the ventilator settings should be adjusted appropriately. The chest is then auscultated bilaterally to be sure there is ventilation of both lungs and all monitoring is evaluated (blood pressure, electrocardiogram, pulse oximeter, ETCO2, etc.). Any concerning changes should be addressed immediately.

Once the patient appears to be stable, arterial blood gas analysis is ideal for accurate titration of ventilator settings. If an arterial blood gas in not available, a venous blood gas can be used to assess PCO_2, and oxygenation is evaluated by pulse oximetry. Venous PO_2 provides minimal guidance in this scenario because it is not a direct reflection of oxygenation (see Chapter 15, Monitoring Tissue Perfusion: Clinicopathologic Aids and Advanced Techniques).

Goals of mechanical ventilation

The goal of ventilator therapy is to maintain acceptable blood gas values with minimally aggressive ventilator settings. The ideal ventilator settings for each individual animal cannot be predicted and are determined through a process of trial and error. The patient should be fully evaluated after every change in ventilator settings, including blood gas analysis if possible. It is advisable to make only one change in ventilator settings at a time to evaluate accurately the effect of each individual change on the patient.

Common blood gas goals of mechanical ventilation are as follows:

- PaO_2 of 80–120 mm Hg (SpO_2 > 95%)
- $PaCO_2$ of 35–55 mm Hg (35–40 mmHg in patients with brain disease)

PaO_2

If the PaO_2 is higher than the desired range (>120–150 mm Hg), the first priority is to decrease the FiO_2 until it is <60%. Once FiO_2 is <60%, more emphasis is placed on reducing PEEP and peak airway pressure. If the PaO_2 is lower than desired (<80 mm Hg), the simplest option is to increase the FiO_2. If there is an acute and severe drop in PaO_2, placing the animal on 100%

oxygen is appropriate until the issue can be evaluated and more definitive therapy can be provided. Ultimately it is hoped that manipulation of ventilator settings will increase the oxygenating efficiency of the lung and allow lowering of the FiO_2. Increases in PEEP and peak airway pressure are the major ventilator setting adjustments that may improve pulmonary oxygenating efficiency. An acute hypoxemic episode in a patient that was previously not hypoxemic is a life-threatening complication that requires immediate intervention. See the troubleshooting section later in this chapter.

$PaCO_2$

The $PaCO_2$ depends primarily on effective alveolar minute ventilation, which in turn is the product of the effective tidal volume and the respiratory rate. If the $PaCO_2$ is higher than the desired range, the respiratory rate or tidal volume or both should be increased and the patient reevaluated. If the $PaCO_2$ is too low, the respiratory rate and/or tidal volume should be decreased. An abrupt increase in $PaCO_2$ in the ventilator patient may indicate a life-threatening complication. See the troubleshooting section.

Record keeping

An essential aspect of management of the ventilator patient is detailed record keeping. This allows evaluation of patient progress and a review of patient responses to changes in ventilator settings. Hourly recording of patient vital signs, blood pressure, pulse oximeter, and end tidal carbon dioxide readings are ideal. Current ventilator settings should be recorded at the time of every blood gas measurement and every time a change in ventilator settings is made. All ventilator settings and patient values are worth recording, but the most important ones are listed in Box 27.1.

Box 27.1 Minimum recommended ventilator settings and patient values to record

- FiO_2
- Mode of ventilation
- Peak inspiratory pressure
- Tidal volume
- Respiratory rate
  - Machine set rate
  - Total rate
- Minute ventilation
- I : E ratio
- Positive end expiratory pressure

Complications of mechanical ventilation

Hemodynamic compromise

Positive pressure ventilation can reduce cardiac output in some patients. The increases in intrathoracic pressure from ventilation can reduce systemic venous return. Although animals with more aggressive ventilator settings are of more concern for developing negative cardiovascular effects, animals with significant lung disease tend to have such stiff lungs that very little of the positive pressure applied to the lungs is transmitted to the cardiovascular system. Hemodynamic compromise secondary to positive pressure ventilation is mainly a problem for animals with concurrent hypovolemia or vasodilation. Frequent, if not constant heart rate and blood pressure monitoring is recommended for all ventilator patients. Fluid and drug therapy should be given as appropriate if evidence of hypovolemia or hypotension develop.

Ventilator-associated pneumonia

In human medicine, ventilator-associated pneumonia (VAP) has been reported to occur in 10%–48% of patients and leads to an increase in mortality.[2] Endotracheal intubation compromises the normal upper airway defenses, and bacteria from the oral cavity can migrate down the airway to the lungs. This problem can be exacerbated by aspiration of oral secretions or gastric contents.[2] VAP is recognized when new pulmonary infiltrates develop ≥48 hours after beginning ventilation. Decreases in oxygenation, changes in white blood cell count, and a fever are also common findings. Prevention of VAP includes maintaining careful oral hygiene including chlorhexidine rinses and using a sterile technique when handling the circuit or endotracheal or tracheostomy tube.[4,5] The fewer times the circuit is disconnected the better. It is now recommended to replace ventilator circuits only every 5 days (earlier if gross contamination is evident).[2] Many VAP infections have been found to come from the hands of caregivers; for this reason, wearing gloves and frequent handwashing are strongly recommended for all ventilator patients. Wearing gloves should be considered mandatory when dealing with the oral cavity.

Ventilator-induced lung injury

Ventilator-induced lung injury (VILI) describes pulmonary damage that occurs as a result of the action of mechanical ventilation. In addition to increasing pulmonary pathology, in human medicine VILI has been found to increase the incidence of multiple organ dysfunction and patient mortality. It is believed that pulmonary inflammation resulting from VILI leads to the elaboration of inflammatory mediators that can enter the systemic circulation and amplify the systemic inflammatory response, which leads to subsequent organ damage.

There are several mechanisms by which VILI can occur. The two major mechanisms are overdistension of the lung by excessive tidal volumes and repetitive alveolar collapse in patients with lung disease on inadequate PEEP.[2] Manipulation of ventilator settings should always be focused on the use of the least aggressive settings required to keep the patient stable. When the blood gas goals cannot be achieved despite the use of high airway pressures and PEEP, a valid alternative is to change the blood gas goals for the patient. For example, many patients tolerate a PaO_2 of 60 mm Hg and PCO_2 of 60–70 mm Hg, which may be preferable to exposing the patient to higher ventilator settings.

Oxygen toxicity

Oxygen toxicity occurs when animals are exposed to excessive oxygen that overwhelms their natural antioxidant systems. Clinically oxygen toxicity causes pulmonary damage, and in neonates it can lead to retinal dysplasia.[6] Oxygen toxicity is not just a product of the level of oxygen administered; it is also related to the duration of oxygen exposure. The general recommendation for dogs and cats is to avoid the administration of 100% oxygen >12–24 hours, and in situations of long-term oxygen therapy, the FiO_2 should be maintained at <60%. In animals with severe lung disease, it may be very difficult to lower the FiO_2 to ≤60%. It is hoped that by manipulation of ventilator settings and accepting lower PaO_2 levels, FiO_2 will be able to be reduced in the ventilator patient.

Pneumothorax

A pneumothorax can occur in the ventilator patient when alveolar rupture leads air to escape from the lung and accumulate in the pleural space. Although pneumothorax is a feared complication when high airway pressures are used, studies in human patients have not been able to prove there is any association between airway pressure and the occurrence of pneumothorax.[7,8] The incidence of pneumothorax does seem to vary with the nature of the lung disease present. Overdistension of the lung is thought to be the major cause of pneumothorax. Hence restricting tidal volume, especially in patients with lung disease, is currently recommended.

Pneumothorax can be rapidly progressive in the ventilator patient, so it is imperative that it is recognized early. Acute onset of an elevated $PaCO_2$ and a falling

PaO_2 is a common early warning sign. Airway pressure would be expected to increase if a pneumothorax occurs in a patient being ventilated with volume control; tidal volume would decrease if using pressure control ventilation. Auscultation may reveal decreased lung sounds, but this may be difficult to appreciate in the ventilated patient. Thoracic radiographs provide a definitive diagnosis but are often impractical. Thoracic ultrasound can also be helpful in identifying a pneumothorax. Ultimately a pneumothorax can be rapidly fatal in the ventilator patient, and if there is any doubt that one is present, a diagnostic thoracocentesis should be performed immediately. If a pneumothorax is detected, unilateral or bilateral chest tubes will be required.

Troubleshooting the ventilator patient

Hypoxemia

Inadequate oxygenation of the ventilator patient is always an extremely concerning complication. If acute desaturation is detected on the pulse oximeter it is ideal, although not always possible to confirm the abnormality with an arterial blood gas. Acute desaturation of a ventilator patient that was previously oxygenating adequately indicates a dramatic decrease in pulmonary function. Potential causes include pneumothorax, machine malfunction or circuit disconnection, and loss of oxygen supply. The FiO_2 should be immediately increased to 100%, the thorax auscultated, and the ventilator function reviewed. If a pneumothorax is suspected, thoracocentesis should be performed immediately.

A gradual decline in oxygenating efficiency of the lung is not uncommon in the ventilator patient and is more suggestive of progressive pulmonary disease such as pneumonia, acute respiratory distress syndrome, or ventilator-induced lung injury than a pneumothorax or machine issue. Progressive lung disease requires increases in PEEP, peak inspiratory pressure, and FiO_2 as indicated by the blood gases.

Hypercapnia

There are numerous possible causes for hypercapnia in the ventilator patient including the following:

- Increased apparatus dead space: excess tubing/connectors between the patient and the ventilator circuit Y-piece
- Endotracheal or tracheostomy tube kink or obstruction
- Incorrect assembly of the ventilator circuit including large airway leaks, obstruction of the exhalation

circuit, or any problem that would prevent effective generation or delivery of a tidal volume
- Pneumothorax
- Increased pulmonary dead space that may occur with overdistension of alveoli or large pulmonary embolism
- Inadequate ventilator settings, in particular inadequate tidal volume, inadequate respiratory rate, or both. Settings that can impair exhalation such as insufficient expiratory time can also cause hypercapnia.

A sudden increase in $PaCO_2$ in a previously stable patient is suggestive of an acute abnormality such as an endotracheal or tracheostomy tube obstruction or dislodgement, ventilator circuit leak, or pneumothorax. If evaluation of the machine and patient rules out major complications, it is to be assumed there is insufficient alveolar minute ventilation, and appropriate changes in the ventilator settings should be made.

Patient-ventilator dyssynchrony ("bucking the ventilator")

When a patient fights, or bucks, the ventilator, it will not be possible to ventilate the animal effectively; this dyssynchrony commonly leads to desaturation and hypercapnia. When patients begin to buck the ventilator, a systematic approach should be taken to determine the nature of the problem. Possible causes include:

- Hypoxemia
  - Loss of oxygen supply, worsening of underlying disease, or development of new pulmonary disease such as pneumothorax, pneumonia or acute respiratory distress syndrome
- Hypercapnia
  - Circuit disconnect/leak, tube obstruction or kink, pneumothorax
- Pneumothorax
  - Typified by a rapidly climbing PCO_2 and a plummeting PaO_2. Need auscultation and potentially thoracocentesis to diagnose
- Hyperthermia
  - Anesthetized animals like to have relatively low temperatures, and even a rectal temperature of 102°F may cause dogs to pant on the ventilator. Active cooling is required to control panting in hyperthermic ventilator patients.
- Patient-ventilator dyssynchrony (inappropriate ventilator settings)
  - Observe when the patient is trying to inhale and exhale; see if it is possible to match that pattern with your ventilator settings

- Inadequate depth of anesthesia
  - Rely on the routine clinical signs of anesthetic depth. This may be the most common cause of bucking, but care should be taken not to increase blindly the anesthetic drug dose when patients begin bucking the machine without fully assessing the patient.

Weaning from ventilation

Weaning from the ventilator is generally a continuous process of gradually reducing the ventilator settings. Often as the patient improves, the mode of ventilation may be changed to one that requires the animal to perform a greater proportion of the work of breathing. Such modes include SIMV and pressure support. If animals have been anesthetized for prolonged periods of time, it may take some time for them to recover (hours to days). This is especially true for patients on pentobarbital infusions. It is important to consider reducing the anesthetic administration or changing to shorter acting anesthetic drugs when the animal begins improving and weaning is becoming a possibility.

Prior to disconnection from the machine the patient must have obtained certain physiologic goals. These include:

- The original disease process is stable or improving
- A normal respiratory drive
- The patient no longer requires significant ventilator support for adequate gas exchange
- Adequate oxygenation (PaO-to-FiO_2 ratio of at least 150–200 is recommended)

Reasons an animal should not be weaned include cardiovascular instability, requirement of high FiO_2 (>60%), high peak inspired airway pressures (>25 cm H_2O), and/or high PEEP levels (>5 cm H_2O).

When a patient has improved sufficiently to consider removing from the ventilator, it is safest to first test if the animal can maintain spontaneous breathing while still intubated. During such a spontaneous breathing trial, the patient requires intense monitoring. The use of CPAP is ideal during a spontaneous breathing trial because the tidal volume, respiratory rate, and end tidal carbon dioxide can be closely monitored. The development of any of the following would indicate that the trial has failed and that positive pressure ventilation should be reinstituted: hypoxemia, hypercapnia, hyperthermia, tachycardia, hypotension, or tachypnea. In human medicine, it is now recommended to perform spontaneous breathing trials daily once the patient qualifies according to the criteria just listed. When the patient can maintain

---

Box 27.2 Suggested standard contingencies for clinician notification for mechanically ventilated patients

- $PaO_2 < 80\,mm\,Hg$ or $SpO_2 < 95\%$
- $PaCO_2$ or $ETCO_2$ or $PvCO_2 > 60\,mm\,Hg$
- Temperature increase $>1°F$
- Persistent tachypnea, panting, fighting ventilator
- Mean arterial pressure $<70\,mm\,Hg$ or systolic arterial pressure $<100\,mm\,Hg$
- Tachycardia
- Urine output $<1\,mL/kg/h$

---

adequate blood gases without anxiety or fatigue, it can be woken up from anesthesia and extubated.

Contingencies

When providing care to the ventilator patient, it is important to recognize abnormalities that warrant contacting the clinician. Contingencies for notifying the clinician vary on a patient-by-patient basis and are an important part of the clinician orders. Box 27.2 lists some standard contingencies for a ventilator patient that may be helpful as a general guideline. It is recommended that clinicians modify these standard contingencies as appropriate for the patient on a daily basis.

Summary

Mechanical ventilation can be a lifesaving intervention for patients with severe lung disease or ventilatory failure. Critical care ventilators offer multiple modes and options for ventilation that allow the operator to tailor therapy to the individual. Although complications certainly exist, proper precautions can help minimize risks.

References

1. Hess DR, Kacmarek RM. Essentials of Mechanical Ventilation. 2nd ed. New York, NY: McGraw-Hill; 2002.
2. MacIntyre NR, Branson RD. Mechanical Ventilation. 2nd ed. St. Louis, MO: Saunders; 2009.
3. The Acute Respiratory Distress Syndrome Network. Ventilation with lower tidal volumes as compared with traditional tidal volumes for acute lung injury and the acute respiratory distress syndrome. N Engl J Med 2000;342:1301–1308.
4. Genuit T, Bochicchio G, Naplitano LM, et al. Prophylactic chlorhexidine oral rinse decreases ventilator-associated pneumonia in surgical ICU patients. Surgical Infect 2001;2:5–18.
5. Fudge M, Anderson JG, Aldrich J, Haskins SC. Oral lesions associated with orotracheal administered mechanical ventilation in critically ill dogs. J Vet Emerg Crit Care 1997;7:79–87.
6. Lumb AB. Nunn's Applied Respiratory Physiology. 6th ed. Philadelphia, PA: Elsevier Butterworth-Heinemann; 2005.
7. Weg JG, Anzueto A, Balk RA, et al. The relation of pneumothorax and other air leaks to mortality in the acute respiratory distress syndrome. N Engl J Med 1998;338:341–346.
8. Anzueto A, Frutos-Vivar F, Esteban A, et al. Incidence, risk factors and outcome of barotraumas in mechanically ventilated patients. Intensive Care Med 2004;30:612–619.

28

Ventilator waveform analysis

Deborah Silverstein

Ventilator waveforms can aid the veterinarian and veterinary technician in adjusting ventilator settings, assessing lung function, troubleshooting problems, understanding the interactions between patient and ventilator, reducing the incidence of complications, fine-tuning the ventilator to decrease the patient's work of breathing, and monitoring patient progress. The three elemental parts to respiratory function monitoring are scalars (also known as waves), loops, and indirect measurements (values that are calculated such as compliance and resistance). A basic understanding of pulmonary physiology and mechanical ventilation is necessary to interpret ventilatory waveforms.

A mechanical ventilator is programmed to deliver a preset pressure, volume, or flow rate; whichever of these is the programmed cause of inspiration is called the **control variable.** The four parameters most useful to examine a mechanical breath include **pressure, volume, flow,** and **time.** The location of the sensors for detecting these variables depends on the ventilator manufacturer and monitoring system used. For example, most ventilators measure pressure, volume, and flow inside the ventilator, but monitoring devices attached to the end of the endotracheal tube can also be used. In general, the closer the sensor is to the patient, the more accurate the measurement because the compliance and resistance of the patient circuit as well as the compressibility of the gas may significantly alter the pressure, volume, and flow values. Utilizing the measured variables, the formation of three scalars can be created: flow versus time, volume versus time, and pressure versus time. Time is typically plotted on the horizontal (x) axis and the other parameter is plotted on the vertical (y) axis. Additional graphs,

such as flow-volume loops or pressure-volume loops plot pressure, volume, and flow against each other but have no time component. The loops can rapidly provide information regarding changes in lung function.

Five basic flow waveforms are most commonly generated by a mechanical ventilator: a rectangular (or "square") wave, an ascending ramp, a descending ramp, a sinusoidal (or "sine") wave, or an exponential decaying waveform (see Fig. 28.1). The control variable and ventilator model used determine the possible options because some modes of ventilation only offer certain waveform characteristics. For example, volume control ventilation typically offers several choices of flow patterns, whereas pressure control ventilation commonly uses either a descending ramp or decaying flow pattern only.

Scalars

A mechanical breath can be divided into six stages (Fig. 28.2a–c):

1. Beginning of inspiration
2. Inspiration
3. End of inspiration
4. Beginning of expiration
5. Expiration
6. End of expiration

Which factor initiates inspiration depends on the triggering mechanism (**trigger variable**) of the ventilator. When using a control mode or in instances where a backup breath is provided by the ventilator, the breath is initiated based on a predetermined amount of lapsed

Advanced Monitoring and Procedures for Small Animal Emergency and Critical Care, First Edition. Edited by Jamie M. Burkitt Creedon, Harold Davis.
© 2012 John Wiley & Sons, Inc. Published 2012 by John Wiley & Sons, Inc.

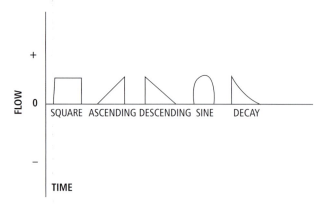

Figure 28.1 The five basic flow waveforms that are most commonly generated by a mechanical ventilator (from left to right): rectangular (or "square") wave, an ascending ramp, a descending ramp, a sinusoidal (or "sine") wave, and an exponential decaying waveform.

time. When using the assist mode or a synchronized intermittent mandatory ventilation (SIMV) mode, the mechanical breath is initiated by the patient's effort and is referred to as a patient triggered or patient-initiated breath. During inspiration, the mechanical breath is delivered and the flow, volume, and pressure of the breath depend on various factors such as airway resistance, lung compliance, type and magnitude of flow, and the delivered volume of each breath. Spontaneous breaths can also be pressure supported to enhance tidal volume.

The attending veterinarian determines the cycling mechanism (**cycle variable**), or the parameter that is responsible for termination of inspiration. Possible choices include volume cycling, pressure cycling, time cycling, and flow cycling.

Typically, when inspiration ends, the expiratory phase begins. There are specific instances, however, when the expiration valve does not open even though inspiratory gas flow has stopped (e.g., when inspiratory pause or inflation hold controls are activated). The delivered volume is retained within the lungs in order to obtain static or plateau pressures; delayed opening of the expiratory valve then allows expiration to occur.

Expiration is a passive phenomenon and the properties of expiration are dependent on the resistance of the animal's airways and the artificial airway, as well as pulmonary compliance. The end of expiration is heralded by the beginning of the next breath.

Scalars in different modes of ventilation

The scalar waveforms vary in their appearance depending on the mode of ventilation used. Sample scalars for

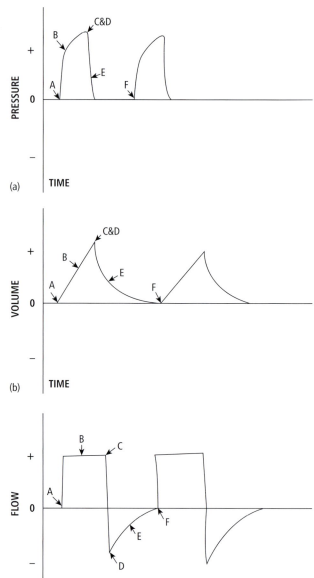

Figure 28.2 (a) The six stages of a mechanical breath as seen in this pressure-time scalar include: A. Beginning of inspiration; B. Inspiration; C. End of inspiration; D. Beginning of expiration; E. Expiration; F. End of expiration. (b) The six stages of a mechanical breath as seen in this volume-time scalar include A. Beginning of inspiration; B. Inspiration; C. End of inspiration; D. Beginning of expiration; E. Expiration; F. End of expiration. (c) The six stages of a mechanical breath as seen in this flow-time scalar include A. Beginning of inspiration; B. Inspiration; C. End of inspiration; D. Beginning of expiration; E. Expiration; F. End of expiration.

the five ventilation modes most commonly used (volume assist/control [A/C], pressure A/C, SIMV, SIMV with pressure support [PS] ventilation, and continuous positive airway pressure [CPAP]), are shown in Figures 28.3–28.7.

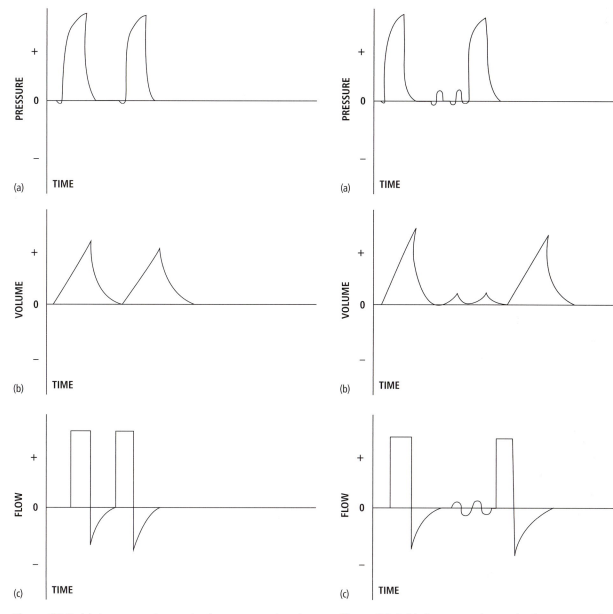

Figure 28.3 (a) A pressure-time scalar from a normal patient receiving volume assist-control mechanical ventilation. (b) A volume-time scalar from a normal patient receiving volume assist-control mechanical ventilation. (c) A flow-time scalar from a normal patient receiving volume assist-control mechanical ventilation.

Figure 28.4 (a) A pressure-time scalar from a normal patient receiving synchronized intermittent mandatory mechanical ventilation. The initial mandatory breath is followed by two spontaneous unsupported breaths and another mandatory breath. (b) A volume-time scalar from a normal patient receiving synchronized intermittent mandatory mechanical ventilation. The initial mandatory breath is followed by two spontaneous unsupported breaths and another mandatory breath. (c) A flow-time scalar from a normal patient receiving synchronized intermittent mandatory mechanical ventilation. The initial mandatory breath is followed by two spontaneous unsupported breaths and another mandatory breath.

Volume assist/control mode of ventilation scalar graphs

Here are some important curve characteristics to note in Figure 28.3 (volume A/C ventilation):

1. The inspiratory time and expiratory time on these graphs corresponds to termination of inspiration and expiration, respectively.

2. A negative tracing below baseline is observed during expiration for the flow/time curve. This is due to the fact that the flow transducer measures inspiratory flow as a positive deflection and expiratory flow as a negative deflection.

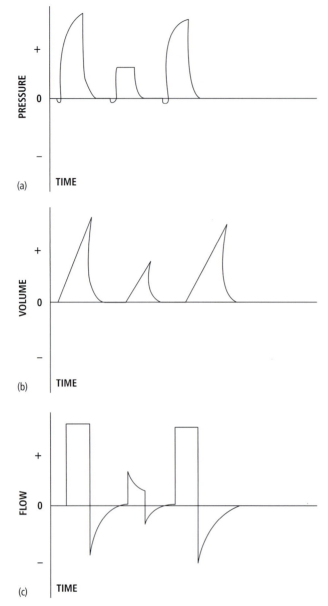

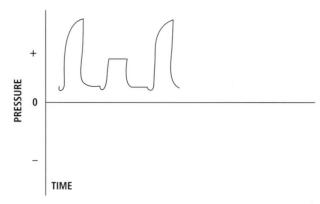

Figure 28.6 A pressure-time scalar from a normal patient receiving synchronized intermittent mandatory mechanical ventilation with pressure support and positive end-expiratory pressure (PEEP). The figure depicts a mandatory breath followed by a spontaneous breath with pressure support and another mandatory breath. PEEP is evident by the elevated baseline pressure.

3. A square flow tracing represents a constant flow pattern.
4. Because flow is constant, the delivery of volume is rectilinear.
5. When the patient triggers an assisted breath, there is a small negative deflection on the pressure/time graph. This bulge occurs as the patient starts to inhale, thus generating negative pressure and flow that is sensed by the ventilator. The initial rise in pressure corresponds to the pressure necessary to overcome airway resistance. After this point, any increase in pressure depends on pulmonary compliance and volume delivered. As the end of the tidal volume is delivered, the pressure wave has flattened because the lungs are almost full.
6. Flow delivery ceases at the end of inspiration because all of the tidal volume has been delivered and the peak inspiratory pressure (PIP) has been achieved.

SIMV mode of ventilation scalar graphs

It is important to note the following in Figure 28.4 (SIMV mode of ventilation):

1. The inspiratory flow tracing during spontaneous breaths is on the positive side of the graph and located in the space between mechanical breaths. During the expiratory phase, the flow is depicted below the baseline.
2. The inspiratory pressure is traced on the negative side of the baseline (unlike flow and volume) and expiration is shown on the positive side of the tracing.
3. The stages of each breath occur in the same order on all three scalars.

Figure 28.5 (a) A pressure-time scalar from a normal patient receiving synchronized intermittent mandatory mechanical ventilation with pressure support. The figure depicts a mandatory breath followed by a spontaneous breath with pressure support and another mandatory breath. (b) A volume-time scalar from a normal patient receiving synchronized intermittent mandatory mechanical ventilation with pressure support. The figure depicts a mandatory breath followed by a spontaneous breath with pressure support and another mandatory breath. (c) A flow-time scalar from a normal patient receiving synchronized intermittent mandatory mechanical ventilation with pressure support. The figure depicts a mandatory breath followed by a spontaneous breath with pressure support and another mandatory breath.

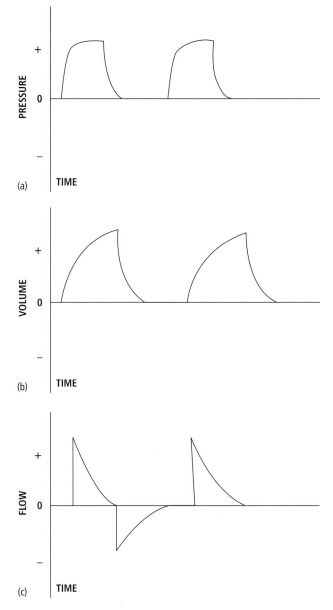

Figure 28.7 (a) A pressure-time scalar from a normal patient receiving pressure controlled mechanical ventilation. (b) A volume-time scalar from a normal patient receiving pressure-controlled mechanical ventilation. (c) A flow-time scalar from a normal patient receiving pressure controlled mechanical ventilation. The expiratory phase of the second breath is not shown here.

SIMV with pressure support scalar graphs

Some important concepts to note in Figure 28.5 (SIMV with pressure support):

1. On the flow/time scalar, the pressure-supported breath delivers a decreasing flow and terminates inspiration when the flow reaches a certain level (also known as flow cycling).

2. A set pressure is maintained throughout the inspiratory phase when a pressure-supported breath is delivered. There is a decrease in pressure down to baseline during the expiratory phase. All breaths are patient triggered in this example, as demonstrated by the small negative deflection at the beginning of inspiration on the pressure-time scalar.

SIMV with pressure-controlled ventilation and continuous positive end expiratory pressure mode of ventilation scalar graphs

Important facts to note in Figure 28.6 (only a pressure-time scalar is shown because the flow-time and volume-time scalars would be identical to those in Fig. 28.5):

1. When positive end expiratory pressure (PEEP) is used, the baseline on the pressure-time graph will be equal to the PEEP value. Upon initiating or increasing PEEP, PIP will also increase.
2. The airway pressure decreases to the new baseline PEEP at the end of expiration.
3. Although not shown, the baseline does not generally change on the flow-time or volume-time scalars when PEEP is begun.

Pressure-Controlled ventilation scalar graphs

Some points to note in Figure 28.7 (pressure-controlled ventilation [PSV]):

1. The ventilator terminates inspiration when a preset time has elapsed. The pressure remains at the set pressure throughout the inspiratory time.
2. The flow decreases to zero on the flow-time scalar before the end of inspiration (before expiration begins).

Diagnosing and Interpreting Auto-PEEP from scalar graphs

Auto-PEEP (also known as intrinsic PEEP or air trapping) often occurs in patients requiring high respiratory rates, high minute volumes, or PEEP settings greater than 10 cm H_2O. In these situations, inspiration begins before a complete expiration has occurred, leading to air trapping within the small airways and increased patient effort required for a patient-initiated breath. Additionally, auto-PEEP leads to flattening of the diaphragm, which decreases the efficiency of diaphragmatic contractions during inspiration. During expiration on the volume-time scalar, the waveform approaches baseline but then starts upward again before reaching baseline (see Fig. 28.8a). When examining the flow-time graph, there is an abrupt movement up to baseline at the end

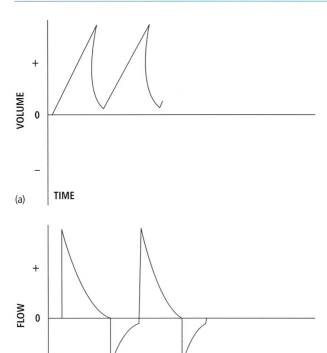

Figure 28.8 (a) A volume-time scalar showing auto-PEEP in an animal with lung disease receiving mechanical ventilation. Note that the waveform approaches baseline but immediately starts upward again before returning to zero. (b) A flow-time scalar showing auto-PEEP in an animal with lung disease receiving mechanical ventilation. Note that there is an abrupt movement up to baseline at the end of expiration, with an immediate increase in inspiratory flow for the next breath before expiration is completed and reaches baseline.

of expiration, with an immediate increase in inspiratory flow for the next breath before expiration is completed and reaches baseline (see Fig. 28.8b).

The presence of auto-PEEP may indicate an airway obstruction. Possible treatment strategies include bronchodilator therapy, placement of a larger endotracheal tube, increasing the inspiratory flow rate (to minimize the ratio of inspiratory to expiratory time), decreasing the tidal volume, or applying extrinsic PEEP. Alternatively, the respiratory rate may be too high (in which case the clinician can decrease the rate while increasing the tidal volume per breath). Sometimes a different mode of ventilation is beneficial in these animals if the troubleshooting methods previously mentioned are not effective.

Occasionally, auto-PEEP is caused by airway collapse, as in patients with chronic obstructive airway disease. In these cases, increasing PEEP may help to prop the airways open and decrease air trapping.

Protocol 28.1 Rapid reference for initial pressure- and flow-time scalar evaluation

Procedure

First look at the pressure-time scalar:
1. Determine the CPAP or PEEP level so baseline pressure is known.
2. Determine whether the patient is triggering any breaths, and identify this on the tracings.
3. Determine the intended shape of the pressure wave (e.g., a flat top is pressure controlled; a "shark fin"–shaped top is volume controlled).

Now look at the flow-time scalar:
1. What is the flow pattern? For example, a square-shaped tracing indicates a volume-controlled breath, but a decelerating shape can be present with any mode.
2. Is the patient air trapping? If expiratory flow does not return to baseline before the next breath begins, air trapping (auto-PEEP) is present.
3. Is the patient triggering breaths? Is the breath controlled, pressure supported, or a compulsory breath during SIMV? For example, the pressure-supported breath has a decelerating flow pattern and has a flat-topped airway pressure wave, and the synchronized breath has a triangular-shaped pressure wave.
4. Is the patient triggering a controlled or supported breath? The main difference between these is the time of the breath because the patient determines the inspiratory time with supported breaths, and therefore the time is variable compared with the identical timeline of a controlled breath.
5. Is the patient synchronizing with the ventilator? If the number of triggering episodes is greater than the number of breaths, asynchrony is present. If the peak flow rate of the ventilator is inadequate, the inspiratory flow will be "scooped" inward and the patient may appear to be fighting the ventilator.

Protocol 28.1 is a rapid reference for initial pressure- and flow-time scalar evaluation.

Pressure-volume and flow-volume loops

These loops are best studied after becoming familiar with the pressure, flow, and volume scalars previously described. Similar to the scalar graphs, both the numeric values and waveform graphs reveal information about the patient. A loop is really just inspiratory and expiratory curves that are connected. These loops allow the clinician to analyze the inspiratory and expiratory phases of each breath using either flow-volume (F-V) or pressure-volume (P-V) tracings. These loops can prove challenging initially because there is no unit of time involved; an entire breath is followed throughout the loop without any reference to the passage of time. Additionally, it is helpful for clinicians to make changes in ventilator and nonventilator treatment variables incrementally so the ventilator waveforms can be used to guide fine-tuning of the ventilator settings and to assess patient changes.

When examining a loop on the monitor screen, the scale of the axes must be set so that the loop images are displayed as large as possible for easy viewing. For example, the slope of the P-V loop, which represents dynamic compliance, is normally around 45 degrees. The clinician can readily observe the slope at a glance to determine whether the dynamic compliance is abnormal.

Unfortunately, there is no convention for how the inspiratory and expiratory limbs of the F-V loops are oriented with respect to the horizontal axis. Traditionally, the F-V loop is displayed with the inspiratory curve below the horizontal axis and the expiratory curve above the axis; however, this is commonly reversed. This chapter depicts the inspiratory curve above the horizontal axis. There is also no consensus as to how the axes should be oriented, but flow is depicted on the vertical scale in this chapter so as to maintain consistency with the scalar previously discussed.

A change in volume in relation to the change in intrapleural pressure is commonly referred to as **compliance.** Figure 28.9 shows how varying degrees of compliance can affect the inspiratory limb of a P-V curve. The largest volume change for a given pressure is obtained at the steepest portion of the curve, typically in the middle (see Fig. 28.10). Spontaneous tidal breathing commonly occurs in this region of the curve, which allows for spontaneous ventilation at the most efficient portion of the curve (where the least pressure change is needed for the greatest volume gain). Pulmonary disease may significantly change the baseline volume or pressure prior to each breath (e.g., due to atelectasis or air trapping) and subsequently decrease ventilatory efficiency by forcing the lung into a less efficient portion of the P-V curve. This leads to a decrease in dynamic and static respiratory compliance and distortion (especially the P-V loop). Table 28.1 lists some common causes of decreased compliance.

Pressure-volume loops

The pressure (horizontal axis) and volume (vertical axis) are typically plotted against each other, and a loop as in Figure 28.11 is generated (**A** represents the inspiratory limb and **B** represents the expiratory limb of the breath).

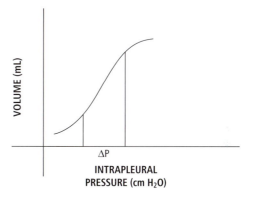

Figure 28.10 A pressure-volume graph from a normal animal receiving mechanical ventilation showing how the largest volume change for a given pressure is obtained at the steepest portion of the curve, typically in the middle.

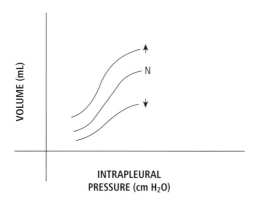

Figure 28.9 A pressure-volume graph from a normal animal receiving mechanical ventilation showing how varying degrees of compliance can affect the inspiratory limb of a pressure-volume curve. N, normal; up arrow, increased compliance; down arrow, decreased compliance.

Table 28.1 Common causes of increased pulmonary resistance and decreased pulmonary compliance in mechanically ventilated animals

Increased Resistance	Decreased Compliance
Bronchospasm	Pleural space disease
Airway secretions	Pulmonary parenchymal disease
Small-diameter endotracheal tube	Single-lung intubation
Mucosal edema of airways	Abdominal distention
	Chest wall disease or deformity

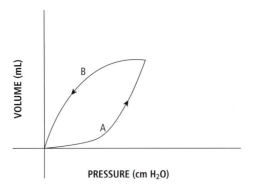

Figure 28.11 A pressure-volume loop from a normal animal receiving mechanical ventilation in which the pressure (horizontal axis) and volume (vertical axis) are plotted against each other and a loop therefore generated. **A** represents the inspiratory limb and **B** represents the expiratory limb of the breath.

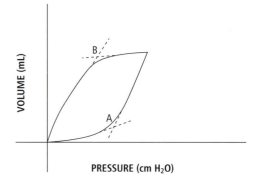

Figure 28.12 A pressure-volume loop from a normal animal receiving mechanical ventilation demonstrating the two inflection points. One point is found during inspiration (A) and the other during expiration (B). Point A is commonly called the lower inflection point and point B, the upper inflection point. If the inflection points are difficult to discern, a straight line can be drawn along the straight portions of the inspiratory and expiratory limbs of the loop, and the point of intersection for the two drawn lines will estimate the inflection point (see dashed lines).

Conceptual renderings of the loop are often elliptical or "football shaped," but the loops are not typically so symmetrical. When a ventilator delivers a "control breath," it is initiated in the lower left-hand corner of the graph and follows the counterclockwise path as indicated by the arrows, eventually returning to the starting point. The upper right corner represents the end of inspiration and the beginning of expiration. This is the point of maximal pressure and volume, and it represents the dynamic compliance of the respiratory system for that breath. Remember that the loop will not begin at zero pressure if PEEP is applied to the patient.

The P-V loop is commonly used to evaluate changes in respiratory compliance. The point of change in the slope of a line is called the **inflection point.** As seen in Figure 28.12, the loop has two inflection points, one during inspiration and one during expiration. Point "A" is commonly called the lower inflection point and point "B" the upper inflection point. If the inflection points are difficult to discern, a straight line can be drawn along the straight portions of the inspiratory and expiratory limbs of the loop, and the point of intersection for the two drawn lines will estimate the inflection point (see dashed lines). When examining a static P-V loop, the inflection points are believed to represent a sudden change in alveolar recruitment during inspiration and derecruitment during expiration. The dynamic P-V loop includes the effect of resistance to flow; the volume increase lags behind the pressure increase and causes a gap between the inspiratory and expiratory curves of the P-V loop. Subsequently, the inflection points obtained from a dynamic P-V loop are difficult to use when setting PEEP or the upper pressure limit.

When an animal triggers a breath spontaneously (in contrast to a controlled breath, which is triggered solely

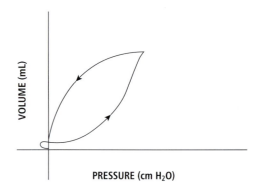

Figure 28.13 A pressure-volume loop from a normal animal that triggers the delivery of an assisted positive pressure ventilation breath (in contrast to a controlled breath that is triggered solely by the timing mechanism of the ventilator). Note the small bulge on the negative side of the pressure axis due to the patient's active inspiratory effort.

by the timing mechanism of the ventilator), there will be a small bulge on the negative side of the pressure axis (see Fig. 28.13) This bulge occurs as the patient starts to inhale, thus generating negative pressure and flow. Spontaneous breaths trace a loop in a clockwise direction (this is discussed further later). If the ventilator senses the patient's effort and begins a machine breath, the line shifts rightward into the positive side of the pressure axis and loops counterclockwise.

Conventionally, compliance is assessed by tracing a line from the beginning to the end of inspiration, with

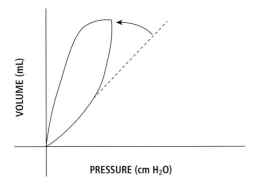

Figure 28.14 A pressure-volume loop from an animal receiving mechanical ventilation with increased compliance. Note how the loop is left-shifted from the 4- degree dotted line.

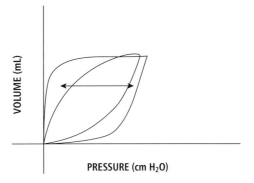

Figure 28.16 Superimposed pressure-volume loops from a mechanically ventilated normal animal (center) and a mechanically ventilated animal with increased airway resistance (outer loop). Note how the increase in airway resistance causes the loop to widen, leading to an increase in the area of the pressure volume loop and an increase in the horizontal distance (arrows).

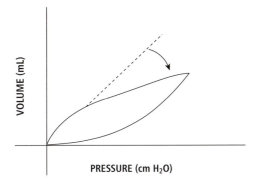

Figure 28.15 A pressure-volume loop from a mechanically ventilated animal with decreased compliance. Note how the loop is right-shifted from the 45-degree dotted line.

a 45-degree angle created to the horizontal axis in a normal animal. An increase in compliance results in a shift to the left of the 45-degree line (see Fig. 28.14) because less pressure is required to produce a given change in lung volume, whereas a decrease in compliance causes a rightward shift in the loop (see Fig. 28.15) because more pressure is required to produce a given change in lung volume. Refer to Table 28.1 for some common causes of decreased respiratory system compliance.

An increase in the width of the loop indicates an increased resistance in the respiratory system. Subsequently, the area of the P-V loop and its horizontal distance increases (see Fig. 28.16). These changes are the result of **hysteresis,** a lag in the change in volume compared with the rate of change in pressure that results from resistance to deformation (elasticity) and resistance of the airways. The rightward shift of the loop indicates that the resistance is creating a decreased com-

pliance effect. It is often easier for the clinician to use the F-V loop to evaluate changes in airway resistance because the changes to the P-V loop can be subtle. However, superimposition of two loops on each other may prove helpful in determining changes in the P-V loop. Using both the F-V and P-V loops is the best way to gauge overall resistance and its changes. Table 28.1 lists some common causes of increased airway resistance.

The work of breathing (WOB) describes the amount of pressure required to move a specific volume of gas. A decrease in compliance or a decrease in functional residual capacity increases the WOB. There are several ways to measure the WOB, but this information focuses on the ventilatory graphics, termed *mechanical WOB*. The patient, ventilator, or both are able to do the WOB. The components of the WOB are shown in Figure 28.17. The WOB to overcome airway resistance is labeled (A) and that required to overcome the elastic nature of the lung is labeled (B). The combination of A and B represent the total mechanical work done during the breath. The WOB equals the area under the changing pressure curve as the volume increases from zero to its peak at the end of inspiration. Most ventilator graphics only display the mechanical work as measured at the endotracheal tube connector, and therefore they do not reveal ventilatory efforts made by the patient. The WOB performed by the patient during the mechanical breaths can be indirectly measured by plotting esophageal pressures because esophageal pressures are a surrogate for measuring intrapleural pressure and intrapleural pressure changes due to patient work.

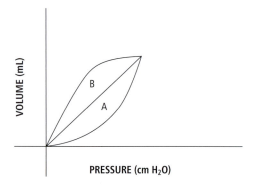

Figure 28.17 A pressure-volume loop from a mechanically ventilated normal animal with the components that determine the mechanical work of breathing (WOB) separated. The WOB to overcome airway resistance is labeled (A), and that required to overcome the elastic nature of the lung is labeled (B). The combination of A and B represent the total mechanical work done during the breath. The WOB equals the area under the changing pressure curve as the volume increases from zero to its peak at the end of inspiration. Most ventilator graphics only display the mechanical work as measured at the endotracheal tube connector, and therefore they do not reveal ventilatory efforts made by the patient. The WOB performed by the patient during the mechanical breaths can be indirectly measured by plotting esophageal pressures.

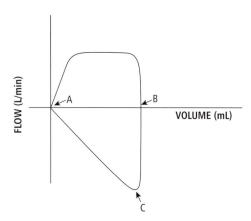

Figure 28.18 A flow-volume loop from a mechanically ventilated normal animal. Point A represents the start of inspiration and point B represents the start of expiration. Point C is showing the peak expiratory flow rate during passive expiration.

Flow-volume loops

The vertical axis of an F-V loop represents flow rate (liters per minute or per second), and the horizontal axis represents volume (milliliters or liters); however, this is not standardized, so it is important to read the axis labels. The inspiratory portion of the F-V loop is above the horizontal axis, and the expiratory portion is below this line in this chapter, but recall that this may be reversed in some graphic displays or references. In Figure 28.18,

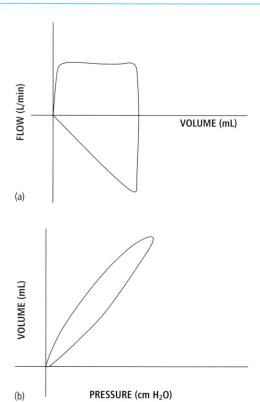

Figure 28.19 (a) A flow-volume loop from a normal animal while receiving positive pressure mechanical ventilation on a machine that delivers constant flow to deliver a breath. Note the square waveform pattern that is displayed. (b) A pressure-volume loop from a normal animal while receiving positive pressure mechanical ventilation on a machine that delivers a constant flow to deliver a breath. This is often the preferred waveform for detecting abnormalities in the P-V loop.

point **A** represents the start of inspiration; point **B** represents the start of expiration. The shape of the F-V curve can be altered by patient changes, ventilator settings, circuit conditions, and the way the ventilator generates and delivers a breath. The transition from inspiration to expiration and back to inspiration is seen where the loop crosses the horizontal axis and the flow rate is transiently zero. The inspiratory curve shape reflects the flow pattern of the ventilator (see note later). The highest point above the x-axis depicts the peak expiratory flow rate (PEFR) during passive expiration (point C in Fig. 28.18). Anything that leads to obstruction of the airways or endotracheal tube influences the shape of this curve, as discussed later.

Important note on flow-volume loops when flow delivery is constant

When the ventilator uses constant flow to deliver a breath, a square waveform pattern is displayed (see Fig. 28.19a).

This results in a constant volume delivery. Although a descending flow pattern may be used more commonly, the square waveform can be more helpful for detecting abnormalities in the P-V loop because the flow and volume delivered are constant (see Fig. 28.19b).

Spontaneous breath loops

Spontaneous breaths create loop waveforms that differ from those produced during positive pressure ventilation. The F-V loop is similar, but the inspiratory curve of a spontaneous breath (above the horizontal axis) is rounded (see Fig. 28.20a). The main difference is a lower peak flow rate during spontaneous breathing. The expiratory waveform (below the horizontal axis) is passive, creating a descending ramp-like shape for both spontaneous and ventilator-created breaths.

The P-V loop during spontaneous respiration is very different than the P-V loop created due to positive pressure. During a spontaneous breath, the negative pressure generated during inspiration causes a leftward bulge of the P-V loop that extends into the negative side of the pressure axis (see Fig. 28.20b). The loop is then traced in a clockwise fashion, and expiration occurs on the positive side of the pressure axis.

Loop interpretation

The interpretation of abnormal loop patterns requires practice and patience. Some of the abnormalities that may be gleaned from analysis of the loops include airway obstruction, the presence of an air leak, or air trapping.

Airway obstruction

The location and severity of airway obstruction determine the changes that result on the F-V loop. Most significant obstructions decrease the PEFR, as seen in Figure 28.21. When the medium and small airways obstruct, the descending segment of the expiratory curve often turns into a more curvilinear shape, referred to as "scooping" (also seen in Fig. 28.21). Comparison of F-V loops over time can help the veterinarian assess the effectiveness of bronchodilator therapy in patients with asthma or bronchospasm. The scooped-out appearance often changes to a more linear shape from the peak expiratory flows down to the end of expiration, reflecting the beneficial effect of therapy in relieving the airway obstruction.

Air leak

The presence of an air leak during a breath is often evident in both the scalar and loop graphs. Leaks may

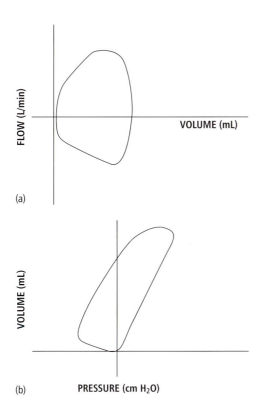

Figure 28.20 (a) A flow-volume loop from a normal animal during a spontaneous breath. The inspiratory curve of the spontaneous breath is above the horizontal axis and appears rounded. (b) A pressure-volume loop from a normal animal during a spontaneous breath. Note that the negative pressure generated during inspiration causes a leftward bulge that extends into the negative side of the pressure axis. The loop continues in a clockwise fashion, and expiration occurs on the positive side of the pressure axis.

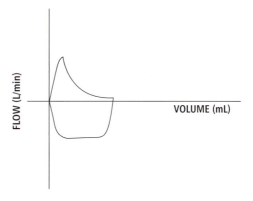

Figure 28.21 A flow-volume loop from a mechanically ventilated animal with airway obstruction. Note the decrease in peak expiratory flow rate (PEFR). The descending segment of the expiratory curve appears more curvilinear, also known as "scooping," which is commonly seen in animals suffering from obstruction of the medium and small airways.

originate from the endotracheal tube cuff, air leaks through chest tubes, or a bronchopleural fistula. The waveform's expiratory volume appears smaller than the inspiratory volume if a leak is occurring during inspiration. If a leak occurs downstream (on the patient side) from the flow transducer used to generate loop graphics, this appears as part of the inspiratory volume in the loop, but the lost volume is not returned through the flow transducer and therefore the loop does not close (see Figs. 28.22a and b). If the delivered inspiratory volume is less than the set volume but has an equivalent expiratory volume, a leak in the ventilator circuit between the flow transducer and ventilator should be suspected.

Air trapping

If the expiratory time is not sufficient or the smaller airways collapse prematurely, air trapping may occur,

causing the expiratory portion of the loop to fall short of baseline (to never reach zero flow rate) prior to beginning the next breath (see Fig. 28.23). It is important to note that the F-V loop for a PSV breath can appear similar to the loop seen with air trapping. The abrupt change in the slope of the loop at the end of inspiration is created when the ventilator cycles from inspiration to expiration based on a preselected flow target. Auto-PEEP is seen as a flow above zero at the end of expiration, however. When looking at the PSV breath using a P-V loop, the inspiratory and expiratory lines typically cross each other at around 2 cm H_2O as the patient makes an effort to inspire during the PSV breath (see Fig. 28.24).

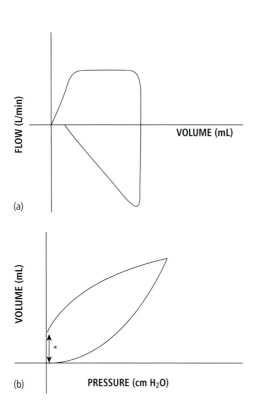

(a)

(b)

Figure 28.22 (a) A flow-volume loop from an animal receiving mechanical ventilation. There is evidence of an air leak downstream (on the patient side) from the flow transducer used to generate the loop. Therefore the lost volume is not returned through the flow transducer upon expiration and the loop does not close. (b) A pressure-volume loop from an animal receiving mechanical ventilation. There is evidence of an air leak downstream (on the patient side) from the flow transducer used to generate the loop. Therefore the lost volume is not returned through the flow transducer upon expiration and the loop does not close. The asterisk represents volume loss.

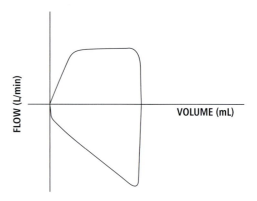

Figure 28.23 A flow-volume loop from an animal receiving mechanical ventilation. The expiratory portion of the loop never reaches a zero flow rate prior to the next breath, indicating the presence of air trapping.

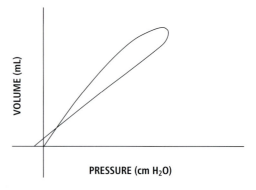

Figure 28.24 A pressure-volume loop from a normal animal receiving a pressure-supported breath. Note how the inspiratory and expiratory lines cross each other at around 2 cm H_2O as the patient attempts to inspire.

Basic pulmonary mechanics measured during mechanical ventilation

To measure compliance of the lungs, a pressure-time scalar is commonly used. Volume control ventilation is used, and once PIP is reached (see Fig. 28.25, point 1), an end inspiratory pause is applied for 0.5–2.0 seconds for only one breath. During the pause there is no flow between the patient and the ventilator, which allows for equilibration between proximal airway pressure and alveolar pressure (Palv). The pressure at the end of the pause is the **peak alveolar pressure,** commonly referred to as the plateau pressure or static compliance (as seen in Fig. 28.25, point 2). The difference between PIP and the peak Palv is due to the resistive properties of the system (either patient airways or artificial airway). The difference between the PIP and end expiratory pressure (EEP; or PEEP if applicable) is referred to as dynamic compliance and is a less accurate measurement of compliance but does not require an inspiratory breath hold. Dynamic compliance is more a measure of impedance because it consists of both resistance and compliance components. The difference between the peak Palv and total PEEP is due to the elastic properties of the system (lung and chest wall compliance).

During pressure control ventilation, PIP and peak Palv may be equal due to the flow waveform that occurs (refer to Fig. 28.7a). Static compliance cannot therefore be determined while a patient is receiving pressure control ventilation (it must be determined while the patient is receiving volume control ventilation). The flow decreases during inspiration and is typically fol-lowed by a period of no flow at the end of inspiration (refer to Fig. 28.7c). During the no-flow time, proximal pressure may be equal to the peak Palv. To determine effective respiratory system compliance, the tidal volume is divided by the difference between PIP and EEP. Dynamic compliance is calculated as PIP minus EEP and includes a component of airway resistance.

The P-V and F-V loops can also be used to assess respiratory system compliance. In Figure 28.26a, a constant flow mode is used and the three F-V loops represent varying compliance levels. The "up" arrow shows increased compliance, the "down" arrow shows decreased compliance, and "N" is normal compliance. Note how the tidal volume increases with increases in compliance. Inspiratory peak flows are fairly constant, but expiratory

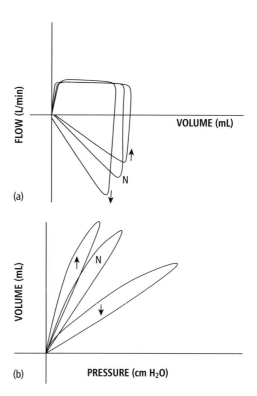

(a)

(b)

Figure 28.26 (a) Flow-volume loops depicting varying levels of compliance in three animals receiving mechanical ventilation with constant flow delivery during inspiration. Increased compliance is evident in the loop marked with an up arrow, decreased compliance in the loop with a down arrow, and normal compliance in the loop marked "N." Note how the tidal volume increases with increases in compliance. (b) Pressure-volume loops depicting varying levels of compliance in three animals receiving mechanical ventilation, as in Figure 28.26a. Increased compliance is evident in the loop marked with an up arrow, decreased compliance in the loop with a down arrow, and normal compliance in the loop marked N. Note the "right shift" of the pressure-volume loop that occurs as compliance decreases.

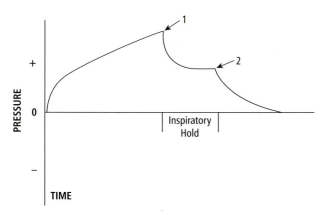

Figure 28.25 A pressure-time scalar during an inspiratory breath hold in a normal animal receiving volume-controlled mechanical ventilation. The peak inspiratory pressure (point 1) is seen prior to the inspiratory breath hold. The plateau pressure, also known as the peak alveolar pressure, is the pressure observed at point 2.

peak flow rates decrease with increases in compliance. Figure 28.26b demonstrates a P-V loop with the same compliance changes as in Figure 28.26a. Airway resistance does not change between the three loops, but notice the "right-shift" of the P-V loop that occurs as compliance decreases. Although not present in this figure, increased hysteresis sometimes accompanies a decrease in compliance.

An increase in inspiratory airway resistance may be subtle on the F-V loop if the driving force of the ventilator is sufficient to overcome the increased resistance, as seen in the loop labeled with the arrow in Figure 28.27a. The loop does reveal a slight decrease in the PEFR and volume compared with the normal (N) curve. The same scenario is seen in the P-V loop of Figure 28.27b, where the expiratory curves are similar, but the volume of the normal curve is again greater than the abnormal curve

and the pressure during inspiration is markedly higher in the abnormal loop labeled with the arrow. Potential causes of increased inspiratory resistance might include patient dyssynchrony with the ventilator, secretions or exudate within the endotracheal tube or large airway, or collapse or a mass of the trachea beyond the length of the endotracheal tube.

Resistance during expiration leads only to a decrease in PEFR, as seen in the loop labeled with the "up" arrow in Figure 28.28a; this pattern is consistent with large airway obstruction. Note there is no scooping on the F-V loop. A small leak is also present as indicated by the shortened return of the abnormal loop. Small airway obstruction leading to increased expiratory resistance, as seen in animals with bronchial collapse or narrowing or emphysema, markedly affects the P-V loop as seen in the loop with the "up" arrow in Figure 28.28b.

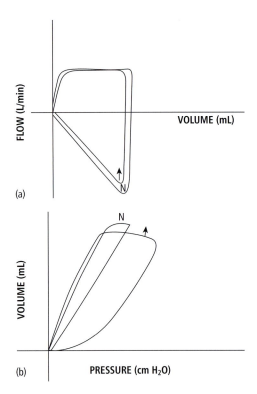

Figure 28.27 (a) Two flow-volume loops from animals receiving mechanical ventilation. The loop labeled with an up arrow depicts the decrease in peak expiratory flow rate and volume in an animal with increased inspiratory airway resistance compared with a normal (N) animal. The changes are subtle because the force of the ventilator is sufficient to overcome the increased resistance. (b) Two pressure-volume loops from animals receiving mechanical ventilation. The loop labeled with an up arrow depicts the decrease in volume and increase in peak pressure in an animal with increased inspiratory airway resistance compared with a normal (N) animal.

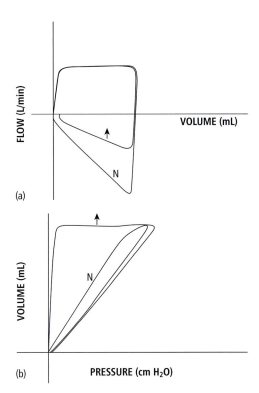

Figure 28.28 (a) Two flow-volume loops from animals receiving mechanical ventilation. The loop labeled with the up arrow shows an increase in expiratory resistance that causes a decrease in the peak expiratory flow rate. The absence of scooping is consistent with a large airway obstruction. A small leak is also present as indicated by the shortened return of the abnormal loop. (b) Two pressure-volume loops from animals receiving mechanical ventilation. Small airway obstruction is evident in the expiratory portion of the loop labeled with an up arrow compared with the normal (N) loop.

Summary

Respiratory waveforms generated during mechanical ventilation can be helpful in bedside patient monitoring. With practice, interpretation of scalars and loops can be a rapid way to evaluate the patient from a distance using graphic information. Please find a set of practice problems to follow.

Practice problems

1. A 20-kg mix breed dog is on its second day on the ventilator for hypoventilation following ventral slot surgery for a cervical disk herniation. You notice that the inspiratory peak pressures have been getting higher and higher during volume-controlled ventilation, so you decide to perform a 1-second inspiratory pause to assess static and dynamic compliance and compare it with yesterday's scalar (A). What is your interpretation of this pressure scalar (B)?

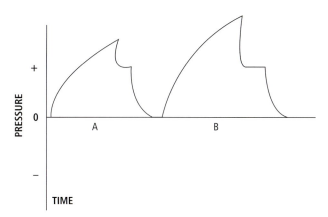

Problem 28.1

   Answer: An increase in PIP with an unchanged pause pressure reveals increased respiratory resistance. Upon changing the endotracheal tube, you find a large blood clot inside.

2. A 5-kg domestic shorthair cat is on volume-controlled ventilation following a severe asthmatic attack. You look at the flow scalar shown here. What is wrong?

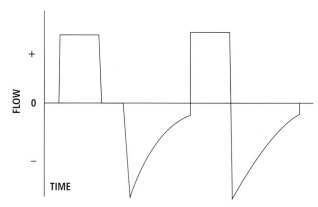

Problem 28.2

   Answer: Remember that the flow pattern does not change with changes in resistance or compliance. The expiratory flow has not reached zero before the next inspiration begins, indicating air trapping and auto-PEEP. A longer expiratory time with or without bronchodilator therapy, especially if peak expiratory flow has declined, may prove helpful.

3. You try switching the cat in problem 2 to pressure-controlled ventilation and get the flow scalar labeled B here and compare it to the normal flow scalar labeled A. Did this change help the cat?

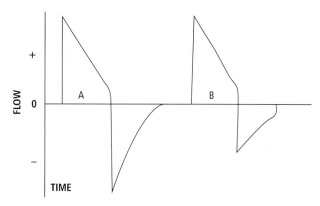

Problem 28.3

   Answer: No. The expiratory flow does not reach zero before the next breath begins, and the decrease in expiratory flow indicates a continued expiratory flow limitation.

4. A 9-year-old Labrador retriever is placed on positive pressure ventilation following a witnessed vomiting and aspiration episode. Following initial setup, you examine the P-V loop. What do you conclude?

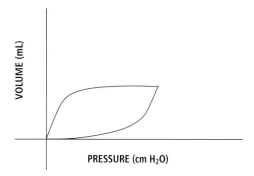

Problem 28.4

   Answer: The slope of the loop is well below 45 degrees and the compliance with and without resistance characteristics of the respiratory system are poor. Perhaps an increase in PEEP is a good place to start to maximize pulmonary function and prevent ventilator-induced lung injury.

5. A 5-year-old Chihuahua is on the ventilator for pulmonary contusions after being hit by a car. Volume-controlled ventilation is being used and you see the F-V loop shown here. What do you suspect?

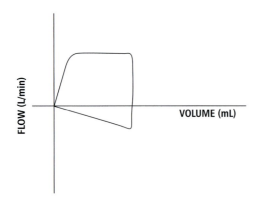

Problem 28.5

Answer: A marked decrease in the expiratory flow rate indicates expiratory flow limitation. Upon examination of the patient, you find no obvious airway obstruction. However, your veterinary technician notices that the water trap in the expiratory limb of the circuit is quite full. Upon emptying the water, the F-V loop returns to normal.

6. This 2-year-old German shepherd required mechanical ventilation for lower motor neuron disease. The dog is currently on SIMV with pressure support, but the clinician reports that the dog is not yet showing any evidence of triggering an assisted or a supported breath. You look at the pressure scalar below and then change a ventilator setting at point A. What did you do?

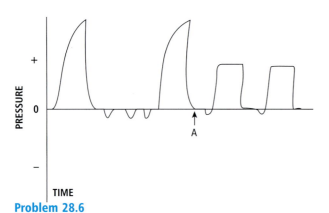

Problem 28.6

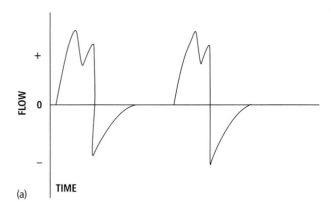

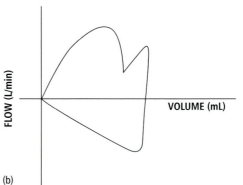

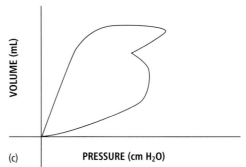

Problem 28.7

Answer: There are negative pressure deflections that are not followed by a delivered pressure support breath, indicating that the trigger sensitivity is set too high. You reduced the trigger sensitivity from 5 L/min to 2 L/min at point A and then observed two pressure-supported breaths.

7. A 10-year-old Siamese cat was placed on pressure A/C ventilation for severe pulmonary parenchymal disease of unknown origin. You look at the cat and the flow scalar (Problem 28.7a), F-V loop (Problem 28.7b), and P-V loop (Problem 28.7c). What do you conclude?

Answer: The cat is making an inspiratory effort toward the end of inspiratory phase of the breath, thus creating a negative deflection in flow and pressure during the normally positive inspiratory time. This is patient-ventilator dyssynchrony and may lead to inadequate inspiratory volumes and poor oxygenation and ventilation. The clinician should try to change the settings to improve patient comfort based on the specific patient, respira-

tory parameters, and blood gas values. For example, an increase in inspiratory pressure, respiratory rate, or flow rate may prove beneficial if the animal has inadequate minute ventilation. Unless the cat appears too lightly anesthetized, it is best to give anesthetics or paralytics only after all other strategies have failed. Dyssynchrony is often the patient's way of telling the clinician that the ventilator settings are inappropriate.

8. A 3-month-old Labradoodle has suspected noncardiogenic pulmonary edema after chewing on an electric cord. The puppy is on pressure-controlled A/C ventilation with PEEP, and the following pressure scalar (Problem 28.8a) and P-V loop (Problem 28.8b) are observed. What might you do after seeing this pressure scalar?

Answer: The spike in the pressure scalar at the beginning of inspiration indicates an excessive flow delivery during a fast rise time. The excessive flow and pressure do not necessarily translate into increased tidal volume delivery and are therefore undesirable. Possible changes that may prove helpful would include

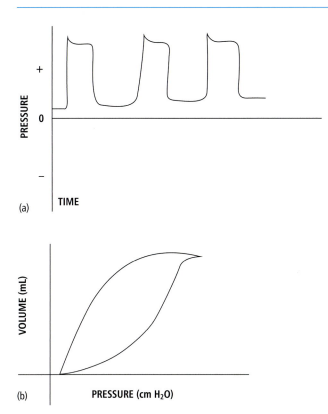

(a)

(b)

Problem 28.8

increasing the rise time (especially if the endotracheal tube is very narrow) or decreasing the flow rate.

Recommended reading

Hess DR, Kacmarek RM. Essentials of Mechanical Ventilation. 2nd ed. New York, NY: McGraw-Hill; 2002.

Oakes D, Shortall S. Ventilator Management: A Bedside Reference Guide. 3rd ed. Orono, ME: Health Educator Publications; 2009.

Tobin MJ. Principles and Practice of Mechanical Ventilation. 2nd ed. New York, NY: McGraw-Hill; 2006.

Waugh JB, Deshpande VM, Brown MK, Harwood R. Rapid Interpretation of Ventilation Waveforms. 2nd ed. Upper Saddle River, NJ: Prentice Hall; 2006.

29

High-frequency ventilation

Jessica Schavone and Elizabeth Rozanski

Intermittent positive pressure ventilation is lifesaving in patients with respiratory or ventilatory failure. In patients with neurologic disease or less severe respiratory disease, adequate ventilation and oxygenation may be achieved without excessive peak inspiratory pressures. In patients with severe pulmonary disease, stiff or noncompliant lungs necessitate the use of higher pressures to achieve adequate tidal volumes. However, ventilation with high inspiratory pressures magnifies lung damage and perpetuates lung injury. High-frequency ventilation (HFV) has been described as a technique to provide ventilation and oxygen supplementation with less **biotrauma** (lung inflammation incited by the overdistention and repetitive opening and closing of lung units). HFV has not been widely adopted in companion animals, although it is wise to be familiar with its background, definitions, applications, indications, and contraindications, as well as the equipment required.

Background

Of interest to veterinary professionals, the ability of the panting dog to remain apparently normoxic initially triggered early interest in the physiology behind HFV as a therapeutic entity. Panting in normal dogs is used for temperature regulation as heat is lost across the respiratory system. The respiratory rate of panting dogs is commonly approximately 300 breaths per minute (5 hertz), which is very close to the resonant frequency of the respiratory system.

The resonant frequency of the respiratory system (RFRS) is the natural frequency of the system at which vibrations will occur with the least amount of energy

being applied. Matching the RFRS is important because it minimizes the energy cost of panting. If dogs pant at a rate that is largely different from the RFRS, it results in heat gain and negates any cooling benefits. This is appreciated in dogs that have an increased respiratory rate from disease because their energy requirements for ventilation can approach 50% of their total metabolic expenditure. In a normal human individual, the work of breathing is fueled by 36–72 calories per day, whereas in a patient with increased respiratory effort, caloric intake of 10 times this may be required to support ventilation. Panting dogs also ventilate adequately; dogs can have adequate gas exchange with these small tidal volumes and rapid respiratory rates.[1] In our lung function laboratory, arterial blood gas samples collected from healthy panting dogs document high PaO_2 values, often greater than 100 mm Hg, and lower $PaCO_2$ levels, often in the 28–32 mm Hg range.

Definitions

High-frequency ventilation (HFV) is any technique that ventilates a patient at a respiratory rate higher than normal for that species, usually >10 times the typical rate. Thus for a dog this would be approximately >200 breaths/min.

High-frequency jet ventilation (HFJV) provides ventilation at rates of 60–400 breaths per minute in people. Inspiration is active; expiration is passive. **High-frequency oscillometric ventilation** (HFOV) provides ventilation at rates >400 breaths/min. In this form, both inspiration and expiration are active, and the gas flow is sinusoidal rather than the triangular flow seen with

Advanced Monitoring and Procedures for Small Animal Emergency and Critical Care, First Edition. Edited by Jamie M. Burkitt Creedon, Harold Davis.
© 2012 John Wiley & Sons, Inc. Published 2012 by John Wiley & Sons, Inc.

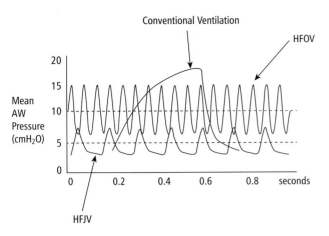

Figure 29.1 Comparison of ventilatory rates and pressure patterns with different ventilatory approaches. AW, airway; HFJV, high-frequency jet ventilation; HFOV, high-frequency oscillometric ventilation. Courtesy of Bunnell Incorporated, Salt Lake City, Utah.

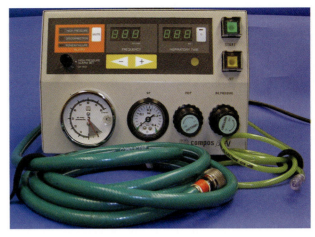

Figure 29.2 High-frequency jet ventilator. The larger green hose coiled on the left of the image is the oxygen input hose. The smaller light green hose coiled on the right is the gas output hose through which HFJV would be delivered to the patient. Note the supply to the patient has a male tubing adapter at the end to attach to a standard vascular catheter or infant feeding tube, which would be inserted into the animal's trachea.

HFJV. See Figure 29.1 for a demonstration of the differences in the rates and pressure tracings for these different forms of ventilation.

Any of these high-frequency ventilation techniques can be combined with positive end-expiratory pressure (PEEP) if needed to help recruit lung units and improve oxygenation. The application of PEEP is often required in patients with significant pulmonary disease but is generally not required when HFV is used for interventional procedures such as routine bronchoscopy.

How High-Frequency ventilation works

Normal conventional mechanical ventilation (CMV) relies primarily on bulk convection and diffusion to eliminate carbon dioxide (CO_2) and to provide oxygenation. In all forms of HFV, convection and molecular diffusion are still the primary mechanisms of gas exchange, but additional mechanisms of CO_2 elimination include Pendelluft ("sloshing" back and forth of gas), Taylor-type dispersion (gas mixing enhanced by turbulence), and asymmetrical gas velocity profiles. These additional effects help HFV to provide adequate ventilation at lower pressures than CMV. Fresh gas is introduced into the system both to displace CO_2-rich gas from the respiratory system and to provide oxygen. This fresh gas is the source of the tidal volume and introduced at an angle into the high-frequency system; thus it is often referred to as **bias flow** because it is introduced "on the bias."

HFJV is often used in tandem with a conventional ventilator (CV), with the CV providing the bias oxygen flow, PEEP, and occasional sighs (larger breaths). An endotracheal tube adaptor is used so the patient does not require reintubation. Ventilation is controlled by altering the rate and peak inspiratory pressure on the jet ventilator. The inspiratory time may be changed but is usually left at 20 ms. As is true of all ventilation (spontaneous as well as mechanical), the volume of the breath in milliliters is determined by the relationship between the pressure difference between the airway opening and the intrapleural cavity and the compliance (the ease of distension) of the lung. Expiration is passive. Sighs are often provided by the CV at 2–10 breaths/min. The ventilatory pressure waveform in HFJV is peaked (see Fig. 29.1). Figure 29.2 depicts a jet ventilator.

High-frequency oscillometric ventilation is provided with a piston and diaphragm, which makes both inspiration and expiration active. There is no need for a CV. The inspiratory-to-expiration ratio is usually fixed at 1:2, although it may be adjusted. The mean airway pressure (mPaw) and oxygen concentration can be adjusted. The pressure waveform in HFOV is sinusoidal (see Fig. 29.1).

Major applications and indications

Overall, HFV is considered beneficial because it uses smaller tidal volumes and it improves ventilation-perfusion matching in the lungs. The alveoli remain in a relatively constant region on the pressure-volume curve, which may minimize biotrauma.

Practically, HFV has found clinical application in two major areas: in neonatal medicine in people and for supportive ventilation during interventional procedures in human and veterinary medicine. HFJV is occasionally used in human adult medicine for patients with severe lung disease, although a multitude of clinical trials have failed to identify a survival benefit with acute respiratory distress syndrome (ARDS).

Human neonatal medicine is the current primary focus of the clinical use of HFV. Techniques for the support of critically ill and premature neonates have improved tremendously in the past 30 years with the advent of surfactant therapy and other advances. Current recommendations for ventilation of neonates include consideration of transition to HFJV or HFOV when peak inspiratory pressures exceed 25 cm H_2O, if tidal volume >6 mL/kg is required, if rapid respiratory rates are required, if air leak syndrome is present, if extracorporeal membrane oxygenation is being considered, or in extreme prematurity.[2] The use of HFV is advised when high respiratory rates are required because CVs are not responsive at such rates, and air trapping (auto-PEEP) is a potential concern due to breath stacking (see Chapter 27, Mechanical Ventilation, and Chapter 28, Ventilator Waveform Analysis, for more information). HFOV is emerging as the more popular method of HFV in neonates.

Interventional procedures commonly use HFJV to provide adequate oxygenation during a procedure when a routine endotracheal tube is not practical. Some veterinary internists and criticalists use this technique during bronchoscopy or other airway manipulations. HFV is used during bronchoscopy through a catheter placed with its tip at the level of the midtrachea or carina, depending on the area being evaluated. Some veterinary pulmonologists simply provide supplemental oxygen during the procedure rather than jet ventilation.

The goals for both HFJV and HVOV are maintenance of optimal lung volume and adequate blood gases. For HFJV, lung volume is primarily maintained by PEEP, which limits the need for high peak inspiratory pressures. As with all ventilators, the training and skill set of those using the ventilator is far more important than the specific type of ventilator chosen.

Patient assessment is similar to that performed during other forms of ventilation. By nature, these are critically ill animals, and minute-to-minute assessments may be required. As in CMV, oxygenation goals may be reduced, such that an $SpO_2 \geq 88\%$ could be acceptable. Depending on the technique used, capnometry may or may not be possible (see Chapter 26, Capnography); standard capnographic waveforms would not be expected due to the very rapid respiratory rate.

Contraindications

There are minimal absolute contraindications to HFV. The major one is lack of familiarity with the equipment and monitoring techniques. Asthma is occasionally listed as a contraindication, although newer studies have suggested this is incorrect. The initial fears were based on the potential for air trapping or hyperinflation because lungs with a delayed time constant (high resistance/low compliance) do not have as a favorable response to HFV.

Veterinary studies

Although HFV and airway pressure release ventilation (APRV) have been used extensively in research settings,[3] there are no clinical descriptions of their use in dogs or cats with naturally occurring acute lung injury. Jet ventilation is used during bronchoscopy procedures by some clinicians,[4] and there exists a report of a premature foal supported by HFJV.[5] Due to the propensity of the dog to pant, it is conceivable that this would be a favorable ventilation scheme in dogs with ARDS.

Other novel ventilation strategies

APRV is another alternative method of ventilation that is occasionally used in a similar patient population as HFOV. Although a complete review is beyond the scope of this chapter, the basics are as follows. The patient is maintained with a high level (10–20 cm H_2O) of continuous positive airway pressure; this pressure is periodically reduced and the baseline pressure falls for 0.5 seconds before returning to the baseline high pressure. If the patient is apneic, this method is similar to an inverse-ratio, pressure-limited ventilation. The goal of this technique is to provide near-permanent recruitment of all available lung and to improve oxygenation.

Summary

HFV, particularly HFOV, is an exciting and possibly underutilized option for ventilatory support in dogs with acute lung injury. Future studies would be helpful to determine if HFV is more effective than CMV in companion animal medicine, particularly in ARDS.

References

1. Meyer M, Hahn G, Piiper J. Pulmonary gas exchange in panting dogs: a model for high frequency ventilation. Acta Anaesthesiol Scand 1989;33(Suppl 90): 22–27.

2. Courtney SE, Asselin JM. High-frequency jet and oscillatory ventilation for neonates: which strategy and when? Respir Care Clin North Am 2006;12(3):453–67.

3. Bednarski RM, Muir WW. Hemodynamic effects of high-frequency oscillatory ventilation in halothane-anesthetized dogs. Am J Vet Res 1989;50(7):1106–1109.

4. Johnson LR, Drazenovich TL. Flexible bronchoscopy and bronchoalveolar lavage in 68 cats (2001–2006) J Vet Intern Med 2007;21(2):219–225.

5. Bain FT, Brock KA, Koterba AM. High-frequency jet ventilation in a neonatal foal. J Am Vet Med Assoc 1988;192(7):920-922.

Recommended reading

Hess DR, Kacmarek RM. High frequency ventilation, partial liquid ventilation, and tracheal gas insufflation. In: Hess DR, Kacmarek RM, eds. Essentials of Mechanical Ventilation. 2nd ed. New York, NY: McGraw-Hill; 2002:361–369.

Ritacca FV, Stuart TE. Clinical review: high-frequency oscillatory ventilation in adults—a review of the literature and practical applications. Crit Care 2003;7(5):385–390.

Stawicki SP, Goyal M, Sarani B. Analytic reviews: High-frequency oscillatory ventilation (HFOV) and airway pressure release ventilation (APRV): a practical guide. J Intensive Care Med 2009;24(4):215–229.

30

Pleural space drainage

Rosemary Lombardi, Emily Savino, and Lori S. Waddell

- The pleural space is a potential space that can be occupied by air or fluid in certain disease states, and evacuation of this space may be necessary to relieve respiratory distress.
- Drainage can be accomplished either by thoracocentesis or thoracostomy tube placement, depending on the rate of reaccumulation of air or fluid.
- If air or fluid is reaccumulating rapidly, a chest tube drainage system with continuous suction should be used.
- Thoracostomy tube management requires 24-hour supervision and strict aseptic handling to prevent life-threatening complications.

The pleural space is a potential space that can be occupied by tumor, fluid, air, or abdominal organs. Drainage of the pleural space is indicated for patients with pleural fluid or air accumulation. The choice of technique, either thoracocentesis or thoracostomy tube placement, depends on a number of factors, including the patient's stability, the rate and recurrence of reaccumulation of air or fluid, and the underlying disease process. Pleural effusion can be secondary to a wide variety of disease processes and may be characterized as exudate, transudate, chylous, or hemorrhagic. These may be caused by a variety of disease processes. Septic exudative effusions are seen with pyothorax, which may arise secondary to penetrating chest wounds, hematogenous spread, extension from adjacent structures or fascial planes, aspirated foreign bodies, ruptured pulmonary abscesses, ruptured esophagus, and

iatrogenic causes. Nonseptic exudates can occur from infection with feline infectious peritonitis virus. Chylous effusions can be caused by trauma, neoplasia, cardiac disease, and idiopathic disease. Transudates (pure and modified) are most often caused by right-sided congestive heart failure but can also develop or be exacerbated by factors such as hypoproteinemia or vasculitis. They can be seen in patients with sepsis or pancreatitis and in patients with pulmonary thromboembolism. Neoplasia and lung lobe torsions may also cause a modified transudate. Hemothorax can be caused by trauma, as a result of a coagulopathy, or may be caused by neoplasia.

Blunt thoracic trauma can result in rupture of the lung and cause air leakage from the alveoli or airways into the pleural space, resulting in collapse of the lung lobes. Pneumothorax is the most common complication of blunt trauma to the chest in dogs.[1] Pneumothorax can also occur spontaneously, most commonly secondary to air leakage from ruptured bullae or blebs. Spontaneous pneumothorax has also been associated with leakage of air from sites of pulmonary abscessation, primary and metastatic pulmonary neoplasia, foreign body migration, pneumonia, and feline asthma. In addition, parasitic disease such as *Dirofilaria*, *Paragonimus*, and *Filaroides osleri* have been associated with acute pneumothorax in dogs.[2] Physical examination findings include dull lung sounds and often dull heart sounds. If the lung sounds are dull ventrally, a pleural effusion should be suspected, whereas dullness dorsally is usually associated with a pneumothorax. The respiratory rate is

Advanced Monitoring and Procedures for Small Animal Emergency and Critical Care, First Edition. Edited by Jamie M. Burkitt Creedon, Harold Davis.
© 2012 John Wiley & Sons, Inc. Published 2012 by John Wiley & Sons, Inc.

often increased, and the respiratory pattern is short and shallow when there is significant pleural space disease present.

Thoracocentesis

Thoracocentesis is a quick and relatively easy method of removing air or fluid from the pleural space. If a patient is in respiratory distress and pleural effusion or pneumothorax is suspected, thoracocentesis should be performed before radiographs to optimize patient stability. Thoracocentesis can be both diagnostic and therapeutic. When either air or fluid is found, the chest cavity should be evacuated, which often eliminates the patient's respiratory distress.

Indications

Patients that present after thoracic trauma such as after being hit by a car, sustaining bite wounds, or falling from a height may develop pneumothorax, so if dull lung sounds are auscultated and the patient is in respiratory distress, thoracocentesis is indicated. Blunt trauma may also cause a hemothorax, which can be diagnosed by thoracocentesis, and, if severe enough, treated by thoracocentesis. If dull lung sounds after trauma are caused by a diaphragmatic hernia and displacement of abdominal organs into the thoracic cavity, gastrointestinal contents may be aspirated via thoracocentesis. Although not ideal, the patient will require surgery to repair the hernia, and the chest and abdomen can be flushed thoroughly at that time to remove any contamination. Additionally, those that have undergone positive pressure ventilation have an increased risk for pneumothorax and warrant thoracocentesis if they develop signs of respiratory distress, hypoxemia, or poor ventilation. Thoracocentesis is also useful for removal of fluid, both to stabilize the patient's respiratory status and to obtain samples for analysis for diagnostic purposes. This can be useful even in cases with small pleural effusions that are not causing significant clinical signs. When fluid is obtained, it should be saved for fluid analysis, and culture and sensitivity if indicated. If a severe coagulopathy is present, thoracocentesis is contraindicated because of the risk of creating a potentially life-threatening hemothorax. Efforts should be made to correct the coagulopathy prior to thoracocentesis, if possible.

Procedure for thoracocentesis

Thoracocentesis (Protocol 30.1) is an essential skill because it can be both therapeutic and diagnostic for patients with pleural space disease. The required equipment is listed in Box 30.1. Extension tubing is used when tapping with a needle to prevent movement of the needle while in the chest as the three-way stopcock is operated. A short over-the-needle catheter can be used to reduce the risk of laceration of the lung or blood vessels, but these often kink once the stylet is removed, negating any benefits that they may have. Cardiovascularly sparing sedation may be needed depending on the patient's stability and temperament. Oxygen supplementation should be provided if the patient is in respiratory distress. With an assistant restraining the animal (preferably in sternal recumbency or standing), the appropriate rib space should be clipped and aseptically prepped. The patient's comfort level often determines which position is best, as well as if air or fluid is expected to be aspirated. If air is expected, sternal or lateral recumbency work because the air will rise to the top of the chest in either position. If fluid is to be aspirated, sternal recumbency is best because the fluid will be in the ventral portion of the pleural space and can most easily be reached with the patient in sternal recumbency (or standing). When pleural fluid is expected, the seventh or eighth intercostal space is recommended, at approximately the costochondral junction. If air is expected, a more dorsal approach, about a third of the way down the chest, in the eighth or ninth intercostal space is used (about halfway between the spine and costochondral junction) (see Fig. 30.1). Sterile gloves should be worn for the insertion of the appropriate size needle or butterfly catheter. Large dogs may require a 1.5-inch needle to penetrate the chest wall, whereas a ¾ or ⅞-inch butterfly needle is sufficient for most cats and small dogs. The needle tip should be placed just cranial to the rib to avoid intercostal blood vessels and nerves that are located caudally, and gently inserted into the thorax perpendicular to the chest wall with the bevel of the needle pointing up while carefully observing the hub of the needle and extension tubing for any signs of fluid. Once through the chest wall, the needle can be directed either dorsally (if air is expected) or ventrally (if fluid is expected) so that the needle is almost parallel to the chest wall (see Figs. 30.2a–c).

If a small amount of frank blood is suddenly and unexpectedly aspirated from the thorax, or if the lungs can be felt rubbing against the tip of the needle, the procedure should be stopped and the needle removed and replaced at a slightly different location. If a large amount of blood is withdrawn from the thorax, 1–2 mL should be placed in a red top tube to see if the blood clots. Blood from a hemothorax should not clot within the tube, whereas blood from the heart or a blood vessel should clot normally, providing there is no significant concurrent coagulopathy. If any other fluid type is seen in the hub of the needle, aspiration of fluid should

Protocol 30.1   Procedure for Thoracocentesis

Items Required
- Clippers
- Surgical scrub
- Large syringe (10–60 mL)
- Sterile gloves
- Three-way stopcock
- Extension tubing
- Needle or a butterfly catheter
  - Large dogs: 1.5-inch needle or even longer catheter
  - Medium dogs and large cats: 1-inch needle or catheter
  - Cats and small dogs: ¾- to ⅞-inch butterfly needle
- Bowl and tubes for samples including one with EDTA and one without anticoagulant (if tapping for fluid)

Procedure
1. Gather supplies
2. Perform hand hygiene and don clean examination gloves.
3. Position patient, preferably in sternal recumbency or standing. Lateral recumbency is also acceptable for pneumothorax. The patient's comfort should help determine which position is used.
4. Have assistant available to restrain patient or give sedation as needed. In many cats, a minimal restraint technique is preferred and generally better tolerated.
5. Clip and aseptically prepare the appropriate rib space:
   a. If expecting fluid, the seventh or eighth intercostal space, at approximately the level of the costochondral junction.
   b. If expecting air, the eighth or ninth intercostal space approximately a third of the way down the chest (about halfway between the spine and costochondral junction).
6. Perform hand hygiene and don sterile gloves.
7. Insert the appropriate size needle or butterfly catheter slowly perpendicular to the chest wall, just cranial to the rib to avoid intercostal blood vessels.
8. Once through the chest wall, the needle can be directed either dorsally (if air is expected) or ventrally (if fluid is expected) so that the needle is almost parallel to the chest wall.
9. Observe hub of needle for any signs of fluid.
   a. If small amount of frank blood is aspirated suddenly or unexpectedly or if lungs can be felt rubbing against needle, it should be removed and replaced at a slightly different location.
   b. If large amount of blood is obtained, place 1–2 mL in a blood collection tube that does not contain anticoagulant, to evaluate for clotting.
   c. Blood from hemothorax should not clot; blood from the heart or a blood vessel should clot normally, if patient does not have a significant coagulopathy.
   d. For any other fluid, aspiration should continue until no more can be removed.
10. Directing the needle ventrally, rolling the patient slightly to the side that thoracocentesis is being performed, and re-aspirating from a more ventral location can facilitate removal of as much fluid as possible.
    a. Fluid is saved for fluid analysis, cytology, and possibly culture.
11. Aspiration of air will turn the tubing a slightly foggy white color as the warm, humid air from the thoracic cavity encounters the room temperature tubing.
12. Aspirate until negative pressure is reached.
    a. If negative pressure is never obtained, a tension pneumothorax may be present, and chest tubes with continuous suction are needed (see section on thoracostomy tube placement).

continue until no more fluid can be removed. If the patient will tolerate it, the needle can be directed ventrally while the patient is rolled slightly to the side that thoracocentesis is being performed, and re-aspirating from a more ventral location can facilitate removal of as much fluid as possible. Any fluid obtained should be saved for fluid analysis, cytology, and possibly culture. If air is aspirated from the thorax, it usually turns the butterfly tubing a slightly foggy white color as the warm, humid air from the thoracic cavity encounters the room temperature tubing and condensation occurs. If air is aspirated, continue aspiration until negative pressure is reached. If negative pressure is never obtained, a tension pneumothorax may be present, and placement of a chest tube(s) with application of continuous suction is recommended. Thoracocentesis is relatively quick (<5 minutes), although it can be prolonged if a large amount of fluid or air needs to be removed or if the effusion has a lot of fibrin or is very pocketed.

> **Box 30.1** Equipment for thoracocentesis
>
> - Clippers
> - Surgical scrub
> - Large syringe (10–60 mL)
> - Three-way stopcock
> - Extension tubing and a needle or a butterfly catheter
> - Bowl and tubes for samples including one with EDTA and one without anticoagulant (if tapping for fluid)

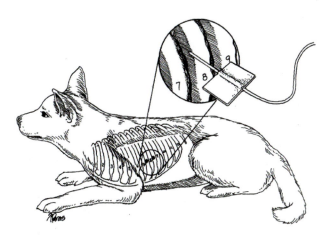

Figure 30.1 Schematic showing thoracocentesis in a dog in sternal recumbency using a butterfly catheter. The needle is inserted in the eighth intercostal space.

Complications

Complications of thoracocentesis can include iatrogenic pneumothorax from lung laceration, intrathoracic hemorrhage from laceration of blood vessels, or reexpansion pulmonary edema in situations of chronic pleural effusions. Thoracocentesis without confirmation of pleural space disease with thoracic radiographs risks tapping an empty pleural space. Although this can lead to iatrogenic pneumothorax or hemorrhage, these are relatively uncommon complications and usually self-limiting in patients with normal lungs. Severe pneumothorax is much more common after thoracocentesis in patients with severe chronic pulmonary pathology. Acute death from the stress of restraint is also possible. Appropriate sedation may reduce these risks, but care should be taken in choosing drugs with minimal respiratory suppression. After thoracocentesis, the patient should be monitored for reoccurrence of respiratory distress that may indicate return of either air or fluid to the pleural space or the development of an iatrogenic pneumothorax or hemothorax (less common).

Thoracostomy tube

Indications

Indications for a thoracostomy tube (chest tube) include recurrent pneumothorax requiring repeated thoracocentesis, tension pneumothorax, pyothorax, rapidly forming pleural effusion, and postoperative management of thoracotomy patients. A tension pneumothorax occurs as air progressively accumulates in the pleural space through a one-way valve leak of the lungs or airways. This leads to pressure atelectasis of the lungs and decreased venous return to the heart. A tension pneumothorax can cause fatal respiratory arrest in

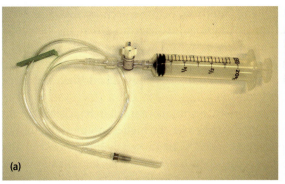
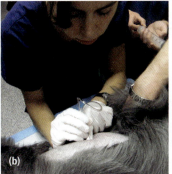
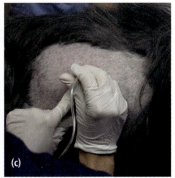

Figure 30.2 (a) Equipment for thoracocentesis using a 1-inch, 22-gauge needle; an extension set; a three-way stopcock; and a syringe. (b) Thoracocentesis in a bearded collie that presented with a spontaneous pneumothorax. Note that the ninth intercostal space is being tapped, a third of the way down the chest (about halfway between the spine and costochondral junction) because air is expected. (c) Close-up of thoracocentesis in the bearded collie. The needle is inserted with the bevel of the needle up.

seconds to minutes. If a tension pneumothorax is present, thoracocentesis and chest tube placement should be performed immediately. The other indications for chest tube placement usually allow a more relaxed, less emergent approach to placement.

Thoracostomy tube placement allows for either frequent intermittent evacuation of the pleural space or continuous evacuation of the chest if attached to continuous suction. Similar to thoracocentesis, a major contraindication for thoracostomy tube placement is a severe coagulopathy, which should be corrected prior to placement of a thoracostomy tube, if possible.

Chest tubes should be placed under cardiovascularly sparing sedation or intubation and general anesthesia. If the patient is unstable, it should be intubated so the airway is controlled. The patient's oxygenation should be monitored with pulse oximetry during placement.

Positive pressure ventilation worsens a closed pneumothorax, so if the patient requires ventilation, the chest cavity should be evacuated while preparing for the procedure, either with continuous thoracocentesis or via an open pneumothorax. An open pneumothorax may be created by inserting a catheter into the thoracic cavity or a mini thoracotomy. If a tension pneumothorax is present, continuous evacuation of the pleural space via thoracocentesis will be needed until the tube is in place.

Thoracostomy tube placement

Box 30.2 lists the equipment needed for chest tube placement. To secure the connections of the chest tube, catheter adapter, and three-way stopcock, 20-g orthopedic wire or zip ties may be used. Bandaging material should also be available.

There are a variety of commercially available thoracostomy tubes made of silicone or polyvinyl that are

---

Box 30.2 Equipment for thoracostomy tube placement

- Clippers
- Surgical scrub
- Surgical blade
- Local anesthetic
- Small surgical pack
- Suture material
- An assistant (if possible)
- Thoracostomy tube
- Catheter adapter (or Christmas tree adapter)
- Chest tube clamp
- Three-way stopcock
- Injection caps
- 20-g orthopedic wire or zip ties to secure connections

---

packaged with stylets. These are the easiest to place and typically have a radiopaque line that allows for easier visualization on radiographs. Red rubber tubes can also be used but are more difficult to place (must use surgical technique) and are more likely to collapse. The size of the tube should be based on the size of the patient and if air or fluid is expected. Smaller tubes can be used for aspiration of air. If fluid is expected to be aspirated through the chest tube, larger sized tubes are used, but care should be taken not to place a tube as large or larger than the patient's intercostal space because it will likely cause increased discomfort. If the fluid is thick or loculated, extra drainage holes can be made in the tube prior to placement with a scalpel blade, making sure the holes are less than 50% of the diameter of tube. If the fenestrations are more than 50% of the diameter, or are made too close together, there is risk of the distal portion of the tube breaking off and requiring surgical removal.

Two common techniques for placement of a thoracostomy tube are described: noninvasive surgical (Protocol 30.2) and trocar (Protocol 30.3) methods. Both methods require the same approach.

Noninvasive surgical method

The patient should be placed in lateral recumbency, and the lateral thorax should be shaved from just caudal to the scapula to the last rib and from dorsal spine to ventral midline. The area should be aseptically prepared (Fig. 30.3a) and draped. The chest tube should be loosened from the stylet if a stiletted tube is being used. For dogs, 0.25–1.0 mL of 0.25% or 0.5% bupivacaine can be injected into the subcutis and intercostal muscles at the planned tube insertion site, or alternatively, an intercostal nerve block can be performed by injecting 0.25–1.0 mL of 0.25% or 0.5% bupivacaine per site just ventral and caudal to the transverse processes of the thoracic vertebrae/head of ribs one space cranial and caudal, and at the site of insertion. Before injecting, always aspirate back into the syringe to determine that the needle is not in an artery or vein. The total dose of bupivacaine should not exceed 3 mg/kg. Small dogs should receive 0.25 mL/site, medium-size dogs 0.5 mL/site, and large dogs 1.0 mL/site.[3]

For the surgical technique, a small stab incision should be made in the skin over the highest point of the thorax at intercostal space 9–10 (about halfway between the spine and costochondral junction). The skin should be stretched forward by an assistant (Figs. 30.3a and b) to allow the chest tube to be placed in intercostal space 7–8, causing a tunnel under the skin of two to three intercostal spaces. Blunt dissection with hemostats through the intercostal muscles and parietal pleura is used to enter

Protocol 30.2 Noninvasive surgical method of chest tube placement

Items Required
- Clippers
- Surgical scrub
- Surgical blade
- Local anesthetic
- Small surgical pack
- Suture material
- An assistant (if possible)
- Thoracostomy tube
- Catheter adapter (or Christmas tree adapter)
- Chest tube clamp
- Three-way stopcock
- Injection caps
- 20-g orthopedic wire or zip ties to secure connections

Procedure
1. Gather supplies
2. General anesthesia or sedation. General anesthesia allows for more control of patient's respiratory function and is preferred.
3. Place patient in lateral recumbency.
4. Clip the lateral thorax from just caudal to the scapula to the last rib and from dorsal spine to ventral midline.
5. Aseptically prepare.
6. Perform hand hygiene and don sterile gloves.
7. Drape the area.
8. Loosen stylet from chest tube. Extra holes can be carefully made in the chest tube to aid drainage if fluid is present in pleural space. The holes are made with a scalpel blade and should not exceed 50% of the diameter of tube to prevent tube breakage within the thoracic cavity.
9. Make a small stab incision in the skin over the widest point of the thorax when the patient is in lateral recumbency at intercostal space 9–10 (about halfway between the spine and costochondral junction).
10. Pull the skin cranially (assistant) to create tunnel and allow the chest tube to be placed in intercostal space 7–8.
11. For dogs, 0.25–1.0 mL of 0.25% or 0.5% bupivacaine (maximum total dose of 3 mg/kg) can be injected into the subcutis and intercostal muscles at the planned tube insertion site. Alternately, an intercostal nerve block can be performed by injecting 0.25–1.0 mL of 0.25% or 0.5% bupivacaine per site just ventral and caudal to the transverse processes of the thoracic vertebrae/head of ribs one space cranial and caudal, and at the site of insertion. Before injecting, always aspirate back into the syringe to determine that the needle is not in an artery or vein. Small dogs should receive 0.25 mL/site, medium dogs 0.5 mL/site, and large dogs 1.0 mL/site.[3]
12. Bluntly dissect into the pleural space using hemostats, and then spread them wide enough to allow the tube to be passed through the hole created. Insert the tube and stylet into the pleural space and advance cranio-ventrally 1–2 inches, holding the tube parallel to the thoracic wall. The tube should then be fed off the stylet cranio-ventrally. Tubes without trochars can also be placed using this technique.
13. Stop positive pressure ventilation while inserting the tube, to allow lungs to deflate and decrease risk of trauma to lungs.
14. Assess placement of the tube by using the stylet to measure the distance the tube has been advanced within the thorax.
15. Connect the tube to a three-way stopcock and injection caps or a pleural drainage system.
16. As soon as the tube is in place, aspirate the air or fluid present.
17. Once finished aspirating, place chest tube clamp on tube.
18. Secure to the skin with a purse-string suture around the tube at the entry site and a Chinese finger trap suture pattern.
19. Place sterile dressing and light bandage.
20. Secure tube connection with orthopedic wire or zip ties.
21. Perform thoracic radiographs (two orthogonal views) to check tube(s) placement.

Protocol 30.3 Trocar method of chest tube placement

Items Required
See the supplies required in Protocol 30.2.

Procedure
1. Gather supplies
2. Provide sedation or anesthesia if possible.
3. Initial preparation as previously described (Protocol 30.2).
4. Incise just the skin, tunnel the tube subcutaneously two to three rib spaces, and then position it perpendicular to the chest wall and grasp in a tight fist to only allow 1–2 inches of the tube to penetrate the chest (to prevent iatrogenic trauma from the tube penetrating too deeply).
5. Bluntly strike the top of the tube with the palm of other hand, popping the tube through into pleural space.
6. Lower the tube, decreasing the angle of insertion as the tube is advanced slightly. Once an additional 1–2 inches of the tube and stylet are in the chest, the tube is slid off the stylet, directing it cranially and ventrally.
7. Assess placement of the tube by using the stylet to measure the distance the tube has been advanced within the thorax.
8. Connect the tube via an adapter piece to a three-way stopcock and injection caps or a pleural drainage system.
9. As soon as the tube is in place, aspirate the air or fluid present.
10. Once finished aspirating, place chest tube clamp on tube.
11. Secure to the skin with a purse-string suture around the tube at the entry site and a Chinese finger trap suture pattern.
12. Place sterile dressing and light bandage.
13. Secure tube connection with orthopedic wire or zip ties.
14. Perform thoracic radiographs (two orthogonal views) to check tube(s) placement.
15. This is a very rapid placement technique but is not recommended unless in an emergency situation with no other options, due to increased risk of iatrogenic trauma

the thorax (Fig. 30.3c). Then, without removing the hemostats, the tip of the chest tube is placed into the thorax at a right angle to the chest wall (Fig. 30.3d). During this part of the procedure, the anesthetist should cease positive pressure ventilation to allow lung deflation, therefore decreasing the chance of iatrogenic trauma to the lungs. Then the end of the tube is lowered to decrease the angle of insertion and allow the tube to be placed along the inside of the thoracic wall, and the tube and stylet are advanced in a cranio-ventral direction as the tube is fed off the stylet (Fig. 30.3e). The tube is generally advanced toward the thoracic inlet. Placement of the tube can be assessed using the stylet to measure the distance that the tube has been advanced within the thorax, or if using a red rubber catheter, by using another catheter of the same size. The tube is sutured in place with a purse-string around the base of the tube and a Chinese finger trap (Fig. 30.3f). This suture pattern helps prevent the tube from slipping out of the thoracic cavity by tightening if the tube is pulled. This is accomplished by first suturing with a single knot to the patient's skin just cranial to the purse-string suture, leaving both ends of the suture long, and then crossing the ends of the suture beneath the chest tube, making a single throw on top of the tube, then repeating this pattern five to six

times, finally tying off the suture. This allows the suture to climb the tube in a crisscross pattern. The tube is then connected via an adapter piece to a three-way stopcock with injection caps and clamped with a chest tube clamp or connected to a pleural drainage system for continuous suction (see Figs. 30.3a–g). The tube is covered with a sterile dressing and light bandage. Both lateral and ventrodorsal or dorsoventral thoracic radiographs should be taken to confirm the cranial and ventral position of the tube(s) (see Figs. 30.4a and b).

Trocar method

The trocar technique is an alternative technique that is more rapid but also has more risk of complications. This method requires the same initial approach as the surgical method in that it begins with a stab incision through only the skin over the widest point (about halfway between the spine and costochondral junction) of the thorax when the patient is in lateral recumbency at intercostal space 9–10. The tube is then tunneled subcutaneously two rib spaces cranial to the skin incision. The tube is then positioned perpendicular to the chest wall and grasped tightly, in the surgeon's fist, so that only an additional 1–2 inches of the tube will be available to

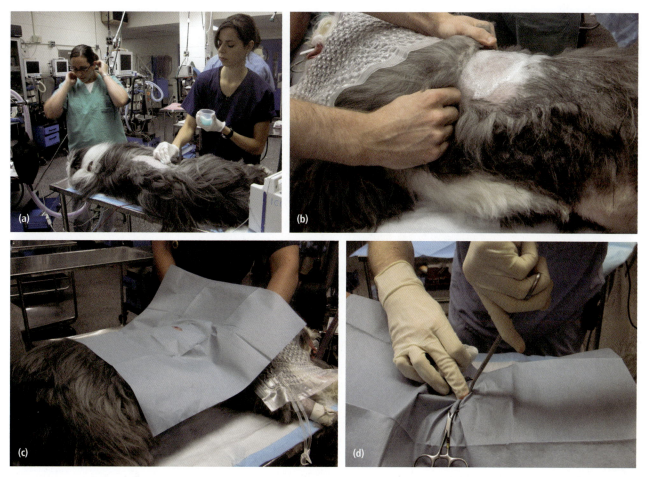

Figure 30.3 (a) A bearded collie is anesthetized, placed in lateral recumbency, and has had the lateral chest clipped and aseptically prepared in preparation for thoracostomy tube placement. (b) An assistant pulls the skin cranially to create the subcutaneous tunnel for the thoracostomy tube. (c) The chest is draped, and an incision approximately 1 cm in length is made between the 9th and 10th ribs, approximately a third of the way down the chest. (d) Carmalt clamps are used to bluntly dissect through the chest wall. Carmalt clamps were chosen because of the size of this patient. (e) The thoracostomy tube is inserted into the chest between the jaws of the Carmalt. (f) The thoracostomy tube is introduced into the pleural space while still on the trocar, angled to become more parallel with the chest wall, advanced several centimeters, and then the tube is fed off the stylet. (g) The thoracostomy tube is secured with a purse string suture around the tube and then a Chinese finger trap pattern to prevent the tube from slipping.

penetrate into the thoracic cavity. The top of the tube is struck bluntly with the palm of other hand, popping the tube through intercostal musculature and the pleura, into the chest cavity. The tube is then lowered, decreasing the angle of insertion as the tube is advanced slightly. Once 1–2 inches of the tube and stylet are in the chest, the tube is slid off the stylet, directing it cranially and ventrally. The tube is then connected and secured as described earlier for surgical placement.

Complications that can occur with the trocar technique include impaling the heart or lungs with the tube (especially if the hand at the distal end of the tube slips), pulmonary contusions, and placement of the tube into the abdominal cavity. This technique is generally not used unless it is an emergency situation with no other

options, and it is never recommended in cats due to their more compliant chest walls. With either method of placement, pain management is very important for patients with chest tubes. See the section on pain management later in this chapter.

Thoracostomy tube maintenance

Management of a thoracostomy tube requires 24-hour monitoring because of the risk of tube detachment, which could create a fatal open pneumothorax. The tube should be capped with a three-way stopcock fitted with injection caps. The three way stopcock must be positioned "off" to the patient when not in use. The chest tube itself should also be clamped using a chest tube

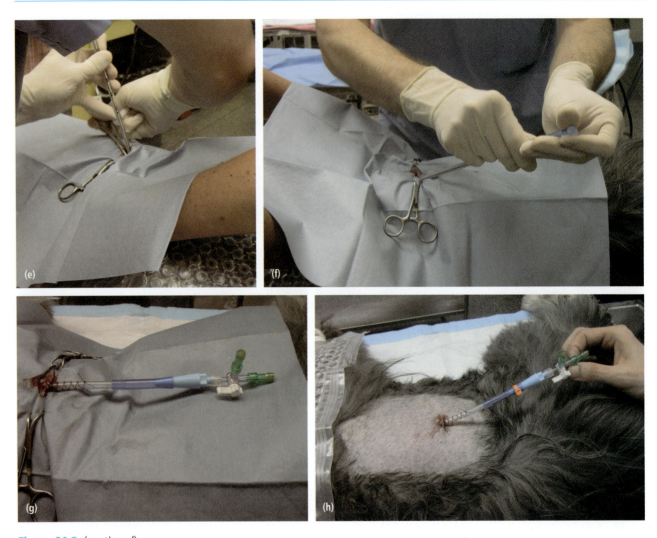

Figure 30.3 (*continued*)

clamp in the event that the three-way stopcock becomes detached from the chest tube (Fig. 30.5). The tube should be removed as soon as possible to reduce discomfort and the risk of nosocomial infection. The chest tube should also be checked daily for any evidence of migration.

Strict aseptic technique must always be practiced whenever handling the thoracostomy tube and evaluating the tube insertion site. The prophylactic use of antibiotics is not recommended.[4] The thoracostomy tube insertion site should be evaluated at least once daily for any signs of inflammation or infection including redness, pain, heat, swelling, subcutaneous emphysema, and/or purulent discharge. The integrity of the purse string, Chinese finger trap, and any sutures used to fix the thoracostomy tube to the body wall should also be noted. The presence of subcutaneous emphysema or seroma formation around the insertion site should be documented in the patient's medical record. An increasing amount of subcutaneous emphysema or an enlarging

seroma may indicate that the chest tube has migrated out of the pleural space. The chest tube may be secured to the patient in a variety of ways such as wrapping the chest tube with bandage material, using a stockinette, or using 1-inch white tape to make butterfly tags that can be sutured to the patient's skin to help prevent accidental removal of the tube. Additionally, an Elizabethan collar may be necessary to prevent the patient from removing the chest tube. The condition of the chest tube bandage should be monitored several times throughout the day for strikethrough. Soiled or damp bandages should be changed immediately. Failure to remove damp bandage material may allow bacteria from the patient's surroundings to wick through the bandage material toward the thoracostomy tube insertion site. The pleural space may be evacuated either by continuous suction drainage or intermittent manual evacuation. In general, if continuous suction is not being used, the thoracostomy tube should be manually evacuated every 4–6 hours. Each time the tube is aspirated, the pleural space

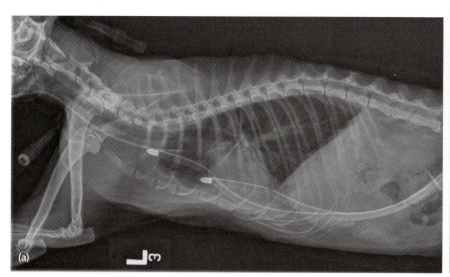
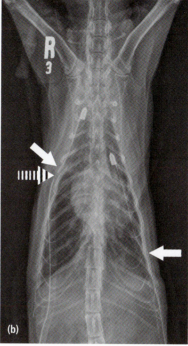

Figure 30.4 (a) Lateral radiograph of a cat with pyothorax to check placement of bilateral thoracostomy tubes. (b) Ventrodorsal radiograph of the same cat. Both views are needed to confirm correct placement. Note the left thoracostomy tube enters the chest too cranially (solid white arrows show where tubes enter thoracic cavity), at the fourth intercostal space, and it has one fenestration outside the pleural space (striped arrow). This tube should be repositioned.

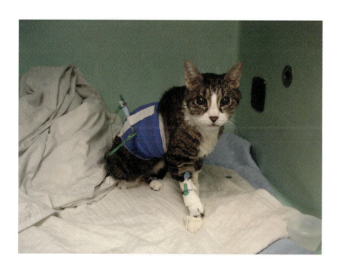

Figure 30.5 Use of orthopedic wire to secure thoracostomy tube, clamp, three-way stopcock, and injection caps to prevent accidental uncapping and iatrogenic pneumothorax.

should be evacuated until negative pressure is obtained, except in patients in which reexpansion pulmonary edema is a concern. This is most commonly a concern in cases that have had prolonged pleural space disease such as a postoperative chronic diaphragmatic hernia

patient. In these cases, the pleural space should not be fully evacuated initially, allowing the lungs to reinflate gradually and reducing the risk of pulmonary edema. Depending on the patient's disease, the tube may need to be evacuated more or less frequently. Indications for more frequent evacuation of the patient's thoracostomy tube include increased respiratory rate and effort, dyspnea, diminished breath sounds on chest auscultation, and/or the patient's posture (i.e., orthopnea).

During evacuation of the chest tube, the tubing should be evaluated to ensure that there are no leaks in the system, kinks, or accumulation of fibrin material or other proteinaceous material in the tubing. An unnoticed kink or accumulation in the chest tube yields negative pressure on aspiration. This "false" negative pressure is misleading and leads to the incorrect assumption that the pleural space has been evacuated. If the tube is clogged, the tube can be aseptically flushed, with strict attention to aseptic technique, with a small amount of sterile 0.9% saline to try to dislodge the blockage.[5]

A loose connection within the evacuation system can lead to the incorrect assumption that the patient has a continuous pneumothorax or has developed a pneumothorax if this was not the patient's initial problem. To check the chest tube for leaks, first all connections on the chest tube and three-way stopcock should be tightened. A chest tube clamp should be placed on the chest tube proximally. If all connections are tight and the chest tube is clamped, aspiration should yield negative pressure. If air is obtained on aspiration, there is a leak in the system. All connections should be rechecked, and the chest tube should be evaluated for any small holes or cracks. If repeated attempts to evacuate the thoracostomy tube fail to yield negative pressure and a leak is not identified during inspection of the system, continuous suction drainage may be indicated.

After manually evacuating a thoracostomy tube and achieving negative pressure, the patient's clinical status should be reassessed. Any increase in respiratory rate and effort, orthopneic posture, or diminished lung sounds on auscultation may warrant further diagnostics such as pulse oximetry, arterial blood gas analysis, and/or thoracic radiographs. Radiographs may demonstrate tube malposition leading to unaspirated fluid or air in the pleural space or the presence of pulmonary parenchymal disease. Other causes of increased respiratory rate and effort such as pain should also be considered.

The amount of air and/or fluid obtained from the chest tube should be monitored daily. The tube should be removed once there is negative pressure in the chest on several consecutive aspirations or the fluid obtained on aspiration decreases significantly. Normally, small volumes of fluid (up to 1–2 mL/kg/day) are generated as a result of the body's natural inflammatory response to a foreign object (thoracostomy tube) in the pleural space.[6] In general, if aspiration of the tube yields little to no air and no greater than 2–4 ml/kg of pleural fluid over a 24-hour period, the tube can be removed. If it is suspected that air or fluid remains in the chest despite repeated chest tube aspirations yielding negative pressure, diagnostic imaging such as thoracic ultrasound (for fluid) or thoracic radiographs are indicated to determine if a new chest tube needs to be placed and the old chest tube removed.

When the thoracostomy tube is removed, it should be pulled in a rapid, smooth motion. Removal may be uncomfortable for the patient so analgesia should be considered before removing. The thoracostomy tube insertion site should be left to heal by second intention; no sutures are generally needed. The site should be covered with a light bandage including a nonadherent pad.[5]

Chest tube drainage systems

Chest tube drainage systems are indicated when large quantities of air or fluid are accumulating in the pleural space rapidly. This prevents the patient from developing respiratory distress between aspirations of the tube, and it also may aid in healing of the lung if a pneumothorax is present. In cases of pneumothorax, the lungs should be kept fully inflated to allow the lung to heal in its normal expanded position. Otherwise, each time the chest tube is aspirated, the lung will reinflate from a relatively collapsed position, which may cause the seal to break apart. For patients with pyothorax that are producing a large volume of effusion, continuous drainage of the pleural space is indicated to reduce the amount of purulent material in the chest cavity.

Continuous suction drainage systems

Active drainage of the pleural space can be accomplished by connecting the patient to a continuous suction source and a drainage system. The various drainage systems are based on the three-bottle system (Fig. 30.6). In this model, the first bottle acts as a fluid trap, the second bottle provides the underwater seal, and the third bottle regulates the amount of suction that is applied to the pleural space. The three-bottle system is cumbersome and can be difficult to use because the bottles are hard to transport and maintain in the upright position.[6]

For ease of use, the commercially available continuous chest drainage systems combine the three-bottle

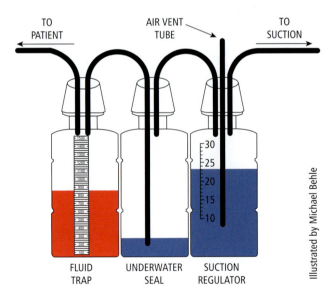

Figure 30.6 Schematic of a three-bottle system for continuous drainage of a chest tube. The chamber on the left accumulates and measures the volume of fluid from the pleural space. The middle chamber is the water seal to prevent air from flowing backward into the patient's pleural space, and the chamber of the right is the suction control chamber. It is the depth of the vent tube below the water level that determines the amount of suction.

Protocol 30.4 Setting up a continuous chest drainage system

Items Required
- Continuous chest drainage system (Thora-Seal III and the Pleurovac)
- Christmas tree adapter
- Short piece of sterile nonconductive connecting tubing (6-mm diameter)
- Sterile water
- Y connector (optional)
- Suction source

Procedure
1. Place the suction unit on a flat surface, and secure if needed to prevent it from falling over.
2. Pour water into the water seal chamber to the level indicated on the unit, then pour water into the suction control chamber to the required level (usually 15-20 cm of water).[5,6]
3. Remember, the level of water in the suction control chamber determines the level of suction, not the vacuum meter.
4. Connect drainage tubing to the chest tube, and connect the suction tubing to the vacuum source, then unclamp the chest tube(s) to allow evacuation of the pleural space.
5. Two chest tubes can be connected into one chest drainage system by using a Y connector (Figure 30.7) and a piece of 6-mm diameter sterile nonconductive connecting tubing.

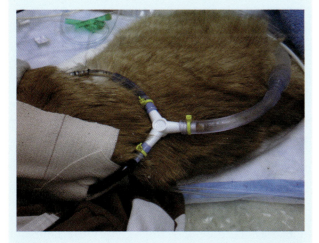

Figure 30.7 A sterile plastic Y piece and tubing are used to connect bilateral chest tubes to a single drainage system.

system into one compact plastic unit (Protocol 30.4). The left-most section of the unit is the collection chamber. The patient's chest tube connects to the collection chamber of the drainage unit via the included tubing and tube adapter in most cases. If the chest tube is small, the adapter may be too large to connect to it and a Christmas tree adapter and a short piece of sterile nonconductive connecting tubing (6-mm diameter is commonly used, available from Medline Industries, Mundelein, IL) may be needed to attach to the tubing adapter. Fluid from the chest tube collects in this chamber, which allows for easy measurement and recording of the amount of drainage. The middle chamber of the chest drainage system provides the water seal. The purpose of the water seal is to allow air to exit from the pleural space on exhalation while preventing air from flowing backward through the tubing and into the pleural cavity. It is recommended that the water seal chamber be filled with sterile water up to the 2-cm line, so a 2-cm water seal is established. To maintain an effective seal, it is important to keep the chest drainage unit upright at all times and to monitor the water level in the water seal because it may evaporate. Bubbling in the water seal chamber is caused by air flowing from the tubing into the chamber. This can indicate air is being removed from the patient's pleural space or that there is a leak in the system. The amount of air bubbling in this chamber cannot be quantitated but does allow a subjective evaluation of the amount of air coming off the pleural space. The right-most chamber of the unit is the suction control chamber. Traditional chest drainage units regulate the amount of suction by the height of the column of water in the suction control chamber. It is important to remember that it is the height of the water, not the setting of the suction source, that limits the amount of suction transmitted to the pleural cavity. The recommended height of water is 15–20 cm.[5,6] The unit is then attached via a 6-mm diameter sterile nonconductive connecting tubing to a suction source such as wall suction or a portable suction machine like the Schuco Vac (Allied Healthcare Products, Inc., St. Louis, MO).

A few brand-name units are commonly used in critical care. Some examples include the Thora-Seal III (Kendall, Watertown, NY) and the Pleurovac (Teleflex Medical, Research Triangle, NC). Another disposable drainage system that incorporates suction into the unit is the Thorovac (AN-50) (Andersen Products, Haw River, NC), which may be a good alternative if no central suction is available.

The chest drainage system must be kept on a flat, level surface. If the unit is not level, it could disrupt the water seal. The gentle bubbling causes evaporation of the water in the chambers over time. It is necessary to check the water levels every few hours to ensure the proper water seal and suction. Careful inspection of all chest tube connections to the chest drainage system is warranted to avoid potential leaks. The system can be checked for leaks by briefly clamping off the chest tube and watching for bubbling in the water seal chamber. If bubbles are still occurring in the water seal chamber while the chest tube is clamped, there is a leak in the system distal to the clamp. All connections should be checked, and then the process should be repeated.

The chest drainage tubing should be checked for kinks. Any fluid that accumulates in the tubing should periodically be encouraged to flow into the collection chamber by elevating the tubing (but not above the level of the chest tube) so gravity will aid in its drainage. The fluid collection chamber has a capacity of approximately 2000 mL, depending on the type of drainage system. The fluid collection chamber should be monitored closely and emptied or replaced if it becomes filled. Aseptic technique should be used if the collection chamber is emptied. Many units do not allow for emptying, so a new unit is required if the collection chamber fills. If the chest drainage tubing becomes clogged with thick secretions, the chest drainage unit needs to be replaced.

Nonsuction drainage

A passive continuous drainage method is also available. The Heimlich valve consists of a rubber one-way valve inside a plastic tube that connects to a standard chest tube. These units only allow air and fluid to move from the chest into the environment or collection bag. They are not recommended for animals lighter than 15 kg because smaller patients do not generate sufficient increases in intrapleural pressure during exhalation to allow the valve to operate properly. Heimlich valves (Fig. 30.8) are best suited for removal of air from the pleural space because fluid may cause the valve to stick and no longer function.[7] Even when a pneumothorax is the primary problem, small amounts of fluid, blood, or fibrin may cause the Heimlich valve to stick, so they should only be used with constant supervision.

Manual drainage of the thoracostomy tube

Strict attention to aseptic technique must be followed whenever the chest tube is handled or aspirated. The chest tube may be manually evacuated by attaching a chest tube adapter to a three-way stopcock. An empty syringe should be attached to the three-way stopcock, and the stopcock should be positioned in the open position to both the patient and the syringe. Gentle aspiration of the syringe plunger should draw air or fluid from the pleural space into the syringe. The chest tube should be gently aspirated until negative pressure is obtained. Once negative pressure is obtained, the patient should be repositioned and the chest tube reaspirated to determine if changing the patient's position yields any additional air or fluid from the tube. Occasionally, there may be a pocket of fluid that cannot be drained by the chest tube unless the patient is repositioned.

The total amount of air and fluid aspirated from the chest tube should be measured and recorded in the patient's record. Significant changes in the volume of air or fluid aspirated from the patient's thoracostomy tube from one intermittent aspiration to the next should be closely monitored. Decreasing amounts of air and/or fluid may indicate improvement in the patient's pleural space disease; conversely, increasing amounts of air or fluid may indicate a worsening of the patient's pleural space disease. In addition to noting changes in volume of air and fluid aspirated from the pleural space, any gross changes in the appearance of the fluid aspirated (i.e., changes in consistency and color of pleural fluid) should be noted. Fluid analysis may be indicated in the event of increasing volumes of pleural effusion, changes in the appearance of the effusion, or before removing the chest tube if it were placed to drain a pyothorax.

Pain management

Indwelling chest tubes can be very painful; therefore, it is important to provide analgesia to these patients. Bupivacaine 0.5% (Hospira Inc., Lake Forest, IL) can provide local analgesia when administered via the thoracostomy tube at a total dose of 1.5 mg/kg every 6–8 hours for dogs.[8,9] A lower dose of 1 mg/kg every 6–8 hours is recommended for cats.[10,11] Cats are more sensitive to local anesthetics than dogs and should be carefully monitored if they are used. After injecting into the chest tubes, 2–3 mL of sterile 0.9 % NaCl should be used to flush the bupivacaine out of the tube and into the patient's pleural

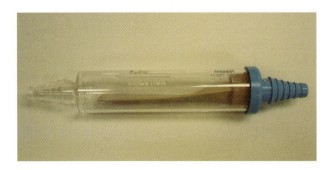

Figure 30.8 A Heimlich valve, which allows for passive continuous drainage of a thoracostomy tube.

space. If a single chest tube is present, placing the patient with the chest tube side down after instillation of bupivacaine may allow for better local analgesia. The bupivacaine dose can be split and given via two tubes in patients that have bilateral thoracostomy tubes. Bupivacaine should not be used in patients that are attached to a chest drainage unit with continuous suction because it will be suctioned back out of the thoracostomy tube immediately after administration. Similarly, the thoracostomy tube should not be aspirated immediately after administration of a local anesthetic. Bupivacaine can sting on initial injection due to the acidity of the solution. Sodium bicarbonate can be used to buffer the solution at a dose of 1 part sodium bicarbonate to 9 parts bupivacaine.[10] If the total volume of bupivacaine or bupivacaine plus sodium bicarbonate is very small, it can be diluted with sterile 0.9% NaCl to a total volume of 10–20 mL, depending on the size of the patient. The use of bupivacaine in animals that have had a pericardectomy is controversial due to the possibility of cardiotoxicity.[12] Injectable opioids offer excellent analgesia but may be associated with decreased respiratory drive at higher doses (See Chapter 43, Systemic Analgesia). The combination of opioids and intrapleural bupivacaine can provide excellent pain relief for most patients. A tranquilizer such as acepromazine (Butler

Animal Health Supply, Dublin, OH) or a benzodiazepine can be administered with an opioid to treat anxiety. It is important to keep patients calm to prevent them from disconnecting the chest drainage system or pulling out the chest tube. Nonsteroidals may also be used for analgesia if the patient has no contraindications (see Chapter 43, Systemic Analgesia).

Handling samples for fluid analysis

Analysis of the pleural fluid may indicate whether the effusion is a transudate, modified transudate, chylous, exudate, neoplastic, or hemorrhagic effusion.[13] A sample of the effusion should be submitted for fluid analysis to aid in identification of the disease process causing the effusion. Fluid analysis should include cell counts, protein concentration, and cytology[8] (See Table 30.1). Fluid should be submitted for bacterial culture (aerobic and anaerobic) if bacteria or suppurative inflammation are seen on cytology or an infectious process is suspected. If a chylothorax is suspected, triglyceride concentrations of both the effusion and serum should be measured and compared.[14] A diagnosis of chylothorax can be made if triglyceride concentrations are greater in the effusion and fluid cytology shows a large number of mature lymphocytes. A sterile red top tube (without

Table 30.1 Pleural effusion types and characteristics[14]

Fluid Type	Appearance	Cell Counts (cells/µL)	Protein Concentration (g/dL)	Triglyceride Present	Cytology
Transudate	Clear, pale yellow	<1500	<2.5	No	Predominately acellular, occasional RBC
Modified transudate	Yellow or pink; clear to slightly cloudy	1500–5000	~3.0	No	Moderately cellular, some RBCs, macrophages, and mesothelial cells
Chylous	Milky/white; turbid	500–20,000	≥3.0	Yes (triglyceride more than serum triglyceride)	Mature lymphocytes, neutrophils, and macrophages
Exudate	Yellow to orange brown	>5000	>3.0	No	Primarily nondegenerate to degenerate neutrophils; bacteria may or may not be present
Hemorrhagic	Red	Resembles peripheral blood	>3.0	Yes. Triglyceride level equal to serum triglyceride level	Resembles peripheral blood

anticoagulant) should be used for cell counts, cytology, and triglyceride levels. Hemorrhagic fluid samples should be submitted in a purple-top tube (with EDTA anticoagulant). An iatrogenic hemothorax may result if the needle used during thoracocentesis made contact with the patient's heart or a blood vessel. Active hemorrhage can be ruled out by placing a small amount of the effusion into a red top tube or a tube with diatomaceous earth and monitoring for clot formation. If samples are to be submitted for culture, a sterile red top tube or anaerobic and aerobic culturettes should be used.

References

1. Spackman CJ, Caywood DD, Feeney DA, Johnston GR. Thoracic wall and pulmonary trauma in dogs sustaining fractures as a result of motor vehicle accidents. J Am Vet Med Assoc 1984;185(9):975–977.

2. Puerto D, Brockman DJ, Lindquist C, Drobatz K. Surgical and nonsurgical management of and selected risk factors for spontaneous pneumothorax in dogs: 64 cases (1986–1999). J Am Vet Med Assoc 2002;220(11):1670–1674.

3. Skarda RT. Local and regional anesthetic and analgesic techniques: dogs and cats. In: Thurmon JC, Tranquilli WJ, Benson, GJ, eds. Lumb & Jones' Veterinary Anesthesia. Baltimore, MD: Williams & Wilkins; 1996:426–447.

4. Luchette FA, Barie PS, Oswanski MF, et al. Practice management guidelines for prophylactic antibiotic use in tube thoracostomy for traumatic hemopneumothorax: the EAST practice management guidelines work group. J Trauma 2000;48(4):753–757.

5. Crowe DT, Devey JJ. Thoracic drainage. In: Bojarab MJ, ed. Current Techniques in Small Animal Surgery. Baltimore: Williams & Wilkins; 1997:403–417.

6. Monnet E. Pleura and pleural space. In: Slatter D, ed. Textbook of Small Animal Surgery. 3rd ed. Philadelphia, PA: Saunders; 2003:387–405.

7. Sigrist NE. Thoracostomy tube placement and drainage. In: Silverstein DC, Hopper K, eds. Small Animal Critical Care Medicine. Philadelphia, PA: Saunders; 2009:134–137.

8. Thompson SE, Johnson JM. Analgesia in dogs after intercostal thoracotomy. A comparison of morphine, selective intercostal nerve block and intrapleural regional analgesia with bupivacaine. Vet Surg 1991;20(1):73–77.

9. Conzemius MG, Brockman DJ, King LG, Perkowski SZ. Analgesia in dogs after intercostal thoracotomy. A clinical trial comparing intravenous buprenorphine and intrapleural bupivacaine. Vet Surg 1994;23:291–298.

10. Hellyer PW, Fails AD. Pain management for the surgical patient. In: Slatter D, ed. Textbook of Small Animal Surgery. 3rd ed. Philadelphia: Saunders; 2003:2503–2515.

11. Torres BT, Radlinsky MG, Budsberg SC. What is the evidence? Surgical intervention in a cat with idiopathic chylothorax. J Am Vet Med Assoc 2009;235(10):1167–1169.

12. Quandt JE, Powell LL, Lee JA. Analgesia in critically ill patients. Compend Contin Educ Pract Vet 2005;27:433–445.

13. Waddell LS, King LG. General approach to dyspnoea. In: King LG, Boag A, eds. BSAVA Manual of Canine and Feline Emergency and Critical Care. 2nd ed. Gloucester, UK: British Small Animal Veterinary Association; 2007:83–113.

14. Macintire DK, Drobatz KJ, Haskins SC, Saxon WD. Respiratory emergencies. In: Troy DB, ed. Manual of Small Animal Emergency and Critical Care Medicine. Baltimore, MD: Lippincott Williams & Wilkins; 2005:115–159.

SECTION IV

Urinary and abdominal

31

Urethral catheterization

Janet Aldrich

Urethral catheterization means to pass a urinary catheter through the urethra into the urinary bladder. It is easy to learn the procedure and, with practice, to perform it safely and quickly. Every catheterization has risks; perform the procedure only when benefits outweigh risks.

We describe methods for catheterization of dogs and cats, both males and females. For female dogs we prefer the digital palpation technique, but we also describe direct visualization methods.

Indications

Indications are to alleviate urethral obstruction, empty the bladder, monitor urine output, get samples for analysis, and aid in diagnostic procedures and urologic surgery.[1] Indwelling urinary catheters should not replace good nursing care to keep patients clean and dry. Urine samples for urine analysis and culture are usually better procured by cystocentesis or voiding.

Urinary catheters

Urinary catheters are made of materials such as silicone, latex, and latex-based with various coatings. Antimicrobial or antiseptic-impregnated and hydrophilic catheters are also available and might reduce infection, but more research is needed.[2] The ideal material does not elicit inflammation, resists kinking, and inhibits bacterial adherence. In an experimental dog model, latex catheters tended to cause more inflammatory changes in urethral cells than did silicone, Teflon-coated latex, and polyvinylchloride catheters.[3] In an extensive review of

scientific studies in humans comparing types of standard catheters (silicone, latex, hydrogel-coated latex, siliconized latex), no catheter was found better than another in reducing bacteriuria.[2] Siliconized catheters may be less likely to cause urethral side effects in men.[2] Silicone catheters resisted kinking better than latex-based catheters.[4] Bacteria colonize indwelling urinary catheters and grow as biofilms embedded in a gel-like polysaccharide matrix. Bacteria growing in the biofilm are resistant to antibiotics. Biofilms in a crystalline form can occlude the catheter lumen. All types of catheters, including those coated with antimicrobials, are vulnerable to biofilm formation.[5] These characteristics are not well studied in dogs or cats, but catheters suitable for use in humans are likely acceptable for our patients as well. General-use catheters such as red rubber, polypropylene, or feeding tubes are also used. Marked bacterial adherence to red rubber catheters compared with other materials has been shown.[6] Its stiffness makes the polypropylene the easiest insert but also the least desirable because it can directly traumatize the urethra and, if left indwelling, can traumatize the bladder wall. An experimental study in cats showed that both polypropylene and polyvinyl catheters caused inflammatory lesions in the urethra and bladder, but polypropylene caused the most lesions.[7]

Design

Foley-type urinary catheters have an inflation balloon at the distal end which, when inflated with sterile water, retains the catheter in the bladder. We prefer these for indwelling use. There are lengths suitable for both males

Advanced Monitoring and Procedures for Small Animal Emergency and Critical Care, First Edition. Edited by Jamie M. Burkitt Creedon, Harold Davis.

© 2012 John Wiley & Sons, Inc. Published 2012 by John Wiley & Sons, Inc.

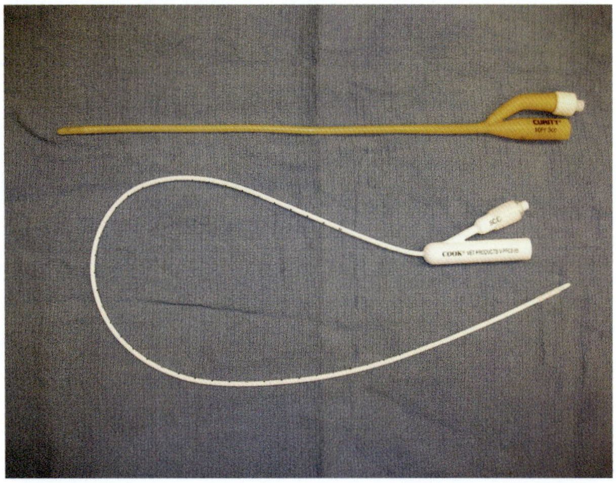

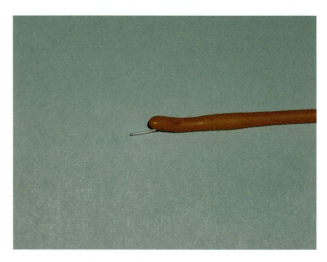

Figure 31.1 Foley catheter in lengths for females (above) and males (below).

Figure 31.2 Stylet protruding from side hole of the catheter.

and females (see Fig. 31.1) and sizes as small as 5F. Some of the smaller catheters for use in females have a stylet.

For male cats, tomcat-style urinary catheters in 3.5F or 5F do not have an inflation balloon and must be sutured in place. Some have a removable stylet. These catheters are either open ended (having a single opening at the tip) or closed ended (having openings along the side). The open-ended catheter allows retrograde flushing of an obstructed urethra. The rounded tip of the closed-ended catheter might reduce urethral trauma. The Minnesota olive-tip urethral catheter is a 22-gauge metal catheter with an olive-shaped open-ended tip. It is inserted into the distal urethra of an obstructed male cat to assist in retropulsion of debris from the urethra into the bladder.

Stylets

A stylet can make it easier to advance a catheter, especially one of small diameter. However, it can cause mucosal trauma or even rupture of the urethra because it allows excessively vigorous efforts to advance the catheter. Also, a stylet can be dislodged during placement attempts such that it exits through a side hole in the catheter, thus preventing passage of the catheter into the urethra and traumatizing the mucosa with the exposed stylet tip (see Fig. 31.2). Use a stylet only with proper caution. Make sure the stylet is properly positioned before attempting insertion. With practice and a good technique, most catheters can be placed without a stylet.

Diameter

We recommend using the smallest diameter catheter that will achieve good urine flow and not kink. Approxi-

mate requirements are 3.5F or 5F for cats or small dogs, 8F for medium dogs, and 8F or 10F for large dogs.

Length

When correctly placed, the catheter tip rests in the bladder near the trigone. As the patient moves or the bladder size changes, the catheter should remain in the bladder (not retract into the urethra) but should not be so far advanced that it contacts the cranial bladder wall.

Closed collection systems

In human medicine it is accepted practice and strongly recommended to connect all indwelling urinary catheters to a sterile closed urine collection system.[1] Closed urine drainage systems facilitate aseptic emptying of the urine from the bag without disconnection from the catheter, have a check valve to prevent retrograde flow of urine from the bag to the bladder, and often include a sampling port for getting urine samples. In veterinary practice, urine collection systems are often created from available materials using a macrodrip set and a sterile empty fluid bag. This is considered an open system because when the fluid bag is filled with urine, it must be disconnected from the tubing and replaced with a new bag. The disconnection carries the risk of introducing bacteria into the system. These systems were reported not to be associated with the likelihood of developing nosocomial bacteriuria in dogs with short-term urinary catheterization, but the authors cautioned that asepsis must be maintained when changing the collection bag.[8,9] These open urine collection systems must not be confused with leaving a catheter unattached to any urine collection system, referred to as an open catheter. Thirty years ago, it was common practice to treat urethral obstruction in male cats by placing an indwelling urinary catheter and not attaching a urine collection system but instead leaving the catheter open to the environment. An experimental study in cats with these open indwelling catheters showed that 20 of 36 developed bacteriuria.[10] We recommend all indwelling catheters be attached to a sterile urine collection system. If an open urine collection system using a sterile empty fluid bag as the reservoir is used, it is essential to maintain sterility in setting up and maintaining the system. The purpose-specific closed urine collection systems have advantages as previously discussed.

Aseptic practice for placement and maintenance

Infection is a complication of urinary catheterization. Bacteria might be introduced into the bladder during catheterization or while maintaining an indwelling system. Organisms can ascend into the bladder from the catheter insertion site or through the catheter lumen from the collection system. In humans, urinary tract infection is the most common hospital-acquired infection, and indwelling urinary catheters are the major associated cause.[2] Onetime urinary catheterization in healthy dogs resulted in catheter-associated urinary tract infection in 20% of female dogs and none of the males.[11] Hospitalized dogs and cats[12,13] or in dogs[8,14–17] with indwelling urinary catheters developed catheter-associated urinary tract infection at a rate from 52% to 10%. Increasing duration of indwelling urinary catheterization increased the risk of catheter-associated urinary tract infection.[14,16,17] In the studies with the lowest catheter-associated urinary tract infection, the authors speculated that their use of a strict protocol to maintain asepsis during insertion and maintenance of indwelling catheters contributed to the lower rate.[8,14] Those protocols are the ones recommended here.

Antibiotic treatment of patients with indwelling urinary catheters is variously reported to increase,[16] decrease,[14] or not affect[17] the development of a urinary tract infection. In human medicine, the Centers for Disease Control and Prevention (CDC) strongly recommends not using systemic antimicrobials routinely to prevent catheter-associated urinary tract infections either with short-term or long-term catheterization.[1] The available evidence does not support administering prophylactic antibiotics for an indwelling urinary catheter but does not preclude administering them for other purposes.

The risk of infection is reduced by proper patient selection, aseptic practices by trained caregivers in insertion and maintenance of indwelling catheters and collection systems, and using indwelling catheters for the shortest time possible. The known risk of catheter-associated urinary tract infections should be considered in patient management after catheter removal.

Protocols

Based on our experience and informed by the CDC 2009 guidelines[1] for prevention of catheter-associated urinary tract infections in humans, we use and recommend the following protocols.

1. Ensure that only properly trained caregivers who know the correct aseptic techniques perform catheter insertion and maintenance.
2. Perform hand hygiene before and after insertion or manipulation of catheter or collection system.
3. Use sterile gloves, drape, and sterile lubrication for insertion.
4. Follow a protocol (preferably written) for catheter insertion and indwelling catheter care to assure consistency in using good technique between caregivers.
5. Use the smallest bore, softest catheter possible consistent with good drainage to minimize urethral and bladder trauma.
6. Secure indwelling catheters to prevent movement and urethral traction.
7. Attach all indwelling catheters to a closed sterile collection system. If breaks in aseptic technique occur, replace the catheter and collection system.
8. For indwelling catheters attached to a sterile collection system, maintain unobstructed flow, keep the catheter and collecting tubes from kinking, and keep the collecting bag lower than the bladder to prevent retrograde urine flow. For closed systems, empty the collecting bag regularly using a clean container, avoid splashing, and prevent contact of the collecting bag drainage tube with the collecting container. For open systems, follow aseptic technique when breaking the line to replace the urine collection bag. Use sterile gloves and gowns as needed for aseptic technique and for protection of caregivers if public health considerations are present.
9. Do not change indwelling catheters and drainage bags at fixed intervals but rather based on clinical indications such as infection, obstruction, or compromise of the closed collection system.

10. Do not irrigate the bladder or collection system with antiseptics or antimicrobials without specific indication.
11. Use good nursing care to minimize contamination of the catheter and periurethral area from contact with soiled hospital surfaces, wound discharges, or feces.

Catheter placement

Catheter placement must be according to good aseptic practice taking into consideration the patient, environment, operator, and equipment. Assemble the material for placement before beginning the procedure (Protocol 31.1). The procedure varies according to species and gender. A summary of the steps is provided for female dog or cat (Protocol 31.2), male dog (Protocol 31.3) and male cat (Protocol 31.4).

Catheter selection

Measure from the vulva or prepuce to the bladder to determine the length of catheter needed. The bladder can be located by palpation or estimated to be just cranial to the pubis. Alternatively, estimate the bladder position as the cranial aspect of the proximal femur with the patient in lateral recumbency and the limb in neutral position. Select the softest, smallest diameter catheter that will serve the purpose.

Protocol 31.1 Preparation of materials for urinary catheter placement

Items Required
- Urinary catheter in sterile wrap.
- If using Foley catheter: sterile syringe containing sterile water for balloon inflation
- If catheter will be indwelling: sterile urinary collection system, cable ties
- Sterile barrier drape
- Sterile gloves
- Examination gloves
- Clean gauze pads soaked in chlorhexidine (or other surgical) scrub
- Clean gauze pads soaked in water to rinse off the scrub
- 0.05% chlorhexidine solution
- Sterile syringe to use to flush with chlorhexidine solution
- Sterile lubricant
- For females: sterile 2% lidocaine jelly and sterile syringe for injecting jelly into vestibule
- Clippers
- Tape
- If catheter will be indwelling: suture material, instruments, and cable ties for securing catheter and collection system

---

Protocol 31.2 Patient preparation and urinary catheter placement using digital technique in female dog or cat

Items Required
- See Protocol 31.1 for appropriate supplies

Procedure
1. Ensure that only properly trained caregivers perform catheter insertion and that sterility is maintained throughout.
2. Sedate patient if indicated.
3. Position the patient.
4. Determine the length of catheter needed to reach the bladder by measurement on the patient.
5. Clip hair to maintain an adequate hair-free zone adjacent to the vulva.
6. Perform hand hygiene and don clean examination gloves.
7. Wash off visible dirt.
8. Perform surgical scrub of the skin surrounding the vulva; rinse off the scrub with water.
9. Flush the vulva and vestibule five times with 0.05% chlorhexidine solution.
10. Instill sterile 2% lidocaine jelly into the vestibule.
11. Operator dons sterile gloves.
12. Position barrier drape to provide adequate sterile field.
13. Remove catheter from sterile wrap.
14. If the catheter has a stylet, verify that it is in the correct location.
15. If using Foley catheter, test the balloon.
16. Sterilely mark the catheter or otherwise indicate the length needed to reach the bladder.
17. Lubricate the end of the catheter.
18. Lubricate the operator's gloved palpating finger.
19. Insert the gloved palpating finger between the labia of the vulva.
20. If patient size permits, advance the finger to palpate the urethral papilla.
21. If patient size does not permit advancing, leave the finger between the labia of the vulva.
22. Insert the catheter ventral to the finger and advance into the urethra and bladder.
23. If urine is not obtained, verify the proper placement of the catheter in the bladder or reposition if needed.
24. Withdraw the palpating finger without disturbing the placement of the catheter.
25. Inflate the Foley balloon if using a Foley catheter.
26. If the catheter is to be indwelling, attach a sterile collection system; secure the catheter and the collection system to prevent urethral traction and catheter movement.

Sedation

Sedation is usually needed for cats, not usually for dogs. However, patient compliance is important to success, and therefore sedation or anesthesia should be provided as indicated.

Protocol 31.3 Patient preparation and urinary catheter placement in male dog

Items Required
- See Protocol 31.1 for appropriate supplies

Procedure
1. Ensure that only properly trained caregivers perform catheter insertion and that sterility is maintained throughout.
2. Position the patient.
3. Determine the length of catheter needed to reach the bladder by measurement on the patient.
4. Clip hair to maintain an adequate hair-free zone adjacent to the opening of the prepuce.
5. Perform hand hygiene and don clean examination gloves.
6. Wash off visible dirt.
7. Perform surgical scrub of the skin surrounding the prepuce; rinse off the scrub with water.
8. Flush the prepuce five times with 0.05% chlorhexidine solution.
9. Assistant extrudes the penis and maintains it in that position until catheter is placed.
10. Perform surgical prep of the extruded penis with 0.05% chlorhexidine solution.
11. Operator dons sterile gloves.
12. Position barrier drape to provide adequate sterile field.
13. Remove catheter from sterile wrap.
14. If using Foley catheter, test the balloon.
15. Sterilely mark the catheter or otherwise indicate the length needed to reach the bladder.
16. Lubricate the end of the catheter.
17. Insert the catheter into the penis and advance it into the bladder.
18. Verify correct position of catheter in the bladder, and reposition if needed.
19. Inflate the Foley balloon if using a Foley catheter.
20. If the catheter is to be indwelling, attach a sterile collection system; secure the catheter and the collection system to prevent urethral traction and catheter movement.

Protocol 31.4 Patient preparation and urinary catheter placement in male cat

Items Required
- See Protocol 31.1 for appropriate supplies

Procedure
1. Ensure that only properly trained caregivers perform catheter insertion and that sterility is maintained throughout.
2. Sedate the patient if indicated.
3. Position the patient.
4. Determine the length of catheter needed to reach the bladder by measurement on the patient.
5. Clip hair to maintain an adequate hair-free zone adjacent to the opening of the prepuce.
6. Perform hand hygiene and don clean examination gloves.
7. Wash off visible dirt.
8. Perform surgical scrub of the skin surrounding the prepuce; rinse off the scrub with water.
9. Flush the prepuce five times with 0.05% chlorhexidine solution.
10. Have an assistant extrude the penis and maintain it in that position until catheter is placed.
11. Perform surgical preparation of the extruded penis with 0.05% chlorhexidine solution.
12. Operator dons sterile gloves.
13. Position barrier drape to provide adequate sterile field.
14. Remove catheter from sterile wrap.
15. Sterilely mark the catheter or otherwise indicate the length needed to reach the bladder.
16. Lubricate the end of the catheter.
17. Insert the catheter into the penis and advance toward the bladder while putting traction on the penis in a caudal direction to straighten the sigmoid flexure.
18. Verify correct position of catheter in the bladder; reposition if needed.
19. If the catheter is to be indwelling, attach a sterile collection system; secure the catheter and the collection system to prevent urethral traction and catheter movement.

Patient preparation

Clip hair from the perivulvar or peripreputial area to establish a 5-cm hair-free zone that can be cleaned and to allow for insertion of sutures if needed. Take care to avoid damage to the skin during clipping. Local irritation causes discomfort, potentially increases risk of skin infection, and decreases patient tolerance of the indwelling catheter. Clean the skin that has been clipped with an antiseptic scrub such as chlorhexidine scrub and rinse well with tap water. Do not contact mucosal surfaces with the scrub.

Next use 5–10 mL of 0.05% chlorhexidine solution (add 6.25 mL of 2% chlorhexidine to 250 mL sterile water) as an antiseptic solution to flush the vulva and vestibule or prepuce five times. Sterile water or saline, or another antiseptic solution at concentrations suitable for mucosal contact, could be used as the flush. The remaining portion of the sterile solution is stored for subsequent use in catheter care if the catheter is to be indwelling.

In males, after positioning the patient and extruding the penis, gently clean the area of the external urethral orifice with the solution. Thereafter do not allow the penis to retract into the prepuce until the catheter has been placed into the bladder and will not be further advanced.

Catheter preparation

While maintaining sterility, mark the catheter or otherwise indicate the spot where it will exit the body when the tip is in the bladder. During insertion it is easy to lose track of how much catheter has been inserted. If a flexible catheter curls up in the bladder, it can form a knot that requires surgical removal.

If using a Foley catheter with a balloon, test the balloon before insertion (see Fig. 31.3). The inflation

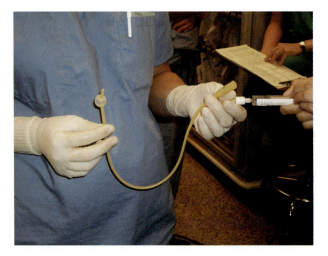

Figure 31.3 Test the balloon of the Foley before placing the catheter.

port is imprinted with the amount of sterile water required. Follow the manufacturer's directions regarding the fluid and volume for inflation. Under or overinflation can cause an asymmetrical balloon that can deflect the catheter tip and cause occlusion or irritation of the bladder wall. Water is recommended because saline can cause crystal formation in the balloon and prevent deflation of the balloon at the time of removal. Inflation with air causes the balloon tip to float in the urine.[18] To test the balloon, fill a syringe with the recommended amount of water and attach it to the inflation port. Inflate and verify that the balloon maintains inflation; then deflate the balloon. The proper method to deflate the balloon is to attach the empty syringe to the inflation port and let the fluid drain without aspirating. If the balloon does not deflate, reseat the syringe firmly and try again.

Lubrication and local anesthesia

In males, apply lubricant to the tip of the catheter and the tip of the extruded penis. As the catheter is passed, continue to apply lubricant on the catheter at the tip of the penis.

In females we have found that both local anesthesia and lubrication are important to improve patient compliance. After aseptic preparation we use 2% lidocaine jelly to get both. While maintaining sterility, fill a syringe barrel with a suitable volume of sterile lidocaine jelly, replace the plunger, and gently insert the catheter tip between the labia and into the vestibule. Then inject the jelly. Lidocaine is absorbed through the mucosa, so limit the total amount to 0.2 mL of 2% lidocaine jelly per kilogram. Wait 10 minutes for the lidocaine to take effect. If you plan on using a speculum or otoscope cone technique for placing the catheter, lubricate the instrument and catheter tip, but do not fill the vestibule with lubricating jelly because it will obscure visualization of the urethral papilla.

Species- and gender-specific instructions

This section outlines instructions for catheter placement in female dogs (digital, speculum, and otoscope cone techniques), female cats or small female dogs, male cats, and male dogs. If the catheter is to be indwelling, see the section "Indwelling Catheters" for instructions on securing and maintaining the catheter and collection system.

Female dog

Female catheterization is a skill that takes concentration, correct technique, and some practice. The required skills are similar to those needed to place a venous catheter dependably. In both cases the target is identified by knowing the relevant anatomy and by palpation. In both cases, one must line up the catheter carefully along the long axis of the structure one is attempting to enter (vein or urethra), and the catheter tip must be directed downward. Small controlled motions are better than large ones. As with any procedure, it is important to know when to stop and seek assistance. The patient is the primary concern.

We prefer the digital technique with the patient comfortably restrained in lateral recumbency. This has been successfully used in our hospital and taught in wet labs for many years. Other techniques using a speculum or otoscope cone are less well tolerated by the patient and require specialized equipment. However, it is valuable to know more than one way of performing a procedure, and so we also describe these techniques.

Anatomy

The relevant anatomy from caudal to cranial is the vulva, vestibule, and vestibulovaginal junction (see Fig. 31.4). The vagina is cranial to this junction and not entered during this procedure. When attempting to enter the vestibule, avoid the clitoris, which is in a blind ending pouch located just inside the labia of the vulva (see Fig. 31.5). The urethral opening is in the vestibule on the ventral midline at or just caudal to the vaginovestibular junction. Various strips and bands of tissue can form strictures in the vestibule or, uncommonly, in the vulva. They may prevent digital palpation. Nonetheless, the catheter can usually be successfully placed by directing it without palpation as described in the section for small dogs.

Digital technique
Positioning

Sedation is not usually required if the patient is compliant. Position the patient in lateral recumbency. For a right-handed operator, position the patient in right lateral recumbency and use the right hand for palpation. Let the pelvic limbs rest in a relaxed, normal position. Move the tail out of the way, but do not elevate it because that position can narrow the vulvar opening and make entering through it more difficult.

Palpation

First, familiarize yourself with the anatomy in this patient by palpation. In this procedure, you are not palpating in the vagina but rather in the vestibule. Insert the palpating finger under the dorsal fold of the vulva in a vertical (not horizontal) orientation, and direct it vertically toward the spine so the fingertip passes under the dorsal fold and avoids the clitoris. Then change the angle to horizontal and advance the finger cranially into the vestibule until the vestibulovaginal junction is palpated as a circumferential thickening that usually does not allow passage of the palpating finger into the vagina. This is a normal structure, not a stricture. With the fingertip in contact with the vestibulovaginal junction, move the fingertip ventrally and caudally to palpate on the ventral midline for the urethral papilla as a soft mound of tissue surrounding the urethral opening, about 0.5 cm caudal to the vestibulovaginal junction in a moderate-size dog. It may be obvious or subtle. It is not absolutely necessary to palpate the papilla because the correctly directed catheter will enter it if the catheter

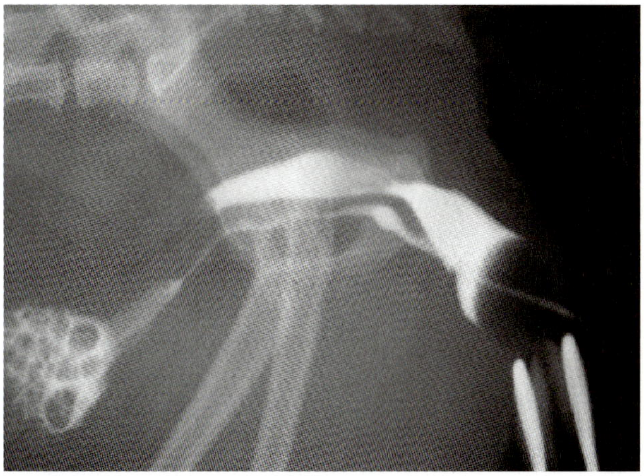

Figure 31.4 Contrast vaginourethrogram showing the relevant anatomy in the female dog.

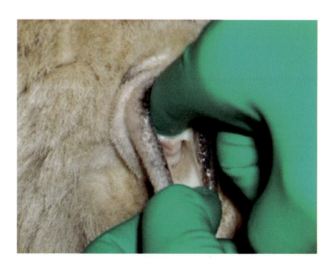

Figure 31.5 The clitoris is in a blind ending pouch, which must be avoided when inserting the finger into the vestibule.

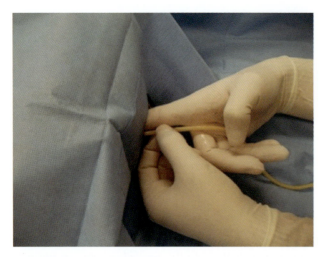

Figure 31.6 Digital technique for inserting urinary catheter in a female dog. Note the angle of the right index finger to help direct the catheter ventrally. The left hand holds the catheter very close to the vulva and makes advancing motions to push the catheter forward. No stylet in needed with this technique.

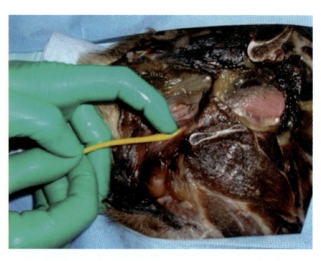

Figure 31.8 Cadaver preparation of sagittal section of female dog. The catheter has just contacted the urethral papilla and the finger is being flexed to help advance the catheter. (See text for description of this technique.)

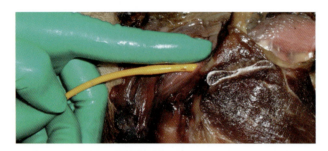

Figure 31.7 Cadaver preparation of sagittal section of female dog. The urethral papilla is seen just cranial to the tip of the catheter. Note that the guiding finger is not pressing down on the urethral papilla. To do so is likely to close off the papilla and prevent the catheter from entering.

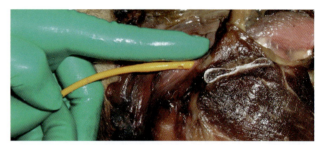

Figure 31.9 Cadaver preparation of sagittal section of female dog. The catheter has now entered the urethral papilla and can be advanced into the bladder.

is properly aligned and moved forward exactly along the ventral midline.

Placing the catheter with digital technique

Once you have familiarized yourself with the anatomy, withdraw the palpating hand and use that hand to grasp the catheter near the tip. Use the other hand to keep the length of the catheter aligned along the midline. With the palpating hand, reenter the vestibule as before, taking the catheter tip along (see Fig. 31.6). Use the palpating finger to guide and the other hand to push the catheter. Make sure not to twist or turn the hand as you maneuver the catheter in. Position the catheter tip in the vestibule caudal to the perceived location of the urethral papilla and exactly on the midline. Place the palpating finger back into position over the papilla (but not compressing

it), and check the position of the finger and catheter to assure all is aligned along the midline. Use the nonpalpating hand to keep that portion of the catheter protruding from the vulva lined up along the midline. It is better if the catheter enters between the dorsal, not the ventral aspect of the labia of the vulva because this will help direct the catheter ventrally. Let the tip of the palpating finger hover over the urethral papilla, and gently advance the catheter using the other hand (see Fig. 31.7). When you think the catheter tip is near to engaging the slit of tissue that is the urethral papilla, flex the palpating finger, press very gently down on the catheter just behind the tip, and extend the finger to push the catheter tip cranially under the slit of tissue (see Fig. 31.8). Attempt to move the catheter only a few millimeters at a time. Think of sliding a piece of cooked spaghetti along the top of a wet surface. The idea is to get the catheter tip to engage the slit of tissue that is the papilla instead of moving over it (see Fig. 31.9). Be sure the palpating finger is not pressing down on the urethral papilla because that pressure will close the opening. Other operators insert the palpating finger firmly into the vestibulovaginal junction to close it off and prevent the catheter from entering it. They use the other hand to advance the catheter and let the catheter tip engage the papilla on its own.

The catheter tip will either slip into the urethral papilla and ideally enter the urethra or slide over the top of it and move cranially toward the vestibulovaginal junction. With experience, you will be able to discern the friction as the catheter passes through the urethra compared with the relatively free passage if it slips over the papilla and moves forward in the vestibule. If it seems the catheter has entered the papilla, continue to advance it in small increments until the tip of the catheter has reached the premeasured distance to the bladder or until there is good urine flow.

Verify catheter placement

If urine is not obtained (and the bladder is known to contain urine), palpate along the length of the catheter in the vestibule from caudal to cranial to determine its location. If the catheter has entered the urethra, you will feel the catheter disappear into a hole on the ventral surface of the vestibule, and no catheter will be palpable cranial to the hole. If the catheter has passed over the papilla, you will be able to palpate it going through the vestibulovaginal junction or curling up in the vestibule. If the catheter needs to be repositioned, pay particular attention to meticulous technique in aligning the entire catheter along the midline and keeping it on the midline as you advance it. Be sure to withdraw it sufficiently caudally to ensure that the urethral papilla has not already been passed before the catheter is advanced again. If you are not sure of the location of the papilla, just advance the catheter on the midline in small increments. If the catheter is correctly oriented, it is likely to engage the urethral papilla on its own.

If you think the catheter tip is in the bladder, but no urine is flowing, attach a sterile syringe to the catheter and gently aspirate for urine or infuse sterile saline and aspirate. If injected fluid comes back around the vulva, the catheter tip is likely in the vestibule and must be repositioned. One can also place an ultrasound probe over the bladder and either see the tip of the catheter in the bladder or see the flow of fluid as it is flushed through the catheter.

Speculum or otoscope cone technique

Preparation is as described for the digital technique except the vestibule is not filled with sterile anesthetic lubricant because that would obscure visualization. Lubricate the device and the catheter before insertion.

Positioning

Sedation is frequently required for this technique. The patient may be positioned in lateral or sternal recumbency. Some operators place the patient sternally and drape the pelvic limbs over the end of a table.

Speculum

A separate light source is needed, preferably a headset. The correct orientation for a speculum is with the handles pointing up (toward the spine), not down. This allows an assistant to grasp the handles once the speculum has been inserted into the vestibule with the assistant's hand out of the way of the operator.

Otoscope cone

Attach the cone to the otoscope handle in the usual way, and use the handle to manipulate the cone into the vestibule. Visualize the urethral papilla, pass the catheter through the cone, and advance it into the urethral papilla. Once the catheter is placed into the bladder and the cone removed from the handle, the cone is left on the portion of the catheter outside the body because the attachment end of the catheter will not fit through the cone. Although this may look a little odd, it does not cause problems, and the cone is retrieved when the catheter is removed.

Placing the catheter

Insert the speculum (in closed position) or otoscope cone between the labia of the vulva, directing it first vertically to avoid the clitoris and then horizontally to enter the vestibule. If using a speculum, open the blades and have an assistant hold it in position. Look through the device and locate the urethral papilla as a slit of tissue on the ventral floor of the vestibule slightly caudal to the vestibulovaginal junction. Because you will not be able to touch the catheter tip to guide it into the papilla, a stylet will be required unless you are using a catheter made of stiff material, such as polypropylene.

Insert the catheter between the blades of the speculum or through the otoscope cone and advance it into the urethral papilla and into the bladder. If you cannot see the papilla, you may still be able to place the catheter by gently advancing the catheter tip into the mucosal tissue in the area where the papilla should be located, in other words, by using the tip of the catheter as a probe to identify the papilla. When the catheter tip is positioned in the bladder, inflate the balloon if there is one, and gently withdraw the catheter to seat the balloon at the neck of the bladder. Withdraw the device. If using an otoscope, disconnect the cone from the handle and leave the cone on the catheter outside the body.

Female cat or small female dog

If the patient is too small to allow digital palpation of the urethral papilla, the catheter can nonetheless usually be placed successfully.

Anatomy

The relevant anatomy for cats is as described for female dogs, except the urethra opens to the floor of the vestibule in a groove that actually facilitates catheterization.

Positioning

Sedation is usually required in female cats. Position the patient in lateral recumbency. For cats, some operators prefer dorsal recumbency with the pelvic limbs drawn cranially to expose the vulva. However, this position tends to decrease the opening of the vulva and can make it more difficult to insert the catheter into the vestibule.

Placing the catheter

Follow the preceding instructions for preparation for insertion. Then gently separate the labia of the vulva and pass the catheter between the most dorsal aspects of the labia, directing it to the ventral midline aiming toward the bladder (see Fig. 31.10). Even in small patients, the operator can usually insert at least the tip of the finger

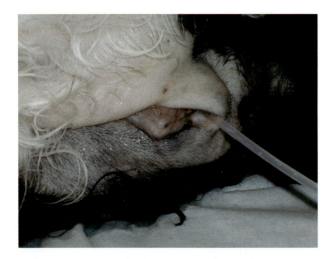

Figure 31.10 Urinary catheter placed by blind (without internal palpation) technique. Note that the catheter is entering between the dorsal aspect of the vulva to facilitate directing it ventrally to engage the urethral papilla.

between the labia to help direct the catheter ventrally. The urethral papilla is very close to the vulva, and most missed insertions occur because the catheter tip has already passed the urethral opening before it is properly positioned on the ventral midline. The operator can usually feel the slight resistance as the catheter tip enters the urethra. Advance the catheter into the bladder.

Verify catheter placement

If you think the catheter tip is in the bladder but no urine is flowing, attach a sterile syringe to the catheter and gently aspirate for urine or infuse sterile saline and aspirate. If injected fluid comes back around the vulva, the catheter tip is likely in the vestibule and must be repositioned. You can also place an ultrasound probe over the bladder and either see the tip of the catheter in the bladder or see the flow of fluid within the bladder as it is flushed through the catheter.

Male cat

Many male cats in need of a urinary catheter have urethral obstruction caused by some form of feline lower urinary tract disease. Sometimes the obstructing material is at the distal tip of the penis and can be relieved by gently massaging the most distal part of the penis to dislodge obstructing substances. If successful, this will result in immediate urine flow because of increased pressure from the overdistended bladder.

Anatomy

The prepuce is a short haired sheath facing caudally and covering the nonerect penis. When the penis is extruded sufficiently, the reflection of the prepuce off the surface of the penis about 1–1.5 cm from the tip can be seen.

The penis is directed caudo-ventrally and covered by the prepuce. Penile barbs are visible near the tip of the penis in the noncastrated male.

In its course from the bladder to the tip of the penis, the urethra has a marked sigmoid flexure near the penis. To pass a catheter up the urethra, the penis must be drawn caudally to straighten out the urethra.

Positioning

Sedation is usually required. Position the patient in lateral or dorsal recumbency. In dorsal recumbency, the pelvic limbs can be drawn cranially to expose the prepuce.

The goal is to extrude the penis caudally and horizontally out of the prepuce and keep it in this position as the catheter is passed. To extrude the penis, gently grasp the prepuce with thumb and finger and press gently onto the ischial arch to provide a firm base for the procedure and to align the penis parallel to the spine. If the penis is extruded facing in a ventral direction, it will be difficult to pass the catheter. Then gently move the prepuce cranially to expose the penis. The penis should now be extruded far enough to see the reflection of the prepuce off its surface about 1–1.5 cm from the tip. Hold all structures in a horizontal straight line with the tip of the penis facing caudally, not ventrally. The operator can digitally grasp the penis near the reflection of the prepuce to stabilize it or can use an instrument to grasp the preputial tissue (not the penile tissue) at the site of its reflection off the penis. Insert the lubricated catheter into the tip of the penis, and gently advance into the bladder without losing control of the extruded penis. As the catheter is moved cranially, put traction on the penis in a caudal direction to straighten out the flexure in the urethra. Otherwise, the catheter might not advance into the bladder. Once the catheter is positioned properly in the bladder, let the penis withdraw into its normal position within the prepuce.

Male dog

Anatomy

The prepuce is the tubular sheath of integument covering the nonerect penis. The penis in nonerection is entirely withdrawn into the prepuce. Within the penis, the os penis bone surrounds the dorsal surface of the urethra. The distal end of the os penis has a fibrocartilaginous projection that is slightly curved ventrally.

Positioning

With the male dog in left lateral recumbency the assistant stands at the patient's spine with the patient's head on the assistant's left, reaches over the abdomen, presses the left hand against the body wall at the place where the prepuce reflects from the ventral body wall, and exerts pressure caudally. With the right hand, the assistant grasps the os penis through the prepuce at the most proximal aspect (meaning away from the tip) of the os penis and pushes the penis out of the prepuce while moving the left hand more caudally to stabilize it and keep the penis as parallel to the spine as possible. The penis must now be held in this position and not allowed to withdraw into the prepuce while the catheter is being placed. Gently wipe the tip of the penis with 0.05% chlorhexidine solution.

Placing the catheter

Gently insert the catheter tip into the fibrocartilaginous projection of the os penis and then direct it ventrally to enter the urethra. Advance the catheter into the bladder.

Orienting the catheter in a direction parallel to the body wall and slightly ventrally once the fibrocartilaginous tip has been negotiated facilitates passage. The penis must remain exposed during catheter passage to assure that the catheter tip is entering the penis and to prevent contamination of the catheter. Resistance is usually felt as the catheter tip enters the os penis because it is narrow at this site and again as the catheter changes direction at the ischial arch and passes through the prostatic section of the urethra. Use the softest catheter possible to ease passage and minimize discomfort. Advance the catheter into the bladder.

Indwelling catheters

Securing the catheter and collection system

Once the catheter is properly placed, it must be secured if it is to remain indwelling. For Foley catheters with a balloon, the inflation port is imprinted with the amount of sterile water required. Fill a syringe with this amount and firmly attach it to the inflation port. Slowly inflate the balloon and gently withdraw the catheter to seat the balloon at the neck of the bladder. If the patient exhibits any discomfort during inflation, the balloon may be in the urethra. Deflate the balloon, reposition the catheter, and try again.

Catheters without an inflation balloon must be secured at the site where the catheter exits the body to keep the catheter tip in the bladder. To do this, first dry the catheter and apply adhesive tape butterfly on the catheter where it exits the vulva or prepuce. Catheters can easily slip through a tape butterfly unless the tape is kept closely adhered to the catheter surface so we recommend placing an encircling suture around the catheter. Insert the needle through the tape as close as possible to the catheter, draw some suture material through, and insert the needle up through the tape on the opposite side of the catheter. Tie the suture securely but do not occlude the catheter. To secure the adhesive butterfly to the patient, we recommend placing stay sutures in the patient and then suturing the adhesive butterfly to them.

All indwelling catheters must be attached to a sterile collection system. Cable ties are useful to provide extra security, especially between the catheter and the collection system. Secure a portion of the collection system tubing to the patient's leg, tail, or ventral abdomen (using tape or sutures) to prevent dislodging or discomfort caused by pulling on the catheter as the patient moves.

Management of indwelling urinary catheter and collection system

Make sure the personnel handling catheters and collection systems are properly trained and perform hand hygiene before and after handling the system. Inspect the system several times a day. Make sure all connections are secure. Use good nursing care to minimize contamination of the catheter and periurethral area from contact with soiled hospital surfaces, wound discharges, or feces. Maintain unobstructed flow, keep the catheter and collecting tubes from kinking, and keep the collecting bag lower than the bladder to prevent retrograde urine flow.

Catheter care

Perform catheter care every 8 hours or whenever the system is visibly soiled. Use surgical scrub followed by water rinse to clean any visible soiling on the exposed portion of the catheter, the collection system, or the patient's skin in the perivulvar or peripreputial area. Do not let scrub contact mucosal surfaces. Wipe the exposed portion of the catheter and the skin of the perivulvar or peripreputial area with 0.05% chlorhexidine solution. This solution can be that saved from the preparation

for catheter placement as described earlier. Flush the prepuce or vulva and vestibule five times with the 0.05% chlorhexidine solution.

Emptying or changing the urine collection bag

Wash hands and put on examination gloves. Use gowns and barriers as needed for aseptic technique or if public health considerations are present. For closed systems, drain the urine into a clean container. Do not let the drainage tube contact the container, and avoid splashing. Close the drainage tube.

For open systems assemble the needed materials to replace the bag and maintain sterility. Disconnect the full bag from the macrodrip and sterilely attach an empty sterile fluid bag.

Do not change indwelling catheters and drainage bags at fixed intervals but rather based on clinical indications such as infection, obstruction, or compromise of the closed collection system (see Protocol 31.5).

Protocol 31.5 Indwelling catheter maintenance

Items Required
- Water
- Gauze pads
- Surgical scrub
- Sterile syringe
- Examination gloves
- 0.05% chlorhexidine solution
- Sterile empty fluid bag for a collection system or sterile closed urinary collection bag (optional)

Procedure
1. Gather supplies.
2. Ensure that only properly trained caregivers perform the procedure.
3. Perform hand hygiene before and after handling the catheter or collection system.
4. Inspect the catheter and collection system several times a day.
5. Make sure the catheter and the collection system are properly secured.
6. Minimize contamination of the catheter, collection system, and periurethral area from contact with soiled hospital surfaces, wound discharges, or feces.
7. Maintain unobstructed flow; prevent kinking.
8. Keep collection bag lower than the patient to prevent retrograde flow of urine.
9. Perform catheter care every 8 hours or whenever the system is visibly soiled.
10. Perform hand hygiene and don clean examination gloves.
11. Use surgical scrub followed by water rinse to clean soiling on catheter, collection system, or the perivulvar or peripreputial area as needed.
12. Wipe the exposed portion of the catheter and the skin of the perivulvar or peripreputial area with gauze sponges soaked in 0.05% chlorhexidine solution.
13. Clean the perivulvar or peripreputial area with 0.05% chlorhexidine-soaked gauze sponges and flush the vulva and vestibule or prepuce with 0.05% chlorhexidine solution.
14. Empty or change the urine collection bag as needed.
15. Perform hand hygiene and don clean examination gloves.
16. For the closed system, open the urine drainage spout and drain the urine into a container. Avoid touching the container with the drainage tubing and avoid splashing. Close the urine drainage tube.
17. For the open system, disconnect the full bag from the macrodrip and sterilely attach an empty sterile fluid bag.

Retropulsion for urethral obstruction

Retropulsion is the process of expanding the urethra with fluid to flush an obstructing substance retrograde and deposit it back into the bladder. It is not desirable to use a catheter to force an obstructing substance retrograde because this may damage or even rupture the urethra. Retropulsion is most commonly needed in males and required uncommonly in females because their urethra is shorter and of larger diameter. The goal of retropulsion is to expand the diameter of the urethra with fluid to suspend the obstructing substance in a fluid column that will carry it back into the bladder. Be aware that the urethra can be ruptured by overly aggressive flushing technique or by overly aggressive attempts to advance the catheter against an obstruction.

We suggest the following steps.

1. The procedure can be painful. Provide pain control and sedation as indicated. The relaxation of the urethra that occurs during general anesthesia might be needed for difficult obstructions.
2. Evaluate bladder size to determine whether it would be safe to add more fluid. If not, perform cystocentesis before retropulsion. If performed correctly (small-gauge needle inserted as atraumatically as possible), cystocentesis even of a distended bladder is probably lower risk than adding fluid to an already pathologically distended bladder.
3. Fill a syringe (5- to 20-mL size) with sterile saline for flush.
4. Follow all the protocols as previously described to maintain sterility. Pass the catheter as far as possible up the urethra. If the catheter cannot be advanced far enough to seat it inside the urethra, try a smaller or stiffer catheter. Remember that in male cats the penis must be pulled caudally to straighten the sigmoid flexure in the urethra before the catheter can be passed. For male cats, an olive-tip catheter or a 22-gauge venous catheter (with the stylet removed) may be easier to place in the most distal urethra. Once the obstruction is relieved, a regular catheter can be placed indwelling.
5. Attach the syringe to the end of the catheter.
6. Occlude the tip of the penis around the catheter with digital pressure to prevent the flush from flowing back out.
7. Briskly inject flush while gently advancing the catheter. If the catheter can be advanced, continue to inject fluid until the catheter tip is in the bladder. Keep track of the amount of flush injected, do not overdistend the bladder, and decompress the bladder by cystocentesis if needed.

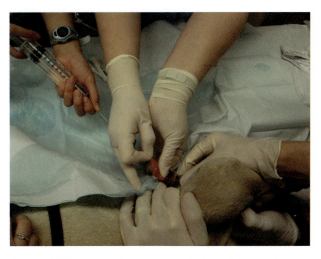

Figure 31.11 Retropulsion with occlusion of the urethra per rectum in a male dog.

For male dogs, a supplement to retropulsion as described earlier is to also occlude the urethra proximal to the obstruction (see Fig. 31.11). Follow steps 1–6. To occlude the urethra proximal to the obstruction, an assistant inserts a gloved finger into the rectum and occludes the urethra by pressing it down onto the pelvic floor. In a large dog, two fingers may be inserted to better trap the urethra against the pelvis. Briskly inject 5–20 mL of the flush, depending on the patient's size. The assistant occluding the urethra must be able to feel the urethra dilate. The assistant then abruptly releases the urethral occlusion as injection of flush continues and the operator attempts to advance the catheter.

If unsuccessful, and the patient is not already anesthetized, consider providing anesthesia before retrying the procedure (Protocol 31.6).

Unable to deflate the foley balloon

The correct method for deflating a Foley balloon is as follows. Attach a Luer slip syringe to the catheter valve. Allow the pressure in the balloon to force the saline into the syringe to deflate the balloon completely. Do not apply aspirating pressure at this time. If the balloon does not deflate, reseat the syringe gently and try again. If unsuccessful, reposition the patient; ensure there is no traction on the catheter, and then try again. If the balloon still does not deflate apply gentle, slow aspiration, remembering that the rapid or forceful aspiration can collapse the inflation tube and prevent balloon deflation. If the balloon cannot be deflated, cut the channel through which the balloon was inflated to allow fluid to egress, which will deflate the balloon.

Protocol 31.6 Retropulsion

Items Required
- See Protocol 31.1 for appropriate supplies
- Sterile flush solution
- Several sterile syringes (for flushes)
- Two assistants

Procedure
1. Gather necessary supplies.
2. Ensure that only properly trained caregivers perform the procedure and that sterility is maintained throughout.
3. Consider sedation or anesthesia if catheter placement has been difficult.
4. Evaluate bladder size. Perform decompressive cystocentesis if needed.
5. Assure that sufficient personnel are available to perform the various aspects of the procedure (catheter insertion by operator, flushing the catheter by assistant 1, in male dogs, digital occlusion of the proximal urethra per rectum (if needed) by assistant 2, and patient restraint).
6. Follow procedure for catheter insertion and advance the catheter gently until the obstruction is reached. For male cats, be sure the penis is always under traction in a caudal direction to straighten out the sigmoid flexure in the urethra.
7. Operator occludes tip of penis around the catheter to prevent backflow of flush.
8. Assistant 1 injects sterile flush briskly while operator gently attempts to advance the catheter.
9. For male dogs, occlusion of the urethra per rectum can be used.
   a. Assistant 2 inserts a gloved finger into the rectum and prepares to apply firm digital pressure on the proximal urethra to occlude it.
   b. Repeat step 5.
   c. Assistant 2 firmly occludes the urethra per rectum.
   d. Assistant 1 injects flush briskly and continues injecting.
   e. Assistant 2 feels the urethra dilate and abruptly releases the pressure while assistant 1 continues the flush and the operator attempts to advance the catheter.
10. If unsuccessful and the patient is not yet anesthetized, consider anesthesia before repeating the procedure.

References

1. Centers for Disease Control and Prevention. Guideline for prevention of catheter-associated urinary tract infections 2009. Washington, DC: Department of Health and Human Services; 2009.

2. Schumm K, Lam TBL. Types of urethral catheters for management of short-term voiding problems in hospitalized adults. Cochrane Database Syst Rev 2008;2:CD004013.

3. Nacey JN, Delahunt B, Tulloch AG. The assessment of catheter-induced urethritis using an experimental dog model. J Urol 1985;134(3):623–625.

4. Lawrence EL, Turner IG. Kink, flow and retention properties of urinary catheters part 1: conventional Foley catheters. J Mater Sci Mater Med 2006;17:147–152.

5. Stickler DJ. Bacterial biofilms in patients with indwelling urinary catheters. Nature Clin Pract Urol 2008;5:598–608.

6. Roberts JA, Kaack MB, Fussell EN. Adherence to urethral catheters by bacteria causing nosocomial infections. Urology 1993;41(4):338–342.

7. Lees GE, Osborne CA, Stevens JB, et al. Adverse effects caused by polypropylene and polyvinyl feline urinary catheters. Am J Vet Res 1980;41:1836–1840.

8. Sullivan LA, Campbell VL, Onuma SC. Evaluation of open versus closed urine collection systems and development of nosocomial bacteriuria in dogs. J Am Vet Med Assoc 2010;237(2):187–190.

9. Barrett M, Campbell VL. Aerobic bacterial culture of used intravenous fluid bags intended for use as urine collection reservoirs. J Am Anim Hosp Assoc 2008;44:2–4.

10. Lees GE, Osborne CA, Stevens JB, et al. Adverse effects of open indwelling urethral catheterization in clinically normal male cats. Am J Vet Res 1981;42:825–833.

11. Biertuempfel PH, Ling GV, Ling GA. Urinary tract infection resulting from catheterization in healthy adult dogs. J Am Vet Med Assoc 1981;178(9):989–991.

12. Barsanti JA, Blue J. Edmunds J. Urinary tract infection due to indwelling bladder catheters in dogs and cats. J Am Vet Med Assoc 1985;187(4):384–388.

13. Lippert AC, Fulton RB, Parr AM. Nosocomial infection surveillance in a small animal intensive care unit. J Am Anim Hosp Assoc 1988;24:627–636.

14. Smarick SD, Haskins SC, Aldrich J, et al. Incidence of catheter-associated urinary tract infection among dogs in a small animal intensive care unit. J Am Vet Med Assoc 2004;224:1936–1940.

15. Ogeer-Gyles J, Mathews K, Weese JS, et al. Evaluation of catheter-associated urinary tract infections and multi-drug-resistant *Escherichia coli* isolates from the urine of dogs with indwelling urinary catheters. J Am Vet Med Assoc 2006;229(10):1584–1590.

16. Bubenik LJ, Hosgood GL, Waldron DR, et al. Frequency of urinary tract infection in catheterized dogs and comparison of bacterial culture and susceptibility testing results for catheterized and noncatheterized dogs with urinary tract infections. J Am Vet Med Assoc 2007;231:893–899.

17. Bubenik L, Hosgood G. Urinary tract infection in dogs with thoracolumbar intervertebral disc herniation and urinary bladder dysfunction managed by manual expression, indwelling catheterization or intermittent catheterization. Vet Surg 2008;37:791–800.

18. Smith JM. Indwelling catheter management: from habit-based to evidence-based practice. Ostomy Wound Manage 2003;49(12):34–45.

32

Urinalysis in acutely and critically ill dogs and cats

David J. Polzin and Carl A. Osborne

Value of urinalysis

Urinalysis is a useful, cost-effective, and typically noninvasive means of evaluating the cause and status of various syndromes affecting the urinary system and other body systems. The primary indications for routine urinalysis are as an aid in the search for diagnosis of various diseases, to screen patients for asymptomatic diseases, to monitor the biologic behavior of diseases (i.e., reversible versus irreversible and progressive versus nonprogressive), and to monitor the safety and efficacy of various therapies. It is also important to recall that serum creatinine and urea nitrogen concentrations should generally be interpreted in light of a concurrently determined urine specific gravity (SG) value (obtained before initiating fluid or diuretic therapy).

For patients in which urinary disease is suspected, a complete urinalysis can help verify or eliminate rule-outs, including primary kidney disease (acute or chronic), impaired urine concentrating ability, bacterial urinary tract infection, renal tubular acidosis, Fanconi syndrome, cystinuria, urinary tract neoplasia, urolithiasis, and idiopathic cystitis.

In patients with nonurinary disorders, detection of abnormal findings by urinalysis may indicate the systems or organs affected and dictate the need for further evaluation. Urinalysis findings that may be associated with nonurinary diseases include diabetes mellitus, central diabetes insipidus, hepatic failure, severe hemolytic disease, and systemic acidosis.

Serial urinalyses can be used to monitor patient response to therapy, and to detect relapses or recurrences of various diseases. Urinalyses may also be used to monitor the safety of drugs. For example, evidence of gentamicin-induced nephrotoxicity may be obtained by serial evaluation of urine sediment for casts, monitoring urine SG for impaired tubular function, and watching for the onset of normoglycemic glucosuria. Also, serially collected urine samples may be monitored for increases in urine enzyme concentrations.

Basic urinalysis

What is a complete urinalysis?

A complete routine urinalysis consists of the evaluation of several physical and chemical properties of urine, estimation of its solute concentration, and microscopic examination of urine sediment. We recommend that all of these tests be performed because they aid in semiquantitation and localization of abnormal findings and in refinement of problems. For example, interpretation of the results of chemical tests and sediment examination is aided by knowledge of urine SG.

The value of light microscopic examination of urine sediment in the interpretation of urinalyses is comparable to light microscopic examination of blood smears in the interpretation of hemograms. Meaningful interpretation of physical (color and turbidity) and chemical (protein, occult blood, and pH) test results of routine urinalysis depends on knowledge of the composition of urine sediment. For example, a moderate degree of proteinuria in the absence of significant numbers of white cells and red blood cells usually indicates proteinuria due to glomerular disease. However, a moderate degree of proteinuria associated with pyuria and hematuria is

Advanced Monitoring and Procedures for Small Animal Emergency and Critical Care, First Edition. Edited by Jamie M. Burkitt Creedon, Harold Davis.
© 2012 John Wiley & Sons, Inc. Published 2012 by John Wiley & Sons, Inc.

Box 32.1 Necessary equipment for performing a urinalysis

Equipment:
   Centrifuge
   Refractometer
   Microscope
   Optional: Automated dipstick reader
Disposables:
   Vessels for collection of urine (clean, ideally sterile,
      opaque, and with tight-fitting lids to prevent
      evaporation)
   Urine dipsticks
   Conical centrifugation tubes
   Disposable pipettes
   Glass slides and coverslips
   Sediment stain (optional)
   System (e.g., forms) for reporting results

---

consistent with an inflammatory response located some-where along the urinary and/or genital tracts. Likewise, a moderate degree of proteinuria associated with hematuria is consistent with hemorrhage located somewhere along the urinary and/or genital tracts.

Laboratory equipment

Minimum equipment for urinalysis (Box 32.1) includes a centrifuge, a refractometer, and a microscope. An automated dipstick reader is optional. Disposables required include vessels for collection of urine (clean, ideally sterile, and with tight-fitting lids to prevent evaporation), urine dipsticks, conical centrifugations tubes, disposable pipettes, glass slides, and cover slips. Sediment stain is optional.

Sample handling

Urine should be collected and stored in an appropriate container (as just described) with a tightly closed lid. Evaporation of water, changes in pH, degradation of casts, formation of crystals, and other changes in physical properties may occur if urine is allowed to remain exposed to air and room temperature for extended periods of time.[1] In addition, urine dipsticks are designed to be used for urine at or near room temperature. As a consequence, urine samples should ideally be analyzed within 60 minutes of collection. If analysis cannot be completed within 30 minutes of collection, the sample should be held at 4°C and brought back to room temperature just before the analysis.

In most cases, urine is best collected by cystocentesis because this minimizes contamination of the sample from outside the urinary tract. Samples collected by cys-tocentesis may be contaminated by small amounts of blood during bladder puncture; thus this method of collection may be suboptimal for investigating patients with mild hematuria. Urine may also be collected by midstream voiding or by urinary catheterization. These samples are more likely to be associated with extra-urinary contamination from the genitalia or skin. Because the method of collection may influence the results of the urine sediment examination, the method of urine collection should always be reported on the urinalysis report.

The complaint for which the patient is being seen should be considered when selecting the method of urine collection. Collection of urine by catheterization may be imprudent when the patient has sustained trauma to the caudal portion of the body, and cystocentesis may be problematic in patients suspected of having a coagulopathy.

Useful test methods and how to perform them

Urinalysis consists of four components: (1) determination of color and turbidity by visual inspection, (2) chemical analysis using multitest dipsticks, (3) measurement of urine SG by refractometry, and (4) microscopic examination of the urine sediment.[1] All four components should always be performed to maximize the value of urinalysis.

Urine chemistries are most often performed using reagent strips (dipsticks). Normally, the reagent strip is immersed in well-mixed urine before it is centrifuged and rapidly withdrawn. The strip is then tapped against the side of the vessel to remove excess urine. The dipstick should then be oriented parallel to the table surface (horizontally) to avoid contamination of fluid and reagents between different test pads on the strip. Color changes on the reagent strip should be compared with the manufacturer's provided color scale at the proper time interval following immersion in urine.

Tests commonly included on reagent dipsticks include urine pH, glucose, ketones, bilirubin, occult blood, protein, urobilinogen, nitrites, leukocyte esterase, and SG. Dipstick tests for nitrituria, leukocyte esterase, and SG are inaccurate in dogs and cats and should not be used; urobilinogen is a poor test and should be ignored.[1] The nitrituria strip, designed to detect bacteriuria in humans, does not consistently detect bacteriuria in dogs and cats. The leukocyte esterase strip, designed to detect pyuria, is specific but insensitive for pyuria in dogs. However, preliminary studies suggest that in dogs a positive leukocyte esterase test predicts a positive urine culture.[1] In cats, the leukocyte esterase test is usually positive and of no diagnostic value. SG test pads have been found to be unreliable in dogs and cats and only measure SG values up to about 1.025 to 1.030, which is inadequate for assessing adequate urine-concentrating ability in dogs and cats.[1]

Urine PH

Reagent strips detect urine pH in the range of 5 to 8.5 visually and 5 to 9 instrumentally. However, the reliability of this test has been challenged, particularly when the urine pH is close to neutral. Reagent strips reportedly may overestimate urine pH in dogs and may yield an alkaline pH in urine that is slightly acid.[3] When accurate urine pH measurement is important, a pH meter should be used. Relatively inexpensive handheld instruments are available. Accurate urine pH is important in diagnosing and managing urolithiasis and renal acidification disorders (e.g., renal tubular acidosis). Although urine pH may provide a crude index of body acid-base balance, it should not be used in lieu of blood gas analysis when acid-base abnormalities are suspected.

Urine glucose

Canine and feline urine are normally negative for glucose as measured by glucosuria reagent strips. A positive test for glucosuria may result from hyperglycemia, acute stress (primarily cats), or renal glucosuria. Determining the blood glucose concentration usually identifies the cause. Persistent or marked hyperglycemia and glucosuria are consistent with diabetes mellitus, whereas persistent glucosuria absent hyperglycemia confirms renal glucosuria, a form of renal tubular disease. Renal glucosuria may occur either as a congenital defect or with renal tubular injury as in toxic or ischemic acute kidney injury (AKI). Some cats exhibit transient mild glucosuria associated with stress. Blood glucose concentrations in these cats may be normal to moderately elevated. Because serum fructosamine concentration reflects blood glucose concentrations over an extended period of time, it may be used to differentiate stress-associated glucosuria from diabetes mellitus.

The "transport maximum" or threshold for glucosuria in normal dogs is about 170 to 180 mg/dL; cats have a higher transport maximum of about 260 to 310 mg/dL. As a consequence, mild hyperglycemia may occur without glucosuria.[1] Refrigerated urine samples should be brought to room temperature before testing for glucosuria or false-negative results may occur.

Urine ketones

Ketonuria is always considered abnormal in dogs and cats. Most often, ketonuria occurs concurrently with glucosuria and is associated with diabetic ketoacidosis.

Ketonuria absent glucosuria most likely results from excess lipid catabolism (lipolysis), typically in fasting or anorectic patients.

Reagent strips for ketonuria only detect acetoacetate and acetone but not β-hydroxybutyrate. As a consequence, under certain circumstances, such as concurrent lactic acidosis, patients with ketoacidosis may test negative for ketones using the reagent strip. If this condition is suspected, adding a few drops of hydrogen peroxide to a urine specimen facilitates nonenzymatic conversion of β-hydroxybutyrate to acetoacetate that can be detected.[4]

Urine bilirubin

Bilirubin reagent pads may be unreliable as screening tests in dogs because of a high percentage of false-positive and false-negative results in this species. This is true because, in addition to simple glomerular filtration, the canine kidney produces bilirubin and causes it to appear in urine. In contrast, positive bilirubin test results in cats are usually indicative of underlying disease. The sensitivity of bilirubinuria as an indicator of diseases associated with icterus in cats results in part from the fact that the feline renal threshold for bilirubin is nine times higher than in dogs.[5] Thus, in cats, detection of bilirubinuria by routine urinalysis may precede clinical recognition of jaundice. Nonetheless, lack of bilirubinuria does not exclude disorders associated with bilirubin metabolism in either species, so positive or negative urine bilirubin test results should be evaluated in conjunction with other clinical findings.

In dogs, urine SG may be helpful in interpreting the clinical importance of bilirubinuria. A low concentration of bilirubin in highly concentrated urine with a high urine SG (e.g., 2+ bilirubin with a urine concentration of 1.045) is less likely to be of clinical significance than a low concentration of bilirubin in less concentrated urine with a lower urine SG (e.g., 1+ bilirubin with a urine SG of 1.015).

Urine occult blood

The reagent pad for occult blood is highly sensitive and reacts to hemoglobin, myoglobin, and, to a lesser degree, red blood cells. Interpretation of a positive occult blood test requires examination of the urine sediment for evidence of red blood cells. If red blood cells or ghost cells are present in the urine sediment, then hematuria is present. Very dilute or alkaline urine may promote red blood cell lysis, and the lysed cells may be difficult to find. Absent red blood cells, a positive test may indicate the presence of either myoglobin or hemoglobin. If the patient's plasma has a pink or red discoloration, hemoglobinuria should be suspected. The plasma becomes pink because free hemoglobin in plasma binds to haptoglobin until haptoglobin is fully saturated; only unbound hemoglobin enters the glomerular filtrate and final urine. However, myoglobin is freely filtered by the glomerulus and does not remain in the plasma in sufficient quantity to color the plasma. Thus colorless plasma suggests myoglobin.

The most common cause for a positive occult blood test is hematuria (discussed in the urine sediment section). Hemoglobinuria suggests hemolytic anemia, whereas myoglobinuria suggests rhabdomyolysis or myositis. If apparent hemoglobinuria persists with no evidence of hemolytic anemia, it should be pursued as hematuria.[2]

Urine protein

Proteinuria reagent strips are quite sensitive for detecting proteins in urine, particularly albumin. They are used to screen for pathologic proteinuria of any origin; however, small amounts of protein in urine are considered normal. Proteinuria is an important sign of kidney disease in dogs and cats; however, urinary tract hemorrhage and inflammation at any point along the urinary tract may also be associated with proteinuria. Results of the urine sediment are useful in differentiating these conditions. In patients with pyuria, it is necessary to first eliminate pyuria (e.g., antibiotics for urinary tract infection [UTI]) and then reevaluate the patient for proteinuria. It usually requires grossly visible hematuria to cause even a small increase in proteinuria.

Urine reagent strips provide a semiquantitative estimate of the magnitude of proteinuria. It is difficult to extrapolate the clinical implications of a positive proteinuria dipstick from just the dipstick reaction and urine SG. To confirm the clinical importance of a positive protein dipstick obtained on a patient without pyuria, hematuria, or bacteria, it is necessary to measure the urine protein-to-creatinine ratio (UPC; see later). The UPC should probably be performed on dogs with 1+ or greater proteinuria (especially when the urine SG is 1.012 or lower).[6] Proteinuria of any magnitude should prompt consideration of performing the UPC in cats.

Depending on the magnitude of proteinuria (based on the UPC), pathological proteinuria may result from renal tubular or interstitial disorders (mild proteinuria; UPC values less than about 2.5) or glomerular diseases (potentially any magnitude of proteinuria but especially when UPC exceeds about 2.5). Moderate to marked increases in proteinuria are consistent with protein-losing nephropathies that may be associated with the nephrotic syndrome.

Urine sediment examination

Handling of urine and preparation of slides

The urine sediment should be examined (Protocol 32.1) as quickly as possible after collection of urine. The ability to recognize casts, crystals, and cellular components may degrade with extended storage of the urine sample. Casts, cells, and oxalate crystals may be of great significance in identifying disease processes commonly seen in emergency and critical care patients.

Protocol 32.1 Procedure for urine sediment examination

Items Required
- Centrifuge
- Microscope
- Vessels for collection of urine (clean, ideally sterile, opaque and with tight-fitting lids to prevent evaporation)
- Conical centrifugation tubes
- Disposable pipettes
- Glass slides and cover slips
- Sediment stain (optional)

Procedure
1. Collect urine specimen in an appropriate container.
2. Mark the container with appropriate identification.
3. If analysis cannot be performed within 30 minutes, refrigerate the sample.
4. Thoroughly mix specimen; then transfer a standard amount (we use 5 mL) to a conical tip centrifuge tube.
5. Centrifuge the sample for 3 to 5 minutes at 450 g (1500 to 2000 rpm)
6. Remove supernatant using a transfer pipette or decanting, and save for chemical analysis. Allow a standard amount (about 1/2 mL) to remain in the conical tip centrifuge tube.
7. Thoroughly resuspend the urine sediment in the remaining urine supernatant by agitation or "finger-flipping" of the tube.
8. Transfer a drop of reconstituted sediment to a microscope with a transfer pipette, and place a coverslip over it.
9. Subdue the intensity of the microscope light by lowering the condenser and closing the iris diaphragm.
10. Systematically examine the entire specimen under the coverslip with the low power objective, assessing the quantity and type (casts, cells, crystals, etc.) of sediment.
11. Examine the sediment with the high power objective to identify the morphology of the elements and to detect bacteria.
12. Record the results.

The urine sample should be thoroughly mixed, then examined for color and turbidity. Before centrifugation of the sample, the reagent dipstick should be immersed in the well-mixed urine (see later) and the urine SG measured.

A pellet of sediment is then prepared by centrifuging 3 to 5 mL of urine at 1500 to 2000 rpm for 5 minutes[2] Accurate interpretation of the urine sediment is greatly influenced by the urine volume, speed, and time of centrifugation because these factors will affect the numbers of solid particles that appear in the urine sediment (the quantity of urine used should be reported if the volume centrifuged was less than 3 mL). If the urine was visibly hemorrhagic or very turbid prior to centrifugation, the dipstick examination should be repeated on the centrifuged sample. Most of the supernatant may be decanted off leaving approximately 0.5 mL in the centrifugation tube.

The sediment is then resuspended in the remaining supernatant. A drop of this fluid is then placed on a slide and covered with a cover slip. After dimming the light intensity of the microscope, the sediment should be examined under low power (10×) for casts, crystals, and cells. Identification of cell types and detection of bacteriuria is performed under high power (40×). The number of red and white blood cells should be counted and reported as the number per high power field (hpf). The number of bacteria observed under high power field is semiquantitatively reported as trace, moderate, or many.

Although many clinical pathologists and laboratory technicians prefer to examine urine sediment unstained, less experienced viewers may find examination of stained preparations more interpretable. Urine sediment stains that may be mixed with the urine sediment resuspension before applying a drop of the mixture to a slide are available commercially. Although stains seemingly facilitate visualization of the sediment, they may dilute the material on the slide, vary in stain quality, contaminate the slide, or add stain precipitate that may be confused with bacteria.[2] As a consequence, it is prudent to also examine unstained slides if stained urine sediment slides are to be used. A recent study reported that air-dried modified Wright-stained preparations of urine sediment improved sensitivity, specificity, and positive predictive value for detecting bacteriuria.[7]

Specific findings

Cells

Low numbers of erythrocytes (less than 5/hpf) may be seen in normal urine; slightly higher numbers may be seen in samples obtained by cystocentesis due to iatrogenic hemorrhage. Increased numbers indicate

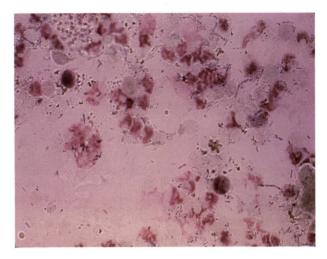

Figure 32.1 Bacteria and degenerating white blood cells (×250) (Gram stain).

hemorrhage from anywhere in the urinary tract upstream from the urine collection site. Important rule-outs for hematuria include uroliths, trauma, neoplasia, hemorrhagic diathesis, infectious or noninfectious inflammation, and, in cats, idiopathic cystitis. Less common causes may include renal cysts or infarcts, urinary parasites, strenuous exercise, and glomerular disease. Urine may also become contaminated with blood arising from the prostate in males or estrus in females. Blood originating from the prostate may reflux into the bladder, thus being present even in urine obtained by cystocentesis.

Leukocytes also may be found in low numbers (less than 3/hpf) in normal urine. Increased numbers of white blood cells (pyuria) indicate inflammation, most frequently due to urinary tract infection (see Fig. 32.1). Therefore, finding pyuria indicates the need for urine culture. Urinary calculi and neoplasia may also cause pyuria. Preputial or vaginal secretions may contaminate samples not obtained by cystocentesis. Absence of pyuria does not eliminate the possibility of urinary tract infection.

Small numbers of epithelial cells may be seen in normal urine. Cells may be transitional cells, squamous epithelial cells, or, rarely, renal tubular cells. High numbers of any type of epithelial cells or atypical epithelial cells are abnormal and indicate the need to evaluate the patient for possible urinary tract neoplasia.

Organisms

It is abnormal to observe any organisms (bacteria or fungal organisms) in urine samples obtained by cystocentesis (see Fig. 32.1). However, small numbers of organisms may be observed in samples collected from unclean surfaces (e.g., floor, tabletop, or litter box), particularly if the urine is allowed to sit at room temperature for an extended period. In addition, debris or stain sediment may be erroneously mistaken for bacteria. Greater than 10^4 rods/mL or 10^5 cocci/mL must be present before they can be readily identified in the urine sediment; therefore, absence of bacteriuria on the urinalysis does not rule out bacterial infection.[2] A urine culture obtained by cystocentesis is the gold standard for confirming the presence or absence of UTI and should be considered for all patients suspected of having a UTI.

Casts

Casts are cylinder-shaped structures that form in the lumens of the renal tubules. The presence of increased numbers of casts is called cylindruria. Up to two hyaline or granular casts per low power field in moderately concentrated urine (urine SG values greater than 1.025)

may be normal in otherwise normal dogs and cats.[2] When present in increased numbers, casts provide evidence supporting a diagnosis of kidney disease, although they are only sporadically observed. They are often shed in "showers" and thus may be present in one urine sample yet absent in a subsequent sample. Examination of fresh urine is most likely to yield casts because they tend to degenerate the longer urine is stored before examination. Vigorous shaking of the urine sample may also promote disruption of casts. Casts may be less visible in alkaline urine.

Casts are classified as cellular, granular, waxy, or hyaline (see Fig. 32.2a–d) Cellular casts may include renal tubular, red blood cells, or white blood cells and indicate epithelial injury, hemorrhage, or inflammation, respectively, occurring within the kidneys and particularly within the renal tubules. Granular casts are composed of degenerating cells, proteins, and other

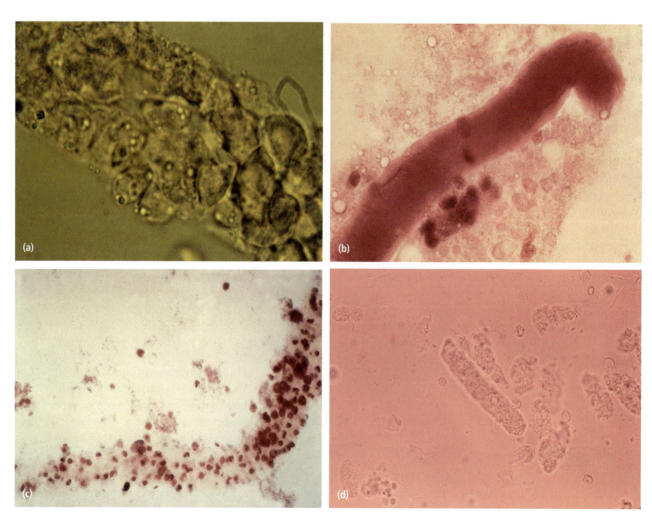

Figure 32.2 (a) Cellular cast (×250) (unstained); (b) hyaline cast (×104) (Sedi-Stain); (c) white cell cast (×104) (Sedi-Stain); (d) granular cast and various cells (×160) (unstained).

substances and indicate renal tubular epithelial injury and necrosis. Granular casts may degenerate over time into waxy casts. Hyaline casts are observed with proteinuria or diuresis.

Crystals

A variety of crystals may be found in urine. The more common types include calcium oxalate, struvite, ammonium urate, and cysteine. Fresh urine should be used when investigating crystalluria; evaporation, cooling, and changes in pH may influence crystal formation when samples are not fresh. Crystalluria does not indicate the presence of uroliths; however, it may indicate that conditions suitable for the formation of uroliths exist in the patient. Although the crystal type often predicts the composition of uroliths that are present, the crystal type alone may not accurately predict the chemical composition of uroliths if conditions (e.g., diet, drugs) have changed since formation of the uroliths.

When crystals are present, it is important to attempt to identify the chemical composition of the crystals. The morphology of the crystals is useful in determining crystal composition (see Fig. 32.3a–f). Further, crystal composition may suggest possible diagnoses. For example, the presence of calcium oxalate crystals in animals with AKI suggests ethylene glycol intoxication. The presence of ammonium urate crystals in breeds other than Dalmatians prompts consideration of hepatic failure. The presence of cystine crystals confirms the presence of the renal tubular defect cystinuria. The presence of struvite crystals may be an incidental finding.

Neoplastic cells

Neoplastic cells may occasionally be suspected by urinalysis. When neoplastic cells are suspected, a large volume of urine should be collected, immediately centrifuged, and a slide prepared from the resulting sediment. The slide should be allowed to dry and then stained with new methylene blue or Wright-Giemsa. However, cytologic findings of such preparations should be interpreted with caution because urine itself, inflammation associated with UTI, and radiographic contrast material may all induce changes in cell morphology that may mimic neoplastic change.

Evaluation of urine concentration

Specific gravity

Although SG does not directly measure the concentration of urine, so to speak, it does reflect the relative relationship between solute and water in urine. The SG of a solution is the density of the solution. The density of a substance is the ratio of its mass (weight) to its volume. Density of urine reflects the total mass of all solutes per unit volume of solution. Stated in another way, urine SG is the ratio of the density (or weight) of urine to the density (or weight) of an equal volume of distilled water, both measured at the same temperature.

The SG of water is 1.000 under conditions of standard temperature and pressure. If the density of urine were equal to the density of water, the SG value would be 1. However, it is physiologically impossible for the kidneys to excrete pure water. Urine is denser than water because it is composed of water and various solutes of different densities. Therefore, urine always has an SG greater than 1.

Because SG is a measurement of density, it is affected by the number of solute particles present; however, it is also affected by the molecular weight of each solute present. Therefore, there is only an approximate relationship between SG and total solute concentration. Thus, two dogs with the same SG may have different osmolalities (see later) if the solutes in their urine differ.

Each type of solute has its own characteristic effect on the SG of urine. Urine samples having equivalent numbers of solute molecules per unit volume may have different SG values if different mixtures of solutes are present. For example, equal numbers of molecules of sodium chloride, albumin, and glucose all have a different quantitative effect on SG. Looking at this illustration in a slightly different context, addition of either of (1) 0.147 g of sodium chloride, (2) 0.27 g of glucose, and (3) 0.4 g of albumin to 100 mL of urine will increase urine SG by 0.001.

Methods/equipment

Refractometry is the preferred method for measuring urine SG. Small handheld refractometers calibrated to determine urine SG are commonly used. The basic components of clinical laboratory refractometers consist of a prism, a liquid compensator, and a chamber cover designed to direct a specific wave length of light (usually 589 nm) onto a calibrated scale.

High-quality refractometers typically provide reproducible results. They have an adjustable scale and contain a built-in mechanism for temperature correction (from 60°F to 100°F). However, many refractometers acquire an increasing error with increasing amounts of solids. Ideally, refractometers should be calibrated by the manufacturer for the species being studied by using urine samples of known SG. Therefore, dog and cat urine

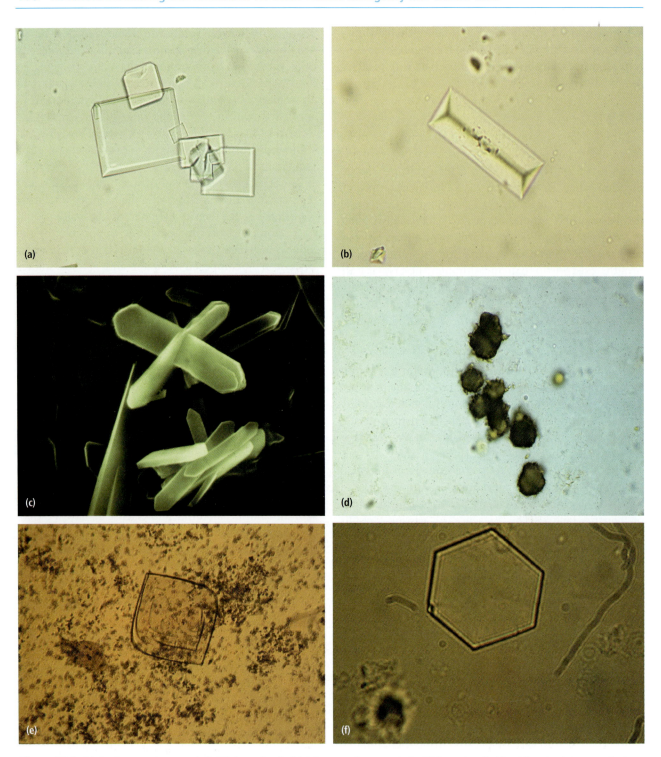

Figure 32.3 (a) Canine struvite crystals (×40) (unstained); (b) feline struvite crystals (×40) (unstained); (c) calcium oxalate monohydrate (×40) (unstained); (d) "Thorn-apple" ammonium urate crystals (×40) (unstained); (e) uric acid and amorphous urate crystals (×25) (unstained); (f) cystine crystals (×250) (unstained).

require different scales. Those designed for physicians are calibrated for human urine. If a refractometer designed for use in humans is used for cat urine, the measured SG will be falsely elevated. This error becomes more pronounced as urine becomes more concentrated.[8]

Urine dipsticks commonly include a pad for measuring urine SG. However, the dipstick method is an unreliable method for measuring urine SG in dogs and cats and should not be used in these species.[1]

Osmolality

The clinical unit of osmotic concentration is the milliosmole, defined as the quantity of a substance that dissociates to produce one millimole of particles in solution. The size of these particles does not determine osmotic concentration—only the number of particles matters. By contrast, the SG of a solution is affected by both molecular size (weight) and the number of particles. Thus SG and osmolality measure different although related characteristics of urine.

The concept of osmolality may be explained by considering the effects of relatively large albumin particles (molecular weight: 68,000), much smaller glucose molecules (molecular weight: 180), and tiny sodium chloride molecules (NaCl; molecular weight: 58) on the osmolality of urine. Does albumin, glucose, or NaCl have the greater effect on osmolality? Because albumin does not dissociate in urine to form an increased quantity of solute, 1 mmol of albumin provides 1 mOsm of solute. Likewise, 1 mmol of glucose provides 1 mOsm of solute because glucose does not dissociate in urine to form an increased quantity of solute. But 1 g/dL of glucose has a greater effect on osmolality than 1 g/dL of albumin because the number of particles in 1 g/dL of glucose is many times greater than the number of particles of albumin in 1 g/dL. What about NaCl? In urine, 1 mmol of NaCl dissociates to form 2 mmol (one sodium ion and one chloride ion) in solution. Thus a 1 g/dL solution of NaCl has many hundred times the osmotic activity of a 1 g/dL solution of albumin because undissociated and dissociated NaCl contributes many small molecules in large numbers while the same weight of protein contributes half the number of molecules. However, because of their high molecular weight, protein molecules could substantially affect SG measurements. When urine contains 1 g/dL of protein, 0.003 must be subtracted from the observed SG. In contrast, the effect of 1 g/dL of protein on urine osmolality is negligible (less than 1 mOSM/kg).

Methods/equipment

In clinical medicine, the osmotic concentration of solutions is usually measured with instruments that determine freezing points (freezing point osmometers) or vapor pressure (vapor pressure osmometers). Commercially manufactured osmometers determine osmolality by measuring relative changes in freezing point or vapor pressure of unknown solutions, utilizing standard solutions as reference points. Currently available equipment uses microprocessors to provide rapid digital readout of data on samples as small as 0.2 mL. See Chapter 51,

Osmolality and Colloid Osmotic Pressure, for more information about osmometers.

Measurement of urine osmolality provides information that is more closely related to renal concentrating capacity than SG or refractive index. Osmometers provide more accurate assessment of osmolality than refractometers. However, compared with refractometers, osmometers are expensive.

Application/interpretation

Measurement of urine concentration, either directly by osmometry or indirectly by evaluation of urine SG, is the primary method used to evaluate the kidney's "response ability" to concentrate (remove water in excess of solute) or dilute (remove solute in excess of water) urine according to varying needs. Thus it is an index of tubular reabsorption. Knowledge of urine osmolality or SG is extremely helpful when attempting to differentiate the underlying cause(s) of polyuria and when localizing the pathophysiologic mechanisms of azotemia (prerenal versus renal azotemia).

Isosthenuria means the urine concentration (osmolality) is the same as plasma osmolality (typically 280 to 300 mOsm/L). SG values between 1.008 and 1.012 are generally regarded as isosthenuric. Hypersthenuria, indicating the ability to concentrate urine (excrete less water than solute), includes urine osmolalities in excess of the plasma osmolality (or greater than 300 mOsm/L) or urine SGs of 1.013 or greater. Hyposthenuria, indicating the ability to dilute urine (excrete more water than solute), includes urine osmolalities below the plasma osmolality (or less than 280 mOsm/L) or urine SGs 1.007 or less.

Urine SG is used as the primary test for differentiating prerenal azotemia from renal azotemia. In a dehydrated or azotemia dog, a urine SG value of 1.030 or greater is interpreted as "adequate urine concentrating ability" and supports a diagnosis of prerenal azotemia. The critical value indicating adequate urine concentrating ability in cats is 1.035. Urine SG values below these critical values suggest a defect in urine SG and would be consistent with primary renal azotemia. Causes other than kidney disease may also be responsible for impaired urine concentrating ability.

Another major indication for routine evaluation of urine SG involves interpretation of other tests that are part of the complete urinalysis. Correct interpretation of other urinalysis test results depends on knowledge of SG (or osmolality) because the SG value provides information regarding the ratio of solutes to solvent (water). Semiquantitative interpretation of other test results is unfeasible in randomly obtained urine samples without knowledge of SG. Consider proteinuria as an example. Does 2+ proteinuria at a SG of 1.010 reflect an equal or greater loss of protein than a 2+ proteinuria at SG of 1.050? The answer is obvious. There is more protein in the less concentrated sample. The same concept is applicable to interpretation of positive test results for glucose, ketones, bilirubin, occult blood, and constituents in urine sediment.

Evaluation of urine electrolytes

Methods/equipment

Potassium and sodium may be measured in serum, plasma, or urine by ion-specific potentiometry or dry reagent methods. Chloride may be measured in serum, plasma, or urine by ion-specific potentiometry, dry reagent methods, spectrophotometry, colorimetric titration, or coulometric-amperometric titration.

Application/interpretation

Measurements of urinary electrolytes may play an important role in the diagnosis and management of a variety of disorders. They may be examined as concentrations, 24-hour excretions, or fractional excretions. It is important to understand that there are no fixed normal values for electrolyte excretions because the kidneys vary their rate of excretion to match net dietary intake and endogenous production as well as metabolic needs. For example, a well-hydrated individual may be expected to excrete approximately the same amount of sodium in the urine as is ingested (24-hour excretion); however, urinary excretion of the same amount of sodium would be inappropriate in a volume-depleted individual.[4]

Urine sodium concentrations ("spot samples") are commonly used to detect volume contraction in humans. Specifically, urine sodium concentrations below 20 mEq/L generally suggest volume contraction. Because dogs and cats concentrate urine well beyond values achieved by humans, urine concentration is often used to provide the same volume estimate. However, in patients with impaired urine concentrating ability, a low urine sodium concentration implies the presence of volume depletion. A limitation in this application of urine sodium concentration as a measure of volume status is that defective renal tubular sodium reabsorption can be associated with a high rate of sodium excretion despite volume depletion. This may occur in patients with hypoadrenocorticism, advanced kidney disease, or patients receiving diuretics. Similarly, the rate of water excretion may influence urine sodium concentration. A well-hydrated patient with diabetes insipidus and a very low urine SG may have a very low urine sodium concentration due to a dilutional effect. Similarly, a patient with a very high urine SG due to volume contraction may have a relatively high urine sodium concentration due to the low water content of the urine. The effect of urine water excretion can be compensated for by calculating the fractional excretion of sodium (FE_{Na}).

FE_{Na} is calculated using the following equation[1]:

$$FE_{Na}(\%) = [(U_{Na} \times P_{Cr})/P_{Na} \times U_{Cr})] \times 100$$

In this equation, U_{Na} and P_{Na} are urine and plasma sodium concentrations, respectively, and P_{Cr} and U_{Cr} are plasma and urine creatinine concentrations, respectively. The FE_{Na} is most commonly applied in patients with AKI. In humans, volume contraction is typically associated with FE_{Na} values less than 1%; AKI is associated with values in excess of 2%–3%.[4] The major limitation to the use of FE_{Na} is that it depends on the amount of sodium filtered by the kidneys. Values for FE_{Na} confirming the diagnosis of AKI versus volume contraction have not been validated for dogs and cats.

Urine potassium and chloride excretion are less often likely to be helpful compared with sodium. In patients with hypokalemia, urine excretion may help determine whether hypokalemia results from excessive loss of potassium in urine. Ideally this would be established by comparing daily potassium intake to daily urinary potassium excretion. "Spot" urine potassium concentration measurements are unreliable, and FE_K is influenced by the amount of potassium filtered by the kidneys. Because the kidneys would normally readily excrete excess potassium, a defect in potassium excretion is presumed in patients with chronic hyperkalemia.

Urine chloride excretion generally parallels urine sodium excretion, so it is seldom measured. However, in patients with metabolic alkalosis and alkaline urine pH, urine sodium may be high because sodium is excreted as sodium bicarbonate. In this setting, finding that urine chloride excretion is low provides evidence of volume contraction.

Urine creatinine

Methods/equipment

Urine creatinine is usually measured by photometric methods using an autoanalyzer. A dipstick method for

---

[1]The fractional excretion of any electrolyte may be calculated by substituting the plasma and urine concentrations of the electrolyte in question for P_{Na} and U_{Na} in the fractional excretion equation.

measuring urine creatinine to determine the urine protein creatinine ratio is available.

Utility

Daily creatinine production, and thus daily urine excretion in urine, is essentially constant. Thus 24-hour urinary excretion of creatinine may be used to compare the completeness of 24-hour urine collections because they should vary little from day to day. Because the concentration of any substance excreted in urine may vary either by the quantity of substance excreted or the concentration of urine, the ratio of the concentration of the substance (e.g., protein or cortisol) to the urine creatinine concentration may be used to correct for variation in urine concentration. This correction works because the effect of changes in urine concentration on any given substance will parallel changes in urine creatinine concentration. Urine creatinine concentration is also used in measurement of glomerular filtration rate (GFR).

Urine protein concentration

UPC (measured as milligrams per deciliter) divided by urine creatinine concentration (also in milligrams per deciliter) will yield a unit-less figure that estimates the daily excretion of protein in urine. The UPC is considered to be normal in dogs and cats when it is less than 0.2. Values greater than 0.4 in cats and 0.5 in dogs are considered to be abnormal and are interpreted as proteinuria. Values between these two ranges are considered borderline proteinuria. The UPC is usually performed on a "spot" urine collection and has been shown to be a reasonable estimate of 24-hour urine protein excretion in dogs and cats. However, day-to-day variation may be substantial in proteinuric dogs.[9]

The UPC ratio is only valid in assessing proteinuria in patients with an inactive urine sediment and sterile urine. Thus a urinalysis and, ideally, a urine culture, should be examined at the time that the UPC is measured.

Measurement of glomerular filtration rate

Because creatinine is excreted almost exclusively by glomerular filtration, creatinine clearance (C_{Cr}) is suitable for measuring GFR. This is the formula for creatinine clearance:

$$C_{Cr} = U_{Cr} * V/P_{Cr}/BW_{kg}$$

Where U_{Cr} is the urine creatinine concentration, P_{Cr} is the plasma creatinine concentration, V is the urine flow in milliliters per minute, and BW_{kg} is the body weight in kilograms.

Endogenous creatinine clearance is measured using the patient's own creatinine already in the body. A timed urine collection is made (often 24 hours, but it can be shorter). Then the volume of urine collected, the duration (time in minutes) of the collection, the patient's body weight, and the creatinine concentrations of the urine and the patient's blood (ideally at the midpoint of the urine collection) are determined. The urine flow (V) is the volume of urine divided by the duration of the collection in minutes. From this data, the GFR can be calculated using the preceding formula. Normal values fort endogenous creatinine clearance in dogs and cats are approximately 2 to 5 mL/min/kg.

Exogenous creatinine clearance methods and creatinine disappearance curves may also be used to determine GFR; however, a safe, reliable source of creatinine solution for injection is not currently available commercially.

Measurement of creatinine clearance assumes that the patient's GFR is stable. If the patient's GFR is actively changing, such as with AKI or changes in renal perfusion, the results obtained are likely to be unreliable.

Specialized urine tests specific to estimated creatinine clearance

Urine enzymes (enzymuria)

Early detection of AKI has the potential to minimize development of irreversible renal injury by facilitating early therapeutic and/or prophylactic intervention. Unfortunately, the usual measures of kidney dysfunction such as serum creatinine and urea nitrogen concentrations and urine SG are relatively insensitive; they may not become abnormal until later in the course of disease when reduction of approximately 67%–75% in GFR has occurred. Urinary casts may be an earlier sign of AKI but were reportedly been detected in only 30%–40% of dogs with AKI.[10] In contrast, increases in the activities of certain urine enzymes have been shown in dogs and cats to occur before changes in blood urea nitrogen, serum creatinine, urine protein-to-creatinine ratio or urine SG are detectable.[11-15]

Urine enzymes are early and sensitive markers of proximal renal tubular injury in dogs and cats. Gamma-glutamyl transpeptidase (GGT) activity and N-acetyl-β-glucosaminidase (NAG) are the most commonly measured urine enzymes in dogs and cats. Urine enzyme levels are usually reported as the ratio of urine enzyme activity to urine creatinine concentration. The usual method for using urine enzymes to detect AKI is to obtain a baseline value and compare it with subsequent changes in serially measured values. Typically a two- to threefold increase from baseline values is interpreted as evidence of AKI.

Recently, reference ranges for urine GGT-to-creatinine and NAG-to-creatinine ratios have been reported for dogs; 1.93 to 28.57 U/g for GGT/creatinine and 0.02 to 3.63 U/g for NAG.[16] There was an effect of sex on NAG/creatinine values with a range of 0.02 to 3.65 U/g for males and 0.002 to 2.31 for females. Urine GGT values were significantly lower when urine pH was lower than 7.0. Absent a baseline determination, urine enzyme/creatinine values may be compared with these reference values to assess for evidence of AKI; however, the accuracy and sensitivity of this approach has not been reported.

Ideally, urine enzymes should be measured shortly after collection. If there is a delay in analysis, urine should be refrigerated (up to 8 hours for GGT determinations). Urine pH may influence enzyme stability and should be measured simultaneously with urine enzymes to optimize their interpretation; GGT degrades more quickly in acid urine, whereas NAG degrades more quickly in alkaline urine.

There are at least two settings where measurement of urine enzymes may be particularly useful in emergency and critical care patients. The first is acute presentation of a dog or cat that may have been exposed to a nephrotoxic insult (e.g., nonsteroidal anti-inflammatory drug overdosage), and the second is in the hospital setting where iatrogenic AKI may occur (e.g., aminoglycoside therapy or postanesthesia). In the first setting, collection of a baseline value upon admission to the hospital followed by serial monitoring provides the most sensitive and early means of establishing whether AKI is developing. In the second setting, baseline values may be obtained before beginning the intervention with collection of serial enzymuria determinations to assess for development of AKI.

Toxins

Urine may provide a basis for screening for some toxins and drugs. Generally, as much urine as is available should be collected and frozen for submission for toxicologic examination. Among the substances that can be tested for in urine are acetaminophen, alkaloids (strychnine, nicotine, caffeine, theobromine), amphetamines, arsenic, barbiturates, benzodiazepines, cannabis, cocaine, codeine, cyanide, glycols, heroin, lead, mercury, metaldehyde, morphine, nonsteroidal anti-inflammatory drugs, oleander, paraquat, phencyclidine, sympathomimetics, thallium, tranquilizers, and others.

References

1. Osborne CA, Stevens JB. Urinalysis: A Clinical Guide to Compassionate Patient Care. Shawnee Mission, KS: Bayer Corporation; 1999.
2. Barsanti J, Lees G, Willard M, Green R. Urinary disorders. In: Willard MD, Tvedten H, eds. Small Animal Clinical Diagnosis by Laboratory Methods. 4th ed. Philadelphia, PA: WB Saunders; 2004:135–164.
3. Johnson K, Lulich J, Osborne C. Evaluation of the reproducibility and accuracy of pH-determining devices used to measure urine pH in dogs. J Am Vet Med Assoc 2007;230:364–369.
4. Rose BD, Post TW. Clinical Physiology of Electrolyte and Acid-Base Disorders. 5th ed. New York, NY: McGraw-Hill; 2001:601.
5. Wamsley H, Allerman R. Complete Urinalysis. 2nd ed. Gloucester, UK: British Small Animal Association; 2007:87–116.
6. Zatelli A, Paltrinieri S, Nizi F, et al. Evaluation of a urine dipstick test for confirmation or exclusion of proteinuria in dogs. Am J Vet Res 2010;71:235–240.
7. Swenson C, Boisvert A, Kruger J, et al. Evaluation of modified Wright-staining of urine sediment as a method for accurate detection of bacteriuria in dogs. J Am Vet Med Assoc 2004;224:1282–1289.
8. George J. The usefulness and limitations of hand-held refractometers in veterinary medicine: an historical and technical review. Vet Clin Pathol 2001;30:201–210.
9. Nabity MB, Boggess MM, Kashtan C, Lees GE. Day-to-day variation of the urine protein: creatinine ratio in female dogs with stable glomerular proteinuria caused by X-linked hereditary nephropathy. J Vet Intern Med 2007;21:425–430.
10. Vaden SL, Levine J, Breitschwerdt EB. A retrospective case-control of acute renal failure in 99 dogs. J Vet Intern Med 1997;11:58–64.
11. Greco DS, Turnwald GH, Adams R, Gossett KA, Kearney M, Casey H. Urinary gamma-glutamyl transpeptidase activity in dogs with gentamicin-induced nephrotoxicity. Am J Vet Res 1985;46(11):2332–2335.
12. Grauer GF, Greco DS, Behrend EN, Mani I, Fettman MJ, Allen TA. Estimation of quantitative enzymuria in dogs with gentamicin-induced nephrotoxicosis using urine enzyme/creatinine ratios from spot urine samples. J Vet Intern Med 1995;9(5):324–327.
13. Rivers BJ, Walter PA, O'Brien TD, King VL, Polzin DJ. Evaluation of urine gamma-glutamyl transpeptidase-to-creatinine ratio as a diagnostic tool in an experimental model of aminoglycoside-induced acute renal failure in the dog. J Am Anim Hosp Assoc 1996;32(4):323–336.
14. Sato R, Soeta S, Miyazaki M, et al. Clinical availability of urinary N-acetyl-beta-D-glucosaminidase index in dogs with urinary diseases. J Ved Med Sci 2002;64(4):361–365.
15. Sato R, Soeta S, Syuto B, Yamagishi N, Sato J, Naito Y. Urinary excretion of N-acetyl-beta-D-glucosaminidase and its isoenzymes in cats with urinary disease. J Ved Med Sci 2002;64(4):367–371.
16. Brunker JD, Ponzio NM, Payton ME. Indices of urine N-acetyl-beta-D-glucosaminidase and gamma-glutamyl transpeptidase activities in clinically normal adult dogs. Am J Vet Res 2009;70(2):297–301.

33

Peritoneal dialysis

Diane M. Welsh and Mary Anna Labato

Dialysis is defined as the transfer of water and solute from one compartment to another across a semipermeable membrane, governed by diffusion, convection, and ultrafiltration. In peritoneal dialysis (PD) the peritoneum serves as the semipermeable membrane between the peritoneal cavity and blood in the peritoneal capillaries. *Diffusion* is the random movement of molecules from an area of high concentration of the molecule in question to an area of low concentration of that molecule. *Osmosis* refers to the movement of water from an area of low solute concentration to an area of high solute concentration. For diffusible molecules the process of solute diffusion and osmosis ultimately results in equal concentrations on both sides of the membrane. *Ultrafiltration* is the movement of water across the semipermeable membrane caused by differences in hydrostatic pressure or osmolality in the two solutions. Removal of excess fluid from the patient is referred to as ultrafiltration that is accomplished in PD by instilling fluid into the peritoneal cavity that is of a higher osmolality than plasma. *Convection* takes place when solutes are carried along with the bulk flow of water during ultrafiltration. Convection does not play an important role in PD.

Indications

The primary indication for PD in veterinary medicine is acute kidney injury (AKI), which is the sudden inability of the kidneys to regulate solute and water balance. AKI can also be defined as the rapid deterioration of kidney function resulting in the accumulation of nitrogenous wastes such as creatinine and urea.[1] AKI includes oliguric or anuric renal failure, AKI with severe uremia that is unresponsive to fluid therapy, and postrenal uremia resulting from ureteral obstruction or a rupture in the urinary collecting system.[2] Even though PD is less efficient than hemodialysis (HD) in correcting uremia, there are still some definite therapeutic advantages. PD is technologically simple, relatively inexpensive, and more efficacious in removing uremic middle molecules that are molecules in the 500- to 15,000-Da range including parathyroid hormone, leptin, β-2-microglobulin, tumor necrosis factors, and many others. PD is very labor intensive, however. HD is more efficacious in altering water and solute balance but does require a high level of technological expertise along with expensive equipment and supplies.

PD can also be used for the treatment of toxicities where the offending toxin is diffusible across the peritoneal membrane; such toxins include ethylene glycol and its toxic metabolites, ethanol, and barbiturates. Hyperkalemia, hypercalcemia, the metabolites and neurotransmitters responsible for the clinical signs of hepatic encephalopathy, and resistant metabolic acidosis are responsive to PD therapy. Volume overload, as occurs with heart failure, can also be treated with PD using a hypertonic dialysate to remove excess body water. Hypothermia, hyperthermia resulting from heat stroke, and pancreatitis can also benefit from peritoneal lavage, using solutions and techniques similar to those used in PD.

The how's of peritoneal dialysis

The basic equipment needed for PD (Box 33.1) consists of items that are readily available in most practices

Advanced Monitoring and Procedures for Small Animal Emergency and Critical Care, First Edition. Edited by Jamie M. Burkitt Creedon, Harold Davis.
© 2012 John Wiley & Sons, Inc. Published 2012 by John Wiley & Sons, Inc.

Box 33.1 Items required for performing peritoneal dialysis

- Peritoneal dialysis catheter
- Dialysate
- Three-way stopcock
- Fluid warmer
- Sterile collection bags
- Sterile drip sets/IV fluid lines (2)
- Infusion pump (not required but helps ensure volume accuracy of infusions)
- Minute timer (not required but helps in keeping on schedule)

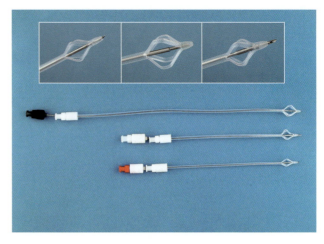

Figure 33.1 Stamey Prepubic Percutaneous catheter (Cook Medical, Inc.).

except for the catheters. The equipment that will be needed include a peritoneal dialysis catheter, dialysate, sterile collection bags, sterile intravenous (IV) fluid lines, a three-way stopcock, and a fluid warmer.

Catheter types

There are many different types/brands of peritoneal dialysis catheters. Most are variations of a fenestrated silicone tube, with or without Dacron cuffs (Invista, Wichita, KS) to promote fibrous attachments at the peritoneal and cutaneous exit sites. For acute short-term PD, a percutaneous prepubic cystotomy tube catheter can be used (see Fig. 33.1). These are generally only functional for 12–36 hours, depending on how long it takes for them to become occluded with omentum that will restrict flow of dialysate out of the body. Due to the high incidence of omentum occluding the catheter, it is highly recommended to perform a surgical omentectomy when placing the long-term peritoneal dialysis catheter.

There are a variety of straight and curled catheters with straight and flexed necks for long-term use (see Fig. 33.2). The two catheters that have been most successful in veterinary medicine for long-term use are the Fluted-T catheter and the Missouri catheter.[2–4] The pediatric lengths are best used in cats and ferrets. When it is believed PD will be performed for longer than 24 hours, a surgically placed catheter should be utilized if possible. Although some catheters such as the Fluted-T and the Missouri Swan Neck curled catheter have been designed to be placed either via laparoscope or blind trocarization in humans, based on our experience it is preferable to place these catheters surgically in dogs and cats.

The Quinton Swan Neck Peritoneal Dialysis Curl Catheter (Kendall/Tyco Healthcare) with two felt cuffs, ranging in size from 38.9 cm (infant) to 43 cm (pediatric) or the Quinton Swan Neck Missouri Peritoneal

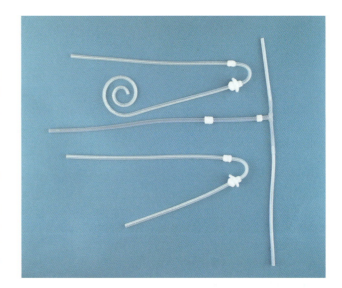

Figure 33.2 Various PD catheters (Kendall/Tyco Healthcare).

Dialysis Curl Catheter (Kendall/Tyco Healthcare) with two felt cuffs ranging in length from 38 cm, 44.5 cm, and 62.2 cm are the catheters that we have recently found to be the most successful for long-term applications (see Table 33.1). The Missouri variety also has a hard silicone bead in addition to the felt cuffs. The bead is positioned just inside the peritoneum to prevent dialysate leakage. The felt cuff is positioned just outside the peritoneum and is sutured to the rectus muscle. Fibroblasts grow into the fibers of the felt cuff to anchor the catheter. A second cuff in the subcutaneous tissue is designed to seal the exit site, helping to prevent bacteria from entering

Table 33.1 Catheter manufacturers

Catheter	Manufacturer
Stamey Percutaneous Suprapubic Catheter	Cook Medical, Inc. 800–457–4500 www.cookmedical.com
• Ash Advantage T-Fluted PD Catheter • SWAN NECK Missouri and SWAN NECK CURL CATH Peritoneal Catheters • QUINTON Tenckhoff Peritoneal Catheters	Kendall/Tyco Healthcare (a division of Covidien) 800–962–9888 www.Kendallhq.com/healthcarecatalog.asp Medigroup, Inc. 800–323–5389 www.medigroupinc.com Medcomp 215–256–4201 www.medcompnet.com
Blake Silicone Drain	Johnson and Johnson Gateway www.jnjgateway.com/home

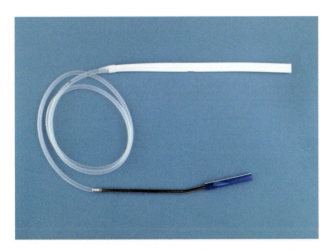

Figure 33.3 Blake surgical drain (Johnson and Johnson Gateway).

into the catheter tract. However, catheters that are surgically placed and have the previously mentioned silicone bead will need to be surgically removed. PD catheters that are placed percutaneously have the advantage of not requiring surgical removal.

Other devices that may be used in an emergency situation as PD catheters are the Blake surgical (Johnson & Johnson, Arlington, TX) drain, biliary drainage catheters, and the Jackson-Pratt drain.[5–7] Although not specifically designed for PD, the Blake surgical drain functions in a manner similar to the fluted-T catheter and has been used for PD in human infants and cats[6,7] (see Fig. 33.3).

Site selection and preparation and fluid selection

In the emergency situation when a percutaneous PD catheter is being placed, the animal should be administered light sedation with a local anesthetic block. The patient should have the abdomen shaved and aseptically cleaned as for a surgical procedure. A stab incision should be made 3–5 cm lateral to the umbilicus. The side does not matter; however most right-handed individuals tend to place the catheter on the left side. Insert the trocar toward the pelvis and inguinal canal. Tunnel subcutaneously for several centimeters and then insert through the abdominal muscles into the abdomen. The catheter is advanced over the trocar until it is fully in the abdominal cavity. Ideally the subcutaneous tunnel should create a snug fit. Use a purse-string suture pattern to secure the catheter. Alternatively, a small percutaneous chest tube may be used such as a Mila Percutaneous Chest Tube (Mila, Erlanger, KY).

When long-term use of a PD catheter is expected, surgical placement is highly preferable. Omentectomy is necessary to provide adequate exchanges if treatment is anticipated to last greater than 48 hours. The curled tip should be positioned in the inguinal area. The fluted aspect of the Fluted-T catheter is placed against the parietal peritoneum and oriented in a cranial to caudal plane. It is placed in a paramedian location with the long aspect directed toward the inguinal ring. The subcutaneous tunnel should be such that there is a gentle bend in the catheter that does not kink and that exits caudally and off midline by 3–5 cm. When a cuffed catheter is used, the cuffs should be soaked in sterile saline before placement to remove air and facilitate fibroblast cuff invasion. The inner cuff is placed in the rectus muscle, and the other cuff is placed in the subcutaneous tunnel. A tight subcutaneous tunnel with fibrous ingrowths into the cuff decreases the incidence of dialysate leak.[1,8–11]

Dialysate solutions

Commercially prepared dialysate solutions containing various concentrations of dextrose are available (Baxter, Deerfield, IL). Dialysis for removal of solutes is generally performed using 1.5% dextrose. Dialysates containing 2.5% and 4.25% dextrose are used in moderate to severely overhydrated patients. Dialysate solutions are buffered, slightly hyperosmolar crystalloid solutions designed to pull fluid, creatinine, urea, electrolytes, and phosphates from the plasma into the dialysate while providing diffusible buffer and other needed compounds such as magnesium and calcium.[12]

Hyperosmolar dextrose-containing dialysate solutions are effective for minimizing edema in overhydrated patients and for enhancing ultrafiltration (removal of water) in all patients. Hypertonic dextrose appears to favor capillary vasodilation and promotes solute drag. A 1.5% dextrose dialysate is used in dehydrated or normovolemic patients. The 2.5% and 4.25% dialysates should be used in mildly to severely overhydrated patients. Intermittent use of a 4.25% dialysate solution may increase the efficiency of dialysis in all patients.[2] Heparin (250–1000 U/L) should be added to the dialysate for the first few days after catheter placement to help prevent occlusion of the catheter by fibrin deposition.[2,5] This heparin is minimally absorbed by the patient's circulation and unlikely to prolong clotting times.[2,5,13–15] The dialysate should be warmed to 38°C to improve permeability of the peritoneum. The dialysate line should be placed in a fluid warmer to help maintain this temperature.

In an emergency situation where there is no commercially prepared dialysate solution available, a suitable dialysate solution can be made by adding dextrose to lactated Ringer solution. Osmolality should closely approximate that of the patient and the dextrose concentration should be at least 1.5%. Adding 30 mL of 50% glucose to 1 L of lactated Ringer solution will result in a 1.5% dextrose solution (see Box 33.2).

Box 33.2 Recipe for homemade dialysate solution

1 L lactated Ringer solution
30 mL 50% dextrose
Mixing both together will yield a 1.5% dialysate solution

Catheter management

To try to avoid catheter-related infection, the catheter and all lines should be maintained as aseptically as possible. The first step after catheter placement is to wrap the catheter exit site with a sterile bandage and connect the catheter to the input and output lines that are the sterile IV fluid lines. From this point on all manipulations of the lines, daily bandage, and line changes (Box 33.3) should be performed with the clinician and technician wearing sterile surgical gloves. When handling the patient including physical examinations, treatments, and when taking the patient outside or to other areas within the hospital, examination gloves should be worn.

An important aspect of catheter management is proper bandaging of the exit site and stabilization of the exiting catheter lines. The items needed are listed in Box 33.3 and shown in Fig. 33.4.

Box 33.3 Items needed for catheter and line care

Three-way stopcock
2- to 4-inch conforming gauze bandage
2- to 4-inch cast padding
2- to 4-inch conforming flexible bandaging material (e.g., VetWrap or CoFlex)
Porous tape
Waterproof tape
Two sterile drip lines
One sterile collection bag (size depends on size of patient and volume of exchanges)
Small sterile gauze squares
Povidone iodine

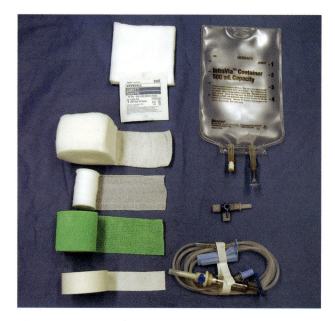

Figure 33.4 PD supplies.

To wrap the catheter in place you will need to cover the exit site of the catheter with a piece of sterile gauze. Making a cut into the middle of the gauze square and then position the catheter into the middle of this works well. Wrap the cast padding around the abdomen of the pet without kinking or occluding the catheter, trying to keep the catheter in line with the way it is exiting the body. Then add a layer of conforming gauze bandage and finish with a layer of the flexible bandaging material, again making sure to not kink or occlude the catheter in any way. A layer of 4-inch porous tape may need to be applied around the cranial aspect of the bandage to help keep it from sliding. Half of the tape should be on the animal and half of the tape should be on the bandage.

Once the bandage is applied, the input and output lines should be connected. In a sterile manner a three-way stopcock is attached to the end of the catheter. The heparinized dialysate solution is spiked with a drip set; if using a fluid pump to control and monitor your infusions, it should be a pump drip set. Prime the line with dialysate. Attach this drip line to the T-side of the three-way stopcock. A second drip set (regular, not pump set) should be spiked into a sterile empty collection bag. The other end of this drip line is attached to the last remaining side of the stopcock. This line should be positioned so that it is a straight route from the patient's dialysis catheter through the stopcock into the outflow bag. These lines should be labeled "inflow" and "outflow," and the drainage bag should be labeled "effluent or outgoing dialysate" (see Fig. 33.5). At our institution we soak three small gauze squares with either povidone iodine or chlorhexidine solution. These squares are going to be wrapped around each connection of the stopcock and secured with waterproof tape.

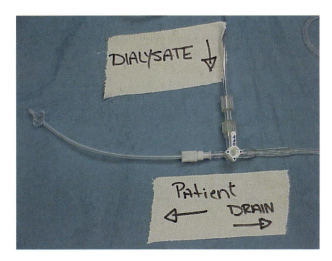

Figure 33.5 PD "Y" setup.

The abdominal bandage should be removed and reapplied every 24 hours. The exit site of the catheter should be inspected for any redness, swelling, discharge, catheter slippage, or any other abnormalities and should be brought to the doctor's attention. The outflow line and used dialysate collection bag should be changed every 24 hours. The dialysate fluid bag and inflow line should also be changed every 24 hours as well. If the dialysate bag is lasting less than 24 hours, only the bag needs to be changed at that time, and then both bag and lines changed at the 24-hour time point. These should all be done as aseptically as possible wearing sterile gloves. If possible the patient should also have a urinary catheter in place. This line should be labeled "urine," and the collection bag should also be labeled "urine." The urinary collection system should be wiped down with a dilute chlorhexidine solution every 4–8 hours.[16,17] We recommend that the exposed part of the PD catheter and the inflow and outflow lines should also be wiped down with a dilute chlorhexidine solution every 4–8 hours. At our hospital the indwelling urinary catheter is changed every 48 hours to lessen the risk of nosocomial infections.

It is very important not to instill cool or even room temperature dialysate into the patient. Instilling even room temperature dialysate into a patient will dramatically and sometimes detrimentally lower the body temperature. There are a number of ways to warm the dialysate. A fluid line warmer on the end of the inflow line between the stopcock and fluid bag can be used. It is important to make sure that it will sufficiently warm the fluid at the rate at which the fluid is being infused. A drawback to this method is that it is another apparatus on the fluid line, which requires a line long enough to wind through the fluid warmer. Another drawback is the extra weight pulling on the catheter, especially if the patient is mobile. The other way to heat the dialysate fluid is to wrap the dialysate fluid bag in a heating blanket. The drawback to this method is that the fluid in the line cools down during the dwell and drain period. Thus with small infusion volumes, the cool inline dialysate fluid could amount to a large portion of the total infusion. A combination of the inline and around-the-bag fluid warming techniques is an ideal option.

Once everything is attached, secured, and labeled, exchanges may begin. Beginning exchanges are generally done hourly. Sterile gloves should be worn when handling the pet and/or lines in any manner. The total dialysate dose is usually infused over 10–20 minutes, depending on the volume and speed at which it can be given. Generally there is a 30- to 40-minute dwell followed by a 10- to 20-minute drainage period. Initially, this exchange procedure is generally repeated every hour.

At the beginning of every exchange, 2 mL of dialysate should first be flushed through the stopcock and into the outflow bag.[18–20] This is referred to as the drain first protocol. This is to rinse any potentially trapped bacteria that might be sitting in the stopcock into the outflow line and not into the patient. This amount should not be included in the measured "in" and "out" volumes (explained later). To infuse this first 2 mL of fluid, the stopcock should be turned "off" to the patient. This is where a fluid pump comes in handy for accuracy in delivery of the proper infusion amounts, and this also avoids having to disconnect the lines, which increases the possibility of introducing contamination. Program the pump to deliver 2 mL; when that 2 mL has been flushed through the stopcock, turn the stopcock "off" to the outflow bag. Program the pump to deliver the prescribed amount of infusion over the prescribed time. When the infusion is complete, turn the stopcock "off" to the patient. The patient is now "dwelling" because dialysate fluid is dwelling within the peritoneal space. At the end of the dwell time the stopcock is now turned "off" to the fluid pump or dialysis inflow line. Fluid (dialysate) should now flow freely from the patient into the outflow line and effluent collection bag. Occasionally fluid will not flow freely. Poor fluid efflux generally occurs if the catheter was placed percutaneously and it has become occluded by omentum. Even with a surgically placed catheter in an omentectomized animal, there are times that fluid will not drain freely. To help with this, try manipulating the patient's position. If it is a small dog or cat, try picking the animal up and rotating its position, right to left, or head up and then tail up. At the completion of the drain period, another exchange will be repeated. The type of dialysate, the amount infused, and the dwell and dry times are collectively referred to as the *dialysis prescription*. A *dialysis cycle* refers to how often exchanges occur. These may be hourly (initially in the acute setting) or may consist of dwell times ranging from 1 to 12 hours chronically. More often in the chronic situation dwell times may last 2–4 hours with 4- to 6-hour dry times (peritoneal cavity devoid of dialysate solution) in between exchanges.

Monitoring

Accurate and complete recordkeeping is a critical aspect of the peritoneal dialysis procedure. The following values should be recorded hourly with a running total.

    IV fluids in (including all medications and fluids)
    Dialysate in
    Dialysate out
    Urine out

A flow sheet is very helpful in recording and tracking these values (see Table 33.2).

At the end of a cycle record the IV fluids given (if any) over the previous hour, the dialysate amount that was infused at the beginning of the dwell period that is now ending, the amount of dialysate that just drained out of the patient, and the amount of urine that has accumulated over the last hours (if any) are inserted into the flow sheet. This allows the clinician to track the current volumes of dialysate in and out, as well as the total fluid volumes in and out (including IV fluids and urine output). When and if the exchanges go to every 2 hours or longer, the orders are modified to quantify all the data at the end of the exchange for the designated number of hours' worth of values.

Depending on how the patient responds to treatment, the exchanges can be varied in many ways. The dwell time can be lengthened or shortened. The dialysate solution can be changed to a different percentage of dextrose. Commercially available dialysate solutions contain dextrose of 1.5%, 2.5%, and 4.25%. Initially the 2.5% or the 4.25% dialysate solution is usually used. The higher concentrations are used to remove water by ultrafiltration and correct overhydration and to more efficiently use the principles of diffusion and convection to correct electrolyte and acid-base abnormalities or when effluent dialysate volume is inadequate due to severe hyperosmolality. The 1.5% dialysate solution is the most commonly used solution for maintenance PD.

Additional monitoring

As well as accurate records of the patient's ins and outs during PD, there are many other parameters that are essential to monitor. The patient's weight should be recorded twice a day, before an infusion of dialysate (in a dry state). Monitoring the patient's weight is another way of monitoring the volume status. Rapid decreases in weight may be an indicator that the patient is becoming volume depleted, or it may indicate successful fluid removal from an overhydrated pet. Acute increases in body weight may be an indication, for instance, that an oliguric patient is in jeopardy of developing volume overload.

Blood pressure should be monitored every 6–8 hours, to ensure that the patient is not becoming either hypo- or hypertensive.

The patient's temperature should be monitored three to four times a day. This should be done at least once right after dialysate infusion to determine if the exchanges are affecting the body temperature.

Renal and electrolyte values should be monitored. Initially these values should be checked two to three

Table 33.2 PD flow sheet

Date	Dialysate #	Please Note AM or PM. Also Note Date on Each Sheet	Dwell Time	Outflow Time	Dialysate Volume In	Dialysate Volume Out	Current Exchange Net Balance of Dialysate Only (Volume Out Minus Volume In = Balance)	Running Total of Balance of Dialysate Only	IV Fluids In	Urine Out	Total Fluids In	Total Fluid Out	Current Exchange Fluid Difference (Total Fluid in Minus Total Fluids Out = Fluid Diff)	Running Total of Fluid Difference	Exchange	Comments
	1	Inflow Time													1	
	2														2	
	3														3	
	4														4	
	5														5	
	6														6	
	7														7	
	8														8	
	9														9	
	10														10	

times on the first day and then daily. The goal is to correct the uremia and electrolyte abnormalities but not too quickly. For example, if a drop in blood urea nitrogen of more than 50% of the starting value occurred on day 1 of treatment, the frequencies of exchanges would be decreased from hourly to every 4 hours.

Heart rate and respiratory rate and effort should be monitored every 1–2 hours. It should be noted if there is any increase in respiratory rate and effort and how this correlates to the dialysate infusion. Too much distension of the peritoneal cavity with dialysate will put pressure on the diaphragm, making respirations difficult. Increases in heart rate and respiratory rate and effort can also be signs of hypovolemia, volume overload, or pain.

Complications

Some of the potential problems that could occur while performing peritoneal dialysis include outflow problems, dialysate leakage, hypo/hyperthermia, hypokalemia, hypoalbuminemia, infection, volume overload, and dysequilibrium. As noted earlier, the most common cause of an outflow problem is clogging of the catheter with omentum. The best way to avoid this complication is to perform an omentectomy at the time of surgical placement of the catheter. If dialysate efflux is poor, one can try to improve it by altering the animal's position or manually maneuvering the patient about if it is small enough. Standing the patient on its rear limbs with its head elevated or elevating the pelvis with the thoracic limbs on the ground may move dialysate about the abdomen and encourage drainage through the catheter. Another potential way to clear an outflow problem that may be from omentum covering the drainage holes along the catheter is to instill a small amount of dialysate solution back into the abdomen and see if this dislodges whatever is there and allow for a more effective drainage. Sometimes this is successful, but often once the catheter is clogged with omentum it is difficult to correct. Another potential cause of slow fluid outflow may be a kink in the catheter or drainage tubing. Kinks are fairly easy to find and remedy if they are outside the patient's body. Manually inspect all lines leading from the patient to the collection bag, and remedy any kinks or occlusions. If there are no occlusions in the distal lines but fluid efflux remains poor, the patient's body bandage should be unwrapped and the catheter exit site inspected to make sure it has not become kinked at the exit site. Unfortunately, line kinks within the patient are difficult to distinguish from omental clogging. However, if dialysate flows freely into the patient but efflux is slow, an omental clogging problem is probably more likely than an internal kink, which should lead to difficulty with both fluid

ingress and egress. Missouri Swan Neck catheters help reduce and prevent kinking in the patient's subcutaneous tissues because of these catheters' preformed bend.

Dialysate leakage into the subcutaneous tissue usually through the abdominal incision site is another problem that occurs commonly. The Missouri PD catheters (with the silicone bead) and felt cuffs may help decrease this problem. Generally, when a PD catheter is placed, the patient needs the therapy as soon as possible; however, if it is possible to delay the first exchange for 12–24 hours, it may help the site to "seal up" and therefore minimize leakage. In our experience if treatment cannot be delayed, then infusing small volumes (10 mL/kg) with each exchange for the first 12 hours seems to provide some benefit in lessening the potential for dialysate leakage. The most frequent complication at our institution is dialysate leakage into the subcutaneous tissue. A total of 62% of cats with percutaneously placed catheters experienced subcutaneous leakage and 50% of cats with surgically placed catheters had subcutaneous leakage.[21] Dialysate leakage can be minimized by ensuring a closely apposed abdominal incision closure (simple interrupted suture pattern only), starting the initial exchange volumes at a quarter of the calculated infusion amount, and if leakage does occur, intermittently wrapping the limbs to promote mobilization of the edema. Additionally, if subcutaneous leakage occurs, the dialysate solution should be changed to the lowest possible osmolality formulation available; otherwise the hyperosmolar glucose solution in the dialysate will continue to bring body water with it into the subcutaneous tissue.

Hypothermia can be prevented by adequate warming of the dialysate solution before instillation into the patient. Also, providing the patient with external warming support, such as a hot water blanket, can help prevent hypothermia. Regular temperature monitoring is crucial to maintaining an appropriate body temperature in the PD patient. One would think that this would be an easy task, but it is not, due to the constant changes in the patient's treatment (inflow versus dwell versus outflow) all affecting the body temperature. An increase in body temperature may be a sign of infection or peritonitis and should be thoroughly investigated. One of the best ways to prevent infection related to PD is to be extremely careful when changing dialysate bags so as not to introduce any bacteria into the bag.

Hypokalemia and hypoalbuminemia may both develop in patients undergoing PD. Therefore, both serum potassium and albumin concentrations should be monitored daily. Hypokalemia develops due to the nature of diffusion of this across the semipermeable membrane from the patient into the dialysate and then loss into the used dialysate solution.

Protein losses can be clinically important in patients undergoing PD.[22] Losses may increase dramatically (50%–100%) when peritonitis is present. Hypoalbuminemia was the most common complication in a review of PD cases in dogs and cats, with 41% of animals affected.[23] In another study 16% of cats developed hypoalbuminemia.[21] Hypoalbuminemia may be the result of low dietary protein intake, gastrointestinal or renal protein loss, loss into the dialysate itself as a result of chronic inflammatory changes in the peritoneum, uremic catabolism, and concurrent diseases. Usually the animal can maintain a normal serum albumin concentration if nutritional intake is adequate. However, adequate enteral nutrition may be difficult to achieve in uremic patients. Supportive measures to maintain positive nitrogen balance often must be utilized. Nutritional support includes feeding tubes, partial or total parenteral nutrition, and the technique of PD using 1.1% amino acid solutions.[5,24–27] Gastrostomy and jejunostomy tubes are contraindicated during PD because of increased risk of infection and abdominal wall exit site dialysate leaks.

The prevalence of peritonitis in veterinary patients on PD has previously been reported as higher (22%) than that reported for humans (15%).[23,28] Additionally, exit site infection is a troublesome problem in humans.[29] In recent studies at our institution, peritonitis was not identified in any of the PD cases in dogs reviewed during a 4-year period and was reported in only 1 of 22 cats (2.5%) over a 5-year period.[21,30] The most common source of peritonitis is contamination of the bag spike or tubing by the handler, although intestinal, hematogenous, and exit site sources of infection do occur.[29] It is important to recognize pericatheter leaks to minimize exit site sources of infection.[5] Peritonitis is diagnosed when two of the following three criteria are recognized: (1) cloudy dialysate effluent, (2) greater than 100 inflammatory cells per microliter of effluent or positive culture results, and (3) clinical signs of peritonitis. In our practice the incidence of peritonitis has dramatically decreased with the use of the closed Y-system and drain first protocol.

Dialysis dysequilibrium is a rare complication characterized by dementia, seizures, or death. If it occurs, dysequilibrium is usually seen during early exchanges. Dialysis dysequilibrium is seen most commonly in patients with extreme azotemia, acidosis, hypernatremia, or hyperglycemia. Rapid removal of urea and other small solutes causes influx of water into brain cells and neurologic dysfunction.[2] Other compounds such as idiogenic osmoles are thought to play a role, as may paradoxical intracellular acidosis.[31] If evidence of dysequilibrium occurs, the dialysate prescription should be adjusted to remove urea and small solutes at a slower rate (i.e., fewer exchanges or longer dwell times). If signs of disequilibrium occur, the patient should be treated with mannitol 0.5–1 g/kg as an IV bolus and diazepam 0.1–1 mg/kg IV if seizures occur.

Contraindications to peritoneal dialysis

There are few situations in which PD is absolutely contraindicated. In humans these include peritoneal adhesions that prevent fluid distribution throughout the peritoneal cavity and pleuroperitoneal leaks that would result in pleural effusion and respiratory compromise. Adhesions are not often seen in dogs and cats. Diaphragmatic or peri-cardiodiaphragmatic hernias are seen in animals and could result in respiratory or cardiac dysfunction. However, there was an early report of the use of pleural dialysis in two dogs with acute kidney injury.[32] PD is contraindicated in severe catabolic states in which marked hypoalbuminemia exists because large amounts of protein can be lost through the peritoneum during dialysis exchanges. Marked ascites, obesity, recent abdominal surgery, bowel distention, or abdominal masses may interfere with catheter placement or adequate volume exchanges and are relative contraindications for PD.[11]

The future of peritoneal dialysis

Most of this chapter has referred to the care and treatment of the patient with an acute reversible kidney injury; however, it is possible that continuous ambulatory PD could become a viable treatment option for chronic renal disease. With a dedicated owner that is not inhibited by the medical treatment, this could be an option for those in end-stage kidney failure where transplantation or HD is not an option. It would require a close working relationship between the owner and the hospital staff to maintain aseptic techniques as well as daily bandage changes and care of the catheter and patient.

Summary

PD is a viable option for the treatment of acute kidney injury in animal patients. It is a technically simple yet labor-intensive therapy that could be utilized by many veterinary practitioners. The objectives of PD are to resolve the clinical signs of uremia, reduce azotemia, and to correct electrolyte, fluid, and acid-base abnormalities until the kidneys can recover sufficiently to maintain these values themselves. The main indication for the discontinuation of PD is when the animal has changed from an anuric or oliguric state to a polyuric state and azotemia has improved or stabilized. PD is also a realistic treatment for dialyzable toxin exposure.

References

1. Labato MA. Strategies for management of acute renal failure. Vet Clin North Am 2001;31(6):1265–1287.
2. Ross LA, Labato MA. Peritoneal dialysis. In: DiBartola SP, ed. Fluid Electrolyte and Acid-Base Disorders in Small Animal Practice. 3rd ed. Philadelphia, PA: WB Saunders; 2006:635–649.
3. Stone RW. A protocol for peritoneal dialysis. J Vet Crit Care 1985;8(1):2.
4. Ash SR, Janle EM. T-fluted peritoneal dialysis catheter. Adv Perit Dial 1993;9:223.
5. Dzyban LA. Labato MA, Ross LA, et al. Peritoneal dialysis: a tool in veterinary critical care. J Vet Emerg Crit Care 2000;10:91.
6. Dzyban LA, Labato MA, Ross LA. CVT update: Peritoneal dialysis. In: Bonagura JD, ed. Kirk's Current Veterinary Therapy. Vol 13. Philadelphia, PA: Saunders; 2000:859.
7. Boysen SR, Dorval P. Management of acute renal failure in cats using peritoneal dialysis: a retrospective study of six cases (2003–2007). J Feline Med Surg 2009;11(2):107–115.
8. Langston C. Advanced renal therapies: options when standard treatments are not enough. Vet Mod 2003;98:999.
9. Department of Health and Human Services. Fact sheet: Infection control for peritoneal dialysis (PD) patients. Atlanta, GA: Centers for Disease Control and Prevention; September 2005:1–4.
10. Peppelenbosch A, van Kuijk WHM, Bouvy N, et al. Peritoneal dialysis catheter placement technique and complications. NDT Plus 1 2008(Suppl 4):23–28.
11. Labato MA. Peritoneal dialysis in emergency and critical care medicine. Clin Tech Small Anim Pract 2000;15(3):126–135.
12. Lane IF, Carter LJ. Peritoneal dialysis and hemodialysis. In: Wingfield W, ed. Veterinary Emergency Medicine Secrets. Philadelphia, PA: Hanley and Belfus; 1997:350.
13. Lane IF, Carter LJ, Lappin MR. Peritoneal dialysis: an update on methods and usefulness. In: Bonagura JD, ed. Kirk's Current Veterinary Therapy. Vol 11. Philadelphia, PA: WB Saunders; 1992:865–870.
14. Cowgill LD. Application of peritoneal dialysis and hemodialysis in the management of renal failure. In: Osborne CA, ed. Canine and Feline Nephrology and Urology. Baltimore, MD: Lea and Febiger; 1995:573.
15. Sjoland JA, Pederson RS, Jespersen J, Gram H. Intraperitoneal heparin reduces peritoneal permeability and increases ultrafiltration in peritoneal dialysis patients. Neprol Dial Transplant 2004;10:1264–1268.
16. Smarick SD, Haskins SC, Aldrich J. Incidence of catheter-associated urinary tract infection among dogs in a small animal intensive care unit. JAVMA 2004;224(12):1936–1940.
17. Ogeer-Gyles J, Mathews K, Weese JS. Evaluation of catheter-associated urinary tract infections and multi-drug resistant Escherichia coli isolates from the urine of dogs with indwelling urinary catheters. JAVMA 2006;229(10):1584–1590.
18. Maiorca R, Vonesh EF, Cavalli P, et al. A multicenter, selection-adjusted comparison of patient and technique survivals on CAPD and hemodialysis. Perit Dial Int 1991;11:118–127.
19. Maiorca R, Cancarini G. Experiences with the Y-system. Contemp Issue Nephrol Perit Dial 1990;22:167–190.
20. Rippe B. Peritoneal dialysis: principles, techniques and adequacy. In: Feehally J, Floege J, Johnson RJ, eds. Comprehensive Clinical Nephrology. 3rd ed. Philadelphia, PA: Elsevier; 2007:979–990.
21. Cooper RL, Labato MA. Peritoneal dialysis in cats with acute kidney injury: 22 cases (2001–2006). J Vet Intern Med 2011;25(1):14–19.
22. Young GA, Brownjohn AM, Parsons FM. Protein losses in patients receiving continuous ambulatory peritoneal dialysis. Nephron 1987;45:196–201.
23. Crisp MS, Chew DJ, DiBartola SP, et al. Peritoneal dialysis in dogs and cats: 27 cases (1976–1987). J Am Vet Med Assoc 1989;195:1262.
24. Kopple JD, Bernard D, Messana J, et al. Treatment of malnourished CAPD patients with an amino acid based dialysate. Kidney Int 1995;7:1148.
25. Jones M, Hagan T, Boyle CA, et al. Treatment of malnutrition with 1.1% amino acid peritoneal dialysis solution: results of a multicenter outpatient study. Am J Kidney Dis 1998;32:761–769.
26. ter Wee PM, van Ittersum FJ. The new peritoneal dialysis solutions: friends only, or foes in part? Nature Clin Pract Nephrol 2007;3(11):604–612.
27. Tjiong HL, Rietveld T, Wattimenn JC, et al. Peritoneal dialysis with solutions containing amino acids plus glucose promotes protein synthesis during oral feeding. Clin J Am Soc Nephrol 2007;2:24–80.
28. Tzandoukas AH. Peritonitis in peritoneal dialysis patients: an overview. Adv Renal Replace Ther 1996;3(3):232–236.
29. Peng SJ, Young CS, Ferng SW. The clinical experience and natural course of peritoneal catheter exit site infection among continuous ambulatory peritoneal dialysis patients. Dialysis Transplant 1998;27(2):71–78.
30. Beckel N, O'Toole T, Rozanski E, et al. Peritoneal dialysis in the management of acute renal failure: five dogs with leptospirosis. J Vet Emerg Crit Care 2005;15(3):201–205.
31. Ali, II, Pirzala NA. Neurologic complications associated with dialysis and chronic renal insufficiency. In: Henrich WL, ed. Principles and Practice of Dialysis. 3rd ed. Philadelphia, PA: Lippincott Williams & Wilkins; 2004:502–512.
32. Shahar R, Holmberg DL. Pleural dialysis in the management of acute renal failure in two dogs. J Am Vet Med Assoc 1985;187:952.

34

Technical management of hemodialysis patients

Karen Poeppel and Cathy Langston

Hemodialysis is a therapy by which blood is removed from the patient, run through an artificial kidney called a dialyzer where uremic toxins are removed, and then returned to the patient (Fig 34.1). Removal of these toxins is achieved by diffusion across a semipermeable membrane in the dialyzer. Blood is circulated on one side of the membrane, and a balanced electrolyte solution called dialysate is circulated on the other side of the membrane. Molecules small enough to pass through the pores in the membrane move from the side with higher concentration to the side with lower concentration. Used dialysate, which is on the opposite side of the semipermeable membrane from the patient's blood and contains the patient's uremic waste products, is then washed down the drain. Blood continuously circulates in this loop for the duration of the dialysis treatment, usually 4 to 5 hours for intermittent hemodialysis (IHD). This way the entire blood volume of the patient is treated many times over while minimizing the actual volume of blood in the extracorporeal circuit at any given time. Vascular access for this circuit is obtained by placing a large double-lumen catheter into the jugular vein. In addition to removing uremic waste products, hemodialysis can restore appropriate patient hydration via ultrafiltration, as well as electrolyte and acid-base balance via diffusion or convection. Ultrafiltration is the removal of excess patient fluid from the vascular compartment and is achieved when a pump on the side of the outgoing dialysate creates a negative pressure across the semipermeable membrane in the dialyzer.

Intermittent hemodialysis is a renal replacement therapy performed for a set period of time per day, generally 3 days per week during the maintenance phase of treatment. Continuous renal replacement therapies (CRRTs) exist that rely on the same concepts of diffusion, ultrafiltration, and convection across an extracorporeal semipermeable membrane. As the name implies, patients are treated continuously rather than intermittently. There are increasingly more veterinary facilities that provide CRRT. Full discussions of veterinary CRRT are published elsewhere.[1,2] Many concepts to be discussed in this chapter hold true for both intermittent and continuous therapies, but key differences are discussed when appropriate.

Patient selection

Acute kidney failure

There are a number of indications for IHD (see Box 34.1), but in veterinary medicine IHD is used most commonly to treat patients with acute kidney injury or failure.[3,4] Standard medical therapy should always be attempted before initiating hemodialysis, but a certain number of patients do not respond adequately. Presence of uremic signs, progressive azotemia, or azotemia that does not improve over a 24-hour period with standard medical therapy is an indication for dialysis. Anuria or oliguria is often present in patients with more severe renal injury. Life-threatening volume overload can develop in these patients as a result of aggressive intravenous (IV) fluid diuresis, excessive volumes of medications, or total or partial parenteral nutrition. In the absence of urine production, the body has very limited methods of removing extra fluid, so hemodialysis is indicated to remove the accumulated fluid.[3–5]

Advanced Monitoring and Procedures for Small Animal Emergency and Critical Care, First Edition. Edited by Jamie M. Burkitt Creedon, Harold Davis.
© 2012 John Wiley & Sons, Inc. Published 2012 by John Wiley & Sons, Inc.

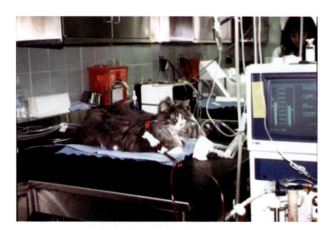

Figure 34.1 A cat being dialyzed. Patients are not sedated for dialysis treatments.

Box 34.1 Indications for hemodialysis

Azotemia refractory to conventional medical management
Severe electrolyte or acid-base disturbances
Life-threatening volume overload
Toxicities and drug overdoses
Chronic kidney failure

Anuric or oliguric patients, patients with severe renal impairment, and patients receiving overly aggressive potassium supplementation are at risk of hyperkalemia. Emergency treatment (i.e., insulin, dextrose, bicarbonate) only shifts the potassium to the intracellular space, but if urine production cannot be established, there is no way for the patient to excrete the excess potassium. Hemodialysis is indicated in these patients to remove the potassium.[3,6]

In all cases of acute renal injury, the ultimate goal of dialytic therapy is to provide a supportive therapy to allow time for the kidneys to recover sufficiently so dialysis can be discontinued.[5] Renal recovery generally takes at least a few weeks, and sometimes months, so without dialytic therapy the patient would die of uremic complications before renal recovery could occur. Of the patients who survive, a certain percentage have full renal recovery, some no longer require dialysis but have renal insufficiency, and the final group remain dialysis dependent for the remainder of their lives.

Chronic kidney failure

Hemodialysis can also be used to treat patients with chronic kidney failure.[5] In these patients there is no hope for renal recovery because the disease is degenerative. Therefore the patients are dialysis dependent for the remainder of their lives. Chronic dialysis is indicated when medical management fails to control uremic symptoms, which include vomiting, nausea, anorexia, and weakness.

It is not uncommon for patients with end-stage chronic kidney disease to present in an acute uremic crisis. In this setting treatment progresses similarly to treatment for acute renal injury until the crisis is stabilized. The difference is that the owner and the medical staff know the patient will always be dialysis dependent, so they can make decisions accordingly. It would not be prudent to treat a chronic kidney failure patient in the long term with CRRT because an intermittent therapy would be the only mode of treatment that would allow the patient to leave the hospital.

Toxin removal

Finally, hemodialysis can be used to treat certain intoxications and drug overdoses. For effective removal by dialysis, the substance must be small enough to pass through the semipermeable membrane, and it cannot be protein bound or sequestered in extravascular tissues.[3–5] The dialysis treatment must be initiated before the toxin causes irreversible damage to the patient. Antifreeze (ethylene glycol), alcohol, and digoxin are a few substances that can be effectively removed by dialysis. For a more complete list, see Box 34.2.

Hemodialysis is superior to CRRT for clearing most toxins because diffusion happens much more quickly in the dialyzer during an IHD treatment than it would during a CRRT treatment. A continuous therapy may be beneficial for removal of toxins that have a high postdialysis rebound, meaning they are sequestered in the extravascular space and diffuse more slowly into the blood compartment.[7]

Patient considerations

Hemodialysis involves prolonged and intimate operator contact with the patient. It would be unsafe for both the patient and technician to treat an aggressive patient. Repositioning of the catheter or patient for continuous blood flow is frequently necessary. Inability to handle the patient can lead to inadequate dialysis treatment, significant blood loss from clotting in the dialyzer, physical harm to the technician, or inadvertent dialysis catheter removal. Sedation for 4 to 5 hours daily is likely counterproductive to renal recovery.

Patients weighing less than 2.5 kg are difficult to treat due to their low blood volume. The smallest priming volume available for the extracorporeal circuit is 68 mL, so treatment of a patient smaller than 2.5 kg would require priming the circuit with blood from the blood

Box 34.2 Substances removed by dialysis[5]

Alcohols	Anticonvulsants	Mexiletine
Ethanol	Gabapentin	Nitroprusside
Ethylene glycol	Phenobarbital	Procainamide
Methanol	Phenytoin*	Sotalol
Analgesics/anti-inflammatory	Primidone	Tocainide
Acetaminophen	Antifungals	Chelating agents
Aspirin	Dapsone	Deferoxamine
Mesalamine (5-ASA)	Fluconazole	EDTA
Morphine*	Flucytosine	Penicillamine
Pentazocine	Antineoplastics	Immune suppressants
Antibacterials	Busulfan	Azathioprine
Amikacin	Carboplatin	Methyl prednisolone
Amoxicillin (most penicillins)	Cytarabine*	Miscellaneous
Cephalexin	Cyclophosphamide	Allopurinol
Cefotetan	Fluorouracil (5-FU)	Ascorbic acid
Cefoxitin	Ifosfamide	Carisoprodol
Ceftriaxone	Methotrexate	Chloral hydrate
Chloramphenicol	Mercaptopurine	Chlorpheniramine
Gentamicin	Antivirals	Diazoxide
Imipenem/Cilastatin	Acyclovir	Foscarnet
Kanamycin	Famciclovir	Iohexol
Linezolid	Valacyclovir	Iopamidol
Nitrofurantoin	Zidovudine	Lithium
Ofloxacin	Cardiac/vasoactive drugs	Mannitol
Metronidazole	Atenolol	Metformin
Sulbactam	Bretylium	Minoxidil
Sulfamethoxazole	Captopril	Octreotide
Sulfisoxazole	Enalapril	Ranitidine
Trimethoprim	Lisinopril	Theophylline
Vancomycin*	Metoprolol	Caffeine

*High-flux dialysis only.

bank. There are limited situations in which this should be attempted.

Equipment

Machines

The IHD and CRRT machines used in veterinary medicine are all manufactured for human use. In the United States, most units performing IHD or CRRT use either Gambro or Fresenius machines (see Fig. 34.2). Machines for CRRT are significantly different in appearance than IHD machines (see Fig. 34.2C) and are not discussed in this chapter. Regardless of the model or manufacturer, all modern IHD machines have certain common characteristics. First, they all contain a display screen. This screen displays the current operating mode (such as "setup," "autotest," "dialysis"), all options available in that mode, treatment parameters, alarm conditions, and any necessary instructions. During the dialysis treatment, the screen also displays treatment status information such as time remaining in treatment, total fluid removed, and liters of blood processed (passed through the dialyzer).

IHD machines house a dialysate proportioning system. This system mixes incoming purified water with the appropriate volume of bicarbonate and electrolyte concentrate solutions to create dialysate. It is essential for patient safety that the dialysate is proportioned consistently and accurately to the operator's specifications. To that end, the machines also have sensors to assure the dialysate meets concentration and temperature requirements.

Each machine has a blood pump and clamps for the blood lines. There are housings for the blood cartridge, blood lines, and dialyzer. The vast majority of patients are anticoagulated with heparin to prevent blood clotting in the extracorporeal circuit, so all modern dialysis

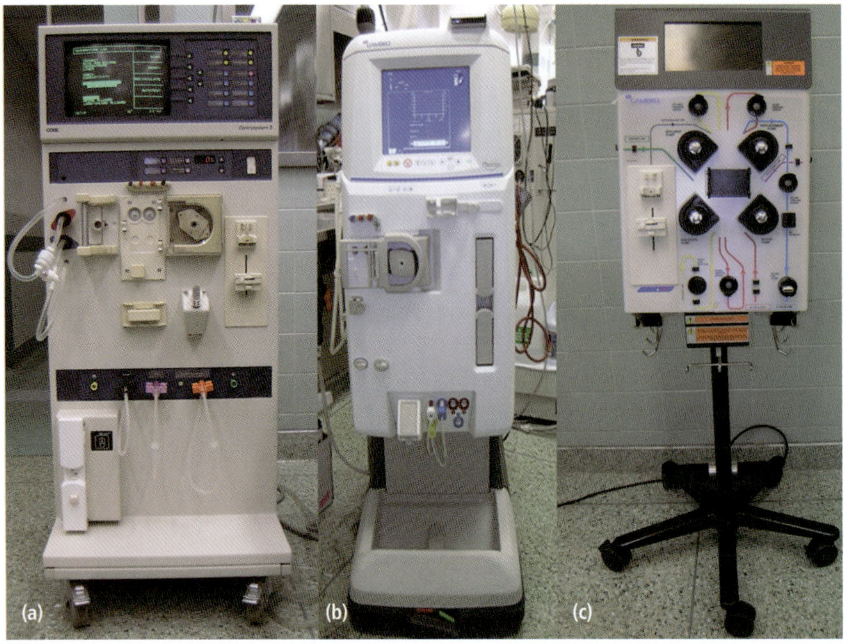

Figure 34.2 (a) Centrysystem 3 hemodialysis machine; (b) Phoenix hemodialysis machine; (c) Prisma CRRT machine. All three are manufactured by Gambro.

machines have a built-in syringe pump for heparin administration.

Finally, the machines contain a number of additional sensors that monitor for pressure changes in the extracorporeal circuit, air in the return line, blood leaks in the dialyzer, and other unsafe conditions. In any alarm situation, the machine automatically takes actions to ensure patient safety. For example, if a problem is detected in the dialysate, dialysate is diverted from the dialyzer so as not to affect the patient, but the blood continues to circulate to minimize the chances of clotting. If a problem is detected in the extracorporeal circuit, the blood pump stops and a clamp shuts on the return line to prevent further removal of blood from the patient or unsafe return of blood to the patient. In extreme situations, the machine requires the operator to perform an emergency stop treatment procedure.

Water treatment system

A water treatment system is essential to providing a safe hemodialysis treatment. The patient is exposed to roughly 20 gallons of water in the form of dialysate in an average dialysis treatment, so even trace amounts of impurities can have detrimental effects.[8–10] Water treatment systems vary in size and water output, from a small unit that fits the back of a dialysis machine (see Fig. 34.3A) to an entire room full of equipment that provides water for up to 30 dialysis machines (see Fig. 34.3B), but

they all have certain common features. A typical system contains a mixing valve (to blend hot and cold water to the optimal temperature), sediment filter (to remove debris), ion exchange tank (to remove calcium and magnesium), carbon tanks (to remove organic components), and reverse osmosis or deionization (to remove any remaining contaminants and ions). Daily monitoring of the product water is required to assure patient safety. The technician performing the hemodialysis treatment generally performs this task.

Extracorporeal circuit

The extracorporeal (EC) circuit used in IHD consists of a blood cartridge, blood tubing, and the dialyzer. Infusion lines are generally built in to the cartridge for fluids, medications, and heparin. The entire EC circuit is discarded at the end of each dialysis treatment. In human medicine dialyzers are reused, although this practice is on the decline; in veterinary medicine, reuse is not cost effective. The EC circuits used in veterinary medicine are manufactured for human use, so generally neonatal and pediatric sizes are used. Adult sizes are used for the largest patients (see Table 34.1).

The variation in length and diameter of the tubing allows for maximal blood flow in larger patients and minimal priming volumes in smaller patients.

A number of different dialyzers are used for veterinary patients, but they all have certain common charac-

Table 34.1 Recommended extracorporeal volumes[3]

	Body Weight (kg)	Dialyzer Volume (mL)	Total Extracorporeal Volume (mL)	% Blood Volume
Cats, dogs	<6	<20	<60	13–40
Cats	>6	<30	<70	<23
Dogs	6–12	<45	<90	9–19
Dogs	12–20	<80	100–160	6–17
Dogs	20–30	<120	150–200	6–13
Dogs	>30	>80	150–250	6–10

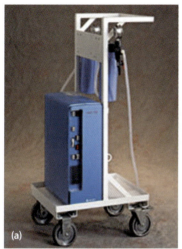 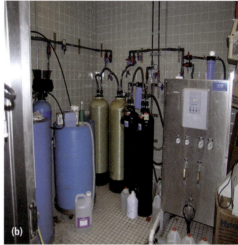

Figure 34.3 (a) A portable reverse osmosis unit that fits the back of a hemodialysis machine. (b) Water treatment system with, from left to right, an ion exchange tank, carbon tanks, backup deionization tanks, and the reverse osmosis system. Not pictured are the mixing valve and sediment filter.

teristics. They are a hollow fiber design, which means the semipermeable membranes form thin straw-like tubes through which the blood passes. The dialysate then bathes these blood-filled fibers (see Fig. 34.4).

This design allows for smaller priming volumes than other dialyzer configurations, and it also provides greater membrane surface area for greater efficiency.

Dialyzer membranes are made of either natural or synthetic material. The natural fiber membranes are generally less expensive than synthetic membranes, but they are more likely to induce thrombosis and bioincompatability reactions. Synthetic membranes usually have larger pore sizes, which allow for better clearance of middle molecular weight uremic toxins in addition to small molecule clearance. They are also reportedly more biocompatible and less thrombogenic than the natural fiber membranes.[11,12] Synthetic membranes are now predominantly used in veterinary medicine.

Dialyzers come in a variety of different sizes. Priming volumes for dialyzers commonly used in veterinary

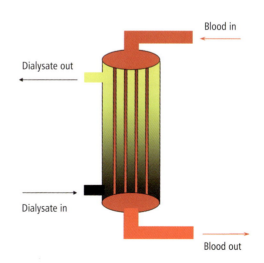

Figure 34.4 Diagram of a hollow fiber dialyzer. Countercurrent flows of blood and dialysate allow for more effective clearance of waste products.

medicine range from 28 mL to more than 150 mL. The larger dialyzers have more membrane surface area, so they are more efficient at clearing waste products, and the smaller dialyzers, although less efficient, allow for treatment of very small patients because of the small priming volumes.

Catheters

Consistent long-term vascular access is key in providing adequate dialytic therapy via intermittent and continuous modes. In veterinary medicine this is almost always achieved by placing a double-lumen catheter into the jugular vein.[5,12,13] The catheter should be large enough to supply a blood flow between 80 and 125 mL/min in cats or small dogs and between 250 and 500 mL/min in medium or large dogs. This generally means placing the largest bore catheter that will fit into the patient's vein. A number of different catheters manufactured for human dialysis patients are suitable for veterinary use. Most of these catheters have two lumens, referred to as the arterial lumen and the venous lumen. Because of the location of the catheter, all blood flowing through it is venous blood, so the terminology has to do with the direction of blood flow with relation to the patient and the dialysis machine. The arterial lumen is the access, so blood flows through it from the patient to the extracorporeal circuit, and the venous lumen is for return of blood to the patient from the dialysis machine. The ends of the lumens are staggered to reduce the reuptake of "clean" blood by the arterial lumen (called access recirculation). The tip of the arterial lumen is proximal to the tip of the venous lumen (see Fig. 34.5).

Dialysis catheters are referred to as temporary (nontunneled) or permanent (tunneled). Temporary catheters are noncuffed, tapered at the tip, and usually placed percutaneously. These catheters are meant to stay in place for only a few weeks. In most cases, temporary catheters are the appropriate choice, as long as chronic dialysis therapy is not anticipated. Permanent catheters have an external cuff, frequently are blunt at the end, and they must be placed surgically. The catheter is tunneled in a subcutaneous pocket that extends from the skin exit site to the vessel before being inserted into the vessel. The subcutaneous pocket is a few centimeters in length, and the external cuff of the catheter is positioned in this pocket. Fibroblasts attach to the cuff, which secures the catheter in the pocket and creates a physical barrier inhibiting bacteria around the skin exit site from moving along the catheter and into the vessel. These catheters can stay in place 1 to 2 years and are the preferred choice for a patient receiving chronic dialysis.[5,12]

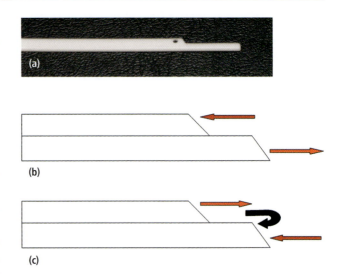

Figure 34.5 (A) Picture of the actual tip of a hemodialysis catheter demonstrating the staggered lumens. (B) Diagram indicating preferred direction of blood flow in to the proximal lumen and out of the distal lumen. (C) Diagram showing how access recirculation occurs when blood flows in to the distal lumen and out of the proximal lumen.

Several double-lumen or multilumen catheters are adequate for small patients (Mila, Arrow). These catheters are designed to be placed percutaneously and are used as temporary dialysis catheters. The proximal lumen is used as the arterial (access) lumen, and the distal lumen is used as the venous (return) lumen. In multilumen catheters, the medial lumen(s) can be used when one of the other lumens fails. Use of a multilumen catheter is not recommended for dialysis because the more lumens in a catheter, the smaller the size of each lumen, and therefore the slower the blood flow. Also, use of a catheter smaller than 7F is not recommended for the same reason, although a smaller catheter can be placed when there is no other option. Examples of various sizes of dialysis and multilumen catheters, as well as their respective blood flows, are listed in Table 34.2.

Placement

As previously discussed, hemodialysis catheters can be placed percutaneously or surgically, depending on the type of catheter and the personnel involved. Strict attention to aseptic technique during placement is mandatory for both temporary and permanent catheters.[14] These catheters are generally placed in a clean procedure room with restricted traffic. All personnel involved in the procedure should wear caps and masks. A large barrier drape and sterile gloves are necessary. Because of the "springiness" of the guidewire, a surgical gown is

Table 34.2 Common hemodialysis catheter specifications and approximate blood flow rates*

Manufacturer	Type	Lumens	French Size	Length (cm)	Max Qb (mL/min)
Quinton PermCath	Cuffed	2	15	45	370
Quinton PermCath	Cuffed	2	15	40	400
Quinton PermCath	Cuffed	2	15	36	410
MedComp Pediatric	Cuffed	2	8	18	120
Hohn	Cuffed	2	7	36	30
MedComp Temporary	Noncuffed	2	11.5	24	360[‡]
Mila	Noncuffed	2	7	20	
[†]Arrow	Noncuffed	2	7	20	100
[†]Arrow, 20 ga lumen	Noncuffed	3	5.5	13	40
[†]Arrow, 22 ga lumen	Noncuffed	3	5.5	13	20
[†]Arrow, 20 ga lumen	Noncuffed	3	5.5	8	50
[†]Arrow, 22 ga lumen	Noncuffed	3	5.5	8	30
[†]Intracath through the needle	Noncuffed	1	19 ga	30.5	20

*Maximum blood flows determined *in vitro* using canine packed red blood cell solution (29% packed cell volume). Arterial chamber pressure maintained at −250 mm Hg or higher. Maximum blood flow rates *in vivo* may be lower.
[‡]Maximum blood flow determined *in vivo*.
[†]Not designed for dialysis.

recommended to decrease the risk of contaminating it during placement. Permanent catheters are placed with a surgical technique and so should be placed in an operating room.

The person placing the catheter must be skilled and should use the method with which he or she is most comfortable. In addition to dialysis personnel, emergency and critical care personnel are often equally skilled at placing percutaneous catheters. A dialysis nephrologist, criticalist, or surgeon may have the most experience in placing a permanent dialysis catheter. In some cases catheter placement is facilitated by a cutdown procedure to isolate the vessel, followed by the percutaneous technique.

Sedation or anesthesia is often needed for catheter placement. Some compliant or severely depressed animals may only require a local anesthetic. A short-acting or reversible drug can be used for percutaneous placement. General anesthesia should be used if catheter placement is expected to be problematic, and it is required for placement of a permanent, tunneled catheter.

Location

The jugular veins are the only vessels large enough for a dialysis catheter in most animals because of the catheter size needed relative to patient size. All attempts should be made to preserve at least one jugular vein in any patient that may eventually need hemodialysis. There is no documented difference in veterinary medicine

between the right and left jugular vein in regard to the dialysis treatment aside from individual preference during placement.

The tip of the catheter should be positioned at the junction of the cranial vena cava and the right atrium to provide maximum blood flow. Whether placed percutaneously or surgically, fluoroscopy can be used during the procedure to assure proper placement.[14] If fluoroscopy is not used, a postprocedure radiograph should be taken. In either case, blood flows are evaluated by rapidly aspirating blood into a 10-cc or 12-cc syringe before the procedure is complete. Blood should flow from both lumens with ease to determine the final position of the catheter.

Care and maintenance

The dialysis catheter should be handled in an aseptic fashion at all times. The catheter should only be handled by personnel trained in dialysis catheter care, and it should not be used for purposes other than dialysis. Each time the catheter is unwrapped for treatment, the catheter exit site should be cleaned and assessed (see Fig. 34.6). The bandaging material should be changed as needed if it becomes wet, blood soaked, or otherwise compromised.[13–15] If dialysis is not being performed, the catheter locking solution (see later) should be changed at least every 3 to 4 days, and the exit site can be cleaned at that time. Guidelines for accessing the catheter for dialysis treatments or changing the catheter locking solution are outlined in Protocol 34.1.

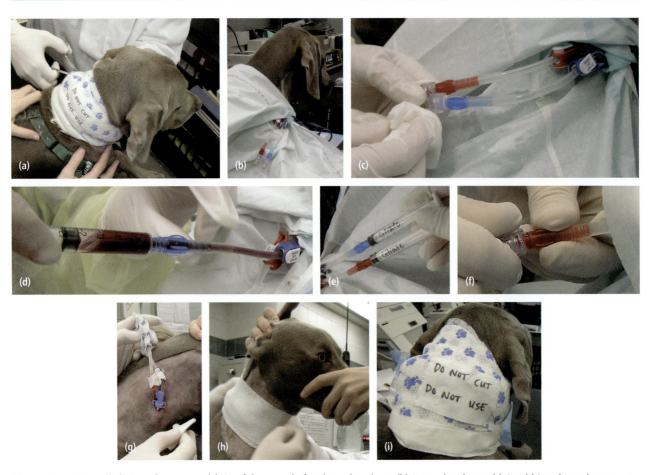

Figure 34.6 Hemodialysis catheter care. (a) Careful removal of catheter bandage. (b) Draped catheter. (c) Scrubbing the catheter ports. (d) Aspirating the anticoagulant lock. (e) Replacing the anticoagulant locks. (f) Placing caps on the catheter. (g) Secured catheter ports. (h) Wrapping the catheter. (i) Final bandage with reminder not to use the catheter.

When the catheter is not in use, it is wrapped securely to protect it from dislodgement or inadvertent opening. The wrap should completely cover the catheter, and the catheter should not be accessed regularly for heparinized saline flushes. Instead, an anticoagulant locking solution is placed in each lumen to prevent clotting between dialysis treatments. The locking solution has historically been sodium heparin (500 to 5000 U/mL), but a number of recent studies have shown that sodium citrate, at a 4% or higher concentration, is as effective an anticoagulant as heparin, does not stimulate biofilm production, is bacteriostatic, and is less expensive than heparin.[16–18] For that reason, our facility has changed the catheter locking protocol to use 4% sodium citrate instead of sodium heparin. Higher concentrations of citrate can be used but create a risk of hypocalcemia if inadvertently flushed into the patient.[19] Each dialysis catheter has the exact volume of the two lumens printed on the catheter and/or in the package insert, which informs the handler of the volume of anticoagulant solution to instill.

Performing hemodialysis

Hemodialysis machine preparation

The structure and function of dialysis machines was described earlier; the following is instruction regarding the steps necessary to prepare a machine for a hemodialysis treatment. Each model of dialysis machine has a specific and detailed setup protocol, but all include these same general steps.

First, the water treatment unit is turned on and any daily water testing is done. Then the dialysis machine is turned on and the acid and bicarbonate concentrate containers are attached. The machine runs through a series of internal tests as the dialysate is being proportioned. During this time, the EC circuit is loaded onto the machine. The next step is to prime the EC circuit, which on some machines can be done immediately, and on others must wait until the internal tests are complete or the dialysate is ready. Priming involves filling with saline all sections of the EC circuit that will contain

Protocol 34.1 Hemodialysis catheter care

Items required
- Bandage scissors
- Two sterile barrier drapes
- Clean examination gloves
- Surgical mask
- Surgical scrub and solution (chlorhexidine or Betadine)
- Sterile gauze pads
- Syringes
- Heparinized saline
- Injection caps
- Antiseptic cream
- Porous tape
- Cohesive bandage (Vetwrap)
- Cast padding
- Conforming bandage

Procedure
1. Gather materials.
2. Perform hand hygiene.
3. Unwrap catheter bandage by cutting bandage on opposite side of neck from where catheter is (Fig. 34.6A).
4. Clean area around catheter exit site.
5. Assess catheter exit site for redness, swelling, odor, or discharge, and assess subcutaneous tunnel for signs of infection or excess bruising.
6. Remove cohesive bandage and the tape that is on the clamps.
7. Place a sterile barrier around catheter to prevent ports from touching fur or skin (Fig. 34.6B).
8. Don a surgical mask and exam gloves (mask and gloves should be worn from here until you begin wrapping the catheter again).
9. Perform a surgical-type scrub on both ports, extending from the clamps to the tops of the injection ports (Fig. 34.6C).
10. Spray ports with dilute Nolvasan (Pfizer Animal Health, NY) or Betadine.
11. Place another sterile barrier around catheter.
12. Have two squares of *sterile* gauze within reach, as well as all syringes that are needed.
13. Open arterial/proximal port by removing injection cap.
14. Wipe port opening with sterile gauze.
15. Withdraw the exact volume (the exact volume for each side is printed on the catheter) of the lumen and discard. This is the locking solution, so you must *never* flush the catheter first (Fig. 34.6D).
16. Flush lumen with 6 cc fresh (prepared within 24 hours) heparinized saline or normal saline.
17. Repeat steps 13–16 on the venous/distal side.
18. Replace the locking solution by injecting the exact volume of each lumen (Fig. 34.6E).
19. Place a new injection cap on each lumen (Fig. 34.6F).
20. At this point, you can remove your gloves and mask.
21. Tape both clamps shut.
22. Place a piece of cohesive bandage around both ports.
23. Place a gauze square with an antiseptic cream over the catheter exit site (Fig. 34.6G).
24. Wrap catheter with cast padding, conforming bandage, and then a flexible cohesive bandage. Wrap tightly enough that the bandage stays in place but not too tightly (Fig. 34.6H).
25. Place a strip of porous white tape around both ends of bandage to anchor it to skin and prevent slipping. This is especially important for active animals.
26. Place a final piece of tape with the words "DO NOT CUT/ DO NOT USE" on the outside of the wrap (Fig. 34.6I).

blood, thus removing all air. Air removal is essential because blood that comes into contact with any trapped air will be more likely to clot.

Once the EC circuit is filled with saline, the machine is put through a recirculation phase. The arterial and venous patient lines are connected to each other, and the saline is then circulated throughout the loop created by the EC tubing and the dialyzer. The purpose of this phase is to remove any residual substances from the manufacturing and sterilization process of the dialyzer and tubing.[20] During recirculation, the blood pump is running quickly, so saline flow through the EC circuit is rapid. This aids in propelling any remaining air bubbles from the dialyzer fibers or the sides of the blood tubing into the pressure chambers, which also act as air traps. The recirculation phase usually takes from 15 to 30 minutes. With most machines, there is no one specific point during setup at which the treatment parameters (treatment time, fluid to be removed, dialysate concentration, anticoagulant protocol) must be set. Each hemodialysis unit, though, should have an established protocol that defines when these parameters are set to ensure that they are set appropriately for each treatment.

When the recirculation phase is complete, the saline in the tubing and dialyzer is flushed out by the priming solution. The priming solution is the fluid given to the patient to replace the volume of blood removed when the dialysis treatment begins. The blood pump is used to flush the EC circuit with twice the priming volume, using the desired priming solution (e.g., 0.9% NaCl, hetastarch solution). At this point, some machines are ready to start a treatment. Other machines need to run through another set of internal tests before they are ready.

Patient preparation

Patient preparation includes an assessment of a standard set of pretreatment parameters as well as preparation of the hemodialysis catheter. Parameters to be assessed prior to each dialysis treatment should include a blood pressure, heart rate, packed cell volume (PCV), total protein (TP), body weight, temperature, activated clotting time (ACT) or other measure of coagulation, and the patient's attitude, mentation, and hydration status. If the systemic arterial blood pressure is less than 80 mm Hg systolic, we generally recommend use of pressor agents to increase blood pressure before initiating hemodialysis. If the blood pressure cannot be maintained above 80 mm Hg, the patient can experience life-threatening hypotension when the dialysis treatment is started. In our experience, if the PCV is not at least 20% in dogs or 18% in cats, a blood transfusion will likely benefit the patient. The body weight and TP will help assess the patient's hydration, and the weight pre- and posttreatment will aid in assessing fluid balance during the dialysis treatment because any weight changes in that short a period of time are due to fluid gain or loss. Finally, the ACT will help to determine how much heparin to give the patient initially, and how much to infuse during the dialysis treatment.

Prior to each dialysis treatment, a set of serum biochemical parameters is generally measured that includes at the least urea, creatinine, phosphorus, and potassium concentrations. It is not always essential to have these results before starting the dialysis treatment, but it is often useful to see the results within an hour of beginning treatment. Remeasuring these same parameters at the end of the treatment provides a useful method of determining the adequacy of the dialysis treatment, which is discussed in the monitoring section of this chapter.

The hemodialysis catheter needs to be prepared with great care. As discussed previously, only properly trained personnel should handle this catheter. The catheter should be opened using the same protocol as for changing the locking solution (Protocol 34.1). After the locking solution is removed, blood samples for pretreatment blood work are taken through the catheter. The loading dose of heparin can be administered through the catheter at this time if prescribed.

Starting treatment

When both the machine and the patient are ready, it is time to connect the patient and start dialyzing. The arterial patient line of the EC circuit is connected to the proximal lumen of the dialysis catheter, and the venous patient line of the EC circuit is connected to the distal lumen of the catheter. This connection should be covered with gauze soaked in antiseptic to minimize contamination during the treatment. The patient lines are anchored to the patient in some manner (attached to harness or thoracic limb) to prevent excess pressure directly on the dialysis catheter.

As the blood is removed from the patient through the arterial EC circuit line, the priming solution is infused into the patient through the venous EC circuit line. The blood is removed slowly to try to prevent a sudden drop in blood pressure. The blood will fill more and more of the EC circuit and eventually fill the dialyzer. A key is pressed to start the dialysis treatment when blood has filled the dialyzer. When this key is selected, treatment time begins to count down, heparin infusion begins, programmed fluid removal begins, and any other programs that run during the dialysis treatment will begin.

Ending treatment

The dialysis machine alerts the operator when the specified treatment time is finished. The operator can elect to end the treatment early, usually in emergency situations. Generally about 10 minutes before the end of treatment, the catheter is prepared for disconnection by uncovering and scrubbing the connection site. The procedure is the same as for opening the catheter. When treatment time is complete, blood for posttreatment lab work is drawn. The exact time of sampling (i.e., immediately, 2 minutes after treatment ends) and site of sampling (i.e., EC circuit, dialysis catheter) may vary between different dialysis units but should be consistent within a unit. Then the patient's blood is returned in a procedure called rinseback. Most commonly the arterial patient line is attached to saline. The blood pump is started, and the saline is drawn in so that it flushes the blood from the EC circuit back into the patient. In specially monitored situations, the arterial line can be left open to the air without attaching the saline bag, if there is a concern about volume overload in the patient, but this risks creating a massive air embolus for the patient. When rinseback is complete, the locking solution is infused into both lumens of the dialysis catheter and the catheter is wrapped. Finally, posttreatment patient parameters, which are the same as pretreatment parameters, are assessed and recorded.

Monitoring during the hemodialysis treatment

There are a number of patient and machine parameters that should be monitored throughout the hemodialysis treatment (Box 34.3). The following is a summary of the parameters that are routinely measured; additional parameters may need to be assessed in individual patients. These parameters are recorded in the patient chart.

Blood pressure

Blood pressure may decrease for a variety of reasons, including acute decrease in effective circulating blood volume associated with filling the EC circuit with blood, inflammatory reactions associated with exposure of blood to the dialysis membrane, rapid ultrafiltration, excessive ultrafiltration, and bleeding from excessive anticoagulation or uremic thrombocytopathy. The patient's underlying disease can also lead to hypotension.

The frequency of blood pressure monitoring depends on the circumstances, and certainly patients with unstable or marginal blood pressure measurements or those developing clinical signs of hypotension should be monitored frequently. In our dialysis unit, blood pressure measurements generally are taken 15 and 30 minutes after starting the dialysis treatment and then every 30 minutes thereafter.

Coagulation

When blood is removed from the patient and circulated through the extracorporeal tubing and dialyzer, it usually clots within an hour in the absence of an anticoagulant. The vast majority of intermittent hemodialysis treatments are performed using heparin as the anticoagulant. The ACT is generally used to monitor heparin therapy. As previously mentioned, the ACT is assessed prior to starting treatment, and this value is used to determine the initial heparin dose. The ACT should be checked 30 minutes after starting dialysis to determine if a dose adjustment is necessary.[21] The normal range for ACT is 80 to 100 seconds in dogs and 100 seconds in cats (Poeppel and Bogue, unpublished data, Animal Medical Center, 1998). The target ACT during a dialysis treatment is 1.6 to 2 times normal.[4] If the ACT is in the target range and no dose adjustments are needed, it is monitored hourly thereafter. The ACT is measured 30 minutes after any dose adjustment. Although partial thromboplastin time evaluates the arm of the coagulation cascade affected by heparin, it has not been used clinically to monitor heparin therapy in dialysis patients.

For patients where systemic anticoagulation is contraindicated, regional citrate anticoagulation can be used. This involves infusing citrate into the blood as it is removed from the patient and simultaneously infusing calcium into the patient at a rate calculated to exactly chelate the citrate as it is returned to the patient. This process is more labor intensive than heparin anticoagulation and the infusion rates are not as clearly defined for veterinary patients as they are for heparin therapy, so citrate anticoagulation is not recommended for intermittent hemodialysis treatments unless necessary.

Regional citrate anticoagulation may become the preferred method of anticoagulation in continuous therapies because continuous systemic anticoagulation is more problematic than intermittent. Citrate anticoagulation is contraindicated in patients with severe liver failure due to their inability to metabolize citrate.[4]

Box 34.3 Parameters to monitor during dialysis

Recommended	Optional*
Blood pressure	Blood volume
Heart rate	Hematocrit (inline)
Ultrafiltration rate	Temperature
Blood flow/Access pressures	Oxygen saturation
Heparin rate	
Activated clotting time	
Adequacy	

*Based on patient status.

Access pressure and blood flows

The pressure transducers that attach to the blood cartridge allow the dialysis machines to determine pressure in the arterial and venous tubing segments. The dialysis technician should monitor these pressures throughout the treatment. The arterial access pressure is negative when the blood pump is running. The access pressure will be excessively negative if the arterial lumen of the dialysis catheter is functioning poorly. Causes of poor function include kinking, being lodged against the vessel wall, or partial occlusion by a thrombus. Venous access pressure is positive when the blood pump is running. This access pressure will be excessively positive if there is an obstruction to the return of blood to the patient. High venous access pressure could be due to kinking or thrombosis of the venous lumen of the dialysis catheter or a clot obstructing the filter in the venous chamber.

In addition, two specific values are routinely measured for each dialysis treatment. One is the maximum blood flow maintained during the treatment. If this value decreases over time, it may indicate impending catheter malfunction. The other value is the blood flow at a certain arterial access pressure, for example at −200 mm Hg. If the blood flow at this same pressure decreases over time, it may also indicate an impending problem with the catheter. Blood flow can be affected by other factors, such as the patient's blood pressure and intravascular volume, which must be taken into account when blood flows are being evaluated. These factors have usually stabilize within the first week of dialytic therapy.

Hematocrit

The patient's hematocrit is measured at the beginning and end of every dialysis treatment. An inline hematocrit monitor (Crit-Line, HemaMetrics, Kaysville, UT) records real-time hematocrit throughout the dialysis treatment. This information, although not essential, is very helpful in some cases. The hematocrit tends to drop at the beginning of the treatment because the patient's blood volume is diluted with the priming solution. Blood transfusions are sometimes administered during a dialysis treatment, so an inline monitor immediately displays the efficacy of the transfusion. Finally, if fluid therapy is required to maintain blood pressure during the dialysis treatment, the inline monitor provides information that helps the clinician avoid severe hemodilution.

Blood volume

Changes in blood volume during a dialysis treatment can be measured using the inline hematocrit monitor also. Presuming that the red blood cell mass remains constant (i.e., there is no ongoing bleeding or blood administration), any changes in the hematocrit reflect changes in plasma volume. An increase in hematocrit concentration indicates plasma volume removal (via ultrafiltration), whereas a decrease in hematocrit concentration would be expected if fluid is being administered at a rate exceeding fluid removal via ultrafiltration. A rapid decrease in intravascular volume may precipitate symptomatic hypotension. Generally it is not advisable to have more than a 10% decrease in blood volume within an hour.[3,4] Some of the newest dialysis machines include an integrated hematocrit monitor so that an external monitor is not necessary.

Oxygenation

It is not always necessary to measure oxygen saturation in a stable patient undergoing hemodialysis, but it is generally part of the overall treatment plan in the unstable patient or the patient with respiratory or cardiovascular compromise. It can be useful to measure oxygenation in patients receiving aggressive ultrafiltration because a decrease in oxygen saturation is often a precursor to a decrease in blood pressure.[3] An inline hematocrit monitor measures the oxygen saturation of the blood in the extracorporeal circuit, which in veterinary patients is central venous blood. This is an effective method of measuring changes in oxygen saturation that can adversely affect the patient's blood pressure. The inline monitor is convenient because the sensor is attached to the tubing and thus is not dislodged by patient movement.

Adequacy

The adequacy of dialysis treatments, meaning the amount of waste product that has been cleared from the patient, should be measured, if not for every dialysis treatment then on a routine basis (i.e., weekly). By tracking adequacy, the dialysis team is assured that the patient is receiving the prescribed dose of dialysis. A complete discussion of dialysis adequacy is beyond the scope of this chapter, so only the two most commonly used methods are briefly discussed here. More detailed discussions have been published for IHD.[3,22,23]

The most straightforward method of measuring adequacy is by calculating the urea reduction ratio (URR), which is calculated by subtracting the posttreatment blood urea nitrogen (BUN) from the pretreatment BUN and then dividing that value by the pretreatment BUN. The URR typically exceeds 90% except during the initial few dialysis treatments for each patient.

The most common measure of dialysis dose in human hemodialysis is Kt/V, in which K is a clearance constant of the dialyzer, t is time on dialysis, and V is volume of distribution.[24] The constant K for each dialyzer is calculated in vitro under specific conditions and is published on the package insert. The actual K during the treatment can be calculated using the blood flow and the simultaneous BUN of blood flowing into and out of the dialyzer. Most newer dialysis machines have a program that measures a treatment Kt/V, so this may become the most common measure of adequacy in veterinary medicine as well.

Other parameters

Any patient parameters that are monitored in the intensive care unit or patient ward should also be monitored during hemodialysis. Examples are continuous electrocardiogram or temperature monitoring, pulse oximetry for arterial oxygen saturation, and urine output.

Recordkeeping

Recordkeeping for a hemodialysis treatment should be thorough and descriptive. This entails documenting the dialysis prescription itself, a summary of what was accomplished during the treatment, patient or machine complications, all values obtained while monitoring the patient, and any medical treatments done on the patient during dialysis. As with any monitoring record, the best way to assure all parameters are recorded is to have a template for recording. This template can be a preprinted form or a computer database. It is essential that the dialysis technician performing the treatment maintain meticulous records to keep track of what parameters work best for a particular patient and to aid in troubleshooting if problems should arise.

Complications and special considerations

Patients with kidney failure severe enough to require hemodialysis are complex patients, and case management is rarely straightforward. Patients exhibit the usual manifestations of uremia commonly encountered in uremic patients managed with traditional medical therapies. Hemodialysis patients may also develop complications directly related to the dialytic therapy. Finally, the clinician may encounter long-term complications of uremia that are rarely seen because of limited patient survival time with traditional medical therapy of the end-stage renal failure patient. This section focuses mainly on complications directly related to dialysis therapy.

Technical complications

Technical complications due to machine errors or malfunctions are rare because of the number of redundant monitors and alarms built into modern hemodialysis machines. When they occur, they may range from mild to devastating problems. Complications related to the water treatment system include chemical or infectious contamination.[8,10] It is therefore essential to maintain and monitor the function of both the dialysis machine and the water treatment system to achieve peak performance. The operator must also have superb knowledge of the machines so as to be able to troubleshoot quickly during a dialysis treatment to prevent minor problems from escalating. The hemodialysis technician is generally responsible for maintaining the dialysis equipment and monitoring dialysis treatments.

Operator errors can also occur, and the number and severity depend on a variety of factors, including the training and experience of the operator, the work environment, and some patient factors. Again, it is important to have highly trained personnel to minimize these errors and their consequences.

Hypotension

A decrease in blood pressure is common at the start of a hemodialysis treatment.[13] The volume of blood required to fill the extracorporeal circuit in relationship to the patient's total blood volume can be considerable, up to 40% in smaller cats (Table 34.1). Priming the extracorporeal circuit with a colloid (i.e., 3% Dextran-70, or a 50:50 mixture of 0.9% NaCl and hetastarch) helps mitigate the drop in blood pressure in cats and small dogs but is not generally necessary for medium to large dogs (in which a saline prime suffices). Most patients are able to autoregulate and return blood pressure to almost baseline values within 30 to 60 minutes of the start of dialysis, but some cannot. These patients may require intervention if the blood pressure drops too low. The blood pressure generally returns to predialysis values when all of the patient's blood is returned at the end of the dialysis treatment.

Exposure of the blood to a bioincompatible dialyzer membrane can activate the complement and coagulation cascades, releasing several mediators that may cause hypotension.[25,26] Use of synthetic membranes can minimize this problem. Rapid ultrafiltration may lead to hypotension, if the rate of removal from the vascular compartment exceeds the capacity for refilling from the interstitial compartment. Monitoring blood volume (e.g., with an inline hematocrit monitor) may predict symptomatic hypotension, allowing intervention before hypotension occurs.[3,4] If hypotension develops, decreasing or stopping ultrafiltration (temporarily or for the duration of the treatment), small boluses of crystalloid or colloidal solutions, or use of pressor drugs may be used to correct the blood pressure.

Dialysis disequilibrium syndrome

Dialysis disequilibrium syndrome (DDS) is a syndrome induced by rapid, or highly efficient, dialysis in severely azotemic patients. The cause of this syndrome is not well described, but it results secondary to the development of cerebral edema induced by rapid changes in the osmolality of the blood.[3,4,27] It is most likely to occur during the first few dialysis treatments when uremia is more severe. However, DDS can occur at any time, even with chronic dialysis.

Clinical signs of DDS include agitation, disorientation, seizures, vomiting, coma, and death. Dogs usually have premonitory signs such as restlessness in a previously quiet dog. Cats frequently have no noticeable premonitory signs and may rapidly go from a normal appearance to a coma-like state. Dialysis disequilibrium syndrome may occur at any time during dialysis or up to 24 to 48 hours after dialysis.[3] Therefore, it is essential that patients be monitored for signs of DDS continually for a full day after each of the first few dialysis treatments. The signs of DDS may reverse entirely within a few hours, particularly if the signs are mild or treatment for DDS was started early. More severe signs may persist for up to 24 hours. Some patients do not regain consciousness or die acutely.

Treatment of DDS involves dissipating the blood-brain osmotic gradient by infusing osmoles into the bloodstream. Mannitol is the most commonly used treatment in veterinary hemodialysis.[3] Hypertonic saline has the same short-term effect as mannitol but creates an undesirable sodium load. Some dialysis machines have the capacity to increase the sodium concentration of the dialysate quickly, to cause rapid diffusion of sodium from dialysate into the bloodstream, having the same effect as an IV bolus of hypertonic saline.

Prevention of DDS is clearly desirable. Mannitol may be given prophylactically in high-risk patients such as severely uremic patients (BUN >150 mg/dL), small patients (<5 kg), or those with preexisting central nervous system disease. The dose is administered 30 to 45 minutes after the start of dialysis for the first one to three treatments.[3,15] Sodium profiling, in which the dialysate sodium is initially higher and gradually decreases during the treatment, is another preventive measure. Sodium profiling is a specific program set on the dialysis machine when prescribed.

Other preventive measures include decreasing the efficiency of hemodialysis during the first few treatments. Methods of accomplishing this goal include slowing blood flows, shortening treatment times, reversing the dialysate lines so dialysate flows concurrent to blood, and reversing the arterial and venous ports on the catheter to increase recirculation. Continuous therapies, with slower dialysate flow rates and generally slower blood flow rates, theoretically have a lower risk of inducing DDS.

Hemorrhage

Anticoagulation is necessary during hemodialysis, so a risk of hemorrhage is present. Mild forms may involve bleeding from the skin exit site of the dialysis catheter or other insertion sites. Internal bleeding, including bleeding from gastric ulceration, central nervous system hemorrhage, or massive pulmonary hemorrhage, have been encountered.[28] Discontinuation of the anticoagulant (usually heparin), administration of a reversal agent (i.e., protamine sulfate for heparin), and red cell or plasma transfusion may be required. Bleeding problems can be minimized by careful control of anticoagulation and minimizing sources of bleeding. It is best not to do any procedures, place catheters, or even pierce the skin in any manner immediately before or after a dialysis treatment.

To prevent or minimize hemorrhage after the hemodialysis treatment, heparin is stopped 30 minutes before the end of treatment. The patient should receive no needle sticks for 8 hours after the treatment. Even removal of a catheter can lead to excessive bleeding in a heparinized patient. All procedures such as thoracocentesis or feeding tube placement should be performed at least 8 hours after the dialysis treatment. Surgeries or more invasive procedures are best scheduled on nondialysis days. If the patient requires a treatment or procedure that could cause bleeding within the 8-hour period, a reversal agent (such as protamine sulfate) should be used.

Respiratory complications

Mild to severe hypoxemia is common during dialysis both in human and animal patients. Contact of blood with the dialyzer membrane activates the alternate complement pathway. This causes leukocyte and platelet aggregation in the pulmonary microvasculature that interferes with oxygen diffusion.[29] The maximal effect of this is seen within 30 to 60 minutes of the start of dialysis and resolves within 120 minutes after discontinuation of dialysis. Therefore, oxygen therapy that began during a dialysis treatment may need to be continued for a few hours after the treatment, but improvement is expected. Some patients come to dialysis with respiratory compromise from pulmonary edema or pleural effusion resulting from volume overload. Pulmonary hemorrhage is common in dogs with leptospirosis.[30]

Gastrointestinal complications

Anorexia, nausea, and vomiting are common complications of renal failure but also may be seen at the start of hemodialysis secondary to diversion of blood flow from the gastrointestinal tract caused by hypotension, bioincompatibility reactions to the membrane, or contaminants in the dialysate. Dialysis disequilibrium can also cause centrally mediated nausea and vomiting.[31] Using slow blood flow rates at the beginning of dialysis treatments with a gradual increase to the prescribed rate minimizes these signs and patient discomfort. It is not standard to fast a patient the morning of a hemodialysis treatment, but it is advisable to allow at least an hour between feeding and initiation of dialysis in case one of these complications arise. If the patient routinely vomits at the start of dialysis regardless of preventive measures, a morning fast may be considered.

Thrombosis

Catheter

Catheter thrombosis may be intraluminal or extraluminal. It can occur at any time but is uncommon within the first week after catheter placement unless there have been major problems with anticoagulation in that time period.[14] Intraluminal thrombosis can affect catheter flow when severe enough. Treatment options for intraluminal thrombosis are limited. Aggressive flushing of the affected lumen may restore blood flow but usually does not remove all remnants of thrombi. Mechanical disruption of thrombi by feeding a stylet into the lumen may be slightly more effective. Despite the ever-present risk of inducing significant or fatal thromboembolic complications with these maneuvers, rarely have we encountered clinically detected problems. A thrombolytic agent such as tissue plasminogen activator can be instilled in the catheter for a period of time. This seems to be effective in the short term, but treatment frequently needs to be repeated within a week (unpublished data, K. Poeppel, Animal Medical Center, 2008). Thrombolytic therapy should be initiated as soon as aggressive flushing is not effective so that thrombi do not continue to grow and completely obstruct the catheter. If these measures are unsuccessful, the affected catheter can be replaced as a last resort. A percutaneous catheter is relatively easy to replace over a guidewire with no or minimal sedation.[12,32] Replacement of a tunneled catheter requires heavy sedation or general anesthesia and is technically more difficult. Both techniques carry a risk of contamination of the new catheter if the exit site or tunnel are infected, and they are more likely to result in loss of the vessel. If the catheter cannot be replaced due to technical issues or other factors, a new catheter may be placed in the opposite jugular vein. Extraluminal thrombosis can be even more troublesome. A thrombus may be attached to the outside of the catheter, but it can act as a flap or ball valve that occludes catheter flow. Aggressive flushing may remove the thrombus if the attachment is weak. Thrombolytic therapy may not be very effective because it is hard to direct this therapy to an extraluminal thrombus. Systemic thrombolytic therapy can lead to uncontrollable hemorrhage.[5] Replacement of the affected catheter is the last option, which carries with it the risk that the thrombus will be stripped off the catheter during removal and enter the patient's circulation.

Systemic

Patients who have hemodialysis catheters in place for more than 2 weeks are at risk of developing a right atrial thrombus. Pulmonary thromboembolism from platelet aggregation or thrombus formation induced by the catheter can cause acute onset of mild to severe dyspnea during or between dialysis treatments.[4,13]

Prevention

Patients with indwelling hemodialysis catheters routinely receive low-dose aspirin therapy to prevent systemic thrombus formation. As previously mentioned, the catheter lumens are filled with an anticoagulant lock between dialysis treatments to prevent intraluminal thrombosis.

Infection

There are multiple potential sites of infection in the hemodialysis patient. Uremia decreases immune function, and indwelling catheters (vascular or urinary) and feeding tubes are potential portals of entry for bacteria.[33,34] Other open sites, such as surgical incisions or pressure sores, are possible entry sites for bacteria as well. Finally, the dialysis catheter and the extracorporeal circuit are potentially large sources of bacteria. If bacteria from any site enters the vascular system, they can then reach the dialysis catheter and adhere to it. Once bacteria adhere to the dialysis catheter, they can produce a biofilm that adheres to the walls of the catheter and protects the bacteria from removal or destruction. Then the only way to eliminate all bacteria is to remove the dialysis catheter.[5,14]

For this reason extra vigilance is required to prevent infections from developing in hemodialysis patients. All drugs and flushes given through any catheter should be freshly prepared (we prefer less than 24 hours old). Aseptic technique must be maintained for catheter placement, feeding tube placement, and other procedures. Urinary catheters are typically removed once hemodialysis has been initiated. Examination gloves are worn when setting up the dialysis machine, and examination gloves and a surgical mask are worn when accessing the dialysis catheter. Finally, as mentioned previously, only trained personnel should handle the dialysis catheter.

Edema

Volume overload may manifest as pulmonary edema, pleural effusion, ascites, and generalized peripheral edema. Ultrafiltration during dialysis and careful attention to fluid balance can help minimize this problem.[3,12] The problem may persist longer in anuric or oliguric patients than nonoliguric or polyuric patients. Facial, intermandibular, and forelimb edema may occur in dogs over time and can be severe. Edema in these specific locations may be an indication of partial cranial vena caval occlusion by the catheter itself or thrombosis or stenosis induced by the catheter.[5] In many dogs, hypoalbuminemia is a concurrent problem due to ongoing renal albumin loss, loss in the extracorporeal circuit, gastrointestinal loss, and suppressed synthesis due to systemic inflammation. Hypoalbuminemia can exacerbate edema formation.

Malnutrition

Malnutrition is common in uremic patients due to uremia-induced gastrointestinal complications and high metabolic needs associated with acute renal failure and other critical illness. Early and aggressive nutritional support is prudent. It is unclear how to determine the exact protein requirements of the acute renal failure patient.[35,36] Certain amino acids are lost during the dialysis treatment, particularly taurine and carnitine, so patients on long-term dialysis therapy should receive taurine and carnitine supplementation.[37]

Nausea, vomiting, and the dialysis treatments themselves can interfere with feedings, which adds to the problem of malnutrition. A feeding tube is often placed at the time of dialysis catheter placement to allow early nutritional support. Nausea and/or vomiting can often be alleviated by medications and control of uremia via hemodialysis. Patients do not need to be fasted before dialysis treatments, and feedings scheduled during dialysis should not be skipped unless necessary. If feedings have to be missed during a treatment, they can be supplemented when dialysis is complete.

Aluminum toxicity

Aluminum is used in many municipal water treatment plants as one stage of the water purification process. If the hemodialysis water treatment process is not sufficient, trace amounts of aluminum can appear in the dialysate. Aluminum-containing phosphate binders provide an additional and greater source of aluminum. Acute aluminum toxicity can occur if water treatment is inadequate, but it is generally encountered only after long-term exposure with chronic dialysis. Aluminum accumulation can lead to a microcytic, hypochromic anemia. Clinical signs associated with aluminum toxicity include neurologic or neuromuscular signs including mild weakness, paresis, dullness, obtundation, or coma. There have been two cases of hemodialysis-related aluminum toxicity reported in veterinary medicine.[38]

Anemia

Small amounts of blood are lost with each dialysis treatment, and this combined with any gastrointestinal losses and iron deficiency leads to anemia in almost all dialysis patients.[39] Patients receiving dialysis treatment for more than 2 to 3 weeks generally require iron supplementation and some erythropoietin hormone replacement therapy such as darbepoetin (Aranesp, Amgen, Thousand Oaks, CA).

Medication dosing

It is often necessary to adjust the dose and timing of medications given to a patient receiving hemodialysis. Many drugs are removed from the blood during dialysis, some to a significant degree.[40] For this reason, it is best to give all once-a-day medications in the evening. It also may be necessary to withhold a medication until after dialysis or to supplement the dose when dialysis is complete.[41] This may be particularly important when administering antibiotics, pain medications, cardiac medications, or antiseizure medications.

Patient care

The typical IHD treatment lasts from 4 to 5 hours, which means an animal is away from the patient care ward for a significant period of time. In addition to feedings and medication, therapies such as peripheral catheter care, wound management, turning, bathing, and physical therapy may be indicated during this time. Considerations must be made to determine if these therapies are safe to perform while the patient is undergoing hemodialysis.

During an IHD treatment, patients are essentially tethered to the hemodialysis machine because the blood lines of the EC circuit are attached to the dialysis catheter. The hemodialysis machine must remain connected to the incoming water source, so it is not freely mobile. This means the patients are not free to walk around to urinate, defecate, and exercise during the dialysis treatment, so it is beneficial to allow ambulatory patients time to walk outside or around a room before and after the treatment.

Patients are generally anticoagulated during an IHD treatment, so any therapies that have the potential to cause bleeding, such as wound debridement or nail trims, should be avoided. Peripheral catheter care should be avoided if there is a high probability that the catheter will be removed. Gentle wound cleaning and application of topical ointments is acceptable.

Patient temperament will dictate whether or not certain therapies, such as oral medication administration, can be performed. The dialysis catheter is unwrapped during hemodialysis, so any therapy that would cause the patient to struggle and possibly damage or remove the catheter must be done only after the catheter has been safely wrapped.

Finally, dialysis catheter flow can dictate how much the patient should be moved. A well-placed catheter in a medium to large patient often flows very well when the patient is in a variety of different positions. In this case, turning the patient, expressing the bladder, doing passive range-of-motion exercises, and any similar therapy is unlikely to pose problems while the patient is undergoing hemodialysis. Changes in intrathoracic pressure can affect catheter flow, so coupage is not recommended until after the treatment. Catheter flow problems can occur in any patient during any given treatment, so the hemodialysis technician often determines on a day-to-day basis how much to allow or prevent movement of a patient. There will be times when it is best to keep the patient very still throughout the entire hemodialysis treatment.

Outcomes

Overall, 40%–60% of veterinary patients with acute uremia treated with hemodialysis survive.[4] In recent studies, the reported survival rates for acute kidney injury (AKI) from infectious causes were 58%–100%.[42–44] Hemodynamic and metabolic causes of AKI had a 40%–72% survival rate.[44,45] Only 20%–40% of patients with AKI from toxic causes survive.[42,44] Of the patients receiving hemodialysis that do not survive, about half of those die or are euthanatized due to extrarenal conditions (e.g., pancreatitis, respiratory complications). About a third of nonsurvivors are euthanized due to failure of recovery of renal function. Ongoing uremic signs, dialysis complications, and unknown causes

> **Box 34.4** Summary
>
> - Hemodialysis is a method of clearing the blood of uremic toxins when the kidneys are not functioning properly.
> - Patients with acute renal injury, chronic renal disease, toxicities, and fluid or electrolyte imbalances are candidates for hemodialysis.
> - Hemodialysis requires equipment that must be maintained and operated by highly trained personnel.
> - Patients receiving hemodialysis can experience complications directly related to treatment in addition to complications related to their disease.
> - Overall survival of hemodialysis patients is 40%–60%.

account for the remaining patient deaths. As with patients treated medically, approximately half of hemodialysis patients regain normal renal function (defined by normal serum creatinine concentration) and half have persistent chronic kidney disease.[4]

Summary

Box 34.4 provides a summary of the chapter. Intermittent hemodialysis is a highly advanced therapy used primarily to treat patients with kidney disease. For patients with acute kidney injury, IHD is initiated when medical management fails, and it is a means of stabilizing the patient long enough to allow for renal repair. For patients with chronic kidney failure, IHD is a method of extending the animal's life. Intermittent hemodialysis can also be used to remove excess fluids or electrolytes, restore acid–base balance, or treat toxicities and drug overdoses.

Overall survival rate of animals undergoing IHD for acute kidney failure is 40%–60%. The patient population in this case generally has a prognosis of 0% survival without some type of renal replacement therapy. Hemodialysis is therefore a viable alternative to euthanasia for veterinary patients.

References

1. Acierno MJ. Continuous renal replacement therapy. In: Bartges JW, Polzin DJ, eds. Nephrology and Urology of Small Animals. West Sussex, UK: Wiley-Blackwell; 2011, pp. 286–292.
2. Acierno MJ, Maeckelbergh V. Continuous renal replacement therapy. Compend Contin Educ Pract Vet 2008;30:264–280.
3. Cowgill LD, Francey T. Hemodialysis. In: DiBartola SP, ed. Fluid, Electrolyte, and Acid-Base Disorders in Small Animal Practice. 3rd ed. Philadelphia, PA: Saunders Elsevier; 2006;650–677.
4. Langston CE. Hemodialysis. In: Bonagura JD, Twedt DC, eds. Current Veterinary Therapy. Vol 14. Philadelphia, PA: Saunders; 2009:896–890.

5. Fischer JR, Pantaleo V, Francey T, et al. Veterinary hemodialysis: advances in management and technology. Vet Clin North Am Small Anim Pract 2004;34:935–967.

6. Zawada ET. Indications for dialysis. In: Daugirdas JT, Ing TS, eds. Handbook of Dialysis. 2nd ed. Boston: Little, Brown; 1994:3–9.

7. Kitiyakara C, Winchester JF. Use of dialytic techniques for drug overdose. In: Nissenson AR, Fine RN, eds. Dialysis Therapy. 3rd ed. Philadelphia, PA: Hanley & Belfus; 2002:523–528.

8. Van Stone JC. Hemodialysis apparatus. In: Daugirdas JT, Ing TS, eds. Handbook of Dialysis. 2nd ed. Boston: Little, Brown; 1994:30–52.

9. Ward RA. Water treatment for in-center hemodialysis including verification of water quality and disinfection. In: Nissenson AR, Fine RN, eds. Dialysis Therapy. 3rd ed. Philadelphia, PA: Hanley & Belfus; 2002:55–60.

10. Ward RA. Water treatment equipment for in-center hemodialysis: including verification of water quality and disinfection. In: Nissenson AR, Fine RN, eds. Handbook of Dialysis Therapy. 4th ed. Philadelphia, PA: Saunders Elsevier; 2008:143–156.

11. Hoenich NA, Ronco C. Biocompatibility of dialysis membranes. In: Nissenson AR, Fine RN, eds. Handbook of Dialysis Therapy. 4th ed. Philadelphia, PA: Saunders Elsevier; 2008:279–294.

12. Langston CE. Hemodialysis. In: Bartges JW, Polzin DJ, eds. Nephrology and Urology of Small Animals. West Sussex, UK: Wiley-Blackwell; 2011:255–285.

13. Cowgill LD, Elliott DA. Hemodialysis. In: DiBartola SP, ed. Fluid Therapy in Small Animal Practice. 2nd ed. Philadelphia, PA: WB Saunders; 2000:528–547.

14. White JJ, Oliver MJ, Schwab SJ. Temporary vascular access for hemodialysis. In: Nissenson AR, Fine RN, eds. Handbook of Dialysis Therapy. 4th ed. Philadelphia, PA: Saunders Elsevier; 2008:23–36.

15. Langston CE. Hemodialysis. In: Bartges JW, Polzin DJ, eds. Nephrology and Urology of Small Animals. West Sussex, UK: Wiley-Blackwell; 2010:255–285.

16. Grudzinski L, Quinan P, Kwok S, et al. Sodium citrate 4% locking solution for central venous dialysis catheters—an effective, more cost-efficient alternative to heparin. Nephrol Dial Transplant 2007;22:471–476.

17. Shanks RMQ, Sargent JL, Martinez RM, et al. Catheter lock solutions influence staphylococcal biofilm formation on abiotic surfaces. Nephrol Dial Transplant 2006;21:2247–2255.

18. Lok CE, Appleton D, Bhola C, et al. Trisodium citrate 4%—an alternative to heparin capping of haemodialysis catheters. Nephrol Dial Transplant 2007;22:477–483.

19. Polaschegg HD, Sodemann K. Risks related to catheter locking solutions containing concentrated citrate. Nephrol Dial Transplant 2003;18:2688–2690.

20. Hoenich NA, Ronco C. Selecting a dialyzer: technical and clinical considerations In: Nissenson AR, Fine RN, eds. Handbook of Dialysis Therapy. 4th ed. Philadelphia, PA: Saunders Elsevier; 2008:263–278.

21. Groman RP. Anticoagulation in hemodialysis. Proceedings of the Advanced Renal Therapies Symposium 2008: 50–52.

22. Francey T. Dialysis Quantification and Adequacy. Proceedings of the Advanced Renal Therapies Symposium 2006; CD-ROM.

23. Palevsky PM. Intensity of continuous renal replacement therapy in acute kidney injury. Semin Dialysis 2009;22:151–154.

24. Gotch F. Urea kinetic modeling for guiding hemodialysis therapy in adults In: Nissenson AR, Fine RN, eds. Handbook of Dialysis Therapy. 4th ed. Philadelphia, PA: Saunders Elsevier; 2008:297–309.

25. Jaber BL, Pereira BJG. Biocompatibility of hemodialysis membranes. In: Pereira BJG, Sayegh MH, Blake P, eds. Chronic Kidney Disease, Dialysis, & Transplantation. 2nd ed. Philadelphia, PA: Elsevier Saunders; 2005:363–387.

26. Cheung AK. Hemodialysis and hemofiltration. In: Greenberg A, ed. Primer on Kidney Diseases. 4th ed. Philadelphia, PA: Elsevier Saunders; 2005:464–476.

27. Kotanko P, Levin NW. Common clinical problems during hemodialysis. In: Nissenson AR, Fine RN, eds. Handbook of Dialysis Therapy. 4th ed. Philadelphia, PA: Saunders Elsevier; 2008:407–417.

28. Langston CE. Hemodialysis in dogs and cats. Compend Contin Educ Pract Vet 2002;24:540–549.

29. DeBroe ME. Haemodialysis-induced hypoxaemia. Nephrol Dial Transplant 1994;9:173–175.

30. Greenlee JJ, Bolin CA, Alt DP, et al. Clinical and pathologic comparison of acute leptospirosis in dogs caused by two strains of Leptospira kirschneri serovar grippotyphosa. Am J Vet Res 2004;65:1100–1107.

31. Cowgill LD, Langston CE. Role of hemodialysis in the management of dogs and cats with renal failure. Vet Clin North Am Small Anim Pract 1996;26:1347–1378.

32. Mokrzycki MH, Lok CE. Traditional and non-traditional strategies to optimize catheter function: go with more flow. Kidney Int 2010;78:1218–1231.

33. Chew DJ. Fluid therapy during intrinsic renal failure. In: DiBartola SP, ed. Fluid Therapy in Small Animal Practice. 2nd ed. Philadelphia, PA: WB Saunders; 2000:410–427.

34. Vanholder R, Glorieux G. Uremic toxicity. In: Pereira BJG, Sayegh MH, Blake P, eds. Chronic Kidney Disease, Dialysis, & Transplantation. 2nd ed. Philadelphia, PA: Elsevier Saunders; 2005:87–121.

35. Druml W. Nutritional support in patients with acute renal failure. In: Molitoris BA, Finn WF, eds. Acute Renal Failure: A Companion to Brenner and Rector's The Kidney. Philadelphia, PA: WB Saunders; 2001:465–489.

36. Cowgill LD, Francey T. Acute uremia. In: Ettinger SJ, Feldman EC, eds. Textbook of Veterinary Internal Medicine. 6th ed. Philadelphia, PA: Elsevier Saunders; 2005:1731–1751.

37. Fischer JR. Chronic hemodialysis and its complications. Proceedings of the Advanced Renal Therapies Symposium 2006; CD-ROM.

38. Segev G, Bandt C, Francey T, et al. Aluminum toxicity following administration of aluminum-based phosphate binders in two dogs with renal failure. J Vet Intern Med 2008;22:1432–1435.

39. Paganini EP. Hematologic abnormalities. In: Daugirdas JT, Ing TS, eds. Handbook of Dialysis. 2nd ed. Boston: Little, Brown; 1994:445–468.

40. Karriker MJ. Drug dosing in renal failure and the dialysis patient. Proceedings of the Advanced Renal Therapies Symposium 2006.

41. Langston CE. Special problems in dialysis patients. Proceedings of the Advanced Renal Therapies Symposium 2004.

42. Langston CE, Cowgill LD, Spano JA. Applications and outcome of hemodialysis in cats: a review of 29 cases. J Vet Intern Med 1997;11:348–355.

43. Francey T, Cowgill LD. Use of hemodialysis for the management of ARF in the dog: 124 cases (1990–2001) [abstract]. J Vet Intern Med 2002;16:352.

44. Pantaleo V, Francey T, Fischer JR, et al. Application of hemodialysis for the management of acute uremia in cats: 119 cases (1993–2003) [abstract]. J Vet Intern Med 2004;18:418.

45. Fischer JR, Pantaleo V, Francey T, et al. Clinical and clinicopathological features of cats with acute ureteral obstruction managed with hemodialysis between 1993 and 2004: a review of 50 cases [abstract]. 14th ECVIM-CA Congress, Barcelona, Spain. 2004.

35

Peritoneal evaluation

Linda Barton and Amanda Adams

Dogs and cats with abnormalities of the peritoneal cavity, often characterized by abdominal pain, represent a common emergency presentation. In general, abdominal pain is caused by capsular stretch of solid organs or distention, traction, or forceful contractions of hollow organs. Additionally, inflammation and ischemia cause the production of proteinases and other vasoactive substances that can stimulate abdominal nerve endings. Specific disorders that commonly present as an "acute abdomen" are listed in Table 35.1.

Diagnostic procedures used to evaluate the peritoneal cavity include physical examination with thorough abdominal palpation, abdominal imaging (radiographs, ultrasound, computed tomography), and evaluation of peritoneal fluid obtained by abdominocentesis, diagnostic peritoneal lavage, or from a previously placed abdominal drain. Additionally, intra-abdominal pressure can be monitored in patients at risk for the development of intra-abdominal hypertension.

Physical examination

Physical examination with an emphasis on careful abdominal palpation is the initial step in evaluation of the peritoneal cavity. The abdomen should be examined systematically starting with the spinal column and abdominal wall before evaluation of the deeper structures. Direct palpation of the spine and body wall will aid in the differentiation of back and/or muscle pain from conditions affecting the peritoneal structures. The integrity of the abdominal wall should be carefully evaluated to rule out penetrating injuries. Abnormalities in the contour of the abdomen suggest distention and/or enlargement of intra-abdominal structures or accumulation of fluid and/or air in the peritoneal cavity.

Gentle persistent digital pressure should be used to evaluate the size and position of organs and for the presence of abdominal masses. Pain should be noted and localized. Pain localized to the upper right quadrant suggests a pancreatic, duodenal, or pyloric abnormality. Caudal abdominal pain is associated with prostatic disease, pyometra, uterine torsion, cryptorchid testicle torsion, and abnormalities of the urinary bladder and urethra. Diffuse abdominal pain suggests peritonitis or involvement of a significant portion of the intestinal tract.

Percussion, striking the body wall with short sharp blows and noting the tone of the resultant sound, aids in the detection of a fluid wave or gas accumulation with the peritoneal cavity or within a distended hollow viscus. Abdominal auscultation has been recommended to detect hypermotility or ileus but lacks reliability.

A rectal examination should be done to evaluate for the presence of abnormal stool, especially melena or frank blood. In male dogs, the prostate gland should be assessed for size, symmetry, and presence or absence of pain.

Abdominal imaging

Survey abdominal radiographs should be obtained in any patient presenting with abdominal pain. The abdominal and extraabdominal structures should be evaluated in a systematic fashion. Deviation from normal density, shape, size, and/or location of abdominal organs may provide clues to abnormalities in the peritoneal

Advanced Monitoring and Procedures for Small Animal Emergency and Critical Care, First Edition. Edited by Jamie M. Burkitt Creedon, Harold Davis.

© 2012 John Wiley & Sons, Inc. Published 2012 by John Wiley & Sons, Inc.

Table 35.1. Differential diagnosis for acute abdomen

Digestive system
Gastric dilatation +/− volvulus
Gastrointestinal perforation (secondary to foreign body, neoplasia, or dehiscence)
Gastroenteritis (dietary indiscretion, viral, toxic, bacterial)
Intestinal obstruction (secondary to foreign body, intussusception, neoplasia)
Gastrointestinal ulceration
Constipation/obstipation
Pancreatitis +/− pancreatic abscess

Hepatobiliary System
Acute hepatitis (toxic, infectious)
Cholangiohepatitis
Cholecystitis
Hepatic abscess
Biliary obstruction

Genitourinary System
Pyometra
Metritis
Uterine torsion
Ovarian cyst
Ovarian neoplasia
Prostatitis/prostatic abscess
Prostatic cyst
Prostatic neoplasia
Testicular torsion
Acute nephrosis
Acute nephritis-pyelonephritis
Urinary calculi (renal, ureteral, cystic, urethral)
Ureteral obstruction (neoplasia, stricture, calculi)
Urethral obstruction (neoplasia, stricture, calculi)
Renal neoplasia

Hematopoietic System
Splenic torsion
Splenic mass
Splenic rupture (trauma, neoplasia)

Peritoneum, Mesentery, and Abdominal Wall
Peritonitis (septic, chemical secondary to urine or bile leakage)
Mesenteric lymphadenopathy/lymphadenitis
Mesenteric volvulus
Adhesions with organ entrapment
Strangulated abdominal wall hernias

Extra-abdominal
Intervertebral disk disease
Discospondylitis
Myositis
Steatitis

cavity. Radiographs are most valuable in detecting distention of a hollow viscus and are less useful in detecting solid organ injury or dysfunction. The retroperitoneal space should also be carefully evaluated. Decreased visualization of the kidneys, distention, or a streaky appearance of the retroperitoneal space is seen with abnormal fluid accumulation (urine, blood) or a space-occupying mass in the retroperitoneum. Differentials for decreased detail in the peritoneal space include free abdominal fluid, lack of abdominal fat, and carcinomatosis.

Intestinal gas patterns should be evaluated. Ileus, resulting in the accumulation of fluid and gas within the intestine, may be seen with a number of conditions. Segmental ileus supports a diagnosis of intestinal obstruction. In dogs, bowel obstruction is considered likely if the internal diameter of a small bowel segment is four times or more the width of a rib, two times or more the width of a vertebral body, or if the ratio of the diameter of the bowel to the height of the narrowest point of the body of L5 is >1.6.[1] In cats, a ratio of the maximum diameter of small intestine to the height of the cranial endplate of the second lumbar vertebra ≥2.5 was most often associated with intestinal obstruction.[2] Additionally, all small bowel loops should be of a similar diameter. The presence of "two populations" of small bowel, where one segment is 50% larger than the other segment of small bowel, strongly suggests bowel obstruction secondary to a foreign body, neoplasia, or intussusception. Generalized small bowel distention can be associated with a distal bowel obstruction or with a number of nonobstructive conditions that cause generalized ileus. An upper gastrointestinal (GI) positive contrast study may be needed to make a definitive diagnosis of GI obstruction in a patient with generalized ileus. Barium sulfate provides the highest diagnostic quality contrast study, but because of its propensity to cause severe intraperitoneal inflammation and granuloma formation if leakage occurs, its use is controversial when gastric or intestinal perforation is suspected or surgery is anticipated.[3] Iodine-based contrast media (Hypaque [sodium diatrizoate, Nycomed, Princeton, NJ], Gastrografin [meglumine diatrizoate, Bracco Diagnostics, Princeton, NJ]) can be used; however, the quality of the study is reduced. When performing a contrast study, it is important to use an adequate amount of the contrast agent. Low-volume administration causes inadequate filling and a nondiagnostic study. The recommended dose of barium (60% wt/wt) is 5–10 mL/kg for large dogs and 10–12 mL/kg for small dogs and cats given per os or by orogastric tube.[1]

The radiograph should be examined for the presence of free gas in the peritoneal cavity. In the standard lateral view, free gas can be most easily detected between the stomach or liver and the diaphragm. The sensitivity for detecting free gas can be increased by positioning the patient in left lateral recumbency and taking a horizontal beam radiograph focused at the least dependent area of the abdomen. The presence of free peritoneal gas in a patient with no previous open abdominocentesis or recent abdominal surgery indicates a penetrating injury of the abdominal wall, rupture of a hollow viscus, or the presence of gas-producing microorganisms in the peritoneal cavity and is considered a surgical emergency.

Abdominal ultrasound

Abdominal ultrasound can be used to further evaluate the peritoneal structures. Ultrasound provides valuable information about the abdominal viscera, lymph nodes, and vascular structures. Ultrasound is superior to radiography to evaluate solid organ structure and abnormalities in blood flow to organs (for instance, as seen with splenic torsion). In the emergency setting, abdominal ultrasound is often most useful to aid in the detection and collection of small volumes of free abdominal fluid. It is important to remember that diagnostic accuracy is operator dependent. However, it has been shown that clinicians with limited ultrasonographic experience can reliably detect free abdominal fluid using a simple protocol involving assessment at four defined sites in the abdomen.[4]

Abdominal fluid analysis

The detection, collection, and analysis of free abdominal fluid are extremely useful in peritoneal evaluation.

Abdominocentesis

Blind abdominocentesis, also known as abdominal paracentesis, is a simple way to obtain an abdominal fluid sample for evaluation. The procedure is performed with manual restraint, eliminating the need for sedation or anesthesia. The veterinary team should prepare for the procedure and have all necessary equipment in place before attempting abdominocentesis. The procedure is detailed in Protocol 35.1. Either a closed needle or open needle technique can be used. The open needle technique reduces the chance of omentum or viscera occluding the needle, but it may introduce free air into the abdominal cavity. Ideally an open abdominocentesis should be performed after abdominal radiographs have been obtained to prevent misinterpretation of iatrogenically introduced abdominal free air. There are minimal associated risks, but risks may be increased in patients with a coagulopathy, or with marked organomegaly or distention of an abdominal viscus. The procedure is

simple and specific but not sensitive. It has been estimated that 5–6 mL of fluid per kilogram body weight within the abdominal cavity is required to obtain fluid by blind centesis.[5] Ultrasound guidance increases the sensitivity of the procedure by allowing the clinician to view and aspirate small accumulations of fluid.

Diagnostic peritoneal lavage

If no fluid can be obtained by abdominocentesis and abdominal pathology is highly suspected, diagnostic peritoneal lavage (DPL) can be performed to obtain abdominal fluid samples for evaluation. The technique is described in Protocol 35.2. The procedure is performed with local anesthesia with or without sedation. General anesthesia should be avoided; turgid abdominal musculature will facilitate catheter placement. There are a number of different commercially available multifenestrated catheters that can be used including peritoneal dialysis catheters, chest tubes, or abdominal drainage catheters. Alternatively, readily available over-the-needle catheters, red rubber catheters, or large single-lumen intravenous catheters can be used if additional fenestrations are added. Figure 35.1 illustrates the technique for creating additional fenestrations.

Generally diagnostic peritoneal lavage is reserved for patients where free abdominal fluid is strongly suspected but cannot be recovered by other methods. In our experience this technique is seldom required in patients that have been adequately fluid resuscitated if ultrasound is available to enhance the detection of small fluid pockets. The patient's urinary bladder should be emptied either by voiding or manual expression to avoid accidental puncture. Other complications include omental obstruction of the DPL, catheter fenestrations, and incomplete fluid retrieval. Contraindications for DPL include pregnancy, marked organomegaly, cardiovascular or respiratory compromise that can be exacerbated by large-volume lavage, diaphragmatic hernia, previous celiotomy, or patients suspected to have abdominal adhesions.

Fluid analysis/evaluation

Gross, cytologic, and biochemical evaluation of peritoneal fluid collected either by centesis or peritoneal lavage can provide important diagnostic clues in the patient with abdominal pain, especially if peritonitis is suspected. Evaluated parameters and their clinical associations are summarized in Table 35.2.

The peritoneal fluid sample should be separated into one tube containing ethylenediaminetetraacetic acid (EDTA) to prevent clotting and another tube containing no additives. The additive-free tube will be used for

Protocol 35.1 Abdominocentesis

Items Required
- Clippers
- Surgical scrub, alcohol, and gauze sponges for skin preparation
- Sterile gloves
- Blood tube with EDTA additive (lavender-top tube)
- Blood tube with no additive (red-top tube)
- Needles: 20 or 22 gauge, 1.5–2 inches long. Needle size should be based on the patient's size and body wall thickness. Alternately, an over-the-needle catheter of similar size may be used.
- Several ≥3 cc syringes for aspiration of sample
- Ultrasound for guidance: optional

Procedure
1. Gather supplies.
2. Place patient in left lateral recumbency or in a standing position. Positioning in left lateral recumbency may be most effective to avoid inadvertent puncture of the spleen
3. Clip and scrub the ventral abdomen.
4. Perform hand hygiene and done sterile gloves.
5. Insert the needle or catheter just cranial or caudal to the umbilicus 1–2 cm to the right of midline.
    a. Closed technique: The needle or catheter is attached to a syringe before penetration into the abdominal cavity.
    b. Open technique: An unattached needle or catheter is inserted into the abdominal cavity.
6. Once the bevel of the needle has been advanced through the skin and body wall (depth of needle insertion is relative to patient size), pull back on the plunger of the syringe to apply suction if using the closed technique. If using the open technique, observe for a flash of fluid in the hub of the needle.
    a. If using an over-the-needle catheter, after the catheter is inserted into the abdominal cavity, remove the stylet and collect the sample.
7. If blood is aspirated, the needle should be removed from the abdomen and the sample placed in a red-top tube and observed for clot formation.
    a. Blood from inadvertent laceration of a vessel or organ will clot.
    b. Hemorrhagic free abdominal fluid will not clot.
8. Allow fluid to drip into sterile collection tubes or apply gentle suction with a syringe to collect sample. The fluid should be collected into sterile tubes for further analysis.
9. If no fluid is retrieved:
    a. Gently twist the needle within the abdomen and if needed advance the needle.
    b. Consider four quadrant centesis, ultrasound guidance, or diagnostic peritoneal lavage.

Four Quadrant Centesis Technique:
1. Place patient in left lateral recumbency.
2. Clip and scrub the ventral abdomen 4 inches cranially and caudally from the umbilicus and laterally to the mammary chain on either side. Perform hand hygiene and don sterile gloves
3. Using the umbilicus as a center point, divide the abdomen into four quadrants and sample the right cranial, left cranial, right caudal, and left caudal quadrants as directed in the abdominocentesis protocol.
    a. Use caution to avoid superficial and deep epigastric vessels that lie parallel and in the vicinity of the mammary chain.
4. Continue collection of sample as described in the Abdominocentesis protocol.

biochemistries and cultures because EDTA is bacteriostatic. To prevent contamination by sample handling, any microbial cultures should be performed aseptically, immediately after fluid sampling. Slides should be made soon after fluid collection to prevent degeneration of cells in the fluid.

Color and clarity should be noted before additional sample handling occurs. Peritoneal fluid color can range from colorless to red tinged, red, white, yellow, brown, and anything in between. Fluid color is not specific for, but could indicate an organ system as the primary cause for the effusion. Red-colored fluid suggests intra-abdominal hemorrhage. Green-tinged fluid is seen with bile leakage. Clarity of the fluid is noted as clear to slightly turbid or turbid. The degree of turbidity indicates the presence of cellular material and other particulate matter. Foul-smelling fluid is associated with anaerobic infection.

Protocol 35.2 Diagnostic peritoneal lavage

Items Required
- Clippers
- Surgical scrub, alcohol, and gauze sponges for skin preparation
- Sterile gloves
- Sterile drape
- 2% lidocaine
- No. 11 scalpel blade
- Sterile 10- to 14-gauge catheter for abdominal drainage
    - Various "tubes" can be used including multifenestrated peritoneal dialysis catheters, chest tubes, or abdominal drainage catheters. Alternatively, over-the-needle catheters, red rubber catheters, or large single-lumen intravenous catheters can be used if additional fenestrations are added. See Figure 35.1.
- Warm, sterile 0.9% sodium chloride fluid (attached to intravenous [IV] drip set)
- Sterile collection system (IV drip set, three-way stopcock, collection bag)

Procedure
1. Gather supplies.
2. Ensure that the urinary bladder is empty (manual expression or catheterization).
3. Place patient in left lateral recumbency.
4. Clip and surgically prepare a wide area around the umbilicus.
5. Place drape fenestration centered at the umbilicus.
6. Instill local anesthetic in the skin and down to the peritoneum.
7. Catheter placement will vary depending on the type of drainage catheter used.
    a. Trochar type catheter (or over-the-needle catheter):
        i. Create a small stab incision (no larger than the diameter of the catheter) in the skin 2–3 cm caudal to the umbilicus and 1–2 cm lateral to midline.
        ii. Introduce the trochar and catheter through the body wall at a 45° angle directed caudal dorsally (toward the coxofemoral joint).
        iii. Advance the catheter off the trochar ensuring that all of the fenestrations are within the peritoneal cavity.
    b. Catheters may also be introduced by the Seldinger and peel-away methods (See Chapter 4, Catheterization of the Venous Compartment, for more information).
8. If no fluid is obtained when the catheter is placed, the abdomen is lavaged by instillation of 20 mL/kg of warm 0.9% sodium chloride through the catheter and into the peritoneal cavity.
    a. While the fluid is being infused, the patient should be monitored carefully for signs of respiratory distress and/or discomfort.
9. Clamp the infusion set.
10. The patient's abdomen should be gently agitated to assure movement of the saline within the cavity.
11. After several minutes, open the infusion set and allow the fluid to drain through the catheter by gravity into a sterile collection bag. Collect samples in sterile empty and EDTA-containing tubes for evaluation.
12. If the catheter is being used for continuous abdominal drainage (such as may be the case for a uroabdomen), the catheter should be sutured in place and covered with a sterile dressing. See Chapter 55, Care of Indwelling Device Insertion Sites, for more information.

Peritoneal fluid packed cell volume (PCV) and total protein should be measured. A PCV >5% in centesis fluid is suspicious for abdominal hemorrhage. Following peritoneal lavage, the amount of blood in the abdomen can be estimated by the following formula[5]:

$$x = L \times V/P - L, \tag{35.1}$$

where x = amount of blood in the abdominal cavity; L = PCV of the returned lavage fluid; V = volume of lavage fluid infused into the abdominal cavity; and P = PCV of the peripheral blood before intravenous infusion of fluids.

Normal peritoneal total protein should be <2.5 g/dL.

Total nucleated cell counts can be estimated by running the sample through the in-house complete blood count machine, or estimated microscopically by trained personnel. See Chapter 52, Cytology, for more information. Samples that are clear or slightly turbid may have a low cellularity and thus may require

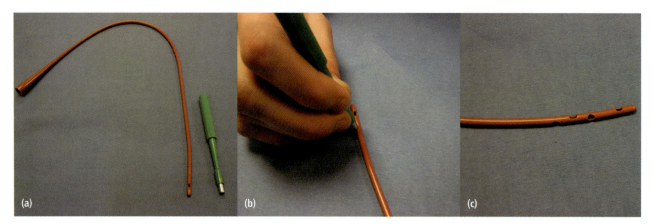

Figure 35.1 How to create additional fenestrations in a silicone or rubber tube. (A) Pick the appropriate tube size for your patient (10–14 gauge for DPL). Obtain a sterile 2- or 4-mm biopsy punch. (B) Lay the tube flat on a sterile field and press the punch firmly onto the very edge of the tube. Roll the tube a third turn, and make another fenestration at least ¾ inches above the last fenestration. (C) The DPL catheter following the addition of the fenestrations.

   In the authors' experience, tube integrity becomes compromised (kinking, breaking) when fenestrations are larger than a third of the circumference of the tube or if the fenestrations are made too close together. Personnel should practice this technique prior to the procedure or have an additional tube available in the event a mistake is made.

Table 35.2. Abdominal fluid analysis

Parameter	Interpretation
PCV (free fluid) >5%	Significant intra-abdominal hemorrhage
WBC >5000/mm³, neutrophils	Peritoneal inflammation
Intracellular bacteria	Bacterial peritonitis
Degenerative neutrophils	Suppurative peritonitis
Plant/vegetable fibers	Gastrointestinal leakage
Neoplastic cells	Intra-abdominal neoplasia
Creatinine	Fluid: serum ratio >2:1 indicates uroabdomen
Potassium	Fluid: serum ratio >1.4:1 indicates uroabdomen
Bilirubin	More than peripheral blood indicates bile peritonitis
Amylase	More than peripheral blood indicates pancreatitis
Glucose	≥20 mg/dL lower than in peripheral blood suggests septic peritonitis
Lactate	≥2.5 mmol/L higher than in peripheral blood suggests septic peritonitis in dogs

centrifugation before microscopic evaluation. Normal abdominal fluid contains <1000 nucleated cells/mm³. Cytology includes evaluation for degenerate or toxic neutrophils, intracellular bacteria, neoplastic cells, bile stain or crystals and any other abnormalities. An elevated white blood cell (WBC) count (>5000 nucleated cells/mm³) indicates an inflammatory process. Increased numbers of neutrophils and degenerate neutrophils support a diagnosis of peritonitis. Intracellular bacteria can be seen with septic peritonitis. Leukocyte morphology and the presence of bacteria are more important than absolute leukocyte numbers. Identification of a large number of bacteria with no WBC is seen with inadvertent aspiration of the GI tract. Gram staining of

septic effusions will assist with empirical selection of antibiotics.

   Based on the patient's physical examination, history, and suspected disease, specific chemistry analysis on the sample may be indicated. In most cases, the peritoneal chemistries are compared with a simultaneously collected peripheral blood sample. Abdominal fluid bilirubin higher than the bilirubin in the peripheral blood is diagnostic for bile peritonitis.[6] The gold standard for differentiating septic peritoneal effusions from inflammatory nonseptic processes such as pancreatitis is the identification of intracellular bacteria in the fluid. Intracellular bacteria are not always seen in patients with septic peritonitis, especially if the patient has been receiving antibiotic therapy or there is a walled-off process such as a hepatic abscess. Comparison of blood glucose in the peripheral blood and abdominal effusion can be helpful in differentiating septic for nonseptic effusions. Peripheral blood glucose ≥20 mg/dL higher than peritoneal fluid glucose has been shown to be highly predictive of septic peritonitis in dogs and cats.[7]

Similarly, lactate concentrations greater in abdominal fluid than in peripheral blood (blood-to-peritoneal fluid lactate concentration difference less than −2.0 mmol/L) is predictive of septic peritonitis in the dog, but not in the cat.[7,8]

Intra-abdominal pressure monitoring

Abdominal pressure can be measured in patients at risk of intra-abdominal hypertension (IAH). Elevated pressure in the abdomen is referred to as IAH, whereas pathologic derangements that occur as a result of IAH are referred to as the abdominal compartment syndrome (ACS). IAH is caused by tissue edema or free fluid collecting in the abdominal cavity. Elevated pressure in the closed abdominal space can compromise perfusion to the abdominal organs and adversely affect outcome.

IAP is most commonly measured in veterinary patients via a catheter placed in the urinary bladder (Fig. 35.2). The technique is relatively easily and described in Protocol 35.3. Measurements can be taken in either lateral or sternal recumbency, but the position should be consistent with serial measurements as IAP is affected by body position. The measured value has also shown to be affected by the volume of saline instilled into the urinary bladder, body condition, and by the presence of abdominal wall or detrusor muscle contractions.

Reported normal intra-abdominal pressure in dogs is 0–7.5 cm H_2O.[9] Rader and Johnson reported a median IAP in healthy cats of 7 cm H_2O but showed that patient struggling significantly increased the measured value.[10] Severe elevations in IAP can result in decreased renal blood flow, decrease in celiac and portal blood flow, diminished ventilatory function, and decreased cardiac output and stroke volume. In humans, consensus guidelines for management of IAH and ACS have been developed. Similar recommendations do not exist for veterinary patients.

Summary

Abnormalities of the peritoneal cavity and intra-abdominal structures are common in veterinary patients. Physical examination, abdominal imaging, evaluation of peritoneal fluid, and monitoring of intra-abdominal

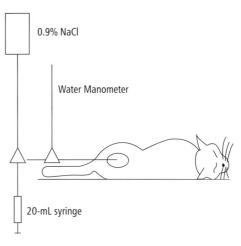

Figure 35.2 Measurement of intra-abdominal pressure in a cat. Reprinted from the Journal of Veterinary Emergency and Critical Care 2011;20(4); p. 388.

Protocol 35.3 Abdominal pressure measurement

Items Required
- Sterile gloves
- Foley urethral catheter
- Sterile urine collection system
- Two three-way stopcocks
- Water manometer
- 35- to 60-mL syringe
- Sterile saline
- Intravenous (IV) administration set

Procedure
1. Gather supplies.
2. Perform hand hygiene and don sterile gloves.
3. A Foley catheter should be aseptically placed with the catheter tip located just inside the trigone of the urinary bladder and connected to a sterile urine collection system, with two three-way stopcocks incorporated into the collection system.
4. Attach a water manometer to the first upright stopcock.
5. Attach the syringe and IV fluid bag to the second stopcock for filling the manometer and infusion of the bladder.
6. Place the patient in lateral or sternal recumbency.
7. Empty the urinary bladder.
8. Instill 0.5–1.0 mL/kg of sterile saline into the urinary bladder.
9. The manometer should be zeroed to the patient's midline and filled with sterile saline.
10. Close the stopcock to the fluid source to allow the meniscus in the manometer to equilibrate to the pressure within the urinary bladder.
11. The measurement should be taken 30–60 seconds after instillation of the saline into the bladder to allow for detrusor muscle relaxation and in the absence of active abdominal contractions.

pressure are essential components of peritoneal evaluation.

References

1. Mathews K, Halling K, Nykamp S. Acute abdomen. In: Mathews K, ed. Veterinary Emergency Critical Care Manual. 2nd ed. Guelph, Ontario, Canada: LifeLearn; 2006:26–27.
2. Adams WM, Sisterman LA, Klauer JM, et al. Association of intestinal disorders in cats with findings of abdominal radiography. J Am Vet Med Assoc 2010;236:880–886.
3. Riedesel RA. The small bowel. In: Thrall DE, ed. Textbook of Veterinary Diagnostic Radiology. 4th ed. Philadelphia, PA: Saunders; 2002:641–642.
4. Boysen S, Rozanski EA, Tidwell ES, et al. Evaluation of a focused assessment with sonography for trauma protocol to detect free abdominal fluid in dogs involved in motor vehicle accidents. J Am Vet Med Assoc 2004;225:1198–1204.
5. Fossum TW. Surgery of the abdominal cavity. In: Fossum TW, ed. Small Animal Surgery. 3th ed. St. Louis, MO: Mosby; 2007: 332–335.
6. Ludwig LL, McLoughin MA, Graves TK, Crisp MS. Surgical treatment of bile peritonitis in 24 dogs and 2 cats: a retrospective study (1987–1994). Vet Surg 1997;26:90–98.
7. Bonczynski JJ, Ludwig LL, Barton LJ, et al. Comparison of peritoneal fluid and peripheral blood pH, bicarbonate, glucose, and lactate concentration as a diagnostic tool for septic peritonitis in dogs and cats. Vet Surg 2001;32:161–6.
8. Levin GM, Bonczynski JJ, Ludwig LL, et al. Lactate as a diagnostic test for septic peritoneal effusions in dogs and cats. J Am Anim Hosp Assoc 2004;40;364–371.
9. Conzemius MG, Sammarco DE, Holt DE, et al. Clinical determination of preoperative and postoperative intra-abdominal pressure in dogs. Vet Surg 1995;24(3):195–201.
10. Rader RA, Johnson JA. Determination of normal intra-abdominal pressure using urinary bladder catheterization in clinically healthy cats. J Vet Emerg Crit Care 2010;20(4):386–392.

36

Specialized gastrointestinal techniques

Lisa Smart

Gastric intubation

The two basic goals for intubation of the gastrointestinal tract are removing the contents or administering medications. Although many of these techniques are used routinely in veterinary emergency medicine, all of these procedures have the potential for complication, and the veterinarian should always ask if the benefits of the procedure outweigh the risks.

Orogastric intubation

Orogastric intubation involves inserting a tube through the oral cavity down to the stomach.

Indications

The indications for orogastric intubation include decompression of gastric dilation, removal of ingested toxins, and administration of medications. Possible complications include damage to, or perforation of, the esophagus or gastric wall, regurgitation and aspiration of gastric contents, and complications related to sedation or general anesthesia. The risk of complications related to sedation or anesthesia may be increased if the animal is showing clinical signs of intoxication. Although in my experience, these complications are uncommon if the correct technique is followed, the true incidence of these complications has not been reported in the veterinary literature.

Technique

Determine if the patient is an appropriate candidate for decompression and whether sedation or anesthesia is required for that particular patient. Choose a single-lumen orogastric tube (OGT) with the largest diameter that will reasonably fit within the patient's esophagus (see Fig. 36.1). Measure the length of tube that will be required to pass into the stomach, which is the distance from the nares to the last rib (see Fig. 36.2). Mark the tube with either tape or black marker.

Unroll approximately 30 cm from a roll of adhesive bandage material, such as Elastoplast (Beiersdorf, Hamburg, Germany), and leave this attached to the roll. With someone restraining the dog's head from behind, place the roll of bandage into the dog's mouth so that the hole in the roll faces the pharynx, hold the mouth closed, then wrap the free end of the bandage around the dog's muzzle to hold the roll in place. If the dog starts to regurgitate or vomit, the roll can be removed quickly out of the mouth rostrally without the need to unwrap the bandage from around the muzzle. Lubricate the end of the OGT and slowly feed the tube through the hole in the middle of the bandage roll (see Fig. 36.3). Aim to push the tube through the animal's left dorsal aspect of the pharynx to avoid intubating the larynx. Try to advance the tube when the dog swallows. Leave the other (distal) end of the tube below the level of the animal in a collection container, so that any fluid within the tube will start draining by gravity. Location of the tube within the esophagus must be confirmed by one or more of the techniques described (see Box 36.1). If there remains any doubt as to whether the tube is in the trachea as opposed to the esophagus, remove the tube and start again.

Once the location of the tube within the esophagus is confirmed, advance the tube gently up to the mark previously made on the tube (see Fig. 36.4). In the case of

Advanced Monitoring and Procedures for Small Animal Emergency and Critical Care, First Edition. Edited by Jamie M. Burkitt Creedon, Harold Davis.
© 2012 John Wiley & Sons, Inc. Published 2012 by John Wiley & Sons, Inc.

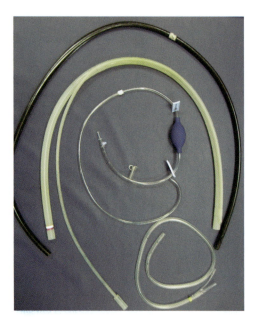

Figure 36.1 Various tubes used in gastrointestinal techniques. Large black tube: Simple orogastric tube stained with activated charcoal. Large white tube: Double-lumen orogastric tube used for gastric lavage. Small bottom tube: Orogastric tube with fenestrations and intraluminal side port for flushing; suitable for smaller patients or for enemas. Clear tube with blue bulb: Enema tube with insufflation bulb to aid flushing.

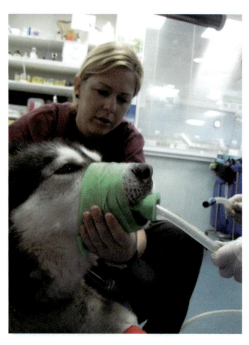

Figure 36.3 Advancement of an orogastric tube through the middle of a bandage roll. The bandage roll serves as a mouth gag and allows gastric intubation in a conscious dog.

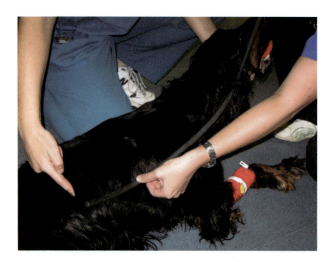

Figure 36.2 Measurement of the length of tube needed for orogastric intubation in this dog. Note the distal end of the tube is measured to the final rib.

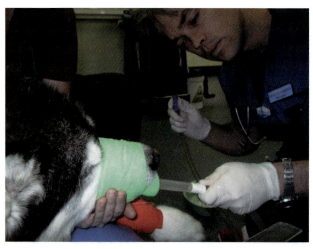

Figure 36.4 Orogastric intubation. Once the tube has been advanced to the mark made on the tube (white tape), the person is then listening for gas escaping from the tube to indicate that it is in the stomach.

gastric dilation and volvulus (GDV), if there is resistance, apply gentle pressure with a twisting motion to aid entry through the cardia. If there is still resistance, sterile gauze may be placed over the end of the tube, to protect the operator's mouth from contamination, and a small amount of air blown into the tube while gently

advancing it. If the tube still cannot be passed into the stomach in a patient with GDV, then the stomach should be trocarized percutaneously to relieve tension on the fundus (see later for technique); the tube will often then pass more easily. If there is no flow into the collection container below the level of the patient, gentle ballotte-

Box 36.1 Techniques to distinguish between intubation of the esophagus/stomach and trachea

Indications that the tube is within the esophagus or stomach:
- Seeing the presence of esophageal fluid or gastric reflux fluid in the tube. The fluid should look like saliva as well as any other substances such as ingesta, bile pigment, or blood.
- Palpation of the tube on the left side of the neck, separate from the trachea, confirms its placement in the esophagus.
- Either a rush of gas or gastric fluid will confirm its location in the stomach. Air blown into the tube by the operator with simultaneous stethoscope auscultation of borborygmus within the stomach also confirms its location.

Indications that the tube is within the trachea:
- If humidified air is seen within the tube during each exhalation, the tube may be within the trachea.
- Coughing, although the absence of coughing does not confirm placement within the esophagus.
- The tracheal rings may be felt as vibrations along the tube if the tube is passed down the trachea.
- A capnometer may be placed at the end of the tube; the presence of an increase in carbon dioxide while the dog exhales confirms its location in the trachea.
- If placing a nasogastric tube, intubation of the trachea is likely if a copious amount of air is aspirated via syringe from the end of the tube.

ment of the abdomen may help to dislodge an obstruction. If there is still no flow, 10–60 mL of water can be infused into the tube to flush any obstruction (see Gastric Lavage technique).

Before removing the tube, tightly kink the tube 10–15 cm from the operator's end. Hold the tube firmly in this kinked position while removing the tube to prevent fluid leaking out as it is removed from the esophagus and pharynx. The technique used for orogastric intubation is also described in Protocol 36.1.

Nasogastric intubation for gastric decompression

Nasogastric intubation involves placing a tube through the nasal cavity down into the stomach.

Indications

Nasogastric intubation may be useful in patients that are experiencing significant discomfort due to gastric dilation (GD), secondary to either aerophagia or gastric fluid accumulation. This technique is not appropriate

Protocol 36.1 Orogastric intubation

Items Required
- Sedation or general anesthetic supplies with appropriate monitors, as indicated
- OGT appropriate for patient size
- Adhesive medical tape or dark marking pen
- Roll of adhesive bandaging material
- One tube of aqueous lubricant
- Collection container for gastric material
- Trocarization materials, if GDV
- Assistants: at least one

Procedure
1. Collect necessary supplies.
2. Measure the length of tube from the nares to the last rib. Mark the tube with either tape or black marker.
3. Unroll approximately 30 cm from a roll of adhesive bandage material and leave this attached to the roll.
4. Assistant restrains the dog's head from behind. Decompressor places the bandage roll into the dog's mouth so that the hole in the roll faces the pharynx.
5. Hold the mouth closed around the bandage roll and wrap the free end of the bandage around the muzzle.
6. If the dog starts to regurgitate or vomit, remove the roll quickly from the mouth rostrally.
7. Lubricate the OGT end and slowly feed the tube through the hole in the middle of the bandage roll. Advance the tube through the animal's left dorsal pharynx to avoid the larynx. Try to advance the tube when the dog swallows. Leave the other (distal) end of the tube below the level of the animal in a collection container.
8. Confirm location of the tube within the esophagus. If there remains any doubt as to whether the tube is in the trachea, remove the tube and start again.
9. Once the location of the tube within the esophagus is confirmed, advance the tube gently to the mark previously made on the tube. In the case of GDV, if there is resistance, apply gentle pressure with a twisting motion to aid entry through the cardia.
10. If the tube still cannot be passed into the stomach in a patient with GDV, consider percutaneous gastric trocarization to relieve tension on the fundus; the tube will often then pass more easily. If there is no flow into the collection container below the level of the patient, gentle ballottement of the abdomen may help to dislodge an obstruction. If there is still no flow, 10–60 mL of water can be infused into the tube to flush any obstruction.
11. Before removing the tube, tightly kink the tube 10–15 cm from the operator's end. Hold the tube firmly in this kinked position while removing the tube to minimize fluid leakage into the airways as it is removed.

Box 36.2 Nasogastric intubation for gastric decompression

Indications

Gastric dilation caused by aerophagia or gastric stasis *and* one of the following:
- Increased work of breathing
- Frequent regurgitation
- Signs of nausea, such as hypersalivation and frequent swallowing
- Signs of abdominal pain on palpation
- Intra-abdominal pressure >20 cm H_2O with no other underlying cause

Contraindications
- Respiratory distress, whereby the stress of placing an NGT may worsen the patient's condition
- Cats with aerophagia
- Coagulopathy
- Thrombocytopenia (<50,000/μL)

---

for the management of engorgement (see later). Placement of a nasogastric tube (NGT) in cats for aerophagia is not recommended because stress will usually exacerbate the cause of aerophagia. However, if an NGT is already in place for enteral nutrition, it may be used for gas evacuation in the cat. Discretion should be used as to whether or not the patient will benefit from NGT placement for the purpose of gastric decompression, and the procedure should be aborted if the patient shows signs of respiratory distress during the procedure. See Box 36.2 for a list of indications and contraindications.

For the patient with GD secondary to gastric stasis, intermittent emptying of stomach contents every 6–8 hours via a NGT may decrease the incidence of vomiting and abdominal discomfort. Gastric pH may also be monitored by this procedure to evaluate the efficacy of antacid therapy, and the NGT may be used for enteral feeding (see Chapter 40, Assisted Enteral Feeding). Removal of large amounts of gastric fluid may contribute to fluid and electrolyte losses; therefore monitoring of serum electrolytes and acid base status is recommended in these patients. It is unknown whether the presence of a NGT through the lower esophageal sphincter promotes reflux of gastric contents into the esophagus.

Technique

The technique for placing an NGT has been covered elsewhere (see Chapter 40, Assisted Enteral Feeding). The NGT can be used in conscious animals; however,

sedation should be used in most cases of gaseous GD because placement of the NGT can be stressful and exacerbate aerophagia. Once the NGT is in place, gentle suction should be applied to evacuate air or fluid until negative pressure is reached. Blockages of the NGT with food material or thick saliva may impede evacuation; therefore, intermittent flushing of the NGT with 3–5 mL of water or air may be necessary. Record volumes of fluid removed so that fluid balance of the patient can be monitored.

Considerations for the GDV patient

Risk factors for, presentation of and management of shock in the patient with GDV have been reviewed elsewhere.[1,2] Diagnosis of GDV may be confirmed by the presence of a dorsally displaced pylorus on a right lateral abdominal radiograph.[3]

Analgesia/sedation

Moderate to severe vasoconstrictive shock in animals with GDV is due to lack of venous return from the caudal half of the body, leading to decreased cardiac output and organ ischemia, including the myocardium. Therefore shock fluid therapy is a priority in these patients. Analgesia should also be given as soon as possible, not only for the patient's well-being but also to aid orogastric intubation by providing sedation. Suitable analgesics to give during the fluid resuscitation and decompression phase of managing GDV include pure μ-opioid agonists such as morphine, oxymorphone, hydromorphone, and methadone. Partial μ-agonists, such as buprenorphine, may also be used but may not provide adequate analgesia. Nonsteroidal anti-inflammatory drugs and corticosteroids should not be used in GDV patients due to adverse effects such as decreased gastric perfusion and decreased renal blood flow.

To facilitate orogastric intubation, additional sedation may be given, although it is usually not needed. A combination of opioids and benzodiazepines, such as diazepam or midazolam, usually suffices. Indicators of perfusion, such as heart rate, capillary refill time, mucous membrane color and femoral pulse quality, should be monitored during sedation and procedures that follow. There is an increased risk of ventricular arrhythmias due to decreased myocardial perfusion;[4,5] therefore, an electrocardiogram should be performed if an irregular heart rhythm is detected. Although these dysrhythmias do not usually require treatment, presurgical ventricular arrhythmias are associated with gastric necrosis and increased mortality.[6,7] However, most dysrhythmias in

GDV patients occur after surgery, and one study showed that the presence of arrhythmias during hospitalization was not associated with outcome.[8] The patient's stomach should be decompressed by either orogastric intubation or trocarization (see later) before general anesthesia is induced.

Trocarization

Gastric trocarization, also referred to as gastrocentesis or gastric needle decompression, is often required in the patient with GDV because orogastric intubation is difficult or impossible in the presence of severe gastric distention (see technique for orogastric intubation). Gastric trocarization often decreases the time to gastric decompression and therefore may decrease the risk of gastric necrosis. The risk of gastric perforation due to trocarization is small, and studies that include trocarization as a part of the gastric decompression protocol do not report the presence of gastric perforation on exploratory laparotomy.[7–11] One study used trocarization alone for presurgical decompression, without orogastric intubation, and reported a low overall mortality rate of 10%.[7]

Technique for trocarization

Choose a tympanic area on the lateral abdomen, which is usually the left dorsolateral abdomen just caudal to the last rib. Clip the area and prepare aseptically. Perform hand hygiene and don sterile gloves. Insert a 16-gauge over-the-needle catheter at a right angle to the abdominal wall, with the bevel facing up, into the abdomen. Once gas flow is heard or gastric fluid is seen in the hub, advance the catheter off the stylet into the abdomen up to the hub of the catheter. Remove the stylet. Hold the catheter in place with a sterile hand and allow the gas to passively escape until the abdomen becomes flaccid or noticeably reduced in size (see Fig. 36.5). If the catheter becomes occluded, it may be withdrawn slowly from the abdomen until gas flow resumes or the catheter comes out. Never advance the catheter back into the abdomen. Do not ballot the abdomen with catheters in place because it may dislodge them from the stomach and contaminate the abdomen. If the flow of gas from the first catheter is insufficient, a second catheter may be placed near the first using the same technique. Once the abdomen has reduced in size, orogastric intubation may be attempted again in a gentle manner to fully evacuate the stomach. Any catheters used for trocarization should be removed before repeat orogastric intubation. Detailed instructions for gastric trocarization are also available in Protocol 36.2.

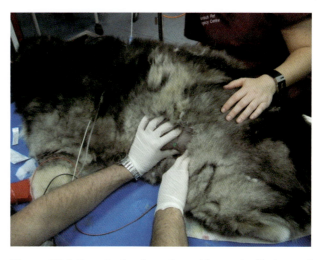

Figure 36.5 Trocarization in a dog with gastric dilation and volvulus. An 18-gauge catheter (note green hub) has been placed in the region of most tympany and is facilitating gas escape from the stomach.

Conservative management of GDV

There is a low chance of a good long-term outcome after decompression only for a GDV patient. Funquist and Garmer[12] first described conservative therapy as a means of spontaneous repositioning of GDV. Their protocol consisted of initial decompression, including trocarization and orogastric intubation. The dog was hospitalized for a minimum of 12 hours, and decompression was performed every 1–2 hours. Using this protocol, 10 of 14 dogs survived. Of these 10 dogs, 4 had surgery within 16 days, 3 had a repeat GDV in 3 months, and 3 were symptom free at 3–4 months. In a subsequent study,[13] spontaneous repositioning occurred in 11 of 21 dogs that received decompression (orogastric intubation and trocarization). Two different sized gastric tubes, one reinforced with a guidewire, were used simultaneously to fully evacuate the stomach. Of the 11 dogs, 3 died within 3 days, all with evidence of gastric necrosis on necropsy. Follow-up was available for 6 of the 8 dogs that survived the initial GDV; 4 of these dogs had repeat GDV within 7 months. The same author also described a technique for active nonsurgical repositioning using a stomach tube with an inflatable balloon on the end and fluoroscopy. Reposition was possible in all animals but outcome was unavailable.

A retrospective study from 1985 to 1989 included 103 GDV cases that received decompression only.[14] Sixty-six percent survived initial treatment, and 99% of these dogs had recurrence within 1 year. A more recent study[11] included 134 cases of GDV, of which 33 received conservative management only, as spontaneous repositioning after decompression was confirmed by abdominal

Protocol 36.2 Gastric trocarization

Items Required
- Clippers with clean blade
- Surgical scrub
- Long 16-gauge over-the-needle catheter
- Sterile gloves

Procedure
1. Collect necessary supplies.
2. Choose a tympanic area on the lateral abdomen, which is usually the left dorsolateral abdomen just caudal to the last rib.
3. Clip the area and prepare aseptically.
4. Perform hand hygiene and don sterile gloves.
5. Insert a 16-gauge over-the-needle catheter at a right angle to the abdominal wall, with the bevel facing up, into the abdomen. Once gas flow is heard or gastric fluid is seen in the hub, advance the catheter off the stylet up to the hub of the catheter. Remove the stylet.
6. Hold the catheter in place with a sterile hand and allow the gas to passively escape until the abdomen becomes flaccid or noticeably reduced in size.
7. If the catheter becomes occluded, it may be withdrawn slowly from the abdomen until gas flow resumes or the catheter comes out. Never advance the catheter back into the abdomen. Do not ballot the abdomen with catheters in place because it may dislodge them from the stomach and contaminate the abdomen.
8. If the flow of gas from the first catheter is insufficient, a second catheter may be placed near the first using the same technique.
9. Once the abdomen has reduced in size, orogastric intubation may be attempted again. Any catheters used for trocarization should be removed before repeat orogastric intubation.

radiography. Within an 8-month period, 25 dogs had a recurrent GDV (2 died and 6 had recurrent GDV within 2 days of the first GDV event), giving a recurrence rate of 81.8%. Given this information, although repositioning of the torsed stomach is possible with decompression only, recurrence is likely if gastropexy is not performed. Also, if there is gastric necrosis present and only conservative therapy is provided, the patient is likely to suffer a painful demise. Conservative treatment should only be undertaken for GD in the absence of volvulus; however, gastropexy should still be considered in breeds at high risk of subsequent GDV. Immediate surgical intervention of GDV after decompression is recommended to improve the chance of survival.

Considerations for engorgement

Engorgement with subsequent GD is a normal occurrence for carnivores because they are designed to eat large amounts in one sitting. However, cases of engorgement associated with clinical signs are usually secondary to ingestion of large amounts of dry commercial dog food, which absorbs fluid and slowly expands in the stomach, leading to gross distension of the stomach and considerable abdominal pain. A diagnosis of engorgement is confirmed by evidence of a dilated ingesta-filled stomach in its correct anatomic position on a right lateral abdominal radiograph. There have been no studies published assessing the efficacies of various treatment options for engorgement; therefore the following recommendation is based on my clinical experience. Cases of engorgement that do not have signs of obstructive shock can be treated with intravenous fluid therapy to maintain hydration and analgesia. Tachycardia is usually present in these patients, which resolves with analgesia. The risk of gastric rupture with this method of conservative management is low. Gastric lavage is rarely successful because the OGT becomes obstructed with food material, and the patient has an increased risk of complications, such as aspiration, if sedation is performed. Emesis is not indicated, as gastric contraction against the bulk of dry food may lead to gastric mucosal tear. Aspiration is also a risk after emesis. If the animal does have signs of obstructive shock (poor venous return to the right side of the heart due to compression of the abdominal veins as a result of gastric dilation), then aggressive shock fluid therapy should be followed by either gentle gastric lavage (see later) or gastrotomy. Gastrotomy is also indicated if the dog has ingested a substance that has solidified, such as polyurethane adhesive (Gorilla Glue, Gorilla Glue Inc., Ohio), which does not have a chance of passing through the intestinal tract.

Gastrointestinal decontamination

Gastrointestinal decontamination (GID) for ingested toxins includes emesis, gastric lavage, whole bowel irrigation (WBI), enema, and activated charcoal administration. In human medicine, the routine use of GID has become controversial due to a lack of evidence that GID has a significant impact on patient outcome, except for specific indications addressed later.[15–17] Often the time between ingestion and GID being performed in human emergency departments is beyond the time at which GID may be useful. Despite the American Academy of Clinical Toxicology concluding that no method of GID should be performed routinely in the management of the poisoned patient, its widespread use has continued at the hospital level.[15] No studies in veterinary medicine have been conducted to assess whether or not GID changes patient outcome for routine poisoning cases; however, it still remains as the current recommendation for ingested toxins within certain guidelines.[18–20] Veterinary poisoning cases differ from human cases in that there may be a large volume of toxin within the gastrointestinal tract, and the time to presentation may be shorter; therefore there still remains a role for GID in veterinary medicine, despite the lack of scientific evidence that it has an impact on outcome. Clinicians should ask themselves these three questions before performing GID, according to the "gastrointestinal decontamination triangle" published by Bailey[21]:

1. Is the ingested toxin likely to cause significant effects?
2. Is GID likely to change outcome?
3. Do the risks of GID outweigh the potential benefits in this particular patient?

Indications and technique for emesis have been covered elsewhere[18–20] and are not addressed in this textbook.

Gastric lavage

Gastric lavage (GL) involves orogastric intubation and removal of gastric contents. In clinical studies in human medicine, GL has shown no clear benefit over activated charcoal administration alone.[15,16] However, there still remain some indications for this procedure in veterinary medicine.

Indications

GL is indicated for intoxication cases where the amount of toxin ingested is potentially harmful, it was ingested within 1 hour of performing GL, and emesis cannot be achieved due to altered mentation or other neurologic signs (see Box 36.3). If the patient has already vomited after ingestion of the toxin, GL is unlikely to recover a significant amount of toxin. One exception is where there has been a large amount ingested, such as in snail pellet ingestion.

The risks of GL include those associated with general anesthesia, aspiration, and gastrointestinal tract trauma. The incidence of esophageal or gastric perforation secondary to GL is unknown in veterinary medicine but rarely occurs in human medicine,[16] and the same is likely true for veterinary patients. It is not necessary to perform GL in a case of food engorgement (see Considerations for Engorgement). It is also contraindicated to perform GL for animals that have ingested caustic or volatile substances, due to the risk of esophageal reflux, and

---

> **Box 36.3** Gastric decontamination procedures
>
> **Gastric lavage**
>
> **Indications:**
> - Toxin ingested within 1–2 hours and emesis contraindicated
> - Large volume of ingested toxin, such as snail bait pellets
>
> **Contraindications:**
> - Food engorgement
> - Ingestion of caustic or volatile substances
> - Ingestion of a small number of tablets or capsules
>
> **Nasogastric intubation**
>
> **Indications:**
> - Large volume of liquid toxin
> - Ingestion of caustic substances (in conjunction with endoscopy)
>
> **Contraindications:**
> - Respiratory distress, whereby the stress of placing an NGT may worsen the patient's condition
> - Cats with aerophagia
> - Coagulopathy
> - Thrombocytopenia (<50,000/μL)

---

subsequent esophageal damage and aspiration. These patients also have an increased risk of esophageal and gastric perforation.

If the animal has ingested a small volume of toxin, such as a small number of tablets or capsules, then GL is unlikely to be rewarding, and activated charcoal administration alone should be considered instead.

Technique

Refer to the protocol for orogastric intubation for insertion and removal of the OGT. The patient must always be orotracheally intubated with an appropriately inflated cuff and placed in lateral recumbency before lavage is performed. With the OGT in place, use room temperature water to lavage the stomach by use of a siphon or stomach pump. Although it is stated as common practice[18–20] to use approximately 5–10 mL/kg of water for each cycle, more is usually needed to lavage the stomach adequately, and I commonly use up to 20–30 mL/kg per cycle to achieve mild gastric distension on abdominal palpation. After instilling a volume of water, allow the effluent to passively drain, aided by gentle ballottement of the abdomen. A double-lumen tube can also be used to aid continuous drainage of the stomach

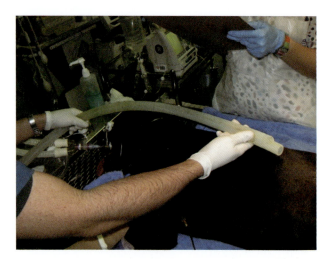

Figure 36.6 A double-bore tube used for gastric lavage, with ingress (smaller bore) and egress (larger bore) ports. The tube is being measured to the last rib to determine the length needed for gastric intubation.

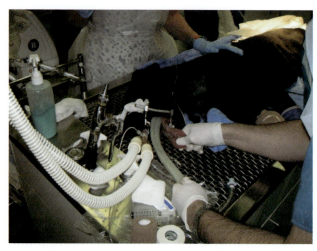

Figure 36.7 Insertion of a double-bore orogastric tube for gastric lavage.

while flushing (see Figs. 36.1, 36.6, 36.7, and 36.8). Never attach a hose to the tube to instill water or attach suction to the end to empty the stomach. This may cause trauma to the gastric wall. It is useful to record the volume of the effluent water to monitor the degree of water ingestion and avoid hyponatremia. Check that the cuff of the endotracheal tube is still adequately inflated, and then shift the patient into the other lateral recumbency. Again check the endotracheal tube position and cuff inflation. Repeat the lavage as above.

If activated charcoal administration is indicated, it may be instilled in the stomach before removal of the tube; however, be careful not to significantly distend the stomach because this leads to increased risk of aspiration during anesthetic recovery. It seems reasonable to limit the dose of activated charcoal to 2–3 mL/kg while under anesthesia. Kink the tube when removing. Keep the patient tracheally intubated with an inflated cuff until it is able to maintain sternal recumbency and is swallowing. This may reduce the risk of aspiration. It is not advised to delay extubation in cats due to risk of laryngospasm; therefore, activated charcoal should either not be given after lavage or the dose reduced. The technique for gastric lavage is described in detail in Protocol 36.3.

Nasogastric intubation for decontamination

Nasogastric intubation (NGI) may be useful for removal of large volumes of liquid toxin in which emesis is contraindicated (see Box 36.3). It will only be useful within 30 minutes of ingestion unless delayed gastric emptying

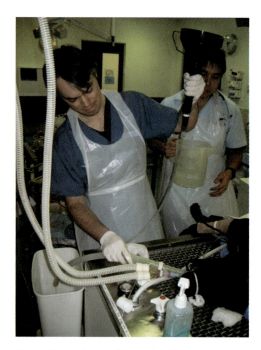

Figure 36.8 Gastric lavage for snail pellet ingestion. A double-bore tube is being used. A funnel (black) is attached to the ingress tube while water flows out of the stomach through the egress tube into a receptacle (white).

is present. The NGT can then be used for activated charcoal administration (see later).

In humans with caustic substance ingestion, endoscopy for identification of perforations and placement of an NGT is a part of routine management because the NGT reduces the incidence of esophageal stricture

Protocol 36.3 Gastric lavage

Items Required
- All equipment for orogastric intubation
- Siphon or stomach pump
- Room temperature water
- Cuffed endotracheal tube of appropriate size
- Examination gloves and other supplies to keep operator clean
- All anesthetic supplies, including appropriate monitoring tools

Procedure
1. Collect necessary supplies.
2. Anesthetize and orotracheally intubate the patient with an appropriately inflated cuff. Place patient in lateral recumbency before lavage is performed.
3. Please refer to Protocol 36.1 for orogastric intubation for instructions on insertion and removal of the OGT.
4. With the OGT in place, use room temperature water to lavage the stomach by use of a siphon or stomach pump. Use a minimum of 5–10 mL/kg of water for each cycle, up to 20–30 mL/kg per cycle, to achieve mild gastric distention on abdominal palpation.
5. After instilling a volume of water, allow effluent to passively drain, aided by gentle ballottement of the abdomen.
6. Record the volume of infused and effluent water to monitor the degree of water ingestion and avoid hyponatremia.
7. Check that the cuff of the endotracheal tube is still adequately inflated, and then shift the patient into the other lateral recumbency.
8. Recheck the endotracheal tube position and cuff seal.
9. Repeat the lavage as above.
10. If activated charcoal administration is indicated, instill before removal of the tube, taking care not to significantly distend the stomach.
11. Kink the tube when removing.
12. Keep the patient tracheally intubated with an inflated cuff until it is able to maintain sternal recumbency and is swallowing.

development and allows enteral nutrition.[22;23] The presence of an NGT through the lower esophageal sphincter does not appear to increase complications related to esophageal ulceration in humans, likely due to the small bore of the tube. The NGT may also aid in dilutional therapy of the caustic substance if the animal will not drink water or milk, by instilling small amounts down the NGT. This is in contrast to gastric lavage, which, as stated previously, is contraindicated in caustic substance ingestion.

Activated charcoal administration

Indications

The indications for activated charcoal administration have been covered elsewhere.[20] The absorption of many ingested toxins is decreased by activated charcoal if the charcoal is given within 2 hours of toxin ingestion. Activated charcoal may be beneficial greater than 2 hours postingestion for toxins that undergo enterohepatic recirculation or for delayed release capsules.

Contraindications of activated charcoal administration include oral administration in patients with abnormal mentation, hydrocarbon ingestion, and gastrointestinal tract perforation.

Techniques

Voluntary consumption

Some dogs, especially puppies, will drink activated charcoal suspension if it is mixed with canned commercial food or water. Often, though, they will not consume the required dose and one of the other techniques here may need to be used.

Syringe feeding

Animals may be restrained and force-fed activated charcoal with a syringe. The risks include undue stress and aspiration, especially if the solution is administered with pressure. The solution is given by dribbling small amounts in the commissure of the animal's mouth and allowing them time to swallow. Gloves and gowns will need to be worn as it becomes quite messy. Another technique for larger dogs is to place the sleeve of a disposable gown over the dog's head, allowing only the nose and mouth to protrude, leaving the eyes covered (see Fig. 36.9). The person can then stand behind the

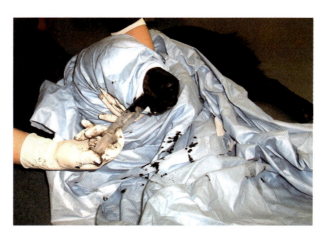

Figure 36.9 Administration of activated charcoal by syringe feeding. The disposable gown over the head prevents the dog from seeing the advancing syringe and keeps the animal clean.

dog, gently restraining the head, and dribble the solution in the corner of the dog's mouth slowly and patiently. Because the eyes are covered, the dog does not try to get away from the syringe and often just accepts administration of the suspension. Also, the gown keeps the rest of the dog clean.

Nasogastric tube

NGTs can be useful for slow activated charcoal administration. The technique of placing an NGT has already been covered.

Orogastric tube

In some poisoning cases, an OGT has been placed for GL. Activated charcoal may be administered into the stomach via an OGT at the end of a procedure. However, be aware that as the animal recovers from sedation or anesthesia, there is a significant risk of aspiration. Therefore only small volumes (2–3 mL/kg) should be instilled into the stomach at this point in time. Prelavage administration of activated charcoal, to decrease intestinal absorption of toxin that may be pushed into the duodenum during lavage, has shown no benefit over postlavage administration in preliminary clinical studies in human medicine.[16]

Catharsis

Catharsis involves the use of an orally administered, osmotically active, nonabsorbed substance to speed transition of a toxin through the gastrointestinal tract. Cathartics such as sorbitol are often combined with activated charcoal in commercially available suspensions. There is little evidence in human and veterinary literature for the benefit of catharsis as a part of GID.[19] However, a single dose is often used with few side effects. Multiple doses are not recommended because cathartics may contribute to excessive fluid and electrolyte losses.

Enemas

Indications

Enemas are used to relieve constipation and for GID. They can also be used in the treatment of hepatic encephalopathy.

Techniques

Constipation

An enema is required if there is distension of the colon with hard, dry feces and the animal is straining to defecate. If there are hard feces in the rectum only, a small amount of lubricant administered by syringe into the

rectum may help passage. Alternatively, commercially available micro-enemas, containing osmotically active substances and lubricant, may be used to relieve mild cases of constipation. If there is gross distension of the colon with hard feces, then a complete enema will need to be performed. The animal, in some cases, will need to be sedated. Rehydration fluid therapy should also be included in the treatment plan.

To perform an enema, pass a lubricated soft red rubber catheter or similar tube (see Fig. 36.1) to the level of the midabdomen and gently infuse 5–10 mL/kg of warm water into the colon and allow time for the animal to defecate voluntarily.[24] Other substances can be added to the enema solution, such as lubricant, lactulose (5–10 mL), or mineral oil (5–10 mL) to aid the removal of feces. The enema can be repeated if the colon is not emptied by voluntary defecation.

If the performance of a simple enema is not successful in relieving the patient's constipation, manual fecal extraction may be needed. The dog or cat should be anaesthetized and orotracheally intubated to avoid pain and stress, and to reduce the risk of aspiration because manipulation of the colon may induce vomiting. Repeat the enema as above and gently palpate the colon via external abdominal palpation to help break up the feces and move them into the rectum, where they can be removed digitally. Be careful with the use of instruments to aid extraction, such as sponge forceps, because they can cause perforation of the colon.

Enema for GID

Colonic enemas can be useful in the management of ingestion of large amounts of toxin. In particular, enemas using colonic lavage techniques are useful for removing snail pellets from the colon. The technique is similar as described earlier; however, the animal is anaesthetized and the cycle repeated until the effluent is clear. It is usually performed at the same time as GL. To perform an enema for GID, lubricate a tube of similar size to an OGT and feed up through the rectum to the level of the transcending colon (midabdomen) (see Fig. 36.10). If there is resistance during passage of the tube, do not force the tube any further into the colon. Siphon water by gravity feed into the colon, allowing the effluent to pass around the tube. This cycle is repeated until the effluent is clear.

Whole bowel irrigation

WBI, also known as a through-and-through enema, involves oral administration of large quantities of an iso-osmotic polyethylene glycol electrolyte solution to irrigate the entire gastrointestinal tract to prevent

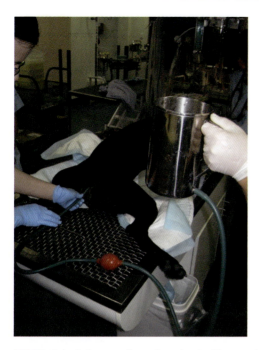

Figure 36.10 Colonic lavage of a patient that had ingested snail pellets. The green pellets can be seen around the perianal area. The enema tube (green) is being inserted into the rectum. Note the use of a gravity feed for flushing (metal container) and the orange bulb within the tubing, which can be used to increase pressure during flushing.

absorption of a toxin. It is also used to prepare the colon for colonoscopy and surgery, at a dose of up to 100 mL/kg in divided doses, several hours apart.[25,26] The technique for GID in human pediatric medicine is to administer the solution via a nasogastric tube at approximately 100–500 mL/hour until the rectal effluent is clear.[27] This method is rarely used in human and veterinary medicine for GID but may be considered for large ingestions of sustained-release drugs or iron tablets, or packets of illicit drugs, which would be a rare scenario for veterinary medicine. Although one study in dogs showed improved evacuation of paraquat with WBI compared with no GID,[28] there is little evidence in the literature supporting its clinical efficacy in removing toxins or improving outcome. Benefits exceeding that of activated charcoal alone are questionable, even in ingestion of sustained-release drugs.[29]

Contraindications include gastrointestinal perforation or gross hemorrhage, ileus, intractable vomiting, or cardiovascular instability. Risks include electrolyte and fluid losses, abdominal pain, vomiting, and aspiration. Major complications have been reported in the veterinary literature associated with the use of polyethylene glycol preparations for colonoscopy, which included fatal aspiration and gastrointestinal hemorrhage.[26]

Retention enema

Retention enemas use substances such as lactulose that are not absorbed by the colon. Hence they are retained in the colon and may encourage water movement into the colon by osmosis. This method is most commonly used for treatment of hepatic encephalopathy. Lactulose reduces absorption of ammonia from the colon by lowering colonic pH and by osmotic catharsis.[30]

The most common technique is to instill 5–10 mL/kg of a 30% lactulose solution into the colon, leave for 20–30 minutes, and then flush out using warm water. A routine enema (such as that described for constipation) may also suffice for treatment of hepatic encephalopathy.

Use of rectal catheters

Recumbent patients with liquid diarrhea pose many nursing challenges in terms of cleanliness and prevention of wound infection. Each institution has its own technique of keeping patients and bedding clean, including absorbent products, skin barrier creams, and frequent washing of the rear end. It remains difficult, though, to keep the area clean and prevent contamination of surgical wounds. These patients also inevitably develop perineal dermatitis and ulceration due to fecal scalding and frequent abrasive cleaning.

In human medicine, rectal Foley catheters, or rectal tubes, are used to collect feces over a short-term period.[31] These are wide-bore tubes, with or without an inflatable balloon on the distal end, connected to a collection system similar to a closed urinary collection system. See Protocol 36.4 for a detailed description of rectal catheter placement. The risks of using these tubes include colonic or rectal ulceration, pressure necrosis of the bowel wall, or obstruction of the tube leading to colonic distension and possibly perforation.[31] Humans can also develop temporary or permanent anal sphincter incompetence with prolonged use. For these reasons, use of these tubes is falling out of favor in human medicine despite the low rate of complication in short-term use. Rectal tubes are now being replaced with fecal or bowel management systems such as the Flexi-seal Fecal Management System (ConvaTec, NJ) and the Zassi Bowel Management System (Zassi Medical Evolutions, Florida) that can be used for up to 29 days.[32] These tubes have a collapsible neck proximal to the inflation balloon, the transsphincteric zone, which allows the anal sphincter to maintain tone. They also contain multiple lumens, which allow irrigation of the colon, and a retention cuff to allow retention enemas. Bowel management systems are still relatively invasive, however, and sporadic reports of rectal trauma associated with these devices are now

Protocol 36.4 Rectal catheter insertion

Items Required
- Examination gloves
- Aqueous lubricant
- Foley catheter of appropriate size (24–28F)
- Syringe filled with 0.9% NaCl for balloon inflation
- Adhesive medical tape
- Closed collection system for fecal collection

Procedure
1. Collect necessary supplies.
2. Perform a digital rectal examination in the patient to ensure there is no obstruction.
3. Inflate the catheter's balloon with saline to ensure integrity. No more than 10–20 mL should be used to inflate the balloon, depending on the size of the catheter. The balloon should be no wider than slightly larger than the anus in the dog.
4. Lubricate the catheter and gently insert into the rectum so that the tip lies several centimeters beyond the anal sphincter.
5. Slowly inflate the balloon to the predetermined volume, watching the animal for signs of discomfort. Stop inflating the balloon if the patient shows signs of distress.
6. Attach the catheter to the collection system. Tape the catheter and collection system to the tail of the animal.
7. If the catheter becomes repeatedly blocked with solid fecal material or repeatedly comes out of the patient, it should be removed.
8. The balloon should be deflated and reinflated every 6–12 hours.
9. The catheter should be removed if bleeding becomes evident.

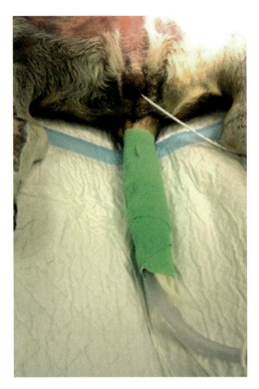

Figure 36.11 Urogenital region of a dog after a motor vehicle accident. The dog is in dorsal recumbency. A rectal Foley catheter can be seen exiting the anus of the dog (yellow tube), which has been taped securely to the tail. The collection system can be seen exiting the distal end of the tail wrap. A rectal Foley catheter was placed to prevent diarrhea contaminating the perivulvar area and the urinary catheter (white tube).

Box 36.4 Rectal tube placement

Indications:
- Recumbent patients with large volume of liquid diarrhea
- Postoperative patients with loose stool that are at high risk of infection from fecal contamination

Contraindications:
- Rectal bleeding or compromised rectal or colonic mucosa
- Patients with bleeding disorders
- Patients with formed stool
- Use beyond 24 hours

emerging.[33,34] See Box 36.4 for a list of indications and contraindications for rectal tube placement.

No studies have evaluated the risk of use of rectal tubes in veterinary medicine; however, use of rectal tubes for less than 24 hours likely carries a low risk as it does in human postoperative patients.[35] I have used this method in many patients and found it useful (see Fig. 36.11). No doubt the newer bowel management systems may also prove useful in veterinary medicine in the future. The same considerations of complications should be applied to veterinary patients as it is in human medicine.

Rectal Foley catheters are also used in human medicine to remove some rectal foreign bodies, such as bottles or jars.[36] Feeding the balloon past the foreign body and injecting some air through the catheter disrupts the vacuum created around the foreign body (see Protocol 36.4 for more information). The balloon can then be used to pull the foreign body out of the rectum. Although rectal foreign bodies are rarely seen in veterinary medicine, they may present as a result of animal abuse.

References

1. Broome CJ, Walsh VP. Gastric dilatation-volvulus in dogs. N Z Vet J 2003;51(6):275–283.

2. Volk SW. Gastric dilatation-volvulus and bloat. In: Silverstein DC, Hopper K, eds. Small Animal Critical Care Medicine. St. Louis MO: Saunders; 2009:584–588.

3. Hathcock J. Radiographic view of choice for the diagnosis of gastric volvulus. J Am Anim Hosp Assoc 1984;20:967–969.

4. Horne WA, Gilmore DR, Dietze AE, Freden GO, Short CE. Effects of gastric distension-volvulus on coronary blood flow and myocardial oxygen consumption in the dog. Am J Vet Res 1985;46(1):98–104.

5. Schober KE, Cornand C, Kirbach B, Aupperle H, Oechtering G. Serum cardiac troponin I and cardiac troponin T concentrations in dogs with gastric dilatation-volvulus. J Am Vet Med Assoc 2002;221(3):381–388.

6. Brourman JD, Schertel ER, Allen DA, Birchard SJ, DeHoff WD. Factors associated with perioperative mortality in dogs with surgically managed gastric dilatation-volvulus: 137 cases (1988–1993). J Am Vet Med Assoc 1996;208(11):1855–1858.

7. MacKenzie G, Barnhart M, Kennedy S, DeHoff W, Schertel E. A retrospective study of factors influencing survival following surgery for gastric dilatation-volvulus syndrome in 306 dogs. J Am Anim Hosp Assoc 2010;46(2):97–102.

8. Brockman DJ, Washabau RJ, Drobatz KJ. Canine gastric dilatation/volvulus syndrome in a veterinary critical care unit: 295 cases (1986–1992). J Am Vet Med Assoc 1995;207(4):460–464.

9. Hammel SP, Novo RE. Recurrence of gastric dilatation-volvulus after incisional gastropexy in a rottweiler. J Am Anim Hosp Assoc 2006;42:147–150.

10. Wagner AE, Dunlop CI, Chapman PL. Cardiopulmonary measurements in dogs undergoing gastropexy without gastrectomy for correction of gastric dilatation-volvulus. J Am Vet Med Assoc 1999;215(4):484–488.

11. Meyer-Lindenberg A, Harder A, Fehr M, Luerssen D, Brunnberg L. Treatment of gastric dilatation-volvulus and a rapid method for prevention of relapse in dogs: 134 cases (1988–1991). J Am Vet Med Assoc 1993;203(9):1303–1307.

12. Funkquist B, Garmer L. Pathogenetic and therapeutic aspects of torsion of the canine stomach. J Sm Anim Pract 1967;8:523–532.

13. Funkquist B. Gastric torsion in the dog: non-surgical reposition. J Sm Anim Pract 1969;10:507–511.

14. Eggertsdóttir AV, Moe L. A retrospective study of conservative treatment of gastric dilatation-volvulus in the dog. Acta Vet Scand 1995;36(2):175–184.

15. Greene S, Harris C, Singer J. Gastrointestinal decontamination of the poisoned patient. Pediatr Emerg Care 2008;24(3):176–185.

16. Heard K. The changing indications of gastrointestinal decontamination in poisonings. Clin Lab Med 2006;26:1–12.

17. Krenzelok EP. New developments in the therapy of intoxications. Toxicol Lett 2002;127:299–305.

18. Luiz JA, Heseltine J. Five common toxins ingested by dogs and cats. Compend Contin Educ Vet 2008;30(11):578–588.

19. Cope RB. Current methods for emergency decontamination for acute small animal poisoning. Aust Vet Pract 2004;34(1):23–31.

20. Rosendale ME. Decontamination strategies. Vet Clin North Am Small Anim Pract 2002;32:311–321.

21. Bailey B. Gastrointestinal decontamination triangle. Clin Toxicol 2005;43:59–60.

22. Arevalo-Silva C, Eliashar R, Wohlgelernter J, Elidan J, Gross M. Ingestion of caustic substances: a 15-year experience. Laryngoscope 2006;116:1422–1426.

23. Mamede RCM, De Mello Filho FV. Treatment of caustric ingestion: an analysis of 239 cases. Dis Esophagus 2002;15:210–213.

24. Washabau RJ, Holt DE. Diseases of the Large Intestine. In: Ettinger SJ, Feldman EC, eds. Textbook of Veterinary Internal Medicine. 6th ed. St Louis, MO: Elsevier; 2005.

25. Burrows CF. Evaluation of a colonic lavage solution to prepare the colon of the dog for colonoscopy. J Am Vet Med Assoc 1989;195(12):1719–1721.

26. Leib MS, Baechtel MS, Monroe WE. Complications associated with 355 flexible colonoscopic procedures in dogs. J Vet Intern Med 2004;18:642–646.

27. [No authors listed]. Position paper: whole bowel irrigation. J Toxicol Clin Toxicol 2004;42(6):843–854.

28. Mizutani T, Yamashita, M, Okubo N, Tanaka N, Naito H. Efficacy of whole bowel irrigation using solutions with or without absorbent in the removal of paraquat in dogs. Hum Exp Toxicol 1992;11:495–504.

29. Lapatto-Reiniluoto O, Kivisto KT, Neuvonen PJ. Activated charcoal alone and followed by whole-bowel irrigation in preventing the absorption of sustained-release drugs. Clin Pharmacol Ther 2001;70(3):255–260.

30. Cash WJ, McConville P, McDermott E, McCormick PA, Callendar ME, McDougall N. I. Current concepts in the assessment and treatment of hepatic encephalopathy. Q J Med 2010;103:9–16.

31. Beitz JM. Fecal incontinence in acutely and critically ill patients: options in management. Ostomy Wound Manage 2006;52(12):56–58.

32. Rees J, Sharpe A. The use of bowel management systems in the high-dependency setting. Br J Nurs 2009;18(7):S19–S24.

33. Sparks D, Chase D, Heaton B, Coughlin L, Metha J. Rectal traums and associated hemorrhage with the use of the ConvaTec Flexi-Seal fecal management system: report of 3 cases. Dis Colon Rectum 2010;53(3):346–349.

34. Page BP, Boyce, SA, Deans C, Camilleri-Brennan J. Significant rectal bleeding as a complication of a fecal collecting device: report of a case. Dis Colon Rectum. 2008;51(9):1427–1429.

35. Gurjar S, Forshaw MJ, Ahktar N, Stewart M, Parker MC. Indwelling trans-anastomotic rectal tubes in colorectal surgery: a survey of usage in UK and Ireland. Colorectal Dis 2007;9(1):47–51.

36. Kann B. Anorectal foreign bodies: evaluation and treatment. Semin Colon Rectal Surg 2004;15(2):119–124.

37

Postoperative peritoneal drainage techniques

Margo Mehl

There are numerous indications for abdominal drainage, some of which include peritonitis, uroperitoneum, increased abdominal pressure, and peritoneal dialysis. The type of peritoneal drainage chosen by the overseeing clinician depends on the primary disease process. The techniques for postoperative peritoneal drainage discussed in this chapter include maintaining an open abdomen, closed-suction abdominal drains, and intermittent drainage using a percutaneous catheter. Several types of passive drains, such as Penrose drains or dialysis catheters, have been described for use in abdominal drainage. These passive drains rely on gravity and are less effective and associated with higher complication rates compared with other abdominal drainage techniques. I do not recommend their use for abdominal drainage.

Open abdominal drainage suture

The underlying cause of contamination must be determined and controlled, the abdominal cavity copiously lavaged, and then open peritoneal drainage techniques can be used.[1] In all patients with open abdominal drainage it is ideal to have an indwelling urinary catheter to prevent urine soiling the abdominal bandages and to allow for the measurement of urine output. The technique for open abdominal drainage involves leaving a gap in the midline abdominal wall closure. This is accomplished by loosely suturing the ventral rectus sheath in close proximity while not pulling the suture tight. The span of the gap in the midline abdominal closure depends on the size of the patient but generally ranges from 1 to 4 cm (Fig. 37.1A). This space or gap in

the abdominal wall closure allows for fluid to drain easily out of the peritoneal cavity. Ideally, the suture chosen is monofilament and suture bites are close together to prevent bowel or organ strangulation. A detailed description of the surgical technique for performing open abdominal drainage is outside the scope of this chapter but has been described in several surgical textbooks such as *Slatter's Textbook of Small Animal Surgery*, 3rd edition, or *Fossum's Small Animal Surgery Textbook*, 3rd edition.

After the abdominal wall is loosely closed, a sterile nonadherent dressing is applied over the incision. The second layer (Fig. 37.1B) is a thicker and more absorbent sterile layer, and the third layer is usually one or more sterile towels. The bandage is then secured in place with a stretchy bandage material that wraps around the patient's body. There are many good material choices for the external bandage layers, some of which include 3M Vetrap, cling gauze, and Elastikon elastic tape. Additionally, per the clinician's request, a water barrier layer (Fig. 37.1C) may be incorporated into the bandage layers before the final layer is placed (Fig. 37.1D). The bandage should extend far enough cranially and caudally to assure coverage of the incision even with bandage migration. The abdominal bandage should be changed once or twice a day depending on fluid production and strikethrough of the bandage. It is important to remember that a patient with open peritoneal drainage does not require an increased level of analgesics. Certainly, most patients managed with open peritoneal drainage have significant systemic disease and have recently undergone a laparotomy; these conditions are indications for pain medications, but the technique of leaving the abdominal

Advanced Monitoring and Procedures for Small Animal Emergency and Critical Care, First Edition. Edited by Jamie M. Burkitt Creedon, Harold Davis.
© 2012 John Wiley & Sons, Inc. Published 2012 by John Wiley & Sons, Inc.

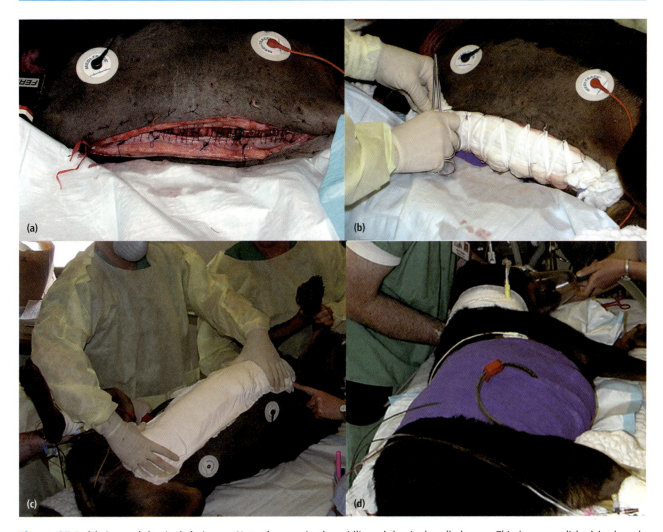

Figure 37.1 (a) Open abdominal drainage. Note the gap in the midline abdominal wall closure. This is accomplished by loosely suturing the ventral rectus sheath in close proximity. The span of the gap in the midline abdominal closure generally ranges from 1 to 4 cm. (b) The second layer, a thicker and more absorbent sterile layer (laparotomy pads) is applied. To secure the pads, sutures are preplaced along the length and on each side of the incision. The pads are held in placed with umbilical tape tied through the stay sutures. (c) An infant diaper is used as a water barrier layer and is incorporated into the bandage layers before the final layer is placed. (d) An elastic bandage wrap is applied as the final layer.

wall slightly open does not increase the patient's level of pain.

Changing the abdominal bandages

In a patient with open abdominal drainage, the bandages should be monitored for strikethrough and changed one or two times per 24 hours. The bandages should be weighed before and after removal to estimate ongoing fluid loss, which should be taken into account when calculating a patient's fluid requirement. When weighing the bandages and converting weight into volume, the bandages should first be weighed prior to placement and then when removed the bandages should

be reweighed. The weight of the wet bandages minus the weight of the dry bandage will give you the fluid weight. One gram of fluid is equivalent to 1 mL in volume, and this quantity should be recorded as a fluid loss in the patient's daily record. Changing the bandages involves the following steps (Protocol 37.1): First, the patient often requires sedation, the choice of which depends on the cardiovascular status of the patient. Second, any person handling the bandages should wear sterile gloves and use aseptic technique. The patient may have the bandage changed either while in a standing position with support or while in dorsal or lateral recumbency. Each layer is carefully removed, and then the midline

Protocol 37.1 Open abdominal drainage: changing the bandages

Items Required
- Sterile gloves
- Sterile nonadherent bandage material(Kendall Telfa dressing pad)
- Sterile absorbent layer (Curity laparotomy sponges)
- Sterile surgery towels
- Outer nonsterile gauze (dry cast padding)
- Elastic tape (Johnson & Johnson Elastikon elastic tape or 3M Vetrap)
- Optional: water-impermeable barrier in the bandage (Ioban drapes, potty training pads, or infant diapers)

Procedure
1. Sedate and position the patient.
2. Perform hand hygiene.
3. Don sterile gloves using aseptic technique.
4. Carefully remove bandages and weigh them.
5. Visually evaluate midline incision to make sure no bowel loop or intra-abdominal structure is outside of the peritoneal cavity.
6. Place sterile nonadherent bandage material over the incision.
7. Place second layer of sterile thicker more absorbent bandages material.
8. Place sterile surgery towels.
9. Incorporate water impermeable layer as needed.
10. Use outer nonsterile layers to secure the bandage to patient.

incision is visually evaluated to make sure no bowel loop or intra-abdominal structure is outside of the peritoneal cavity. Then the bandage is replaced in the same order as previously described: (1) sterile nonadherent bandage material over the incision (i.e., Kendall Telfa dressing pad, (2) sterile, thicker more absorbent layer (i.e., Curity laparotomy sponges), (3) sterile surgery towels, and (4) outer nonsterile layers including gauze and 3M Scotch-cast dry cast padding and elastic tape (Johnson & Johnson Elastikon elastic tape) or 3M Vetrap to secure the bandage around the patient. Some clinicians advocate including a water-impermeable barrier in the bandage, such as 3M Ioban drapes, potty training pads, or infant diapers, which would decrease contamination wicking from the exterior into the peritoneal cavity. Ideally, the bandage is changed before strikethrough occurs; however, if the situation arises in which the bandage cannot be changed that often, then a water-impermeable barrier incorporated into the bandaging layers will assist in preventing outer contamination

wicking from the environment into the patient's peritoneal cavity.

When the volume of fluid produced within the abdominal cavity has significantly decreased and the cytologic characteristics of that fluid indicate the abdominal cavity is free of infection (i.e., nontoxic neutrophils, no intracellular bacteria), the overseeing clinician will recommend closure of the abdominal wall.

The patient undergoes an anesthetic procedure for closure of the abdominal incision. At the time of closure, I recommend reexploring the abdominal cavity, copiously lavaging the abdominal cavity, and obtaining aerobic and anaerobic cultures.

Complications of open abdominal drainage predominantly include hospital-acquired infections and loss of plasma proteins.[1,2] The risk of hospital-acquired infections can be reduced if aseptic techniques are always instituted for bandage changes and during abdominal wall closure. The clinician should expect loss of plasma proteins such as albumin that maintain oncotic pressure; fluid therapy that supports oncotic pressure should be used as needed. Additionally, these patients with ongoing protein loss may benefit from enteral feeding and thus may have an esophageal or nasogastric feeding tube in place.

Closed-suction drains

The use of closed-suction drains allows the clinician to close the abdominal cavity and may be associated with less protein loss than open abdominal drainage. Closed-suction drains may still be associated with hospital-acquired infections, although potentially to a lesser degree than with open peritoneal drainage.[3] The disadvantage of the closed-suction drains technique is it does not allow the clinician to reexplore or reevaluate the abdominal cavity. Closed-suction drains permit measurement of fluid production in the peritoneal cavity and also allow for cytologic evaluation. The presence of a drain in a body cavity will stimulate fluid production; therefore waiting for cessation of fluid production before drain removal is unnecessary. The time at which to remove the abdominal drains is guided by when the cytology demonstrates the abdominal cavity is free of infection and when the fluid production has decreased to <2.2–5 mL/kg/day.[4,5]

A number of closed-suction drains are available. All of these drains aim to increase the surface area for drainage and reduce the incidence of drain obstruction with omentum, other tissue, or cellular debris. Closed-suction drains can be placed in a closed manner (see later), but I advocate placing the drains surgically. Placing the drains surgically allows for evaluation of the abdominal

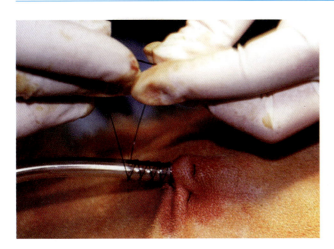

Figure 37.2 Once the drains are placed and exiting through the abdominal cavity, they are secured with a anchoring suture pattern, such as a finger trap pattern.

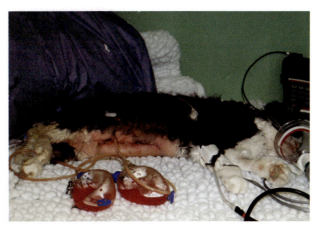

Figure 37.3 Jackson Pratt drains, a closed drainage system, is used in a cat following abdominal surgery.

cavity and treatment of the primary disease. Also, closed placement of abdominal drains can cause damage to intra-abdominal organs. After the abdominal cavity has been explored and the cause of contamination controlled, the drains are placed away from the midline incision, either laterally or cranial or caudal to the incision. The drains should never exit through the midline abdominal incision. The size of the drain and the number of drains placed is determined by the weight of the patient. I advocate using two drains in a cat or small dog (<10 kg) and three to four drains in larger patients. Once the drains are placed and exiting through the abdominal cavity, they are secured with am anchoring suture and a finger trap pattern (Fig. 37.2) up the tubing of the drain, not so tight as to occlude the drain. Once the abdominal cavity is closed, the drain tubing should be attached to a vacuum-assisted chamber that has an antireflux valve, to collect fluid and reduce the risk of ascending infection (Fig. 37.3). In the absence of a commercial product, an active drainage system can be constructed by connecting the intra-abdominal drain to an extension set with a needle attached, or a butterfly needle, which is then inserted into a large vacuum blood collection tube to generate negative drain pressure. This technique is further described in O'Dwyer's *Wound Management in Small Animals: A Practical Guide for Veterinary Nurses and Technicians.* Once drains are secured in place, the drain exit holes are covered with a sterile bandage and an abdominal bandage to reduce hospital contamination.

Managing the closed-suction drains

The vacuum created by the reservoir does not pull as effectively once the drain reservoir expands with fluid.

Therefore, it is recommended to empty the drain reservoir when it is approximately two-thirds or more full. Wear examination gloves when handling the drains. The reservoir bulb is disconnected from the drain tubing, and both openings/surfaces are wiped with isopropyl alcohol prior to collecting or emptying fluid. All fluid collected is measured and cytology is performed every 24–48 hours. The drain exit sites from the abdominal cavity should be evaluated for infection or fluid accumulation and addressed as indicated. These drain exit sites should also be cleaned daily with an antimicrobial scrub, wiped with sterile saline, and rebandaged with new clean dressings (Protocol 37.2). As previously stated, all drains produce some amount of fluid; therefore the drains are removed when the patient's clinical status improves, the fluid production decreases to an acceptable level, and the cytology of the fluid collected shows no evidence of infection. The patient does not often require additional analgesics for drain removal. The drains are gently pulled from the abdominal cavity and the exit holes are evaluated; if no evidence of infection is seen, the holes can be covered with a sterile dressing.

Percutaneous catheter drainage

Abdominal drainage can be achieved by percutaneous drain placement. This technique can be used to assist with abdominal fluid collection, rapid decompression of large abdominal effusions, or to stabilize a patient prior to surgical intervention such as in the case of a uroabdomen. Peritoneal dialysis catheters can also be placed in this manner. This therapy is described in Chapter 33, Peritoneal Dialysis. Percutaneous catheter drainage is

Protocol 37.2 Closed suction drain management

Items Required
- Closed suction drain (Jackson-Pratt)
- Examination gloves
- Alcohol-soaked gauze pad
- Laboratory specimen tubes and culturette (optional)
- Graduated cylinder
- Surgical scrub
- Sterile saline
- Materials for light dressing

Procedure
1. Gather materials.
2. Empty drain reservoir when the bulb is two-thirds full.
3. Perform hand hygiene and don examination gloves when handling the drains.
4. Disconnect the reservoir bulb from drain tubing and wipe both openings with isopropyl alcohol prior to emptying or collecting fluid.
5. Measure all fluid collected; cytology may be performed.
6. Evaluate drain exit sites from the abdominal cavity.
7. Clean drain exit sites daily with an antimicrobial scrub, wiped with sterile saline, and keep bandaged with light clean dressings.
8. When closed suction drains are no longer needed, drains can be removed by gently pulling drain tubing from the abdominal cavity.
9. Once drains are removed, evaluate exit holes and apply dressings as needed.

not indicated for treatment of septic peritonitis because ongoing contamination of the abdomen would not be controlled. There are a number of catheters available on the market that could be placed in a closed manner or via a mini laparotomy. A fenestrated catheter is likely to be more effective than a nonfenestrated catheter because it is less likely to be occluded by omentum or other tissue. There are commercially available fenestrated catheters (Cook peritoneal dialysis catheters), or alternatively a regular over-the-needle catheter or red rubber tube can be fenestrated for this purpose. It is essential to be very careful when fenestrating these catheters to avoid weakening the integrity of the catheter and maintaining sterility. Fenestrations are made with a scalpel blade and should be staggered and each hole less than the diameter of the catheter.

A closed method of placement can be used with any over-the-needle type catheter, and local anesthetic can be infused into the site prior to placement. The catheter is placed through the abdominal wall, with careful technique to avoid damage to intra-abdominal structures. The site of placement is best identified with ultrasound

guidance. In the absence of ultrasound the catheter is usually placed caudal to the umbilicus in an effort to minimize the chance of puncturing the liver or spleen. A mini laparotomy technique can also be used for placement of catheters, and it allows use of catheters without a trocar, such as a red rubber tube. The mini laparotomy technique requires strict asepsis, and a small incision is made on the ventral midline. Through the skin incision the linea alba is accessed, and a stab incision is made through a tented portion of the linea alba. The catheter is introduced through a separate skin opening and associated subcutaneous tunnel and then passed into the previously made stab incision through the linea alba. The small midline approach incision is closed, and then the skin incision is closed in a routine manner. The catheter is secured with a purse-string suture and finger trap suture pattern, making sure it is not occluding the catheter lumen. Lastly, a sterile dressing is applied over the catheter exit site.

Managing a fenestrated catheter

The management of a percutaneously placed catheter is similar to those techniques previously described. Intermittent or continuous drainage can be utilized, and the person handling the catheter should always wear examination gloves and use aseptic techniques. Wipe the opening to the catheter with isopropyl alcohol before aspirating and use sterile syringes and tubing.

Conclusion

Managing peritoneal drainage is a key step in treating patients with abdominal disease. Effective nursing care with abdominal drainage techniques will maximize the therapeutic benefits of abdominal drainage and minimize complications.

References

1. Staatz Aj, Monnet E, Seim HB III. Open peritoneal drainage versus primary closure for the treatment of septic peritonitis in dogs and cats: 42 cases (1993–1999). Vet Surg 2002;31:174–180.
2. Parsons KJ, Owen LJ, Lee K, Tivers MS, Gregory SP. A retrospective study of surgically treated cases of septic peritonitis in the cat (2000–2007). J Small Animal Pract 2009;50:518–524.
3. Mueller MG, Ludwig LL, Barton LJ. Use of closed-suction drains to treat generalized peritonitis in dogs and cats: 40 cases (1997–1999). J Am Vet Med Assoc 2001;6:789–794.
4. Miller CW. Bandages and drains. In: Slater DH, ed. Textbook of Small Animal Surgery. Vol 1. 3rd ed. Philadelphia, PA: WB Saunders; 2003:244–249.
5. Fossum TW. Surgery of the lower respiratory system: pleural cavity and diaphragm. In: Fossum TW, ed. Small Animal Surgery. 3rd ed. St. Louis, MO: Mosby; 2007:901.

SECTION V

Nutrition

38

Nutritional requirements in critical illness

Daniel L. Chan

Basic physiology of malnutrition in critical illness

Appropriate nutritional support has long been considered essential for the recovery of critically ill human patients. Although there is convincing evidence of the deleterious effects of malnutrition in people, the optimal nutritional strategies for critically ill animals remain controversial and largely unknown. Despite the lack of definitive answers, it must be emphasized that recommendations for nutritional support of critically ill animals are based on having a good understanding about the disease processes involved and the limited information available. The fact that there is limited information available should not discourage the implementation of nutritional support for critically ill animals. In fact, with proper patient selection, sound nutritional planning, and careful monitoring, nutritional support can be an integral part in the successful recovery of many critically ill animals.

The metabolic responses to illness or severe injury are complex and place critically ill animals at high risk for malnutrition and its deleterious effects. These effects, which are likely to have a negative impact on overall survival, include alterations in energy and substrate metabolism, compromised immune function, and impaired wound healing.[1–3] Although generalizations tend to oversimplify complex systems, the concept of "ebb/flow" offers a basic description of the metabolic response to critical illness or severe injury. According to this model, there is an initial hypometabolic response ("ebb phase"), followed by a period of a more prolonged course of hypermetabolism ("flow phase"). The ebb phase refers to a period of hemodynamic instability associated with decreased energy expenditure, hypo-thermia, mild protein catabolism, decreased cardiac output, and poor tissue perfusion. Without intervention, this instability may progress to a state of refractory or irreversible shock characterized by severe lactic acidosis, decreased tissue perfusion, multiple organ failure, and death. Nutritional intervention during the ebb phase is associated with a high risk for complications such as electrolyte abnormalities, which may result in further detrimental effects to some critically ill animals.[4–7] Following successful resuscitation, patients enter the flow phase, during which profound metabolic alterations occur. Increases in energy expenditure, glucose production, insulin and glucagon concentrations, cardiac output, and profound protein catabolism are the hallmarks of this response.[1,4,8] Provision of nutritional support during this stage of illness can attenuate and sometimes reverse the detrimental effects of malnutrition.[9]

One of the major metabolic alterations associated with critical illness involves body protein catabolism, in which protein turnover rates may become markedly elevated. Whereas healthy animals primarily lose fat when deprived of sufficient calories (simple starvation), sick or traumatized patients catabolize lean body mass when they are not provided with sufficient calories (stressed starvation).[8,9] During the initial stages of fasting in the healthy state, glycogen stores are used as the primary source of energy. Within days, a metabolic shift occurs toward the preferential use of fat deposits, sparing catabolic effects on lean muscle tissue. In diseased states, the inflammatory response triggers alterations in cytokines and hormone concentrations, which rapidly shifts metabolism toward a catabolic state. Glycogen stores are quickly depleted, especially in strict carnivores such as the cat, and this leads to an early

Advanced Monitoring and Procedures for Small Animal Emergency and Critical Care, First Edition. Edited by Jamie M. Burkitt Creedon, Harold Davis.
© 2012 John Wiley & Sons, Inc. Published 2012 by John Wiley & Sons, Inc.

mobilization of amino acids from muscle stores. Because cats undergo continuous gluconeogenesis, the mobilization of amino acids from muscles is more pronounced than that observed in other species. In both cats and dogs, continued inadequate food intake leads to further changes in metabolism where the predominant energy source is derived from accelerated proteolysis, which in itself is an energy-consuming process. Muscle catabolism that occurs during stress provides the liver with glucogenic precursors and other amino acids for glucose and acute-phase protein production.[8,9] The resultant negative nitrogen balance or net protein loss has been documented in critically ill dogs and cats.[10,11] One study in particular estimated that 73% of hospitalized dogs across four different veterinary referral centers were deemed to be in a negative energy balance.[12] The consequences of continued lean body mass losses include negative effects on wound healing, immune function, strength (both skeletal and respiratory), and ultimately on overall prognosis.[9,13]

It is becoming increasingly more evident that the metabolic consequences of critical illness are part of an integrated response to the initial insult, driven in part by cytokines and counterregulatory hormones.[6,8] These mediators may result in changes in energy expenditure, substrate metabolism, and body composition. The most well-known cytokine to affect metabolism is perhaps tumor necrosis factor-α, which is responsible for increased energy expenditure, hepatic gluconeogenesis, protein breakdown, activation of the hypothalamic-pituitary-adrenal axis, lipolysis, and peripheral insulin resistance.[6]

Due to the metabolic alterations associated with critical illness, and in part due to an inability or reluctance of many critically ill dogs and cats to ingest sufficient calories, this patient population is at increased risk for rapid development of malnutrition. Given the serious sequelae of malnutrition, preservation of lean body mass or reversal of deteriorating nutritional status via nutritional support is paramount.

Rationale for providing nutrition in critical illness

Identification of overt malnutrition in animals can be challenging because there are no established criteria of malnutrition in companion animals. In dogs, a period as short as 3 days of anorexia has been documented to produce metabolic changes consistent with starvation in people.[14] In cats, detectable impairment of immune function can be demonstrated in healthy individuals subjected to acute starvation by day 4, and therefore, nutritional support should be also considered in any ill

cat with inadequate food intake for more than 3 days.[15] The need to implement a nutritional intervention becomes more urgent when a dog or cat has not eaten for more than 5 days because by this time there are detectable changes in metabolism and immune function directly related to prolonged period of poor food intake.[14,15]

However, even in patients with severe malnutrition, the immediate therapy of critically ill patients should focus on resuscitation, stabilization, and identification of the primary disease process. As steps are made to address the primary disease, formulation of a nutritional plan should strive to prevent (or correct) overt nutritional deficiencies and imbalances. By providing adequate energy substrates, protein, essential fatty acids, and micronutrients, the body can support wound healing, immune function, and tissue repair. A major goal of nutritional support is to minimize metabolic derangements and catabolism of lean body tissue. During hospitalization, repletion of body weight is not the top priority because regaining body weight is best achieved once the animal has recovered from the primary disease. Therefore, there is little justification to feed excessive amounts of calories to critically ill animals.

Nutritional assessment

The formal assessment of patients in terms of their nutritional needs and what precautions need to be considered in formulating a plan is referred to as "nutritional assessment." Because all nutritional support techniques carry some risk of complications, appropriate patient selection is crucial in ensuring the full benefits of nutritional support. Careful patient selection is the first step in performing nutritional assessment. This subjective clinical assessment process remains the predominant method of identifying malnourished patients that require immediate nutritional support as well as identifying patients that are not currently malnourished but where nutritional support is aimed at preventing the development of malnutrition.[16,17] The next step in nutritional assessment involves assessing how urgently nutritional support is required. This involves taking into account obvious indicators of malnutrition including unexpected weight loss more than 10% body weight, poor hair coat quality, muscle wasting, signs of inadequate wound healing, hypoalbuminemia, lymphopenia, and coagulopathy.[17] However, these abnormalities are not specific to malnutrition and often do not occur early in the process. In addition, fluid shifts may mask weight loss in critically ill patients, highlighting the need to assess body condition as well. For example, fluid retention in the form of peripheral edema or ascites increases

---

Box 38.1 Nutritional assessment

- Does the patient show clinical signs consistent with overt malnutrition?

    Evidence such as >10% loss in body weight in past month, loss of lean body mass, poor hair coat quality, and nonhealing wounds are consistent but not specific to malnutrition. It is also important to note current body weight and perform assessment of body condition.
- Does the patient have risk factors for development of malnutrition?

    Anorexia >3 days, presence of serious inflammatory condition (e.g., sepsis, pancreatitis), structural impediments for voluntary eating (e.g., severe injury to mouth or jaw, megaesophagus), intestinal dysfunction (vomiting, regurgitation, gastric paresis, ileus, diarrhea), presence of condition known to increase metabolic rate (e.g., burns).
- Is the patient cardiovascularly stable, properly hydrated, and with acid-base and electrolyte disturbances addressed?

    Feeding patients before addressing these disturbances puts them an increased risk for complications.
- Which route of nutrition is the most appropriate?

    Patients should be carefully evaluated for the ability to tolerate enteral nutrition. This involves considering the oral, esophageal, gastric, and enteric feeding depending where abnormalities are noted. Only when it is not feasible to feed via some segment of the gastrointestinal tract should parenteral nutrition be considered. For patients being considered for parenteral nutrition, feasibility for placing central venous catheters safely and making note of obvious contraindications for feeding parenterally (e.g., providing high dextrose to patient with uncontrolled diabetes, high lipid concentration to patients with severe hypertriglyceridemia, high protein infusion to encephalopathic patients).
- How can nutritional support be safely initiated?

    After devising a plan to meet the patient's nutritional needs, provision of nutrition should have the initial target of meeting 100% of the patient's calculated resting energy requirement (RER) within 48–72 hours. During first day of nutritional support, aim to start with 30%–50% RER and increase by 10%–20% in each subsequent day as long as the patient shows no complication related to feeding.
- How patients with nutritional support be monitored?

    Basic monitoring includes daily checks in body weight, vital signs, the appearance of all sites relating to catheters and feeding tubes, bandaging of catheters and tubes. In patients with previous metabolic disturbances, daily checks of electrolytes and biochemical profiles may be indicated. Body condition should be checked weekly, and patients with continued decline in body condition should be fed greater amounts of calories, provided they tolerate the increase in feeding. Patients that do not tolerate increases in feeding should be evaluated for other interventions (e.g., use of prokinetics). Patients with metabolic abnormalities such as hyperglycemia or hyperlipidemia following initiation of nutritional support should be evaluated for either reformulation in composition of diet provided or treated with insulin or heparin, respectively.
- What should be looked for when reassessing patients?

    Basic considerations include whether patient continues to require nutritional support or if the animal can consume approximately 70% of RER voluntarily. Animals eating voluntarily can be transitioned from assisted feeding to voluntarily oral feeding.

    Other considerations involve how much to feed: Patients with continuing signs of lean body mass loses should be fed more (increase calories provided by 20% if tolerated), and animals that have recovered the weight lost can be transitioned to their normal feeding regimen.

---

overall body weight, despite continued lean muscle mass losses. Given the limitations of performing nutritional assessment, the expeditious identification of risk factors that may predispose patients to malnutrition is crucial. These risk factors include anorexia lasting longer than 3 days, serious underlying disease (e.g., trauma, sepsis, peritonitis, or pancreatitis), and large protein losses (e.g., protracted vomiting, diarrhea, protein-losing nephropathies, protein-losing enteropathies, draining wounds, or burns).

Nutritional assessment also allows identification of factors that can have an impact on the nutritional plan, such as the identification of electrolyte abnormalities, hyperglycemia, hypertriglyceridemia, or hyperammone-mia, or comorbid illnesses (e.g., renal or hepatic disease) that should lead to alterations of the composition of the diet used. In summary, nutritional assessment involves performing a risk assessment of a patient in terms of its nutritional status and the considerations required in providing safe and effective nutritional support. An outline of the nutritional assessment process is listed in Box 38-1.

Nutritional plan

The key to successful nutritional management of critically ill patients lies in the proper diagnosis and treatment of the underlying disease. Another crucial factor is the selection of the appropriate route for nutritional support. Providing nutrition via a functional digestive system is the preferred route of feeding, and so particular care should be taken to evaluate whether the patient can tolerate enteral feedings. Even if the patient can only tolerate small amounts of enteral nutrition, this route of feeding should be pursued and supplemented with parenteral nutrition as necessary to meet the patient's nutritional needs. In some circumstances feeding patients enterally may seem to be contraindicated (e.g., animal anesthetized for mechanical ventilation, animals with upper airway dysfunction; however, there is a strong argument that in such a situation there should be some consideration for feeding enterally but that the compromised area is avoided). Ventilated human patients are commonly fed via nasogastric tubes, and there is no reason a similar approach could not be pursued in companion animals receiving mechanical ventilation. Patients with severe laryngeal or esophageal dysfunction could be fed via gastrostomy or enteric feeding tubes. On the basis of the nutritional assessment, the anticipated duration of nutritional support, and the appropriate route of delivery (i.e., enteral or parenteral), a nutritional plan is formulated to meet the patient's nutritional needs.

The first steps of instituting nutritional support include achieving hemodynamic stability, restoring proper hydration status, and correction of electrolyte or acid-base disturbances.[17] Beginning nutritional support before these abnormalities are addressed can increase the risk of complications (e.g., regurgitation, vomiting, hypotension) and, in some cases, further compromise the patient.[4-7] For example, feeding leads to mesenteric vasodilation, which could compromise systematic mean arterial pressure in some patients. It should be emphasized that this strategy is *not* counter to the concept of "early nutritional support," which has been documented to result in positive effects in several animal and human studies.[18-22] Early nutritional support advocates feeding as soon as possible after achieving hemodynamic stability rather than delaying nutritional intervention for several days.[19,20] Implementation of the nutritional plan should be gradual, with the goal of reaching target level of nutrient delivery in 48 to 72 hours. Rapid feeding has several potential complications. First, animals that have not eaten for several days have significant delays in gastric emptying and compromised overall intestinal motility. In some patients, this situation leads to significant ileus. Feeding these patients rapidly leads to abdominal pain, distension, and potentially vomiting and regurgitation. Second, because of various hormonal disturbances associated with poor food intake (e.g., low insulin, high glucagon, high cortisol), there is a

potential for severe metabolic derangements such as refeeding syndrome whereby a sudden spike in insulin concentrations leads to life-threatening electrolyte abnormalities.

Nutritional requirements

Whereas the protein requirements of critically ill people have been determined based on nitrogen balance studies, this information is not readily available in critically ill animals. One method of estimating the extent of amino acid catabolism is to measure urinary urea nitrogen content. Although measurement of urinary urea nitrogen in critically ill dogs has been shown to be a feasible tool in assessing nitrogen balance in an experimental setting, further studies are warranted to better characterize the protein requirements of critically ill animals seen in practice.[10,11] A recent study[23] demonstrated significant changes in amino acid status in critically ill dogs; however, further studies are required to determine if correction of these amino acid changes is beneficial.

Currently, it is generally accepted that hospitalized dogs should be supported with 4–6 g of protein/100 kcal (15%–25% of total energy requirements); cats are usually supported with 6–8 g of protein/100 kcal (25%–35% of total energy requirements).[24] Patients with protein intolerance (e.g., hepatic encephalopathy, severe azotemia) should receive reduced amounts of protein. Similarly, patients with hyperglycemia or hyperlipidemia may require decreased amounts of these nutrients. Other nutritional requirements depend on the patient's underlying disease, clinical signs, and laboratory parameters.

When an animal is unable to synthesize adequate amounts of a nutrient and must rely on dietary sources, that nutrient is qualified as *essential*. However, during certain conditions including critical illness, nutrients usually considered nonessential become in short supply due to increased demands. These nutrients have been termed *conditionally essential*, and glutamine is one such example. A number of recent human studies have evaluated the modulation of disease with these so-called nonessential nutrients such as such as glutamine, arginine, omega-3 fatty acids, and nucleotides.[7,10,25-29] Although study results have been mixed, glutamine supplementation has been associated with the most beneficial results.[7,25,26,28-30] Glutamine is the primary energy source for enterocytes and cells of the immune system, and its supplementation may attenuate gastrointestinal permeability and improve overall immune function.[26,27,29] In select populations of critically ill people, supplementation with either enteral or parenteral glutamine has been shown to reduce infectious complications and improve survival.[28,29] Studies in dogs and cats have failed to demonstrate clear benefits of glutamine supplementation.[30,31] Nevertheless, it is increasingly evident that the requirements of specific nutrients during critical illness may be considerably different than those in health. Future studies are warranted to evaluate whether "critical care diets" designed for dogs and cats should be enriched with these conditionally essential nutrients.

Calculation of nutritional requirements

Ideally, nutritional support should provide ample substrates for gluconeogenesis, protein synthesis, and adenosine triphosphate (ATP) production necessary to maintain homeostasis. Ensuring that enough calories are being provided to sustain critical physiologic processes such as immune function, wound repair, and cell division and growth would necessitate the actual measurement of the patient's total energy expenditure. However, precise measurements of energy expenditure (i.e., calorimetry) in clinical veterinary patients are still in the developmental phases. The basic premise of calorimetry is to measure the total heat lost by an animal, as a reflection of total energy produced by metabolism. With direct calorimetry, the animal is placed in an airtight insulated chamber, and precise thermal measurements are made of the chamber. This method is only suitable for experimental models because clinical cases would not be able to be managed in this environment. Indirect calorimetry, in contrast, is more commonly used in human hospitals and by veterinary clinical researchers to extrapolate energy requirements. This method provides a noninvasive means of estimating energy expenditure by measuring the rate of oxygen consumption and the rate of carbon dioxide production and applying the obtained values to a mathematical equation known as the Weir formula.[32,33] Because consumption of oxygen and production of carbon dioxide can directly be related to glucose, protein, and fat metabolism, energy expenditure can be calculated from the measured variables. However, indirect calorimetry also requires specialized equipment, so-called metabolic carts, making the technique available only in a few select sites. Oxygen and carbon dioxide exchange is measured with a hood, canopy, or expiratory collection device. These systems are portable and easier to use in clinical situations than previous calorimetry units where the patient needed to be confined within the divide. A few studies have used indirect calorimetry to estimate energy expenditure in select populations of clinical veterinary patients, but the use of mathematical formulas currently remains the most practical means of estimating a patient's energy requirement[33,34](see Box 38.2).

> **Box 38.2** Estimating total daily energy requirements in dogs and cats
>
> RER (kcal/day) = $70 \times$ (current body weight in kg)$^{0.75}$
>
> For animals weighing between 2 and 30 kg: RER (kcal/day) = $(30 \times$ current body weight in kg) + 70

Results of indirect calorimetry studies in dogs support the recent trend of formulating nutritional support to meet resting energy requirements (RER) as a starting point, rather than more generous illness energy requirements, which require multiplying resting or even maintenance energy requirements by an illness factor.[35] RER is defined as the number of calories required for maintaining homeostasis at rest in a thermoneutral environment while the animal is in a postabsorptive state.[36,37] Although several formulas are proposed to calculate the RER, a widely used allometric formula can be applied to both dogs and cats of all weights. For animals weighing between 2 and 30 kg, there is also a linear formula that provides reasonable estimation of RER (See Box 38.2).

Until recently, it was recommended to multiply the RER by an illness factor between 1.0 and 2.0 to yield an Illness Energy Requirement (IER), to account for increases in metabolism associated with different diseases and injuries. However, less emphasis is now being placed on such subjective and extrapolated factors, and the current recommendation is to use more conservative energy estimates (i.e., start with the animal's RER) to avoid overfeeding. Overfeeding can result in metabolic and gastrointestinal complications, hepatic dysfunction, and increased carbon dioxide production.[4,7]

It should be emphasized that these general guidelines should be used as starting points, and animals receiving nutritional support should be closely monitored for tolerance of nutritional interventions (see the section on complications of providing nutrition in the critically ill). Continual decline in body weight or body condition should prompt the clinician to reassess and perhaps modify the nutritional plan (e.g., increasing the number of calories provided by 25%).

Nutritional requirements in special cases

Much remains unclear regarding the nutritional requirements of critically ill animals in general. In certain circumstances assumptions are made that nutritional requirements in animals are similar to people afflicted with similar diseases. However, it is important to recognize that there may be significant species and disease differences that make direct comparisons or extrapolations less applicable. For example, pancreatitis in people is often related to gallstones or alcoholism. Because pancreatitis in animals is often related to high-fat diets or is idiopathic, the nutritional requirements for the treatment of this disease in each species are likely different.

Burns

Experimental data suggest dramatic changes in energy requirements in animals with thermal burns; however, there are virtually no clinical data to support this notion. In experimental models, dogs with thermal burns experienced increased energy requirements, accelerated gluconeogenesis, glucose oxidation, lipolysis, and increased amino acid oxidation.[38,39] In the absence of definitive data to suggest otherwise, current recommendations are to start nutritional support as soon as it is deemed safe and initially target RER but to continually reassess the patient as energy requirements may exceed $2 \times$ RER. The goal of aggressive nutritional support is to optimize protein synthesis and preserve lean body mass. Feeding at least 6–7 g protein per 100 kcal (25%–35% of total energy) may be necessary. It is unknown whether nutrients such as glutamine and arginine would provide extra benefits in this patient population.

Tetanus

Another population that may merit more vigilant attention to energy requirements is dogs with tetanus. A recent study demonstrated that despite feeding a median of $1.4 \times$ RER, dogs lost a median of 5% body weight during the course of hospitalization.[40] It is proposed that increased muscle activity in this disorder increased energy requirements despite the fact that dogs were mostly recumbent and had limited physical activity.

Sepsis

Animals with sepsis are perhaps another population whereby nutritional requirements may be altered. The intense inflammatory response, coupled with changes in substrate handling, likely alters the metabolic rate and nutrient requirements. Experimental data in dogs suggest that during the early phase of sepsis, energy expenditure may increase by 25%, which appears to be accompanied by an increase in oxidation of free fatty acids and triglycerides.[41] However, it is also recognized that energy expenditure can be quite variable in sepsis and may even decrease in septic shock.[42] Depending on the etiology of sepsis (e.g., septic peritonitis, pyothorax), protein requirements may also dramatically increase, and therefore general nutritional recommendations for animals with septic peritonitis may involve initially feeding at RER with 35% of total calories derived from protein, 40% from fats, and 25% from carbohydrates.[24] Further studies are warranted to determine if these recommendations are optimal for clinical veterinary patients with sepsis.

Complications of providing nutrition in the critically ill

Body weights should be monitored daily in critically ill animals. However, the clinician should take into account fluid shifts in evaluating changes in body weight. For this reason, assessing body condition scores is very important. The use of the RER as the patient's caloric requirement is merely a starting point; however, there is growing evidence that this conservative approach or even feeding less than RER may be preferable in the critically ill patient.[43] The number of calories provided may need to be increased to keep up with the patient's changing needs, typically by 25% if well tolerated. In patients unable to tolerate the prescribed amounts (i.e., start to vomit), the clinician should consider reducing amounts of enteral feedings and supplementing the nutritional plan with some form of parenteral nutrition.

Possible complications of enteral nutrition include mechanical complications such as clogging of the feeding tube or premature tube removal by the patient. Metabolic complications of enteral or parenteral feeding include electrolyte disturbances, hyperglycemia, fluid volume overload, and gastrointestinal signs (eg, vomiting, diarrhea, cramping, bloating).

In rare instances, a condition known as refeeding syndrome may develop. This syndrome occurs when severely malnourished patients are fed perhaps too aggressively, and the sudden increase in insulin concentrations results in severe hypophosphatemia, hypokalemia, and hyperglycemia. During prolonged fasting, cells become metabolic inactive, and sudden reintroduction of substrates leads to rapid synthesis of ATP, leading to consumption of phosphate, leading to severe hypophosphatemia. Other electrolytes such as potassium and magnesium also translocate intracellularly in response to insulin. Recommendations for reducing the risk for the developing refeeding syndrome include gradually introducing feeding and decreasing the proportion of calories derived from carbohydrates.

In critically ill patients receiving enteral nutritional support, the clinician must also be vigilant for the development of aspiration pneumonia. Monitoring parameters recommended for patients receiving enteral nutrition include daily checks on body weight, serum electrolytes, feeding tube patency, the appearance of feeding tube stoma site, gastrointestinal signs (eg, vomiting, regurgitation, diarrhea), and signs of volume overload or aspiration pneumonia.

Possible complications associated with parenteral nutrition include sepsis (such as seen with catheter infections, contamination of the parenteral solution bag), mechanical complications associated with the catheter and lines (obstructed catheters, line breakage), thrombophlebitis, and metabolic disturbances related to the composition of the parenteral nutrition solution (hyperglycemia, electrolyte shifts, hyperammonemia, and hypertriglyceridemia). Avoiding serious consequences of complications associated with parenteral nutrition requires early identification of problems and prompt action. Frequent monitoring of vital signs, catheter-exit sites, and routine biochemistry panels may alert clinician to developing problems. The development of persistent hyperglycemia during nutritional support may require adjustment to the nutritional plan (e.g., decreasing dextrose content in parenteral nutrition) or administration of regular insulin. This obviously necessitates more vigilant monitoring.

With continual reassessment, the clinician can determine when to transition patient from assisted feeding to voluntary consumption of food. The discontinuation of nutritional support should only begin when the patient can consume approximately its RER without much coaxing.

Summary

- Nutritional support of the critically ill patient should be considered an essential part of the overall treatment plan.
- Metabolic responses to illness or severe injury place critically ill patients at high risk for development of malnutrition.
- Consequences of malnutrition include altered substrate metabolism, compromised immune function, impaired wound healing, and potentially increased mortality.
- Energy expenditure in critically ill animals may vary considerably depending on the patient, underlying disease, and illness severity; therefore initial nutritional support should target RER.
- Specific nutritional requirements for critically ill dogs and cats have not been determined, but recommended levels of protein provision include feeding 4–8 g protein/100 kcal or 25%–35% of total calories derived from protein.
- Before implementation of nutritional support, patients must be cardiovascularly stable and have hydration, acid-base, and electrolyte abnormalities addressed first.

- Monitoring of patients receiving nutritional support is extremely important because this population is prone to various metabolic complications.
- Upon reassessment, nutritional support may be increased, decreased, or discontinued depending on patient response and disease progression.
- With appropriate patient selection, accurate nutritional assessment, and careful execution of the nutritional plan, nutrition can play an instrumental role in the successful recovery of many critically ill patients.

References

1. Thatcher CD. Nutritional needs of critically ill patients. Compend Cont Educ Pract Vet 1996;18:1303–1313.
2. Lippert AC, Fulton RB, Parr AM. Retrospective study of the use of total parenteral nutrition in dogs and cats. J Vet Intern Med 1993;7:52–64.
3. Zsombor-Murray E, Freeman LM. Peripheral parenteral nutrition. Compend Contin Educ Pract Vet 1999;21:512–523.
4. Barton RG. Nutrition support in critical illness. Nutr Clin Pract 1994;9:127–139.
5. Biffl WL, Moore EE, Haenel JB, et al. Nutrition support of the trauma patient. Nutrition 2002;18: 960–965.
6. Wray CJ, Mammen JM, Hasselgren P. Catabolic response to stress and potential benefits of nutrition support. Nutrition 2002;18:971–977.
7. Nitenberg G. Nutritional support in sepsis: still skeptical? Curr Opin Crit Care 2000;6:253–266.
8. Biolo G, Toigo G, Ciocchi B, et al. Metabolic response to injury and sepsis: changes in protein metabolism. Nutrition 1997;13:52S–57S.
9. Roberts SR, Kennerly DA, Keane D, et al. Nutrition support in the intensive care unit: adequacy, timeliness, and outcomes. Crit Care Nurse 2003;23:49-57.
10. Michel KE. Nitrogen metabolism in critical care patients. Vet Clin Nutr 1998;1:20–22.
11. Michel KE, King LG, Ostro E. Measurement of urinary urea nitrogen content as an estimate of the amount of total urinary nitrogen loss in dogs in intensive care units. J Am Vet Med Assoc 1997;210:356–359.
12. Remillard RL, Darden De, Michel KE, et al. An investigation of the relationship between caloric intake and outcome in hospitalized dogs. Vet Ther 2001;2:301–310.
13. Marik PE, Zaloga GP. Early enteral nutrition in acutely ill patients: a systematic review. Crit Care Med 2001;29:2264–2270.
14. Owen OE, Richard GA, Patel MS, et al. Energy metabolism in feasting and fasting. Adv Exp Med Biol 1979;111:169–188.
15. Freitag KA, Saker KE, Thomas E, et al. Acute starvation and subsequent refeeding affect lymphocyte subsets and proliferation in cats. J Nutr 2000;130:2444–2449.
16. Marks SL. Enteral and parenteral nutritional support. In: Ettinger SJ, ed. Textbook of Veterinary Internal Medicine. 5th ed. Philadelphia, PA: Elsevier; 2000:275–283.
17. Michel KE. Prognostic value of clinical nutritional assessment in canine patients. J Vet Emerg Crit Care 1993;3:96–104.
18. Heyland DK. Enteral and parenteral nutrition in the seriously ill, hospitalized patients: a critical review of the evidence. J Nutr Health Aging 2000;4:31–41.

19. Lewis SJ, Egger M, Sylvester PA, et al. Early enteral feeding versus "nil by mouth" after gastrointestinal surgery: systematic review and meta-analysis of controlled trials. BMJ 2001;323:773–776.

20. Bisgaard T, Kehlet H. Early oral feeding after elective abdominal surgery—what are the issues? Nutrition 2002;18: 944–948.

21. Zaloga GP, Bortenschlager L, Black KW, et al. Immediate postoperative enteral feeding decreases weight loss and improves healing after abdominal surgery in rats. Crit Care Med 1992;20(1): 115–119.

22. Chiarelli A, Enzi G, Casadei A, et al. Very early nutrition supplementation in burned patients. Am J Clin Nutr 1990; 51:1035–1039.

23. Chan DL, Rozanski EA, Freeman LM. Relationship among plasma amino acids, C-reactive protein, illness severity, and outcome in critically ill dogs. J Vet Intern Med 2009;23:559–563.

24. Hurley KJ, Michel KE. Nutritional support of the critical patient. In: King LG, Boag AK, eds. BSAVA Manual of Canine and Feline Emergency and Critical Care. 2nd ed. BSAVA, Gloucester, UK: BSAVA; 2006:327–338.

25. Conejero R, Bonet A, Grau T, et al. Effect of a glutamine-enriched enteral diet on intestinal permeability and infectious morbidity at 28 days in critically ill patients with systemic inflammatory response syndrome: a randomized, single-blind, prospective, multicenter study. Nutrition 2002;18:716–721.

26. Wernerman J, Hammarqvist F. Glutamine: a necessary nutrient for the intensive care patient. Int J Colorectal Dis 1999;14: 137–142.

27. Mazzaferro E, Hackett T, Wingfield W, et al. Role of glutamine in health and disease. Compend Contin Edu Pract Vet 2000;22:1094–1101.

28. Goeters C, Wenn A, Mertes N, et al. Parenteral L-alanyl-L-glutamine improves 6-month outcome in critically ill patients. Crit Care Med 2002;30:2032–2037.

29. Novak F, Heyland DK, Avenell A, et al. Glutamine supplementation in serious illness: a systematic review of the evidence. Crit Care Med 2002;30:2022–2029.

30. Marks SL, Cook AK, Reader R, et al. Effects of glutamine supplementation of an amino acid-based purified diet on intestinal mucosal integrity in rats with methotrexate-induced enteritis. Am J Vet Res 1999;60:755–763.

31. Lana SE, Hansen RA, Kloer L, et al. The effects of oral glutamine supplementation on plasma glutamine concentration and PGE2 concentration in dogs experiencing radiation-induced mucositis. Int J Appl Res Vet Med 2003;1:259–265.

32. Osborne BJ, Saba AK, Wood SJ, et al. Clinical comparison of three methods to determine resting energy expenditure. Nutr Clin Pract 1994;9:241–246.

33. Ogilvie GK, Salman MD, Kesel ML, et al. Effect of anesthesia and surgery on energy expenditure determined by indirect calorimetry in dogs with malignant and nonmalignant conditions. Am J Vet Res 1996;57:1321–1326.

34. Greco DS, Rosychuk AW, Ogilvie GK, et al. The effect of levothyroxine treatment on resting energy expenditure of hypothyroid dogs. J Vet Intern Med 1998;12:7–10.

35. Walton RS, Wingfield WE, Ogilvie GK, et al. Energy expenditure in 104 postoperative and traumatized injured dogs with indirect calorimetry. J Vet Emerg Crit Care 1996;6:71–99.

36. Raffe MR. Total parenteral nutrition. In: Slatter D, ed. Textbook of Small Animal Surgery. 2nd ed. Philadelphia, PA: WB Saunders; 1993:78–81.

37. Freeman LM, Chan DL. Parenteral and enteral nutrition. Compend Stand of Care: Emerg Crit Care Med 2001;3:1–7.

38. Tredget EE, Yu YM. The metabolic effects of thermal injury. World J Surg 1992;16:68–79.

39. Wolfe RR, Durkot MJ, Wolfe MH. Effect of thermal injury on energy metabolism, substrate kinetics, and hormonal concentrations. Circ Shock 1982;9(4):383–394.

40. Adamantos SE, Chan DL. Adequacy of nutritional support in dogs with tetanus [abstract]. Proceedings of the British Small Animal Veterinary Congress, Birmingham, UK, 2008.

41. Shaw JH, Wolfe RR. A conscious septic dog model with hemodynamic and metabolic responses similar to responses of humans. Surgery 1984;95:553–561.

42. Tappy L, Chiolero R. Substrate utilization in sepsis and multiple organ failure. Crit Care Med 2007;35:S531–S534.

43. Jeejeebhoy KN. Permissive underfeeding of the critically ill patient. Nutr Clin Pract 2004;19:477–480.

39

Enteral diets for critically ill patients

Sally C. Perea

When selecting an enteral diet, there are a variety of factors to consider, including route of delivery, nutritional status, and underlying disease. Veterinary products designed for enteral feeding of critically ill patients are limited, but using options such as blended canned slurries, home-cooked formulations, and human enteral products can help to tailor the diet to the patient's individual needs.

Nutrient considerations for critical care diets

Energy

The goal of nutrition support in critically ill patients is to provide an appropriate level of energy to limit the loss of lean body mass and sustain critical physiologic processes such as immune function and wound healing. Because individual energy needs vary, the ideal method to determine energy expenditure in hospitalized patients is by indirect calorimetry.[1] However, indirect calorimetry is costly and unavailable in most veterinary hospitals; therefore, calculated requirements remain the most practical tool to estimate energy needs. During hospitalization, patients' energy needs are estimated to be equivalent to their calculated resting energy requirement (RER). Multiple RER equations have been recommended, but exponential equations using the patient's metabolic body weight are the most accurate:

$$RER = 70 \times \text{body weight in kg}^{0.75}$$

The use of illness energy factors is no longer recommended because multiplying RER by these factors gen-

erally results in overestimation of true energy needs in hospitalized patients and may lead to complications associated with overfeeding.[2]

Protein

Similar to energy needs, protein needs in critically ill patients should be focused on minimizing muscle catabolism and maintaining lean body mass. A healthy animal under conditions of starvation adapts by decreasing muscle breakdown and converting to the use of fatty acids and ketones for energy. However, in critically ill patients, muscle catabolism is not appropriately down-regulated, and elevations in endogenous corticosteroids, catecholamines, and inflammatory cytokines promote a hypercatabolic state.[3] In critically ill dogs, urinary nitrogen excretion has been shown to be two to six times the obligatory nitrogen excretion reported in healthy dogs, demonstrating the significant protein catabolism occurring in these patients.[4] Furthermore, the amino acids generated from muscle breakdown are primarily used for gluconeogenesis and production of acute-phase proteins, whereas synthesis of other selected proteins (such as albumin, transferrin, prealbumin, retinol-binding protein, and fibronectin) is actually decreased.[5]

Standard dog and cat foods meeting average protein needs generally provide between 20% and 30% and 30%–35% protein on a metabolizable energy (ME) basis, respectively. Foods that provide protein levels near the higher end of this range are generally preferred for most critically ill patients; however, the appropriate level of dietary protein also depends on individual patient needs and underlying disease. Animals with renal disease

Advanced Monitoring and Procedures for Small Animal Emergency and Critical Care, First Edition. Edited by Jamie M. Burkitt Creedon, Harold Davis.
© 2012 John Wiley & Sons, Inc. Published 2012 by John Wiley & Sons, Inc.

or hepatic encephalopathy should be provided with reduced protein levels, whereas growing animals and patients with significant protein losses (i.e., patients suffering from burns) may require increased protein levels.

Fat

Foods designed for critically ill patients are generally higher in fat to promote an increased energy density. Because problems with volume intolerance can arise when initiating enteral feeding, higher fat levels are used to help maximize energy delivery while limiting the required volume.

Average adult dog and cat dry foods generally range from 20% to 35% fat ME; critical care enteral foods range from 45% to 68% fat ME. Animals that have been without food for more than 3 days are using primarily endogenous fat for energy, making the transition to a higher fat food a fairly smooth transition for most patients. However, because of the high fat content of critical care diets, caution should be used when refeeding a patient with a condition associated with fat intolerance, such as hyperlipidemia, pancreatitis, or lymphangectasia. For patients such as these, a lower fat canned food slurry or home-cooked diet slurry can be used.

Carbohydrates

Dietary carbohydrates help to provide needed energy and spare the use of protein for gluconeogenesis. Carbohydrates also help to reduce the proportion of calories coming from fat, which can be helpful in patients with fat intolerance. However, carbohydrates are not a required nutrient, and for some patients, a lower carbohydrate diet may provide some benefits.

Patients experiencing hyperglycemia is one example where limiting dietary carbohydrates may be helpful. Hyperglycemia has been a topic of interest in both human and veterinary patients in recent years, with studies showing increased risk of mortality in human, canine, and feline critically ill patients with hyperglycemia.[6-8] Although hyperglycemia is more commonly seen as a metabolic complication in patients receiving parenteral nutrition, hyperglycemia has been reported in a feline patient with pancreatitis following implementation of enteral nutrition.[9]

Hyperglycemia in critically ill cats is also commonly seen prior to nutritional intervention; therefore, careful monitoring and adjustment of treatment protocols is recommended as nutrition support is implemented in these patients. Critically ill cats have been shown to have significantly higher glucose, lactate, cortisol, glucagon, and norepinephrine concentrations, and

significantly lower insulin concentrations when compared with controls.[10] These findings are consistent with those from human studies, showing higher concentrations of counterregulatory hormones and insulin resistance in critically ill patients.[11,12] Further research in this area is needed to determine the most appropriate management strategies for hyperglycemic veterinary patients. However, maintaining tighter glycemic control in patients receiving nutritional support may help to improve patient outcome.

Amino acids

Many critical care foods are enriched with selected amino acids, such as branched chain amino acids, arginine, and glutamine.

The branched chain amino acids valine, leucine, and isoleucine are metabolized by skeletal muscle, whereas other amino acids are metabolized by the liver.[13] For this reason, some foods designed for critically ill patients are supplemented with branched chain amino acids to supply energy for lean body tissue and help maintain lean body mass. A recent study in critically ill dogs showed that concentrations of branched chain amino acids were significantly higher in survivors compared with nonsurvivors.[14] Similarly, the ratio of branched chain amino acids to aromatic amino acids was also significantly higher in surviving dogs. This study supports the nutritional philosophy of supplementing with branched chain amino acids in critically ill patients; however, no studies have been conducted to date evaluating the efficacy of supplementation and its impact on patient outcome.

Because branched chain amino acids are not metabolized in the liver, they also have a theoretical benefit in patients with liver disease and hepatic encephalopathy. Similar to the study in critically ill dogs, it is known that the ratio of plasma branched chain amino acids to aromatic amino acids is decreased with declining liver function.[15] However, although branched chain amino acids have many theoretical benefits, studies evaluating their use in dogs with hepatic encephalopathy have failed to demonstrate measurable benefits.[16]

Glutamine is another amino acid commonly incorporated into critical care diets. Glutamine is preferentially used by enterocytes as an energy source, and it may help to promote the health of the small intestine and reduce the risk of bacterial translocation. In addition, glutamine is also used as a fuel source by immune cells and may aid in improving the patient's immune response. Despite the numerous theoretical benefits of glutamine supplementation, clinical studies evaluating its impact on outcome have been mixed.

Studies evaluating the use of glutamine-supplemented enteral diets in veterinary patients are limited. One study evaluating a glutamine-enriched enteral diet for cats with experimentally induced gastrointestinal disease did not find a significant clinical benefit.[17] Another experimental study evaluating radiation injury in dogs also failed to show a benefit of glutamine supplementation.[18]

Recent studies in experimental animals have demonstrated that glutamine supplementation helps to maintain mucosal barrier function, but other studies evaluating hospitalized surgery and trauma patients have failed to demonstrate a benefit on outcome.[19,20] Human studies evaluating free glutamine versus glutamine-rich protein supplementation have shown that feeding glutamine from complete protein sources is more efficacious in increasing mucosal glutamine concentrations.[21] Further studies are needed to determine how to most effectively use glutamine in enteral diets for critical care patients.

Arginine is another amino acid that may provide benefits in critically ill patients. Arginine is an essential amino acid for dogs and cats but is not normally essential in humans. In recent years arginine has gained attention in human medicine as "conditionally essential" during periods of stress due to its important roles in wound healing, immune function, and nitric oxide synthesis.[22] Recent studies in humans and rodents have demonstrated that arginine-supplemented enteral support can help to improve wound healing, decrease length of hospital stay, and change cytokine expression from a pro- to an anti-inflammatory profile.[23,24] Arginine supplementation has not been evaluated in veterinary critical care patients, but studies showing lower plasma arginine levels in critically ill dogs and dogs with early chronic valvular disease suggest that arginine supplementation may be beneficial.[14,25]

Other nutrients

Like supplemental amino acids, many of the other enhanced nutrients in critical care diets have theoretical benefits but have not been evaluated in critically ill dogs or cats. Antioxidants may benefit by counteracting the generation of free radicals associated with inflammation or reperfusion injury. Increased levels of long-chain omega-3 polyunsaturated fatty acids (PUFAs) can aid in modulating inflammatory reactions associated with underlying inflammatory processes. Finally, the addition of prebiotics, such as fermentable fibers and oligopolysaccharides, may be beneficial in critically ill animals that have a compromised gastrointestinal tract by promoting production of short-chain fatty acids and energy for colonocytes.

Enteral diets

Liquid enteral diets

Liquid enteral diets are required when feeding through a nasoesophageal or jejunostomy feeding tube. Liquid enteral diets can be categorized as polymeric or elemental formulations. Polymeric formulations are composed of proteins, carbohydrates, and fats in a high molecular weight form. Technically, a true "elemental" formulation would be comprised of free amino acids, monosaccharides, and fatty acids; however, true elemental formulations are rare, and many human formulations are more often "semi-elemental," containing hydrolyzed proteins, di- and tripeptides, disaccharides, oligosaccharides, and/or dextrin. Elemental diets have the advantage of requiring little to no digestion, which is ideal for patients with severe gastrointestinal disease, short bowel syndrome, or those being fed at the level of the jejunum. The potential disadvantage of elemental formulations is that some may have a higher osmolality when compared with polymeric formulations.

Studies in human patients with pancreatitis receiving jejunal enteral nutrition have shown that both polymeric and semi-elemental formulations are well tolerated; however, some advantages were seen with semi-elemental formulations including reduced length of hospital stay and less marked weight loss.[26] Currently available liquid canine and feline enteral foods are limited to polymeric formulations; therefore, if an elemental formulation is desired, a human product would be required (Table 39.1).

Although the selection of liquid enteral foods designed for dogs and cats is limited, available liquid commercial diets generally meet the needs of most hospitalized patients. For those patients that may require a lower fat content, or semi-elemental or hydrolyzed ingredients, a human liquid diet or enteral formulation may be used. It should be noted that human liquid products often contain vitamins and minerals but are not necessarily complete and balanced to meet the nutrient needs of dogs and cats. This is especially true in cats, in which protein and amino acid supplementation is generally required to meet protein and essential amino acid needs.

Canned enteral diets

Canned foods for critical care veterinary patients are designed to be highly digestible, energy dense, and provide a moderate to high protein content. Diets may be enriched with additional nutrients such as antioxidants, specific amino acids (arginine, glutamine, branched chain amino acids), omega-3 fatty acids, prebiotics, and soluble or insoluble fibers. These canned diets are also designed with a smooth consistency that

Table 39.1 Liquid and canned enteral foods[*]

	Caloric Distribution			Energy Density	Osmolality
	Protein %	Fat %	Carbohydrates %	kcal/oz or mL	mOsm/kg H$_2$O
Canine/Feline Critical Care Canned Formulas					
Hill's Prescription Diet a/d	33	55	12	32.7	–
Iams Maximum-Calorie	29	68	3	55.5	–
Royal Canin Recovery RS	40.7	57.5	1.8	32.9	–
Liquid Veterinary Foods					
CliniCare Canine/Feline Liquid Diet[a]	30	45	25	1.0	315
CliniCare RF[a]	22	57	21	1.0	235
PetAg EnteralCare HLP Liquid[b]	34	45	21	1.2	312
PetAg EnteralCare MLP Liquid[b]	27	52	21	1.2	256
Liquid Human Foods					
Ensure[a]	14.4	21.6	64	1.06	620
Ensure High Protein[a]	21.2	23.9	54.9	0.97	610
Nestlé Impact[c]	22	53	25	1.0	375
Human Semi-Elemental Foods					
Vital HN[a]	16.7	9.5	73.8	1.0	500
TwoCal HN[a]	16.7	40.1	43.2	2.0	725

[*]Nutrient and caloric composition of products as of March 2010.
[a]Abbot Laboratories, Abbot Park, IL.
[b]PetAg, Hampshire, IL.
[c]Nestlé HealthCare Nutrition, Minnetonka, MI.

facilitates syringe feeding through a feeding tube. These products can generally be delivered through a 12–14F feeding tube without additional water dilution; however, they generally need to be slightly warmed and mixed well to facilitate delivery. Current commercially available canned enteral foods for dogs and cats are outlined in Table 39.1.

Canned food blended slurries

Blended canned foods can be used when feeding through an esophagostomy or gastrostomy tube. Food provision through feeding tubes is discussed in detail in Chapter 40, Assisted Enteral Feeding. The use of blended canned slurries helps immensely to expand the dietary options and allows the diet to be more easily tailored to the pet's specific dietary needs. To achieve the highest possible energy density, it is recommended to slowly add water to the slurry while blending until a smooth consistency that can be delivered through the tube is achieved. Once an appropriate consistency has been achieved, the energy density and moisture level of the slurry can be determined, and feeding volumes can be calculated (Box 39.1).

Guidelines for the amounts of water needed to create blended slurries of common canned foods, and their resulting energy density and moisture levels, are outlined in Table 39.2. These guidelines were determined by testing the minimum amount of water needed to add to each canned food for delivery through a 12F feeding tube for feline foods and a 14F feeding tube for canine foods. Water was slowly added to the canned diet until a smooth texture was achieved, and the final mixture was allowed to blend for up to 5 minutes to ensure that all particles were finely blended and distributed. The final slurry should be tested through a feeding tube of the same size being used in the patient to ensure that the slurry can be easily delivered and does not require additional dilution (see Fig. 39.1).

Home-cooked diet blended slurries

Home-cooked (or hospital-cooked) blended slurry formulations can be helpful when commercially available products do not meet the needs of the patient (Fig. 39.2). Dietary fat intolerance is one of the most common complications that leads to the need for a home-cooked formulation. Highly digestible/low-fat,

Box 39.1 Enteral feeding worksheet

Step 1: Calculate patient's resting energy requirement
Resting energy requirement (RER) = $70 \times$ body weight in kg$^{0.75}$
$$= \text{kcal/day}$$

Step 2: Calculate energy density of blended slurry
$$\frac{\text{Energy provided by of canned food (kcal)}}{\text{Volume of final slurry (mL)}} = \frac{\text{kcal}}{\text{mL}}$$

Step 3: Calculate feeding daily volume
$$\frac{\text{RER (kcal/day)}}{\text{Energy density of slurry (kcal/mL)}} = \text{mL slurry/day}$$

Day 1 = 25–33% × total mL slurry/day = total day 1 volume (mL)

Day 2 = 50–66% × total mL slurry/day = total day 2 volume (mL)

Day 3 = 75–99% × total mL slurry/day = total day 3 volume (mL)

Day 4 = 100% × total mL slurry/day = total day 4 volume (mL)

Step 4: Calculate water contribution from blended slurry
% moisture of canned food × g/can = water from food (mL)

water from food (mL) + water added to slurry (mL)
= total water volume (mL)

$$\frac{\text{total water volume (mL)}}{\text{slurry volume (mL)}} = \text{\% moisture of final slurry}$$

mL slurry fed daily × % moisture of final slurry
= total water delivered daily (mL)

Step 5: Calculate additional water needs
Patient's water requirement (mL) minus water delivered from blended slurry (mL) = additional water needed daily (mL)

uncommon ingredient/low-fat, and renal disease/low-fat canine and feline formulations are outlined in Tables 39.3 to 39.8. The ingredients in these formulations are designed to be simple, and require minimal preparation in a hospital setting.

When preparing these slurries, the water should be slowly added to the mixture during the blending step because adding the water all in the beginning step can result in a soupy blend, leaving fragments of rice or other ingredients that are not well blended. A slightly longer blending time than required for the canned food slurries is also recommended for the home-cooked formulations (minimum of 5 minutes). Allowing ample time for blending helps ensure that the ingredients are broken down and smoothly distributed throughout the mixture.

Preparation instructions for blended slurries

Measure out the ingredient amounts and add to a blender. Add a fourth of the recommended water amount and beginning to blend the mixture, adding an additional fourth of water every 30 seconds until the full amount has been added. Blend the mixture for an additional 4–5 minutes, and test the final slurry to ensure that it can easily be delivered through the appropriate feeding tube size. If needed, additional water can be added to create a more dilute mixture for easier delivery. If additional water is added, slurry energy density and moisture content should be recalculated to reflect the new slurry volume. Unused slurry may be stored in the refrigerator for a later feeding; however, the slurry may require reblending and heating to room temperature to regain a smooth and fluid consistency prior to feeding. Tightly covered slurry should be discarded after 3 days to prevent spoilage.

Supplements

When using a supplement, it is important to consider the impact on the overall balance of the diet. When adding more than 10% of the total calories from a supplemental ingredient, additional nutrients such as vitamins and/or minerals may be required to ensure that minimum nutrient requirements are met. For short-term in-hospital management (less than 1–2 weeks), adding additional vitamins and minerals to create a complete and balanced formulation may not be necessary. However, for patients that require long-term enteral nutrition support, a consultation with a board-certified veterinary nutritionist is recommended to ensure that the diet formulation is complete and balanced (Table 39.9) for long-term feeding.

Fat supplements

Oils can be added to solutions to increase fat and energy density, as well as provide specific fatty acids of interest. Vegetable oils, such as corn and canola oil, can be used to increase both total dietary fat and linoleic acid levels of the diet; fish oils can be used to provide long-chain omega-3 polyunsaturated fatty acids.

Carbohydrate supplements

Light corn syrup is an energy-dense, highly digestible carbohydrate ingredient that can be added to formulations to boost energy density without increasing the fat level. The addition of light corn syrup can be very helpful to boost calories for canine formulations but are not recommended for feline formulations due to the fructose content. As an alternative, glucose or

Table 39.2 Canned foods and blended slurry guidelines[*,†]

	Caloric Distribution			Energy Density	Can Size	Water Needed	Energy Density	Final Moisture
	Protein %	Fat %	Carbohydrate %	kcal/oz	oz	mL	kcal/mL	%
Canine Gastrointestinal Formulas								
Hill's Prescription Diet i/d[a]	22.0	32.0	46.0	37.3	13.0	170	0.92	84.5
Iams Low-Resisue[b]	28.0	38.0	34.0	29.6	14.0	120	0.83	85.8
Purina Gastroenteric EN[c]	27.0	29.6	43.3	33.9	12.5	180	0.83	86.7
Royal Canin Digestive Low Fat LF[d]	30.1	15.3	54.6	28.3	13.6	120	0.77	84.1
Royal Canin Intestinal HE[d]	26.5	30.1	43.4	28.3	14.0	200	0.66	84.8
Feline Gastrointestinal Formulas								
Hill's Prescription Diet i/d[a]	29.0	48.0	23.0	29.3	5.5	25	0.92	85.6
Iams Low-Resisue[b]	35.0	34.0	31.0	28.2	6.0	55	0.75	83.4
Purina Dietetic Management DM[c]	46.3	47.1	6.6	35.3	5.5	35	1.08	86.2
Purina Gastroenteric EN[c]	35.0	51.8	13.2	32.5	5.5	30	0.90	75.8
Energy Dense Uncommon Ingredient Formulas								
EVO 95% Duck Canine & Feline Formulas[d]	25.8	69.6	4.5	39.4	5.5	15	1.35	85.4
EVO 95% Venison Canine & Feline Formulas[d]	29.7	64.5	5.8	39.6	5.5	30	1.09	75.8
California Natural Salmon & Sweet Potato Canine Formula[d]	34.6	58.1	7.3	42.0	13.2	100	1.23	87.0

[*]Nutrient and caloric composition of products as of March 2010. Please confirm that nutrient and caloric data is current prior to using these guidelines.
[†]Guidelines developed by Dr. Sally Perea, Davis, CA.
[a]Hill's Pet Nutrition, Inc., Topeka, KS.
[b]The Iams Company, Dayton, OH.
[c]Nestlé Purina, St. Louis, MO.
[d]Royal Canin USA, Inc., St. Charles, MO.
[e]Natura Pet Products, Inc., Davis, CA.

dextrose powders or solutions could be used in cat formulations.

Considerations for specific underlying conditions

When providing assisted enteral feeding to patients with underlying conditions, the nutrient modifications and recommendations mirror those of oral diets. Therefore, efforts should be made to select a food that first addresses the patient's underlying illness, and then consider how to prepare the food for enteral delivery.

Gastrointestinal disease

Highly digestible diets are recommended for patients with underlying gastrointestinal diseases. There are a variety of highly digestible veterinary diets available that serve as excellent choices for blended canned food slurries (Table 39.2). These highly digestible foods general provide moderate protein and fat levels, also making them good choices when looking for a more equally distributed caloric distribution of protein, fat, and carbohydrates compared with some of the critical care formulas.

Adverse reactions to food

For patients with adverse reactions to food such as food allergy dermatitis or inflammatory bowel disease, an uncommon ingredient canned food may be used to create a blended slurry for esophagostomy or gastrostomy feedings. Some energy-dense uncommon ingredient formulas are outlined in Table 39.2. In addition to

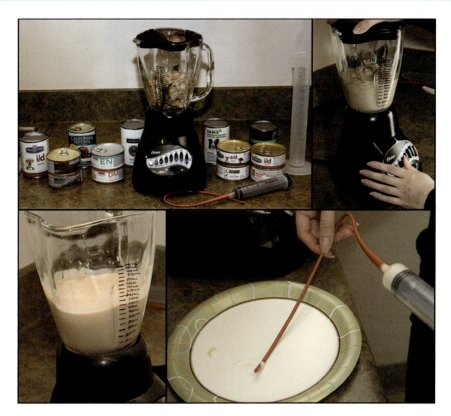

Figure 39.1 Canned food slurries can be used for esophagostomy and gastrostomy enteral feedings. Slowly add water to the canned food slurry and blend mixture for 4–5 minutes until a smooth texture is achieved. For blenders that do not provide volume designations, volumes guidelines can be premeasured and marked on the side of the blender using known volumes of water. Once the slurry has been adequately blended, measure the final slurry volume for energy density calculations. Test the final slurry to ensure that it can be easily delivered through the appropriate feeding tube size.

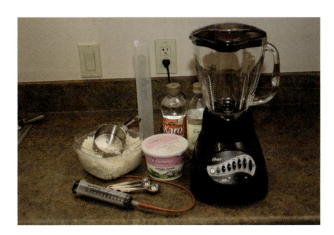

Figure 39.2 Highly digestible low-fat ingredients can be used to create low-fat recipes, and supplemental ingredients can be used to improve energy density of the diet.

these, a variety of veterinary therapeutic uncommon ingredient canned formulations are available. If the patient is currently being managed on an uncommon ingredient food, then a canned food with the same ingredients should be select. For patients recently diag-

nosed with food allergies, or with suspected food allergies, a food with ingredients that the pet has not previously been exposed to should be selected.

Fat intolerance

It should be noted that although canned diets designed for intestinal disease and food allergies generally provide less fat than those designed for critical care, many are still relatively high in fat, especially when compared with their dry food equivalent. For patients with disease conditions related to dietary fat, such as hyperlipidemia, pancreatitis, and lymphangectasia, a lower fat formulation should be selected. Patients with decreased gastrointestinal mobility and cylothorax may also benefit from a low-fat diet.

Because commercial canned foods generally run higher in fat, there are a limited number of low-fat canned food options available for use in a blended slurry. Low-fat home-cooked recipes provided in this chapter can serve as low-fat dietary options when commercial options are unavailable.

Table 39.3 Feline low-fat recipe*

Ingredient	Grams	Amount
Hormel[a] Canned Chicken Breast in water, no salt added	142	1 can (not drained)
White rice, long grain, regular, cooked	118.5	¾ cup
Canola oil	3.4	¾ teaspoon
Nordic Naturals[b] Pet Cod Liver Oil	1.2	¼ teaspoon
Balance IT[c] feline	3.2	6 white scoops
Water (mL)		150
Total recipe kcal		329
Total slurry volume (mL)		400
Total slurry moisture (%)		82
Energy Density of Slurry (kcal/mL)		**0.82**
Caloric Distribution		
Protein % ME		37.58
Fat % ME		20.25
Carbohydrate % ME		42.17

*Guidelines developed by Dr. Sally Perea, Davis, CA.
[a]Hormel Foods Corporation, Austin, MN.
[b]Nordic Naturals, Inc., Watsonville, CA.
[c]Davis Veterinary Medical Consulting, Inc., Davis, CA.

Table 39.4 Feline low-fat uncommon ingredient recipe*

Ingredient	Grams	Amount
Bumble Bee[a] canned crab meat	120	1 6-oz can drained
Betty Crocker[b] Potato Buds, dried potatoes	23	⅓ cup dry amount mixed with equal parts hot water
Canola oil	3.4	¾ teaspoon
Balance IT[c] feline	2.6	5 white scoops
Water (mL)		80
Total recipe (kcal)		202
Total slurry volume (mL)		280
Total slurry moisture		82
Energy Density of Slurry (kcal/mL)		**0.72**
Caloric Distribution		
Protein % ME	40.6	
Fat % ME	20.11	
Carbohydrate % ME	39.28	

*Guidelines developed by Dr. Sally Perea, Davis, CA.
[a]Bumble Bee Foods, LLC, San Diego, CA.
[b]General Mills, Inc., Minneapolis, MN.
[c]Davis Veterinary Medical Consulting, Inc., Davis, CA.

Renal disease

For patients with renal disease, a canned renal food can be used to create a blended slurry for esophagostomy and gastrostomy feedings. If a liquid food is required, CliniCare RF is available for feline patients, but options are limited for canine patients. Some human liquid diets, such as Ensure, are lower in protein but are not phosphorus restricted, making them less than ideal for longer term management.

Liver disease

For patients with hepatic encephalopathy, a canned protein-restricted liver disease food can be used to create a blended slurry for esophagostomy and gastrostomy feedings. Currently available commercially canned veterinary therapeutic foods for the management of hepatic encephalopathy are limited to Hill's Prescription Diet l/d (canine and feline varieties). Although renal failure canned foods are also protein restricted, they generally contain ingredients, such as liver, which are less ideal protein sources for patients with hepatic encephalopathy.

For liver disease patients that are not suffering from hepatic encephalopathy, protein restriction is not necessary or recommended. A standard critical care diet or a highly digestible canned food blended slurry are both acceptable options for these patients.

Initiating nutrition support

Patients should be slowly weaned onto full energy needs, starting at approximately 25%–33% of RER, followed by 25%–33% increases every 12–24 hours until full RER is reached.[27,28] Patients that have been without food for an extended period of time are at an increased risk of developing hyperglycemia or electrolyte abnormalities upon refeeding (i.e., hypokalemia, hypophosphatemia, and hypomagnesemia as well as low thiamin) and may require a slower weaning and increased frequency of monitoring. Once full RER is reached, the patient may be reassessed to determine if increased caloric levels are needed to maintain body weight.

Enteral formulas can be fed via continuous infusion or via intermittent bolus feeding. Esophagostomy and

Table 39.5 Feline low-fat renal recipe*

Ingredient	Grams	Amount
Hormel[a] Canned Chicken Breast in water, no salt added	71	½ can (not drained)
White Rice, long grain, regular, cooked	118.5	¾ cup
Canola oil	3.4	¾ teaspoon
Nordic Naturals[b] Pet Cod Liver Oil	1.2	¼ teaspoon
Balance IT[c] feline-K	4.6	1 yellow and 2 white scoops
Water (mL)		170
Total Recipe (kcal)		262
Total slurry volume (ml)		315
Total slurry moisture (%)		83
Energy Density of Slurry (kcal/mL)		**0.83**
Caloric Distribution		
Protein % ME		25.93
Fat % ME		21.08
Carbohydrate % ME		52.98

*Guidelines developed by Dr. Sally Perea, Davis, CA.
[a]Hormel Foods Corporation, Austin, MN.
[b]Nordic Naturals, Inc., Watsonville, CA.
[c]Davis Veterinary Medical Consulting, Inc., Davis, CA.

Table 39.6 Canine low-fat recipe*

Ingredient	Grams	Amount
Cottage cheese, 2% milk fat	339	1½ cup
White rice, long grain, regular, cooked	158	1 cup
Light corn syrup	85.2	4 tablespoons
Corn oil	4.5	1 teaspoon
Nordic Naturals[a] Pet Cod Liver Oil	1.2	¼ teaspoon
Balance IT[b] canine	11.9	1 black and 7 white
Water (mL)		20
Total recipe (kcal)		801
Total slurry volume (mL)		525
Total slurry moisture (%)		67
Energy Density of Slurry (kcal/mL)		**1.53**
Caloric Distribution		
Protein % ME		26.86
Fat % ME		14.01
Carbohydrate % ME		59.13

*Guidelines developed by Dr. Sally Perea, Davis, CA.
[a]Nordic Naturals, Inc., Watsonville, CA.
[b]Davis Veterinary Medical Consulting, Inc., Davis, CA.

gastrostomy feedings are generally given by intermittent bolus feedings. One clinical study evaluating continuous versus intermittent bolus feedings in dogs with gastrostomy tubes showed no differences in weight maintenance, gastrointestinal-adverse effects, glucose tolerance, nitrogen balance, or feed digestibility.[29] Continuous infusions may be better tolerated for nasoesophageal feedings if large volumes of liquid formulas are required to meet daily energy needs, and they are recommended for jejunal feedings to help minimize malabsorption and diarrhea associated with feeding large volumes of nutrients directly into the jejunum.

If a continuous infusion is not available, bolus feeding may be used. In general, four or more feedings per day are required. The amount fed per feeding should not exceed 5–10 mL/kg of body weight during initial introduction of feedings.[30] Maximum gastric capacities for dogs and cats are reported as high as 45–90 mL/kg body weight.[28] However, meeting the patient's RER should be achievable at volumes far below these maximum capaci-

ties. Feeding boluses should be given slowly to allow for gastric expansion. The patients should be monitored for signs of nausea such as salivating, gulping, or retching during the feeding. If any of these signs develop, the feeding should be temporarily discontinued or stopped. Further details and guidelines for enteral feeding are provided in Chapter 40.

Monitoring

Patients receiving enteral nutrition should be monitored daily for potential complications and to ensure that the nutritional plan is continuing to meet the patient's needs. Daily physical examinations should include assessment of body condition and measurement of body weight. Because of the risk of aspiration and fluid overload, care should be taken to assess respiratory parameters, and thoracic radiographs should be taken if respiratory distress or fever develops at any time during administration. The stoma site of enteral feeding tubes

Table 39.7 Canine low-fat uncommon ingredient recipe[*]

Ingredient	Grams	Amount
Bumble Bee[a] canned crab meat	120	1 6-oz can drained
Betty Crocker[b] Potato Buds, dried potatoes	51.8	¾ cup dry amount
Canola oil	4.5	1 teaspoon
Balance IT[c] canine	4.4	1 black
Water (mL)		150
Total recipe (kcal)		219
Total slurry volume (mL)		460
Total slurry moisture (%)		83
Energy Density of Slurry (kcal/mL)		**0.48**
Caloric Distribution		
Protein % ME		27.77
Fat % ME		16.26
Carbohydrate % ME		55.96

[*]Guidelines developed by Dr. Sally Perea, Davis, CA.
[a]Bumble Bee Foods, LLC, San Diego, CA.
[b]General Mills, Inc., Minneapolis, MN.
[c]Davis Veterinary Medical Consulting, Inc., Davis, CA.

Table 39.8 Canine low-fat renal recipe[*]

Ingredient	Grams	Amount
Hormel[a] Canned Chicken Breast in water, no salt added	71	½ can (not drained)
White rice, long grain, regular, cooked	237	1½ cup
Light corn syrup	63.9	3 tablespoons
Corn oil	6.8	1½ teaspoons
Nordic Naturals[b] Pet Cod Liver Oil	2.5	½ teaspoon
Balance IT[c] canine-K	7.1	2 blue and 1 white scoops
Water (mL)		250
Total recipe (kcal)		638
Total slurry volume (mL)		550
Total slurry moisture (%)		77
Energy Density of Slurry (kcal/mL)		**1.16**
Caloric Distribution		
Protein % ME		12.57
Fat % ME		15.54
Carbohydrate % ME		71.89

[*]Guidelines developed by Dr. Sally Perea, Davis, CA.
[a]Hormel Foods Corporation, Austin, MN.
[b]Nordic Naturals, Inc., Watsonville, CA.
[c]Davis Veterinary Medical Consulting Inc., Davis, CA.

Table 39.9 Nutritionally complete canine formulation[*,†]

Ensure	ProMod[a]	Balance IT[b] Canine	Total kcal	Protein ME (%)	Fat ME (%)	% Carbohydrate ME (%)
1 8-oz bottle	¼ cup (16 g)	1 black scoop (4.4 g)	322	26.1	20.9	53.0
1 8-oz bottle	⅓ cup (22 g)	1 black scoop (4.4 g)	347	29.4	20.7	49.9

[*]Ensure can be supplemented with ProMod protein supplement and Balance IT canine vitamin and mineral supplement to provide a nutritionally complete canine formulation.
[†]Guidelines developed by Dr. Sally Perea, Davis, CA.
[a]Abbot Laboratories, Ross Products Division, Columbus, OH.
[b]Davis Veterinary Medical Consulting, Inc., Davis, CA.

should be cleaned with dilute antiseptic (e.g., chlorhexidine or povidone-iodine) and carefully examined daily for signs of infection.

Serum potassium, magnesium, and phosphorus concentrations should be measured within 12–24 hours of starting enteral nutrition. Daily monitoring of electrolytes should be continued during the weaning on period, and no less than once every other day once at goal rate of infusion for 24 hours for critically ill hospitalized patients. A complete blood count (CBC) and chemistry panel should be measured within 24 hours of instituting enteral nutrition. Continued monitoring of a CBC and chemistry panel every 2–3 days is recommended for critically ill patients.

Acknowledgment

My thanks to Dr. Kari Christianson for her assistance in preparing the canned food blended slurry guidelines and photos.

References

1. Boullata J, Williams J, Cottrell F, et al. Accurate determination of energy needs in hospitalized patients. J Amer Diet Assoc 2007;107(3):393–401.
2. O'Toole E, Miller GW, Wilson BA, et al. Comparison of the standard predictive equation for calculation of resting energy expenditure with indirect calorimetry in hospitalized and healthy dogs. J Amer Vet Med Assoc 2004; 225(1):58–64.
3. Chan DL. Nutritional requirements of the critically ill Patient. ClinTech Small Anim Pract 2004;19(1):1–5.
4. Michel KE, King LG, Ostro E. Measurement of urinary urea nitrogen content as an estimate of the amount of total urinary nitrogen loss in dogs in intensive care units. J Am Vet Med Assoc 1997;210(3):356–359.
5. Gianni B, Toigo G, Ciocchi B, et al. Metabolic response to injury and sepsis: changes in protein metabolism. Nutrition 1997;13(9S):52S–57S.
6. Pyle SC, Marks SL, Kass PH. Evaluation of complications and prognostic factors associated with administration of total parenteral nutrition in cats: 75 cases (1994–2001). J Am Vet Med Assoc 2004;225(2):242–250.
7. Torre DM, deLaforcade AM, Chan DL. Incidence and clinical relevance of hyperglycemia in critically ill dogs. J Vet Intern Med 2007;21(5):971–975.
8. Sleiman I, Morandi A, Sabatini T, et al. Hyperglycemia as a predictor of in-hospital mortality in elderly patients without diabetes mellitus admitted to a sub-intensive care unit. J Am Geriatr Soc 2008;56(6):1106–1110.
9. Jennings M, Center SA, Barr SC, et al. Successful treatment of feline pancreatitis using an endoscopically placed gastrojejunostomy tube. J Am Anim Hosp Assoc 2001;37:145–152.
10. Chan DL, Freeman LM, Rozanski EA. Alterations in carbohydrate metabolism in critically ill cats. J Vet Emerg Crit Care 2006;16(2)(S1):S7–S13.
11. Marik PE, Raghavan M. Stress-hyperglycemia, insulin and immunomodulation in sepsis. Intensive Care Med 2004;30(4):748–756.
12. Zauner A, Nimmerrichter P, Anderwald C, et al. Severity of insulin resistance in critically ill medical patients. Metab Clin Exper 2007;56(1):1–5.
13. Skeie B, Kvetan V, Gil KM, et al. Branch-chain amino acids: their metabolism and clinical utility. Crit Care Med 1990;18(5):549–571.
14. Chan DL, Rozanski EA, Freeman LM. Relationship among plasma amino acids, C-reactive protein, illness severity, and outcome in critically ill dogs. J Vet Intern Med 2009;23:559–563.
15. Zicker SC, Rogers QR. Use of plasma amino acid concentrations in the diagnosis of nutritional and metabolic diseases in veterinary medicine. In: Kaneko JJ, ed. Proceedings of IVth Congress of the International Society for Animal Clinical Biochemistry. 1990:107–121.
16. Meyer HP, Chamuleau RA, Legemate DA, et al. Effects of a branched-chain amino acid-enriched diet on chronic hepatic encephalopathy in dogs. Metab Brain Dis 1999;14:103–115.
17. Marks SL, Cook AK, Reader R, et al. Effects of glutamine supplementation of an amino acid-based purified diet on intestinal mucosal integrity in cats with methotrexate-induced enteritis. Am J Vet Res 1999;60:755–763.
18. McArdle AH. Protection from radiation injury by elemental diet: does added glutamine change the effect. Gut 1994;(Suppl 1):S60–S64.
19. Schulman AS, Willcutts KF, Claridge JA, et al. Does the addition of glutamine to enteral feeds affect patient mortality? Crit Care Med 2005;33:2401–2506.
20. Yang L, Chen Y, Zhang J, et al. Protective effect of glutamine-enriched early enteral nutrition on intestinal mucosal barrier injury after liver transplantation in rats. Am J Surg 2010;199:35–42.
21. Preiser JC, Peres-Bota D, Eisendrath P, et al. Gut mucosal and plasma concentrations of glutamine: a comparison between two enriched enteral feeding solutions in critically ill patients. Nutr J 2003;2:13–17.
22. Michel KE. Interventional nutrition for the critical care patient: Optimal diets. Clin Tech Small Anim Pract 1998;13(4):204–210.
23. De Luis Da, Izaola O, Cuellar L, et al. High dose of arginine enhanced enteral nutrition in postsurgical head and neck cancer patients. A randomized clinical trial. Eur Rev Med Pharmacol Sci 2009;13(4):279–283.
24. Fan J, Meng Q, Guo G, et al. Effects of early enteral nutrition supplemented with arginine on intestinal mucosal immunity in severely burned mice. Clinical Nutr 2010;29(1):124–130.
25. Freeman LM, Rush JE, Markwell PJ. Effects of dietary modification in dogs with early chronic valvular disease. J Vet Intern Med 2006;20:1116–1126.
26. Tiengou LE, Gloro R, Pouzoulet J, et al. Semi-elemental formula or polymeric formula: is there a better choice for enteral nutrition in acute pancreatitis? Randomized comparative study. J Parenter Enteral Nutr 2006;30(1):1–5.
27. Marks SL. The principles and practical application of enteral nutrition. Vet Clin North Am Small Anim Pract 1998;28(3):677–708.
28. Remillard RL, Armstrong PJ, Davenport DJ. Assisted feeding in hospitalized patients: enteral and parenteral nutrition. In: Hand MS, Thatcher CD, Remillard RL, Roudebush P, eds. Small Animal Clinical Nutrition. 4th ed. Topeka, KS: Mark Morris Institute; 2000:351–399.
29. Chandler ML, Guilford WG, Lawoko CRO. Comparison of continuous versus intermittent enteral feeding in dogs. J Vet Intern Med 1996;10(3):133–138.
30. Chan DL. The inappetent hospitalized cat: clinical approach to maximizing nutritional support. J Feline Med Surg 2009;11:925–933.

BISHOP BURTON COLLEGE

40

Assisted enteral feeding

Scott Campbell and Natalie Harvey

Introduction

Adequate nutritional intake is required to support the immune system, wound healing, and intestinal structure and function. As such, animals that have inadequate nutritional intake are at higher risk of infection, wound breakdown, and intestinal villous atrophy.[1]

Enteral nutrition, as opposed to parenteral nutrition, has been associated with improved gut barrier function, a lower incidence of infectious complications, and shorter recovery times in humans.[2] Maintenance of gut barrier function and faster recovery times have also been demonstrated with early enteral nutrition, when compared with nil per os, in dogs with parvoviral enteritis.[3] Early enteral nutrition is recommended as the first choice where possible for these reasons,[2,3] which has given rise to the adage "if the gut works, use it!"[4]

Deciding when to implement nutritional support can be difficult because the ideal time to begin differs for each animal. Indications for nutritional support previously reported in the literature include 3 days of anorexia/withheld food (sooner for puppies, kittens, and overweight cats), body condition score (BCS) of 2 or less on a 5-point scale, 3 or less for dogs and 4 or less for cats on a-9 point scale, weight loss of 10% or greater, and/or hypoalbuminemia.[4]

A thorough diet history (see Box 40.1) is required to accurately assess nutritional adequacy of an animal's diet and whether assisted nutritional support is indicated.[5] Accurately monitoring nutrition during hospitalization will also assist in identification of animals requiring assisted enteral nutrition. This includes recording an initial BCS, the full diet name of the food

to be fed in the hospital, the amount offered and consumed per meal, and body weight daily (considered in relation to hydration status).[6]

The goal for daily caloric intake is the calculated resting energy requirement (RER) while in the hospital (shown below in Box 40.9). The RER has been multiplied by illness energy factors in the past that were extrapolated from human recommendations. Studies by Walton et al[7] and O'Toole et al[8] indicate that the energy requirements of critical care patients are more closely represented by RER. These calculations are a reasonable starting point, and ongoing assessment of the nutritional status of the patient and adjustments to nutritional intake should be performed as required.

Animals that have been anorexic for extended periods are at greater risk of refeeding syndrome. Refeeding syndrome refers to the rapid electrolyte shifts that occur during realimentation, especially with rapidly digestible and absorbable carbohydrates, which can cause muscle weakness and tremors, cardiac arrhythmias, neurologic signs, intravascular hemolysis, and death.[9,10] Initiating feeding slowly at quarters of RER over 4 days (see refeeding schedule below in Box 40.9) with daily monitoring of serum biochemistry can help to detect refeeding syndrome before it becomes critical (see Chapter 38, Nutritional Requirements in Critical Illness, for more details).

A number of factors should be considered when deciding which form of nutritional support to use to meet caloric requirements. These include the following[11]:

- Disease or condition being treated
- Cost

Advanced Monitoring and Procedures for Small Animal Emergency and Critical Care, First Edition. Edited by Jamie M. Burkitt Creedon, Harold Davis.
© 2012 John Wiley & Sons, Inc. Published 2012 by John Wiley & Sons, Inc.

Box 40.1 Core diet history questions

- Is your pet housed indoors, outdoors, or both?
- Please describe your pet's activity level including type, duration, and frequency.
- Do you have other pets?
- Is food left out for your pet during the day or taken away after the meal?
- Does your pet have access to other unmonitored food sources (e.g., from neighbor, other animals, etc.)?
- Who typically feeds your pet?
- How do you store your pet's food?
- Does your pet have confirmed food allergies or difficulty chewing or swallowing?
- Please indicate if your pet has experienced any of the following before today's visit: recent involuntary or unintended weight gain or weight loss, vomiting, diarrhea.
- Have you observed any changes in urination, defecation, drinking, or appetite?
- Please list the brand and product names of all foods, snacks, and treats your pet currently eats.
- Please list other diets and treats your pet has received in the past.
- Please list the name of each additional supplement your pet receives.

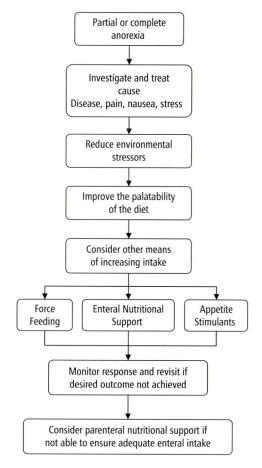

Figure 40.1 Pathway for ensuring adequate nutritional intake.

- Availability of intensive care facilities
- Dietary requirements of the individual animal (e.g., growth, pregnancy, lactation status)
- Anticipated length of feeding assistance needed

Enticing voluntary eating

Measures aimed at improving palatability of the diet and/or offering a variety of different foods are commonly used as the first step in the hope that the animal will consume adequate calories voluntarily. This practice may increase the risk of developing learned taste aversion to multiple foods,[12,13] making it more difficult to feed the animal when it has recovered or to introduce a therapeutic diet to help manage disease states. A more strategic approach to enticing voluntary consumption using a single diet initially and utilizing assisted enteral and parenteral techniques where required is recommended (see Fig. 40.1).

Partial or complete anorexia can have several causes. Pain or nausea can reduce appetite and may be caused by chronic or acute disease, trauma, or medication.[14] Animals should be stabilized first and made as comfortable as possible by treating pain prior to initiating feeding. If the medication used is suspected of causing nausea, an alternative medication should be sought

Box 40.2 Medications that may cause anorexia, nausea and/or vomiting in dogs and cats[15,16]

- Amoxicillin
- Amoxicillin/clavulanate
- Cardiac glycosides
- Cephalexin
- Chloramphenicol
- Erythromycin
- Most chemotherapeutic agents
- Most narcotic analgesics
- Nonsteroidal anti-inflammatory drugs
- Tetracyclines
- Trimethoprim/sulphadiazine
  Adapted from: Michel[15]

where possible.[14] A list of medications that may cause anorexia, nausea, or vomiting in cats is shown in Box 40.2.

Some animals may also experience anorexia secondary to fear and anxiety while in the hospital. Helping a

---

Box 40.3 Environmental stressors that may affect appetite

- Loud noises
- Other animals
- Irregular lighting cycles
- Food bowl near soiled area
- Unfamiliar people/people associated with negative experience(s)
- Unfamiliar food receptacle
- Obstacles to reaching the food

---

pet to feel less stressed in the hospital typically involves attempting to mimic the feeding circumstances of the pet at home.[14] A diet history (see Box 40.1) can provide this information for the hospital staff. A quick reference guide for identifying environmental stressors that may affect appetite is provided in Box 40.3.

Loud noises are common in emergency and critical care wards and should be minimized when offering food to animals. Where this is not practical, moving the animal to a quieter room or place within the hospital during feeding may be beneficial.[14]

Other animals in the immediate environment may also cause stress that affects appetite. Placing a towel, or other sight barrier, over the cage door can help anxious animals, especially cats, to feel less threatened. Moving the animal to another area during feeding may help in this situation as well.

Environmental cues, such as light-dark cycles, may be linked to consumption patterns for some animals. Keeping lighting cycles where animals are housed as normal as possible and keeping feeding times similar to regular feeding times for the individual may help maintain these cues for food consumption.[14,17]

Food acceptance may be decreased by the proximity of the food bowl to areas of defecation or urination, such as litter boxes; thus cages should be cleaned prior to feeding and food bowls placed as far away as possible from litter trays.[14]

Who presents the food and how they present it may also affect food acceptance. People associated with less negative experiences, such as those not required to restrain the animal or give it injections, may have more success encouraging animals to eat.[14] The owner may be encouraged to feed inappetent animals, but they should be instructed on which food or foods to offer and should ideally be monitored while doing so. The type of food receptacle may also be important to the individual; for example, the animal may prefer to consume food from a ceramic plate as opposed to a stainless steel bowl.

Obstacles that may impede an animal from consuming food should be removed or managed where possible. Some animals are unwilling to eat while wearing an e-collar. Where these are removed, the animal will need to be supervised while eating.[14] Animals that have compromised mobility or spinal pain may need the food bowls raised or positioned carefully to ensure the animal can reach the food. Where this is not possible, hand feeding may need to be instituted.[14]

At this point, if the animal still does not consume sufficient calories, the palatability of the diet may be improved. Several factors can affect the palatability of the diet to an animal, including moisture, fat, protein, salt, sugar and other, more intangible, factors of the diet.

Increasing the moisture content of a diet may increase its palatability, although cats raised on a dry diet often develop a learned texture preference for dry foods,[14] in which case increasing food moisture will not help. An effective means of increasing moisture content is to use a canned diet because canned diets typically contain between 70% and 85% moisture on an "as-fed" basis, whereas dry diets typically contain between 7% and 10% moisture on an "as-fed" basis. Canned diets are often higher in protein and fat, and thus should not be used when increasing these nutrients is contraindicated.[14] There can be significant differences between the dry and canned versions of the same therapeutic diet, so even within the same therapeutic food, changing from a dry to a canned formulation should be done with caution. Dry kibble can be soaked to increase the moisture content, but this will not raise the moisture content to the same extent as changing to a canned diet.[14]

Amino acid receptors are the most common taste receptors in cats and dogs. These receptors are particularly responsive to the amino acids L-proline and L-cysteine.[18,19] Beagles have also been shown to select foods with a higher protein level.[20] Increasing the protein content may therefore improve the palatability of the diet. Higher protein content is contraindicated in animals with renal failure or hepatic encephalopathy.[14]

Increasing the fat content of the diet may improve its palatability.[14] This also has the advantage of increasing the energy density of the diet, so less volume of the diet is required to meet energy needs. Many of the therapeutic canned diets are higher in fat content for these reasons. Increasing the fat content is contraindicated in canines with pancreatitis and animals with impaired gastrointestinal motility.[14]

Dogs show a preference for sugars, such as lactose, sucrose, and fructose,[20,21] and adding sugars or syrups to the food to add a sweet flavor can increase the palatability of foods for dogs. Cats do not have sweet receptors and are indifferent to sweetened foods.[18,22] Any sugar or syrup added to the diet should not constitute more than 10% of the total calories to avoid the risk of unbalancing the base diet.[14] Sweetening foods with sugars and other rapidly digestible and absorbable carbohydrates should be avoided in diabetic patients. Artificial sweeteners, such as xylitol, should be avoided because they can cause a hypoglycemic crisis in dogs.[23]

Cats and dogs do not have salt receptors; however, the amino acid receptors are stimulated by high concentrations of sodium chloride.[18] Salt may also increase taste responses to sugar in dogs.[19] Therefore, adding salt or using diets with higher sodium content may improve palatability. Increasing the sodium content of the diet may be detrimental to patients with renal disease or heart disease, particularly those with hypertension, ascites, or edema.[14]

Other intangibles, for example, texture of the diet, mouth feel, and temperature preference, and their influence on food preference is recognized but has not been studied to the same degree as flavor preference. Cats prefer foods near body temperature (38.5°C [101.5°F]), and warming food can increase its olfactory stimulus.[14,24] The mouth feel of the food is also important for cats, and they may reject foods with a powdery or greasy texture or a different kibble shape.[15,24]

If the voluntary enteral daily caloric intake of the animal still does not meet the desired goal, then other means of increasing intake should be considered. Appetite stimulants have limited success in completely anorectic animals but may increase food intake in partially anorectic animals.[25] Because they are less expensive and invasive than tube feeding, appetite stimulants are often tried first where owners are initially unwilling to consider other options. Most of the appetite stimulant medications currently available are short acting. Mirtazapine has become popular recently as an appetite stimulant in cats and dogs because it has a longer duration of action of 24 hours in dogs and 72 hours in cats.[26] If the animal is not consuming enough food to meet its RER with the use of appetite stimulants within 2 days, more aggressive nutritional support is recommended.[25] A list of appetite stimulants currently used and their potential side effects are provided in Box 40.4.

Force feeding, including syringe feeding or placing small boluses of food in the mouth, may be attempted to overcome reduced voluntary intake. Animals that are recumbent must be placed in sternal recumbency before offering food voluntarily or for forced feeding. Many animals find this procedure stressful and may as a consequence develop learned taste aversions. Force feeding is contraindicated in animals that lack a gag reflex and should be discontinued in animals that become fractious or refuse to swallow.[24]

Box 40.4 Appetite stimulant medications for dogs and cats

Drug	Drug Class	Potential Side Effects
Diazepam	Benzodiazepine	Nonpurposeful eating, sedation, exacerbation of hepatic encephalopathy, idiosyncratic hepatic necrosis
Oxazepam	Benzodiazepine	As for diazepam
Flurazepam	Benzodiazepine	As for diazepam
Cyproheptadine	Antihistamine	Excitability, aggression, vomiting
Cyanocobalamin	Vitamin	Not reported
Boldenone	Anabolic steroid	Delayed onset of activity, muscle pain at injection site
Stanozolol	Anabolic steroid	Delayed onset of activity
Nandrolone	Parenteral anabolic steroid	Uncommon
Prednisolone	Corticosteroid	Polyuria/polydipsia, impaired wound healing
Mirtazapine	Tetracyclic antidepressant	Uncommon

Source: References 16, 27, and 28.

If the previously discussed means of increasing food intake have failed, tube feeding may be indicated. Assisted enteral feeding may be considered when the animal is unable or unwilling to consume sufficient calories to maintain weight but has the capability to digest and absorb solutions delivered into the gastrointestinal tract.[5,29]

Tube route selection

The indications, concerns, and contraindications for each assisted enteral feeding tube route are shown in Table 40.1, which can be used to determine which technique to use.

If the tube is likely to be required long term, polyurethane or silicone tubes should be selected, in preference to the red polyvinyl chloride (PVC) tubes, because they do not become brittle or disintegrate in situ when

Table 40.1 Indications, concerns, and contraindications of each tube route

Tube Type	Indications	Concerns	Contraindications
NE/NG	Short-term tube feeding (1–10 days) Functional nasal cavity, pharynx, esophagus, stomach, and intestines High anaesthesia risk	Unable to evaluate gastric residual volumes with NE tube Liquid diets only due to tube size	Vomiting Comatose/Laterally recumbent Respiratory disease Lack of gag reflex Facial trauma involving nose/nasal cavity
E	Medium-term feeding (1–20 wk) Oral trauma/surgery/cancer	Unable to evaluate gastric residual volumes Light anaesthesia required	Vomiting Respiratory disease Megaesophagus Esophageal stricture Impaired wound healing[a]
G	Long-term feeding (months to years) Esophageal disorders Oral surgery/trauma Pancreatitis without vomiting Hepatic lipidosis Specific dietary need	Complications from early inadvertent removal of tube Cost	Anaesthesia risk Impaired wound healing[a] Persistent vomiting
J	Long-term feeding (weeks to months) Resting upper gastrointestinal tract (pancreatitis, recent gastric surgery) Intestinal anastomosis Coma	Cost Limited diet selection Complications from early inadvertent removal of tube Can only use in hospital	Anaesthesia risk Impaired wound healing[a]

[a]Skin and alimentary tract incisions are required to place these tube types.
Sources: References 5, 11, 25, 29, and 30.

exposed to digestive juices.[31] The internal diameter of the polyurethane tubes is slightly larger than the silicone tubes of the same French size because they are stronger with thinner walls. A French (F) unit is equivalent to 0.33 mm and measures the external diameter of the tube.[31]

Nasoesophageal and nasogastric tubes

Placement

Placement equipment and technique for nasoesophageal (NE) and nasogastric (NG) tubes is described in Protocol 40.1 and shown in Figure 40.2.

Correct placement of NG and NE tubes should be verified either with a lateral thoracic radiograph (Fig. 40.2k) or by injecting 3–15 mL of sterile water and assessing for coughing. Injecting 5–10 mL of air and auscultating the cranial abdomen for borborygmus can also be used for NG tubes.[5,11,29]

Feeding

Initiating feeding through NE and NG tubes may begin as soon as the tube position has been confirmed, unless the animal has been sedated.[29] Only liquid enteral diets can be used for NE and NG feeding due to the small diameter of these tubes.[5,25] The amount of the chosen diet to be administered can be calculated using the worksheet below in Box 40.9.

The tube may be flushed with warm water before feeding (3–10 mL) to ensure the tube is patent prior to feeding, and flushing the tube with 5–10 mL of warm water after each meal is essential to prevent a blockage.[33] It is advisable to monitor total fluid intake in renal patients because excessive water administration may lead to electrolyte imbalances. The minimum amount of water required to sufficiently flush the tube differs between the tube size, tube material (smaller lumen for PVC tubes), and the length of tube used. The amount of water needed to flush the tube is not typically printed on product packaging. An identical tube to the one chosen to be placed in the patient can be used to determine the smallest volume of water needed to flush the tube if required.

Food should be warmed to between room temperature and body temperature (20–38°C) prior to feeding. Instill food slowly, up to 3 mL per minute in our

Protocol 40.1 NG and NE tube placement[5,11,24,29,32]

Items Required
- 5–8F, 22- to 43-inch tube for dogs <15 kg and cats
- 8–10F, 43-inch tube for dogs >15 kg
- 2% lidocaine or 0.5% proparacaine
- Water-soluble lubricant or 5% lidocaine ointment
- Superglue or nylon suture material
- Luer slip catheter plug
- Elizabethan collar
- Tape or marker

Procedure
- Gather the equipment needed for placement (see Fig. 40.2a).
- Measure the tube from the nasal meatus to the last rib (region of the stomach) for NG tubes and three-quarters of this distance for NE tubes (see Fig. 40.2b).
- Mark the tube at the measured point with tape or an indelible marker (see Fig. 40.2c).
- Drip a few drops of local anaesthetic into the nostril and allow time for the anaesthetic to take effect (see Fig. 40.2d).
- Generously lubricate the tube (see Fig. 40.2e).

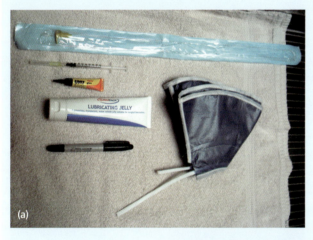
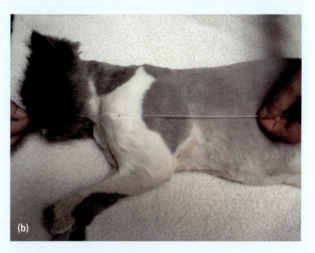

Figure 40.2 (a) Equipment gathered for NE tube placement.   **Figure 40.2** (b) Measuring the length of tube required.

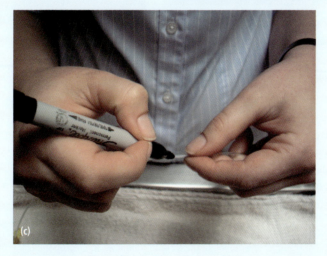

Figure 40.2 (c) Marking the tube at the premeasured length.

(*Continued*)

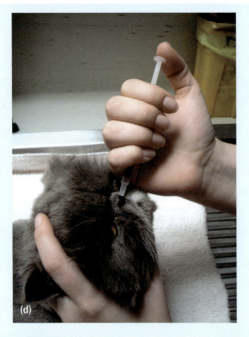

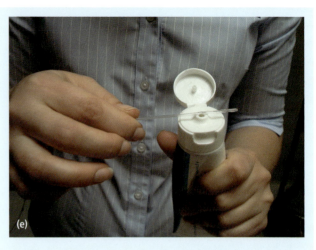

Figure 40.2 (e) Generously lubricating the tube.

Figure 40.2 (d) Placing a few drops of local anaesthetic.

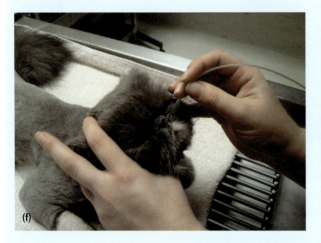

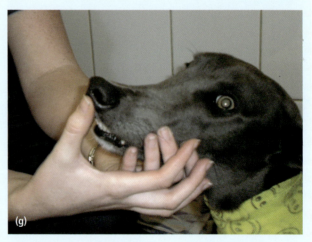

Figure 40.2 (f) Inserting the tube in a caudoventral medial direction into the ventromedial aspect of the nasal cavity.

Figure 40.2 (g) Pushing the nares dorsally in the dog.

- With the animal's head held in a normal static position, insert the tube in a caudoventral medial direction into the ventromedial aspect of the nasal cavity (see Fig. 40.2f).
  - In dogs the external nares are pushed dorsally after the tube has been introduced into the nose (approximately 2.0–3.0 cm) to open the ventral meatus and aid the tube's passage into the oropharynx (see Fig. 40.2g).
- Brace the introducing hand against the animal and introduce the tube in short, well-controlled insertions up to the premeasured mark (see arrow in Fig. 40.2h).
- Secure the tube lateral to the eye or medial to the eye and to the top of the head using superglue or sutures (see Fig. 40.2i).
- Place an Elizabethan collar to prevent removal of the tube by the animal (see Fig. 40.2j).
- Check correct placement by either:
  - Injecting 3–15 mL of sterile water and assessing for coughing
  - Injecting 5–10 mL of air and auscultating the cranial abdomen for borborygmus (NG tubes only)
  - A lateral thoracic radiograph looking for the outline of the feeding tube from the radiopaque strip or contrast media (see Fig. 40.2k)
    - A nasogastric tube should end in the fundus of the stomach
    - A nasoesophageal tube should end in the distal third of the esophagus

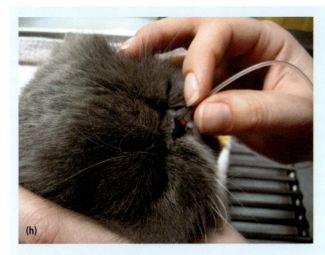

Figure 40.2 (h) The tube inserted up to the premeasured mark.

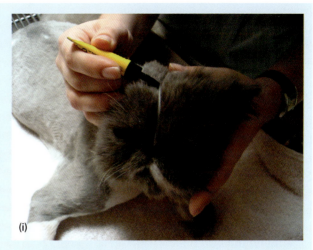

Figure 40.2 (i) Super gluing the tube in place.

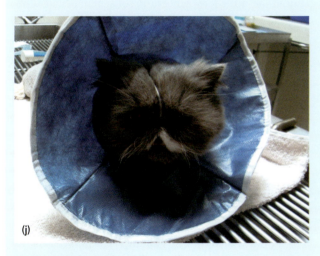

Figure 40.2 (j) An Elizabethan collar placed to prevent removal of the tube by the animal.

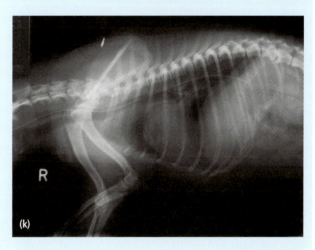

Figure 40.2 (k) Radiograph showing correct placement of a nasogastric tube. (Courtesy University of Queensland Small Animal Clinic Radiology Department.)

experience, to allow gastric expansion, and watch for salivating, retching, or vomiting. If these signs occur, stop feeding. When feeding is resumed, infuse a smaller amount at a slower rate.[24] After feeding, flush the tube as previously described, and close the port at the end of the tube to prevent ingestion of air, which could cause distension and discomfort of the stomach.[33]

Complications and troubleshooting

Placement of the tube in the trachea can be a life-threatening complication. It is advisable to confirm correct placement before initiating feeding.[5] A lateral thoracic radiograph should show a NE tube ending past the heart in the distal third of the esophagus and a NG tube ending in the fundus (see Figure 40.2K).[29]

Epistaxis may occur during tube placement, and the tube can be dislodged by vomiting or sneezing.[5,29] If the technician or veterinarian witnesses the animal vomiting, the position of the tube should be checked. The tube may be visible inside the mouth or protruding from the mouth if it has been dislodged. The mark made during placement should also be checked, or another radiograph may be taken. If the tube has been dislodged, removal and replacement is indicated.

Animals may also develop rhinitis or sinusitis.[5,29] The tube may damage some of the small capillaries in the nasal cavity when being placed, so alternative means of nutritional support should be considered in animals with coagulopathies.

If the animal coughs, vomits, or shows discomfort during flushing, before feeding, or during feeding,

feeding should be stopped and tube position should be checked, ideally with a radiograph.[29] Once the proper tube position is confirmed, feeding can then be restarted at a smaller volume and slower rate of infusion.[24]

Using the correct diet and flushing after each meal will reduce the risk of tube blockage. Using a syringe pump to ensure continuous flow may also help to decrease the risk of the tube becoming blocked.[30] If a tube has become blocked, a solution of 1 crushed tablet of a pancreatic enzyme product (9000 USP units lipase, 57,000 USP units protease, 64,000 USP units amylase), 1 crushed tablet (324 mg or ¼ teaspoon) of sodium bicarbonate and 5 mL of warm water can be injected into the tube with a little pressure and left in the tube for a minimum of 5 minutes and up to 2 hours before attempting further flushing.[34] Other methods that have been used for unblocking feeding tubes are shown in Box 40.5. Alternatively, the blocked tube can be removed and replaced with a new tube if continued assisted feeding is required.

Other authors have indicated that the risk of gastro-esophageal reflux is increased with the use of NG tubes, which may subsequently increase the risk of esophageal strictures.[24,30] There were no reports of this complication in previous studies of the use of NG tubes.[32,39,40] NG tubes are often used where decompression of the stomach is required, and NE tubes are used more routinely for feeding.

Tube removal by the animal is common if appropriate steps are not taken, and it may be prevented by the placement of an Elizabethan collar.[25] Animals may not voluntarily eat with an Elizabethan collar on and need it removed under supervision to encourage voluntary consumption.[29]

Small bowel diarrhea may result from the consistency and/or composition of the diets that can be fed via NE and NG tubes.[29]

Box 40.5 Methods for unblocking feeding tubes

Studies	Method	Outcome
Metheny et al[35] Wilson and Haynes-Johnson[36] Marcuard and Perkins[37]	Water Cranberry juice	Water was more successful at maintaining tube patency. The acidic pH of cranberry juice may precipitate proteins in the feeding formula.
Marcuard and Stegall[34] Marcuard et al[38]	Water Carbonated beverage Pancreatic enzyme solution	The pancreatic enzyme solution was significantly better at clearing an obstruction than water or the carbonated beverages.

Esophagostomy tubes

Placement

The equipment and placement technique of an esophagostomy tube are shown in Protocol 40.2. A photographic sequence demonstrating placement technique is shown in Figure 40.3A–K.

Feeding

Feeding may be initiated when the position of the tube has been confirmed and the animal has recovered from the anaesthetic. The larger diameter of these tubes compared with the NE or NG tubes allows the use of blended or liquid diets.[29,30] The amount of water that needs to be added to the diet will depend on the tube size and the initial composition of the diet; however, enough water should be added to achieve a consistency that allows passage through a syringe tip.[4] See Box 40.9 below for calculating feeding amounts.

Flushing the tube before and after feeding with 5–10 mL of warm water to prevent blockage should be performed, with care in renal patients as previously mentioned for NE and NG tubes.[33] Similar to NE tube feeding, warm the food to between room temperature and body temperature (20–38°C) prior to feeding and infuse slowly. Close the port at the end of the tube after feeding and flushing the tube to prevent ingestion of air that may cause distension and discomfort of the stomach.[33]

Stoma site care

The stoma site should be kept as clean and dry as possible at all times.[33] Checking the stoma site for redness, swelling, heat, and discharge at least daily is recommended. If the site requires cleaning, a sterile saline or a weak chlorhexidine solution may be used. The site should be thoroughly dried after cleaning. For more information on the care of the stoma site, see Chapter 55, Care of Indwelling Device Insertion Sites. A light bandage (e.g., a conforming bandage) may be placed taking care not to occlude the airway.[33]

Complications and troubleshooting

Inadvertent placement in the trachea or periesophageal space may occur, so tube placement should always be confirmed with radiographs (Fig. 40.3H).[29]

Complications include tube displacement from vomiting or removal by the animal.[30] Marking the skin exit point of a tube with a permanent marker when the position is initially radiographed can help to detect subsequent movement of the tube.[42] If the patient is witnessed vomiting, check inside the mouth to visualize if the tube is still

Protocol 40.2 E tube placement[5,41,29,11]

Items Required
- 8–14F tube in cats and small dogs
- 14–20F tube in medium to large dogs
- Right-angled/ curved forceps (Carmalt, Mixter, Schnidt, or Kantrowitz)
- #10 or 11 scalpel blade
- Nylon/polypropylene suture material
- Marker
- Luer slip catheter plug
- Conforming bandage/light bandage material

Procedure
- Anesthetize, endotracheally intubate, and position the animal in right lateral recumbency. Measure the tube from the center of the neck to the eighth to ninth intercostal space and mark with a permanent marker. Clip the left side of the neck and aseptically prepare the area (see Fig. 40.3a)
- Insert the curved forceps (shown in Fig. 40.3b) into the esophagus until the midpoint in the cervical esophagus, and then push outward to tent the skin. Make an incision through the skin over the tip of the forceps and extend the incision through the

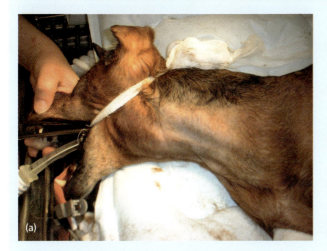

(a)

Figure 40.3 (a) Animal in right lateral recumbency with the left side of the neck clipped and aseptically prepared.

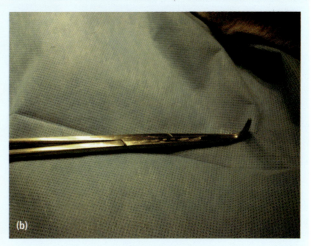

(b)

Figure 40.3 (b) Curved Carmalt forceps.

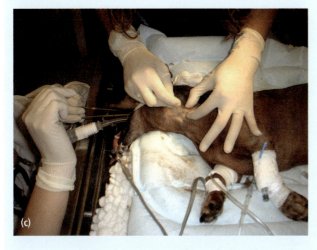

(c)

Figure 40.3 (c) The forceps inserted into the esophagus then pushed outward to tent the skin. An incision is made through the skin over the tip of the forceps.

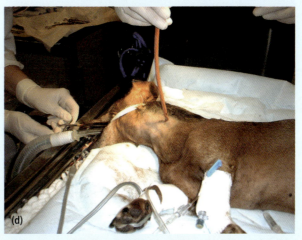

(d)

Figure 40.3 (d) The distal end of the tube grasped in the forceps.

(*Continued*)

subcutaneous connective tissues and wall of the esophagus. The incision should only be large enough to allow the tips of the forceps to be pushed through (see Fig. 40.3c).

- Grasp the distal end of the tube in the forceps, taking care not to catch the tissues in the mouth in the hinge of the forceps (see Fig. 40.3d).
- Pull the distal end of the tube grasped in the forceps rostrally out through the mouth (see Fig. 40.3e).
- Unclamp the distal end of the tube and gently push the distal end caudally. The forceps can be used to direct the tube into the esophagus. The proximal end of the tube can be manipulated to facilitate the progression of the distal end of the tube into the esophagus to prevent the tube from forming hard kinks that could remain during tube advancement (see Fig. 40.3f).
- Once the tube is in place, the proximal end will flip from caudal to cranial. Check that enough of the tube has been inserted to reach the eighth to ninth intercostal space or to the premeasured mark (see Fig. 40.3g).
- Confirm correct tube placement by radiographs. The outline of the tube should be visible and show the tube ending in the distal third of the esophagus (see Fig. 40.3h).
- Place a loose purse-string suture around the tube entrance site (see Fig. 40.3i).
- Place a finger trap suture around the base of the tube where it enters the skin to secure it in place (see Fig. 40.3j, k).

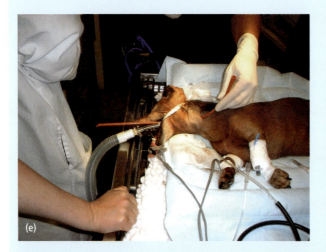

Figure 40.3 (e) The distal end of the tube pulled rostrally out through the mouth.

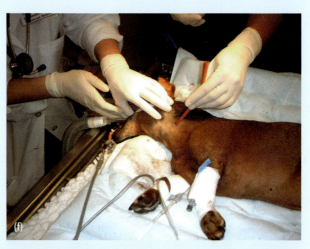

Figure 40.3 (f) The distal end of the tube being pushed caudally while manipulating the proximal end.

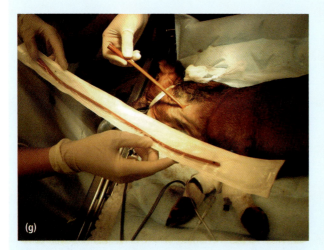

Figure 40.3 (g) The proximal end of the tube has flipped from caudal to cranial. A packaged tube can be used to measure how much of the tube has been inserted.

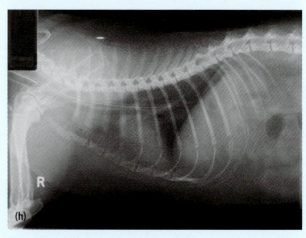

Figure 40.3 (h) Radiograph showing correct placement of an esophagostomy tube. (Courtesy University of Queensland Small Animal Clinic Radiology Department.)

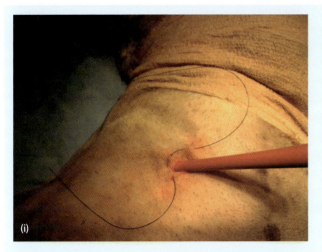

Figure 40.3 (i) A loose purse-string suture around the tube entrance site.

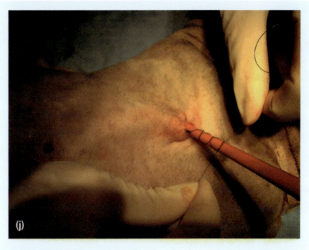

Figure 40.3 (j) Starting the finger trap suture where the tube enters the skin.

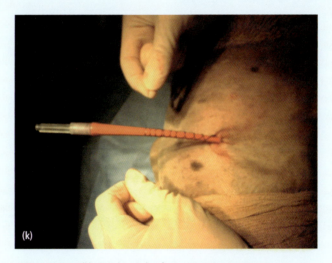

Figure 40.3 (k) Finishing the finger trap suture.

positioned in the esophagus, or alternatively take another lateral thoracic radiograph. If the tube has been dislodged, it should be removed and another placed.

If the patient vomits, salivates, or shows discomfort during feeding, feeding should be stopped. When feeding is resumed, feed a smaller amount at a slower rate and ensure food is freshly prepared and warmed prior to feeding.

Tube blockage can be prevented by using a diet with an appropriate consistency and by flushing with water as mentioned earlier. Only liquid medications should be delivered through the tube where possible. Where tablets are required, these should be crushed to a fine powder, where possible, before mixing with water.[42] Then if a blockage does occur, a solution of 1 crushed tablet of a

pancreatic enzyme product (9000 USP units lipase, 57,000 USP units protease, 64,000 USP units amylase), 1 crushed tablet (324 mg or ¼ teaspoon) of sodium bicarbonate and 5 mL of warm water can be injected into the tube with a little pressure and left in the tube for a minimum of 5 minutes and up to 2 hours before attempting further flushing.[34] Other methods used for unblocking feeding tubes are shown in Box 40.5.

Skin infection or abscessation can occur around the stoma site.[14,29] Any bandages should be removed daily to examine the tube site and appropriate site care administered (see Chapter 55, Care of Indwelling Device Insertion Sites, for more details). Changing the tube from a red PVC tube to a silicone or polyurethane tube can reduce inflammation.[31]

Gastrostomy tubes

Placement

The standard length gastrostomy (G) tubes, which have a length of tubing extending from the skin when placed, are routinely used in veterinary hospitals (Fig. 40.4). Where a G tube is likely to be required long term, a silicone or polyurethane tube should be selected because they do not become brittle or disintegrate in situ when exposed to digestive juices and require less frequent replacement.[31] Low-profile gastrostomy devices are also available, which are designed to sit flush with the skin (see Fig. 40.5).

Some of the positives and negatives of using standard length versus low-profile G tubes are shown in Box 40.6. A full discussion of tube type selection is beyond the scope of this chapter.

A low-profile device can be used to replace a standard percutaneous endoscopic gastrostomy (PEG) tube after 3 months when a permanent stoma has formed.[44,45] Insertion of a one-step low-profile gastrostomy device as the initial G tube was also reported by Campbell et al.[43] and Ferguson et al.[46] Initial placement of a low-profile gastrostomy device may result in lower cost for the owner in the long term because they require only a single anaesthetic and do not require frequent replacement.[43]

G tubes may be placed surgically or percutaneously. Percutaneous placement can be performed blindly or with the use of an endoscope.[27,30] PEG tube placement and blind placement of a G tube is described in Han[29] and Marks.[31] Percutaneous endoscopic placement is routinely performed in many clinics as endoscopes have become more available. The equipment required for percutaneous endoscopic placement is shown in Box 40.7. Surgical placement of a G tube is often used when the animal is undergoing abdominal surgery for another reason and is described in Fossum et al.[47]

Box 40.6 Positives and negatives of standard-length and low-profile gastrostomy devices[43]

	Standard Length	Low Profile
Positives	Lower initial cost Lower cost for short-term use Well tolerated Readily available in most clinics	Less frequent replacement and reduced overall cost for long-term use More aesthetically pleasing to owners Fewer complications (blockage, inadvertent removal)
Negatives	Higher risk of blockage and inadvertent removal	Higher initial cost

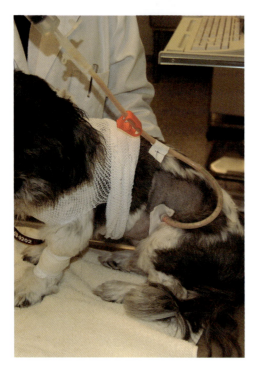

Figure 40.4 Feeding via a gastrostomy tube. (Courtesy Scott Campbell.)

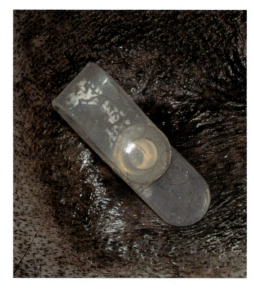

Figure 40.5 Low-profile gastrostomy device. (Courtesy UC Davis Nutrition Support Service.)

> **Box 40.7** PEG tube placement equipment[5,11]
>
> - 20–24F tube
> - Endoscope
> - Endoscope grasping instrument
> - Scalpel blade
> - 14- to 16-gauge needle or catheter
> - 2-0 nylon suture material
> - Catheter guide
> - Sterile lubricant
> - Luer slip catheter plug

> **Box 40.8** J tube surgical placement equipment[11,48]
>
> - 3.5F for <4-kg animals
> - 5F for 4- to 10-kg animals
> - 8F for >10-kg animals
> - #11 scalpel blade
> - 4-0 absorbable suture material
> - 2-0 nonabsorbable suture material
> - Hemostat
> - Luer slip catheter plug

Feeding

Water may be given within 6–12 hours of tube placement, but feeding should not be initiated until 12–24 hours after placement to allow formation of a fibrin seal at the stoma.[5,29] A permanent stoma will form in 7–14 days at the gastrocutaneous junction,[29,30] after which time the tube may be removed.[6]

Diets of gruel consistency can often be fed through PEG tubes.[29] To calculate the feeding amount, see Box 40.9 below. Warm food before feeding, infuse food slowly, and flush with 5–10 mL warm water before and after feeding,[33] with consideration of the possibility of excessive fluid administration in renal patients as previously mentioned. Close the port at the end of the tube after feeding.[33]

Stoma site care

G tube stoma site care is the same as E tube stoma site care, described earlier.

Complications and troubleshooting

Complications that may occur during placement include gastric hemorrhage, splenic laceration, and pneumoperitoneum.[5,30] Complications that may occur after tube placement include vomiting, aspiration pneumonia, inadvertent tube removal, peritonitis, gastric pressure necrosis, tube migration, and infection of the tube site.[29,30]

Pressure necrosis can be prevented by ensuring that the tube can be rotated after it has been placed, with a 5-mm space between the skin and the external flange.[31] Marking the tube at the level of the skin on initial placement with a pen or tape can help to detect subsequent movement of the tube.[31] An Elizabethan collar can be placed to help prevent tube removal by the patient. Where the tube is being removed by another pet in the household, a low-profile device should be considered.

Ultrasound or contrast radiography may be used to confirm displacement of the tube. If inadvertent removal or dislodgement occurs before a stoma has formed, surgical intervention is advised.

Tube obstruction may occur, although it is less likely in larger diameter tubes, and it can be prevented by flushing before and after feeding, blending the diet with sufficient water, only using elixir medications, or thoroughly crushing a mixing medications and flushing well after administration. Antacids and sucralfate have been reported to cause obstruction when administered with enteral formulas because they precipitate.[31] Where a tube has become obstructed, a solution of 1 crushed tablet of a pancreatic enzyme product (9000 USP units lipase, 57,000 USP units protease, 64,000 USP units amylase), 1 crushed tablet (324 mg or ¼ teaspoon) of sodium bicarbonate and 5 mL of warm water can be injected into the tube with a little pressure and left in the tube for a minimum of 5 minutes and up to 2 hours before attempting further flushing.[34] Other methods that have been used for unblocking feeding tubes are shown in Box 40.5.

Infection of the stoma site can be treated by cleaning with a dilute chlorhexidine or Betadine solution and applying an antibacterial cream. More frequent bandage changes should also be considered.[31] Checking the stoma site daily can help to detect infection early.

Jejunostomy tubes

Placement

Jejunostomy (J) tubes are most commonly placed surgically, often in animals that are identified as requiring jejunal feeding and require surgery for other reasons. Surgical placement of J tubes is described in Heuter[48] and Slatter.[49] The equipment used for surgical placement of J tubes is shown in Box 40.8.

Laparoscopic-assisted placement of J tubes has also been used and is an option for J tube placement when

Box 40.9 Calculating feeding amounts worksheet

1. **Calculate resting energy requirement (RER)**
   RER (kcal/day) = $70(BW_{kg})^{0.75}$
   Where BW_{kg} = the animal's current body weight in kilograms
   Calculating on a standard calculator: $\left(\sqrt{\sqrt{(BW*BW*BW)}}\right)*70$
   Alternative formula for animals weighing between 2 and 45 kg = $30(BW_{kg}) + 70$

2. **Calculate energy density of the diet**

$$\text{Energy density (kcal/mL)} = \frac{\text{Total kcal (diet)}}{\text{Total mL (diet + water added)}}$$

3. **Calculate amount to feed per day (in hospital–increase to MER/DER* at home)**

$$\text{Amount to feed (mL/day)} = \frac{\text{RER (kcal/day)}}{\text{Energy density (kcal/mL)}}$$

Refeeding schedule:

	Day 1	Day 2	Day 3	Day 4
Fraction of RER	or 1/3 →	2/3 →	RER	
	1/4 →	1/2 →	3/4 →	RER

4. **Calculate amount to feed per meal**

$$\text{Amount to feed per meal} = \frac{\text{Amount per day}}{\text{Number of meals per day}}$$

NOTE: For constant rate infusion feeding, divide the amount per day by the number of hours that the food will be administered over to establish mL/hour.

5. **Consider when to start offering food orally**

*MER and DER calculations in Hand et al.[24]

the animal does not require a celiotomy for another purpose.[50] A third option is percutaneous endoscopic gastrojejunal (PEG-J) tube placement. This method involves the placement of a PEG tube, through which a J tube is inserted through the pylorus into the proximal jejunum.[48] The advantage of the PEG-J tube is that the J tube can be removed and the animal can be easily transitioned to PEG tube feeding.[51] PEG-J placement is described in Heuter[48] and Jergens et al.[51]

Low-profile jejunostomy devices are also available and may be a feasible option for long-term nutritional support.[52]

J tubes are recommended to be left in place for at least 7–10 days to allow for adhesions to form around the tube site, which help prevent leakage into the abdomen.[30]

Feeding

Feeding may be initiated 12–24 hours after tube placement.[48,27] Due to the small diameter of these feeding tubes, only a liquid enteral diet can be used. A constant rate infusion (CRI) is recommended because bolus feeding may cause cramping and diarrhea.[27] See Box 40.9 to calculate the feeding amount to be provided each day (step 3), and then divide this amount by 24 (hours/day) to get the amount to be infused each hour as a CRI.

Tube and site care

Flush the tube with water every 4 hours and after any disruption in CRI feeding.[42] The syringe and tubing (or other delivery equipment) through which the diet is delivered should be replaced every 24 hours.[30] J tube exit site care is the same as for E tubes, described earlier.

Complications and troubleshooting

Vomiting and osmotic diarrhea are common complications of J tubes, which may be alleviated by decreasing the administration rate or by adding fiber to the liquid diet for diarrhea.[25]

Bacterial growth may occur in the delivery equipment, which can be prevented by replacing this equipment every 24 hours.[30] Blockage of the tube is another common complication, which can be minimized by using suitable diets and flushing the tube well every 4 hours and after any interruption in CRI feeding.[42,30] Previous methods described for unblocking tubes may be used when a tube has become blocked. Alternatively, the tube may be replaced surgically or left in place until a stoma has formed while using parenteral nutrition.

Peritonitis is a serious complication that may occur from leakage of small intestinal contents at the enterostomy site from dislodgement or premature removal of the tube. In nonsurgically placed tubes, retrograde movement may occur, which is best prevented by placing the tube as far into the small intestine as possible on initial placement.[48] PEG-J tubes with a weighted tip have been used in human medicine with the theory that gravity helps to maintain the tube's position. In cats and dogs the weight will have less of an effect on maintaining tube position because of anatomic differences.[48]

Summary

- Adequate nutritional intake is required to support the immune system, wound healing, and intestinal structure and function.
- Obtain a thorough diet history and accurately monitor nutrition during hospitalization for early identification of animals requiring nutritional support.
- RER is the minimum caloric goal for animals in the hospital.
- Use a strategic approach to entice voluntary consumption and reduce the risk of learned taste aversions.
- Tube selection is based on multiple factors, including the disease or condition being treated, functionality of gastrointestinal tract, anticipated length of feeding assistance, and cost of administration.
- Tube position should always be verified prior to initiating feeding.
- Tubes should be flushed with enough warm water to fill the tube prior to feeding if desired and always after feeding to maintain tube patency.

- Ensure that an appropriate diet consistency is used to reduce the risk of tube blockage.
- Always warm food prior to feeding and administer slowly.
- Delivery of medications through E tubes and G tubes should be done with caution.
- Unblocking of tubes may be achieved with warm water or a pancreatic enzyme solution.

References

1. Chan DL. Nutritional requirements of the critically ill patient. Clin Tech Small Anim Pract 2004;19:1–5.
2. Silk DBA. Enteral vs parenteral nutrition. Clin Nutr 2003;22:43–48.
3. Mohr AJ, Leisewitz AL, Jacobson LS, et al. Effect of early enteral nutrition on intestinal permeability, intestinal protein loss, and outcome in dogs with severe parvoviral enteritis. J Vet Intern Med 2003;17:791–798.
4. Delaney SJ, Fascetti AJ, Elliot DA. Critical care nutrition of dogs. In: Pibot P, Biourge V, Elliot D, eds. Encyclopedia of Canine Clinical Nutrition. Aimargues, France: Aniwa SAS on behalf of Royal Canin; 2006:426–450.
5. Ettinger SJ, Feldman ED, eds. Textbook of Veterinary Internal Medicine. 6th ed. St. Louis, MO: Elsevier Saunders; 2005.
6. Wortinger A. Nutrition for Veterinary Technicians and Nurses. Ames, IA: Blackwell; 2007.
7. Walton RS, Wingfield WE, Ogilvie GK, et al. Energy expenditure in 104 postoperative and traumatically injured dogs with indirect calorimetry. J Vet Emerg Crit Care 1998;6:71–79.
8. O'Toole E, Miller CW, Wilson BA, et al. Comparison of the standard predictive equation for calculation of resting energy expenditure with indirect calorimetry in hospitalized and healthy dogs. JAVMA 2004;225:58–64.
9. Justin RB, Hohenhaus AE. Hypophosphatemia associated with enteral alimentation in cats. J Vet Intern Med 1995;8:228–233.
10. Marinella MA. Refeeding syndrome and hypophosphatemia. J Intensive Care Med 2005;20:155–159.
11. Wortinger A. The ins and outs of feeding tubes. Vet Tech 2005;26:11–22.
12. Bernstein IL. Taste aversion learning: a contemporary perspective. Nutrition 1999;15:229–234.
13. Horn CC. Why is the neurobiology of nausea and vomiting so important? Appetite 2008;50:430–434.
14. Delaney SJ. Management of anorexia in dogs and cats. Vet Clin North Am Small Anim Pract 2006;36:1243–1249.
15. Michel KE. Management of anorexia in the cat. J Feline Med Surg 2001;3:3–8.
16. Plumb DC. Plumb's Veterinary Drug Handbook. 6th ed. Ames, IA: Blackwell; 2008.
17. Van Itallie TB. Sleep and energy balance: interactive homeostatic systems. Metabolism 2006; 55:S30–S35.
18. Boudreau JC, Sivakumar L, Thi Do L, et al. Neurophysiology of geniculate ganglion (facial nerve) taste systems: species comparisons. Chem Senses 1985;10:89–127.
19. Bradshaw JW. The evolutionary basis for the feeding behaviour of domestic dogs (*Canis familiaris*) and cats (*Felis catus*). J Nutr 2006;136:1927S–1931S.
20. Tôrres CL, Hickenbottom SJ, Rogers QR. Palatability affects the percentage of metabolizable energy as protein selected by adult beagles. Neurosci Biobehav Rev 2003;133:3516–3522.

21. Ferrell F. Preference for sugars and non-nutritive sweeteners in young beagles. Neurosci Biobehav Rev 1984;8:199–203.

22. Li X, Li W, Wang H, et al. Cats lack a sweet taste receptor. J Nutr 2006;136:1932S–1934S.

23. Dunayer EK. Hypoglycemia following canine ingestion of xylitol-containing gum. Vet Hum Toxicol 2004;46:87–88.

24. Hand MS, Thatcher CD, Remillard RL, et al., eds. Small Animal Clinical Nutrition. 4th ed. Topeka, KS: Mark Morris Institute; 2000.

25. Nelson RW, Couto CG, eds. Manual of Small Animal Internal Medicine. 2nd ed. St. Louis, MO: Elsevier Mosby; 2005.

26. Kuehn NF. North American Companion Animal Formulary. 8th ed. 2008. http://www.vin.com/Members/Drug/NACA.plx?ID=1059 (accessed September 29, 2009).

27. Macintire DK, Drobatz KJ, Haskins SC, et al. Manual of Small Animal Emergency and Critical Care Medicine. Ames, IA: Blackwell; 2006.

28. Quimby JM. The pharmacokinetics of mirtazapine in healthy Cats. In: Proceedings. ACVIM Forum 2009. http://www.vin.com/Members/Proceedings/Proceedings.plx?CID=acvim2009&PID=pr51761&O=VIN (accessed October 1, 2009).

29. Han E. Esophageal and gastric feeding tubes in ICU patients. Clin Tech Small Anim Pract 2004;19:22–31.

30. Wortinger A. Care and use of feeding tubes in dogs and cats. J Am Anim Hosp Assoc 2006;42:401–406.

31. Marks SL. Nasoesophageal, esophagostomy, and gastrostomy tube placement techniques. In: Ettinger SJ, Feldman EC, eds. Textbook of Veterinary Internal Medicine. Vol 1. St. Louis, MO: Elsevier Saunders; 2005:329–336.

32. Abood SK, Buffington CA. Improved nasogastric intubation technique for administration of nutritional support in dogs. JAVMA 1991;199:577–579.

33. Aspinall V. Clinical Procedures in Veterinary Nursing. 2nd ed. Edinburgh, UK: Elsevier Butterworth-Heinemann; 2008.

34. Marcuard SP, Stegall KS. Unclogging feeding tubes with pancreatic enzyme. J Parenter Enteral Nutr 1990;14:198–200.

35. Metheny N, Eisenberg P, McSweeney M. Effect of feeding tube properties and three irrigants on clogging rates. Nurs Res 1988;37:165–169.

36. Wilson MF, Haynes-Johnson V. Cranberry juice or water? A comparison of feeding-tube irrigants. Nutr Supp Serv 1987;7:2324.

37. Marcuard SP, Perkins AM. Clogging of feeding tubes. J Parenter Enteral Nutr 1988;12:403–405.

38. Marcuard SP, Stegall KL, Trogdon S. Clearing obstructed feeding tubes. J Parenter Enteral Nutr 1989;13:81–83.

39. Abood SK, Buffington CA. Enteral feeding of dogs and cats: 51 cases (1989–1991). JAVMA 1992; 201:619–622.

40. Crowe DT. Use of a nasogastric tube for gastric and esophageal decompression in the dog and cat. JAVMA 1986;188:1178–1182.

41. Hackett TB, Mazzaferro EM. Veterinary Emergency & Critical Care Procedures. Ames, IA: Blackwell; 2006.

42. Michel KE. Preventing and managing complications of enteral nutritional support. Clin Tech Small Anim Pract 2004;19:49–53.

43. Campbell SJ, Marks SL, Yoshimoto SK, et al. Complications and outcomes of one-step low-profile gastrostomy devices for long-term enteral feeding in dogs and cats. J Am Anim Hosp Assoc 2006;42:197–206.

44. Bright RM, DeNovo RC, Jones JB. Use of a low-profile gastrostomy device for administering nutrients in two dogs. J Am Vet Med Assoc 1995;207:1184–1186.

45. McCrackin Stevenson MA, Stiffler KS, Schmeidt CW. One-step placement of a percutaneous nonendoscopic low-profile gastrostomy port in cats. J Am Vet Med Assoc 2000;217:1636–1641.

46. Ferguson DR, Harig JM, Kozarek RA, et al. Placement of a feeding button ("one-step button") as the initial procedure. Am J Gastroenterol 1993;88:501–504.

47. Fossum TW, Hedlund CS, Johnson AL, et al. Small Animal Surgery. 3rd ed. St. Louis, MO: Mosby Elsevier; 2007.

48. Heuter K. Placement of jejunal feeding tubes for post-gastric feeding. Clin Tech Small Anim Pract 2004;19:32–42.

49. Slatter D, ed. Textbook of Small Animal Surgery. 3rd ed. Philadelphia, PA: Saunders; 2003.

50. Hewitt SA, Brisson BA, Sinclair MD, et al. Evaluation of laparoscopic-assisted placement of jejunostomy feeding tubes in dogs. J Am Vet Med Assoc 2004;225:65–71.

51. Jergens AE, Morrison JA, Miles KG, et al. Percutaneous endoscopic gastrojejunostomy tube placement in healthy dogs and cats. J Vet Intern Med 2007;21:18–24.

52. Swann HM, Sweet DC, Holt DE, et al. Placement of a low-profile duodenostomy and jejunostomy device in five dogs. J Small Anim Pract 1998;39:191–194.

41

Parenteral nutrition

Jennifer Larsen

Introduction

Malnutrition in hospitalized patients is a problem in veterinary medicine as well as in human medicine. One study showed that positive energy balance (provision of adequate calories to meet >95% of calculated requirements) was only achieved 27% of the time in 276 hospitalized dogs over a total of 821 days.[1] It is known that people whose nutritional needs are not met during a hospital stay suffer from adverse effects, especially a higher complication rate.[2] Despite a paucity of research, inadequate nutritional support for veterinary patients can also be expected to result in poor outcomes.[3] One study showed that hospitalized dogs and cats that received less than a third of their target energy requirements had a higher rate of poor outcomes.[4] In addition, illness and other physiologic stressors are associated with a hypermetabolic state characterized by increases in circulating cytokines, catecholamines, and other stress mediators.[5] These ultimately result in an inflammatory response with undesirable effects including increased protein catabolism and impaired healing ability.[6,7] This preferential catabolism of lean body mass over glycogen and fat stores in animals that are critically ill has a profoundly negative impact on healing, immune function, and recovery from disease and trauma. As such, intervention and provision of appropriate and adequate nutritional support is necessary to promote positive outcomes in veterinary patients.

Indications for parenteral nutrition

Feeding by the enteral route is the preferred method of providing energy and nutrients to maintain the functional integrity of the gastrointestinal tract and prevent dysfunction of the immune barrier.[8–10] The evidence from the human medical literature shows improved outcomes, greater cost effectiveness, and fewer complications when patients are fed enterally.[11–13] However, in many cases enteral feeding is not possible, in particular for patients with an increased risk of aspiration or that are not candidates for feeding tube placement. In some cases bleeding disorders or anesthetic risks preclude the use of most enteral feeding devices.

Careful consideration should be given to the route of nutritional support for any patient that cannot protect its airway. Contraindications of gastrointestinal feeding include protracted vomiting, decreased consciousness, and a decreased or absent gag reflex. Likewise, many patients with severe head trauma, those that need ventilator-assisted respiratory support, those requiring medications that impair consciousness, or those with severe pancreatic or malabsorptive gastrointestinal diseases cannot safely be fed enterally; however, nutritional support is still required. In these patients, parenteral nutrition (PN) is the only way to administer calories and nutrients.

When to initiate support

The ideal time to initiate nutritional support varies by individual and depends on the disease process, prognosis for voluntary intake, when the patient last consumed adequate energy and nutrients, and the animal's body condition. A validated body condition scoring system is well established.[14,15] Such assessment tools should be used routinely in the clinic for monitoring of healthy pets as well as hospitalized patients. For acutely ill or

Advanced Monitoring and Procedures for Small Animal Emergency and Critical Care, First Edition. Edited by Jamie M. Burkitt Creedon, Harold Davis.
© 2012 John Wiley & Sons, Inc. Published 2012 by John Wiley & Sons, Inc.

injured patients in good condition, consideration for providing nutritional support should occur within 3–5 days of anorexia. Longer periods of starvation are certainly of no benefit and carry the risk of negatively impacting immune function, healing, and overall condition.[16] For patients that are more debilitated, are growing, have inadequate muscle mass or adipose stores, have recent or ongoing weight loss, or that are not expected to consume food voluntarily within 2 or 3 days, intervention should be more immediate. Feline patients, which are at risk of hepatic lipidosis from inadequate energy consumption, should also have their nutritional needs addressed within a shorter time frame of 3 days. For all hospitalized cases, the initial medical management plan as well as the owner's cost estimate should consider the need for nutritional support.

How much to feed

For all hospitalized patients, regardless of feeding method, the caloric goal is the provision of resting energy requirement (RER) calculated for the current weight regardless of body condition. RER is the amount of energy needed by a resting, awake animal that is lying down in a thermoneutral environment. The RER is estimated by this equation (see Box 41.1):

$$70 \times \text{body weight in kg}^{0.75}$$

This amount is adequate to maintain weight in a majority of hospitalized patients but may vary in patients that are hypercatabolic or those with high or low body condition scores. Regardless, overfeeding has risks and should be avoided. As such, adjustments based on the individual patient's response are necessary.

Overfeeding can result in hyperglycemia and hyperlipidemia, which are also the most commonly recognized adverse effects in parenterally fed veterinary patients.[17–21] Hyperglycemia has been identified as a risk factor for poor outcome in both human and feline patients,[20,22] and insulin therapy is routinely used in the human intensive care unit to control blood glucose elevation.[23] It is a frequent clinical observation that elevations in blood glucose normalize within 24 hours of beginning the PN infusion without intervention; this has also been reported in the literature.[18] This likely reflects metabolic adaptation to the glucose infusion and underscores the importance of adjusting the rate to the individual patient's tolerance.

I currently recommend that the rate of parenteral administration should initially be 25% of RER. If the formula and feeding rate are well tolerated, the rate should be increased in 25% increments every 4–12 hours depending on patient response, until full RER is successfully reached (Box 41.2). Body weight should be assessed at least once daily, and if PN is used for a prolonged period without complications and weight loss is

---

> **Box 41.1** Examples of calculations for meeting energy requirements with parenteral nutrition
>
> - Equation for resting energy requirement (RER):
>   - $70 \times$ (body weight in kg)$^{0.75}$ = RER in kcal per day
> - For a 35-pound (15.9 kg) canine patient, calculate RER:
>   - $70 \times 15.9 \text{ kg}^{3/4}$ = 557 kcal per day
> - Using a calculator without an exponent function:
>   - Multiply the weight in kilograms by itself three times:
>   - $15.9 \times 15.9 \times 15.9 = 4019.68$
>   - Square root twice = 7.96
>   - Multiply by 70 = 557 kcal per day
> - If the parenteral solution provides 1.15 kcal/mL, the patient needs approximately 484 mL/day or 20 mL/hour.
>   557 kcal per day/1.15 kcal per mL = 484 mL per day
>   484 mL per day/24 hours = 20 mL per hour

> **Box 41.2** Gradually increase to goal rate of parenteral nutrition infusion
>
> - When increasing the infusion rate up to full RER, start with 25%–33% of the rate, and increase by 25%–33% increments every 4–24 hours if tolerated, with blood glucose within target ranges (between 100 and 250 mg/dL).[32]
> - Assess blood lipids, phosphorus, potassium, and magnesium, HCT within 24 hours of initiation of PN.
> - After full infusion rate is achieved, assess at least once daily:
>   - Body weight
>   - Catheter insertion site
>   - Plasma lipemia index
>   - Glucose
>   - Magnesium
>   - Thoracic auscultation
>   - Body temperature
>   - HCT
> - Assess at least every other day:
>   - Phosphorus
>   - Potassium
>   - BUN
>   - Albumin

noted, slowly increasing the rate by 10%–20% increments is reasonable.

Central and peripheral nutrition

Parenteral nutrition is often called "total" ("TPN") or "partial" ("PPN"). The terms TPN and PPN refer to the completeness of the diet with respect to required nutrients or calories. In human medicine, PN is often used for prolonged periods, and the solutions include all required nutrients, including trace elements. In contrast, in veterinary patients, PN is most often used on a short-term basis as a bridge to enteral feeding or voluntary intake. The average length of PN administration in veterinary patients is between 3 and 5 days.[17–20] Further, parenteral veterinary formulations do not typically include the full complement of required nutrients. As such, the nomenclature is more accurate in reference to the route of administration, with central parenteral nutrition (CPN) being administered through catheters that terminate in the caudal or cranial vena cava, and peripheral parenteral nutrition (PPN) being administered through standard short catheters that terminate in peripheral vessels.

Both types of PN are appropriate for delivery of full caloric requirements, despite differences in maximum osmolarity (Box 41.3). Peripherally administered solutions such as PPN should not exceed a maximum of 750 mOsm/L to reduce the risk of phlebitis; however, other characteristics of the formula and its administration (especially pH and flow rate) as well as patient factors contribute to phlebitis risk as well. In contrast, CPN formulas should not exceed 1400 mOsm/L because delivery into a large high-volume and high-flow vessel results in rapid dilution of the solution. Full caloric requirements may be delivered using PPN because PPN

solutions have a higher fat concentration than CPN. Fat contributes more calories per milliliter than protein and carbohydrate, but the osmolarity of the solution is much lower. As such, to achieve appropriately low osmolarity for PPN while maintaining a reasonable caloric density, the proportion of calories from fat must be high (approximately 70%). CPN solutions are typically lower in fat (approximately 50% on a calorie basis).

Composition of the solution

PN solutions are composed primarily of three base elements: amino acid solution, fat emulsion solution, and dextrose solution. The most commonly used amino acid solutions have a concentration of 8.5% and include all amino acids required by dogs and cats except for taurine. Lipid emulsion products are primarily composed of long chain polyunsaturated fatty acids from plant oils. This ingredient is iso-osmolar and can be used in high concentrations in PN while contributing little to the osmolarity of the overall solution. Dextrose solutions are 5% or 50% concentration products typically found in veterinary pharmacies.

In most cases additives providing electrolytes, B vitamins, and trace minerals are also included in the PN formulation. The inclusion of B vitamins in particular is important. With the exception of a small amount of vitamin B_{12} (cobalamin) in the liver, there is no storage of B vitamins in the body. These are important nutrients for metabolism and efficient use of energy, protein, fat, and glucose. Further, B vitamins can be lost in the urine due to their water-soluble nature; this is an important consideration for patients with polyuria secondary to their underlying disease or due to parenteral fluid administration. Other micronutrients are also critical, and some amino acid solutions include electrolytes; however, many clinicians prefer to adjust these more precisely for individual patients by using additives such as potassium phosphate, potassium chloride, magnesium sulfate, and sodium chloride. Any of these can be added to the PN solution or to a crystalloid fluid solution. Other components and additives such as medications should not be introduced into the PN solution unless compatibility can be assured to avoid adverse effects; appropriate resources should be carefully consulted.[24]

Formulations can also be customized in other ways, with modification of the energy distribution of the solution the most common. Specific patient needs can be accommodated by adjusting the proportions of calories coming from protein, fat, and carbohydrate. For example, low-carbohydrate solutions may be useful for patients with compromised pulmonary function and

---

Box 41.3 General characteristics of central and peripheral PN

	Central PN	Peripheral PN
Catheter termination	In vena cava	In peripheral vessel
Osmolarity	<1400/L	<750/L
Energy density	1.0–1.4 kcal/mL	0.7–1.0 kcal/mL
Fat content	~50% of calories	~70% of calories
Delivery of energy requirement	Yes	Yes

hypercapnia, and low-protein solutions are used for patients with hepatic encephalopathy or renal disease. For some patients with severe hepatic disease, fat may be poorly tolerated. Provided that blood lipid clearance is normal, parenteral fat infusions are generally safe for patients with pancreatitis because exocrine pancreatic stimulation results from nutrients in the small intestine. To some extent, the osmolarity and energy density of the solution can also be adjusted to address issues such as phlebitis or volume intolerance.

Compounding PN solutions

Aseptic procedures (see Fig. 41.1) are required for safe compounding of PN solutions (Protocol 41.1). To

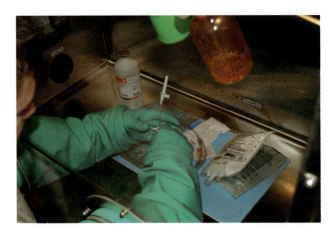

Figure 41.1 To avoid contamination, parenteral nutrition solutions should be mixed in a sterile environment such as an isolation chamber or laminar-flow hood.

Protocol 41.1 Protocol for building PN

Items Required
- Isolation chamber or laminar-flow hood (see Fig. 41.1)
- Empty intravenous (IV) solution bags with attached transfer tubing set and tubing clamps
- Alcohol swabs for cleansing injection ports
- Needles and syringes for additives
- Amino acid solution, lipid emulsion solution, dextrose solution, vitamin B complex, electrolyte additives (potassium chloride or potassium phosphate, magnesium sulfate)
- Sterile gloves

Procedure
1. Gather supplies.
2. Always use sterile technique.
3. Perform hand hygiene and don sterile gloves.
4. Assemble all necessary components and supplies in the chamber or hood (see Fig. 41.4).
5. Hang the dextrose and amino acid solutions, swab the ports, and connect the tubing from the empty IV bag to each container.
6. Open the tubing to mix the specified volumes of dextrose and amino acid solution in the empty bag, and then add the lipid emulsion (or add all three simultaneously with gentle agitation to ensure thorough mixing; do not mix dextrose and lipid together).
7. Clamp and remove the transfer tubing from the IV solution bag.
8. Add any desired additives (potassium phosphate or potassium chloride, B vitamin complex).
9. Limit needlesticks as much as possible.
10. If solution will not be used immediately, omit the additives for refrigerated storage and add them just prior to use.

Box 41.4 Sensitivity factors associated with PN solutions

- Microbial contamination
- Temperature
- pH
- Light
- Oxygen exposure
- Continuous agitation of solution
- Lipid emulsion stability

---

deliver a quality product, the solution must remain both stable and sterile. Because several ingredient components are added to the solution, multiple needlesticks are used, and contamination is possible. Further, the solution itself is a good medium for bacterial growth. The stability of the solution may be impacted not only by microbial contamination but also by storage or transport conditions. Many nutrients are sensitive to temperature, light, and oxygen (see Box 41.4). Degradation or destruction of the solution constituents is possible, in addition to modification of nutrients, as in the case of fatty acid oxidation.

Solution stability may also be impacted due to mixing procedures. Some components of PN solutions may interact with others, or react with additives, which may result in instability of the product. For example, the dextrose and amino acid components should be mixed to allow for pH equilibrium and dilution of cations prior to adding the lipid solution. Alternatively, all three components can be added simultaneously, with gentle agitation to ensure proper homogeneity of the solution. Care should be taken to avoid the mixing of

> **Box 41.5** Signs of lipid instability indicating an unsafe PN solution
>
> - Any change in visual texture
> - Any change in color of solution
> - Yellow steaks in solution
> - Visible oil layer in solution
> - Appearance of particulate matter in solution
> - Any loss of appearance of homogeneity of solution

dextrose and lipid solutions together. The amino acid solution will buffer the low pH of the dextrose solution and protect the lipid component, which is sensitive to excessive acidity as well as higher concentrations of reactive cations such as ionized calcium and magnesium.

PN solutions without electrolyte or micronutrient additives can be premade and stored in the refrigerator for convenience, with the addition of a vitamin B complex injection to the solution just before beginning the infusion. Premade bags without additives may be stable for up to 28 days when stored at refrigerated temperature.[25] If the lipid becomes unstable (referred to as "breaking" or "oiling out"), visible separation, yellow streaking, and/or precipitation of particulate matter can be noted in the solution. PN solutions should always be visually examined prior to infusion and at regular intervals thereafter to assess for breaking and other stability problems. If signs of instability (see Box 41.5) are noted, the animal is at risk of adverse events related to lipid emboli, and the solution should be discontinued and discarded.

There are currently no formal practice guidelines regarding the use of PN from the American Veterinary Medical Association or many state veterinary medical boards. However, as of 2004 the United States Pharmacopeia (USP) Chapter 797 is enforceable by the U.S. Food and Drug Administration and has been adopted by most state pharmacy boards.[26] This statute describes the procedures and requirements for compounding sterile preparations and applies to all settings, veterinary or otherwise. The stringency of enforcement may vary; however, these procedures and guidelines should be followed in all veterinary practices and pharmacies to ensure patient safety.

Among other restrictions and guidelines, USP Chapter 797 guidelines specify the use of a clean room or isolation chamber (such as a laminar-flow hood) to prepare sterile parenteral products (see Fig. 41.1). For most vet-erinary practices, the feasibility of compliance is challenging if not impossible. As such, options for in-house preparation are limited. Large practices or academic institutions typically use isolation chambers or laminar-flow hoods for hand mixing or automatic compounding machines to mix parenteral solutions. Automatic compounders reduce human error, increase efficiency, and improve accuracy of the measurements of each component, but these are not cost effective for most veterinary practices. However, many human home health care pharmacies and hospitals can provide parenteral mixtures for use in almost any veterinary practice. A prescription can be submitted that specifies the type and amounts of lipid solution, amino acid solution, dextrose solution, and vitamins and/or electrolytes to be used to create an appropriate parenteral solution. The product can be sent the same day or overnight to the veterinary practice, making this option economical and practical in most settings.

Maintenance of the infusion and catheter

Peripherally inserted central catheters (PICC lines) are often used in veterinary patients for the administration of CPN; these are inserted in the limbs but are long enough to terminate in the caudal or cranial vena cava. PICC lines in the limbs of veterinary patients may be more difficult to keep clean compared with those in other locations, especially if the bandaging is likely to be exposed to urine, diarrhea, or vomit. Shorter CPN catheters inserted into the jugular vein and that terminate in the cranial vena cava are also common; these typically have multiple lumens so that a dedicated line is possible. Dedicated lines are recommended for PN administration to avoid incompatibility issues with other infused substances, minimize contamination, and maintain line integrity.

Catheters intended for PN infusion use should be placed aseptically, using standard techniques for skin preparation including shaving and proper cleansing. Procedures should also include the use of appropriate barriers (drapes, gloves) as well as proper handling of all equipment (see Chapter 4 for information regarding proper techniques for catheterization of the venous compartment). Catheter maintenance during the infusion period should follow accepted protocols for cleansing and bandaging to avoid contamination and infection (see Chapter 55 for information about care of indwelling device insertion sites). The insertion site should be visually inspected for signs of inflammation and cleansed every 12–24 hours. Catheter removal may be necessary if swelling, redness, or discharge is present,

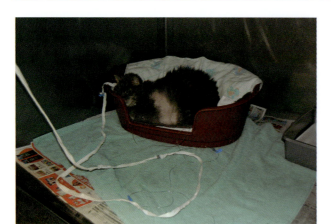

Figure 41.2 The infusion line for parenteral nutrition solutions should be covered to avoid light exposure and potential degradation of nutrients.

and the catheter tip should be cultured whenever infection is suspected.

Due to the sensitivity of some nutrients to ultraviolet light, the solution bag and infusion lines should be kept covered (Fig. 41.2). Amino acids and B vitamins are most susceptible to such degradation. In fact, PN solutions without electrolyte or micronutrient additives can be premade and stored in the refrigerator for convenience, and they may be stable for up to 28 days.[25] After the addition of B vitamins and gentle mixing of the solution, the solution is stable at room temperature during the infusion period for at least 48 hours; continuous agitation is not recommended.[27] The bag should be labeled with the date and time it was hung to ensure that it is discarded after 48 hours along with the entire infusion tubing set (Fig. 41.3). Once the infusion has started, any disconnection of the line should be prevented to maintain sterility. In all cases this means that the bag and line must accompany the patient on walks outside, trips to undergo diagnostic procedures, and to visits with owners. If the line is disconnected anywhere between the bag and the patient's intravenous catheter, the administration set and solution are no longer considered sterile and must be discarded.

Contraindications and Complications

PN should be used cautiously in patients that are volume intolerant. The energy density of the solution is the primary determinant in the infusion rate; if the rate must be decreased to address volume intolerance, full RER may not be delivered. Regardless, the provision of partial energy requirements is preferable to none. Patients with vasculitis or that are septic or hypercoagu-

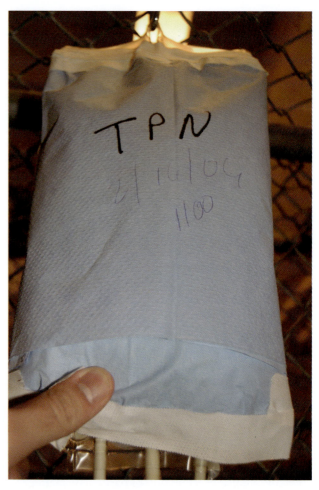

Figure 41.3 Parenteral nutrition solutions should be labeled with the date they are mixed.

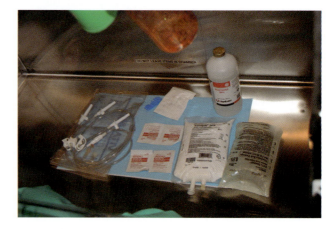

Figure 41.4 Assemble all needed supplies prior to mixing the parenteral nutrition solution.

lable are not ideal candidates for PN. If PN is instituted is such a patient, additional monitoring and precautions may be necessary to reduce complications. All patients should be monitored for metabolic, mechanical, and septic complications (Box 41.6).

Box 41.6 Examples of complications associated with PN administration

- **Mechanical**
  - Catheter dysfunction (dislodgement, occlusion, kinking)
  - Disconnection or leakage of the infusion line
  - Inadvertent removal by the patient
  - Equipment failure (pump dysfunction, etc)
- **Septic**
  - Inflamed catheter insertion site
  - Fever
  - Elevated white blood cell count
  - Positive culture of blood or catheter
- **Metabolic**
  - Abnormalities in serum biochemical values (hyperglycemia, hyperbicarbonatemia, etc.)
  - Lipemic serum (or elevated serum triglyceride concentration)
  - Refeeding syndrome

Box 41.7 Signs of parenteral nutrition intolerance

- Hyperglycemia
- Hyperammonemia
- Hyperlipidemia
- Fluid overload

Box 41.8 Signs of refeeding syndrome

- Hypophosphatemia
- Hypokalemia
- Hypomagnesemia
- Thiamin deficiency
- Fluid imbalance

Metabolic Complications

Commonly Reported Metabolic Complications

Metabolic complications are commonly recognized in veterinary patients, amounting up to 70% of total recorded complications associated with PN in dogs in one study.[18] Hyperglycemia is a common metabolic abnormality in dogs and cats receiving PN.[17–20,28] This has been associated with poor outcome in cats in one study,[20] but no association with mortality in either dogs or cats has been found in other studies.[19,28] Critically ill cats show abnormalities in carbohydrate metabolism associated with hyperglycemia, hyperlactatemia, and hypoinsulinemia,[29] which may contribute to intolerance of dextrose-containing infusions of PN. Indeed, one study documented hyperglycemia in a significant number of critically ill cats (55%) and dogs (26%) prior to PN administration.[28] Despite the consistently high incidence of hyperglycemia reported in veterinary patients both prior to and during PN infusion, the importance of this remains unclear.

Intolerance of PN

Patients that do not appear to tolerate PN (Box 41.7) due to hyperlipidemia, hyperglycemia, or hyperammonemia should be assessed for new or progressing underlying conditions; however, the first steps should include confirmation of proper formulation and mixing of the solution because any errors may result in a drastically different nutritional profile than intended. The formulation calculations should be rechecked, as well as the volume and specifications of the individual components. Once the composition of the solution has been confirmed, measures can be taken to reduce adverse effects. In all cases the infusion rate should be decreased or the infusion discontinued if the adverse effect is severe. In some cases, insulin can be used to control hyperglycemia, and heparin can be used to induce lipoprotein lipase, which increases peripheral uptake of lipids to address hyperlipidemia.

Refeeding Syndrome

Another potential metabolic complication is refeeding syndrome, which can be seen in any animal fed enterally or parenterally after a period of reduced food intake. The syndrome is characterized by hypophosphatemia, hypokalemia, hypomagnesemia, thiamin deficiency, and fluid imbalances (Box 41.8). These aberrations occur as a result of insulin release in response to parenterally or enterally administered calories. During starvation and critical illness, reserves of metabolically important compounds are depleted, and the main energy sources are fatty acids, ketone bodies, and amino acids. Despite normal serum concentrations, the whole-body pool of nutrients such as phosphorus, potassium, magnesium, and thiamin is significantly reduced. When calories are delivered by any route, especially in the form of glucose, the pancreas responds by releasing insulin, and there is a subsequent sudden shift in the substrates used for energy production as glucose becomes abruptly available.

The subsequent binding of insulin to receptors in peripheral tissues causes a phosphorylation cascade to occur intracellularly. This in addition to the upregulation of glycolysis and subsequent production of adenosine triphosphate (ATP; the main energy source for cellular functions) creates a sink such that phosphorus moves intracellularly, depleting the extracellular (plasma) compartment, which can result in clinical signs of phosphorus deficiency, including hemolysis and anemia.

Insulin also promotes a dramatic influx of potassium from the extracellular to the intracellular compartment. This can result in clinically significant hypokalemia manifested by hypotension, neuromuscular dysfunction including weakness and intestinal ileus, cardiac arrhythmias, and arrest. Likewise, magnesium is an important cofactor for the first steps in glycolysis, so that when glucose is being used to produce ATP, there is a sink for magnesium in the intracellular space. Deficiency results in cardiac arrhythmias and neuromuscular signs and can be documented as a decrease in serum ionized magnesium concentration. Hypokalemia may be refractory to treatment with parenteral supplementation unless adequate magnesium concentrations are restored because magnesium closes passive potassium channels in cellular membranes. Lastly, thiamin is important for the metabolism and use of carbohydrates for energy, and many patients may have suboptimal thiamin status from decreased intake and/or increased loss. When demand increases during refeeding, subclinical or clinical thiamin deficiency may result, including severe neurologic abnormalities.

Unlike in humans, refeeding syndrome appears to be uncommon in dogs and cats, and it causes mild to moderate adverse events in veterinary patients. Regardless, in some cases the problem can result in catastrophic complications. Monitoring for such occurrences is cost effective and easily accomplished. Patients with preexisting metabolic derangements such as diabetic ketoacidosis or those with a prolonged history of malnourishment may be at higher risk and should be assessed closely for clinical signs of refeeding syndrome. In such cases, reintroduction of either enteral or parenteral nutrition should be done conservatively, with very gradual increases in the amount provided to assess tolerance and address any potential problems very early (no more than 25% of RER for at least 6–8 hours, in my opinion). Correction of these issues is not costly or difficult, and it undoubtedly improves outcome and reduces morbidity and mortality associated with a useful treatment modality.

Mechanical Complications

Mechanical complications include catheter dysfunction (dislodgement, occlusion, kinking), disconnections in the infusion line, and inadvertent catheter removal by the patient. Such situations occur in patients receiving PN from 9% to 26% of the time.[18–20] Preventing patient access to the catheter site, maintaining appropriate bandaging, and instituting procedures to maintain line integrity during patient care can help reduce the incidence of mechanical complications. Although infusion line obstructions are not commonly encountered, administration sets are available that include inline filters. Occlusions may be due to coalescing fat globules that would indicate an unstable or broken solution. The PN solution should be carefully inspected in the event of an occlusion because significant adverse effects may occur if a broken lipid solution is used.

Septic Complications

Due to the nature of the parenteral solution and the need for direct intravenous access, patients receiving PN are at higher risk of infectious complications. However, septic complication rates in clinical canine and feline patients receiving PN solutions range from 0% to 8%.[17–20,28] These rates are lower than reported in human medicine[30–31] and may be due to attention to proper catheter placement and maintenance and sterile solution preparation as well as the short duration of most infusions. All patients receiving PN solutions should be monitored for catheter insertion site infection, fever, and leukogram abnormalities. If catheter-related sepsis is suspected, the catheter should be removed and cultured to institute appropriate antimicrobial therapy.

Conclusion

PN can be a useful modality for providing nutritional support to critically ill patients unable to tolerate enteral feeding. Proper formulation, compounding, administration, and patient monitoring are necessary to ensure the delivery of a safe and effective product. Metabolic complications are the most frequently documented adverse effects; septic complications are uncommon. PN nutrition can be safely and effectively used in most 24-hour veterinary practice settings (Box 41.9).

Summary

- Critically ill patients are often malnourished or are consuming inadequate diets.

> **Box 41.9** Summary
>
> - Critically ill patients are often malnourished or are consuming inadequate diets.
> - When enteral feeding is impossible or impractical, provision of nutritional support via the parenteral route is indicated.
> - Parenteral feeding is an excellent option for providing adequate amounts of energy to patients with a wide range of needs.
> - Parenteral feeding can be easily utilized in most practice settings, assuming 24-hour monitoring is available.

- When enteral feeding is impossible or impractical, provision of nutritional support via the parenteral route is indicated.
- Parenteral feeding is an excellent option for providing adequate amounts of energy to patients with a wide range of needs.
- Parenteral feeding can be easily utilized in most practice settings, assuming 24-hour monitoring is available.

References

1. Remillard RL, Darden DE, Michel KE, et al. An investigation of the relationship between caloric intake and outcome in hospitalized dogs. Vet Ther 2001;2(4):301–310.
2. Koretz RL, Avenell A, Lipman TO, et al. Does enteral nutrition affect clinical outcome? A systematic review of the randomized trials. Am J Gastroenterol 2007;102(2):412–429.
3. Chan DL, Freeman LM. Nutrition in critical illness. Vet Clin North Am Small Anim Pract 2006;36(6):1225–1241.
4. Brunetto MA, Gomes MOS, Andre MR, et al. Effects of nutritional support on hospital outcome in dogs and cats. J Vet Emer Crit Care 2010;20(2):224–231.
5. Coss-Bu JA, Klish WJ, Walding D, et al. Energy metabolism, nitrogen balance, and substrate utilization in critically ill children. Am J Clin Nutr 2001;74:664–669.
6. Michel KE, King LG, Ostro E. Measurement of urinary urea nitrogen content as an estimate of the amount of total urinary nitrogen loss in dogs in intensive care units. J Am Vet Med Assoc 1997;210(3):356–359.
7. Hasselgren PO, Fischer JE. Muscle cachexia: current concepts of intracellular mechanisms and molecular regulation. Ann Surg 2001;233(1):9–17.
8. Windsor AC, Kanwar S, Li AG, et al. Compared with parenteral nutrition, enteral feeding attenuates the acute phase response and improves disease severity in acute pancreatitis. Gut 1998;42(3):431–435.
9. Braga M, Gianotti L, Gentilini O, et al. Feeding the gut early after digestive surgery: results of a nine-year experience. Clin Nutr 2002;21(1):59–65.
10. Gupta R, Patel K, Calder PC, et al. A randomised clinical trial to assess the effect of total enteral and total parenteral nutritional support on metabolic, inflammatory and oxidative markers in patients with predicted severe acute pancreatitis (APACHE II > or =6). Pancreatology 2003;3(5):406–413.
11. Gramlich L, Kichian K, Pinilla J, et al. Does enteral nutrition compared to parenteral nutrition result in better outcomes in critically ill adult patients? A systematic review of the literature. Nutrition 2004;20(10):843–848.
12. McClave SA, Chang WK, Dhaliwal R, et al. Nutrition support in acute pancreatitis: a systematic review of the literature. J Parenter Enteral Nutr 2006;30(2):143–156.
13. Jeejeebhoy KN. Enteral nutrition versus parenteral nutrition—the risks and benefits. Nat Clin Pract Gastroenterol Hepatol 2007;4(5):260–265.
14. Laflamme DP. Development and validation of a body condition score system for dogs. Canine Pract 1997;22:10–15.
15. Laflamme DP. Development and validation of a body condition score system for cats: a clinical tool. Feline Pract 1997;25:13–18.
16. Freitag KA, Saker KE, Thomas E, et al. Acute starvation and subsequent refeeding affect lymphocyte subsets and proliferation in cats. J Nutr 2000;130(10):2444–2449.
17. Lippert AC, Fulton RB, Parr AM. A retrospective study of the use of total parenteral nutrition in dogs and cats. J Vet Intern Med 1993;7(2):52–64.
18. Reuter JD, Marks SL, Rogers QR, et al. Use of total parenteral nutrition in dogs: 209 cases (1988–1995). J Vet Emerg Crit Care 1998;8:201–213.
19. Chan DL, Freeman LM, Labato MA, et al. Retrospective evaluation of partial parenteral nutrition in dogs and cats. J Vet Intern Med 2002;16(4):440–445.
20. Pyle SC, Marks SL, Kass PH. Evaluation of complications and prognostic factors associated with administration of total parenteral nutrition in cats: 75 cases (1994–2001). J Am Vet Med Assoc 2004;225(2):242–250.
21. Myers CJ, Magdesian KG, Kass PH, et al. Parenteral nutrition in neonatal foals: clinical description, complications and outcome in 53 foals (1995–2005). Vet J 2009;181(2):137–144.
22. van den Berghe G, Wouters P, Weekers F, et al. Intensive insulin therapy in the critically ill patients. N Engl J Med 2001;345(19):1359–1367.
23. Finfer S, Chittock DR, Su SY, et al. Intensive versus conventional glucose control in critically ill patients. N Engl J Med 2009;360(13):1283–1297.
24. Trissel LA, ed. Handbook of Injectable Drugs. 15th ed. Bethesda, MD: American Society of Health-System; 2008.
25. Desport JC, Hoedt B, Pelagatti VV, et al. Twenty-nine day study of stability for six different parenteral nutrition mixtures. Crit Care 1997;1(1):41–44.
26. Pharmaceutical Compounding—Sterile Preparations. Chapter 797. United States Pharmacopoeia (USP). 28th ed. US Pharmacopoeial Convention. Rockville, MD: US Pharmacopoeial Convention Inc; 2004:2461–2477.
27. Thomovsky EJ, Backus RC, Mann FA, et al. Effects of temperature and handling conditions on lipid emulsion stability in veterinary parenteral nutrition admixtures during simulated intravenous administration. Am J Vet Res 2008;69(5):652–658.
28. Queau Y, Larsen JA, Kass PH, et al. Factors associated with adverse outcomes during parenteral nutrition administration in dogs and cats. J Vet Internal Med 2011;25(3):446–452.

29. Chan DL, Freeman LM, Rozanski EA, et al. Alterations in carbohydrate metabolism in critically ill cats. J Vet Emerg Crit Care 2006;16:S7–S13.

30. Roongpisuthipong C, Getupook V, Chindavijak B. Impact of a new guideline for central venous catheter care on sepsis in total parenteral nutrition: experience in Ramathibodi Hospital. J Med Assoc Thai 2007;90(10):2030–2038.

31. Schmitz G, Schädler D, Engel C, et al. Current practice in nutritional support and its association with mortality in septic patients—Results from a national, prospective, multicenter study. Crit Care Med 2008;36:1762–1767.

32. Campbell SJ, Karriker MJ, Fascetti AJ. Central and peripheral parenteral nutrition. WALTHAM Focus 2006;16(3):22–30.

SECTION VI

Analgesia and anesthesia

42

Pain recognition and management

Chiara Valtolina and Robert Goggs

Accurate recognition and effective management of pain are vital to veterinary critical care. Optimal pain control depends on a sound understanding of the physiology of nociception, an ability to recognize pain behaviors, diligent and thorough pain assessment, and an understanding of the principles of multimodal therapy. We must also be cognizant of potential analgesic-related adverse effects in order to recognize and manage them appropriately.

Nociceptive physiology

The International Association for the Study of Pain (IASP) defines pain as an unpleasant sensory and emotional experience associated with actual or potential tissue damage or described in terms of such damage (see Table 42.1).[1] By contrast, **nociception** refers to the unconscious activity induced by a noxious stimulus in specialized receptors, peripheral nerves, and the central nervous system and must not be confused with pain, which is a conscious experience. Nociception typically but not universally causes pain, and pain can occur without nociception.

Pain may be classified as physiologic or pathologic. Nociceptive or **physiologic pain** arises from noxious stimuli associated with the risk of tissue injury. Physiologic pain is proportional to stimulus intensity, transient, and characterized by a high stimulus threshold and narrow localization. Physiologic pain is protective because it induces withdrawal reflexes and avoidance responses but is rare in a clinical setting.[2]

In the clinic, noxious stimuli are persistent and perpetuated by inflammation (inflammatory pain) or nerve injury (neuropathic pain). This type of pain is pathologic and implies tissue damage has already occurred.

Pathologic pain is characterized by a low stimulus threshold and an exaggerated pain response to noxious stimuli (hyperalgesia). Pathologic pain is felt at sites of injury (primary hyperalgesia) and in surrounding areas (secondary hyperalgesia or extraterritorial pain).[3]

Pain may also be classified as adaptive or maladaptive.[4] **Adaptive pain** encompasses nociceptive and inflammatory pain, and it is a normal response to tissue damage and confers tissue protection. Inadequate management of adaptive pain may alter brain and spinal cord function leading to **maladaptive pain,** which does not have protective properties and is challenging to control. The longer the duration of pain, the more likely this switch to maladaptive pain.[4] Intense or prolonged noxious stimuli can alter nervous system function peripherally by decreasing the threshold of nociceptors or centrally by increasing the spinal neuron responsiveness through altered neuronal gene expression.[5]

Pathologic pain is pain that ceases to serve a protective function and becomes maladaptive, degrading health and functional capabilities. Pathologic pain may be acute or chronic. Acute pain is typified by postoperative pain and that associated with inflammatory disease such as pancreatitis. In a study evaluating pain in canine and feline emergency admissions to a teaching hospital, inflammation was identified as the cause in 70% of patients.[6] By contrast, chronic pain persists beyond the time frame expected for a given disease or injury and has been arbitrarily defined as persisting for more than 3–6 months.[1] Chronic pain may arise from sustained noxious stimuli due to ongoing inflammation or may be independent of tissue injury. More than 200 clinical syndromes are associated with chronic pain including cancer, osteoarthritis, and postamputation "phantom limb" syndrome.[1,2]

Advanced Monitoring and Procedures for Small Animal Emergency and Critical Care, First Edition. Edited by Jamie M. Burkitt Creedon, Harold Davis.
© 2012 John Wiley & Sons, Inc. Published 2012 by John Wiley & Sons, Inc.

Table 42.1 Pain definitions

Type of Pain	Definition
Adaptive pain (inflammatory)	Spontaneous pain and hypersensitivity to pain in response to tissue damage and inflammation. Occurs with tissue trauma, injury, surgery. Causes suffering. Responds to treatment.
Adaptive pain (nociceptive)	Transient pain in response to a noxious stimulus. Small aches and pains that are relatively innocuous and that protect the body from the environment.
Allodynia	Pain caused by a stimulus that does not normally result in pain.
Analgesia	Absence of pain in response to stimulation that would normally be painful.
Anesthesia	Medically induced insensitivity to pain. The procedure may render the patient unconscious (general anesthesia) or merely numb a body part (local anesthesia).
Causalgia	A syndrome of sustained burning pain, allodynia, and hyperpathia after a traumatic nerve lesion, often combined with vasomotor and sudomotor dysfunction and later trophic changes.
Distress	Acute anxiety or pain.
Dysphoria	A state of anxiety or restlessness, often accompanied by vocalization.
Hyperalgesia	An increased response to a stimulus that is normally painful.
Hypoalgesia	Diminished pain in response to a normally painful stimulus.
Hyperesthesia	Increased sensitivity to stimulation, excluding the special senses.
Hyperpathia	Painful syndrome characterized by an abnormally painful reaction to a stimulus and an increased threshold.
Maladaptive pain (functional)	Hypersensitivity to pain resulting from abnormal processing of normal input.
Maladaptive pain (central)	Pain initiated or caused by a primary lesion or dysfunction in the CNS. Often called "central pain."
Maladaptive pain (neuropathic)	Spontaneous pain and hypersensitivity to pain in association with damage to or a lesion of the nervous system.
Multimodal analgesia	Use of more than one drug with different actions to produce optimal analgesia.
Neurogenic pain	Pain initiated or caused by a primary lesion, dysfunction, or transitory perturbation in the peripheral or central nervous system.
Neuropathic pain	Pain initiated or caused by a primary lesion or dysfunction in the peripheral or central nervous system.
Nociceptor	A receptor preferentially sensitive to a noxious stimulus or to a stimulus that would become noxious if prolonged.
Nociception	Physiologic component of pain consisting of the processes of transduction, transmission, and modulation of neural signals generated in response to an external noxious stimulus.
Noxious stimulus	A noxious stimulus is one that is damaging to normal tissues.
Paresthesia	An abnormal sensation, whether spontaneous or evoked.
Pain	An unpleasant sensory and emotional experience associated with actual or potential tissue damage.
Preemptive analgesia	Administration of an analgesic before painful stimulation.
Wind-up pain	Heightened sensitivity that results in altered pain thresholds both peripherally and centrally.

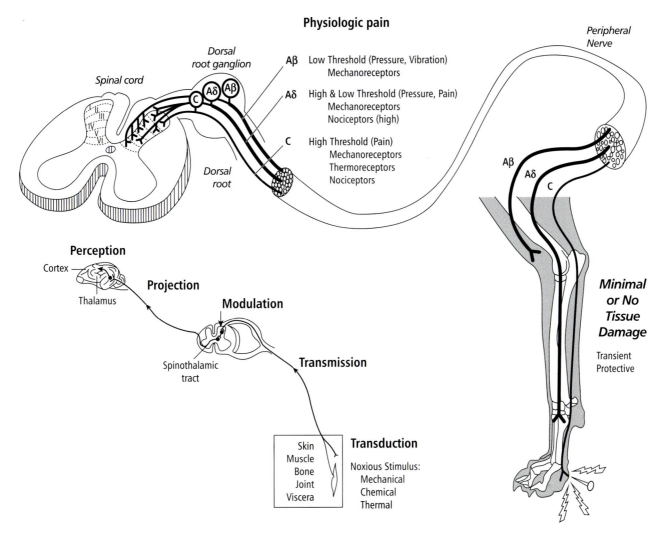

Figure 42.1 Schematic diagram of the pathways of physiologic pain sensation. Minimal or non–tissue-damaging stimuli are transduced by thermal, mechanical, and chemical peripheral nociceptors and transmitted to the dorsal horn of the spinal cord by Aδ and C fibers that release glutamate, activating dorsal horn neuron receptors that mediate reflex responses and transient pain. The pathways of nociception then involve stimulus transduction, transmission, modulation, projection, and perception. Adapted with permission from Muir WW 3rd, Woolf CJ. Mechanisms of pain and their therapeutic implications. *J Am Vet Med Assoc* 2001;219(10):1346–1356.

Nociception

Nociception involves perception of noxious stimuli at the site of injury, transduction into electrical signals, transmission of that signal to the spinal cord, signal modulation by amplification or inhibition, and finally supraspinal conduction and central integration to produce a pain experience unique to the individual (see Fig. 42.1). This multiple component system of transmission and integration also permits modulation of nociceptive information. The gate-control theory of pain modulation caused a revolution when published in 1965.[7,8] This theory suggests that nociceptive signals from the body are modulated by concurrent somatic afferent inputs as well as by descending influences from the brain. The gate-control theory, although simplistic, helps to explain how nociceptive signal propagation dependent on multiple synaptic gates can be modulated, and it illustrates how the brain may exert descending inhibition or facilitation of nociceptive signals.

Peripheral nociception begins with specialized free nerve endings (nociceptors) of primary afferent fibers located in cutaneous tissues, muscle, and viscera. These nociceptors transduce high-threshold stimuli into electrical activity and transmit this information to the spinal cord.[9,10] Nociceptors encode the localization, intensity, and duration of noxious stimuli. Most nociceptors are nonselective ion channels gated by temperature, chemical ligands, or mechanical shearing forces.[4] Once activated, the channels permit Na^+ and Ca^{2+} ion influx, producing an inward depolarizing current, which if of sufficient magnitude, activates voltage-gated Na$^+$ channels, further depolarizing the membrane and initiating bursts of action potentials. These are conducted from the periphery to the central nervous system (CNS) along primary afferent nociceptive fibers.[11] Nociceptors, by virtue of their specificity and threshold, constitute the first and most important filter in nociceptive processing.[10]

Sensory nerve fibers are divided into three groups (see Fig. 42.1). **Aβ fibers** are large myelinated sensory fibers activated by low-intensity stimuli; these fibers normally conduct nonnoxious information (touch, vibration, pressure, and rapid movement). Aδ and C fibers are the principal nociceptive primary afferents responsible for fast and slow pain.[9]

Aδ fibers are small (1–5 μm in diameter), myelinated, rapidly conducting (5–30 ms^{-1}) fibers responsible for the sensation of physiologic pain, fast pain, or "first pain," which is sharp, localized, and transient. Aδ fibers have small receptive fields and specific high-threshold ion channels activated by noxious thermal or mechanical input.[9] **C fibers** constitute most of the cutaneous nociceptive innervations, but they are also found extensively in muscle and viscera. They are small (0.25–1.5 μm in diameter) and unmyelinated with conduction velocities of only 0.5–2 ms. Their receptive fields are large compared with those of Aδ fibers. These characteristics contribute to the nature of pathologic pain, slow pain, or "second pain," which is a poorly localized, dull, aching, or burning sensation that persists despite termination of the noxious stimulus. C fibers are considered polymodal because they can be activated by thermal, mechanical, or chemical stimuli.

Afferent sensory nerve fibers enter the spinal cord via the dorsal nerve root and then separate to innervate second-order neurons within the gray matter. Aδ fibers terminate in laminae I, II, and IIa, whereas C fibers terminate in laminae II, IIa, and V. Sensory fibers synapse first at the level of the dorsal horn of the spinal cord where initial integration and modulation of nociceptive input occurs. Three principal paths are possible. Primary afferents may synapse with local interneurons (excitatory or inhibitory) causing modulation, with neurons involved in segmental spinal reflexes or with neurons that project to supraspinal structures.

Three types of nociceptive neurons project from the dorsal horn to supraspinal centers.[2] **Wide dynamic range** (WDR) **neurons** receive innocuous input from low-threshold Aβ fibers in addition to nociceptive input from Aδ and C fibers. Wide dynamic range neurons respond in a graded manner over large receptive fields and often receive convergent inputs from visceral and **nociceptive-specific** (NS) **neurons**. NS neurons involved in stimulus localization and discrimination have small receptive fields and respond to noxious, mechanical, and thermal stimuli via Aδ and C fibers. Wide dynamic range and NS fibers define the spatial and temporal qualities of pain. NS neurons may be persistently sensitized by repetitive noxious stimuli. Wide dynamic range neurons exhibit prolonged after-response generated by primary afferent input, intensifying and continuing nociceptive transmission.[9] Wide dynamic range and NS neurons project to the reticular formation and thalamus via multiple parallel pathways, including the spinothalamic (STT) and spinocervicothalamic (SCT) tracts and the dorsal column.[2]

Transmission and modulation

Interneuronal transmission in the dorsal horn occurs via excitatory and inhibitory amino acid-mediated signalling.[12] **Glutamate** is the principal excitatory synaptic neurotransmitter in both the spinal cord and brain. Two types of glutamate receptors exist: metabotropic, which are G-protein coupled receptors and ionotropic, which are ligand-gated ion channels. Three types of ionotropic receptor are described: kainate, α-amino-3-hydroxy-5-methylisoxazole-4-proprionate (AMPA), and **N-methyl-D-aspartate** (NMDA) **receptors**. Glutamate initially binds to AMPA receptors inducing ligand-gated sodium and calcium channel activation and rapid depolarization, which then activates NMDA receptors. Normally NMDA receptors are blocked by Mg^{2+} ions, but intense stimuli may remove this blockade. This in turns allows generation of a greater postsynaptic depolarizing response causing pain to remain after the stimulus has disappeared. C fibers also release various neuropeptides, particularly those of the tachykinin family including substance P and the neurokinins. Because these neuropeptides are the mediators of pathologic pain, the development of neuropeptide antagonists offers the hope of improved therapies for chronic pain states.

Nociceptive pathways permeate the medulla, pons, mesencephalon, diencephalon, and cerebrum. Modulation of pain responses occurs on four levels: spinal cord dorsal horn, the rostroventral medulla (RVM) of the brainstem, the periaqueductal grey matter (PAG) in the midbrain, and the thalamocortex. The thalamocortical system produces both the sensory, discriminative aspects of pain and the motivational, behavioral aspects of the pain experience. The thalamus integrates the pain experience with other brain centers. Relay nuclei exist between the thalamus; the limbic system (involved in behavior and emotion), which includes the amygdala (conditioned fear and anxiety); the prefrontal cortex; the hypothalamus (sympathetic autonomic activity); and the PAG (fight-or-flight behavior, stress-induced analgesia).[3] The PAG is a key structure in the endogenous analgesia system consisting of endorphin- and encephalin-containing neurons. Excitatory and inhibitory projections extend from the PAG to the brainstem. The RVM integrates and processes ascending nociceptive information and modulates descending output. Within the RVM, there are unique populations of cells referred to as facilitative and inhibitory or *on* and *off* cells involved in transmission of nociceptive stimuli, nociceptive reflexes, and behavioral responses. These cells are critical in producing hyperalgesia after peripheral tissue injury by maintaining central sensitization. At the level of the spinal cord, high concentrations of gamma-aminobutyric acid (GABA), glycine, serotonin, and the endogenous opioid peptides (encephalin, endorphin) produce inhibition of nociceptive stimulus transmission.

Allodynia

Tissue inflammation may lead to an exaggerated response to noxious stimuli (hyperalgesia) or a reduction in the intensity of the stimulus necessary to induce pain (allodynia).[3] This sensitization is caused by changes in the chemical environment of nociceptor peripheral terminals following release of adenosine triphosphate (ATP) and H^+ and K^+ ions from damaged cells at the site of injury. Proteases, cyclooxygenase-2, and nitric oxide synthase induced by inflammation, together with cytokines, chemokines, serotonin, and histamine produced by recruited inflammatory cells, act synergistically to lower the threshold for Aδ and C-fiber activation.[13] This threshold reduction recruits silent nociceptors producing allodynia.

Central sensitization/"wind-up"

Hypersensitivity also occurs due to dynamic modification of the receptive field properties of dorsal horn neurons in the spinal cord. Temporal summation and cumulative depolarization of dorsal horn neurons causes "wind-up," which is due to NMDA receptor disinhibition. NMDA stimulation leads to intracellular Ca^{2+} mobilization increasing responsiveness to glutamate.[4] Wind-up increases dorsal horn neuron excitability, which in conjunction with decreased spinal cord neuron inhibition creates central sensitization. Peripheral sensitization involves sensitized Aδ and C fibers while central sensitization allows low-threshold Aβ fibers to induce pain by increasing spinal neuron excitability and altering spinal cord sensory processing.

Glial cells, particularly those in the spinal cord, previously thought only to provide neuronal support and nutrition, are now considered key players in the creation and maintenance of pathologic pain states.[14] Glial cell activation due to nerve trauma or inflammation results

in proinflammatory mediator production, which contributes to central sensitization. Furthermore, these cells may also play a role in reducing opioid efficacy.[15]

Importance of pain control

The word *pain* derives from Greek and Latin words meaning punishment or penalty.[16] Numerous definitions of pain exist in the human literature where terms such as *distress, suffering*, and *stress* have been associated with pain.[17] Distress is an aversive state in which the animal is unable to cope effectively and engages in maladaptive behaviors. Suffering is an extremely unpleasant enduring emotional response usually associated with pain, distress, or helplessness.[18] When left untreated, pain may have consequences beyond unnecessary suffering.[19] Pain increases sympathetic tone and causes catecholamine release, resulting in tachycardia, vasoconstriction, decreased gastrointestinal blood flow, and the potential for gastrointestinal ulceration, decreased bladder tone, and increased muscle tone.[2] Pain-induced anxiety and fear enhance sympathetic outflow and may increase blood viscosity, prolong clotting times, and induce fibrinolysis and platelet aggregation. Intense vasoconstriction may lead to decreased tissue oxygen delivery and shock. Pain-induced tachycardia causes an increase in myocardial work and oxygen demand, and high levels of catecholamines predispose to arrhythmias.

Pain activates the renin-angiotensin-aldosterone system and induces the secretion of cortisol, glucagon, antidiuretic hormone, growth hormone, and interleukin-1; it decreases insulin secretion.[2] Increased counterregulatory hormone levels generate a catabolic state characterized by hyperglycemia, proteolysis, lipolysis, sodium and water retention, and decreased glomerular filtration. Such catabolism may have direct consequences for the immune system, decreasing wound healing and reducing an individual's capacity to respond to infection.[20] Pain also reduces appetite, mobility, and leads to postoperative weight loss. Immobility promotes urine and fecal retention.[21]

An important addition to the definition of pain states that "the inability to communicate in no way negates the possibility that an individual is experiencing pain and is in need of appropriate pain relieving treatment."[22] As caregivers we have two important reasons to address pain: a moral and ethical obligation toward animals that are suffering and cannot speak for themselves, and a medical duty to reduce the morbidity and mortality associated with pain. The American College of Veterinary Anesthesiologists (ACVA) states that the prevention and treatment of pain is a central guiding principle of practice,[23] a position embraced by the American

Veterinary Medical Association in 2001.[24] "The AVMA believes that animal pain and suffering are clinically important conditions that adversely affect an animal's quality of life. Drugs, techniques, or husbandry methods used to prevent and control pain must be tailored to individual animals and should be based, in part, on the species, breed, age, procedure performed, degree of tissue trauma, individual behavioral characteristics, degree of pain and health status."

Pain recognition

Effective pain management can only be achieved if pain can be accurately and consistently assessed to enable evaluation of therapeutic response. Pain is considered an individual experience, and the way this experience translates into observable and measurable behavior depends on numerous factors. Animals are unable to describe their pain as humans do, so the potential for observer bias is inherent in any attempt to measure pain in animals.[25]

The assessment and treatment of pain is greatly influenced by knowledge of the specific animal's normal behavior, of normal species behavior, and the caregiver's observational skills and attitude toward pain.[25] It is widely recognized that differences in attitude toward pain and analgesia exist within the veterinary profession.[26–29] These differences appear primarily due to gender and age, with female veterinarians and those recently graduated being more proactive in the evaluation and management of pain.[27]

The difficulties inherent in assessing pain in animals may result in analgesia being withheld inappropriately. Patients may not demonstrate *expected* signs of pain, or assessment may fail to identify these signs. Such problems have been cited by various studies as a major cause of veterinarians withholding analgesia.[30,31] Conversely, analgesia may be administered unnecessarily based on an anthropomorphic evaluation of the animal's condition, a scenario that increases the likelihood of adverse drug reactions.

In human medicine, despite most patients being able to report their pain verbally, the ideal method of pain assessment remains unidentified. Recently the Joint Commission on Accreditation of Healthcare Organizations (JCAHO) adopted pain as the fifth vital sign (after heart rate, respiratory rate, temperature, and blood pressure), which should be assessed by all clinicians.[32] In veterinary medicine, in which our patients are unable to report pain verbally, physiologic and behavioral responses form the basis for pain scoring scales.

Physiologic responses to pain include tachycardia, tachypnea, hypertension, pyrexia, and mydriasis, reflect-ing increased epinephrine, norepinephrine, and cortisol concentrations. These physiologic alterations are also induced by disease processes other than pain, however, making them nonspecific and of limited discriminant value.[25,33] Physiologic parameters may be of use if integrated into a multifaceted scoring system but have limited applicability when used alone.[34] In a study comparing the use of physiological variables and a subjective pain scale to assess pain in dogs after cruciate repair, physiologic variables correlated poorly with the subjective measures of pain.[35] Such limited correlations have led authors to question the validity of incorporating physiologic data into pain scoring systems for veterinary patients.[35,36]

Observational evaluation of animal behavior is an essential part of the assessment of pain but is subject to limitations. Observers must be familiar with the typical behavioral changes associated with pain (see Table 42.2 and Fig. 42.2). Animals undergoing veterinary examination in a strange environment may display altered behaviors that mask signs of pain. It is essential to gain as much information as possible from the primary caregiver regarding the animal's normal behavior prior to attempting pain assessment because an animal's character and temperament influences its response to pain.[37] Changes in behavior secondary to pain may be difficult to distinguish from that due to anxiety. Dogs especially may vocalize, whimper, or become agitated when anxious, and these signs are not pain specific.[37] Attempts to assess pain responses are complicated by the high degree of variation across species, between patients, and within individual patients themselves.

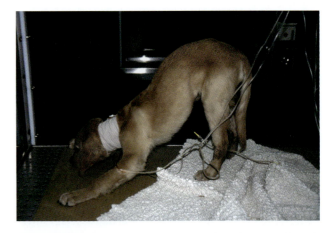

Figure 42.2 A young canine patient in the ICU at Utrecht University with abdominal pain demonstrating a characteristic "prayer" position. This abnormal posture is far more common in dogs than in cats, which tend to adopt a hunched posture or become recumbent and reluctant to move.

Table 42.2 General and species-specific behavioral manifestations of pain

Aspect of Behavior	General
Temperament	A change in temperament becoming aggressive or withdrawn. Aggression in response to forceful movement of painful area. Insomnia.
Vocalization	Vocalization in response to palpation or movement of painful area.
Posture, locomotion	Guarding of the painful area. Severe abdominal pain may result in hunched posture, prayer position, falling and/or rolling. Reluctance to lie down. Trembling; increased muscle tension.
Facial expression	Dull eyes, "staring into space," drooping ears.
Grooming	Decrease of normal grooming, unkempt hair coat. Piloerection. Licking, kicking, biting, or scratching painful area. Self-mutilation if pain is severe.
Activity level	Restlessness or overall decrease in activity level. Failure to use litter box; increased or decreased urination.
Food and water consumption	Decreased.
Aspect of Behavior	Species Specific
Cats	Vocalization is rare. Hissing or growling when approached or handled. Tendency to hide in enclosed space. Tendency to hide painful body parts. Decreased activity, lack of grooming, hunched posture, dissociation from the environment and lack of interaction with severe pain. Aggression if approached or when painful area is manipulated.
Dogs	Attention seeking, whimpering, whining, and howling. Vocalization often stops when animal is comforted. Hunched or "prayer" posture with abdominal pain. Shivering, panting.

Critically ill animals may be unable to display classical signs of pain (see Table 42.2) despite being painful. Critically ill animals may be obtunded, stuporous, or immobile and unable to shift position in response to noxious stimuli. They may not vocalize as otherwise healthy animals would.[21] Caregivers must be aware of the potential for underrecognition of pain causing inadequate analgesia provision in our sickest patients who may be in greatest need. The absence of perceptible behavioral displays associated with trauma or illness may be a factor in undertreatment.

Numerous pain assessment scales have been developed for humans, including the simple descriptive scale (SDS), visual analog scale (VAS), numerical ratings scale (NRS), and the multifactorial pain scale. All have been used and adapted for veterinary patients with variable clinical utility. The number and diversity of pain scales in use demonstrates there are deficiencies in each and suggests that none has been universally adopted. In addition, scales used to evaluate pain in the acute setting may be less useful in the assessment of chronic pain.

The **simple descriptive scale** consists of a number of written statements describing various levels of pain. Each expression is assigned a pain score value. Such scales have been used both for people and for veterinary patients.

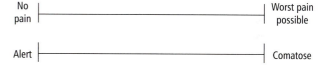

Figure 42.3 Visual analog scales (VAS) for pain and sedation. Observers mark the lines according to their perception of the degree of pain and sedation. The distance in millimeters from 0 to the point of intersection is the VAS score.

Although simple to use, these scales lack sensitivity because of the small number of categories involved.[33]

The **visual analog scale** is a continuous scale designed to allow observers to make a subjective overall judgment about an individual's pain, and because of their simplicity, they can be used for any species. The VAS consists of a 100-mm line, anchored by the descriptor *No pain* at one end with *Unbearable pain*, *Excruciating pain*, or *Worst pain possible* at the opposite end, and it is often combined with concurrent visual analog sedation score (see Fig. 42.3). After watching the animal for a period of time, the observer marks the line according to his or her perception of the degree of pain. The distance in millimeters from 0 to the point of intersection is the VAS pain score. The VAS avoids the need for descriptive terms or for pain to be directly assigned a number. In people, pain scores produced by VAS when used by competent and trained personnel are both reproducible and sensitive. The limitations of the VAS are inherent in the subjective nature of this type of system producing significant interobserver variability.[38] Independent assessors may interpret the upper delimiter differently, and VAS scores may be excessively influenced by easily detectible signs of pain. VAS sensitivity may be increased by using *Worst pain possible for this condition/procedure* as the upper delimiter, but this requires clinical judgment and a degree of anthropomorphism.[35,39]

Numerical rating scales consist of multiple categories with numerical scores used to evaluate patient behavior. Physiologic parameters, typically changes in heart rate, respiratory rate, or temperature by 120% of baseline values, may be included. NRS assume that a change of score from 1 to 2 is equivalent to a change from 2 to 3 and that this correlates with a more painful experience. The categories themselves are not weighted and are assigned equal importance to the overall score, which may be inaccurate. NRS descriptors also lack specificity.[39]

Unfortunately, SDS, VAS, and NRS may all be unreliable in assessing acute pain in dogs in a hospital setting because they are all unidimensional: They measure only the intensity of pain rather than also encompassing its sensory and affective (behavioral) qualities. Pain may be aching, burning, stabbing or stinging—all sensory qualities that affect the way pain is perceived and are independent of intensity. Similarly, pain has affective or behavioral qualities because it is often accompanied by desires to terminate, reduce, or escape its presence. Pain is unpleasant and typically causes behavioral changes designed to ameliorate the experience.

Attempts have been made to overcome this unidimensional limitation by refining the assessed behavioral characteristics and including more objective physiologic data. The **Melbourne Pain Scale (MPS)** developed in the late 1990s consists of six broad categories divided into levels with associated scores.[40] The maximum possible score using this scale is 27. The MPS represents a refinement of the scales previously described but also has limitations. Again, significant interobserver variability occurs and the MPS is insensitive to nonovert behavioral displays as demonstrated by the example of a quiet, depressed, immobile, inappetent amputee suggested by Hansen.[41]

The need to assess the intensity, sensory, and motivational or behavioral aspects of pain formed the basis for the development of **multifactorial pain scales** (MFPS) or **composite measure pain scales** (CMPS), which provide better interobserver repeatability. Two composite pain scales have been described in veterinary medicine. The **Colorado State University Veterinary**

Teaching Hospital Pain Score for Cats and Dogs is based on eight categories of behavioral and physiologic signs.[42] Comfort, movement, appearance, unprovoked behavior, interactive behavior, vocalization, heart rate, and respiratory rate are assessed. Each category is assigned a score of 0–4 according to predefined criteria. The total score is the sum of the category scores. Unfortunately, the detailed rationale for the selection of these categories is obscure, which has limited its use by other researchers working in this field.

The **Glasgow Composite Measure Pain Scale (GCMPS)** designed using psychometric principles (reliability, validity, standardization, freedom from bias) has recently been validated for assessing acute pain in dogs.[43–45] The GCMPS is a behavior-based system based on a structured questionnaire that includes clinical observation, assessment of spontaneous and evoked behavior, and animal–observer interaction. The questionnaire is structured around seven categories: posture, activity, vocalization, attention to wound/painful area, demeanor, mobility, and response to touch. To standardize scoring by multiple observers, each category contains descriptors from which those best matching the dog's behavior are selected (see Table 42.3). Recently a rapid, easy-to-use short form (GCMPS-SF) was developed to facilitate use in a busy clinical setting (see Fig. 42.4).[46]

Assessment of pain in cats can be extremely challenging because behavioral manifestations may be subtle or nonexistent.[47,48] Optimal assessment of pain in cats will require development and validation of behavior-based multidimensional pain measurement tools. Observation of behavior remains the best means of assessing the degree of pain in feline patients (see Fig. 42.5).[49] A VAS that includes physical interaction called the dynamic and interactive visual analogue scale (DIVAS) has been used in cats by several groups to improve sensitivity.[50,51] Most information can be acquired if the animal is observed first from a distance, its response to a person's approach assessed, and finally its response to physical interactions such as stroking or palpation evaluated. Wound sensitivity and response to palpation correlates well with VAS scoring in cats. Manipulation of the affected area appears to be of value in feline pain evaluation.[48]

Future directions in the field of pain assessment may involve computerized behavior and activity monitoring.[41] Such systems have not been clinically validated, however. For now a combination of systems may provide the best all-round pain assessment method for clinical use.

Multimodal analgesia

Multimodal analgesia is an approach to pain relief provision that involves the use of multiple drug types or

Table 42.3 Descriptive terms for the Glasgow Pain Scale

Category	Descriptor	Definition
Posture	Normal	Animal may be in any position, appears comfortable, muscles relaxed.
	Tense	Animal appears frightened or reluctant to move, overall impression of tight muscles; animal can be in any body position.
	Hunched	When animal is standing, its back forms a convex shape with abdomen tucked up, or, back in a concave shape with shoulders and front legs lower than hips.
	Rigid	Animal lying in lateral recumbency, legs extended or partially extended in a fixed position.
Activity	Comfortable	Animal resting and relaxed, no avoidance or abnormal body position evident, or settled, remains in same body position, at ease.
	Restless	Moving bodily position, circling, pacing, shifting body parts, unsettled.
Vocalization	Whimpering	Often quiet, short, high-pitched sound, frequently closed mouth (whining).
	Crying	Extension of the whimpering noise, louder and with open mouth.
	Groaning	Low moaning or grunting deep sound, intermittent.
	Screaming	Continual high pitched noise, inconsolable, mouth wide open.
Attention to wound area	Ignoring	Paying no attention to wound area.
	Rubbing	Using paw or kennel to stroke wound area.
	Looking	Turning head in direction of area of wound.
	Licking	Using tongue to stroke area of wound.
	Chewing	Using mouth and teeth on wound area, pulling stitches.
Demeanor	Bouncy	Tail wagging, jumping in kennel, often vocalizing with a happy and excited noise.
	Content	Interested in surroundings, positive interaction with observer, responsive and alert.
	Quiet	Sitting or lying still, no noise; will look when spoken to but not respond.
	Nervous	Eyes in continual movement, often head and body movement, jumpy.
	Anxious	Worried expression, eyes wide with white showing, wrinkled forehead.
	Fearful	Cowering away, guarding body and head.
	Indifferent	Not responsive to surroundings or observer.
	Disinterested	Cannot be stimulated to wag tail or interact with observer.
	Depressed	Dull demeanor, not responsive, shows reluctance to interact.
	Aggressive	Mouth open or lip curled showing teeth, snarling, growling, snapping, or barking.
Mobility	Normal	Gets up and lies down with no alteration from normal.
	Lame	Irregular gait, uneven weightbearing when walking.
	Reluctant to rise or sit	Needs encouragement to get up or sit down.
	Slow to rise or sit	Slow to get up or sit down but not stilted in movement.
	Stiff	Stilted gait, slow to rise or sit, may be reluctant to move.
Response to touch	None	Accepts firm pressure on wound with no reaction.
	Guard	Pulls painful area away from stimulus or tenses local muscles in order to protect from stimulus.
	Growl	Emits a low prolonged warning sound before or in response to touch.
	Snap	Tries to bite observer before or in response to touch.
	Flinch	Painful area is quickly moved away from stimulus either before or in response to touch.
	Cry	A short vocal response; looks at area and opens mouth, emits a brief sound.

Source: Modified with permission from Holton L, Reid J, Scott E, Pawson P, Nolan A. Development of a behaviour-based scale to measure acute pain in dogs. *Vet Rec* 2001;148(17): 525–531.

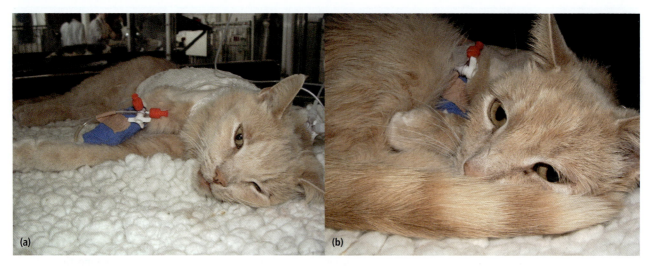

Figure 42.4 Observation of posture and behavior are key components of pain assessment in cats. (a) A feline patient recovering following a thoracotomy. The cat is laterally recumbent, inactive, and disinterested in the environment. (b) The same cat following pain assessment and augmentation of the analgesic plan. The cat appears more comfortable and is seen adopting a more typically feline curled-up pose. Images courtesy of Dr. J. H. Robben (ICU, Utrecht University).

techniques with complementary mechanisms and sites of action within the peripheral and central nervous systems. Some authors have used the term solely in reference to systemic administration of multiple drugs with different mechanisms of action,[52] whereas others refer to systemic drug administration combined with regional anesthesia.[53] The term was introduced in 1991 to describe the combined use of local anesthesia techniques, opioids, and systemic nonsteroidal analgesics to manage pain following colorectal surgery in humans.[54] The aim of this approach is to target different points in the nociceptive pathways so more complete analgesia can be provided while minimizing side effects. One of the driving forces for this approach has been the increase in outpatient surgical intervention in humans, which limits the utility of more conventional opioid and epidural analgesic approaches. Although in-patient surgical procedures are currently the norm in veterinary patients, our patients can still benefit from advances made by our medical colleagues. The multimodal approach uses the additive or synergistic analgesic effects of multiple drug classes, maximizing patient comfort and allowing lower doses of individual analgesic agents to be used, reducing the potential for adverse drug reactions.[55] Effective implementation of multimodal analgesia requires an understanding of physiology and pathophysiology so that complementary drugs and methods can be selected. This approach has been adopted by the medical and veterinary medical professions[53] and was well reviewed in 2008.[56] Limited data are available examining the combined use of opioids with regional anesthesia; however, multiple positive studies in people have been performed using opioids in combination with nonsteroidal agents or with acetaminophen.

Timing of analgesic administration

The optimum definition of preemptive analgesia is disputed, although the pathophysiologic premise is straightforward and theoretically attractive. Preemptive analgesia is an analgesic intervention begun before the onset of noxious stimuli in order to block peripheral and central nociception, thereby preventing postoperative pain amplification.[57] It is hypothesized that inflammation leads to persistent pain elicited by a variety of C fiber–dependent neuropeptides, excitatory amino acids, and mediators including cytokines and prostaglandins. Ongoing nociceptive input modulates the CNS through activation-dependent plasticity resulting in peripheral sensitization, allodynia, and hyperalgesia. Peripheral sensitization paves the way for modulation of central nociceptive pathways by further nociceptive stimulation and sensitization of higher structures. Sensitization causes increased spontaneous activity and afferent responsiveness, reduced threshold, and prolonged discharge after repeated stimulation ("wind-up"). Neuronal plasticity induces "pain memory" allowing a more rapid response from the CNS following future similar stimuli. Maladaptive plasticity thereby leads to central sensitization.[58] NMDA receptors are thought to play a significant role in this process, leading to exploration of the ability of NMDA receptor antagonists such as ketamine to attenuate central sensitization.

SHORT FORM OF THE GLASGOW COMPOSITE PAIN SCALE

Dog's name _____

Hospital Number _____ Date   /   /   Time

Surgery Yes/No (delete as appropriate)

Procedure or condition _____

_____

In the sections below please circle the appropriate score in each list and sum these to give the total score.

A. Look at dog in Kennel

Is the dog?

(i)
Quiet	0
Crying or whimpering	1
Groaning	2
Screaming	3

(ii)
Ignoring any wound or painful area	0
Looking at wound or painful area	1
Licking wound or painful area	2
Rubbing wound or painful area	3
Chewing wound or painful area	4

> In the case of spinal, pelvic or multiple limb fractures, or where assistance is
> required to aid locomotion do not carry out section **B** and proceed to C
> *Please tick if this is the case* ☐ then proceed to C.

B. Put lead on dog and lead out of the kennel.

When the dog rises/walks is it?

(iii)
Normal	0
Lame	1
Slow or reluctant	2
Stiff	3
It refuses to move	4

C. If it has a wound or painful area including abdomen, apply gentle pressure 2 inches round the site.

Does it?

(iv)
Do nothing	0
Look round	1
Flinch	2
Growl or guard area	3
Snap	4
Cry	5

D. Overall

Is the dog?

(v)
Happy and content or happy and bouncy	0
Quiet	1
Indifferent or non-responsive to surroundings	2
Nervous or anxious or fearful	3
Depressed or non-responsive to stimulation	4

Is the dog?

(vi)
Comfortable	0
Unsettled	1
Restless	2
Hunched or tense	3
Rigid	4

© University of Glasgow

Total Score (i+ii+iii+iv+v+vi) = _____

Figure 42.5 Short form of the Glasgow Composite Measure Pain Scale. Copyright 2008 University of Glasgow. Permission granted to reproduce for personal and educational use only. Commercial copying, hiring, lending is prohibited. The short form composite measure pain score (CMPS-SF) can be applied quickly and reliably in a clinical setting and has been designed as a clinical decision-making tool that was developed for dogs in acute pain. It includes 30 descriptor options within 6 behavioral categories, including mobility. Within each category, the descriptors are ranked numerically according to their associated pain severity, and the person carrying out the assessment chooses the descriptor within each category that best fits the dog's behavior/condition. It is important to carry out the assessment procedure as described on the questionnaire, following the protocol closely. The pain score is the sum of the rank scores. The maximum score for the 6 categories is 24, or 20 if mobility is impossible to assess. The total CMPS-SF score has been shown to be a useful indicator of analgesic requirement, and the recommended analgesic intervention level is 6/24 or 5/20.

Kissin in 1994 proposed that preemptive should mean "preventive" rather than simply "before" because ineffective afferent blockade cannot be preemptive even if administered before the noxious stimulus of surgery.[58] Thus the goals of preemptive analgesia are to decrease acute pain after tissue injury, to prevent pain-induced altered sensory processing, and to inhibit the persistence of postoperative pain. The blockade of nociceptive pathways must therefore be maintained from the preoperative stage, throughout surgery, and into the postoperative period.

Multiple nociceptive models in animals confirm the existence of peripheral and central sensitization,[59,60] and there is convincing evidence to support the use of preemptive analgesia in animal models, a subject well reviewed by Woolf and Chong.[61] Agents used within these studies include opioids, local anesthetics, and NMDA receptor antagonists given by a variety of routes. Multiple randomized controlled trials have been conducted in humans with the hope of translating experimental efficacy into clinical benefit. Results of clinical studies assessing preemptive analgesia in people are contradictory, however, and the subject has become controversial.[62]

Since 1995, six notable systematic reviews of preemptive analgesic trials have been published with conflicting results.[63–68] Conflicting results may relate to variations in definition of preemptive analgesia on which the studies were based because this fundamentally affects the methods used.[69] Other potential causes of discrepancy include insufficiency of preemptive analgesic techniques, surgical and anesthetic problems, difficulties assessing outcome and other patient-related factors.[70] Although the systematic review published by Moiniche et al.[66] drew a negative conclusion, publications relating to this study suggest equipoise among anesthesiologists.[71,72]

Clinical veterinary publications describing the use and efficacy of preemptive analgesia are limited and generally involve small sample sizes. Limited information about the efficacy of preemptive analgesia can be gained from these because they too appear to produce conflicting results. A study in cats suggested that meloxicam given preoperatively provides adequate perioperative analgesia for onychectomy.[73] Cats receiving oral or subcutaneous meloxicam preoperatively had significantly fewer signs of pain following ovariohysterectomy, compared with cats receiving oral buprenorphine.[74] However, this study identified no significant difference in VAS scores between groups, only differences in pain scoring that involved an interaction. In addition no difference could be detected when the opioid was administered subcutaneously. A study comparing preemptive extradural morphine with or without bupivacaine involving 265 dogs and cats suggested this technique provided long-lasting analgesia and may be superior to postoperative pain management with opioids and nonsteroidal anti-inflammatory drugs (NSAIDs).[75] A later study of dogs receiving extradural bupivacaine and morphine found that this strategy reduced the neuroendocrine stress response but did not reduce the acute phase response to orthopedic surgery.[76]

Whether preemptive analgesic interventions are more effective than conventional regimens in managing acute postoperative pain remains controversial. Some anesthesiologists now favor use of a multimodal approach to therapy with less concern about the timing of their interventions.[65] Others believe that for a preemptive technique to be effective, it must be multimodal and active before, during, and after surgery.[77,78]

Contraindications and complications of pain management

Recent shifts in veterinarian attitudes toward pain management and the use of the multimodal approach have greatly increased the frequency and diversity of analgesic prescribing. Although concerns about the potential for adverse reactions associated with analgesic administration have been reported,[28,79,80] it is likely these have been overemphasized.[33,81] Despite improvements in our understanding of feline drug disposition, such concerns have slowed progress in provision of pain relief to cats.[49,79,82,83] There is no longer a rationale for withholding analgesics from cats because previously held misconceptions about complications associated with analgesics in the species have been largely discredited.[84,85] But we must remain vigilant for adverse effects in order to manage them correctly.

An **adverse drug reaction** (ADR) is defined as any unexpected, undesirable, or harmful consequence associated with the administration of a medication. ADRs may be common, mild, and reversible or rare, severe, and permanent.[86] As with any medications, analgesic agents have the potential to cause such negative side effects. Indeed in human hospitals analgesics are associated with a large number of adverse effects[87] that can lead to an increase in the duration of stay in the intensive care unit (ICU) or potentially be fatal.[88,89] A prospective study of analgesic prescribing in a veterinary ICU suggested that adverse drug reactions or concerns about side effects affect the prescribing of analgesic medication for small animals.[90] This study observed 272 dogs and 79 cats in a single center over a 2-month period. The authors identified that although 64% of analgesic medication was administered as prescribed, 23% of prescribed doses were reduced or not administered. Dose reductions were primarily due to concerns about levels of sedation, hypotension, and hypothermia associated with analgesic administration.

Although we must consider the potential for ADRs, such concerns should not prevent us from improving efforts to control pain in our patients. A study evaluating a quality control program of analgesic provision to human trauma patients showed that training physicians to monitor and treat ADRs led to an increase in the frequency and appropriateness of drug administration,[91] likely due to increased confidence in analgesic use. It should also be remembered that the risk of analgesic-related complications is reduced in painful patients. We should be vigilant for signs of adverse reactions but proactive in our provision of pain relief because pain itself reduces the likelihood of a successful outcome for our patients.

References

1. International Association for the Study of Pain. Pain terms: a list with definitions and notes on usage. Recommended by the IASP Subcommittee on Taxonomy. Pain 1979;6:249.
2. Lamont LA, Tranquilli WJ, Grimm KA. Physiology of pain. Vet Clin North Am Small Anim Pract 2000;30:703–728.
3. Muir WW 3rd, Woolf CJ. Mechanisms of pain and their therapeutic implications. J Am Vet Med Assoc 2001;219:1346–1356.
4. Woolf CJ. Pain: moving from symptom control toward mechanism-specific pharmacologic management. Ann Intern Med 2004;140:441–451.
5. Pockett S. Spinal cord synaptic plasticity and chronic pain. Anesth Analg 1995;80:173–179.
6. Wiese AJ, Muir WW, Wittum TE. Characteristics of pain and response to analgesic treatment in dogs and cats examined at a veterinary teaching hospital emergency service. J Am Vet Med Assoc 2005;226:2004–2009.
7. Melzack R, Wall PD. Pain mechanisms: a new theory. Science 1965;150:971–979.
8. Melzack R. Recent concepts of pain. J Med 1982;13:147–160.
9. Giordano J. The neurobiology of nociceptive and anti-nociceptive systems. Pain Physician 2005;8:277–290.
10. Woolf CJ, Ma Q. Nociceptors—noxious stimulus detectors. Neuron 2007;55:353–364.
11. Woolf CJ, Salter MW. Neuronal plasticity: increasing the gain in pain. Science 2000;288:1765–1769.
12. Raffe M. Recent advances in our understanding of pain: how should they affect management? Semin Vet Med Surg (Small Anim) 1997;12:75–79.
13. Levine JD, Reichling DB. Peripheral mechanisms of inflammatory pain. In: Wall PD, Melzack R, eds. Textbook of Pain. 4th ed. Edinburgh, UK: Churchill Livingstone; 1999:59–84.
14. Watkins LR, Hutchinson MR, Johnston IN, et al. Glia: novel counter-regulators of opioid analgesia. Trends Neurosci 2005;28:661–669.
15. Hansson E. Could chronic pain and spread of pain sensation be induced and maintained by glial activation? Acta Physiol (Oxf) 2006;187:321–327.
16. Robertson SA. What is pain? J Am Vet Med Assoc 2002;221:202–205.
17. Anil SS, Anil L, Deen J. Challenges of pain assessment in domestic animals. J Am Vet Med Assoc 2002;220:313–319.
18. Chapman CR. Psychological-aspects of postoperative pain control. Acta Anaesthesiol Belg 1992;43:41–52.
19. Siddall PJ, Cousins MJ. Persistent pain as a disease entity: implications for clinical management. Anesth Analg 2004;99:510–520.
20. Hellebrekers LJ. Pathophysiology of pain in animals and its consequences for analgesic drug therapy. In: Hellebrekers LJ, ed. Animal Pain: A Practice-Oriented Approach to an Effective Pain Control in Animals. Ames, IA: Wiley-Blackwell; 2000:71–84.
21. Hansen BD. Analgesia and sedation in the critically ill. J Vet Emerg Crit Care 2005;15:285–294.
22. Merskey H, Bogduk N. Classification of Chronic Pain: Descriptions of Chronic Pain Syndromes and Definitions of Pain Terms. 2nd ed. Seattle, WA: International Association for the Study of Pain; 1994.
23. American College of Veterinary Anesthesiologists' position paper on the treatment of pain in animals. J Am Vet Med Assoc 1998;213:628–630.
24. AVMA adopts position regarding animal pain. J Am Vet Med Assoc 2001;218:1694.
25. Hardie EM. Recognition of pain behaviour in animals. In: Hellebrekers LJ, ed. Animal Pain: A Practice-Oriented Approach to an Effective Pain Control in Animals. Ames, IA: Wiley-Blackwell; 2000:51–70.
26. Coleman DL, Slingsby LS. Attitudes of veterinary nurses to the assessment of pain and the use of pain scales. Vet Rec 2007;160:541–544.
27. Hugonnard M, Leblond A, Keroack S, et al. Attitudes and concerns of French veterinarians towards pain and analgesia in dogs and cats. Vet Anaesth Analg 2004;31:154–163.
28. Lascelles BDX, Capner CA, Waterman-Pearson AE. Current British veterinary attitudes to perioperative analgesia for cats and small mammals. Vet Rec 1999;145:601–604.
29. Raekallio M, Heinonen KM, Kuussaari J, et al. Pain alleviation in animals: attitudes and practices of Finnish veterinarians. Vet J 2003;165:131–135.
30. Capner CA, Lascelles BDX, Waterman-Pearson AE. Current British veterinary attitudes to perioperative analgesia for dogs. Vet Rec 1999;145:95–99.
31. Williams VM, Lascelles BDX, Robson MC. Current attitudes to, and use of, perioperative analgesia in dogs and cats by veterinarians in New Zealand. N Z Vet J 2005;53:193–202.
32. Phillips DM. JCAHO pain management standards are unveiled. Joint Commission on Accreditation of Healthcare Organizations. JAMA 2000;284:428–429.
33. Mathews KA. Pain assessment and general approach to management. Vet Clin North Am Small Anim Pract 2000;30:729–755.
34. Flecknell P. Recognition and assessment of pain in animals. In: Lord Soulsby and Morton D, eds. Pain: Its Nature and Management in Man and Animals. London, UK: Royal Society of Medicine Press; 2001:63–68.
35. Holton LL, Scott EM, Nolan AM, et al. Relationship between physiological factors and clinical pain in dogs scored using a numerical rating scale. J Small Anim Pract 1998;39:469–474.
36. Conzemius MG, Hill CM, Sammarco JL, et al. Correlation between subjective and objective measures used to determine severity of postoperative pain in dogs. J Am Vet Med Assoc 1997;210:1619–1622.
37. Dobromylsky P, Flecknell PA, Lascelles BDX, et al. Pain recognition and pain assessment. In: Flecknell P, Waterman-Pearson AE, eds. Pain Management in Animals. Philadelphia, PA: W.B. Saunders; 2000:53–79.
38. Holton LL, Scott EM, Nolan AM, et al. Comparison of three methods used for assessment of pain in dogs. J Am Vet Med Assoc 1998;212:61–66.
39. Perkowski SZ. Pain and sedation assessment. In: Silverstein DC, Hopper K, eds. Small Animal Critical Care Medicine. St. Louis, MO: Saunders/Elsevier; 2009:696–699.
40. Firth AM, Haldane SL. Development of a scale to evaluate postoperative pain in dogs. J Am Vet Med Assoc 1999;214:651–659.
41. Hansen BD. Assessment of pain in dogs: veterinary clinical studies. ILAR J 2003;44:197–205.
42. Hellyer PW, Gaynor JS. Acute postsurgical pain in dogs and cats. Comp Contin Edu Pract Vet 1998;20:140–153.

43. Holton L, Reid J, Scott EM, et al. Development of a behaviour-based scale to measure acute pain in dogs. Vet Rec 2001;148: 525–531.

44. Morton CM, Reid J, Scott EM, et al. Application of a scaling model to establish and validate an interval level pain scale for assessment of acute pain in dogs. Am J Vet Res 2005;66:2154–2166.

45. Murrell JC, Psatha EP, Scott EM, et al. Application of a modified form of the Glasgow pain scale in a veterinary teaching centre in the Netherlands. Vet Rec 2008;162:403–408.

46. Reid J, Nolan AM, Hughes JML, et al. Development of the short-form Glasgow Composite Measure Pain Scale (CMPS-SF) and derivation of an analgesic intervention score. Anim Welf 2007;16: 97–104.

47. Wright BD. Clinical pain management techniques for cats. Clin Tech Small Anim Pract 2002;17:151–157.

48. Robertson SA. Assessment and management of acute pain in cats. J Vet Emerg Crit Care 2005;15:261–272.

49. Lascelles D, Waterman A. Analgesia in cats. In Pract 1997;19:203–213.

50. Cambridge AJ, Tobias KM, Newberry RC, et al. Subjective and objective measurements of postoperative pain in cats. J Am Vet Med Assoc 2000;217:685–690.

51. Grint NJ, Murison PJ, Coe RJ, et al. Assessment of the influence of surgical technique on postoperative pain and wound tenderness in cats following ovariohysterectomy. J Feline Med Surg 2006;8:15–21.

52. Dahl V, Raeder JC. Non-opioid postoperative analgesia. Acta Anaesthesiol Scand 2000;44:1191–1203.

53. Practice guidelines for acute pain management in the perioperative setting: an updated report by the American Society of Anesthesiologists Task Force on Acute Pain Management. Anesthesiology 2004;100:1573–1581.

54. Dahl JB, Kehlet H. Nonsteroidal antiinflammatory drugs—rationale for use in severe postoperative pain. Br J Anaesth 1991; 66:703–712.

55. Kehlet H, Dahl JB. The value of multimodal or balanced analgesia in postoperative pain treatment. Anesth Analg 1993;77: 1048–1056.

56. Lamont LA. Multimodal pain management in veterinary medicine: the physiologic basis of pharmacologic therapies. Vet Clin North Am Small Anim Pract 2008;38:1173–1186.

57. Kelly DJ, Ahmad M, Brull SJ. Preemptive analgesia I: physiological pathways and pharmacological modalities. Can J Anaesth 2001;48:1000–1010.

58. Kissin I. Preemptive analgesia: terminology and clinical relevance. Anesth Analg 1994;79:809–810.

59. Baumann TK, Simone DA, Shain CN, et al. Neurogenic hyperalgesia: the search for the primary cutaneous afferent fibers that contribute to capsaicin-induced pain and hyperalgesia. J Neurophysiol 1991;66:212–227.

60. LaMotte RH, Shain CN, Simone DA, et al. Neurogenic hyperalgesia: psychophysical studies of underlying mechanisms. J Neurophysiol 1991;66:190–211.

61. Woolf CJ, Chong MS. Preemptive analgesia–treating postoperative pain by preventing the establishment of central sensitization. Anesth Analg 1993;77:362–379.

62. Kissin I. Preemptive analgesia. Why its effect is not always obvious. Anesthesiology 1996;84:1015–1019.

63. Bong CL, Samuel M, Ng JM, et al. Effects of preemptive epidural analgesia on post-thoracotomy pain. J Cardiothorac Vasc Anesth 2005;19:786–793.

64. McQuay HJ. Pre-emptive analgesia: a systematic review of clinical studies. Ann Med 1995;27:249–256.

65. Kelly DJ, Ahmad M, Brull SJ. Preemptive analgesia II: recent advances and current trends. Can J Anaesth 2001;48:1091–1101.

66. Moiniche S, Kehlet H, Dahl JB. A qualitative and quantitative systematic review of preemptive analgesia for postoperative pain relief—the role of timing of analgesia. Anesthesiology 2002;96: 725–741.

67. McCartney CJ, Sinha A, Katz J. A qualitative systematic review of the role of N-methyl-D-aspartate receptor antagonists in preventive analgesia. Anesth Analg 2004;98:1385–1400.

68. Ong CKS, Lirk P, Seymour RA, et al. The efficacy of preemptive analgesia for acute postoperative pain management: a meta-analysis. Anesth Analg 2005;100:757–773.

69. Kissin I. Preemptive analgesia. Anesthesiology 2000;93: 1138–1143.

70. Grape S, Tramer MR. Do we need preemptive analgesia for the treatment of postoperative pain? Best Pract Res Clin Anaesthesiol 2007;21:51–63.

71. Hogan QH. No preemptive analgesia: is that so bad? Anesthesiology 2002;96:526–527.

72. Gottschalk A, Ochroch EA. Preemptive analgesia: what do we do now? Anesthesiology 2003;98:280–281.

73. Carroll GL, Howe LB, Peterson KD. Analgesic efficacy of preoperative administration of meloxicam or butorphanol in onychectomized cats. J Am Vet Med Assoc 2005;226:913–919.

74. Gassel AD, Tobias KM, Egger CM, et al. Comparison of oral and subcutaneous administration of buprenorphine and meloxicam for preemptive analgesia in cats undergoing ovariohysterectomy. J Am Vet Med Assoc 2005;227:1937–1944.

75. Troncy E, Junot S, Keroack S, et al. Results of preemptive epidural administration of morphine with or without bupivacaine in dogs and cats undergoing surgery: 265 cases (1997–1999). J Am Vet Med Assoc 2002;221:666–672.

76. Sibanda S, Hughes JM, Pawson PE, et al. The effects of preoperative extradural bupivacaine and morphine on the stress response in dogs undergoing femoro-tibial joint surgery. Vet Anaesth Analg 2006;33:246–257.

77. Redmond M, Florence B, Glass PS. Effective analgesic modalities for ambulatory patients. Anesthesiol Clin North Am 2003;21:329–346.

78. Pogatzki-Zahn EM, Zahn PK. From preemptive to preventive analgesia. Curr Opin Anaesthesiol 2006;19:551–555.

79. Dohoo SE, Dohoo IR. Factors influencing the postoperative use of analgesics in dogs and cats by Canadian veterinarians. Can Vet J 1996;37:552–556.

80. Watson ADJ, Nicholson A, Church DB, et al. Use of antiinflammatory and analgesic drugs in dogs and cats. Aust Vet J 1996;74:203–210.

81. Dyson DH. Analgesia and chemical restraint for the emergent veterinary patient. Vet Clin North Am Small Anim Pract 2008;38:1329–1352.

82. Fink-Gremmels J. Implications of hepatic cytochrome P450-related biotransformation processes in veterinary sciences. Eur J Pharmacol 2008;585:502–509.

83. Lascelles BDX, Court MH, Hardie EM, et al. Nonsteroidal antiinflammatory drugs in cats: a review. Vet Anaesth Analg 2007;34:228–250.

84. Attard AR, Corlett MJ, Kidner NJ, et al. Safety of early pain relief for acute abdominal pain. BMJ 1992;305:554–556.

85. Brock N. Treating moderate and severe pain in small animals. Can Vet J 1995;36:658–660.

86. Kalso E, Edwards J, McQuay HJ, et al. Five easy pieces on evidence based medicine (5). Trading benefit against harm-pain relief vs. adverse effects. Eur J Pain 2002;6:409–412.

87. Bates DW, Cullen DJ, Laird N, et al. Incidence of adverse drug events and potential adverse drug events—implications for prevention. JAMA 1995;274:29–34.

88. Vargas E, Terleira A, Hernando F, et al. Effect of adverse drug reactions on length of stay in surgical intensive care units. Crit Care Med 2003;31:694–698.

89. Lazarou J, Pomeranz BH, Corey PN. Incidence of adverse drug reactions in hospitalized patients—a meta-analysis of prospective studies. JAMA 1998;279:1200–1205.

90. Armitage EA, Wetmore LA, Chan DL, et al. Evaluation of compliance among nursing staff in administration of prescribed analgesic drugs to critically ill dogs and cats. J Am Vet Med Assoc 2005; 227:425–429.

91. Ricard-Hibon A, Chollet C, Saada S, et al. A quality control program for acute pain management in out-of-hospital critical care medicine. Ann Emerg Med 1999;34:738–744.

43

Systemic analgesia

Sarah L. Haldane and Michelle Storay

Pain can occur in small animal critical care patients as a result of trauma, disease, or surgery. The detrimental effects of pain include tachycardia, altered respiration, aggravation of the sympathoadrenal response, and alterations in mental status. These effects are of particular concern in patients with circulatory shock or critical illness because essential body systems can be further compromised by effects of pain. Pain can lead to alterations in glucose metabolism, increase protein catabolism, impair wound healing, and severely compromise the ability of a patient to recover from severe illness or trauma.[1]

Although analgesia is an essential component of therapy for many patients, we must remember that every analgesic medication has both beneficial and adverse effects. The object of a balanced analgesic regime is to combine medications so as to provide the best pain relief with the least complications. To choose the most appropriate medications to give an individual patient, a basic knowledge of their effects on essential organ systems is required.

Opioids

Opioids are generally the drugs of first choice for pain relief in critical patients. Box 43.1 provides a glossary. They can be used for mild to severe pain, and the range of medications within this class of drugs allows for flexibility in route and frequency of administration. Opioids exert their analgesic effects by activating opioid receptors that are located within the brain, spinal cord, and peripheral neurons. There are three main categories of opioid receptors. They are known as mu (μ), kappa (κ),

and delta (δ), and each has differing clinical effects when activated (Table 43.1). Because every opioid activates each of the receptors to a different degree, the activity of each of the opioids can vary in terms of strength of analgesia, degree of sedation, and adverse effects (see Box 43.2). Opioids can be generally classified into (1) pure μ receptor agonists, (2) partial μ receptor agonists, (3) mixed agonist-antagonist drugs and (4) opioid antagonists.

The pure μ receptor agonists include morphine, fentanyl, oxymorphone, hydromorphone, and methadone (Table 43.2). These drugs have strong analgesic effects and can be used for patients with moderate to severe pain. Analgesia provided by μ agonists is dose related; increased dose increases analgesia. Similarly, the incidence of adverse effects increases when higher doses are administered.

Buprenorphine is a partial μ agonist opioid with a long duration of action. It has a high affinity for the μ receptor but only moderate efficacy. It is an antagonist at κ receptors. Butorphanol is a mixed agonist-antagonist drug because it acts as a κ agonist and μ antagonist. This drug has limited analgesic activity and duration, and it is used primarily for its sedative effects.[3] Opioid antagonists include naloxone and naltrexone. They have very high affinity for opioid receptors, so they block the effects of any of the agonist opioids.

Analgesic effects

Opioids have a central analgesic effect that works within the brain and the spinal cord to reduce transmission of pain signals. There are also opioid receptors located on the presynaptic terminals of the peripheral nociceptors.

Advanced Monitoring and Procedures for Small Animal Emergency and Critical Care, First Edition. Edited by Jamie M. Burkitt Creedon, Harold Davis.
© 2012 John Wiley & Sons, Inc. Published 2012 by John Wiley & Sons, Inc.

Table 43.1 Opioid receptors

	Location	Analgesic Effects	CNS Effects	Respiratory Effects	Gastrointestinal Effects
Mu (μ)	Brain (medial thalamus) Brainstem	Supraspinal analgesia	Euphoria, sedation, dependence	Respiratory depression	Decreased gastrointestinal motility
Kappa (κ)	Brain (diencephalon, including limbic system) Brainstem Spinal cord	Spinal analgesia	Sedation, dependence, dysphoria	Dyspnea, respiratory depression	
Delta (δ)	Brain	Possible pro-nociceptive effects. May be important in development of tolerance to opioids	Dysphoria		
Sigma (σ)	No longer considered opioid receptors				

Box 43.1 Glossary

Afferent: Conducting inward from a given organ (usually with regard to nerves or blood vessels)
Antinociceptive: Reduction in the transmission of painful stimuli through a nociceptor
Efferent: Conducting outward from a given organ
Neurotransmitter: Any specific chemical that is released by a presynaptic neuron and crosses the synapse to stimulate or inhibit the postsynaptic cell
Nociceptor: A peripheral nerve that transmits painful stimuli
Opiate: Naturally occurring alkaloids such as morphine
Opioid: All substances that act at opiate receptors
Postsynaptic: The distal side of the synapse
Presynaptic: The proximal side of the synapse
Supraspinal: All of the central nervous system above the vertebral column
Synapse: The junction between two nerve cells or a nerve cell with a muscle, gland, or receptor cell

Box 43.2 How strong is your opioid?

The **affinity** of an opioid is a measure of how strongly it interacts and binds with its receptor.
   The **efficacy** is a measure of the strength of the effect the drug has after binding to its receptor.
   The **potency** of a drug is the amount of drug required to produce an effect. For example, fentanyl is a more potent drug than morphine because a much smaller amount (micrograms rather than milligrams) is required to activate its receptor.
   An **agonist opioid** binds strongly to the receptor and stimulates them to high activity. These drugs are considered to have both affinity and efficacy. However, agonist opioids with high potency need only a small dose to active the receptor, whereas those with low potency need a larger dose to exert the same effects.
   An **antagonist opioid** binds to the receptor (has high affinity) but does not stimulate the receptor (no efficacy). Its antagonist action comes from binding to the receptor as it stops other opioids from exerting their effects.
   A **partial agonist opioid** has affinity but less efficacy than pure agonists; they bind strongly to opioid receptors but have a weaker effect on them.[2]

When opioid receptors are activated, they inhibit the transmission of painful stimuli through these fibers. In addition, activation of receptors in the brain decreases the amount of the neurotransmitter gamma-aminobutyric acid (GABA) that is released from neurons. GABA is an inhibitory neurotransmitter that reduces the production and release of a stimulatory neurotransmitter, dopamine. Therefore, because stimulation of opioid receptors causes less GABA to be released, there is an increase in available dopamine. Dopamine is responsible

for the pleasurable sensation associated with opioid administration.[2]

Central nervous system effects

Opioids act in the central nervous system (CNS) to cause sedation. They are often used as premedication agents

Table 43.2 Opioid agonist and antagonist drugs

Opioid	Agonist Activity	Antagonist Activity	Dose in Dogs	Dose in Cats	Notes
Morphine	μ κ δ		0.1–0.5 mg/kg IM, SC q4–6h CRI: 0.1–0.2 mg/kg/h	0.1 mg/kg IV, IM, SC q4–6h	Histamine release if given IV, leading to vasodilation. Panting.
Fentanyl	μ		2–5 μg/kg IV, IM, SC then CRI 2–10 μg/kg/h	2–5 μg/kg IV, IM, SC then CRI 2–10 μg/kg/h	
Remifentanil	μ		0.1–0.5 μg/kg/min	0.1–0.5 μg/kg/min	
Hydromorphone	μ (δ)		0.1–0.2 mg/kg IV, IM, SC q4–6h	0.1 mg/kg IV, IM, SC q4–6h	Panting
Oxymorphone	μ		0.1–0.2 mg/kg IV, IM, SC q4–6h	0.1 mg/kg IV, IM, SC q4–6h	Panting
Methadone	μ	NMDA receptor	0.1–0.5 mg/kg IV, IM, SC q4–6h	0.1–0.2 mg/kg IV, IM, SC q4–6h	Panting
Buprenorphine	μ	κ	0.01–0.02 mg/kg IV, IM, SC q6–8 h[50]	0.01–0.02 mg/kg IV, IM, SC, oral q6–8h[45]	Dysphoria, euphoria (cats), mydriasis
Butorphanol	κ	μ	0.1–0.4 mg/kg IV, IM, SC 0.5–1 mg/kg PO q6–8h	0.1–0.4 mg/kg IV, IM, SC	Sedative effects much longer duration (2–4 h) than analgesic effects (30 min)
Codeine	μ		0.5–2 mg/kg PO q6–12 h	0.5–2 mg/kg PO q6–12h	Care with products that contain paracetamol in dogs. Do not use these products in cats.
Naloxone		μ κ δ	0.04 mg/kg IV IM SC	0.04–0.1 mg/kg IV	Can be given via endotracheal tube during cardiopulmonary resuscitation
Naltrexone		μ κ δ	1–2 mg/kg PO once daily	25–50 mg/kg PO once daily	Bitter taste

IV, intravenous; IM, intramuscular; SC, subcutaneous; PO, per os; CRI, intravenous constant rate infusion.

prior to anaesthesia and have an anaesthetic-sparing effect in addition to their analgesic activity.[4–6] Opioids can also be effective in reducing anxiety in stressed animals or patients with respiratory compromise.

Chronic administration or high doses of opioids can lead to dysphoria and, in some cases, vocalization. These side effects usually resolve if the patient is changed to a different opioid medication or to a lower dose of the same medication.[3]

Cardiovascular effects

Administration of opioids at therapeutic doses has little clinical effect on the cardiovascular system.[7] Opioids are considered relatively safe drugs in cardiovascularly compromised patients. However, if these medications are administered at high doses, in combination with sedative drugs or to nonpainful patients, bradycardia can develop.[3,7] Opioid-induced bradycardia is vagally mediated, so it can be effectively treated with atropine or glycopyrrolate. In most cases, the effects of pain counteract the bradycardia, so if a low heart rate is evident, it is an indication that the patient's degree of pain has reduced and the opioid dose can usually be decreased.

In feline studies, both morphine and fentanyl have been shown to cause pulmonary vasodilation, so opioids have been recommended for use as anxiolytic agents in patients with congestive heart failure.[8,9]

Respiratory effects

At high doses, opioids can cause respiratory depression. This effect tends to be more marked when patients are being treated with concurrent sedative or anaesthetic agents. Respiratory depression occurs soon after bolus administration of opioid drugs, but tolerance to the respiratory effects develops quickly, so that repeated or long-term opioid use has little effect on the respiratory system.[3]

Morphine, methadone, oxymorphone, and hydromorphone have all been associated with panting in dogs. Panting usually starts soon after administration of the medications and tends to be transitory.[10,11] Panting may also contribute to the decrease in body temperature seen in dogs after opioid administration because heat loss via the respiratory system is a major factor in canine thermoregulation.[10]

Many opioid drugs have a cough suppressant (antitussive) effect, making them useful for bronchial disease or tracheitis.[12] They also reduce laryngeal sensitivity, increasing the ease of tracheal intubation and prolonging a patient's tolerance of endotracheal intubation after anaesthesia.

Renal effects

Administration of μ agonist opioids has been shown to cause decreased urine output from the kidneys. The exact mechanism for this is unknown.[13] Their use has also been associated with urinary retention in the bladder due to an increase in urethral sphincter smooth muscle tone.[3]

Gastrointestinal effects

Two of the most common and most undesirable effects of opioid administration are nausea and vomiting. These effects occur due to stimulation of the chemoreceptor trigger zone (CRTZ) in the brain. The CRTZ lies outside the blood-brain barrier (BBB), so is rapidly penetrated by any drug within the plasma. The vomiting center lies inside the BBB. Interestingly, stimulation of the opioid receptors in the vomiting centre has an antiemetic effect. Because opioids easily cross the BBB, they can counteract the initial vomition impulse and have an ongoing antiemetic effect. This explains the clinical syndrome where patients vomit soon after administration of opioids but do not continue to vomit despite the ongoing analgesic activity of the drugs.[14] Animals are also more likely to vomit when higher doses of μ agonist opioids are used than when partial agonist or mixed agonist-antagonist drugs are administered.

Opioids can cause decreased gastric emptying and alter intestinal motility, which may lead to intestinal ileus or constipation.[3,7,14,15] These events are also mediated through opioid receptors in the CNS.[14] Decreased intestinal motility, in combination with opioid-induced sedation, can contribute to a patient's lack of appetite, which is a common complication of prolonged illness in small animal patients.

Hepatic effects

Opioids are primarily metabolized in the liver, although some extrahepatic metabolism does occur.[10] Animals with hepatic insufficiency may require lower doses of opioids to achieve adequate analgesia. The sedative effects of opioids may be pronounced in patients with hepatic dysfunction.

Opioids that do not require hepatic metabolism (e.g., remifentanil) or with a short duration of action administered as a constant rate infusion (e.g., fentanyl, sufentanil, alfentanil) are the most appropriate choice for patients in hepatic failure so that the dose administered can be titrated to achieve adequate analgesia with minimal sedation.

Effects on body temperature

In dogs, μ agonist opioids such as morphine and hydromorphone have been shown to reduce body temperature by altering the central thermoregulatory set point.[10] In cats, opioid administration has been associated with postanesthetic hyperthermia. In one retrospective study, 47% of 125 cats became hyperthermic at least once within a 20-hour period after anaesthesia and opioid administration. In 2 of 125 cats, palliative therapy did not reduce the rectal temperature, and naloxone was administered. In both cats, naloxone was effective in reducing temperature. The mechanism for opioid-induced hyperthermia in cats is not known. It does not tend to be responsive to the antipyretic effects of nonsteroidal anti-inflammatory drugs.[16]

Opioid tolerance and addiction

With prolonged administration, opioids become less effective as analgesic agents in a phenomenon known as opioid tolerance. Doses often need to be increased markedly to maintain analgesia in patients that require opioids for more than a few days, and in experimental trials, tolerance has been shown to begin after a single dose of opioid. The mechanisms associated with development of tolerance are complex; tolerance is mediated in part by the opioid receptors themselves. With chronic activation the μ receptors become less sensitive to opioid binding, grow less effective in reducing transmission of pain signals, and, in some cases, internalize within the cell membrane and become inaccessible to circulating opioids. As μ receptors become resistant to opioids, δ opioid receptors are upregulated. It has been hypothesized that δ receptors can be coupled to μ receptors and that activation of δ receptors actually decreases the effectiveness of μ receptor stimulation. N-methyl-D-aspartate (NMDA) receptor activation also contributes to opioid tolerance by increasing production of pronociceptive neurotransmitters.[17,18]

Similar mechanisms lead to development of opioid dependency and withdrawal. Stimulation of δ receptors and upregulation of the NMDA receptors lead to increased pain sensation, so patients become uncomfortable and disoriented if opioid therapy is rapidly withdrawn. In human patients the adverse sensation when opioids are withdrawn and the pleasurable sensation (mediated by dopamine) associated with opioid use can lead to addiction.[2,17,18]

Use of a balanced analgesic regime (multimodal analgesia) can be effective in preventing development of opioid tolerance in critical care patients. To reduce symptoms of opioid withdrawal in veterinary patients, abrupt cessation of opioid analgesia should be avoided. Instead, weaning the patient from a pure μ agonist drug to a partial agonist such as buprenorphine or tramadol is recommended.

Regulations involved in clinical use of opioids

The term *controlled drugs* refers to drugs of addiction or high abuse potential that are supplied to registered practitioners for medical use. Opioids are classified as controlled drugs because they have the potential to produce addiction in people. Legislative requirements for controlled drugs vary slightly from country to country and state to state. An overview of the general legislative requirements is provided here; however, reference should be made to the specific country or state's individual legislation for full details.

Supply of controlled drugs

Licensed wholesalers or pharmacists must only supply drugs to an authorized or licensed person. Details of registered practitioners and/or license numbers are required to be recorded by the supplier.

Storage requirements

Controlled substances must be stored in a securely locked, substantially constructed cabinet or safe, fixed to the floor or wall. Controlled drugs should not be stored with any items other than other drugs of dependence. The receptacle should be kept locked at all times other than when in immediate use with access only by authorized personnel.

Recordkeeping requirements

A drug registry must be maintained in a form that shows the balance remaining after each dose is administered or supplied and cannot be altered without detection. A separate page is required for each drug and for each different formulation of the drug. The date, patient's name, owner's name, amount of the drug dispensed, balance and details of the prescribing veterinarian and signature are the minimum inclusions required on a drug register. Details of incoming stock, date, invoice number, supplier, and the balance of stock are also required. Records are to be retained for periods of 2–3 years in most countries and must be readily available for the regulatory authorities should an audit occur.

Disposal

The legal requirements for the disposal of controlled drugs varies; however, disposal generally needs to be witnessed and cosigned on the drug register along with the quantity of drug disposed.

Systemic administration of opioids

Opioids can be administered parenterally via the intravenous, intramuscular, and subcutaneous routes.[11] In general, the route of administration has little effect on the incidence of side effects; however, morphine administered by intravenous bolus to dogs has been associated with rapid histamine release, which causes vasodilation and potentially hypotension.[19,20] Morphine is usually administered intramuscularly to dogs or very slowly via the intravenous route. Most opioids can be administered by either intermittent bolus injections or as a constant rate infusion (CRI). Longer acting opioids (such as buprenorphine) are rarely given as a CRI, although this is the primary method of administration of very short-acting opioids (such as fentanyl).

Transdermal patches can be used to provide long-term administration of an opioid at a constant rate. Fentanyl is often administered via this route, and buprenorphine patches are also available. Onset of action can take 12–18 hours for fentanyl patches, and duration of action is 2–3 days. Because there is significant interindividual variation in the plasma concentration of fentanyl reached when transdermal patches are applied, the patient's comfort level should continue to be monitored while the patches are in place.[21,22] Effective administration of the drug can be adversely affected by the loss of adherence of the patch. Fentanyl from the patches can also be absorbed transmucosally, so patients should not be allowed to lick or chew the patch.[23]

Most opioids are relatively ineffective if given orally because they are subject to a strong "first-pass" effect, meaning they are absorbed from the gastrointestinal tract and metabolized in the liver to inactive substrates before ever entering the systemic circulation. Opioids that can be used as oral medications in dogs and cats include codeine and butorphanol. An oral form of morphine is available but has varying absorption in dogs and thus is difficult to dose effectively. The doses required for oral administration are up to 10 times higher than those given parenterally. The main adverse effect of orally administered opioids is constipation.

Injectable preparations of buprenorphine are also well absorbed through the oral mucosa in cats. This is an effective route of administration in this species as long as the drug is not swallowed into the digestive tract. To prevent this, the buprenorphine should be squirted under (rather than on top of) the tongue.

An experimental trial showed that this route is also effective for administration of buprenorphine to dogs; however, it did cause them to salivate excessively.[24,25]

Morphine

Morphine is the prototypical μ agonist opioid. It is an excellent analgesic and sedative in both dogs and cats. Although it has been previously associated with hyperexcitability in cats, at currently recommended therapeutic doses these effects are rarely, if ever, witnessed. It can cause vomiting after bolus administration and in some cases is used as an emetic agent. Bradycardia, gastrointestinal stasis, constipation, reduced urine output, and urinary retention have all been associated with morphine administration. Morphine is metabolized in the liver; codeine and hydromorphone are two of the metabolites produced. Intravenous morphine administration can cause histamine release in dogs (see the section on systemic administration of opioids).[2,4,13,14,26–32]

Fentanyl, remifentanil, sufentanil, and alfentanil

Fentanyl is approximately 80 times more potent than morphine and binds very strongly to the μ opioid receptor. It is also an extremely effective sedative. It has a rapid onset of action and rarely causes gastrointestinal side effects such as vomiting or nausea. Administration can lead to bradycardia and decreased temperature. Fentanyl can have respiratory depressant effects similar to morphine[33] and, although these effects are relatively minor at therapeutic doses,[34] fentanyl's rapid onset can result in acute onset of hypoventilation.[35] Fentanyl's duration of action is very short, and so it is primarily used as a CRI or administered in a transdermal patch. Aside from decreased nausea, the primary advantage of using fentanyl as a CRI is the ability to rapidly change the dose and hence the analgesic and sedative effects. Fentanyl can be used during anaesthesia to reduce the requirement for gaseous anaesthetic agent[5] and is often used in combination with other sedatives for patients requiring mechanical ventilation.

Remifentanil is an ultra-short-acting opioid with a half-life of 3–6 minutes. It can be used as an anaesthetic-sparing agent and analgesic in small animal patients. Its primary advantage is that it is broken down by cholinesterase enzymes in the bloodstream, so it does not rely on hepatic or renal function. Also, with such a short half-life, it is very easy to rapidly change the plasma level of the drug, which can be of benefit in animals that have cardiac or respiratory dysfunction.[36–38]

Sufentanil and alfentanil are very rapid-acting derivatives of fentanyl. Both have anaesthetic-sparing effects and sedative and analgesic efficacy in small animal patients, and they both allow rapid recovery from anaesthesia. Both drugs can cause bradycardia in dogs but have minimal effect on heart rate in cats. In clinical trials, alfentanil was associated with hypotension when administered with propofol as total intravenous anaesthesia, but this effect was not seen when it was administered with isoflurane.[39]

Oxymorphone and hydromorphone

Oxymorphone and hydromorphone are semisynthetic μ agonist opioids with similar analgesic efficacy to morphine.[10,11] Although they can display a similar range of adverse effects to morphine, the incidence of occurrence is reduced. Histamine release is not associated with administration of either of these drugs.[19] Hydromorphone has a shorter half-life than morphine in dogs, and it has been suggested that more frequent dosing (every 2 hours) or continuous infusion would be required to maintain serum levels of this drug.[40] However, in both canine and feline clinical trials, hydromorphone appears to have a similar duration of both sedative and analgesic action as oxymorphone (4–6 hours).[6,41,42]

Methadone

Methadone is a synthetic μ agonist opioid that also has antagonist activity at NMDA receptors. Activation of NMDA receptors is intrinsic to development of opioid tolerance as well as increasing the pain response at the level of the spinal cord. NMDA antagonists can decrease spinal sensitization ("wind-up") and prevent tolerance to opioids. Methadone has a prolonged duration of activity and good oral availability in human patients; the oral form is used to treat heroin addiction in people.[2] In dogs and cats, the duration of action of methadone is much shorter, similar to that of morphine, and it is used primarily as a parenteral analgesic for acute pain in these species.

Pethidine (meperidine)

Pethidine is μ agonist opioid that has excellent analgesic activity. It has a short duration of action (45–60 minutes) and is associated with a relatively high incidence of dysphoria.[43]

Buprenorphine

Buprenorphine is a partial agonist (see Box 43.2) at μ receptors and an antagonist at κ receptors. It is effective in dogs for mild to moderate pain.[2] Buprenorphine appears to have better analgesic efficacy in cats than dogs and can also cause euphoria and mydriasis in feline patients.[43–45] It has not been associated with postanesthetic hyperthermia in cats unlike the pure μ agonist opioids.[16]

It has a long duration of activity in comparison with other opioids and can be used to wean patients from full μ agonist opioids because it has a greater affinity for the μ receptors. This can be an undesirable effect if buprenorphine is given to a patient with severe pain because it will blunt the effects of any other opioids that are subsequently administered for the duration of its activity (6–12 hours).[46] Buprenorphine causes minimal sedation compared with full μ agonists and has less of an inhibitory effect on the gastrointestinal tract, so it does not have such an appetite suppressant effect in small animal patients.[45]

Butorphanol

Butorphanol is a κ agonist and provides good sedation with minimal cardiovascular or respiratory effects. It is a weak analgesic with a short duration of activity. The duration of analgesic effect is 1–2 hours; its sedative effects last 2–4 hours.[46–48] Its analgesic and sedative activities have a "ceiling" effect, whereby increasing the dose of the medication will not increase the efficacy. It can antagonize the effects of pure μ agonist opioids if they are used in combination.[49]

Butorphanol is an excellent antitussive agent, so is often used as a short-term agent to control coughing. It also has some antiemetic effects. Side effects of butorphanol are primarily dysphoria.

Codeine

Codeine has a higher oral availability than any of the other opioids. It has weak activity at the μ receptors. Codeine is used infrequently in veterinary medicine for chronic pain or as an antitussive agent.[12] The main adverse effect of codeine is constipation, making it a difficult drug to use long term. It can also cause vomiting, even at low doses, due to stimulation of the CRTZ.[2]

Naloxone and naltrexone

These drugs have antagonist activity at μ, κ, and δ receptors. Naloxone has a short duration of action and poor oral availability, so is used primarily as a parenteral agent for opioid overdose or to rapidly reduce the effects of opioids in patients at risk of respiratory or cardiac arrest. Naltrexone has good oral availability and a long duration of action, so it is more frequently used in human patients recovering from opioid dependence than in veterinary medicine. It is sometimes effective for behavioral disorders such as tail chasing and excessive licking in dogs and cats.

Tramadol

Tramadol is a unique centrally acting analgesic that has multiple mechanisms of action. It is a codeine analog and has some activity at μ opioid receptors. It also has a centrally acting GABA inhibiting effect. In addition, tramadol has activity at α-2 adrenergic receptors and serotonin receptors, preventing norepinephrine and serotonin reuptake, respectively.[30,51,52]

Opioid effects

Tramadol has a weak affinity for μ and δ opioid receptors.[51] The mu receptor activation provides some of its analgesic activity, as well as mild sedation and respiratory depressant effects.[51–55] It is metabolized in the liver to an active metabolite (O-dimethyl-tramadol) that binds to opioid receptors with a higher affinity than the parent drug.[52] These metabolites are produced in most species of animals but in differing amounts. This variance in production of metabolites, as well as differences in elimination half-life and time to maximum plasma concentration, is responsible for the species variation in duration of action of tramadol.[52,54,56]

Despite its weak affinity for μ receptors, tramadol has not been associated with dependence in people and is not scheduled as a controlled drug.

Route of administration

Oral and intravenous forms of tramadol are available, although at the time of writing only the oral form was available in the United States. Although maximum plasma concentration is reached more quickly when the drug is given intravenously, the oral form is rapidly absorbed from the gastrointestinal tract. The oral medication comes in tablets, capsules, and liquid form, making it easy to dose in any size cat or dog. It is generally prescribed in an intermediate-release (IR) form that can be administered two to three times a day. There is also a sustained-release (SR) form that is used for once-daily dosing in human patients. Dogs metabolize tramadol rapidly, so SR tablets still need to be given twice a day in this species. Additionally, administration of the SR tablets to dogs provides a lower maximum plasma concentration of tramadol than the IR tablets, and it takes more time to achieve maximum plasma concentration.[51,54] Tramadol has a longer elimination half-life in cats than dogs (3.4 hours vs. 1.7 hours); however, time to maximum plasma concentration is similar.[52,54]

Clinical efficacy of tramadol

In one study, the analgesic effect of tramadol was compared with morphine after ovariohysterectomy in dogs. In this study, tramadol provided similar analgesia with less respiratory depression than morphine.[30] Epidural tramadol has also been evaluated in dogs after tibial plateau leveling osteotomy (TPLO). In this study the analgesic effects of intravenous tramadol outweighed those of epidural administration.[57] Tramadol has been shown to produce significant analgesic effects in dogs and has no detrimental effect on renal perfusion in normotensive animals.[58] It also reduces the minimal alveolar concentration (MAC) of sevoflurane in anaesthetized cats.[59] However, it is less effective than opioid drugs as a sedative in dogs.[29]

There are few side effects noted with clinical use of tramadol in dogs and cats. Administration of tablets and liquid can cause excessive salivation due to their bitter taste. Dispensing the liquid into a gelatin capsule can reduce this effect and allow for easier administration; however, this needs to be done just prior to giving the medication or the liquid will permeate through the capsule. Seizures have been associated with the use of tramadol in people, but this has not been reported in veterinary medicine. Tramadol can be administered to both dogs and cats. The dose in dogs is 2–4 mg/kg every 8–12 hours. In cats, a dose of 1–2 mg/kg every 12 hours is used.

Nonsteroidal anti-inflammatory drugs

NSAIDs are a diverse group of medications that act to decrease the production of inflammatory mediators at the site of tissue injury. Inflammatory mediators increase transmission of pain signals by stimulating previously unaffected nociceptors surrounding the area of injury.

COX 1 and COX 2

After a tissue has been damaged, arachidonic acid is released from cell membranes, precipitating a chain of events known as the arachidonic acid cascade. The family of inflammatory mediators derived from arachidonic acid are known as eicosanoids. Two enzyme groups act to metabolize arachidonic acid: the lipoxygenases (LOX) and the cyclo-oxygenases (COX). Products from the LOX cascade include leukotrienes and chemotactic factors. Products of the COX cascade include prostaglandins, prostacyclin, and thromboxanes.

NSAIDs are potent inhibitors of prostaglandin production. In some situations, this can have adverse consequences because many prostaglandins have protective or homeostatic functions. Some prostaglandins are required for normal function of the gastrointestinal tract, brain, kidneys, and reproductive system. These prostaglandins required for normal homeostasis are continuously produced, and so they are known as constitutive prostaglandins. Other prostaglandins are produced in response to tissue injury, and these are known as inducible prostaglandins. Inducible prostaglandins act to escalate the inflammatory response and increase peripheral nerve sensitization; they also have protective actions and play a role in tissue repair.[60,61]

Prostaglandins are produced by the COX pathway. There are two main COX enzymes: COX-1 and COX-2. A COX-3 enzyme also exists in the CNS and is discussed later (see Box 43.9 below). Initially, COX-1 was thought to be responsible for production of all constitutive prostaglandins and COX-2 for all the inducible prostaglandins. More recently, it has been determined that both COX enzymes produce protective and inflammatory prostaglandins.[61] COX-1 is important in normal homeostatic function of the gastrointestinal tract, kidneys, and primary hemostasis.[60] COX-2 plays an important role in gastric mucosal healing and has homeostatic mechanisms in the normal brain, kidney, and reproductive systems. COX-2 also catalyzes production of prostacyclin, and a balance exists between this anticoagulant molecule and the procoagulant thromboxane A_2 regulated by COX-1.[61–63]

NSAIDs are described as nonspecific or dual acting if they inhibit both COX-1 and COX-2. Aspirin is the classic example of a dual-acting NSAID. Because the COX-2 enzyme has been more closely associated with the inflammatory response, COX-2-selective drugs (see Box 43.3) have been manufactured. The aim of these medications is to reduce inflammatory prostaglandin production via COX-2 inhibition, with relatively less suppression of COX-1. It is important to realize that all COX-2 inhibitors will still inhibit COX-1 to some degree.

> **Box 43.3** COX-2 drugs and terminology
>
> NSAIDs are often described with reference to their relative ability to suppress COX-2 rather than COX-1. This has given rise to a number of different terms, including **COX-2-preferential** (for drugs with 5–20 times higher selectivity for COX-2 than COX-1) or **COX-2-specific** medications (for drugs with 50–100 times higher selectivity for COX-2 than COX-1).
>
> However, because all the COX-2 suppressing drugs still have some ability to suppress COX-1, the term *COX-2-specific* is an incorrect description of their action. And as clinical trials have shown no difference in adverse effects between drugs with a 5-fold selectivity versus those with a 100-fold selectivity for COX-2, there is no real requirement to differentiate between them. Thus the term ***COX-2 selective*** is now used for this entire class of drugs.[64]

Veterinary COX-2-selective NSAIDs include carprofen, meloxicam, deracoxib, and firocoxib. Dual-acting NSAIDs include ketoprofen and tepoxalin, which also have LOX-suppressing effects.

Analgesic effects

There is considerable proof of the efficacy of analgesia in dogs and cats provided by new-generation NSAIDs. NSAIDs provide peripheral analgesia and, unlike opioids, are very effective at reducing pain during movement. They also have a mild antagonistic effect at NMDA receptors. The analgesic effects of many NSAIDs, including carprofen, ketoprofen, meloxicam, deracoxib, tepoxalin, and firocoxib (Table 43.3), have been favorably compared with opioid administration in various studies of osteoarthritic and surgical pain.[43,44,47,65–72]

NSAIDs are nonaddictive and nonsedating, so animals often feel better and are more alert on these medications than when being treated with opioid analgesics.[43,44,47,65–78] Individual animals may respond better to one NSAID than another, so if analgesia is not adequate with one NSAID, it is often worth trialing a different nonsteroidal medication. However, different NSAIDs should never be used in combination because the risk of adverse effects greatly outweighs the potential benefits and a "washout period," where no anti-inflammatory medications are administered, of 5–7 days (or 7–10 days for aspirin) is recommended if changing from one NSAID to another.[79]

Adverse effects

In healthy dogs, most new-generation NSAIDs have a wide margin of safety. Few NSAIDs are licensed for use in cats and none for long-term use. Chronic use or overdose of new-generation prescription NSAIDs in small animals has been reported to cause adverse effects, but the risk is much less than with older generation NSAIDS, such as flunixin, indomethacin, ibuprofen, or naproxen. However in animals with perfusion deficits, gastrointestinal, renal, or hepatic disease or with disorders of primary coagulation, NSAID administration can have significant detrimental effects.

Gastrointestinal effects

Gastric ulceration is a common side effect of NSAID administration with prolonged use, high doses, or administration to hypovolemic or inappetent animals.[79,80] COX-1 induced prostaglandins in the gastric mucosa have protective effects because they increase gastric mucus production and enhance local blood flow. COX-2 is induced once damage has occurred to the intestinal mucosa and produces prostaglandins that play an important role in mucosal healing.[60,62,80–82] Thus COX-2 suppression can delay ulcer healing. It has been suggested that NSAIDs may also reduce ulcer healing by

Table 43.3 NSAID doses

	Dog	Cat
Carprofen	2–4 mg/kg/d IV, SC, PO	2–4 mg/kg SC, PO once
Deracoxib	2 mg/kg PO q24h	
Firocoxib	5 mg/kg PO q24h	
Ketoprofen	1–2 mg/kg IV, SC then 1 mg/kg PO for no longer than 5 d	1–2 mg/kg IV, SC then 1 mg/kg PO for no longer than 5 d
Meloxicam	0.1 mg/kg IV, PO then 0.01–0.03 mg/kg PO q24h	0.1 mg/kg IV, PO once, then 0.01–0.03 mg/kg PO every 1–2 d[102]
Tepoxalin	10 mg/kg PO q24h	

methods other than reduction in prostaglandin synthesis.[83] Some NSAIDs, such as aspirin, also cause direct injury to the gastric mucosa by disruption of surface phospholipids.[62]

Despite their increased safety margin, adverse gastrointestinal effects are still the most common side effect of COX-2 preferential NSAIDs.[72,73,79,80] In one experimental study assessing long-term NSAID use, carprofen had the lowest incidence of gastrointestinal side effects when compared with meloxicam, ketoprofen, flunixin meglumine, and etodolac. Multiple endoscopic and mucosal permeability studies have been performed evaluating the effects of short-term NSAID use, and no significant adverse effects have been found. However, due to the nature of these studies, only a few dogs were assessed in each, making it difficult to evaluate the importance of their findings.[83,85–89]

Both deracoxib and meloxicam have been associated with gastrointestinal perforation in dogs. In most cases the drugs were administered at higher than recommended dosages (greater than 2 mg/kg for deracoxib or 0.1 mg/kg for meloxicam) or were administered concurrently with a corticosteroid or another NSAID.[90–92]

The incidence of these highly undesirable side effects means that client education is vitally important if patients are discharged with NSAIDs for administration at home. The dose and duration of administration should be carefully explained, and clients should be advised not to administer the medications if their pet is not eating, has vomiting or diarrhea, or if they see hematochezia or melena. NSAIDs should never be administered concurrently with other NSAIDs or with corticosteroids.

Renal effects

When perfusion to the kidney declines, glomerular filtration rate (GFR) decreases accordingly. The juxtaglomerular apparatus in the kidney releases prostaglandins that act to vasodilate the afferent renal arteriole to maintain renal blood flow and GFR. This effect is mediated by both COX-1 and COX-2 enzymes.[93] When NSAIDs are administered to hypovolemic or dehydrated patients, the prostaglandin-mediated effect of local vasodilation is diminished or lost. Significant damage to the kidneys can result, and in severe cases, this can lead to acute renal failure. COX-2-selective medications may increase the relative production of thromboxanes, which have local vasoconstrictive effects and can exacerbate renal damage. Ketoprofen, carprofen, and tepoxalin at therapeutic doses have all been shown to have little effect on renal perfusion in healthy anaesthetized dogs.[94–96] However, overdose or accidental ingestion of large doses of NSAIDs can lead to acute renal failure despite normal blood volume.[79]

Hepatic effects

Like most medications, NSAIDs are metabolized in the liver. Their use has been associated with an increase in liver enzymes and hepatocellular injury in some patients. This toxicity is not dependent on dose or duration of treatment so is classified as an idiosyncratic reaction. In one report describing hepatoxicity secondary to carprofen administration, there was a marked similarity in the course of disease in Labrador retrievers, which may indicate a possible underlying genetic basis in this breed. However this result may have been biased by the large number of Labradors that require NSAID administration for degenerative joint disease.[97] Due to the risk of hepatic toxicity, NSAID administration is not recommended for animals with concurrent hepatic disease.

Coagulation effects

Prostacyclin (PGI_2) is produced from epithelial cells via COX-2 synthesis and acts to inhibit platelet aggregation and cause vasodilation. Conversely, COX-1 mediates production of thromboxane A_2 (TXA_2) from platelets, and it increases platelet aggregation and causes vasoconstriction.[98] The balance between TXA_2 and PGI_2 is important in maintaining a functional coagulation system.

Aspirin is the most effective NSAID at reducing platelet aggregation because it binds permanently to platelets and decreases TXA_2 production for the life of the platelet. Conversely, the COX-2 selective coxib class of drugs has been associated with increased risk of thrombosis-related cardiac events in humans.[99] This led to the recommendation that aspirin be used in conjunction with coxib drugs, a combination that can cause significant gastrointestinal side effects.[62,80] In veterinary medicine, ketoprofen, carprofen, tepoxalin, meloxicam, and deracoxib have been studied to assess their affects on primary hemostasis. Ketoprofen and carprofen have been associated with decreased platelet function and deracoxib with potential for increased thrombosis in experimental trials; however, there are no published reports of clinically relevant hemostatic complications in dogs or cats.[84,96,98,100]

Drug interactions with NSAIDs

Concurrent administration of an NSAID with corticosteroids or other NSAIDs significantly increases the risk of gastrointestinal and renal injury.[79,90,101] Administration of COX-2 inhibitors will also delay healing of gastrointestinal ulcers.[82,83] Concurrent administration of aspirin with other NSAIDs or corticosteroids increases the risk of bleeding and gastrointestinal injury (due to both COX inhibition and direct mucosal injury).[62,80,101]

NSAIDs will displace other highly protein-bound drugs from plasma proteins, leading to their enhanced bioavailability and possibly toxic plasma concentrations. These include other anti-inflammatory agents, warfarin, phenytoin, penicillins, and sulfonamide antibiotics. NSAIDs may also increase plasma levels of digoxin and can decrease the efficacy of furosemide.

Use of NSAIDS with other nephrotoxic drugs (including aminoglycoside antibiotics) and diuretics (due to risk of hypovolemia) is relatively contraindicated, but studies have not been performed to prove a clinical interaction. Drugs that induce cytochrome P450 metabolic pathway in the liver (e.g., phenobarbitone) can increase NSAID metabolism, reducing their analgesic efficacy.

NSAIDS in the critical patient

NSAID use is contraindicated in patients with hypovolemia or dehydration; gastrointestinal, hepatic, or renal dysfunction; increased sympathetic stimulation (such as in trauma); or cardiac disease (particularly with concurrent administration of furosemide or digoxin). When this population is further expanded to include patients with coagulation disorders, recent history of anti-inflammatory administration or inappetance, it seems that NSAID administration is appropriate in a fairly small proportion of critically ill patients. However, NSAIDs are highly recommended for use in cardiovascularly stable patients that have a functional gastrointestinal tract and normal renal function. This subset of patients would include stable postoperative patients and patients with musculoskeletal injuries that are well perfused, have an adequate urine output, and are eating or receiving enteral nutrition. Their excellent analgesic properties make them indispensable in the critical care pharmacopeia.

The α-2 agonists

The α-2 agonist drugs stimulate the α-2 adrenoreceptors around the body. The most important clinical effects of α-2 agonists include profound sedation, centrally mediated analgesia, and hypotension. The clinical effects of α-2 agonists can be reversed by administration of yohimbine or atipamezole.[103–106]

Analgesic effects

The analgesic effects of α-2 agonists are mediated within both the brain and the spinal cord. Their mechanism of

---

Box 43.4 The α-2 adrenoreceptors and noradrenaline

The α adrenergic receptors are classified into type 1 and type 2. The type 2 receptors are further subdivided into 2A, 2B, and 2C. Stimulation of α-2A and B receptors in the brain and spinal cord inhibits pain sensation and wakefulness. 2C receptors are more often located on peripheral nociceptors, and conversely, stimulation of 2C receptors increases the transmission of painful stimuli. 2C receptors are upregulated after neuronal injury and may have a pro-nociceptive effect in inflammatory and neuropathic pain syndromes.[115]

The α-2 receptors are predominantly stimulated by noradrenaline and can be acted on by direct transmission of noradrenaline across the synaptic cleft or by circulating noradrenaline.[115] The α-2 receptors are found in the vasculature, liver, pancreas, kidney, platelets, adipose tissue, and the eye. They have distinct physiologic function in each of these organs.

Receptors are also found in many areas within the CNS, including the dorsal horn of the spinal cord, the vagus nerve, and the locus coeruleus. The locus coeruleus is a small nucleus within the brainstem that contains a large number of noradrenergic cells. This nucleus is responsible for controlling wakefulness and is also an important mediator of analgesia. Activation of α-2 receptors in this area inhibits impulse transmission, leading to sedation and analgesia.[103]

---

antinociceptive action is complex (see Box 43.4). The α-2 adrenoreceptors also interact with opiate receptors in a synergistic fashion. The combination of α-2 agonists and opioids has an analgesic effect that can last several hours. Unfortunately, the sedative and cardiovascular effects of α-2 agonists limit their general use as analgesics, although the sedation induced makes them very effective as premedication agents.[103–105]

Cardiovascular effects

The α-2 agonists have a two-phase effect on the cardiovascular system. In the first phase, peripheral vasoconstriction and bradycardia are seen. Vasoconstriction is mediated by activation of postsynaptic adrenoreceptors in the peripheral blood vessels. Bradycardia occurs by direct and indirect mechanisms. The direct effect is due to stimulation of the vagus nerve, slowing impulse conduction through the atrioventricular (AV) node in the heart, thereby reducing the rate of ventricular contraction. Indirectly, bradycardia results from the cardiac response to increased systemic vascular resistance, which is to lower heart rate in order to prevent hypertension. During phase two the initial vasoconstrictive response declines and a centrally mediated hypotensive phase predominates, with ongoing bradycardia as well as peripheral vasodilation due to decreased sympathetic stimulation.[103]

The cardiovascular effects of α-2 agonists occur even when the drugs are administered at low doses. In one study of medetomidine in dogs, cardiovascular effects were near maximal at a dose of 5 μg/kg and were not significantly different with doses ranging from 1–20 μg/kg.[107] Therefore, α-2 agonists are not recommended for use in patients with an unstable cardiovascular system, which would rule them out for use in most critically ill patients.

Medetomidine

Medetomidine is a highly selective α-2 agonist that produces profound dose-dependent sedation and analgesia.[31,104,105] The analgesic effects occur 20–60 minutes after a single injection.[31] In combination with an opioid, the analgesic efficacy of medetomidine is enhanced, but there is little improvement in the cardiovascular effects.[108] It is an effective sedative, with doses as low as 1 μg/kg causing a reduction in the amount of induction agent required for anaesthesia.[109] It has also been used as a constant rate infusion for prolonged sedation (doses from 1–3 μg/kg/h), but its analgesic efficacy as a CRI has not been assessed. Even at these low doses, bradycardia and hypotension were noted in patients treated with medetomidine.[110–112] It has been administered in combination with opioids via the epidural route but with minimal improvement in analgesic activity.[113]

The most common use of medetomidine is as a sedative or premedication agent. The dose varies with size of the animal, but generally a dose from 1–10 μg/kg IV or IM is effective in dogs and cats. The low end of the dose range is used if medetomidine is administered in combination with an opioid.[114]

Dexmedetomidine

Medetomidine is a racemic mixture of two compounds: dexmedetomidine and levomedetomidine. Most of the analgesic and sedative effects are due to dexmedetomidine, and it is thought that levomedetomidine interferes with the function of dexmedetomidine. It has been suggested that dexmedetomidine alone will provide more consistent sedation and longer lasting analgesia than medetomidine, and this compound has recently been licensed for use in the United Kingdom, Europe, and the United States as a solo agent.[103–106]

Xylazine

Xylazine is an α-2 agonist medication that is used primarily for sedation in large animal practice. It is no longer recommended for use in small animal patients due to its propensity to cause vomiting as well as severe bradycardia and hypotension.

Adjunctive analgesia

Adjunctive analgesics are medications that have synergistic activity with, or potentiate the effects of, the primary analgesic (usually opioids or NSAIDs). In many cases they have mild analgesic activity on their own, but this is greatly outweighed by the benefit they have in combination with other medications. Because the pain pathway is affected by many different neurotransmitters, mediators, and receptors, it is supremely logical that we need to use analgesics with differing mechanisms of action to treat pain effectively. In addition, a multimodal analgesic approach allows lower doses of primary analgesics to be used, reducing the potential for adverse effects and complications from these drugs.

Multimodal analgesia in its simplest form would combine opioid and NSAID medications because these drugs act at different levels of the pain pathway. For patients with acute pain, combinations of intravenous drugs such as an opioid with ketamine and/or lidocaine can be used as CRIs (see Protocol 43.1). Oral adjunctive agents can be used for chronic, inflammatory, or neuropathic pain. Examples of these include gabapentin, amantadine, and acetaminophen (paracetamol).

Lidocaine

Lidocaine is a sodium channel blocker (see Box 43.5) that is primarily used as a local anaesthetic agent. It is also an effective antiarrhythmic for ventricular tachyarrhythmias because it acts on the fast sodium channels in the myocardial cells. Its mechanism of action when administered as a systemic analgesic is poorly understood. As a sodium channel blocker, it can reduce discharge from injured nociceptors in peripheral tissues and thus decrease the transmission of pain sensation to the spinal cord. Intravenous lidocaine has also been hypothesized to interact with opioid receptors[116] as well as having a systemic anti-inflammatory effect by reducing cytokine production.[117,118]

Lidocaine has been shown to be effective as an adjunctive treatment for neuropathic pain, cancer pain, and postoperative pain in people.[119–121] It has also been reported as an effective preemptive analgesic in dogs during intraocular surgery.[122] Administration of intravenous lidocaine can reduce the duration of postoperative ileus in people and horses.[117,118,120,123,124] This effect may be due to reduction in opioid dose, the anti-inflammatory effect of lidocaine, or the decrease in sympathetic tone that has been associated with lidocaine infusion. Similarly, lidocaine CRI has been associated with a decrease

Protocol 43.1 Constant rate infusion recipes

Morphine,* lidocaine, ketamine CRI for syringe pump infusion

Procedure

1.   Make sure each of your components is compatible with the others. Then determine your dose rate for each component.

Example: Morphine 0.1 mg/kg/h, lidocaine 3 mg/kg/h, ketamine 0.6 mg/kg/h

2.   Calculate the dose per hour for each component required for your patient, based on its body weight. Then, using the concentration of each drug, calculate the rate in milliliters per hour.

  Example: MLK CRI for a dog, body weight 20 kg.
  Morphine 0.1 × 20 = 2 mg/h. Using morphine 10 mg/mL, rate is 0.2 mL/h
  Lidocaine 3 × 20 = 60 mg/h. Using lidocaine 20 mg/mL, rate is 3 mL/h
  Ketamine 0.6 × 20 = 12 mg/h. Using ketamine 100 mg/mL, rate is 0.12 mL/h.

3.   Determine the volume of each component required.

  A 12-hour infusion of this mixture would require:
  2.4 mL morphine (0.2 mL/h × 12 h)
  36 mL lidocaine (3 mL/h × 12 h)
  1.5 mL ketamine (0.12 mL/h × 12 h)

4.   Mix components and determine the rate at which the mixture will be infused.

  The morphine, lidocaine, and ketamine can be mixed together in a syringe and the rate calculated as the sum of the rates for each of the three components.
  In this case, the MLK mixture would be administered at 3.3 mL/h.

Morphine,* lidocaine, ketamine CRI for fluid pump infusion

1.   Make sure each of your components is compatible with the others and with the crystalloid fluid you are using for the CRI. In most cases, 5% dextrose is the fluid of choice for drug infusions.
2.   Determine the dose of each component
  Morphine 0.1 mg/kg/h, lidocaine 2.4 mg/kg/h, ketamine 0.6 mg/kg/h
3.   Draw 65 mL of fluid out of a 500-mL bag of 5% dextrose and discard.
4.   Add 1200 mg (60 mL of 20 mg/mL) lidocaine to the bag.
5.   Add 50 mg of morphine to the bag.
6.   Add 300 mg of ketamine to the bag.
  The resulting mixture contains 0.1 mg/mL of morphine, 2.4 mg/mL of lidocaine, and 0.6 mg/mL of ketamine.
7.   The rate of administration (in milliliters per hour) of the mixture is equal to the body weight of the patient in kilograms.

Example: For a 20-kg patient, run this mixture at 20 mL/h.

*Other opioids (usually μ agonist drugs) can be used in place of morphine in these recipes. The appropriate CRI doses for each should be used (Table 43.2).

Box 43.5 Sodium channel

Sodium channels are ubiquitous throughout the body within cell membranes. Those present in the nerve cell membrane of the peripheral nociceptor are involved in depolarization of the neuron and transmission of the painful stimulus.

---

in length of hospital stay in human patients after abdominal surgery.[117,118,120] It appears to have no effect on thermal pain.[116,125]

Interestingly, lidocaine can provide enduring analgesia far beyond its duration of administration and plasma half-life. In one human study, an 80-minute infusion of intravenous lidocaine provided sustained analgesia for a mean of 8 days.[119] This may have been due to the finding that lidocaine decays much more slowly in the cerebrospinal fluid (CSF) than in plasma.

Bolus dosing or high CRI rates of lidocaine (rates higher than 5 mg/kg/h) have been associated with drowsiness and light-headedness in people.[119] Other infrequent side effects include vomiting or nausea in humans and in dogs.[120] Cats are more prone to neurologic side effects (including seizures) with use of lidocaine, so lower doses are used in this species (Table 43.4).

Table 43.4 Doses for adjunctive analgesic agents

	Dog	Cat
Amantadine	1.25–4 mg/kg PO q12–24 h	3 mg/kg PO q24h
Gabapentin	10 mg/kg PO q12h	10 mg/kg PO q12h
Lidocaine	1.5–3 mg/kg/h (25–50 µg/kg/min) CRI IV	(0.75–1.5 mg/kg/h (12.5–25 µg/kg/min) CRI IV
Ketamine	10–20 µg/kg/min CRI IV	10–20 µg/kg/min CRI IV
Acetaminophen (Paracetamol)	10 mg/kg q12–24h	*Do not use*

Box 43.6 NMDA receptors

N-methyl-D-aspartate (NMDA) receptors are found in the dorsal horn of the spinal cord as well as within the brain parenchyma. When the NMDA receptors in the dorsal horn are activated by peripheral nociceptors, they affect the neurons leading to the brain, making them hyperexcitable and increasing the sensation of pain. This process is known as spinal sensitization, or "wind-up." NMDA receptor activation is also intrinsic to development of hyperalgesia, neuropathic pain, and opioid tolerance.[129,133]

Ketamine

Ketamine is an NMDA receptor antagonist (see Box 43.6). It has dissociative properties that make it useful as an anaesthetic agent in veterinary medicine, particularly in combination with a sedative agent. The analgesic effects of ketamine become apparent at doses far lower than those required for anaesthesia.

Ketamine has been shown to be effective as an adjunctive analgesic and to reduce opioid requirement in human patients after abdominal and orthopedic surgeries.[126–128] In addition it has been used for end-stage cancer pain in pediatric patients.[129] The adverse effects of ketamine in people include hallucination, dysphoria, sleep difficulties, and disorientation.[129]

Ketamine has also been evaluated for use as a perioperative and postoperative analgesic in dogs and has been shown to be effective in improving comfort after both soft tissue and orthopedic surgery.[130,131] Ketamine does not slow gastrointestinal motility, so it can be useful in dogs with postoperative ileus to reduce the opioid requirement.[132] Dysphoria has been noted in some dogs on ketamine infusions.[130,131]

Amantadine

Amantadine is an oral antiviral agent that has some antagonist activity at NMDA receptors. It has been eval-

---

Box 43.7 Gabapentin and neuropathic pain

Neuropathic pain is the result of injury to the nervous system but tends to persist long after the initial injury has healed. It is caused by pathologic changes to the neurons themselves. Changes may be due to reversible alterations in neuronal ion channels and receptors (called modulation) or due to long-term modification in the expression of receptors or structure of the neuron.[143] Neuropathic pain is poorly responsive to NSAIDs, and even opioids have reduced efficacy for this type of pain.

Gabapentin has been shown to be effective in managing neuropathic pain syndromes. It has central actions in both the brain and the spinal cord and peripheral activity in the nociceptors. Structurally, gabapentin is an analog of GABA; however, activation of GABA receptors is not its primary mode of action. It also interacts with the VSCC that are upregulated during modulation in nociceptors and spinal cord neurones (see Box 43.8).[115,144] By inhibiting calcium flux within the neuron, gabapentin reduces release of excitatory neurotransmitters and hence decreases transmission of nociceptive impulses. Gabapentin may also have some NMDA receptor antagonist activity in the spinal cord that can reduce hyperalgesia associated with chronic pain. In addition, it has been shown to act in the locus coeruleus similarly to α-2 receptor agonists to cause centrally mediated analgesia.[144]

---

uated as an effective adjunctive postoperative analgesic in human patients and for refractory osteoarthritis pain in dogs.[133,134]

Gabapentin

Gabapentin is used primarily as an antiepileptic medication in human and veterinary patients but has also been shown to be very effective in the treatment of chronic and neuropathic pain syndromes in people (see Box 43.7).[135]

Gabapentin's primary mechanism of action as an analgesic agent is to block voltage-sensitive calcium

---

Box 43.8 Calcium channels

Throughout the body, there are a many different calcium channels residing within cell membranes. In pain fibers, the voltage-sensitive calcium channels (VSCC) are crucial to transmission of pain sensation through the nerves. As the nerve depolarizes, the voltage along the cell membrane changes and VSCC open, allowing calcium to move into the cytoplasm of the cell. Increased intracellular calcium stimulates the release of excitatory neurotransmitters from the presynaptic terminus. These neurotransmitters then activate further nociceptors to depolarize and continue transmission of the pain signal.[140]

A drug can exert analgesic properties by altering the function of the VSCC. Specific calcium channel blockers including nifedipine and verapamil have been shown to have antinociceptive effects. In addition, these channels are often situated close to an opioid receptor. When an opioid binds to its receptor, the receptor changes shape and can block the VSCC so that calcium cannot move into the cell. Similarly, modulation of nerve fibers with chronic or neuropathic pain can cause α-2 adrenoreceptors in the spinal cord to be coupled with the VSCC, so that α-2 agonist medications have an extra analgesic effect by blocking calcium influx.

Conversely, pain fiber modulation can also lead to alteration of the channels so that activation of opiate receptors will no longer affect the transmission of calcium. This is one reason that opioids become less effective in the treatment of chronic or neuropathic pain.[115,140–142]

VSCCs are also found in the heart, skeletal muscle, kidneys, pancreas, and liver, but there is such significant variation within this family of receptors that drugs that work on one type of VSCC are unlikely to be able to interact with VSCC in other organs, reducing the risk of side effects.

Box 43.9 Acetaminophen and COX-3

A COX variant known as COX-3 has been isolated in the dog's brain and has similar inflammatory and pyretic effects as COX-1 and COX-2. Acetaminophen has been shown to specifically inhibit COX-3, meaning that it has anti-inflammatory and anti-pyretic effects in the brain itself. However, this is still only part of the story about acetaminophen because COX-3 in other species (including humans) does not have the same inflammatory effects as in dogs.[145,146]

channels (see Box 43.8). It has been used in combination with opiates and/or NSAIDs for postoperative analgesia in human patients and has been shown to be an effective analgesic for soft tissue and spinal surgery.[136–138] The combination of gabapentin and NSAIDs tends to provide better analgesia than NSAIDs alone, and use of gabapentin in a balanced analgesic regime can also decrease the postoperative requirement for opioids.[136,137] The main side effect of administration is mild sedation, and this occurred only rarely in clinical trials.

Although gabapentin has been assessed as an antiepileptic agent in dogs, there are no reports of its efficacy as an adjunctive analgesic in veterinary medicine. Experimental data and anecdotal evidence suggest that it has similar clinical effects in small animal patients as in human patients, but further studies need to be performed to determine its effectiveness and optimal dosing regime.[139] The current dose recommendation for chronic pain in both cats and dogs is 10 mg/kg twice daily. I have used higher doses (up to 30 mg/kg three times a day) without causing sedation. The antiepileptic dose is 10–30 mg/kg every 8 hours.[114]

Acetaminophen (paracetamol)

Although acetaminophen is loosely classified within the NSAID class of drugs, it does not have significant anti-inflammatory effects, and its analgesic activity is more effective centrally than peripherally. In dogs, acetaminophen has been shown to have some COX-inhibiting effects in the CNS (see Box 43.9), but it has also been proposed that there are different mechanisms to account for its analgesic and antipyretic effects. One such mechanism is as a serotonin antagonist, by inhibiting 5HT-3 receptors in the brain and inhibiting descending serotonin-dependent pain pathways. Similarly to other NSAIDs, acetaminophen has an antagonist effect at NMDA receptors.[145]

Acetaminophen also inhibits the metabolism of arachidonic acid to COX-2. Acetaminophen partially reduces a free radical iron cation (Fe^{4+}), thereby making it unavailable for use as a cofactor in the metabolism of arachidonic acid. Acetaminophen is more effective in the brain than in other body tissues due to the relatively low amount of COX-2 that is produced in cerebral cells and the low iron stores in the brain. In peripheral tissues, where the arachidonic acid cascade is initiated in a rapid burst of activity and there are far greater stores of iron, the effects of acetaminophen are overwhelmed and are of little consequence to the production of inflammatory mediators.[145]

Acetaminophen can be used at low doses as an adjunctive analgesic in dogs. Acetaminophen is extremely toxic to cats and should not be given under any circumstances.

References

1. Hansen B. Analgesia and sedation in the critically ill. J Vet Emerg Crit Care 2005;15:285–294.

2. Trescot AM, Datta S, et al. Opioid pharmacology. Pain Phys 2008;11:S133–153.

3. Inturrisi C. Clinical pharmacology of opioids for pain. Clin J Pain 2002;18:S3-S13.

4. Ko JC, Weil AB, Inoue T. Effects of carprofen and morphine on the minimum alveolar concentration of isoflurane in dogs. J Am Anim Hosp Assoc 2009;45:19–23.

5. Steagall PV, Teixeira Neto FJ, et al. Evaluation of the isoflurane-sparing effects of lidocaine and fentanyl during surgery in dogs. J Am Vet Med Assoc 2006;229:522–527.

6. Machado CE, Dyson DH, et al. Effects of oxymorphone and hydromorphone on the minimum alveolar concentration of isoflurane in dogs. Vet Anaesth Analg 2006;33:70–77.

7. Dodam J, Cohn L, et al. Cardiopulmonary effects of medetomidine, oxymorphone or butorphanol in selegiline-treated dogs. Vet Anaesth Analg 2004;31:129–137.

8. Kaye AD, Hoover JM, et al. Morphine, opioids, and the feline pulmonary vascular bed. Acta Anaesthesiol Scand 2008;52:931–937.

9. Kaye AD, Hoover JM, et al. Analysis of the effects of fentanyl in the feline pulmonary vascular bed. Am J Ther 2006;13:478–484.

10. Guedes AG, Papich MG, et al. Pharmacokinetics and physiological effects of intravenous hydromorphone in conscious dogs. J Vet Pharmacol Ther 2008;31:334–343.

11. KuKanich B, Schmidt BK, et al. Pharmacokinetics and behavioral effects of oxymorphone after intravenous and subcutaneous administration to healthy dogs. J Vet Pharmacol Ther 2008;31:580–583.

12. Jackson DM. The effect of nedocromil sodium, sodium cromoglycate and codeine phosphate on citric acid-induced cough in dogs. Br J Pharmacol 1988;93:609–612.

13. Anderson MK, Day TK. Effects of morphine and fentanyl constant rate infusion on urine output in healthy and traumatized dogs. Vet Anaesth Analg 2008;35:528–536.

14. Takahashi T, Tsuchida D, Pappas TN. Central effects of morphine on GI motility in conscious dogs. Brain Res 2007;1166:29–34.

15. Wegner K, Robertson S, et al. Pharmacokinetic and pharmacodynamic evaluation of intravenous hydromorphone in cats. J Vet Pharmacol Ther 2004;27:329–336.

16. Niedfeldt RL, Robertson SA. Postanesthetic hyperthermia in cats: a retrospective comparison between hydromorphone and buprenorphine. Vet Anaesth Analg 2006;33:381–389.

17. Christie MJ. Cellular neuroadaptations to chronic opioids: tolerance, withdrawal and addiction. Br J Pharmacol 2008;154:384–396.

18. Bailey CP, Connor M. Opioids: cellular mechanisms of tolerance and physical dependence. Curr Opin Pharmacol 2005;5:60–68.

19. Guedes AG, Papich MG, et al. Comparison of plasma histamine levels after intravenous administration of hydromorphone and morphine in dogs. J Vet Pharmacol Ther 2007;30:516–522.

20. Guedes AG, Rude EP, Rider MA. Evaluation of histamine release during constant rate infusion of morphine in dogs. Vet Anaesth Analg 2006;33:28–35.

21. Egger C, Duke T, et al. Comparison of plasma fentanyl concentrations by using three transdermal fentanyl patch sizes in dogs. Vet Surg 1998;27:159–166.

22. Egger CM, Glerum LE, et al. Plasma fentanyl concentrations in awake cats and cats undergoing anesthesia and ovariohysterectomy using transdermal administration. Vet Anaesth Analg 2003;30:229.

23. Schmiedt CW, Bjorling DE. Accidental prehension and suspected transmucosal or oral absorption of fentanyl from a transdermal patch in a dog. Vet Anaesth Analg 2007;34:70–73.

24. Robertson SA, Taylor PM, Sear JW. Systemic uptake of buprenorphine by cats after oral mucosal administration. Vet Rec 2003;152:675–678.

25. Abbo LA, Ko JC, et al. Pharmacokinetics of buprenorphine following intravenous and oral transmucosal administration in dogs. Vet Ther 2008;9:83–93.

26. Lucas A, Firth A, et al. Comparison of the effects of morphine administered by constant-rate intravenous infusion or intermittent intramuscular injection in dogs. J Am Vet Med Assoc 2001;218:884–891.

27. Robinson E, Fagella A, et al. Comparison of histamine release induced by morphine and oxymorphone administration in dogs. Am J Vet Res 1988;49:1699–1701.

28. Schurig J, Cavanagh R, Buyniski J. Effect of butorphanol and morphine on pulmonary mechanics, arterial blood pressure and venous plasma histamine in the anesthetized dog. Arch Int Pharmacodyn Ther 1978;233:296–304.

29. Monteiro ER, Junior AR, et al. Comparative study on the sedative effects of morphine, methadone, butorphanol or tramadol, in combination with acepromazine, in dogs. Vet Anaesth Analg 2009;36:25–33.

30. Mastrocinque S, Fantoni DT. A comparison of preoperative tramadol and morphine for the control of early postoperative pain in canine ovariohysterectomy. Vet Anaesth Analg 2003;30:220–228.

31. Ueyema Y, Waselau AC, et al. Anesthetic and cardiopulmonary effects of intramuscular morphine, medetomidine, ketamine injection in dogs. Vet Anaesth Analg 2008;35:480–487.

32. Guedes AG, Papich MG, et al. Pharmacokinetics and physiological effects of two intravenous infusion rates of morphine in conscious dogs. J Vet Pharmacol Ther 2007;30:224–233.

33. Chevillard L, Megarbane B, et al. Characteristics and comparative severity of respiratory response to toxic doses of fentanyl, methadone, morphine, and buprenorphine in rats. Toxicol Lett 2009;191:327–340.

34. Lemmens S, Stienen PJ, et al. The cardiorespiratory effects of a fentanyl infusion following acepromazine and glycopyrrolate in dogs. Tijdschr Diergeneeskd 2008;133:888–895.

35. Meert T, Vermeirsch H. A preclinical comparison between different opioids: antinociceptive versus adverse effects. Pharmacol Biochem Behav 2005;80:309–326.

36. Allweiler S, Brodbelt DC, et al. The isoflurane-sparing and clinical effects of a constant rate infusion of remifentanil in dogs. Vet Anaesth Analg 2007;34:388–393.

37. Murrell JC, van Notten RW, Hellebrekers LJ. Clinical investigation of remifentanil and propofol for the total intravenous anaesthesia of dogs. Vet Rec 2005;156:804–808.

38. Musk GC, Flaherty DA. Target-controlled infusion of propofol combined with variable rate infusion of remifentanil for anaesthesia of a dog with patent ductus arteriosus. Vet Anaesth Analg 2007;34:359–364.

39. Mendes GM, Selmi AL. Use of a combination of propofol and fentanyl, alfentanil, or sufentanil for total intravenous anesthesia in cats. J Am Vet Med Assoc 2003;223:1608–1613.

40. KuKanich B, Hogan BK, et al. Pharmacokinetics of hydromorphone hydrochloride in healthy dogs. Vet Anaesth Analg 2008;35:256–264.

41. Machado CG, Dyson DH, Mathews KA. Evaluation of induction by use of a combination of oxymorphone and diazepam or hydromorphone and diazepam and maintenance of anesthesia

by use of isoflurane in dogs with experimentally induced hypovolemia. Am J Vet Res 2005;66:1227–1237.

42. Bateman SW, Haldane S, Stephens JA. Comparison of the analgesic efficacy of hydromorphone and oxymorphone in dogs and cats: a randomized blinded study. Vet Anaesth Analg 2008.

43. Slingsby LS, Waterman-Pearson AE. Comparison of pethidine, buprenorphine and ketoprofen for postoperative analgesia after ovariohysterectomy in the cat. Vet Rec 1998;143:185–189.

44. Dobbins S, Brown NO, Shofer FS. Comparison of the effects of buprenorphine, oxymorphone hydrochloride, and ketoprofen for postoperative analgesia after onychectomy or onychectomy and sterilization in cats. J Am Anim Hosp Assoc 2002;38: 507–514.

45. Steagall PV, Mantovani FB, et al. Dose-related antinociceptive effects of intravenous buprenorphine in cats. Vet J 2009;182: 203–209.

46. Robertson SA, Taylor PM, et al. Changes in thermal threshold response in eight cats after administration of buprenorphine, butorphanol and morphine. Vet Rec 2003;153:462–465.

47. Al-Gizawiy MM, Rude E. Comparison of preoperative carprofen and postoperative butorphanol as postsurgical analgesics in cats undergoing ovariohysterectomy. Vet Anaesth Analg 2004;31: 164–174.

48. Mathews K, Paley D, et al. A comparison of ketorolac with flunixin, butorphanol, and oxymorphone in controlling postoperative pain in dogs. Can Vet J 1996;37:557–567.

49. Lascelles BD, Robertson SA. Antinociceptive effects of hydromorphone, butorphanol, or the combination in cats. J Vet Intern Med 2004;18:190–195.

50. Andaluz A, Moll X, et al. Pharmacokinetics of buprenorphine after intravenous administration of clinical doses to dogs. Vet J 2009;181:299–304.

51. Giorgi M, Saccomanni G, et al. Pharmacokinetic evaluation of tramadol and its major metabolites after single oral sustained tablet administration in the dog: a pilot study. Vet J 2009;180: 253–255.

52. Pypendop B, Ilkiw J. Pharmacokinetics of tramadol, and its metabolite O-desmethyl-tramadol, in cats. J Vet Pharmacol Ther 2007;31:52–59.

53. Teppema L, Nieuwenhuijs D, et al. Respiratory depression by tramadol in the cat: Involvement of opioid receptors. Anesthesiology 2003;98:420–427.

54. KuKanich B, Papich MG. Pharmacokinetics of tramadol and the metabolite O-desmethyltramadol in dogs. J Vet Pharmacol Ther 2004;27:239–246.

55. Wu WN, McKown LA, et al. Metabolism of the analgesic drug, tramadol hydrochloride, in rat and dog. Xenobiot 2001;31: 423–441.

56. McMillan CJ, Livingston A, et al. Pharmacokinetics of intravenous tramadol in dogs. Can J Vet Res 2008;72:325–331.

57. Vettorato E, Zonca A, et al. Pharmacokinetics and efficacy of intravenous and extradural tramadol in dogs. Vet J 2010;183: 310–315.

58. Kongara K, Chambers P, Johnson CB. Glomerular filtration rate after tramadol, parecoxib and pindolol following anaesthesia and analgesia in comparison with morphine in dogs. Vet Anaesth Analg 2009;36:86–94.

59. Ko J, Abbo L, et al. Effect of orally administered tramadol alone or with an intravenously administered opioid on minimum alveolar concentration of sevoflurane in cats. J Am Vet Med Assoc 2008;232:1834–1840.

60. Stenson W. Prostaglandins and epithelial response to injury. Curr Opin Gastroenterol 2007;23:107–110.

61. Wooten JG, Blikslager AT, et al. Cyclooxygenase expression and prostanoid production in pyloric and duodenal mucosae in dogs after administration of nonsteroidal anti-inflammatory drugs. Am J Vet Res 2008;69:457–464.

62. Lichtenberger L, Romero J, Dial E. Surface phospholipids in gastric injury and protection when a selective cyclooxygenase-2 inhibitor (Coxib) is used in combination with aspirin. Br J Pharmacol 2007;150:913–919.

63. Fukata M, Chen A, et al. Cox-2 is regulated by toll-like receptor-4 (TLR4) signaling: role in proliferation and apoptosis in the intestine. Gastroenterology 2006;131:862–877.

64. Vane JR, Warner TD. Nomenclature for COX-2 Inhibitors. Lancet 2000;356:1373.

65. Bosmans T, Gasthuys F, et al. A comparison of tepoxalin-buprenorphine combination and buprenorphine for postoperative analgesia in dogs: a clinical study. J Vet Med A Physiol Pathol Clin Med 2007;54:364–369.

66. Carroll GL, Howe LB, Peterson KD. Analgesic efficacy of preoperative administration of meloxicam or butorphanol in onychectomized cats. J Am Vet Med Assoc 2005;226:913–919.

67. Dzikiti TB, Joubert KE, et al. Comparison of morphine and carprofen administered alone or in combination for analgesia in dogs undergoing ovariohysterectomy. J S Afr Vet Assoc 2006;77: 120–126.

68. Gassel AD, Tobias KM, et al. Comparison of oral and subcutaneous administration of buprenorphine and meloxicam for preemptive analgesia in cats undergoing ovariohysterectomy. J Am Vet Med Assoc 2005;227:1937–1944.

69. Lascelles B, Butterworth S, Waterman A. Postoperative analgesic and sedative effects of carprofen and pethidine in dogs. Vet Rec 1994;134:187–191.

70. Mollenhoff A, Nolte I, Kramer S. Anti-nociceptive efficacy of carprofen, levomethadone and buprenorphine for pain relief in cats following major orthopaedic surgery. J Vet Med A Physiol Pathol Clin Med 2005;52:186–198.

71. Shih AC, Robertson S, et al. Comparison between analgesic effects of buprenorphine, carprofen, and buprenorphine with carprofen for canine ovariohysterectomy. Vet Anaesth Analg 2008;35:69–79.

72. Steagall PV, Taylor PM, et al. Analgesia for cats after ovariohysterectomy with either buprenorphine or carprofen alone or in combination. Vet Rec 2009;164:359–363.

73. Hazewinkel HA, van den Brom WE, et al. Comparison of the effects of firocoxib, carprofen and vedaprofen in a sodium urate crystal induced synovitis model of arthritis in dogs. Res Vet Sci 2008;84:74–79.

74. Lascelles B, Cripps P, et al. Carprofen as an analgesic for postoperative pain in cats: dose titration and assessment of efficacy in comparison to pethidine hydrochloride. J Small Anim Pract 1995;36:535–541.

75. Lascelles BD, Henderson AJ, Hackett IJ. Evaluation of the clinical efficacy of meloxicam in cats with painful locomotor disorders. J Small Anim Pract 2001;42:587–593.

76. Pollmeier M, Toulemonde C, et al. Clinical evaluation of firocoxib and carprofen for the treatment of dogs with osteoarthritis. Vet Rec 2006;159:547–551.

77. Ryan W, Moldave K, Carithers D. Clinical effectiveness and safety of a new NSAID, firocoxib: a 1000 dog study. Vet Ther 2006;7:119–126.

78. Slingsby LS, Waterman-Pearson AE. Postoperative analgesia in the cat after ovariohysterectomy by use of carprofen, ketoprofen, meloxicam or tolfenamic acid. J Small Anim Pract 2000;41: 447–450.

79. Lascelles B, McFarland J, Swann H. Guidelines for safe and effective use of NSAIDs in dogs. Vet Ther 2005;6:237–251.

80. Micklewright R, Lane S, et al. Review article: NSAIDs, gastroprotection and cyclo-oxygenase-II-selective inhibitors. Aliment Pharmacol Ther 2003;17:321–332.

81. Little D, Jones S, Blikslager A. Cyclooxygenase (COS) inhibitors and the intestine. J Vet Intern Med 2007;21:367–377.

82. Tomlinson J, Blikslager A. Role of nonsteroidal anti-inflammatory drugs in gastrointestinal tract injury and repair. J Am Vet Med Assoc 2003;222:946–951.

83. Goodman L, Torres B, Punke J, et al. Effects of firocoxib and tepoxalin on healing in a canine gastric mucosal injury model. J Vet Intern Med 2009;23:56–62.

84. Luna SP, Basilio AC, et al. Evaluation of adverse effects of long-term oral administration of carprofen, etodolac, flunixin meglumine, ketoprofen, and meloxicam in dogs. Am J Vet Res 2007;68:258–264.

85. Briere CA, Hosgood G, et al. Effects of carprofen on the integrity and barrier function of canine colonic mucosa. Am J Vet Res 2008;69:174–181.

86. Craven M, Chandler ML, et al. Acute effects of carprofen and meloxicam on canine gastrointestinal permeability and mucosal absorptive capacity. J Vet Intern Med 2007;21:917–923.

87. Dowers K, Uhrig S, et al. Effect of short term sequential administration of nonsteroidal anti-inflammatory drugs on the stomach and proximal portion of the duodenum in healthy dogs. Am J Vet Res 2006;67:1794–1801.

88. Punke JP, Speas AL, et al. Effects of firocoxib, meloxicam, and tepoxalin on prostanoid and leukotriene production by duodenal mucosa and other tissues of osteoarthritic dogs. Am J Vet Res 2008;69:1203–1209.

89. Sennello K, Leib M. Effects of deracoxib or buffered aspirin on the gastric mucosa of healthy dogs. J Vet Intern Med 2006;20:1291–1296.

90. Lascelles B, Blikslager A, et al. Gastrointestinal tract perforation in dogs treated with a selective cyclooxygenase-2 inhibitor: 29 cases (2002–2003). J Am Vet Med Assoc 2005;227:1112–1117.

91. Enberg T, Braun L, Kuzma A. Gastrointestinal perforation in five dogs associated with the administration of meloxicam. J Vet Emerg Crit Care 2006;16:34–43.

92. Reed S. Nonsteroidal anti-inflammatory drug-induced duodenal ulceration and perforation in a mature Rottweiler. Can Vet J 2002;43:971–972.

93. Jones C, Budsberg S. Physiologic characteristics and clinical importance of the cyclooxygenase isoforms in dogs and cats. J Am Vet Med Assoc 2000;217:721–729.

94. Lobetti R, Joubert K. Effect of administration of nonsteroidal anti-inflammatory drugs before surgery on renal function in clinically normal dogs. Am J Vet Res 2000;61:1501–1507.

95. Bostrom I, Nyman G, et al. Effects of carprofen on renal function and results of serum biochemical and hematologic analyses in anesthetized dogs that had low blood pressure during anesthesia. Am J Vet Res 2002;63:712–721.

96. Kay-Mugford PA, Grimm KA, et al.. Effect of preoperative administration of tepoxalin on hemostasis and hepatic and renal function in dogs. Vet Ther 2004;5:120–127.

97. MacPhail C, Lappin M, et al. Hepatocellular toxicosis associated with administration of carprofen in 21 dogs. J Am Vet Med Assoc 1998;212:1895–1901.

98. Lemke K, Runyon C, Horney B. Effects of preoperative administration of ketoprofen on whole blood platelet aggregation, buccal mucosal bleeding time, and hematologic indices in dogs undergoing elective ovariohysterectomy. J Am Vet Med Assoc 2002;220:1818–1822.

99. Kearney PM, Baigent C, et al. Do selective cyclo-oxygenase-2 inhibitors and traditional non-steroidal anti-inflammatory drugs increase the risk of atherothrombosis? Meta-analysis of randomised trials. Brit Med J 2006;332:1302–1308.

100. Brainard B, Meredith C, et al. Changes in platelet function, hemostasis, and prostaglandin expression after treatment with nonsteroidal anti-inflammatory drugs with various cyclooxygenase selectivities in dogs. Am J Vet Res 2007;68:251–257.

101. Narita T, Sato R, et al. The interaction between orally administered non-steroidal anti-inflammatory drugs and prednisolone in healthy dogs. J Vet Med Sci 2007;69:353–363.

102. Gunew MN, Menrath VH, Marshall RD. Long-term safety, efficacy and palatability of oral meloxicam at 0.01–0.03 mg/kg for treatment of osteoarthritic pain in cats. J Fel Med Surg 2008;10:235–241.

103. Murrell JC, Hellebrekers LJ. Medetomidine and dexmedetomidine: a review of cardiovascular effects and antinociceptive properties in the dog. Vet Anaesth Analg 2005;32:117–127.

104. Gomez-Villamandos RJ, Palacios C, et al. Dexmedetomidine or medetomidine premedication before propofol-desflurane anaesthesia in dogs. J Vet Pharmacol Ther 2006;29:157–163.

105. Granholm M, McKusick BC, et al. Evaluation of the clinical efficacy and safety of intramuscular and intravenous doses of dexmedetomidine and medetomidine in dogs and their reversal with atipamezole. Vet Rec 2007;160:891–897.

106. Granholm M, McKusick BC, et al. Evaluation of the clinical efficacy and safety of dexmedetomidine or medetomidine in cats and their reversal with atipamezole. Vet Anaesth Analg 2006;33:214–223.

107. Pypendop BH, Verstegen JP. Hemodynamic effects of medetomidine in the dog: a dose titration study. Vet Surg 1998;27:612–622.

108. Kuo WC, Keegan RD. Comparative cardiovascular, analgesic, and sedative effects of medetomidine, medetomidine-hydromorphone, and medetomidine-butorphanol in dogs. Am J Vet Res 2004;65:931–937.

109. Ko JC, Payton ME, W et al. Effects of intravenous diazepam or microdose medetomidine on propofol-induced sedation in dogs. J Am Anim Hosp Assoc 2006;42:18–27.

110. Grimm KA, Tranquilli WJ, et al. Cardiopulmonary effects of fentanyl in conscious dogs and dogs sedated with a continuous rate infusion of medetomidine. Am J Vet Res 2005;66:1222–1226.

111. Ethier MR, Mathews KA, et al. Evaluation of the efficacy and safety for use of two sedation and analgesia protocols to facilitate assisted ventilation of healthy dogs. Am J Vet Res 2008;69:1351–1359.

112. Silva C, Hatschbach E, et al. Continuous infusion in adult females dogs submitted to ovariohysterectomy with midazolam-xylazine and/or medetomidine pre-treated with methotrimeprazine and buprenorphine. Acta Cir Bras 2007;22:272–278.

113. Pacharinsak C, Greene SA, et al. Postoperative analgesia in dogs receiving epidural morphine plus medetomidine. J Vet Pharmacol Ther 2003;26:71–77.

114. Plumb D. Plumb's Veterinary Drug Handbook. 5th ed. Ames, IA: Blackwell Publishing; 2005.

115. Pertovaara A. Noradrenergic pain modulation. Prog Neurobiol 2006;80:53–83.

116. Bach FW, Jensen TS, et al. The effect of intravenous lidocaine on nociceptive processing in diabetic neuropathy. Pain 1990;40:29–34.

117. Herroeder S, Pecher S, et al. Systemic lidocaine shortens length of hospital stay after colorectal surgery: a double-blinded, randomized, placebo-controlled trial. Ann Surg 2007;246:192–200.

118. Kuo CP, Jao SW, et al. Comparison of the effects of thoracic epidural analgesia and I.V. infusion with lidocaine on cytokine response, postoperative pain and bowel function in patients undergoing colonic surgery. Br J Anaesth 2006;97:640–646.

119. Sharma S, Rajagopal M, et al. Phase II pilot study to evaluate use of intravenous lidocaine for opioid-refractory pain in cancer patients. J Pain Symptom Manage 2009;37:85–93.

120. Marret E, Rolin M, et al. Meta-analysis of intravenous lidocaine and postoperative recovery after abdominal surgery. Br J Surg 2008;95:1331–1338.

121. Tremont-Lukats IW, Hutson PR, Backonja MM. A randomized, double-masked, placebo-controlled pilot trial of extended IV lidocaine infusion for relief of ongoing neuropathic pain. Clin J Pain 2006;22:266–271.

122. Smith L, Bentley E, et al. Systemic lidocaine infusion as an analgesic for intraocular surgery in dogs: a pilot study. Vet Anaesth Analg 2004;31:53–63.

123. Brianceau P, Chevalier H, et al. Intravenous lidocaine and small-intestinal size, abdominal fluid, and outcome after colic surgery in horses. J Vet Intern Med 2002;16:736–741.

124. Malone E, Ensink J, et al. Intravenous continuous infusion of lidocaine for treatment of equine ileus. Vet Surg 2006;35:60–66.

125. Pypendop B, Ilkiw J, Robertson S. Effects of intravenous administration of lidocaine on the thermal threshold in cats. Am J Vet Res 2006;67:16–20.

126. Aveline C, Gautier JF, et al. Postoperative analgesia and early rehabilitation after total knee replacement: a comparison of continuous low-dose intravenous ketamine versus nefopam. Eur J Pain 2009;13:613–619.

127. Chazan S, Ekstein MP, et al. Ketamine for acute and subacute pain in opioid-tolerant patients. J Opioid Manag 2008;4:173–180.

128. Yamauchi M, Asano M, et al. Continuous low-dose ketamine improves the analgesic effects of fentanyl patient-controlled analgesia after cervical spine surgery. Anesth Analg 2008;107:1041–1044.

129. Conway M, White N, et al. Use of continuous intravenous ketamine for end-stage cancer pain in children. J Pediatr Oncol Nurs 2009;26:100–106.

130. Sarrau S, Jourdan J, et al. Effects of postoperative ketamine infusion on pain control and feeding behaviour in bitches undergoing mastectomy. J Small Anim Pract 2007;48:670–676.

131. Wagner AE, Walton JA, et al. Use of low doses of ketamine administered by constant rate infusion as an adjunct for postoperative analgesia in dogs. J Am Vet Med Assoc 2002;221:72–75.

132. Fass J, Bares R, et al. Effects of intravenous ketamine on gastrointestinal motility in the dog. Intensive Care Med 1995;21:584–589.

133. Pozzi A, Muir W, Traverso F. Prevention of central sensitization and pain by N-methyl-D-aspartate receptor antagonists. J Am Vet Med Assoc 2006;228:53–60.

134. Lascelles BD, Gaynor JS, Smith ES, et al. Amantadine in a multimodal analgesic regimen for alleviation of refractory osteoarthritis pain in dogs. J Vet Intern Med 2008;22:53–59.

135. Serpell M, Group NPS. Gabapentin in neuropathic pain syndromes: a randomised, double-blind, placebo-controlled trial. Pain 2002;99:557–566.

136. Turan A, Karamanlıoglu B, et al. Analgesic effects of gabapentin after spinal surgery. Anesthesiology 2004;100:935–938.

137. Parsa A, Sprouse-Blum A, et al. Combined preoperative use of celecoxib and gabapentin in the management of postoperative pain. Aesthetic Plast Surg 2009;33:98–103.

138. Gilron I, Orr E, et al. A placebo-controlled randomized clinical trial of perioperative administration of gabapentin, rofecoxib and their combination for spontaneous and movement-evoked pain after abdominal hysterectomy. Pain 2005;113:191–200.

139. Meymandi M, Sepehri G. Gabapentin action and interaction on the antinociceptive effect of morphine on visceral pain in mice. Eur J Anaesthesiol 2008;25:129–134.

140. McCormack K. Fail-safe mechanisms that perpetuate neuropathic pain. Pain: Clin Updates 1999;7:1–4.

141. Assi A. The influence of divalent cations on the analgesic effect of opioid and non-opioid drugs. Pharmacol Res Commun 2001;43:521–529.

142. Mahani S, Vahedi S, et al. Nifedipine potentiates antinociceptive effects of morphine in rats by decreasing hypothalamic pituitary adrenal axis activity. Pharmacol Biochem Behav 2005;82:17–23.

143. Woolf C, Salter M. Neuronal plasticity: increasing the gain in pain. Science 2000;288:1765–1768.

144. Hayashida K, Obata H, et al. Gabapentin acts within the locus coeruleus to alleviate neuropathic pain. Anesthesiology 2008;109:1077–1084.

145. Anderson B. Paracetamol (acetaminophen): mechanisms of action. Pediatric Anesthesia 2008;18:915–921.

146. Botting R, Ayoub S. COX 3 and the mechanism of action of paracetamol (acetaminophen). Prostaglandins Leukot Essent Fatty Acids 2005;72:85–87.

44

Local analgesia

Vicki L. Campbell and Amy Rodriguez

Indications for local analgesia

Local analgesia is an underused technique that can greatly enhance the overall analgesia in a patient, can lead to use of less systemic drugs, and may be used in situations in which sedation, heavy systemic analgesia, or anesthesia is contraindicated.[1] Many animals that present to the emergency department are in shock, and those that are not in decompensated shock may be in compensated shock.[2] Those in compensated shock are able to compensate because their sympathetic nervous system is maintaining their blood pressure and helping to maintain their oxygen delivery.[3] In the intensive care unit, critically ill animals are dynamic with potentially minute-to-minute changes in cardiac output, blood pressure, and oxygen delivery. Almost all sedatives, analgesics, and anesthetics blunt the sympathetic nervous system to some extent.[4–20] This effect puts animals in the emergency department and critical care unit at risk for decompensation when receiving systemic drugs for analgesia, sedation, or anesthesia. Local analgesic techniques may aid in decreasing systemic drug requirements in these patients.[1] Although shock patients in general are at risk for systemic decompensation with systemic sedatives and anesthetics, there are specific conditions in which these drugs should be particularly avoided or delayed if at all possible. Specific examples include head trauma, pulmonary contusions, pneumothorax, myocardial contusions (and subsequent arrhythmias), diaphragmatic hernia, liver fractures, splenic fractures, urinary tract rupture, severe anemia/hypoproteinemia, and neurologic abnormalities. Avoidance of anesthesia and sedation in these situations is beneficial because anesthetic drugs can worsen/induce

arrhythmias, positive pressure ventilation may contribute to or worsen pneumothorax, lungs that have pulmonary contusions are more prone to atelectasis and subsequent hypoxemia, anesthetic drugs can alter blood flow to the brain and worsen head trauma/neurologic status, urinary tract injuries may cause severe life-threatening electrolyte disturbances (especially hyperkalemia), and liver/spleen fractures may lead to intraoperative hemorrhage and hypotension.[14,15,17,18] In addition, many anesthetic drugs are protein bound and become more bioavailable in animals that are acidotic, a common consequence of shock and trauma.[7,14,15,18] Avoidance of anesthesia until full assessment and proper resuscitation is attained is critical. However, sometimes sedation or anesthesia in these patients cannot be avoided. Use of local analgesic techniques in these life-threatening situations frequently decreases the need for systemic drug use and makes for a safer overall procedure.[1]

Because local anesthetics directly block nerve impulses, they decrease pain in an alternative way compared with systemic analgesics.[8,21] When used preemptively, this decreases the likelihood of wind-up of the pain pathways, ultimately helps prevent hyperalgesia, and aids in the multimodal approach to patient analgesia.[8]

Drug choices

Drug selection (see Table 44.1) is an important part of the local anesthetic protocol. Local anesthetics work by blocking nerve impulses.[7,8,21] At a cellular level this occurs by blocking sodium channels in the nerve membrane.[8] When sodium is blocked, the nerve cannot

Advanced Monitoring and Procedures for Small Animal Emergency and Critical Care, First Edition. Edited by Jamie M. Burkitt Creedon, Harold Davis.

© 2012 John Wiley & Sons, Inc. Published 2012 by John Wiley & Sons, Inc.

Table 44.1 Listing of various drug dosages for local anesthetic use (for continuous epidural drug protocol, see the section on epidural)

Drug	Dosage	Use
Lidocaine	1–2 mg/kg	Short-acting analgesia for local infiltration, intrapleural and intraperitoneal blocks, and occasionally epidural use
Bupivicaine	1–2 mg/kg	Longer acting analgesia for local infiltration, intrapleural, intraperitoneal, and epidural use
Dexmedetomidine	0.001–0.005 mg/kg	Epidural, intraarticular, or perineurally
Preservative-free morphine	0.1 mg/kg	Epidural
Fentanyl	0.01 mg/kg	Epidural
Buprenorphine	0.003–0.006 mg/kg	Epidural

conduct an impulse, and therefore no sensation can be transmitted. Local anesthetics cause analgesia but also can cause complete loss of motor function depending on the properties of the drug, location, myelination of the nerve, dose, and size of the nerve fibers.[22] Generally, local anesthetics cause nerve blockade in a particular order by first numbing pain, then warmth, touch, deep pressure, and finally motor function.[22] However, large peripheral nerves are an exception to this and tend to have motor blockade before sensory blockade, as well cause proximal extremity analgesia prior to distal extremity blockade.[22] Local anesthetic drugs differ in their side effects, onset of action, and duration of action. Consideration of these drug factors should influence drug selection.[23]

Lidocaine

Lidocaine is a commonly used local anesthetic that belongs to the amino amide group, meaning it is generally biotransformed by liver microsomal enzymes.[22] It is available in concentrations of 0.5% to 5% with or without epinephrine.[22] In addition to the injectable lido-caine, various forms of lidocaine can also be found: dermal patches, oral gels, topical gels, and nasal sprays. Lidocaine has an onset of action of 5–10 minutes and duration of action of 60–120 minutes.[22] Dosing of lidocaine for local infiltration is generally 1–2 mg/kg in both dogs and cats.[7] Adverse drugs reactions are uncommon when lidocaine is used as a local anesthetic. Most reactions are associated with accidental intravenous (IV) injections, so care should be taken to avoid this when local effects are the goal. In dogs, intravenous administration of lidocaine at a dose of 22 ± 6.7 mg/kg induces convulsions and other signs of central nervous system (CNS) toxicity, such as salivation and muscle tremors.[24] In cats, intravenous administration of lidocaine at a dose of 11.7 ± 4.6 mg/kg induces convulsions.[23] Based on these results, dogs should not exceed a dose of 12 mg/kg IV, whereas cats should not exceed a dose of 6 mg/kg IV.[23] Lidocaine with epinephrine should not be used in distal extremities due to vasoconstriction and potential tissue necrosis.[25]

Bupivacaine

Bupivacaine hydrochloride is a long-acting local anesthetic that also belongs to the amino amide group and is four times more potent than lidocaine.[22] It comes in three different concentrations, 0.25%, 0.5%, and 0.75%, available with or without epinephrine. Bupivacaine has an onset of action of 20–30 minutes and duration of action of 180–480 minutes. Dosing of bupivacaine is 1–2 mg /kg, which is similar to lidocaine even though it is four times more potent. Therefore, caution must be taken if repeat doses are necessary because the CNS toxic dose of bupivicaine is much lower than lidocaine at 5 mg/kg.[24] Bupivacaine is contraindicated for IV regional anesthesia (IVRA) because of the potential risk of tourniquet failure and systemic absorption of the drug. It should be clarified that although bupivicaine has a greater arrhythmogenic effect than lidocaine, it has been shown to cause less hypotension systemically than lidocaine in the cat.[26] Additionally, on an equipotent basis, the seizure threshold is similar for both bupivacaine and lidocaine.[26] Accidental IV injection of bupivacaine is cardiotoxic and may lead to death; therefore, aspiration before injection is crucial. Bupivacaine with epinephrine should not be used on distal appendages due to its vasoconstrictive properties and the potential for tissue death.[25]

α-2 adrenergic agonists

The α-2 adrenergic agonists, such as dexmedetomidine, are typically used systemically for sedation and analgesia. However, there are α-2 receptors present in the spinal cord (epidurally and intrathecally) that are crucial in the pain pathways.[8] These can be stimulated by epidural or intrathecal infiltration of α-2 agonists, although systemic uptake is always a possibility and must be anticipated.[8] The use of α-2 adrenergic receptor agonists (in combination with amino amide local anesthetics or locally administered opioids) is a useful adjunct in optimizing local anesthetic technique for intra-articular pain control.[27] The use of these drug combinations produces a synergistic analgesic effect and is partly due to norepinephrine inhibition at the nerve endings.[8] The α-2 agonists also enhance peripheral nerve blockade when combined with amino amide local anesthetics.[8] This enhancement is multifactorial but is mostly due to enhanced nerve blockade. Adding α-2 agonists to brachial plexus, intercostal, and dental nerve blocks can enhance the analgesia of these procedures.[8] Doses of dexmedetomidine vary depending on the regional block being performed. The doses range from 0.001 to 0.005 mg/kg.[8] Adverse effects should be anticipated when using an α-2 adrenoceptor agonist as a local anesthetic. Systemic effects to watch for include cardiovascular and respiratory effects, such as bradycardia, decreased cardiac output, and decreased respiratory rate.[6,7]

Opioids

Regional anesthesia, affecting a large part of the body or blocking many nerves, can be enhanced with administration of opioids (preservative-free morphine, fentanyl, or buprenorphine) when combined with an amino amide local anesthetic.[8] Opioid administration alone into the epidural or intra-articular space or in combination with α-2 agonists also are acceptable local analgesia techniques.[8] The onset of action for most regional blocks is 30–60 minutes. The duration of action is approximately 18 hours when using preservative-free morphine, and the duration and extent of analgesia can be extended when using drugs in combination.[8] Adverse effects of opioids when used in this route of administration are rarely problematic.[28] Urine retention is possible after epidural morphine administration, and the bladder may need to be manually expressed or catheterized.[28] Other effects such as sedation, vomiting, defecation, constipation, and histamine release may be appreciated but are uncommon.[28] In regard to histamine release, pretreatment with an antihistamine is usually not indicated unless mast cell tumors are of concern. If degranulation of a mast cell tumor is of concern, pretreatment with diphenhydramine at 1–2 mg/kg intramuscularly is recommended.

Local blocks

Specific local blocks are discussed in the following sections. There are various ways to approach each technique, and common sense is important when choosing to use a local anesthetic block. Many of the blocks require general anesthesia, which may be contraindicated in the emergency patient. Additionally, local anesthetics in and of themselves can be painful, so keep this in mind when performing the blocks. Some authors recommend combining sodium bicarbonate with the local anesthetic to reduce the pain of injection; however, this can decrease the efficacy of the local anesthetic and thus is not discussed in this chapter.[22] Lastly, it is imperative that the patient be monitored for proper analgesia after a local block is performed because the block may not have worked properly or may not last as long as anticipated. The technician and clinician should have a standardized method of evaluating the patient for pain. Most hospitals have a systematic approach for assessing pain in their patients. Listed are a few examples that can be readily implemented. Palpate or gently apply pressure to the affected area, watch for a reaction, such as withdrawing the limb, whimpering, or vocalization, the patient looking at the affected area or seeming concerned. Other signs to observe are increases in heart rate, an overall sense of uneasiness, not being able to get comfortable, and vocalization of pain. Cats frequently exhibit pain by not moving or hiding in the back of a cage. Therefore, systemic pain medications are still required in these situations, as well as when the local anesthetic wears off. It should be noted that subcutaneous injection of local anesthetics has a much lower risk of toxicity than intrapleural or intraperitoneal injection due to differences in systemic absorption. This must be kept in mind when total and repeat doses are calculated.

Local infiltration, incisional blocks, ring blocks

Indications

Local infiltration, incisional blocks, and ring blocks are the simplest to perform of all the blocks (Protocols 44.1–44.3). They are infiltrative blocks at the site of the wound/incision and help control the pain associated with wound debridement and management. Such blocks may reduce the need for heavy sedation when repairing a laceration in an animal that is in compensated shock. The most common indications for these blocks in the emergency setting are lacerations, wounds, incisions, toe wounds and amputations, and tail wounds and amputations.

Protocol 44.1 Local infiltration/line block

Procedure
1. Clip affected area.
2. Aseptically prepare area.
3. In one syringe, prepare mixture of 2% lidocaine 1–2 mg/kg and 5.0% or 7.5% bupivacaine 1–2 mg/kg (bupivacaine with epinephrine is suitable, as long as it is not a distal extremity). The volume needed depends on the size of the area being blocked. Alternatively, this block may be performed with single agent lidocaine or bupivicaine at the above doses.
4. With a syringe attached to a 25-gauge, ⅝-inch or a 22-gauge, 1-inch needle, insert needle subcutaneously, aspirate, inject mixture as you withdraw needle, and make a small bleb.
5. Repeat this procedure around the target area, in a rectangular or circular pattern. Make sure to split the dose of your drug equally throughout the area. It is always a good idea to anticipate how big of an area you will be blocking so that you do not exceed your total dose.
6. If your target area is a surgical incision, inject mixture along the incision, using either a 25-gauge, ⅝-inch or a 22-gauge, 1-inch needle (size depends on the size of the animal).
7. It is ideal to make these injections before the surgical process had begun; however, these blocks are still beneficial if done after the surgical procedure.
8. Alternatively, you can use a 22-gauge, 1.5- to 3.0-inch spinal needle (length depends on size of incision). Insert entirety of spinal needle under the skin, aspirate, and inject mixture as you remove the needle from the skin.

Protocol 44.2 Ring block

Procedure
1. Clip area distal to affected area, 360°.
2. Aseptically prepare site.
3. Prepare mixture of 2% lidocaine 1–2 mg/kg and 7.5% bupivacaine 1–2 mg/kg in a single syringe. Alternatively, this block may be performed with single agent lidocaine or bupivicaine at the above doses.
4. With the syringe attached to a 25-gauge, ⅝-inch needle, insert needle subcutaneously.
5. Aspirate; inject mixture as you remove the needle from the skin until a small bleb is formed.
6. Reinsert needle through first bleb, the area of skin that is already desensitized, and inject in the neighboring skin.
7. Repeat steps until you have injected around the circumference of the affected limb.

Protocol 44.3 Soaker catheters

Procedure
1. Soaker catheters can be placed in the subcutaneous tissue for local infiltration when closing an incision for repeat or continuous local anesthetic infiltration.
2. Aseptically prepare site.
3. Place soaker catheter in the subcutaneous space.
4. Suture in place using a Chinese finger trap technique.

Contraindications

There are few contraindications to these simple blocks. There is some evidence that local anesthetics can interfere with wound healing, which should be kept in mind.[29,30] Additionally, if an area is infected, ring blocks and local infiltration should probably be avoided.

Complications

Infection, pain on injection, decreased wound healing,[29,30] drug reaction, bleeding, ineffective block, and clogging of the catheter if using a soaker catheter are possible complications.

Intrapleural blocks
Indications

Intrapleural blocks are usually performed through a chest tube (see Fig. 44.1) that has already been placed and is the mainstay of intrapleural blocks in veterinary medicine (Protocol 44.4). The use of a syringe and needle directly through the thoracic wall can be used to infiltrate the pleural space. However, this direct technique is rarely used and not discussed further.

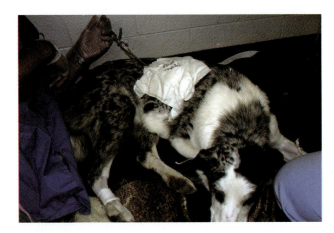

Figure 44.1 Intrapleural block. A dog receiving an intrapleural block through a chest tube.

Protocol 44.4 Intrapleural block

Procedure

1. Aseptically prepare chest tube for injection.
2. Aspirate and remove any fluid or air from the pleural space through the chest tube.
3. Slowly inject a combination of 1 mg/kg of lidocaine mixed with 1 mg/kg of bupivacaine. Your total dosage should not exceed 2 mg/kg. If you prefer to use a single agent, inject 2 mg/kg of lidocaine or 1.5 mg/kg of bupivicaine.[32,33] If bilateral chest tubes are placed, simply divide the drug in half and administer one half of the drug into each chest tube. The bupivacaine alone may sting if it is not given with the lidocaine. Lidocaine alone will only last 30–60 minutes, whereas addition of bupivacaine will extend the analgesia to 4–6 hours.
4. Follow the injection with 5 mL of sterile saline or air to clear the chest tube of the local anesthetic and ensure dispersion into the thoracic cavity.
5. The block may be more effective if you lay the animal down in lateral recumbency for 10–15 minutes after the block, with the affected side down.

Contraindications

Flail chest may be a contraindication because the body wall may not be intact and the local anesthetic may leak into the subcutaneous space. There is no evidence that intrapleural lidocaine or bupivicaine at therapeutic doses given to patients with pericardectomy increases the risk of dysrhythmias.[31]

Complications

Complications include pain on injection, incomplete block, cardiac toxicity, and pyothorax.

Intercostal nerve blocks

Indications

Intercostal nerve blocks (Protocol 44.5) can be performed on any intercostal nerve and generally block structures as far as two rib spaces caudal to the block. These can be useful for broken ribs or cranial abdominal pain.[33]

Contraindications

Flail chest and infection are contraindications for this procedure.

Complications

Pneumothorax and bleeding are the complications.

Protocol 44.5 Intercostal nerve blocks

Procedure

1. Two adjacent intercostal spaces (see Figs. 44.2 and 44.3) both cranial and caudal to the incision or area of discomfort must be blocked due to the nerve supply overlap.[33]
2. Using a 90° angle, insert a 25-gauge, ⅝-inch or a 22-gauge, 1-inch needle through the skin caudal to the rib near the intervertebral foramen.
3. Aspirate, and if no blood is withdrawn, then inject 0.5–1.0 mL 7.5% bupivacaine (volume depends on the size of the animal) at each site. Your total dosage should not exceed 2 mg/kg.

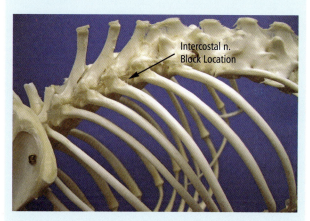

Figure 44.2 Intercostal nerve block. Location of the intercostal nerve on a dog skeleton.

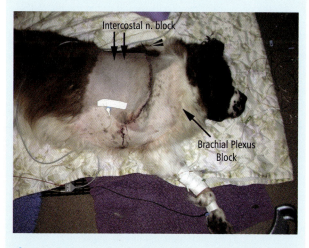

Figure 44.3 Intercostal nerve block and brachial plexus block. Examples of the location of an intercostal nerve block and brachial plexus block on a live dog. The brachial plexus block is performed medial to the shoulder joint with the needle inserted caudally toward the costochondral junction of the ribs.

Protocol 44.6 Brachial plexus block without the use of a nerve locator

Procedure

1. With the patient in lateral recumbency, affected leg up, clip area medial to the shoulder joint.
2. Aseptically prepare site.
3. After washing hands and while donning sterile gloves, insert a 22-gauge, 1.5- to 3.0-inch spinal needle (depending on size of patient) medial to the shoulder joint with the needle pointing caudally toward the costochondral junction of the ribs (Fig. 44.3) and the shaft of the needle parallel to the vertebral column.
4. Once needle is fully inserted, aspirate. If no blood is noted, inject bupivacaine, 2 mg/kg, 7.5% concentration, as you slowly withdraw needle.[3]

Protocol 44.7 Brachial plexus block with the use of nerve locator

Procedure

1. Clip area medial to the shoulder joint.
2. Aseptically prepare site.
3. Attach nerve locator surface electrode to patient.
4. Prime insulated needle delivery set with 7.5% bupivacaine, about 0.5 mL or until bupivacaine is observed at the tip of your needle.
5. Using sterile gloves, insert insulated needle (size 40 mm, 80 mm, or 100 mm, depending on patient size; the distal tip of the needle should lie just caudal to the spine of the scapula) medial to the shoulder joint with the needle pointing caudally toward the costochondral junction of the ribs and the shaft of the needle parallel to the vertebral column.
6. Once the needle is placed through skin, attach the nerve locator to the uninsulated part of the needle.
7. Turn nerve locator on and apply settings at 1 mA (2 Hz).
8. Continue to insert the needle until you obtain contractions of the biceps brachii muscle and flexion of the elbow.
9. Once desired effect is obtained, slowly decrease nerve locator setting until you achieve same muscle contraction and elbow flexion at a mA of 0.5. If the technician is getting a positive stimulation at 0.2 mA, it may indicate an intraneural needle placement.
10. Aspirate. If no blood is observed, inject bupivacaine (2 mg/kg, 7.5% solution) slowly. There should be no resistance while injecting the bupivacaine.
11. Once nerve twitch dissipates, slowly withdraw needle while still injecting bupivacaine as the needle is removed.[34]

Protocol 44.8 Intraperitoneal block

Procedure

1. Position the animal in lateral recumbency.
2. Aseptically prepare site around the umbilicus.
3. Using a 90° angle, insert a 22-gauge, 1 or 1½-inch needle through the skin just ventral to the umbilicus until the needle is within the peritoneal cavity. Depending on the thickness of the subcutaneous tissue, a 1-inch needle usually penetrates into the peritoneal cavity. Usually there is a small loss of resistance as the needle breaks through the parietal peritoneum.
4. Aspirate once in the abdominal cavity. If fluid is aspirated, then do not inject. Commonly the spleen or bladder is hit accidentally with the needle and the procedure needs to be redirected. An ultrasound machine is helpful to determine if fluid is already present within the abdominal cavity prior to injection to know if fluid is expected on aspiration. If no fluid is aspirated or known fluid is present via ultrasound verification, inject 0.5–1.0 mL 7.5% bupivacaine diluted into 9 mL of 0.9% NaCl (amount of bupivacaine depends on the size of the animal). Your total dosage should not exceed 2 mg/kg.

Brachial plexus block

Indications

The brachial plexus nerve block is for procedures occurring distal to the elbow (Protocols 44.6 and 44.7).

Contraindications

Injuries or procedures proximal to the elbow, coagulopathy, and thrombocytopenia are the contraindications. General anesthesia is usually required, so this block may be of limited use in the emergency patient.

Complications

Hemorrhage, incomplete nerve block, and brachial plexus nerve damage are the complications.

Intraperitoneal blocks

Indications

Most intraperitoneal blocks (Protocol 44.8) are performed in animals that have severe abdominal pain secondary to pancreatitis.

Contraindications

Septic abdomen, abdominal wall hernia, thrombocytopenia, and coagulopathy are all contraindications.

Complications

Failure of blockage due to dilution of the local anesthetic within the peritoneal cavity, pain on injection, septic abdomen, and hemoabdomen are complications.

Infraorbital, mandibular, and mental nerve blocks

Indications

The infraorbital nerve block (Protocol 44.9) numbs the maxilla on the side of the block, including the teeth cranial to the maxillary first molar.[35] The mandibular nerve block (Protocol 44.10) numbs the mandible cranial to the injection site, including the teeth and tongue on the affected side.[35] The mental nerve block (Protocol 44.11) numbs the skin, bone, and teeth of the mandible cranial to the second premolar on the ipsilateral side (Fig. 44.4A).[35]

Contraindications

The mandibular nerve block frequently needs to be done under anesthesia and therefore has limited value in the emergency patient. The infraorbital nerve block and mental nerve block should be performed under heavy sedation. Mental nerve blocks for dental work involving symphyseal fractures may not cause complete analgesia of the symphyseal fracture site because the mental nerve innervates the lateral mandible.[8,35]

Complications

Incomplete nerve block, hemorrhage, and permanent nerve damage are complications. Permanent nerve damage could cause lip drooping and numbness, which could cause self-trauma if the animal accidentally bites or chews its lip.

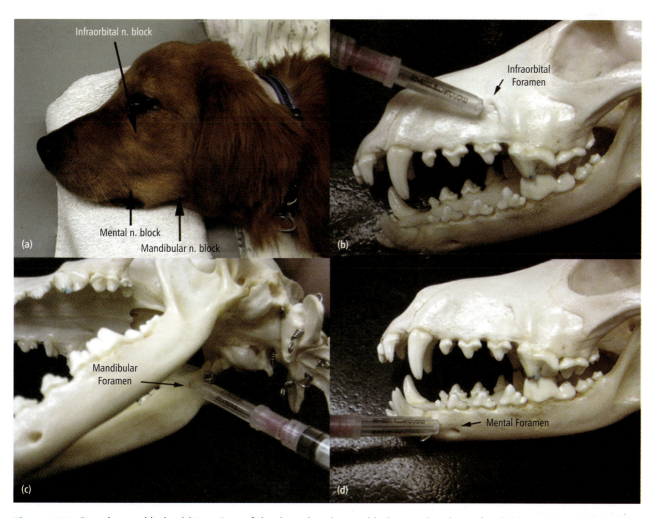

Figure 44.4 Dental nerve blocks. (a) Locations of the three dental nerve blocks on a live dog: infraorbital, mental, and mandibular nerve blocks. (b) Infraorbital block. Skull picture depicting location of the infraorbital foramen. (c) Mandibular block. Skull picture depicting location of the mandibular foramen. (d) Mental block. Skull picture depicting location of the mental foramen.

Protocol 44.9 Infraorbital block (see Fig. 44.5)

Procedure
1. Aseptically prepare site.
2. Lift the patients lip and palpate the infraorbital foramen, which can be located dorsal to the rostral edge of the upper forth premolar (see Fig. 44.4B).
3. Using 1–2 mL of 2% lidocaine or 7.5% bupivacaine, or a mixture of both, insert a 22-gauge, 1-inch needle (or 25-gauge, ⅝-inch needle, depending on the size of the patient) into the infraorbital space.
4. Once you have entered the infraorbital space, insert the entirety of the needle, and aspirate; if no blood is observed, inject desired drug.

Protocol 44.11 Mental block

Procedure
1. The mental foramen is caudal and ventral to the canine tooth (see Fig. 44.4D).
2. Insert a 25-gauge, ⅝-inch needle intraorally, parallel to the teeth, rostral to the mental foramen.
3. Aspirate; if no blood is observed, inject 0.5–1.0 mL of 2% lidocaine or 0.5–1.0 mL of 7.5% bupivacaine or a mixture of both. Do not exceed a total dose of 2 mg/kg.

Protocol 44.10 Mandibular block

Procedure
1. Place your patient in lateral recumbency with the affected side up.
2. Open the patient's mouth and advance your index finger on the medial aspect of the ramus of the mandible, to the palpable lip of the mandibular foramen, which is caudal to the third molar (see Fig. 44.4C). The mandibular nerve is usually palpable at this point.
3. With your index finger in place, using aseptic technique, use your other hand on the exterior of the mouth, at the point of the mandibular foramen. Under the jaw insert a 25-gauge, ⅝-inch, or a 22-gauge, 1-inch needle (size of needle depends on size of patient) at the lower angle of the jaw slightly rostral to the angular process on the medial aspect of the ramus. You should be able to feel the tip of the needle with your index finger that is inside the patient's mouth.[36]
4. Once the needle has been palpated, aspirate; if no blood is observed, inject 1–2 mL of 2% lidocaine or 1–2 mL 7.5% bupivacaine, or a mixture of both, remembering not to exceed a total dose of 2 mg/kg.

direct nerve injury are contraindications. Complications: include hemorrhage, incomplete block, and nerve damage.

Epidural and epidural catheter

Indications

Epidural blocks (Protocols 44.14–44.16) can be performed when a patient has pelvic limb pain, abdominal pain, thoracic pain, or thoracic limb pain.

Contraindications

Local infection, systemic infection, severe pelvic fractures that disrupt the anatomy, coagulopathy, thrombocytopenia, and hypotension are contraindications. This procedure must be performed under general anesthesia.

Complications

Complications include infection, bleeding, incomplete block, urine retention if using opioids, and intercostal nerve root paralysis if using a large volume and a local anesthetic is included. It is recommended that the concentration of bupivacaine not exceed 0.25% if the catheter placement is near the thoracic vertebrae.[28]

Troubleshooting

If an epidural catheter stops functioning, first radiograph the animal to determine if placement of the catheter is correct. Fluoroscopy may be more helpful than a radiograph because of the ability to move the animal around to help determine placement. If the catheter appears in place, attempt to gently flush with sterile saline. If this does not work, then attempt flushing with saline as the epidural catheter is slowly removed. Do not force or advance the epidural catheter back in once it has been removed from the epidural space. The epidural catheter should be removed and placement of a new catheter may be placed.[28,36,38]

Femoral and sciatic nerve block

Indications

The femoral and sciatic nerve blocks (Protocols 44.12 and 44.13) are useful for procedures including the stifle and distal to the stifle.

Contraindications

Infection at the injection site, coagulopathy, thrombocytopenia, inability to use contralateral hind limb, and

Protocol 44.12 Femoral nerve block with the use of a nerve locator

Procedure
1. Place patient in lateral recumbency with the affected leg up (Fig. 44.5).
2. Abduct leg at a 90° angle and extend caudally.
3. Clip and aseptically prepare the area.
4. Attach the nerve locator surface electrode to the patient.
5. Prime the insulated needle delivery system with bupivacaine.
6. Using aseptic technique, palpate the femoral artery. The nerve lies underneath the medial belly of the sartorius muscle and is about 0.5–1.0 cm deep.
7. Using a 40-mm insulated needle, insert the needle cranial to the femoral artery and medial to the sartorius muscle.
8. Once you have entered the skin, place the nerve locator on the uninsulated part of the needle.
9. Turn the nerve locator on and place at a setting of 1–2 mA (2 Hz).
10. The needle should be advanced toward the iliopsoas muscle at a 20–30° angle.
11. Recall that the nerve lies underneath the medial belly of the sartorius muscle and is about 0.5–1.0 cm deep.
12. Once you observe twitches of the quadriceps muscle and extension of the stifle, slowly start to decrease the setting on the nerve locator until you achieve the same desired effect. Your goal is to achieve this desired effect at 0.5 mA. If you are still getting a twitch below 0.5 mA, you increase the risk of an intraneural injection, which is not desirable and may cause neuritis of nerve damage.
13. Aspirate; if no blood is present, inject 0.1 mL/kg of 7.5% bupivacaine. The injection should be smooth and without resistance. If you are having difficulty injecting the drug, the needle may be in the nerve.
14. Slowly withdraw the needle. If you are still obtaining the desired effect on the nerve locator, aspirate; if no blood is present, inject again testing for resistance. If no resistance is appreciated, inject the remainder of the drug.[37]

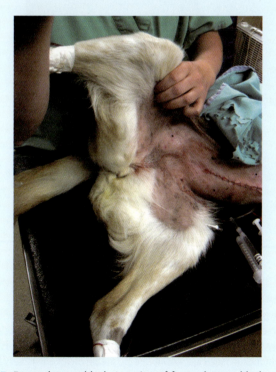

Figure 44.5 Femoral nerve block. Location of femoral nerve block on up leg.

Protocol 44.13 Sciatic nerve block with the use of a nerve locator

Procedure
1. Place the patient in lateral recumbency with the affected leg up.
2. Palpate the ischiatic tuberosity and the greater trochanter of the femur (see Fig. 44.6).
3. Clip and aseptically prepare the site.
4. Attach the nerve locator surface electrode to the patient.
5. Prime the insulated needle delivery system with bupivacaine.
6. Insert a 40-mm insulated needle perpendicular to the skin with an ever so slight angle between the ischiatic tuberosity and the greater trochanter.
7. Attach the nerve locator to the uninsulated part of the needle.
8. Turn the nerve locator on at 1–2 mA (2 Hz).
9. Slowly advance the needle until you get dorsiflexion or plantar flexion of the foot. Once flexion is noted, start to decrease the setting of the nerve locator until you get the same desired effect at 0.5 mA. A positive stimulation <0.5 mA may indicate an intraneural needle placement.
10. Aspirate; if no blood is observed; inject 0.05 mL/kg of 7.5% bupivacaine. There should be no resistance on injection. If you are having difficulty injecting the drug, the needle may be in the nerve. Slowly withdraw the needle. If you are still obtaining the desired effect on the nerve locator, aspirate; if no blood is present, inject again testing for resistance. If no resistance is appreciated, inject the remainder of the drug.[37]

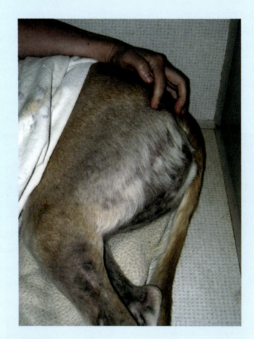

Figure 44.6 Sciatic nerve block. Location of sciatic nerve block on a live dog.

Protocol 44.14 Epidural

Procedure
1. The patient should be placed in either sternal or lateral recumbency depending on the operator's preference. Some people extend the pelvic limbs cranially to possibly increase the size of the epidural space; this is a personal preference.
2. Clip an area at the lumbosacral junction (see Figs. 44.7A and B). Sterile technique is very important in this procedure, so clip an adequate area that allows aseptic technique.
3. Aseptically prepare the skin.
4. After washing hands and while donning sterile gloves, palpate the wings of the ilium with your thumb and middle finger. Using the index finger, palpate the spinous process of the seventh lumbar vertebra.
5. Slide the index finger caudally down the spinous process until the lumbosacral space is palpable. A slight divot can usually be palpated here between L7 and S1.

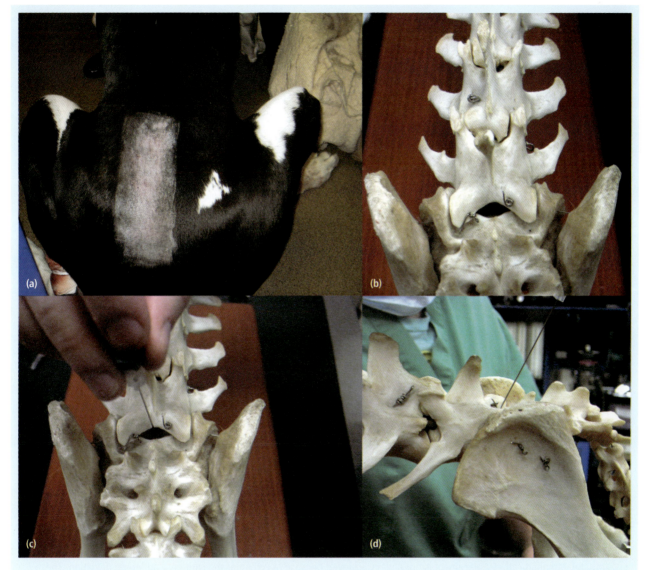

Figure 44.7 Epidural block. (a) Location of an epidural on a live dog. (b) Location of an epidural on a dog skeleton. (c) Location of needle placement on a dog skeleton: dorsal view. (d) Location of needle placement on a dog skeleton: lateral view.

6. Keeping the index finger in place (to maintain positioning), insert a 20- or 22-gauge, 1.5- to 3.0-inch spinal needle (length and size of needle depend on patient size) perpendicular to the skin, ensuring the needle is precisely on midline in 360°.
7. Continue to advance the spinal needle slowly, adjusting the needle angle as needed either cranially or caudally, to ensure proper placement in the epidural space (see Figs. 44.7C and 44.7D).
8. The epidural space sits just ventral to the ligamentum flavum. As the needle is advanced through the ligamentum flavum, usually a "pop" can be felt, although this is not a completely reliable indicator.
9. To ensure correct epidural placement of the needle's tip, remove the stylet, and using a *glass* syringe, which provides little to no resistance, inject a small amount of air (0.25–1.0 mL depending on patient size). While injecting air, there should be no resistance and no back pressure on the plunger of the syringe. If resistance or back pressure on the plunger is appreciated, you are most likely not in the epidural space. Repeat the preceding steps to obtain proper placement.
10. Another method of verifying correct needle placement is by using the "hanging drop" technique. This technique is best performed with the patient in sternal recumbency. Once the needle is placed in the skin, remove the stylet and fill the hub of the needle with saline or local anesthetic. Once you are in the epidural space, the fluid in your needle will drop into the epidural space. This technique is not 100% accurate because tissue plugs can obstruct the needle.

(Continued)

11. Once correct needle placement is verified, examine the needle for blood or cerebrospinal fluid (CSF). If none is observed, gently aspirate the needle to reconfirm absence of blood and CSF.
12. Slowly inject the opioid of choice (refer to Table 44.1). It should inject freely with no resistance, similar to an IV injection. If resistance is experienced, you are most likely not in the epidural space and you will need to repeat the preceding process.
13. Follow the opioid with bupivacaine 7.5%, 0.1–0.4 mg/kg; this too should inject with no resistance. If resistance is noted, you are most likely not in the epidural space and will need to repeat the process.
14. Once you have administered the drugs, remove needle, and place the patient with affected side down, allowing the drugs to disperse to the desired location.[38]

Protocol 44.15 Epidural catheter placement

Procedure
1. Epidural catheter kits are available with most if not all the components needed for the placement of the epidural catheter (see Fig. 44.8).
2. The procedure is fairly similar to that of an epidural, but in place of a regular spinal needle, a Tuohy needle is used. The curved tip of the needle allows the catheter to be passed in the appropriate direction (cranially) after needle insertion.
3. Follow the procedure for performing an epidural injection. However, replace the regular spinal needle with a Tuohy spinal needle.
4. Once in the epidural space, remove the stylet and pass the epidural catheter through the Tuohy needle.
5. The tip of the epidural catheter should be placed in close proximity to the painful area. Therefore, premeasuring the catheter prior to placement is important.
6. Remove the Tuohy needle while leaving the catheter in place.
7. Although not an absolute guarantee of correct placement, a radiograph can be performed to verify placement of the epidural catheter. Intended catheter placement is not always achieved because of coiling of the catheter and lateral deviation. The presence of an epidural catheter decreases the likelihood of failure, but it does not guarantee 100% success. If proper placement was not obtained, repeat steps 1–5.
8. It is important to keep the insertion port of the catheter clean and sterile at all times. The insertion site should be covered with a sterile bandage, and aseptic technique should be used when delivering drugs through the insertion port. Reapplication of a sterile bandage should be applied whenever administration of drugs is performed. The insertion site should be inspected daily for inflammation and infection.

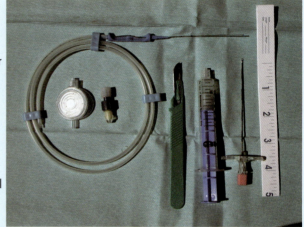

Figure 44.8 Picture of the components of an epidural catheter kit.

Protocol 44.16 Continuous epidural drug infusion[8]

Procedure
1. Dilute preservative-free morphine to 0.5 mg/mL with 0.9% saline.
2. Mix 1 mL of 0.75% bupivicaine with 5 mL of 0.5 mg/mL dilute morphine.
3. Deliver solution at 0.03–0.05 mL/kg/hr.
4. If rear limb paralysis occurs, change concentration of solution to 1 mL of 0.75% bupivicaine in 11 mL of 0.5 mg/mL dilute morphine and deliver at above rate.

Summary

Local analgesia can greatly enhance the overall analgesia in the emergent or critically ill patient. Because local analgesic techniques may aid in decreasing systemic drug requirements, the risk of patient decompensation secondary to sedation, heavy systemic analgesia, or anesthesia is minimized.

References

1. Quandt JE, Rawlings CR. Reducing postoperative pain for dogs: local anesthetic and analgesic techniques. Compendium 1996;18(2):101–111.
2. Kirk RW, Bistner SI. Handbook of veterinary procedures and emergency treatment. 4th ed. Philadelphia, PA: WB Saunders, 1985.
3. Shoemaker WC. Diagnosis and treatment of shock and circulatory dysfunction. In: Shoemaker WC, Ayres SM, Grenvik A, Holbrook PR, eds. Textbook of critical care. 4th ed. Philadelphia, PA: WB Saunders, 2000:85–102.
4. Evans AT. Precautions when using opioid agonist analgesics. In: Haskins SC, Klide AM, eds. The Veterinary Clinics of North America Opinions in Small Animal Anesthesia. Philadelphia, PA: WB Saunders,1992:362–363.
5. Benson GJ, Tranquilli WJ. Advantages and guidelines for using opioid agonist-antagonist analgesics. In: Haskins SC, Klide AM, eds. The Veterinary Clinics of North America Opinions in Small Animal Anesthesia. Philadelphia, PA: WB Saunders, 1992:363–365.
6. Klide AM. Precautions when using alpha-2 as anesthetics or anesthetic adjuvants. In: Haskins SC, Klide AM, eds. The Veterinary Clinics of North America Opinions in Small Animal Anesthesia. Philadelphia, PA: WB Saunders, 1992:294–295.
7. Blaze CA, Glowaski MM. Veterinary Anesthesia Drug Quick Reference. St. Louis, MO: Elsevier Saunders, 2004.
8. Gaynor J, Muir WW. Handbook of Veterinary Pain Management. 2nd ed. St. Louis, MO, Mosby, 2008.
9. Klide AM, Calderwood HW, Soma LR. Cardiopulmonary effects of xylazine in dogs. Am J Vet Res 1975;36(7):931–935.
10. Klide AM. Cardiopulmonary effects of enflurane and isoflurane in the dog. Am J Vet Res 1976;37(2):127–131.
11. Ko JCH, Golder FJ, Mandsager RE, et al. Anesthetic and cardiorespiratory effects of a 1:1 mixture of propofol and thiopental sodium in dogs. J Am Vet Med Assoc 1999;215(9):1292–1296.
12. Kontos HA, Richardson DW, Paterson JL. Vasodilator effects of hypercapnic acidosis on human forearm blood vessels. Am J Physiol 1968;215(6):1403–1405.
13. Kontos HA, Thames MD, Lombana A, et al. Vasodilator effects of local hypercapnic acidosis in dog skeletal muscle. Am J Physiol 1971;220(6):1569–1572.
14. Miller RD. Anesthesia. 5th ed. Philadelphia, PA: Churchill Livingstone; 2000.
15. Muir W, Hubbell J. Handbook of Veterinary Anesthesia. 4th ed. St. Louis, MO: Mosby, 2006.
16. Pypendop B, Verstegen J. Cardiorespiratory effects of a combination of medetomidine, midazolam, and butorphanol in dogs. Am J Vet Res 1999;60(9):1148–1154.
17. Quandt JE, Robinson EP, Rivers WJ, et al. Cardiorespiratory and anesthetic effects of propofol and thiopental in dogs. Am J Vet Res 1998;59(9):1137–1143.
18. Tranquilli WJ, Thurman JC, Grimm KA. Lumb and Jones Veterinary Anesthesia. 4th ed. Baltimore, MD: Lippincott Williams & Wilkins, 2007.
19. Waxman K, Shoemaker WC, Lippmann M. Cardiovascular effects of anesthetic induction with ketamine. Anesth Analg 1980;59(5):355–358.
20. Weiskopf RB, Bogetz MS, Roizen MF, et al. Cardiovascular and metabolic sequelae of inducting anesthesia with ketamine or thiopental in hypovolemic swine. Anesthesiology 1984;60:214–219.
21. Thurmon JC, Tranqulli WJ, Benson GJ. Local and regional anesthetic and analgesic techniques. In: Skarda RT, ed. Essentials of Small Animal Anesthesia & Analgesia. Baltimore, MD: Lippincott, 1999:204–220.
22. Mama KR. Local anesthetics. In: Gaynor J, Muir W, eds. Handbook of Veterinary Pain Management. 2nd ed. St. Louis, MO, Mosby, 2008:221–239.
23. Lemke KA, Dawson SD. Local and regional anesthesia. In: Mathews KA, ed. Veterinary Clinics of North America: Small Animal Practice. Vol. 30. Philadelphia, PA: WB Saunders, 2000:839–850.
24. Liu PL, Feldman HS, Giasi R, et al. Comparative CNS toxicity of lidocaine, etidocaine, bupivacaine, and tetracaine in awake dogs following rapid intravenous administration. Anesth Analg 1983;62:375–379.
25. Benoit PW. Reversible skeletal muscle damage after administration of local anesthetics with and without epinephrine. J Oral Surg 1978; 36:198–201.
26. Chadwick HS. Toxicity and resuscitation in lidocaine- or bupivicaine-infused cats. Anesthesiology 1985;63:385–390.
27. Joshi W, Reuben SS, Kilaru PR, et al. Postoperative analgesia for outpatient arthroscopic knee surgery with intraarticular clonidine and/or morphine. Anesth Analg 2000; 90(5):1102–1106.
28. Hanson BD. Epidural catheter analgesia in dogs and cats: technique and review of 182 cases (1991–1999). JVECCS 2001;11(2):95–103.
29. Zink W, Graf BM. Local anesthetic myotoxicity. Reg Anesth Pain Med 2004;29:333–340.
30. Brower MC, Johnson ME. Adverse effects of local anesthetic infiltration on wound healing. Reg Anesth Pain Med 2003;28:233–240.
31. Bernard F, Kudnig ST, Monnet E. Hemodynamic effects of interpleural lidocaine and bupivicaine combination in anesthetized dogs with and without an open pericardium. Vet Surg 2006;35(3):252–258.
32. Kushner LI, Trim CM, Madhusudhan S, et al. Evaluation of the hemodynamic effects of interpleural bupivacaine in dogs. Vet Surg 1995;24:180–187.
33. Thompson SE, Johnson JM. Analgesia in dogs after intercostal thoracotomy. A comparison of morphine, selective intercostal nerve block, and interpleural regional analgesia with bupivicaine. Vet Surg 1991; 20:73–77.
34. Lemke KA, Creighton CM. Paravertebral blockade of the brachial plexus in dogs. In: Mathews KA, ed. Veterinary Clinics of North America: Small Animal Practice. Vol 38. Philadelphia, PA: WB Saunders, 2008:1231–1241.
35. Beckman B, Legendre L. Regional nerve blocks for oral surgery in companion animals. Compendium 2002;24(6):439–444.
36. Muir WW, Hubbell JA, Skarda RT, et al. Local anesthesia in cats and dogs. In: Muir WW, Hubbell JA, Skarda RT, et al. eds. Handbook of Veterinary Anesthesia. 3rd ed. St. Louis, MO: Mosby, 2000:100–118.
37. International Veterinary Information Service Web site. Campoy L. Fundamentals of regional anesthesia using nerve stimulation in the dog. www.ivis.org (accessed June 2010).
38. Valerde A. Epidural analgesia and anesthesia in dogs and cats. In: Mathews KA, ed. Veterinary Clinics of North America: Small Animal Practice. Vol 38. Philadelphia, PA: WB Saunders, 2008:1205–1230.

45

Monitoring the anesthetized patient

Benjamin M. Brainard and Julie Denton-Schmiedt

Anesthetic monitoring of the critically ill patient is an important aspect of veterinary critical care. No single measured variable provides a full picture of the animal's status; each piece of monitoring data is part of a larger picture, which, taken as a whole, reflects the condition of a patient under general anesthesia. Although single values may be useful, trends of measured physical parameters are more commonly used to guide decisions for anesthetic adjustments. Critically ill patients are either at risk of, or already experiencing, compromise of the body's ability to maintain homeostasis and tissue oxygen delivery. Many of the drugs used for anesthesia contribute directly to additional physiologic derangements that, if left uncorrected, may worsen patient status. In addition, many critically ill animals cannot tolerate high levels of single anesthetic drugs (such as inhalant anesthetics), and the anesthetist must continually monitor the patient's response to ensure that anesthesia and analgesia are adequate for the duration of the procedure, especially when using multiple intravenous (IV) drugs to supplement or maintain anesthesia.

The most common perturbations expected in the anesthetized critical patient are hypoxemia, hypotension, hypoventilation, cardiac arrhythmias, acidosis, and volume overload.

Hypoxemia may be present prior to anesthesia in some cases, and in others it may develop during anesthesia. Common intraoperative events that can result in hypoxemia may be patient related (e.g., pneumothorax, pulmonary embolism, pulmonary edema) or may be machine failure (i.e., inadequate supply of oxygen, malfunctioning flow meter, or a circuit disconnect). Systemic oxygenation can be monitored with arterial blood

gas analysis and estimated with pulse oximetry. Normal oxygen saturation (SO_2) in an animal breathing 100% oxygen should not be less than 98%. An ideal PaO_2 for a patient breathing 100% oxygen is 500 mm Hg, although V/Q mismatch from atelectasis and other causes (e.g., physiologic shunts) usually makes this slightly lower. An SpO_2 below 95% should spur a re-evaluation of the patient for problems that may result in hypoxemia.

Most anesthetic drugs are potent respiratory depressants, and hypoventilation is a common occurrence in the anesthetized or sedated patient. Measurement of ventilation (CO_2 levels) can be accomplished using arterial blood gas analysis and estimated with end-tidal carbon dioxide monitoring ($ETCO_2$). $ETCO_2$ greater than 55 mm Hg is an indication to identify patient problems that may result in decreased tidal volumes (e.g., pneumothorax, unibronchial intubation) and to evaluate the machine for problems such as stuck valves or expired soda lime (this will usually result in an increased inspired CO_2 as well).

Cardiac arrhythmias can be secondary to myocardial hypoxemia or hypoperfusion, or due to systemic acidosis. They can also occur in response to specific anesthetic drugs such as thiopental or ketamine. Electrocardiogram (ECG) monitoring will give information on both cardiac rhythm as well as any conduction disturbances. Some arrhythmias, such as ventricular tachycardia or R on T phenomena, may require drug therapy during the anesthetic period.

Critically ill animals are frequently anesthetized prior to full resuscitation from shock. A shock state represents decreased tissue oxygen delivery and is usually accompanied by a metabolic acidosis. Resuscitation will have

Advanced Monitoring and Procedures for Small Animal Emergency and Critical Care, First Edition. Edited by Jamie M. Burkitt Creedon, Harold Davis.
© 2012 John Wiley & Sons, Inc. Published 2012 by John Wiley & Sons, Inc.

to continue into the anesthetic period, and frequent monitoring of blood gas values and lactate concentration will allow assessment of systemic perfusion and oxygen delivery. Keeping a record of intraoperative blood loss (which is not necessarily represented by packed cell volume/total solids [PCV/TS] measures) will give an indication of the need for transfusions of fresh whole blood or packed red blood cells (RBCs) to maintain oxygen delivery.

Although many critically ill patients will benefit from expanded intravascular volume, some risk hypervolemia from excessive crystalloid administration, and others risk the development of edema if they are hypoproteinemic. In patients who may be at risk for hypervolemia, the placement of a jugular catheter will allow the measurement of central venous pressure (CVP), which estimates the pressure and volume in the right side of the heart. As the CVP approaches 8 cm H_2O, the patient is approaching fluid overload and may be at risk for pulmonary edema and congestive heart failure. Hypoalbuminemic patients can have the colloid osmotic pressure (COP) measured; if the COP is less than 15 mm Hg, it is indicated to include colloid as part of the fluid therapy plan.

The most important tools of the anesthetist are his or her senses. Palpation of the pulse and observation of the mucous membranes give information about perfusion, oxygenation, and blood pressure. Assessment of eye position, jaw tone, and palpebral reflex give information about the patient's anesthetic depth, and auscultation of the Doppler pulse or the ECG beep can alert the anesthetist to the development of cardiac arrhythmias. To supplement the senses and allow objective evaluation of the anesthetized patient, monitoring devices are available.

Anesthetists should place emphasis on physical parameters and physical assessment of the patient. Jaw tone, pulse rate and pulse quality, mucous membrane color, and other types of hands-on information can be much more accurate and important than a number read from a monitoring screen. In addition, the anesthetist should perform a thorough physical examination of the patient and be familiar with the proposed procedure prior to premedication for anesthesia. Table 45.1 lists normal ranges for commonly measured physical examination parameters.

When the anesthetist notes abnormal monitoring values, a series of steps should be followed. First, a brief physical examination should be performed to assess the patient. Second, the abnormal values should be verified (e.g., by readjusting the pulse oximeter probe or repeating a blood pressure). This process should take less than 1 minute to accomplish. With verification of

Table 45.1 Normal values for physiologic parameters in awake dogs and cats

Parameter	Dog	Cat
Heart rate	70–110 bpm	120–200 bpm
Respiratory rate	12–20 breath/min	12–20 breath/min
Rectal temperature	99.5–101.5°F	100–102°F
PaO_2 (at sea level)	85–100 mm Hg	95–115 mm Hg
SpO_2	97%–100%	97%–100%
$PaCO_2$	35–45 mm Hg	30–40 mm Hg
$ETCO_2$	30–40 mm Hg	30–40 mm Hg
Systolic blood pressure	90–140 mm Hg	90–150 mm Hg
Mean blood pressure	60–100 mm Hg	60–100 mm Hg
Diastolic blood pressure	50–75 mm Hg	60–100 mm Hg

abnormal values, specific therapy should be instituted. In the event of problems with oxygenation or ventilation, it should be verified that the anesthetic machine is functioning properly (i.e., that the delivery of oxygen has not been interrupted or that any valves are stuck) and that an acute change has not happened to the patient (e.g., a pneumothorax or pulmonary aspiration). If there is a problem with the machine, an Ambu bag can be used to maintain ventilation while the machine is switched, and anesthesia may be maintained with IV methods.

If hypotension is detected, in addition to verifying proper cuff placement or arterial catheter function, the patient assessment must include an evaluation of the depth of anesthesia. An assessment of the circulating blood volume of the patient should also be made. If hypovolemia is probable, the anesthetist can consider a bolus of IV fluids (either crystalloid or colloid) and should discuss with the surgeon if it is indicated to consider other fluids such as packed RBCs or fresh frozen plasma (or whole blood). The possibility exists in some cases that IV pressor or inotropic agents may be necessary for therapy of intraoperative hypotension.

Anesthesia monitoring record

The physiologic data gathered before, during, and after anesthesia is recorded on the anesthesia monitoring record. This record is a legal document and an important part of the medical record. Anesthesia monitoring sheets for a practice should be standardized with sections for patient name and signalment, and areas for preanesthetic history and laboratory values. This allows quick access of this information during the anesthetic period. A sample anesthetic record is shown in Figure 45.1. Separate sections of the anesthetic record should also be available to describe the type of drugs administered, dosage administered, and the effect on the patient for the premedication, induction, maintenance, and recovery phases of anesthesia. An area for notes or descriptions of events that occurred during the anesthetic episode is also necessary. Documentation should always be in ink and should be as complete as possible. Although some human hospitals and veterinary practices use a computer-based anesthetic record, these are not in widespread veterinary use at this time. A carbon copy form or other mechanism to create a duplicate of the record is also useful. One copy may stay with the record, and another may be catalogued separately in an anesthesia database.

A well-organized record allows veterinary technicians and veterinarians to quickly review the anesthetic record in the event of problems in the perioperative period. Accurate recording of the entire anesthetic episode also provides a reference for future anesthetics in the same patient. If a patient had a previous difficult intubation or adverse reaction to premedicant drugs, a review of the previous anesthetic record will highlight these facts for future anesthetists. For example, if a patient experienced severe hypotension while being anesthetized with propofol, a less vasodilating induction protocol (e.g., using ketamine and diazepam) may be chosen for the next anesthetic. Likewise, if a patient experienced arrhythmias during induction with thiopental, a different induction agent could be chosen. If an animal, after premedication with a potent opioid during a prior anesthetic, became apneic and required immediate intubation, it is indicated to modify future protocols to prevent such an occurrence.

Patient monitoring as it pertains to the anesthetic procedure begins with administration of the premedication drug or combination of drugs. The premedication regimen, route of administration (IM, IV, SC), and the effect of the drugs on the patient should be recorded. Events such as emesis, defecation, bradycardia, excitation, or sedation are particularly important to note. If animals experience emesis prior to the securing of a protected airway, they may be in danger of aspiration pneumonia, and oxygenation will have to be closely monitored in the intra- and postoperative period. As noted earlier, if there are adverse responses to the chosen anesthetic protocol (e.g., respiratory arrest, abnormal excitation, or aggressive behavior), these should be

noted so that similar protocols may be avoided in the future.

Monitoring of the patient continues into induction. The type and amount of induction agent(s) used, as well as route of administration, should be noted. Any adverse effects during induction (e.g., emesis, arrhythmias, hypotension, or excitation) are important to note, in addition to any difficulties associated with endotracheal intubation (this may also be graded on a scale of 1 to 4, with 1 representing a smooth intubation and 4 representing the most difficult intubation). There should be a place on the anesthetic record to note the size of endotracheal (ET) tube used for intubation.

Patient monitoring during the maintenance phase of anesthesia is extremely important, and parameters such as the heart rate, respiratory rate, blood pressure, temperature, end-tidal CO_2, oxygen flow rate, and end-tidal inhalant (if available) or delivered inhalant percentage should be recorded at 5-minute intervals or more frequently. If acute changes occur, these should be noted on the record as well. The type and amount of fluid therapy should also be recorded, in addition to any adjunctive drugs used during anesthesia (e.g., fentanyl or dopamine administered as a constant rate infusion [CRI]). Notes should be made in the anesthetic record about adjustments in fluid therapy, changes in anesthetic depth, changes in position or recumbency, occurrence of reflux, administration of additional drugs, surgical progress, or any other event that occurred during the anesthetic episode. The time of extubation, postoperative analgesic therapy, and other pertinent details are recorded on the recovery section of the sheet. Following extubation, patient monitoring should continue until the body temperature reaches a satisfactory level (>99°F [37.2°C]) and the patient is able to perform purposeful movement such as swallowing. During the recovery phase of anesthesia, measurement of temperature, pulse rate, and respiration rate should take place no less frequently than every 15 minutes.

Physical parameters under anesthesia

Anesthetic depth is most accurately monitored by serial physical examination of the anesthetized patient. Small animal patients progress through a predictable series of physical changes as they become more deeply anesthetized, and they encounter these signs in reverse as they become more lightly anesthetized (see Fig. 45.2). These stages are labeled with Roman numerals: I represents an awake animal through to V, which represents a dangerously deeply anesthetized animal (Fig. 45.2). Because some physical parameters can be similar between animals that are relatively lightly anesthetized and those

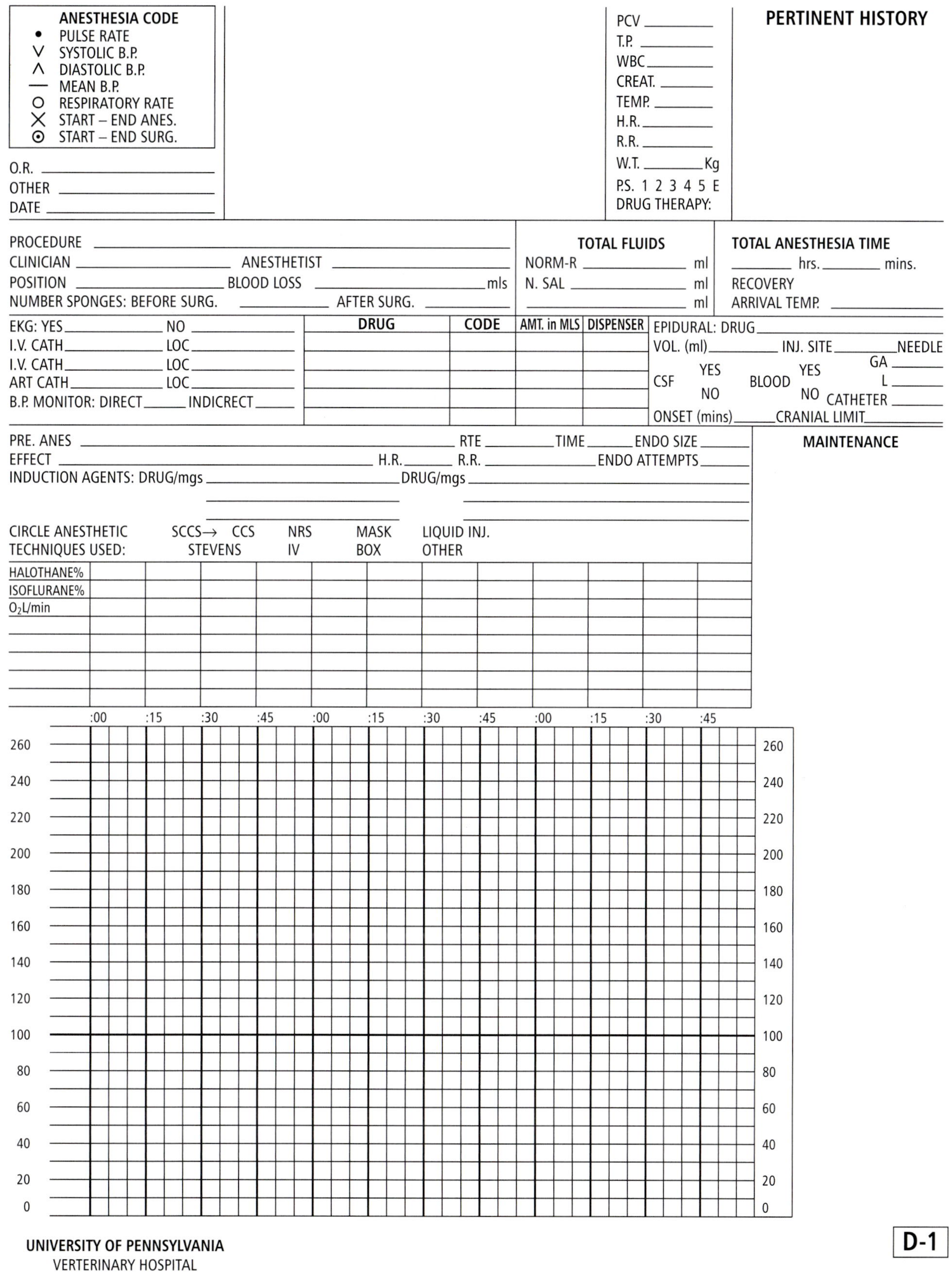

ANESTHESIA CODE
- • PULSE RATE
- V SYSTOLIC B.P.
- ∧ DIASTOLIC B.P.
- — MEAN B.P.
- O RESPIRATORY RATE
- X START – END ANES.
- ⊙ START – END SURG.

O.R. _____
OTHER _____
DATE _____

PCV _____
T.P. _____
WBC _____
CREAT. _____
TEMP. _____
H.R. _____
R.R. _____
W.T. _____ Kg
P.S. 1 2 3 4 5 E
DRUG THERAPY:

PERTINENT HISTORY

PROCEDURE _____
CLINICIAN _____ ANESTHETIST _____
POSITION _____ BLOOD LOSS _____ mls
NUMBER SPONGES: BEFORE SURG. _____ AFTER SURG. _____

TOTAL FLUIDS
NORM-R _____ ml
N. SAL _____ ml
_____ ml

TOTAL ANESTHESIA TIME
_____ hrs. _____ mins.
RECOVERY
ARRIVAL TEMP. _____

EKG: YES _____ NO _____
I.V. CATH _____ LOC _____
I.V. CATH _____ LOC _____
ART CATH _____ LOC _____
B.P. MONITOR: DIRECT _____ INDICRECT _____

DRUG	CODE	AMT. in MLS	DISPENSER

EPIDURAL: DRUG _____
VOL. (ml) _____ INJ. SITE _____ NEEDLE
CSF   YES / NO   BLOOD   YES / NO   GA _____ L _____ CATHETER _____
ONSET (mins) _____ CRANIAL LIMIT _____

PRE. ANES _____ RTE _____ TIME _____ ENDO SIZE _____
EFFECT _____ H.R. _____ R.R. _____ ENDO ATTEMPTS _____
INDUCTION AGENTS: DRUG/mgs _____ DRUG/mgs _____

MAINTENANCE

CIRCLE ANESTHETIC TECHNIQUES USED: SCCS→ CCS   NRS   MASK   LIQUID INJ.
STEVENS   IV   BOX   OTHER

HALOTHANE%											
ISOFLURANE%											
O₂L/min											

:00 :15 :30 :45 :00 :15 :30 :45 :00 :15 :30 :45

260 240 220 200 180 160 140 120 100 80 60 40 20 0

UNIVERSITY OF PENNSYLVANIA
VERTERINARY HOSPITAL

D-1

Figure 45.1 Typical anesthesia record. Note provision of areas for preoperative history and blood work, American Society of Anesthesiologists (ASA) classification, planned procedure, and patient identification. The anesthetist can record the blood pressure and other parameters using the grid and the legend in the upper left corner. There are spaces to note preoperative and induction medications, as well as a space to note the quality of recovery. The open area on the right side allows the anesthetist to take notes during the procedure and is referenced to numbers written on the timeline of the grid. Note also spaces available for notation of SpO₂, ETCO₂, and percentage inhalant administered.

575

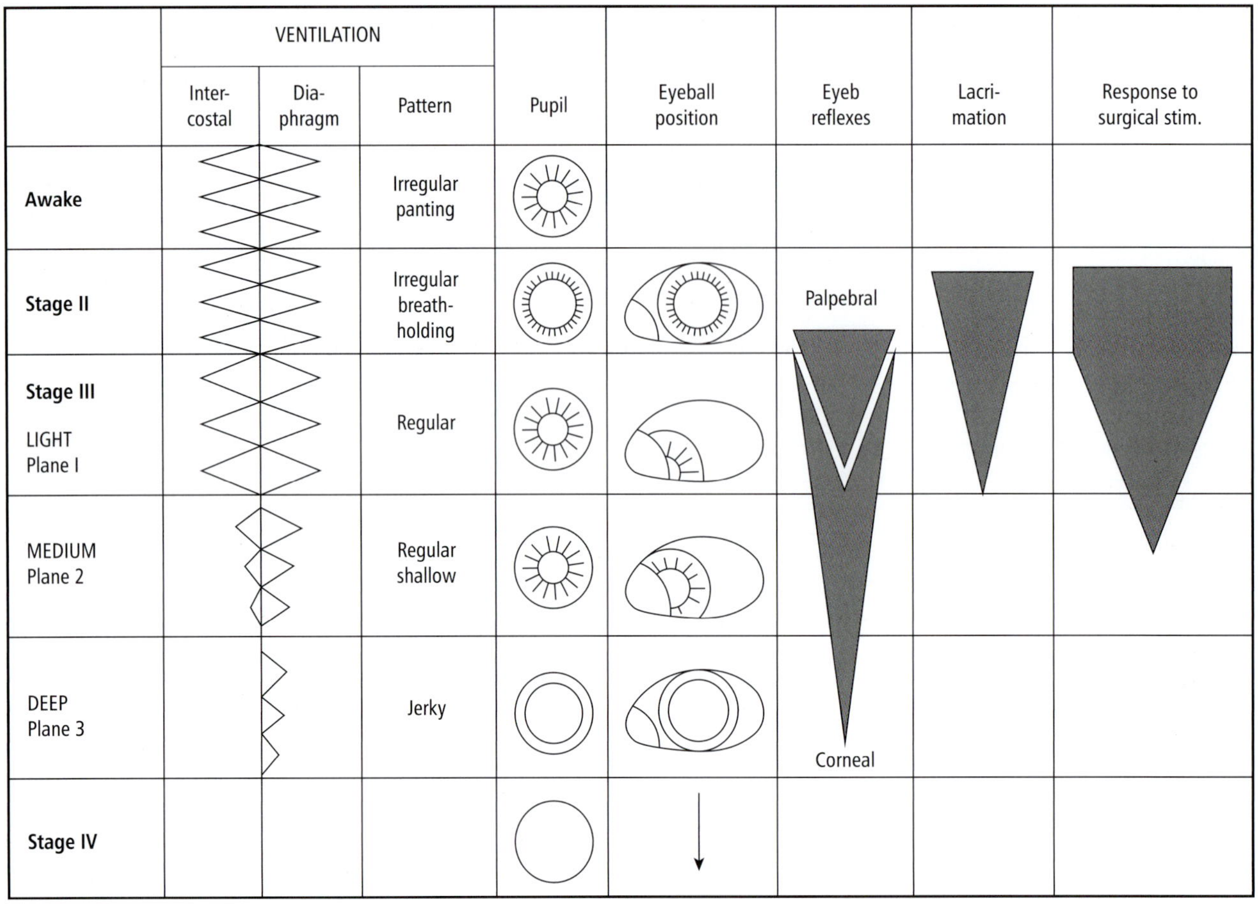

	VENTILATION			Pupil	Eyeball position	Eyeb reflexes	Lacri-mation	Response to surgical stim.
	Inter-costal	Dia-phragm	Pattern					
Awake			Irregular panting					
Stage II			Irregular breath-holding			Palpebral		
Stage III LIGHT Plane I			Regular					
MEDIUM Plane 2			Regular shallow					
DEEP Plane 3			Jerky			Corneal		
Stage IV								

Figure 45.2 A diagram of the physiologic changes that occur in patients as they progress through the stages of anesthesia (noted in the left-hand column). From Hall, Clarke, and Trim, *Veterinary Anaesthesiology,* 10th ed., used with permission.

that are overly anesthetized (e.g., a central eye position), only serial examination will make it possible to accurately assess the patient's depth of anesthesia. For surgical anesthesia, a patient should be in a plane of light to medium stage III anesthesia. Physical parameters should be assessed no less frequently than every 5 minutes in the anesthetized patient.

Eye position

The eye position of an awake animal is a central pupil, which remains constant into light anesthesia. As the patient becomes more deeply anesthetized, the pupil rotates to a ventromedial position and remains this way through moderate anesthesia. As the patient's anesthetic plane deepens, the eye rotates back to a central position. Thus a central pupil in an anesthetized animal can indicate a patient that is either not deep enough for a surgical procedure or one that is excessively deeply anesthetized. Used in combination with other physical examination findings, eye position is an important part of the anesthesia physical examination.

Jaw tone

Jaw tone is a parameter that varies among different canine patients; animals with muscular jaws tend to have higher basal tone and less overall change during anesthesia. In most patients, however, high tone and a tight jaw is associated with lighter anesthetic states that gradually lessens as the animal becomes more deeply anesthetized. Jaw tone is a reliable indicator of anesthetic depth in cats.

Mucous membranes/capillary refill time

Mucous membrane color and capillary refill time (CRT) can allow the anesthetist to estimate perfusion and oxygenation of the anesthetized patient. Well-perfused mucous membranes are pink with a CRT of 1–1.5 seconds. The most accessible mucous membranes to the anesthetist are the gums. Because oxygenated hemoglobin produces the pink color of mucous membranes, factors that affect hemoglobin concentration or saturation of hemoglobin with oxygen can result in changes in the membrane color. In addition, if there is a disturbance that results in decreased blood flow to the gums (i.e., alterations in perfusion), the mucous membrane color may be altered.

Pale mucous membranes are most associated with anemia, and the color can range from a paler pink with moderate anemia to almost white in cases of severe anemia. Other causes of pale mucous membranes include vasoconstriction or hypothermia, both of which result in decreased peripheral perfusion. Decreased perfusion may be physiologic (e.g., response to α-2 agonist drug administration) or may indicate a serious problem (e.g., hemorrhage or cardiac arrest). Membrane color and CRT should be monitored no less frequently than every 5 minutes in pets under anesthesia. Changes in the membrane color should be evaluated in the context of other physical examination and monitoring parameters.

A bluish tinge to the membranes, called cyanosis, indicates a severe decrease in hemoglobin saturation with oxygen. The blue color is due to the presence of deoxyhemoglobin, which is hemoglobin without oxygen molecules attached. In some cases of extremely decreased perfusion (i.e., decompensatory shock), the mucous membranes may also appear to have a blue or purple hue (sometimes described as "muddy"). Cyanosis noted during anesthesia requires immediate action to determine the cause and to restore adequate oxygenation. Possible causes of cyanosis may be due to patient problems (e.g., pneumothorax, pulmonary embolism, aspiration pneumonia) or machine failure (i.e., inadequate supply of oxygen, malfunctioning oxygen flow meter, or a circuit disconnect). Suspected abnormalities derived from mucous membrane assessment should be rapidly confirmed with other methods (e.g., arterial blood gas analysis, pulse oximetry), and the supply of oxygen to the anesthesia machine checked. The bobbin in the oxygen flowmeter will not float if gas is not traveling through the machine (unless it has become stuck). Other variations of mucous membrane color are covered earlier in this book.

Capillary refill time is measured by an initial blanching of the oral mucosa from pressure with a finger and followed by evaluation of the time for the color to return. Normal CRT is 1–1.5 seconds. In animals with pigmented mucous membranes, CRT may be difficult to assess. A slow return of color may indicate impaired systemic perfusion. In animals with pale mucous membranes secondary to vasoconstriction, the CRT may also be slower than normal or difficult to assess. The converse is also true: Animals with vasodilation have bright pink to red mucous membranes. With an increase in cardiac output such as might be seen with compensatory or hyperdynamic shock, the CRT will be faster than normal, usually less than 1 second. The most common reason for brick red membranes and a fast CRT is septic shock.

Response to stimulation

A patient's response to stimulation is decreased with adequate anesthesia. Responses are manifested as increases in sympathetic tone (e.g., tachycardia, hypertension) or a lightening of the anesthetic plane (e.g., an increase in jaw tone). If these responses are seen in response to a surgical or other procedure, there is the possibility that the animal is not adequately anesthetized, and the depth of anesthesia should be verified using other physical examination or monitoring parameters. The use of local anesthetic blocks or total IV anesthesia may result in a patient that retains more tone or reflexes than animals anesthetized with inhalant anesthetic alone.

The palpebral reflex, a blink elicited by light touch over the upper or lower eyelids (or in the medial canthus of the eye), is gradually decreased as the depth of anesthesia increases. In general, for a surgical plane of anesthesia, the reflex may be sluggish but does not need to be absent. The corneal reflex, a withdrawal of the orbit when the cornea is touched, is maintained to even deeper anesthesia. If the corneal reflex is absent, the patient may be overanesthetized or near death.

Heart rate

Cardiac output is the product of heart rate and stroke volume, indicating the amount (volume) of blood pumped from the heart each minute. Stroke volume, the amount of blood pumped with each contraction of the heart, can be difficult to measure directly; therefore, it is important to closely monitor heart rate because it is directly related to cardiac output. An acceptable heart rate under general anesthesia depends on a number of variables including species, patient size, the anesthetic regimen (especially if anticholinergic or α-2 agonist drugs are administered), and the patient's normal heart rate.

There are multiple ways to monitor the heart rate during general anesthesia. The most basic approach is digital palpation of the pulse. The anesthetist palpates the pulse by placing two fingers (not a thumb) over an artery and applying gentle pressure. Pressing down too firmly may occlude or collapse the artery and eliminate the pulse. The most commonly used arteries for digital palpation are the femoral, dorsal pedal, caudal (ventral aspect of the tail), buccal, and lingual arteries (Fig. 45.3). These areas are easily accessible during induction and surgical preparation. When patients are positioned with

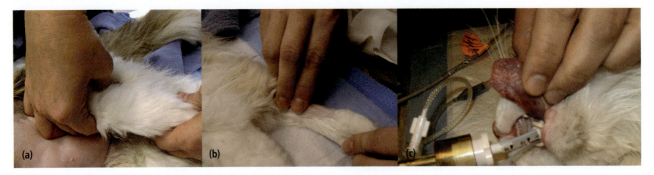

Figure 45.3 Commonly used arteries for digital palpation. (a) Femoral, (b) dorsal pedal, and (c) sublingual.

their head away from the anesthetist, the dorsal pedal, caudal, and femoral arteries are the best choice. However, if the head of the patient is toward the anesthetist, the lingual artery is most accessible. Other palpable pulses are the radial pulse, as well as the apex beat in the thorax. In some cases of cardiac arrhythmias (e.g., ventricular premature contractions [VPC], the palpated pulse rate will differ from the actual heart rate seen on the electrocardiogram (ECG). Arrhythmias will be palpated as weak or irregular pulses and should be verified with other monitoring equipment.

The pulse rate is calculated by counting the pulse over a set number of seconds and multiplying this time by a value to equal 60 seconds. The resulting value is the heart rate in beats per minute (bpm) (see the following equations):

$$\text{No. of beats in 15 seconds} \times 4 = \text{heart rates in bpm}$$

$$\text{No. of beats in 10 seconds} \times 6 = \text{heart rates in bpm}$$

The longer the period of time over which the pulse is counted, the more accurate the recorded pulse rate. It is good practice for the anesthetist to keep a hand on the pulse at all times when not otherwise occupied, to sense the rate and quality of the pulse.

While palpating the pulse, the anesthetist should also note the quality of the pulse. The pulse quality is a subjective value that is not always recorded, but with experience anesthetists may gain valuable information about the patient from pulse palpation. The palpated pulse pressure is the difference between the systolic and diastolic arterial blood pressure. Animals with a large difference in systolic and diastolic blood pressure (due to a lower diastolic or a higher systolic pressure) have a strong or bounding pulse. Bounding pulses may result from conditions such as normovolemic anemia or septic shock (due to excessive vasodilation), and they may give the anesthetist a clue to the underlying condition if these are detected prior to anesthetic induction. If there is a

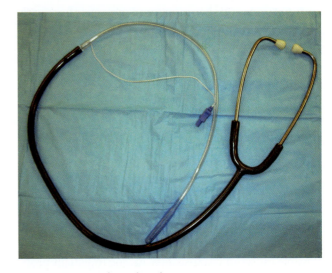

Figure 45.4 Esophageal stethoscope.

low pulse pressure, the animal will have a weak pulse. Weak or "thready" pulses may represent lower mean blood pressure due to poor cardiac output or vessel tone. If weak pulses are palpated, or if pulses become weak during a procedure, a more accurate determination of blood pressure (such as with Doppler or direct arterial pressure monitoring) and re-evaluation of the patient should be performed. Weak pulses may be consistent with hypovolemia, hemorrhage, or decreased cardiac output due to anesthetic drugs or cardiac arrhythmias.[1] Pulse pressure should be evaluated in concert with mucous membrane color and CRT.

Another reliable method for monitoring HR is an esophageal stethoscope (Fig. 45.4). This device is an esophageal probe connected to a listening device. The esophageal probe comes in a variety of sizes and lengths. The probe is connected to either a Doppler unit or standard stethoscope earpieces. After anesthetic induction and endotracheal intubation, the probe is advanced into the esophagus until the heartbeat can be heard. The probe should be advanced only to the point where the heartbeat is clearly heard; additional advancement past this point of maximal intensity may result in the placement of the probe into the stomach and disruption of the lower esophageal sphincter, which may lead to gastroesophageal reflux. Using the stethoscope, heart rate can be directly measured. An advantage of using the esophageal stethoscope is that the heart and lungs may be auscultated constantly and directly. Changes in rate, or in the quality of a heart murmur or lung sounds, may be detected as they happen. Some esophageal stethoscopes are combined with temperature probes and ECG electrodes.

The ECG is used to monitor both the heart rate and rhythm. ECG interpretation is addressed in Chapter 7. A lead II ECG is used to monitor basic cardiac rate and rhythm in small animal patients, and leads may be attached to the patient's skin either using alligator clips or patches with snap leads. In some exotic species, the leads may be attached to the metal part of 25- to 30-gauge needles inserted through the skin. It is not necessary to clip the fur to attach alligator clips, but doing so provides better contact and a better signal. One must apply either alcohol or conductive gel to optimize electrical conduction from the patient's skin to the electrode. Hair must be clipped when using patches, and the area should be wiped with alcohol and allowed to dry before patches are applied to optimize their adherence. Due to evaporation of alcohol or drying of conductive gel, leads may need to be moistened periodically to maintain optimum conductance.

The ECG lead placement is similar to that used for other purposes; however, the standard arrangement may not be possible for some procedures. In the case where the procedure interferes with lead placement (e.g., forelimb amputation), ECG leads should be placed as close to the appropriate area as possible, to maintain the principles of Einthoven's triangle and surgical sterility (see Chapter 6 for more details). It is most important to keep the leads on the correct side of the body and in the correct plane with the heart. Thoracic limb leads can be moved cranially but should not move caudally. Pelvic limb leads may be moved further caudal on the limb.

Respiratory rate

The respiratory rate (RR) can be calculated by observation of the patient or the rebreathing bag. Adequate respiration is essential to a safe and smooth anesthetic episode because anesthesia is most frequently maintained using volatile inhalant gas anesthetics, which can suppress respiratory drive. If a patient is not taking regular breaths with an adequate tidal volume, anesthetic will not be inhaled, and the patient may

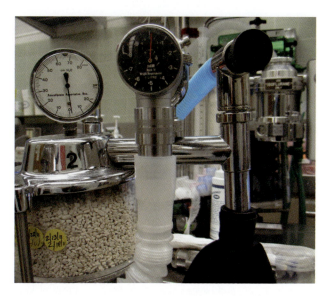

Figure 45.5 A Wright respirometer placed in the expiratory limb of the anesthesia circuit. The respirometer measures tidal volume and respiratory minute volume.

not become anesthetized. Respiratory minute volume (RMV) is the amount of gas exhaled by the lungs over 1 minute and is the product of RR and respiratory tidal volume. The actual RMV can be measured by a respirometer (Fig. 45.5) (e.g., the Wright respirometer) inserted into the anesthetic circuit. Some machines that measure exhaled CO_2 also contain a respirometer feature. The anesthetized patient should take deep breaths at regular intervals. RMV is related to ventilation (and thus arterial CO_2 levels); an increase in RMV results in a decreased arterial CO_2 level, and vice versa. Normal RMV in awake dogs and cats is approximately 200 mL/kg/minute.

Another way to monitor RR is to use an airway monitor. This device produces a humming sound as the patient exhales, which signals to the anesthetist that a respiratory cycle has taken place (i.e., the animal has inhaled and exhaled once). The monitor's sensor is placed in the anesthetic circuit between the ET tube and the wye piece. The sensor is connected to a small speaker, which amplifies the sound of the patient's exhalation. The produced sound does not reflect the quality of ventilation, just the fact that exhalation is taking place. The monitor does not remove any gas samples from the circuit. Modifications to these monitors can make them apnea monitors as well, and some will alarm if the patient has not taken a breath in a specified amount of time. Other monitors, such as the capnograph, also provide an apnea alarm.

The most comprehensive real-time bedside ventilatory monitor is the capnograph. It continuously

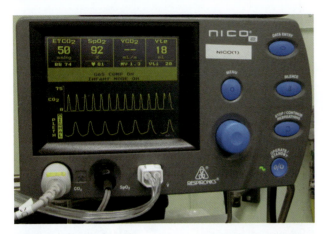

Figure 45.6 The NICO Respiratory Profile Monitor (Phillips-Respironics, Murraysville, PA) a multiparameter monitor that continuously measures and reports inspired and expired PCO_2, respiratory rate, and oxygen saturation. Photo courtesy of Kate Hopper BVSc, PhD, DACVECC.

measures and reports respiratory rate along with inspired and expired PCO_2. Some capnographs (e.g., the Phillips-Respironics, Murraysville, PA) also function as a respirometer (Fig. 45.6); these machines measure tidal volume and can estimate pulmonary compliance, which is an important parameter to monitor in patients requiring long-term ventilation for pulmonary disease (see Chapter 27). The end-tidal carbon dioxide ($ETCO_2$) is a practical estimation of arterial CO_2 and used to monitor ventilation in anesthetized patients. Capnography is covered in depth in Chapter 26.

Hypoventilation (a decreased respiratory minute volume) occurs from a decrease in respiratory rate, tidal volume, or both. Hypoventilation leads to hypercarbia (also called hypercapnia), which is an increase in dissolved carbon dioxide in the blood ($PaCO_2$ or $PvCO_2$). Hypercarbia results in a respiratory acidosis, and as the blood pH decreases, deleterious effects can be seen on vascular tone and cardiac function. High blood levels of CO_2 can also cause narcosis and may result in increased intracranial pressure, cardiac arrhythmias, hypoxemia, and ultimately cardiac arrest.

Decreased respiratory minute volume may be due to a decreased respiratory rate (or complete apnea), seen with patients with an irregular breathing pattern or breathholding, or it may be due to a decrease in tidal volume, despite a normal respiratory rate. If hypercarbia or hypoventilation is identified, the anesthetist must increase the respiratory minute volume, by manually or mechanically ventilating the patient at a steady rate to bring the CO_2 into a normal range. Assisted ventilation may be used to increase the respiratory rate, tidal volume,

or both. Assisted ventilation also increases the inhalant anesthetic delivered to the patient.

When hypoventilation is identified, the anesthetist should first evaluate the patient (Table 45.2), as well as the positioning of the ET tube. Unibronchial intubation occurs when the ET tube is advanced beyond the carina into the bronchus of one of the lung lobes. V/Q mismatch ensues because an entire lung is without effective ventilation. Ideally, the ET tube should be placed so that the distal end of the tube is located in the caudal extrathoracic trachea. If there is a possibility that the tube has been introduced too far into the trachea (resulting in one lung intubation), it may be removed until the cuff of the ET tube is palpated in the caudal extrathoracic trachea. The ET tube cuff should be deflated before readjusting the tube, should adjustment be necessary.

The patient with elevated respiratory minute ventilation is hyperventilating, which causes a decreased PCO_2, called hypocarbia (or hypocapnia). Hyperventilation in the anesthetized patient is most commonly a result of an inadequate anesthetic plane or an elevated body temperature. In some cases where the patient exhibits extreme hypoxia, hyperventilation may be a reflection of hypoxic drive because the need for oxygen overwhelms any depressant effects of anesthetics on the respiratory center. Hyperventilation due to inadequate anesthesia may be accompanied by tachycardia and hypertension. The anesthetist may address this either by increasing ventilation or administered inhalant percentage (both of which provide more anesthetic to the patient), or by administering analgesic drugs (e.g., opioids) to provide additional analgesia.

The normal physiologic response to elevated arterial PCO_2 is an increase in RMV (either by increasing the respiratory rate or tidal volume). This normal response to high $PaCO_2$ is blunted by anesthesia, but an elevated respiratory rate may be seen in patients with a $PaCO_2$ above 65 mm Hg. Due to the effects of anesthesia on the normal responses to PCO_2 as well as effects on RMV (e.g., due to smaller tidal volumes), it is difficult to determine the patient's P_aCO_2 based solely on observation of the respiratory rate; the only true way to assess ventilation is to measure the arterial or venous CO_2 partial pressure.

Malignant hyperthermia (MH) causes increased respiratory rates accompanied by hyperthermia and hypercapnia. Some anesthetic drugs, such as halothane and succinylcholine, have been linked as triggers for MH in susceptible animals. If MH is suspected, anesthesia should be discontinued as soon as possible, the anesthetic lines detached from the ET tube, flushed thoroughly with oxygen, and reattached to the patient. It

Table 45.2 Assessment and approach to common abnormalities in ventilation in the anesthetized patient

Problem	Assessment Steps	Actions
Hypoventilation (PaCO$_2$ or ETCO$_2$ >65 mm Hg)	Is the patient unable to generate an adequate tidal volume by spontaneous ventilation or mechanical ventilation?	Auscult the thorax and rule out pulmonary dysfunction such as a pneumothorax. If tidal volume is limited, consider repositioning the patient or increasing the respiratory rate. Ventilators that deliver a breath to a certain airway pressure will deliver a smaller breath if there is increased pressure in the thorax.
	Is the patient unable to generate an adequate tidal volume by spontaneous ventilation?	Consider the use of a mechanical ventilator for maintenance of anesthesia, or increase the number of assisted breaths delivered to the patient by the anesthetist. If neuromuscular blocking agents (e.g., atracurium) have been used during the procedure, consider reversal.
	Is the patient's level of anesthesia excessive? (see Fig. 45.2)	Efforts should be made to lighten the plane of anesthesia, and if the patient is breathing spontaneously, manual ventilation may be necessary.
	Have potent opiate medications been administered recently?	If anesthetized, increase either tidal volume, respiratory rate, or both. If awake, consider reversal of the opiate medication using naloxone.
	Is there a kink or obstruction in the breathing system?	Inspect the system for kinks or obstructions; address as necessary.
	Is there a leak in the anesthetic system?	Leaks will prevent the delivery of a full tidal volume breath to the patient; if a leak is suspected, it may be necessary to change the tubing, the ventilator bellows, the rebreathing bag, or the entire system. If a leak cannot be readily detected, breathing for the patient with an Ambu bag will allow time to switch out the system and to correct the hypoventilation. It should also be verified that the cuff on the endotracheal tube is adequately inflated.
	Is there a leak in the ventilator bellows?	Leaks in the bellows of a mechanical ventilator will prevent the bellows from returning completely to the full position between breaths. The patient may be hand ventilated using the rebreathing bag or an Ambu bag while the bellows are changed.
	Is the soda lime expired?	Check the soda lime canister for heat and color, as well as the last time the soda lime was changed. Expired or used soda lime will not remove adequate CO$_2$ from the system and may cause it to build up. Switch machines or breathe for the patient with an Ambu bag while the soda lime is changed. Also verify that the soda lime canister is filled correctly; if it is packed too tightly or above the fill line, it may not remove CO$_2$ appropriately. These patients will also have a high inspired CO$_2$ as measured by the capnograph.
	Is there a leak in the valves of the anesthesia machine?	Incompetent inspiratory or expiratory valves will not allow air to travel in a circle system; these patients will also show a high inspired CO$_2$ level.
Hyperventilation (PaCO$_2$ or ETCO$_2$ <25 mm Hg)	Is the respiratory rate or tidal volume excessive? (spontaneous ventilation)	Verify that the patient is adequately anesthetized for the procedure. Verify that the patient's temperature is not elevated.
	Is the respiratory rate or tidal volume excessive? (mechanical ventilation)	If a mechanical ventilator is in use, adjust either the rate or tidal volume to decrease the respiratory minute volume.
	Is the patient hypoxemic?	Assess SpO$_2$ and/or an arterial blood gas to verify patient oxygenation.
Very low ETCO$_2$	Was intubation successful?	Verify that the endotracheal tube is not in the esophagus
Sudden drop in ETCO$_2$	Any acute changes in patient condition?	Severe drops in ETCO$_2$ may reflect circulatory collapse or the occurrence of a pulmonary thromboembolism (PTE). The patient should be assessed for stability immediately and additional diagnostics performed as necessary.
	Is the anesthetic circuit intact?	Evaluate the circuit for any disconnections

may be easier to switch to an unused anesthetic machine. The patient's $ETCO_2$, rectal or esophageal temperature, and oxygenation should be closely monitored. If the temperature rises above 102.5°F, external warming and heat support should be discontinued. If the temperature continues to rise, the patient should be made wet, and a fan used to encourage convective cooling. Dantrolene is a drug that may help to reverse the signs of MH by altering intracellular calcium kinetics. This drug may be given at a dose of 1–10 mg/kg IV. At-risk patients should be treated with dantrolene orally prior to elective surgeries.[2]

$ETCO_2$ is directly proportional to cardiac output and tissue perfusion, except in rare conditions of mitochondrial dysfunction (usually as a result of septic shock). If the respiratory rate and tidal volume have remained the same but the $ETCO_2$ has decreased, the patient is experiencing either a decreased metabolic rate (e.g., due to hypothermia) or a decrease in cardiac output (e.g., due to hemorrhage or arrhythmias). If a sudden decrease in $ETCO_2$ is seen, the anesthetist should evaluate the patient's vital signs immediately to verify adequate perfusion because a precipitous drop in ETCO2 is seen with cardiac arrest. Once it is clear that the patient is not in distress, additional evaluation of the equipment for leaks or disconnections may take place.[3]

Blood pressure

Chapters 8–10 provide an in-depth analysis of the various types of blood pressure monitoring. For the purposes of monitoring the anesthetized patient, the same types of monitors and criteria for evaluation may be used. Although blood pressure is not a direct measure of perfusion in the anesthetized patient, it is the closest and most convenient surrogate measure that we have to determine that organ perfusion is appropriate. Actual perfusion of individual organs is determined by a host of local mechanisms and is extremely difficult to measure, even under experimental circumstances.

In general, mean arterial blood pressure (MAP) of 70–100 mm Hg is acceptable for the anesthetized patient. Systolic arterial blood pressure (SAP) should be between 100 and 140 mm Hg. Diastolic arterial blood pressure (DAP) should be between 40 and 65 mm Hg. A MAP below 60 mm Hg may be associated with decreased perfusion of and oxygen delivery to the kidney and brain.[4] A DAP less than 40 mm Hg may result in poor coronary artery perfusion (the heart is only perfused during diastole), and a decreased oxygen delivery to the heart.[5] In patients who are chronically hypertensive prior to anesthesia (e.g., those with chronic renal disease), an effort should be made to maintain MAP at levels toward the

higher end of the range or toward the normal values for that patient.

Low blood pressure in critically ill patients may be caused by hypovolemia, hemorrhage, a gas-filled viscus (e.g., the stomach in patients with gastric dilatation and volvulus), anesthetic drugs, heart disease, cardiac arrhythmias, or vasodilation (e.g., as a result of vasoplegic shock). Individual patients have individual reasons for hypotension, and the anesthetist's knowledge of the disease state and the patient's physical examination will help to determine therapy and plan a safe anesthetic. As an example, patients with heart disease such as dilated cardiomyopathy may need a positive inotropic drug to support blood pressure by supporting cardiac output. By contrast, a patient that is hypotensive due to hypovolemia may require IV fluid therapy to resolve low blood pressure.

The hypotension associated with anesthetic drugs may have components of myocardial depression and vasodilation, depending on the drug. When hypotension is detected, the anesthetic plane of the patient should be re-evaluated to ensure that they are not too deeply anesthetized (if they are, the anesthetic plane may be lightened). An assessment of the degree of blood or fluid loss should also be undertaken, and if the animal is hypovolemic, an IV bolus of fluids (crystalloid or colloid) may help to restore adequate blood pressures. In cases of excessive vasodilation causing hypotension, pressor drugs such as phenylephrine, dopamine, norepinephrine, or vasopressin may be indicated to cause vasoconstriction.

Although hypertension is uncommon in veterinary patients, it may also have consequences such as retinal detachment or cerebral hemorrhage. Anesthetized animals with a pheochromocytoma may have paroxysmal tachycardias and hypertensive episodes that may merit therapy.

Doppler blood pressure measurement

The most widely used blood pressure monitor is the Doppler flow probe. The Doppler uses a probe containing a piezoelectric crystal. The probe emits sound waves, which are reflected by the RBCs in pulsatile arterial blood. When the sound is reflected from the cells, it is sensed again by the probe, and the shift in the frequency of the sound (due to the movement of the cells) is transduced into an audible signal. The placement of a pneumatic blood pressure cuff and sphygmomanometer proximal to the probe allows the measurement of blood pressure (see Chapter 10). Common areas used for Doppler probe placement in the anesthetized animal are the ulnar artery on the palmar surface of the thoracic limb below the carpus; the dorsal pedal artery on the plantar surface of the pelvic limb; the saphenous artery on the plantar surface of the pelvic limb, proximal to the foot; and the coccygeal artery located on the ventral surface of the tail.

Additional tips for placement of the Doppler probe and selection of pneumatic cuff size are covered in Chapter 10.

For measurement of blood pressure, an appropriate-size blood pressure cuff (ideally with a width that is 40% of the circumference of the limb) is placed proximal to the probe and inflated with the sphygmomanometer until the artery is occluded; this will result in a cessation of the Doppler sound. As the pressure in the cuff is slowly released, the audible signal will return as soon as the cuff pressure is below that of the systolic blood pressure. The anesthetist can repeat this reading as often as desired. Changes in the intensity of sound on the Doppler may be consistent with arrhythmias or a decreased pulse strength (as may occur from sudden hypotension). The placement of the probe and cuff should be checked to verify that nothing has changed after a patient assessment.

An advantage of the Doppler is early detection of decreased flow, along with the ability to hear changes in heart rhythm. A disadvantage is, like the esophageal probe, it becomes difficult to hear once the forced air warming unit is activated, although most Doppler units allow the use of headphones to improve focus on the pulse. Constant air flow from a warming device can also lead to drying of the contact gel; therefore it may be necessary to reapply if the signal fades.

Oscillometric blood pressure measurement

Oscillometric noninvasive blood pressure monitors (e.g., the Cardell [Midmark Corp., Versailles, OH] or Dinamap [GE Healthcare, Wauwatosa, WI]) are excellent tools for monitoring trends in blood pressure in the anesthetized patient. The theory behind these machines is discussed in Chapter 10. Oscillometric monitors are more automated than the Doppler devices. They can be programmed to cycle at various intervals and to give a regular readout of systolic, diastolic, and mean blood pressure. Because these monitors rely on a machine-based interpretation of the blood pressure oscillations, they may be less accurate than the Doppler probe, especially for critically ill patients who may be hypotensive (thus diminishing the strength of oscillations) or in animals experiencing cardiac arrhythmias (the machines require a regular heartbeat to accurately sense oscillations). Unlike the Doppler probe, these machines do not produce an audible signal to reflect heart rate (and in fact may continue to give readings even in the absence of a good pulse). It is thus imperative to compare the machine-read heart rate to a heart rate obtained by another source (e.g., auscultation or ECG). If the heart rate does not match that of the patient, the blood pressure reading should not be trusted. Despite these caveats, the oscillometric blood pressure monitor is a useful tool for monitoring blood pressure in most anesthetized patients.

Direct arterial blood pressure measurement

Direct arterial blood pressure (DABP) is covered in Chapter 9 and considered the gold standard for monitoring arterial blood pressure. Critically ill or emergent patients under anesthesia can experience fluctuations in blood pressure that may not be detectable using intermittent measurement. In these cases, or in cases where it is necessary to use vasoactive drugs to support blood pressure, a direct arterial pressure monitor is ideal. DABP also allows the anesthetist to observe directly the effects of arrhythmias that occur during anesthesia, and it provides a simple way to obtain samples for blood gas analysis. Direct arterial catheters for use during anesthesia may be placed in the metatarsal, caudal, or auricular arteries. The femoral artery may also be used but is associated with more complications on catheter removal.

Oxygen saturation

Monitoring oxygen saturation is imperative in the anesthetized patient. Oxygen saturation is a measure of how much oxygen the hemoglobin in the blood is carrying, described as a percentage of the maximum it could carry, and it is an important component of oxygen content. Adequate oxygen content in the arterial blood, in combination with cardiac output, determines oxygen delivery to tissues.

Oxygen saturation is usually monitored with a pulse oximeter. Pulse oximetry is covered extensively in Chapter 21. The most common site for placement of the pulse oximeter probe in the anesthetized patient is the tongue or lips. If the tongue cannot be used, the probe can be placed on an area of thin skin such as the skin between the toes, the abdomen, or on the vulva or prepuce. Using the transmission (clip) probe, the tissue must be thin enough to allow the probe to pass light through the tissue to the sensor on the other side of the clip. Reflectance probes may be used rectally or on thin areas of skin to obtain a saturation reading without using the clip.

The pulse oximeter provides an oxygen saturation reading given as a percentage, a pulse waveform, and a

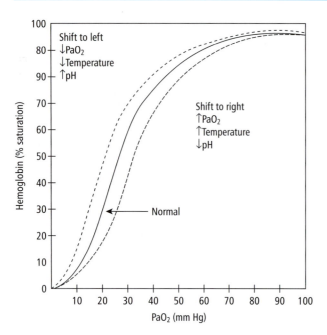

Figure 45.7 Oxyhemoglobin dissociation curve.

heart rate. The oxygen saturation is related to the dissolved oxygen content (PaO_2) by the oxyhemoglobin dissociation curve (Fig. 45.7) (Chapter 21). Normal hemoglobin is expected to be 100% saturated with oxygen at a PaO_2 of 95–100 mm Hg (most normal animals breathing room air have a PaO_2 of 80–100 mm Hg and an SpO_2 of 96%–100%). Under anesthesia and breathing 100% oxygen, an animal's PaO_2 is expected to be greater than 500 mm Hg. Consequently, an anesthetized animal with normal lung function is expected to have a PaO_2 of 99%–100% (hemoglobin cannot be saturated more than 100% with oxygen).

If SpO_2 readings below 98% are obtained in the anesthetized patient breathing 100% oxygen, there is a problem with oxygenation in the patient. In the event of low SpO_2, the patient and subsequently the anesthesia circuit should be inspected for causes of the abnormal reading.

A patient breathing 100% oxygen that has a PaO_2 of 200 mm Hg will have the same SpO_2 as a patient with a PaO_2 of 500 mm Hg, but the first patient may have some significant lung pathology (preventing a normal PaO_2), which may become relevant during anesthesia recovery when the patient needs to breathe room air. For this reason, the pulse oximeter does not replace arterial blood gas analysis but is useful for a continuous estimate of oxygen saturation.

Many critically ill patients may have compromised lung function, whether it is due to primary lung pathology such as pneumonia or due to decreased lung func-

tion from pleural effusion or ascites (which decrease the ability to fully expand the lungs). Animals that have been recumbent frequently develop atelectasis, or lung collapse, on the dependent side. Atelectasis causes a ventilation/perfusion mismatch and decreases the ability of the animal to oxygenate the blood. Atelectasis may also develop during surgery when the patient is immobile for a period of time. If atelectasis occurs during anesthesia, oxygenation during the recovery period may be affected. The pulse oximeter is thus a valuable tool not only during anesthesia but also into the recovery period.

Significant changes in oxygen saturation rarely occur acutely. It is thus important to watch the overall trend of the readings. A gradual decrease in saturation will be clear on the anesthesia monitoring sheet. Changes in saturation may be accompanied by changes in other parameters, such as respiratory rate or ETCO2, and can help the anesthetist determine the possible cause and treatment. A common cause of hypoxemia may be incorrect ET tube placement. If the patient is intubated, the correct placement and patency of the tube should be verified. It is possible for the ET tube to become clogged with blood or mucus during anesthesia, especially in patients undergoing thoracic surgery, or in those with pneumonia. Other causes of a low intraoperative pulse oximeter reading include the development of a pneumothorax (which will be accompanied by hypotension and tachycardia) and the development of atelectasis (which will cause a slower decrease in SpO_2).

When a low SpO2 is detected, it is important to check the patient (Table 45.3) and to verify that the anesthesia machine is providing adequate oxygen. If surgery is occurring, verify that there is not a chance of an iatrogenic pneumothorax or excessive hemorrhage. If the patient is set up on a mechanical ventilator, switch to manual breaths; this will allow an increase in respiratory rate and tidal volume, and it will also give an idea of the pulmonary resistance. If it is very difficult to inflate the lungs when squeezing the rebreathing bag, a pneumothorax may be present. If atelectasis has caused the low SpO2, administration of a slightly larger tidal volume (15–20 mL/kg) for two to three breaths or held for 10–15 seconds may help to open the collapsed alveoli (this is also called a recruitment maneuver). If these actions do not improve oxygenation, other rule-outs, such as pulmonary thromboembolic disease, should be considered. If it is possible, confirmation of a low SpO_2 with an arterial blood gas is indicated because this will give an actual measure of PaO_2.

The pulse oximeter is an indirect indicator of peripheral perfusion; when vasoconstriction results in decreased peripheral perfusion, the probe may be unable

Table 45.3 Assessments and actions for patients with a low pulse oximeter reading (SpO$_2$ <95%) under anesthesia[a]

Problem origin	Assessment	Action
Respiratory system	Has the patient experienced an adverse pulmonary event?	Auscult the chest to rule out presence of pneumothorax, congestive heart failure, or other lung/pleural space disease. If pneumomediastinum is suspected, radiographs may be necessary for diagnosis.
	Is the patient intubated properly? Verify endotracheal intubation using a laryngoscope.	Reintubate if necessary.
	Is the airway patent? Are there kinks or obstructions in the breathing circuit?	Address as necessary, potentially switching machines or breathing circuit
	Is oxygen still being supplied to the circuit (check that the flowmeter bobbin is still floating)?	If oxygen supply has been depleted, use Ambu bag or other device to breathe for the patient while a new source is established.
	Has unibronchial intubation occurred?	If the endotracheal tube has been inserted too far into the bronchial tree, slowly back it out until breath sounds can be auscultated bilaterally
Circulatory system	Does the patient have a pulse?	Palpate pulse, or verify heart beat using stethoscope, esophageal stethoscope, or Doppler flow probe.
	Is the patient hypotensive?	Measure blood pressure and adjust anesthetic protocol to alleviate hypotension.
	Is the patient peripherally vasoconstricted?	If the vasoconstriction is related to administered drugs, consider alternative protocols or alternative placement of the pulse oximeter probe. If high doses of pressors are used, it may be difficult to achieve an accurate pulse oximeter reading.
Other patient factors	Is the patient hypothermic?	Vasoconstriction that may accompany hypothermia may result in a variable pulse oximeter reading; the patient should be aggressively rewarmed if the temperature is <96°F
	Is the tongue (or other probe site) dry?	Moistening the tongue with warm water or saline may allow the pulse oximeter to generate a more accurate reading.
	Is the patient moving/seizuring/shivering?	Calming the patient and limiting movement will allow the pulse oximeter to focus on the arterial pulse.
	Has the probe been placed on pigmented skin?	Attempt to locate a probe site that is not pigmented.
Environmental factors	Is the probe in direct line of the surgical or fluorescent lights?	Try to cover the probe site or redirect the lights to eliminate interference from room lighting.

[a]Factors are generally listed in order of importance, with emphasis on an immediate physical examination and patient assessment, and secondarily addressing possible machine malfunction.

to sense a strong enough pulse, and the monitor may display errors, noise, or incorrect values. This may also happen in the context of severe hemorrhage; the compensatory vasoconstriction and decreased perfusion to the periphery will impair the pulse available for the pulse oximeter to monitor. It is imperative to always compare the pulse reported by the pulse oximeter to another reliable measure of the patient pulse to ensure that the machine is focusing on the correct pulse.

Whereas vasoconstriction will affect the pulse oximeter reading, anemia will not, unless it is very severe (<10%). In addition, fluorescent surgical or overhead lights may affect the ability of the pulse oximeter to register an accurate pulse. If the probe is positioned on the tongue, the signal may become attenuated as the tongue becomes dry from exposure during the anesthetic. For a more in-depth discussion of possible artifacts and errors in pulse oximetry, refer to Chapter 21.

Temperature

The temperature of an anesthetized patient affects heart rate, RR, blood pressure, and oxygen saturation. Patients should be kept as close to normothermic as possible during anesthesia. This not only helps maintain normal physiology during anesthesia; it also correlates to a decreased recovery time.[6] It is also easier to maintain a patient's temperature in the normal range than it is to warm the animal up after it has become severely hypothermic. Monitoring temperature is done using either a rectal thermometer or an esophageal temperature probe.

Maintaining normal body temperature under anesthesia is challenging. The patient is breathing cold dry gas, is often exposed to the room temperature, and is frequently lying on a cold table, all of which contribute to conductive heat loss. Steps that can be taken to minimize loss of body heat include the use of warm water circulating blankets, forced air warming units (e.g., Bair Hugger), the administration of warm IV fluids and placing warm (100–103°F) water bottles around the patient. Some procedures make patient warming difficult. For prolonged radiologic procedures, such as myelography or computed tomography (CT), forced-air warming units and water blankets can interfere with imaging. In magnetic resonance imaging (MRI) units, both metal monitoring devices and metal probes are contraindicated due to interference with the magnet. In these cases, blankets placed over the patient can help to minimize heat loss but are not as effective as active warming devices. Whenever active warming devices of any kind are used, patient temperature *must* be closely monitored to ensure the patient is not overheated. If a patient is to undergo many procedures during which it is exposed to room temperature for long periods of time (e.g., wound debridement, central line placement), a radiant heat source may be used; these ceramic heaters warm the environment around the patient and limit radiant and convective heat loss. Because they are located over the patient, they are not suitable for use during surgery that involves an open body cavity. These devices usually are required to be placed a certain distance (usually about 90 cm) above the patient to prevent burns. Some (e.g., Radiant Heater, Fisher-Paykel, Auckland, NZ) are also equipped with a thermometer feedback system that adjusts the radiant temperature based on the skin temperature of the patient.

Hyperthermia may cause complications as well. When using active warming devices, the temperature setting should be lowered or use discontinued altogether when a patient is at or near normal temperature because the animal's temperature may continue to rise after cessation of active warming. Should a patient become hyperthermic and the cause is determined to be other than MH (by evaluation of $PaCO_2$ and blood lactate), cool the patient slowly. The forced air warming unit can be switched to a cool setting, and the warm water blanket should be turned off. If the patient is already recovered from anesthesia, it may be placed on a cool surface like a metal cage floor, and all blankets should be removed. Continue to monitor temperature every 15 minutes until the patient's temperature has normalized. Opioids may also be associated with the development of postoperative hyperthermia in cats. This hyperthermia may be treated in a similar manner to other causes of hyperthermia, and it may also respond to low doses of naloxone (this therapy may also reverse the analgesia) but is usually self-limiting.[7]

End-tidal inhalant concentrations

In a similar manner to CO_2, the partial pressure (usually expressed as a percentage of alveolar gasses) of inhalant anesthetic circulating in a patient is essentially equivalent to the amount that is exhaled. This is particularly true for commonly used veterinary anesthetics such as isoflurane and sevoflurane. By comparing the exhaled percentage of inhalant anesthetic to the dose required for anesthesia (usually a multiple of the minimum alveolar concentration, or MAC), objective data can be obtained as to the degree of anesthesia provided by inhalant drugs at any given time. This is a similar concept to the measurement of plasma drug levels after administration of an injectable drug. The MAC values for the commonly used anesthetic agents are given in Table 45.4.

Machines that measure end-tidal inhalant concentrations (Fig. 45.8A) are attached to the anesthetic circuit by tubing that will constantly aspirate small amounts (50–150 mL/minute) of gas from the system into the machine (Fig. 45.8B). Once in the machine, the percentage of inhalant in the aspirated gas is determined and reported. Many different companies manufacture machines to determine end-tidal inhalant concentrations, and these monitors frequently measure $ETCO_2$ as well. Manufacturers include Datex-Ohmeda (GE Healthcare, Wauwatosa, WI), SurgiVet (Waukesha, WI), and Criticare Systems (Waukesha, WI).

Table 45.4 MAC values for veterinary species

Species	Isoflurane	Sevoflurane	Desflurane
Cat	1.7%	3.1%	10.3%
Dog	1.3%	2.1%	7.2%

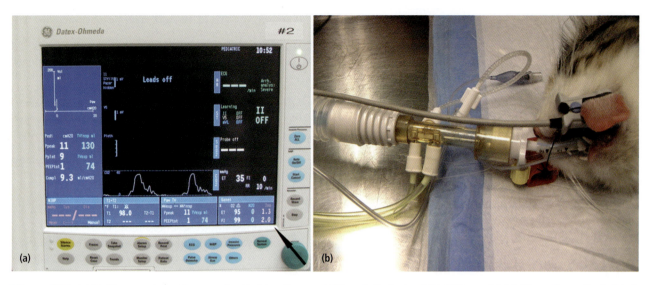

Figure 45.8 (a) Multiparameter patient monitor that has the capabilities of displaying ECG, SPO$_2$, end-tidal CO$_2$, and anesthetic inhalant concentrations. The percentage of inhaled anesthetic is displayed (black arrow). (b) The adapter placed in the anesthetic circuit that continually aspirates small amounts of gas from the system. Once in the machine, the percentage of inhalant in the aspirated gas is determined and reported.

The use of analgesic drugs such as the opioids and α-2 agonists decrease the amount of inhalant anesthetic necessary to maintain anesthesia (i.e., they reduce the effective MAC of the inhalants). In this context, monitoring of the ET inhalant can show the effects of premedicant drugs and constant rate infusions given during anesthesia. If animals have been adequately premedicated and have intraoperative analgesia provided by other drugs, the overall requirement for inhalant anesthetic is decreased (i.e., the MAC is effectively lowered). Because of this, it is recommended that the ET inhalant be used as a guide, but it is more important to rely on the patient's physical examination signs of anesthesia (discussed earlier), rather than trying to target an actual MAC value for each patient.

The inhalant concentration is directly related to the appearance of side effects from inhalant anesthetics. As the inspired concentration of inhalant increases, changes such as hypotension and hypoventilation become more pronounced. From this perspective, the ET inhalant concentration can be a very good way to avoid overdoses of inhalant anesthetic and at the same time predict that adequate anesthesia is present. In critically ill patients, the side effects of inhalant anesthetics may be magnified, and sometimes only a fraction of the MAC dose (if any at all) may be used safely. In addition, patients with diseases such as septic shock and severe hypovolemia actually have lower MAC values than similar healthy patients. The ET inhalant can help to document the overall dose of anesthetic as well as assess any residual anesthetic in the patient if administration is discontinued.

Central venous pressure

Because many conditions in the critically ill patient are associated with hypo- or hypervolemia, and some may require large amounts of IV fluids during anesthesia, it is desirable in some patients to follow the CVP during anesthesia. CVP monitoring, described in Chapter 11, is indicated to monitor intravascular volume status in any animal at risk of hypervolemia (e.g., heart disease or acute renal failure) or in animals who may lose a large amount of blood or require large amounts of infused IV fluids during the surgical procedure.

CVP in the anesthetized patient is expected to range from 0 to 10 cm H$_2$O or 0 to 7 mm Hg. If the patient is undergoing positive pressure ventilation, the pressure during inspiration may raise the measured CVP. Consequently, the CVP measurement should be taken during the expiratory phase. In patients that are anesthetized and receiving mechanical ventilation using positive end-expiratory pressure (PEEP), this pressure will also be transmitted to the CVP and should be taken into account when evaluating the measured pressure. Thoracoscopic procedures may also result in erroneous CVP readings, depending on the amount and pressure of gas instilled into the thoracic cavity. Laparoscopy results in variable changes in CVP.

Occasionally, the same setup used for CVP monitoring may be used to measure portal pressures in patients anesthetized for surgical ligation of portosystemic shunts. The same tools, a transducer, pressure (low-compliance) tubing, and monitor (or water manometer) should be available to allow this pressure measurement (see Chapter 11).

Anesthesia in the critically ill patient can be challenging due to the sensitive nature of the cardiorespiratory systems and the possibility for decompensation. With appropriate monitoring equipment and regular attention paid to physical examination parameters, changes may be recognized early, and interventions may be subsequently taken to restore homeostasis.

References

1. Aldrich J. Global assessment of the emergency patient. Vet Clin North Am Small Anim Pract 2005;35(2): 281–305.

2. Rosenberg H, Davis M, James D, et al. Malignant hyperthermia. Orphanet J Rare Dis 2007;2:21–41.

3. Hartsfield SM. Anesthetic machines and breathing systems. In: Tranquilli WJ, Thurmon JC, Grimm KA, eds. Lumb and Jones' Veterinary Anesthesia and Analgesia. 4th ed. Ames, IA: Blackwell Publishing; 2007:453–494.

4. Earle SA, de Moya MA, Zuccarelli JE, et al. Cerebrovascular resuscitation after polytrauma and fluid restriction. J Am Coll Surg. 2007;204(2):261–275.

5. Farhi ER, Canty JM Jr, Klocke FJ. Effects of graded reductions in coronary perfusion pressure on the diastolic pressure-segment length relation and the rate of isovolumic relaxation in the resting conscious dog. Circulation 1989;80(5):1458–1468.

6. Pottie RG, Dart CM, Perkins NR, et al. Effect of hypothermia on recovery from general anaesthesia in the dog, Aust Vet J 2007;85(4):158–162.

7. Posner LP, Pavuk AA, Rokshar JL, Carter JE, Levine JF. Effects of opioids and anesthetic drugs on body temperature in cats. Vet Anaesth Analg 2010;37(1):35–43.

46

Nursing care of the long-term anesthetized patient

Yekaterina Buriko and Bridget Lyons

Basic indications for long-term anesthesia

A small group of veterinary patients require long-term anesthesia during their hospitalization. The three major groups of patients in this category are patients that require positive pressure ventilation due to inability to oxygenate or ventilate appropriately, endotracheal (ET) intubation for large airway disease (tracheal collapse), and those that require general anesthesia for control of refractory seizures. Typical indications for positive pressure ventilation include arterial partial pressure of oxygen (PaO_2) less than 60 mm Hg with oxygen supplementation, hypoventilation with partial pressure of carbon dioxide ($PaCO_2$) higher than 60 mmHg, and an unacceptable degree of dyspnea associated with increased work of breathing.[1]

Long-term anesthesia and immobility are associated with a number of complications, affecting nearly all body systems of a patient. Recognizing these effects is of particular importance to a veterinary technician because much of the care is focused on preventing and addressing the complications particular to the anesthetized patient. This chapter focuses on specifics of management of this patient population and describes the complications associated with the key body systems, methods to prevent the complications, and treatment modalities, should a problem arise.

All anesthetized patients require an ET or a tracheostomy tube, as well as indwelling intravenous access as a part of their care. Please refer to Chapters 25 and 55, respectively, for details on artificial airway management and care of indwelling devices.

Physical complications associated with long-term anesthesia and immobility

Immobility complications

Neuromuscular weakness

An inevitable consequence of long-term anesthesia is an extended period of immobility. Prolonged recumbency can result in a plethora of complications, including decubitus ulcers,[1–3] tissue necrosis,[1] peripheral limb edema,[1,3] contracture and stiffening of muscles and ligaments,[1] muscle atrophy,[2,3] nerve damage,[2,3] atelectasis,[1,3] and the accumulation of airway secretions in dependent lung regions.[1,3] Neuromuscular weakness is an entity that is recognized in critically ill human patients. One study demonstrated that 46% of the intensive care unit (ICU) patients evaluated had critical illness–associated neuromuscular abnormalities.[4] Pathophysiology of critical care neuromuscular dysfunction is complex and likely multifactorial. Several factors contribute, such as prolonged immobility, as well as catabolic state that can be caused by malnutrition, systemic inflammation, and metabolic derangements.[5,6] Prolonged immobility is associated with a proinflammatory state that increases the production of reactive oxygen species (ROS) along with simultaneous decrease in antioxidant defense mechanisms.[6] This may result in contractile dysfunction and atrophy, as well as protein loss.[6] In mechanically ventilated patients the neurologic and muscular dysfunction may increase the duration of ventilation, extend the length of stay in the hospital, and prolong recovery time.[5,6] Even though this entity has not been formally

Advanced Monitoring and Procedures for Small Animal Emergency and Critical Care, First Edition. Edited by Jamie M. Burkitt Creedon, Harold Davis.
© 2012 John Wiley & Sons, Inc. Published 2012 by John Wiley & Sons, Inc.

recognized in veterinary medicine, it is likely that a similar disorder exists in the veterinary patient population.

Atelectasis

Atelectasis is a major complication of prolonged immobility, as well as anesthesia.[5,7] Atelectasis refers to the collapse of alveoli secondary to absorption of gas into the bloodstream. This could happen due to mechanical compression of the lung from the weight of the nondependent lung, airway obstruction, or repetitive collapse and reexpansion of lungs during breathing.[7] Atelectasis, when severe enough, may cause hypoxemia by causing ventilation/perfusion mismatch.[5,7] Atelectasis may increase patients' oxygen requirements, thus increasing the chance of oxygen toxicity. If the patient is being mechanically ventilated, atelectasis may increase the possibility of ventilator-induced lung injury because overdistention of aerated lung may occur due to the atelectatic portion of the lung not being ventilated.[5,7]

Ocular complications

Patients that are anesthetized for long periods of time lose the ability to protect their eyes. Patients under continuous sedation show a significantly higher incidence of ocular surface disorders, such as exposure keratopathy and corneal ulceration.[8,9] Peak incidence occurs during the first 2–7 days of hospitalization.[10] One veterinary study found that 5% of mechanically ventilated dogs develop corneal ulcers.[11]

Loss of the blink function and decreased tear production during long-term anesthesia both leave the eye vulnerable. Tears are essential for ocular health and have many functions. These include lubrication of the ocular surface, provision of oxygen to the cornea, and prevention of bacterial colonization.[1,8] An intact corneal epithelium protects the eye from infection.[1] Blinking spreads lacrimal secretions over the ocular surface, moistening the eye.[9] The evaporation of these tears changes the temperature of the surface, making it unfavorable for bacterial growth.[9] When the ocular surface is dry, small corneal defects develop that can lead to exposure keratopathy.[9] A loss of blink also results in incomplete closure of the eye and thus prolonged exposure of the cornea and conjunctiva to the environment.

Complications associated with oral cavity

An anesthetized patient loses the ability to swallow, clean, and protect oral structures from mechanical damage. Healthy animals rely on the endogenous glycoprotein fibronectin in their saliva and on their dental surfaces to help protect the oropharynx from colonization by pathogenic bacteria. Fibronectin is a glycoprotein that functions in prevention of adherence of gram-negative bacteria to cells and tooth surfaces. In critically ill patients that cannot swallow appropriately and lack oral cavity hygiene, fibronectin is degraded by hydrolytic enzymes in saliva and dental plaque. As a consequence, colonization of gram-negative bacteria and the formation of biofilm on the tooth surface occurs.[12] This change in oral flora from gram positive to gram negative occurs in mechanically ventilated human patients within 48–72 hours of ICU admission.[13] These bacteria are frequently the causative agents of ventilator-associated pneumonia (VAP).

Migration of bacteria from the oropharynx to the respiratory tract, as well as aspiration of the contents of the oropharynx are leading causes of VAP.[3] VAP increases both morbidity and the length of ICU stay, as well as cost of hospitalization.[14] Ranulas and oral ulcers are potential complications of long-term sedation and intubation (Figs. 46.1 and 46.2). Ranula refers to the accumulation of salivary gland contents, such as mucin, in the soft tissues surrounding the gland, due to trauma or obstruction to the gland. Oral ulcers are often caused by mechanical injury to the structures of the mouth.[13] Persistent pressure from pulse oximeter probes, mouth gags, ET tube and its tie, applied to the tongue and other soft tissue structures leads to ulceration.[13]

Complications associated with the urogenital tract

Anesthetized patients usually do not voluntarily void their bladders on a regular basis. Urine is irritating to the skin and can cause significant inflammation and scald, if not removed promptly and completely, which can be difficult to accomplish in larger patients. Moreover, if patients under anesthesia urinate, they do not always empty their urinary bladder completely.

Venous stasis

Immobility promotes venous stasis, which may lead to many deleterious effects.[5] Human patients who are immobile are at increased risk of venous thrombosis, which, in turn, increases their risk of pulmonary thromboembolism.[5,15] In addition, direct compression of the venous vasculature may occur from prolonged contact of extremities with bedding, which may contribute to stasis, as well as result in vascular endothelial damage.[5] Vascular compression, in turn, may result in diminished blood supply to the skin and puts immobilized patients at risk of impairment in skin integrity.[16] Skin damage and ulceration are important consequences of prolonged immobility, and they can cause significant mor-

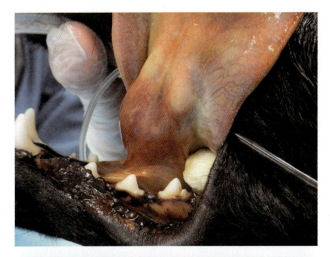

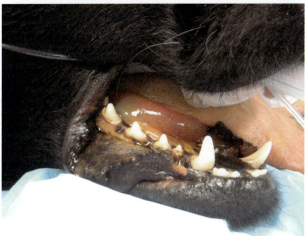

Figures 46.1 and 46.2 Ranulas may form during general anesthesia as a result of trauma to the salivary glands. This may be secondary to equipment in the oral cavity or manipulation of the tongue and the mandible.

bidity. The etiology of skin damage is multifactorial and, in addition to impaired blood supply, includes malnutrition, as well as direct pressure to points of contact during prolonged immobility.[5,17] Skin ulceration may create severe soft tissue damage, cause osteomyelitis of adjacent bones, and may result in systemic infection and sepsis.[5]

Gastrointestinal complications

Gastrointestinal (GI) complications of prolonged anesthesia can be significant, especially during mechanical ventilation. They include splanchnic hypoperfusion and vasoconstriction, as well as diminished GI motility. Patients undergoing mechanical ventilation, particularly those with high levels of positive end-expiratory pressure (PEEP), can experience poor venous return, which

can lead to decreased cardiac output and poor splanchnic perfusion.[18] Poor splanchnic perfusion impairs GI tract and pancreatic function. Mechanical ventilation has also been associated with increased levels of endogenous catecholamines, which can result in splanchnic vasoconstriction and ischemia, making this population of patients at increased risk of GI ulceration and bleeding.[18] Moreover, sedatives, including narcotic agents, further diminish GI motility and therefore contribute to ileus.[5,18] Gut barrier function may be impeded by hypoperfusion, malnutrition, and systemic inflammation. The break in normal gut barrier may result in intestinal bacterial translocation.[18]

Recumbent patient care

The long-term anesthetized patient requires recumbent patient care (Protocol 46.1). Three components contribute to recumbent patient care: proper patient positioning, decubital ulcer prevention and management, and early mobility.

Patient positioning

Patients undergoing long-term anesthesia should be provided with clean, dry, and very well-padded bedding.[1,3] All eliminations have to be cleaned immediately to maintain the skin dry at all times; use of absorbent pads may assist with nursing care. Any bony protuberances should be carefully padded.[19] The extremities should be completely supported at all times and

---

Protocol 46.1 Recumbent patient care

Procedure

To be performed every 4 hours:
1. Perform hand hygiene.
2. Ensure that the bedding is clean, dry, and appropriate for the patient; elevate the head slightly compared to the rest of the body.
3. If the patient is in sternal recumbency, turn hips and reposition the rest of the body slightly; if in lateral recumbency, turn the patient onto the other side.
4. Check for potential sites of ulceration (bony protuberances).
5. If pressure ulcers exist, inspect all dressings to ensure they are clean and cover the wound appropriately.*
6. Perform PROM exercises and massage.

*The pressure ulcer dressing may be changed once to twice daily, depending on the extent of the wound and the amount of exudate produced. Every time the dressing is changed, the size, depth, and extent must be checked.

have contact with a padded surface. A turning schedule should be established early in the patient's care.[20] It is recommended that the animal be turned every 2–4 hours.[1–3] Potential sites for ulcer development should be checked every time a patient is turned.[19] Regular turning is also a key component to the prevention of atelectasis.[3] Compression of dependent lung leads to airway collapse and subsequent perfusion of alveoli that are not ventilated, creating decreased gas exchange and contributing to hypoxemia. Turning the patient shifts the pressure and allows the airways to remain open.

Animals that are anesthetized for long periods of time are most commonly those being mechanically ventilated. In many patients, the need for mechanical ventilation is due to lung pathology and severe hypoxemia. Patients with pulmonary parenchymal disease may not be able to tolerate certain positions, such as lateral recumbency for prolonged periods of time.[1,3] Positioning and turning in these patients may be complicated by their disease process. There is evidence to support sternal positioning as the optimal position for best oxygenation.[21] If an animal is in sternal recumbency, the hips should be turned every 2–4 hours and the position of the rest of the body slightly altered so as to shift pressure points. Oxygenation should be closely monitored after a turn because decompensation may occur during position shifts.[1,7]

VAP is a common complication of long-term intubation. The prone position, as well as placing patients on a 45° angle, may reduce the incidence of VAP in humans; however, such data are not available in our patient population at this time.[22] Elevating the head, as compared with the rest of the body, may be of benefit in dogs and cats.

Decubitus ulcer prevention and management

One of the primary goals of nursing a recumbent patient is the prevention of decubitus ulcers. Decubitus ulcers occur over bony prominences and are the result of soft tissue compression between the bone and a hard surface. Animals that are naturally thin or have a poor body condition are at greater risk for ulcer development.[19] However, any animal that is recumbent for an extended period of time should be considered at risk.

Should a decubitus ulcer develop, it is important that an effort be made to reduce pressure on the site. Ring devices placed around the wound are contraindicated because they contribute to venous congestion and local edema.[20]

The ulcer should be cleaned with a pH-neutral, non-irritating, nontoxic solution, such as saline, and any necrotic tissue debrided.[20] Unless bacterial infection is suspected, chlorhexidine and other antibacterial solutions should be avoided.[20] These agents are toxic to granulomatous tissue and may delay wound healing.[20] Dressings that provide a moist wound environment, keep the skin around the wound dry, control exudate, and eliminate dead space should be chosen.[23] Some examples include moist gauze, hydrocolloid, or calcium alginate dressings.[23] Wet-to-dry dressings are not recommended because they are not continuously moist and therefore not an appropriate wound-dressing selection.[20] The wound should be reassessed with each dressing change to determine whether amendments are needed in the treatment plan as the wound heals or deteriorates. The size, depth, whether debridement is required, and amount of exudate produced by all ulcers should be documented in the medical record each time the wound is evaluated.[20] Adequate nutrient intake and hydration status should be ensured to maximize the potential for wound healing.[24]

Early mobility

A number of serious complications arise from prolonged immobility, such as muscle and ligament contracture, muscle disuse atrophy, and limb edema due to venous stasis. The importance of early mobilization and physical exercise has been highlighted in humans, where trends toward lower mortality, decreased duration of mechanical ventilation, and decreased days in the ICU have been documented, if early mobility is engaged.[6] Feasibility of early mobilization in veterinary patients is of concern, especially in those that are endotracheally intubated and cannot voluntarily move on their own. In these patients, physical exercise regimen should be established and instituted early in the hospitalization to minimize negative effects of immobility. If physical therapy service is available, collaboration with the service may be useful to establish a tailored protocol for the particular patient.

At minimum, physical exercise regimen should include passive range of motion (PROM) exercises and massage. PROM exercises should be performed every 4 hours for 10–15 minutes and ideally involve every joint of the extremities and all of the possible dimensions of movement for the particular joint.[25,26] The joints may be moved separately or concurrently in a motion resembling walking or running.[26] Stretching may also be used. Body massage is useful and may include gentle to deeper stroking, kneading, or skin rolling parallel to the muscle bellies.[25,26] Unfortunately, PROM exercises do not have an effect on muscle atrophy, and exercises that actively engage the muscles are required for better return to function.[26] In select group of patients, active range of motion exercises may be used, if the pet's condition permits. These patients may include animals that are sedated, but not anesthetized, such as those mechanically ventilated via a tracheostomy tube. A wide variety of exercises, from resisted withdrawal to sitting and standing exercises, may be performed, depending on the patient's status.[25,26] In addition, other modalities, such as electrical stimulation, cryotherapy, ultrasound, and heat therapy, may be used, if available.[26]

Eye care

Because the anesthetized patient is unable to produce and spread tear film adequately, protecting the patient's eyes is an essential aspect of nursing care. Eye care (Protocol 46.2) should occur every 2 hours.[1–3,27] Every 2 hours, the eyes should be cleaned with saline-soaked gauze, and artificial tear ointment should be placed in the eyes.[2,3,27] The ointment may be alternated with artificial tear drops.[1] Ideally always, but especially in cases of suspected infections, using dedicated ointment tube for each eye is recommended.[9]

Aerosolization of bacteria occurs during suctioning of the airway and oral cavity.[1,28] Care should be taken not to withdraw the suction catheter near or over the eye.[9,28] Contamination of the eye with the same pathogen causing pneumonia in mechanically ventilated patients has been documented.[28]

Fluorescein staining of the corneas should be performed once daily to check for ulceration.[1–3,27] If detected, a broad-spectrum antibiotic ointment can be used to prevent corneal infection.[1,3,29] If the ulceration does not resolve or improve within 48–72 hours or if there is evidence of progression, such as increased area of stain uptake or depth of the defect, cytology as well as culture and sensitivity testing are indicated to determine the infectious agent.[29] Severe infection may require the hourly application of an antimicrobial agent.[29] Topical atropine is also indicated in the treatment of deep corneal ulcers.[29] Atropine provides analgesia and prevents synechiae formation and barrier.[29] All corneal ulcers and their progression should be documented daily by noting the location, size, and depth of the ulcer in the record.

Chemosis may occur in any patient that is immobilized for prolonged periods of time, and it may be in part responsible for incomplete eye closure and undesired exposure of the cornea and conjunctiva. Decreased drainage, increased vascular permeability, and increased venous pressure contribute to this condition.[9] Incidence is increased in patients who are maintained at a PEEP greater than 5.[28] Periorbital edema and chemosis may also be the result of an overly tight ET tube tie, if tied behind the ears, or the wraps covering central catheters or feeding tubes.[28] Precautions should be taken to avoid edema formation, and steps to resolution of edema should be taken upon its notice. These include carefully monitoring the patient's fluid balance, frequently checking for tightness of the ET tube tie and positioning the patient's head in such a way as to optimize venous return (head slightly higher than the rest of the body, taking care not to occlude the jugular veins).

Oral care

The importance of oral care (Protocol 46.3) in the nursing regimen of patients anesthetized for extended periods of time cannot be stressed enough. Oral care has been documented to decrease the incidence of VAP and therefore is of crucial importance in the management of patients undergoing long-term anesthesia.[14,22,30]

Despite a cuffed ET tube, microaspirations of oral secretions may occur.[14] For this reason, any fluid that pools in the mouth or pharynx should be suctioned every 4–6 hours.[2,3,11,12] The oral cavity may also be rinsed by instilling small amounts (5–20 mL, depending on size of the patient) of sterile saline with a syringe prior to suctioning.[1,3] Care has to be taken to make sure the ET tube is appropriately inflated during rinsing. The oral cavity should also be suctioned prior to adjustment of the ET or tracheostomy tube, reintubation, or a patient position change.[30] It has also been shown that continuous subglottic suctioning, as well as intermittent, regular subglottic suctioning, leads to a reduction in the incidence of VAP.[2,14,30]

Protocol 46.2 Eye care

Procedure

To be performed every 2 hours:
1. Perform hand hygiene.
2. Clean periocular surfaces with saline-soaked gauze.
3. Check eyes for chemosis or inflammation.
4. Ensure that the ET tube tie and any neck wraps are not tight.
5. Place artificial tear ointment in each eye, ideally using a separate designated tube of ointment for each eye. The ointment may be alternated with artificial tear drops.

To be performed every 24 hours:
1. Perform hand hygiene.
2. Fluorescein stain each eye to check for corneal ulcers.
3. If corneal ulcers are visualized, note their location, size, and depth in the progressives section of the medical record.

Protocol 46.3 Oral care

Procedure

To be performed every 6 hours:

1. Remove any pulse oximeter probes, mouth gags, or gauze.
2. Inspect oral cavity for pooling oral secretions, ranulas, and ulcers.
3. Note the approximate size and location of any ulcers or ranulas in the progressives section of the medical record.
4. Check the ET cuff for appropriate inflation.
5. Gently suction the mouth and oropharynx.*
6. Deflate the ET tube cuff, adjust the position of the tube, and reinflate the cuff.
7. Adjust the position of the ET tube tie if needed.
8. Wipe the mucous membranes and tongue with gauze soaked with 0.05% chlorhexidine solution; flush the back of the oral cavity with 0.05% chlorhexidine solution; thoroughly suctioning afterward.
9. Reposition the tongue and wrap in dilute glycerin-soaked gauze.
10. Replace mouth gag and pad teeth with dilute glycerin-soaked gauze.
11. Replace pulse oximeter probe, changing the position of the probe.

*Patients with copious oral secretions and/or persistent regurgitation may require hourly suctioning and/or the placement of an orogastric or nasogastric tube.

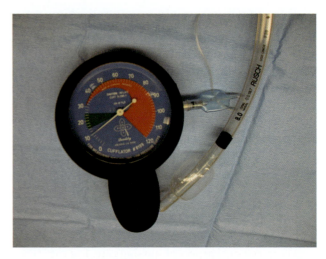

Figure 46.3 Posey Cufflator may be valuable in ensuring appropriate pressure of the ET or tracheostomy tube cuff.

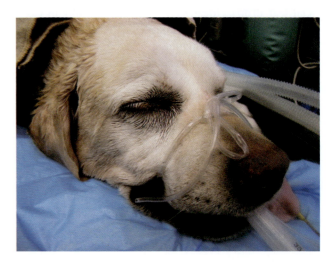

Figure 46.4 Endotracheal tube tie made out of nonporous material, such as IV tubing, reduces the possibility of bacterial contamination.

Although an inflated ET tube cuff may not prevent aspiration, an effort should be made to protect the airway as much as possible by checking that the cuff is appropriately inflated. A Posey Cufflator (J. T. Posey Company, Arcadia, CA) may be used to ensure that the correct pressure is achieved (Fig. 46.3). This device attaches to the ET tube cuff, which allows one to measure the pressure in the cuff while it is being inflated by the bulb of the device. The recommended intracuff pressure is 22–32 cm H_2O. Alternatively, administering a breath while listening for a leak, as the cuff is being inflated by a syringe, can be performed. This ensures that the least amount of air to inflate the cuff sufficiently is instilled, minimizing cuff overinflation. The ET tube cuff should be deflated and the tube's position adjusted every 4 hours to prevent damage to the trachea.[3] When securing the tube, a tie made of a nonporous material is ideal.[3] Cloth that is moistened by oral secretions provides an excellent medium for bacterial growth. As an alternative to muzzle gauze, a tie may be fashioned from IV tubing (Fig. 46.4).[3]

Monitoring equipment, such as a pulse oximeter probe, and the ET tube should be moved every 6 hours.[1,3,11,13] The ET tube tie should be adjusted every 6 hours. A cushion made of saline- or glycerin-moistened gauze should be placed between the tie and the soft tissues it comes into contact with.[3,11,13] If possible, placement of the tongue directly over the teeth should be avoided.[3,11,13] If this is not possible, the teeth should be packed with saline- or glycerin-moistened gauze to reduce trauma (Fig. 46.5).[11] This is especially important in pediatric patients because the primary teeth are sharper than adult teeth.[11] The tongue and other soft tissue structures should be kept moist with gauze soaked

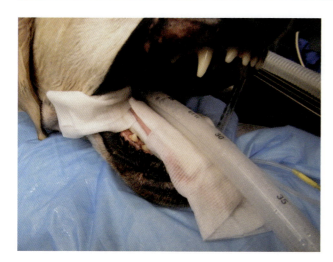

Figure 46.5 Packing of the oral cavity with saline-moistened or dilute glycerin-moistened gauze diminishes desiccation of the mucous membranes and minimizes soft tissue damage that occurs secondary to the equipment, such as ET tube and pulse oximetry monitor.

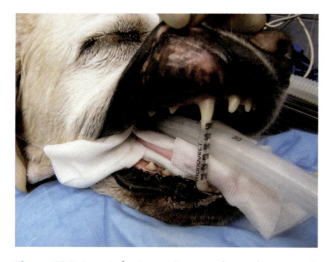

Figure 46.6 A part of a 1-cc syringe may be used as a mouth gag to diminish pressure of the teeth on the tongue.

in dilute glycerin.[1,3,11,13] Any pressure that may have contributed to a lesion should be relieved (Fig. 46.6).

The oral cavity should be decontaminated with a dilute chlorhexidine solution (0.05%) every 6 hours, concentrating on any oral ulceration that may be present.[1,3,12,13] Oral ulcers provide a route for bacteria to enter the systemic circulation, and early and thorough treatment is essential. Chlorhexidine is bacteriostatic and bacteriocidal and has been shown to promote gingival healing.[13] Chlorhexidine use should be instituted

regardless of the presence of ulceration, as a method of selective oral decontamination (SOD). SOD refers to the use of topical antibiotics in the oral cavity and has been shown to reduce mortality in human critical care patients, due to reduction in oropharyngeal bacterial colonization.[13,31]

Persistent regurgitation may further complicate oral care. Aspiration of gastric contents is a cause of VAP.[11] Additionally, regurgitation of gastric contents decreases the pH of the mouth and increases the severity of oral ulcers.[13] A nasogastric or orogastric tube may be passed to relive the stomach of its contents and prevent further regurgitation.

Bladder care

The urinary bladder should be palpated every 4–6 hours and expressed as needed. Urinary catheterization should be considered if effective expression cannot be achieved due to patient's size or bladder dysfunction, or if measuring exact urinary output is important.

Two methods of urinary bladder catheterization are intermittent and indwelling catheter insertion. Decision on which method to used depends on the needs of each individual patient. Urinary tract infection (UTI) is a risk factor for urinary bladder catheterization regardless of the method. Duration of catheterization has been shown to be a more important factor for development of a UTI than the method of catheterization.[32] A Cochrane review reported that the incidence of bacteriuria is higher in the indwelling catheter patient population compared with intermittently catheterized patients; however, some patients with bacteriuria were suspected to have bacterial colonization rather than a symptomatic UTI.[33]

Regardless of the method of catheterization, aseptic technique during catheter placement cannot be overemphasized. Hair should be clipped around the catheter insertion site, and the area should be disinfected with chlorhexidine scrub and rinsed with sterile saline. Sterile gloves and lubricant should be used. A 0.05% chlorhexidine solution is used to flush the vestibule or prepuce prior to the catheter insertion. In females, catheterization is achieved by blind palpation of the urethral papilla or by direct visualization of the urethra using a speculum and a light source. If a Foley catheter is used, the balloon is inflated after the catheter is advanced into the bladder. Afterward, the catheter is gently pulled back until resistance is met. If a different type of indwelling catheter is used, the catheter is sutured in place after measurement has been taken to ensure correct placement. A radiograph should be taken to verify catheter position. Please see Chapter 31 for more details on placement and maintenance of urinary catheters.

Gastrointestinal tract

Patients undergoing long-term anesthesia should be evaluated frequently for abdominal distension, presence of bowel sounds, and frequency of bowel movement.[5] The bowel sounds may be ausculted over the four quadrants of the abdomen with a stethoscope. Frequency varies quite a bit between patients and the relation to a meal, but in general bowel sounds should be auscultated approximately four to five times a minute. If a gastric feeding tube is in place, volume and characteristics of gastric aspirates should be noted in the record. Frequency of gastric tube aspiration varies among patients but typically occurs every 4–6 hours. Prokinetic agents may be considered if significant gastric residuals are present. Human patients undergoing mechanical ventilation are at high risk for development of gastrointestinal ulceration, and they are routinely administered medications aimed at reducing production of gastric acid (H2 blockers, proton pump inhibitors).[34] Whereas the same information is not available in the veterinary population, it is reasonable to believe that the veterinary patients undergoing mechanical ventilation may be at risk for GI ulceration and therefore would benefit from ulcer prophylaxis.

Both diarrhea and constipation may be observed in the patient population under general anesthesia. Care should be taken to keep the anal and perineal area clean and dry; removal of hair may facilitate this and also allow monitoring of the skin for irritation. Careful abdominal palpation should be performed daily to assess for constipation. Enemas may be required to facilitate GI tract emptying.[1]

Techniques to decrease stimulation

Patients undergoing long-term anesthesia are frequently intubated for the duration of the event; however, some may have a tracheostomy tube placed to minimize the amount of sedative and anesthetic agents used, as well as to avoid complications associated with orotracheal intubation, such as oral ulcerations or laryngeal edema. Drugs used to maintain heavy sedation are titrated to the lowest level that is required for immobilization and patient comfort. Occasionally, patients may be rousable and responsive to stimuli. Therefore, several techniques may be used to minimize stimulation. Treatments should be grouped together in such a way that the patient is stimulated as infrequently as possible. Additional sedation may be utilized during periods of stimulation, which may include boluses of injectable anesthetics, opioids, anxiolytics, or tranquilizers. Cotton balls may be placed in the external ear canals to minimize auditory stimuli. This should be noted in the record, so that the cotton can be removed when it is not needed. Ambient noise should be kept as minimal as possible. When not absolutely necessary, lights should be turned down to minimize visual stimulation. When that is not possible, placing a towel over the eyes may aid in reducing stimuli.

Summary

General anesthesia and long-term immobilization may be necessary in a subset of critically ill patients. A number of factors may negatively impact these animals, and vigilant and well-structured nursing care program is paramount in preventing and addressing commonly encountered complications for optimal patient care.

References

1. King LG, Haskins SC. Positive pressure ventilation. In: King LG, ed. Textbook of Respiratory Disease in Dogs and Cats. Philadelphia, PA: Elsevier; 2004:217–229.
2. Hopper K, Clare M. Mechanical ventilation: ventilator settings, patient management and nursing care. Compend Cont Educ Pract Vet 2005:27(4):256–267.
3. Hopper K, Silverstein D. Small Animal Critical Care Medicine. Philadelphia, PA: Saunders, 2008.
4. Stevens RD, Dowdy DW, Michaels RK, Mendez-Tellez PA, Pronovost PJ, Needham DM. Neuromuscular dysfunction acquired in critical illness: a systematic review. Intensive Care Med 2007;33:1876–1891.
5. Brower RG. Consequences of bed rest [review]. Crit Care Med 2009;37(10 Suppl):S422–S428.
6. Truong AD, Fan E, Brower R, Neddham DM. Bench-to-bedside review: mobilizing patients in the intensive care unit—from pathophysiology to clinical trials. Crit Care 2009;13:216–229.
7. Aldrich J. Atelectasis. In: King LG, ed. Textbook of Respiratory Disease in Dogs and Cats. Philadelphia, PA: Elsevier; 2004:465–471.
8. Imanaka H, Taenaka N, Nakamura J, et al. Ocular surface disorders in the critically ill. Anesth Analg 1997;85:343–346.
9. Rosenberg JB, Eisen LA.Eye care in the intensive care unit: Narrative review and meta-analysis. Crit Care Med 2008;36: 3151–3155.
10. Marshall AP, Elliot R, Rolls K, Schacht S, Boyle M. Eye care in the critically ill: clinical practice guideline. Aust Crit Care 2008;21(2):97–109.
11. Hopper K, Haskins SC, Kass PH, Rezende ML, Aldrich J. Indications, management and outcome of long-term positive pressure ventilation in dogs and cats:148 cases(1990–2001). J Am Vet Med Assoc 2007;230(1):64–75.
12. Berry AM, Davidson PM, Masters J, Rolls K. Systematic literature review of oral hygiene practices for intensive care patients receiving mechanical ventilation. Am J Crit Care 2007;16:552–562.
13. Fudge M, Anderson JG, Aldrich J, Haskins SC. Oral lesions associated with orotracheal administered mechanical ventilation in critically ill dogs. J Vet Emerg Crit Care 1997;7(2):79–87.
14. Sierra R, Benitez E, Leon C, Rello J. Prevention and diagnosis of ventilator-associated pneumonia: a survey on current practices in southern Spanish ICUs. Chest 2005;128:1667–1673.

15. Geerts WH, Pineo GF, Heit JA, et al. Prevention of venous thromboembolism: The Seventh ACCP Conference on Antithrombotic and Thrombolytic Therapy. Chest 2004;126:338S–400S.

16. Lindgren VA, Ames NJ. Caring for patients on mechanical ventilation: what research indicates is best practice. Am J Nurs 2005;105(5):50–60.

17. Benbow M. Guidelines for the prevention and treatment of pressure ulcers. Nurs Stand 2006;20:42–44.

18. Mutlu GM, Mutlu EA, Factor P. Prevention and treatment of gastrointestinal complications in patients on mechanical ventilation. Am J Respir Med 2003;2(5):395–411.

19. McCurnin DM, Bassert JM, eds. Clinical Textbook for Veterinary Technicians. Philadelphia, PA: Saunders; 2002.

20. Whitney J, Phillips L, Aslam R, et al. Guidelines for the treatment of pressure ulcers. Wound Repair Regen 2006;14:663–679.

21. McMillan MW, Whitaker KE, Hughes D, Brodbelt DC, Boag AK. Effect of body position on the arterial partial pressures of oxygen and carbon dioxide in spontaneously breathing, conscious dogs in an intensive care unit. J Vet Emerg Crit Care 2009;19(6):564–570.

22. Dodek P, Keenan S, Cook D, et al. Evidence-based clinical practice guideline for the prevention of ventilator-associated pneumonia. Ann Intern Med 2004;141:305–313.

23. Reddy M, Gill SS, Kalkar SR, Wu W, Anderson PJ, Rocho PA. Treatment of pressure ulcers: a systematic review. JAMA 2008;300:2647–2662.

24. Ratliff CR. WOCN's Evidence-based pressure ulcer guideline. Adv Skin Wound Care 2005;18:204–208.

25. Smarick SD, Rylander H, Burkitt JM. Treatment of traumatic cervical myelopathy with surgery, prolonged positive-pressure ventilation, and physical therapy in a dog. JAVMA 2007;230:370–374.

26. Drum MG. Physical rehabilitation of the canine neurologic patient. Vet Clin North Am Small Anim Pract 2010;40:181–193.

27. Marshall AP, Elliot R, Rolls K, Schacht S, Boyle M. Eyecare in the critically ill: clinical practice guideline. Australian Crit Care 2008;21(2):97–109.

28. Cunningham C, Gould D. Eyecare for the sedated patient undergoing mechanical ventilation: the use of evidence-based care. Int J Nurs Stud 1998;35(1–2):32–40.

29. Vygantas KR, Whitley RD. Management of deep corneal ulcers. Compend Cont Educ Pract Vet 2003;25(3):196–205.

30. Chao YFC, Chen YY, Wan, KWK, Lee RP, Tsai H. Removal of oral secretion prior to position change can reduce the incidence of ventilator-associated pneumonia for adult ICU patients: a clinical controlled trial study. J Clin Nurs 2009;18(1):22–28.

31. de Smet AM, Kluytmans JA, Cooper BS, et al. Decontamination of the digestive tract and oropharynx in ICU patients. N Engl J Med 2009;360(1):20–31.

32. Bubenik L, Hosgood G. Urinary tract infection in dogs with thoracolumbar intervertebral disc herniation and urinary bladder dysfunction managed by manual expression, indwelling catheterization or intermittent catheterization. Vet Surg 2008;37(8):791–800.

33. Niël-Weise BS, van den Broek PJ. Urinary catheter policies for short-term bladder drainage in adults. Cochrane Database Syst Rev 2005;20;(3):CD004203.

34. Tauseef A, Harty RF. Stress-induced ulcer bleeding in critically ill patients. Gastroenterol Clin North Am 2009;38:245–265.

SECTION VII

Clinicopathologic techniques

47

Blood sample collection and handling

Lori Baden Atkins

The information obtained from blood sample analysis often plays a critical role in the diagnostic process. For this reason, it is crucial that blood samples be obtained and handled properly to preserve the integrity of the specimen and provide accurate results.

A number of issues can adversely affect the quality of blood specimens. Aggressive collection techniques including rapid aspiration of blood through a small bore needle, prolonged or improper tourniquet use, excessive redirection of the needle, or "fishing," to access a vein, and other practices are frequently associated with poor sample quality. Improper handling issues including failure to invert collection tubes adequately to mix the anticoagulant and blood, improper or delayed centrifugation, inadequate filling of blood tubes, and other handling errors may also have a negative impact on sample quality.

Safety concerns

A number of safety issues need to be considered during collection and handling of blood samples. Conscious patients need to be restrained in a manner that provides for the safety of the person performing the venipuncture, the assistant, and the patient. It is imperative that personnel providing restraint be properly trained in techniques that facilitate control of the patient while minimizing the risk of injury to the animal or staff. Sharps safety practices must be strictly observed to minimize the risk of injury from needles or catheters. Needles should not be recapped and must be disposed of in puncture-resistant biohazard containers. Safety needles and catheters should be used whenever possible. Needleless devices (Fig. 47.1) and ports allow for the administration of fluids and drugs, as well as collection of samples from intravenous (IV) lines and catheters without the risk of a sharps injury.

Aseptic technique should be used when collecting samples, especially in immune-compromised patients. Proper hand hygiene and the use of examination gloves significantly reduces the risk of infection to both the patient and the handler.[1,2] Whenever possible, hair should be clipped and the skin swabbed with antiseptic prior to blood collection.

Once the sample is collected, all tubes must be labeled with the patient's name and identification number. Blood is considered a biohazard; proper packaging is essential for specimens submitted to commercial laboratories. Failure to label or package samples according to the laboratory's specifications may result in rejection of the sample.

Serum and/or plasma must be separated from whole blood by centrifugation. All personnel using the centrifuge should be cognizant of safety and appropriate use guidelines. Ideally, centrifuges should not be operated without a cover or lid in place; when in use, covered centrifuges should never be opened until the rotor has come to a complete stop. Tube caps or stoppers should be securely in place on all samples placed in the centrifuge; any spills need to be cleaned immediately, following all appropriate safety precautions.

Proper venous blood sample collection

Venous blood samples may be collected by direct insertion of a needle into a vein (venipuncture) or by aspiration of blood through an IV catheter.

Advanced Monitoring and Procedures for Small Animal Emergency and Critical Care, First Edition. Edited by Jamie M. Burkitt Creedon, Harold Davis.
© 2012 John Wiley & Sons, Inc. Published 2012 by John Wiley & Sons, Inc.

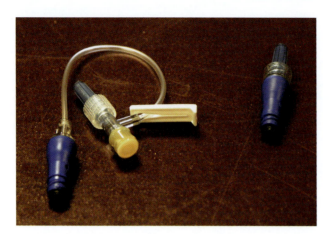

Figure 47.1 Needleless ports.

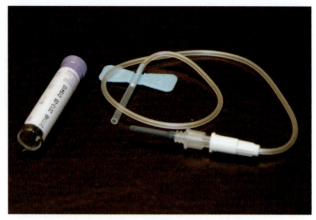

Figure 47.2 Vacutainer System®.

Venipuncture equipment

Several factors play a significant role in the quality of a blood sample, and the person performing the venipuncture should be familiar with these variables to ensure sample quality and achieve accurate results. Needle selection is based on the size and fragility of the vein, the volume of blood required, and the frequency of sampling anticipated. Needle sizes most commonly selected for venipuncture are 18 to 22 gauge; smaller needles ranging from 23 to 28 gauge may be used when veins are extremely small or fragile, or when frequent sampling is required (i.e., bihourly glucose curves). Needles at the larger end of the spectrum are preferred when large sample volumes are required. The size of the needle used for venipuncture is a prime determinant of the rate at which a sample may be aspirated; the larger the needle, the faster the rate. Rapid aspiration of blood through a small-bore needle creates shear forces resulting in hemolysis and may adversely affect test results.

Syringe size is determined by the volume of sample required. The use of large syringes has been associated with application of excessive negative pressure during sample aspiration and may cause hemolysis and vascular collapse. To ensure sample quality, the person performing the venipuncture should apply steady, gentle traction on the syringe plunger in such a manner that the syringe fills at the same rate at which the plunger is retracted. Repetitive application and release of negative pressure on the syringe, or "pulsing," does not increase either the rate or volume of sample collection; this technique causes the vessel to collapse and frequently results in hemolysis.

Alternative venipuncture equipment includes butterfly catheters and Vacutainer (Becton, Dickinson, Franklin Lakes, NJ) systems. Butterfly catheters come in a variety of gauges and can be especially useful in fractious patients or when collecting samples from small or fragile veins. Vacutainer systems (Fig. 47.2) allow blood to be drawn directly into the collection tube(s), facilitating immediate contact with the anticoagulant to help preserve the integrity of the sample.

Table 47.1 Order of draw for venous blood samples[3]

1. Blood culture (yellow or blood culture bottles)
2. Sodium citrate (light blue)
3. Serum or serum separator (SST) (red or red/gray)
4. Heparin or gel separator with heparin (PST) (green or green/gray)
5. EDTA (lavender or pink)
6. Sodium fluoride (gray)

Order of draw

When blood is drawn into multiple blood tubes, it is important that the tubes be collected in a specific order (Table 47.1); filling tubes in the improper order may result in the unintended contamination of the sample with anticoagulants and erroneous results (i.e., false elevation of potassium levels and decreased levels of calcium due to serum or plasma contamination with potassium ethylenediaminetetraacetic acid (K_2EDTA) from the lavender-top tube).

Venipuncture sites

The most common sites for venipuncture include the cephalic, medial saphenous, lateral saphenous, jugular, and femoral veins. Factors influencing site selection

Protocol 47.1 Jugular venipuncture protocol

Procedure
1. The patient is restrained in sternal recumbency with head elevated.
   a. Note: Lateral or dorsal recumbency may be used provided the jugular vein is readily accessible.
2. Clip and prep the area over the jugular according to hospital policy.
3. The person performing the venipuncture occludes the vessel by applying pressure in the jugular furrow lateral to the thoracic inlet.
4. Insert the needle, bevel (opening) up, through the skin and into the vein (~20° angle); once blood is noted in hub, decrease the angle of the syringe and advance the needle ~0.5–1.0 cm into the lumen of the vessel.
5. Apply gentle negative pressure to aspirate blood into the syringe.
6. Once the desired sample volume is obtained, release negative pressure and withdraw the needle from the vein.
7. Apply direct pressure to the venipuncture site for a minimum of 30 seconds or until there is no evidence of continued bleeding.

Protocol 47.2 Cephalic venipuncture technique

Procedure
1. The patient is restrained in sternal recumbency (sitting or standing are also acceptable) with the thoracic limb extended forward.
2. The area over the distal cephalic vein may be clipped or swabbed with isopropyl alcohol according to hospital policy; clipping is often preferred for excessively long or matted hair or when visible dirt is present.
3. The assistant places his or her thumb over the cephalic vein immediately distal to the elbow and applies pressure sufficient to occlude the vessel.
4. The distal portion of the thoracic limb is grasped and traction is applied to minimize movement. The vein may be stabilized by placing the thumb along the lateral aspect of the vein and pulling the skin distally.
5. Insert the needle, bevel (opening) up, through the skin and into the vein (~20° angle); once blood is noted in hub, decrease the angle of the syringe and advance the needle ~0.5–1.0 cm into the lumen of the vessel.
6. Apply gentle suction to aspirate blood into the syringe; release negative pressure once sample is obtained.
7. Release venous occlusion (or tourniquet if used), remove the needle from the vein, and apply direct pressure for 30 seconds or until there is no evidence of continued bleeding.
8. A pressure wrap may be used if bleeding is excessive.

include the sample volume required, the accessibility of the vein, the skill of the person performing the venipuncture, the condition of the skin over the site, and the patient's condition and behavior. When a large sample volume is required, it is generally advisable to select a larger vessel such as the jugular (Protocol 47.1), cephalic, or femoral; lesser volumes may be collected from smaller veins such as the medial or lateral saphenous veins. The vein selected should be easily accessible; excessive probing or redirection of the needle is associated with hemolysis and poor sample quality. To minimize the risk of infection, venipuncture should not be performed at any site where there is evidence of pyoderma or loss of skin integrity.

The patient's condition may play a significant role in the site selection. If there is any concern regarding the patient's coagulation status, samples should be collected from a peripheral vein using a small-bore needle; it has been recommended that samples not be collected from the jugular vein in these patients. Jugular venipuncture is also controversial in patients with head trauma or other neurologic issues because occlusion of the jugular vein may result in a significant increase in intracranial pressure. Trauma patients may have significant injuries, and the person performing the venipuncture should select venipuncture sites with the patient's comfort in mind.

Peripheral venipuncture

Common sites for peripheral venipuncture include the cephalic vein (Protocol 47.2) located on the cranial aspect of the thoracic limb between the elbow and the carpus, lateral saphenous vein located on the lateral aspect of the pelvic limb between the knee and the tarsus, and the femoral or medial saphenous vein located on the medial aspect of the pelvic limb. Although these veins are most commonly used, other peripheral veins including the auricular veins located on the pinna of the ear, sublingual vein located under the tongue (unconscious or sedated patients only), and mammary veins may be accessed when necessary.

Lateral saphenous venipuncture

This site is most commonly used in dogs; in cats the vein is very small and it is rather difficult to draw a sample. The distal lateral saphenous vein is readily visible and accessible but tends to move or "roll" significantly; the proximal portion of the vein is not readily visible but is easily palpated and less prone to movement.

The technique for drawing a blood sample from the lateral saphenous is similar to drawing a cephalic

Protocol 47.3 Femoral or medial saphenous venipuncture technique

Procedure
1. Restrain the patient in lateral recumbency. The assistant holds the distal thoracic limbs in one hand and places his or her forearm against the neck to control the head.
   a. Fractious cats may be more easily handled by grasping the scruff of the neck and bracing a forearm along the spine to provide secure restraint.
   b. Large patients may require two assistants to provide safe restraint.
2. The nondependent pelvic limb is flexed and held tucked against the caudal abdomen with the side of the hand used to occlude the medical saphenous or femoral vein.
3. The venipuncturist grasps the distal portion of the dependent limb to position the extremity for venipuncture.
4. Insert the needle, bevel (opening) up, through the skin and into the vein (~20° angle); once blood is noted in hub, decrease the angle of the syringe and advance the needle ~0.5-1.0 cm into the lumen of the vessel.
5. Apply gentle suction to aspirate blood into the syringe; release negative pressure once sample is obtained.
6. Release venous occlusion (or tourniquet if used), remove the needle from the vein, and apply direct pressure for 30 seconds or until there is no evidence of continued bleeding.
7. A pressure wrap may be used if bleeding is excessive.

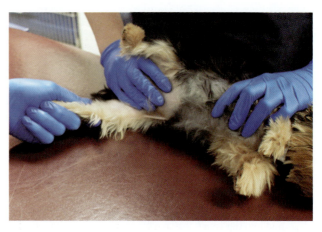

Figure 47.3 Restraint of patient for medial saphenous venipuncture.

sample, but the restraint differs significantly. The patient is restrained in lateral recumbency with the assistant grasping the distal thoracic limbs in one hand and placing their forearm over the patient's neck to control the head. The assistant grasps the nondependent pelvic limb just below the stifle with the free hand to provide restraint and occludes the vessel for venipuncture.

Medial saphenous or femoral venipuncture

The medial saphenous and femoral veins are often the best site for venipuncture (Protocol 47.3) in fractious or uncooperative patients. Again, the technique is similar to cephalic venipuncture, but the restraint (Fig. 47.3) is similar to that used for collection from the lateral saphenous.

Tourniquet use during venipuncture

During venipuncture, a vessel may be occluded by manual pressure or through the use of a tourniquet. The tourniquets most commonly used in veterinary medi-

cine are the Nye tourniquet or the combination of hemostats with either a Penrose drain or a rubber band; both methods are relatively atraumatic and allow quick release. Tourniquet use should be reserved for situations in which manual pressure is insufficient to occlude venous return and allow palpation or visualization of the vein. When a tourniquet is used, in my opinion it should be limited to less than 2 minutes; less than 1 minute is preferred. Significant changes in blood chemistry results including elevations in serum protein, potassium, and lactic acid occur with prolonged tourniquet use.[4]

Blood sample collection from a catheter

Blood samples may be collected from both peripheral and central IV catheters. Hemolysis has been associated with samples collected from IV catheters and appears to be directly proportional to the size of the catheter used. In a study comparing samples collected by venipuncture using a 21-g Vacutainer (Becton, Dickinson, Franklin Lakes, NJ) needle and evacuated sample tubes to samples collected through a peripheral IV catheter at insertion, hemolysis was noted in 3.8% of the samples obtained through venipuncture and in 13.7% of those obtained through a catheter.[5] Further analysis showed that the primary variable was the diameter of the IV catheter as demonstrated by the percentage of hemolyzed samples obtained. Specifically, this study documented that there was no evidence of hemolysis in samples obtained from 16-gauge catheters, whereas all samples drawn from 24-gauge catheters were hemolyzed; a small percentage of samples drawn from cath-

Protocol 47.4 Blood sample collection from an intravenous catheter

Procedure
1. The selected venous access site is clipped and prepped according to hospital policy.
2. The catheter is aseptically placed.
   a. Catheters intended for blood sample collection should not be preflushed to avoid sample dilution.
   b. Hemolysis may be minimized by selection of a large-bore catheter.
3. Attach a syringe (size appropriate for sample volume required) to the hub of the catheter and apply gentle traction to aspirate blood.
   a. It is imperative that the catheter be stabilized throughout the collection procedure.
4. Following sample collection, disconnect the syringe and insert a t-port or male adapter plug into the catheter hub.
5. Flush the catheter with 0.9% sodium chloride or heparinized saline according to hospital policy.
6. Inject the blood sample into the appropriate collection tubes immediately after flushing the catheter.

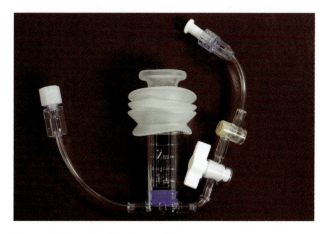

Figure 47.4 Inline blood sampling system.

eters ranging from 18 to 22 gauge also demonstrated hemolysis.[5]

Sample collection from peripheral intravenous catheters

Peripheral catheters are most commonly used for sample collection immediately following catheter placement, which minimizes the number of needlesticks for the patient and possibly expedites sample collection (Protocol 47.4).

Sample collection from central intravenous catheters

Central venous catheters include peripherally inserted central catheters (PICCs), tunneled and nontunneled central catheters, and implanted ports; these devices are frequently used to facilitate serial blood sampling in hospitalized patients. The concerns associated with blood sampling through central lines include an increased risk of catheter complications including infection and occlusion as well as the possibility of inaccurate results due to sample dilution from IV fluids and medications or hemolysis due to improper collection technique.[6] Both the discard method and the push-pull method of sample collection have been shown to yield accurate results when properly performed.

Another method that is very effective for collection of samples from central catheters and arterial lines is the use of an inline sampling system. These systems feature a reservoir, stop cock, and a sampling port (Fig. 47.4); they are connected between the IV line and the catheter. With these devices, "discard" blood is drawn into the reservoir and then returned to the patient without the use of multiple syringes. It is my opinion that the benefits of these devices are a lower risk of catheter-related infections, less blood loss for the patient, and consistent sampling technique.

Discard method

The discard method (Protocol 47.5) involves drawing a volume of blood from the catheter and discarding it to minimize the risk of sample dilution or interfering substances. Significant concerns with this method include iatrogenic anemia as well as an increased risk of catheter-related infections due to the handling of the catheter hub or port.

Push-pull or mixing method[8]

The push-pull (Protocol 47.6) or mixing method of sample collection involves aspiration and injection of blood through the catheter hub or port, followed by sample collection into a fresh syringe. The potential advantages of this method include decreased risk of iatrogenic anemia with frequent sampling and decreased risk of catheter-associated infections through minimizing extraneous handling of the catheter. As in the discard method, all fluids or medications being administered through the catheter are temporarily stopped, and the catheter hub or port is cleaned with antiseptic solution.[8]

Protocol 47.5 Discard method

Procedure
Discontinue administration of all fluids and medications prior to sample collection.
1. Disinfect the catheter hub according to hospital protocol.
2. Flush the catheter with 3-5 mL 0.9% sodium chloride or heparinized saline.
3. Attach a syringe to the catheter hub and aspirate blood.
   a. Minimum of three times: priming volume of the catheter for routine assays.[6]
   b. Six to twelve times: priming volume for coagulation assays.[7]
4. Remove the discard syringe and attach a fresh syringe for sample collection; apply gentle traction to aspirate blood.
5. Depending on the patient's condition, the discard sample may be reinfused.
   a. Preheparinizing the discard syringe will minimize clotting if reinfusion is planned.
   b. Discard samples from an arterial catheter should be reinfused into a venous catheter.
6. Following sample collection, flush the catheter with 3-5 mL 0.9% sodium chloride or heparinized saline according to hospital policy.

Protocol 47.6 Push-pull method

Procedure
1. Discontinue administration of all fluids and medications prior to sample collection.
2. Disinfect the catheter hub according to hospital protocol.
3. Attach a syringe to the catheter hub and aspirate blood (minimum of three times the catheter priming volume).
4. With the syringe still attached to the hub of the catheter, reinfuse the blood.
5. Repeat steps 3 and 4 at least three times.
6. Discard the empty mixing syringe and attach a fresh syringe.
7. Aspirate the required sample volume and inject it into the appropriate blood collection tubes.
8. Following sample collection, flush the catheter with 3-5 mL 0.9% sodium chloride or heparinized saline according to hospital policy.
9. Restart infusion of IV fluids and medications.

Protocol 47.7 Blood culture collection

Procedure
1. It is recommended that a minimum of three samples be obtained from different vascular sites over a period of time.[9]
   a. 10 minutes for critical or septic patients
   b. 24 hours for noncritical patients
2. The general sample volume recommendations are as follows:[9]
   a. Cats and small dogs: 5 mL
   b. Medium dogs: 10 mL
   c. Large dogs: 20 mL
3. Volume must be sufficient for a 1:10 ratio of blood to broth.[9]
4. The venipuncture site is clipped and a surgical scrub is performed over the vein.
5. Disinfect the diaphragm of the culture bottles with 70% isopropyl alcohol or iodine[9] according to hospital policy; allow to air dry.
6. Don sterile gloves to collect the blood sample.
7. Following sample collection, place a new needle on the syringe and inject the blood into the culture bottles, dividing the sample between aerobic and anaerobic media.
   a. Avoid injection of air into the culture bottles.
   b. Invert each bottle two to three times to thoroughly mix the blood and broth.
8. Maintain samples at room temperature; sensitive bacteria may perish under refrigeration.

Blood culture samples

Blood cultures may be helpful to identify causative agents in patients with suspected bacteremia. Samples collected for blood culture (Protocol 47.7) require strict aseptic technique, and proper sample handling is essential for successful culture and accurate results. In most bacteremic patients, the number of organisms in circulation is very small; the volume of blood collected needs to be sufficient to account for the low concentration of bacteria.

The current recommendations are that multiple samples be collected from different vascular sites over a period of several minutes to several hours. Venipuncture is the preferred sample collection method; indwelling catheters have been shown to have a higher percentage of false-positive results due to colonization of the catheter.

Arterial blood sample collection

Arterial blood samples are useful for assessment of oxygenation, ventilation, and acid-base status. These samples may be collected by direct arterial puncture or through an arterial catheter.

A number of arterial blood gas (ABG) syringes prefilled with lyophilized heparin are readily available on the commercial market. These syringes are available in either vented or unvented styles and typically range from 1 to 3 mL in volume. The unvented syringe is handled like a standard syringe; the needle is inserted into the vessel with the plunger positioned at the base of the barrel and then gently retracted to draw blood into the syringe. The vented syringe allows the person performing the venipuncture to position the plunger at the desired draw volume in the barrel; once the needle enters the artery, blood should fill the syringe to the level of the plunger.

Commercial arterial blood gas syringes are preferred for arterial sampling. Blood gas syringes may be created in the hospital by drawing 1000 U/mL heparin into the syringe, allowing it to coat the interior of the barrel, and then expressing the heparin from the syringe prior to sampling. Note that samples obtained using non-ommercial syringes with liquid heparin may lead to dilutional error.[10] To minimize hematoma formation, small-bore needles (25 or 27 gauge) should be used for sample collection.

It is important to note that arterial puncture is considered to be significantly more painful than peripheral venipuncture. It is crucial that the patient be properly restrained for the procedure; the use of a small volume of local or topical anesthetic at the site is often beneficial.

Direct arterial puncture

The dorsal pedal and femoral arteries are most commonly chosen for arterial puncture (Protocol 47.8); on rare occasions samples may be collected from the radial or median arteries, the artery in the pinna of the ear, or from the sublingual artery in anesthetized or unconscious patients. The dorsal pedal artery is the preferred sampling site for me because there appears to be a lesser incidence of mixed arterial/venous samples, and it is relatively easy to apply a pressure bandage following sample collection. The drawback to the dorsal pedal artery is that it is significantly smaller than the femoral artery and may be difficult to access in some patients. The femoral artery is typically easy to palpate and may be easier to access, but it appears more likely to yield mixed samples, and it is difficult to place a pressure bandage to control bleeding following arterial puncture. Arterial sampling should be approached with extreme caution and may be contraindicated in patients with known or suspected coagulopathies.

Arterial catheter sampling

Arterial catheters are placed for the purposes of continuous blood pressure measurements and the repeated

---

Protocol 47.8 Arterial puncture technique

Procedure
1. Restrain the patient in lateral recumbency. The assistant holds the distal thoracic limbs in one hand and places his or her forearm against the neck to control the head.
    a. Large patients may require two assistants to provide safe restraint.
2. The nondependent pelvic limb is flexed and held tucked against the caudal abdomen.
3. Locate the artery by palpation; clip and aseptically prep the area over the vessel.
4. Don exam gloves; palpate and stabilize the artery.
    a. A single digit may be placed directly over the artery; with a heparinized syringe, the needle is advanced into the vessel at a 45° angle directly below the finger, or
    b. A digit may be placed on each side of the artery (~1 inch apart), and the needle is between the fingers and advanced into the vessel at a 90° angle.[11]
5. Following arterial puncture, direct pressure is applied for 5 minutes and the site is closely monitored to ensure there is no continued bleeding.
6. All air is expressed from the syringe immediately after sample collection and the needle is plunged into a rubber stopper or cork.
7. It is recommended that samples be analyzed immediately, but they may be placed in an ice bath for up to 1 hour.[7]

---

sampling of arterial blood. Sampling from an arterial catheter (Protocol 47.9) minimizes the need to perform arterial punctures.

Proper specimen handling

The accuracy of hematology, blood chemistries, and other lab results is directly related to the quality of the sample submitted for analysis. Although the first step in acquiring a high-quality sample requires using appropriate collection techniques as previously noted, the manner in which the sample is handled following collection is equally important.

Handling of venous samples

During or immediately after collection, blood samples should be injected into the appropriate sample tubes for the tests required; all tubes must be labeled with the patient's name and identification number. Each tube needs to be inverted several times to ensure appropriate mixing of the sample. Inversion should be smooth and

Protocol 47.9 Arterial catheter sampling

Procedure
1. Disinfect the sampling port or catheter hub according to hospital protocol.
2. Attach a nonheparinized syringe and aspirate a discard sample.
   a. Minimum of three times: priming volume of the catheter for routine assays.[6]
   b. Six to twelve times: priming volume for coagulation assays.[7]
3. Remove the discard syringe and attach a new heparinized syringe to the catheter; turn the stopcock (if present) to a 45° angle during syringe change.
4. Aspirate sample, disconnect syringe from catheter, and express all air from syringe.
5. Following sample collection, the arterial catheter is flushed with 0.9% sodium chloride or heparinized saline according to hospital protocol.
6. It is recommended that blood gas samples be analyzed immediately, but they may be placed in an ice bath for up to 1 hour.[7]

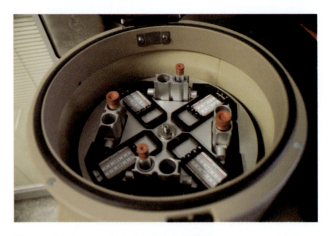

Figure 47.5 Properly balanced centrifuge.

requires a complete turn of the wrist 180° and back.[12] Tubes should never be shaken or mixed aggressively. The number of inversions is dictated by the tube being filled: Serum separator, serum, and clot activator tubes require five inversions; sodium citrate tubes require three to four inversions, and all other additive tubes (EDTA, heparin, plasma separator, etc.) require eight to ten inversions.[12]

Following inversion, Becton, Dickinson recommend that serum and serum separator tubes sit at room temperature for 30 minutes to facilitate adequate clot formation.[12] Plasma separator and all other additive tubes may be submitted for analysis or centrifuged immediately following inversion. Serum and gel tubes should be centrifuged within 2 hours of collection.

Proper centrifugation techniques also play an important role in sample quality. All personnel using the centrifuge should be cognizant of safety and appropriate usage guidelines. Ideally, centrifuges should not be operated without a cover or lid in place. Stoppers should be securely in place on all samples placed in the centrifuge, and any spills must be cleaned immediately.

Centrifuges must be properly balanced (Fig. 47.5) when in use both to obtain quality samples and to promote safety of personnel using the instrument. This is achieved by ensuring that tubes are filled with equal volumes of fluid and placed opposite each other in the centrifuge. If tubes are filled unequally or an uneven number of tubes need to be centrifuged, balance tubes may be used by filling the same size tubes with an equivalent amount of water. Atypical noise or vibration are good indicators that the centrifuge is unbalanced and should be immediately turned off; once the samples are correctly balanced, the centrifuge may be restarted.

Gel tubes include serum separator tubes (SSTs) and plasma separator tubes (PSTs) and should be centrifuged at room temperature at 1000–1300 RCF (relative centrifugal force) or 2000–2500 RPM (rotation per minute) for 10 minutes in a swinging-bucket centrifuge or 15 minutes in a fixed-angle centrifuge.[12] Sodium citrate tubes should be spun at 1500 RCF or about 2500–3000 RPM for 15 minutes; all other tubes (EDTA, heparin, serum, etc.) should be centrifuged at 1300 RCF or 2500 RPM for 10 minutes.[12] To ensure sample quality, it is important to make certain that all similar samples are centrifuged for the same length of time; a packed cell volume (PCV) obtained from a sample centrifuged for 3 minutes may yield significantly different results from one centrifuged for 4 minutes. Following centrifugation, plasma or serum should be immediately removed from the tube and placed in an appropriate sample container labeled with the patient's identification information.

Most serum and plasma samples, once removed from the red blood cells, are stable for up to 8 hours at room temperature or up to 48 hours in the refrigerator; samples needing to be kept beyond 48 hours should be placed in plastic tubes and frozen. Special handling is required for certain specimens. Adrenocorticotropic hormone (ACTH), angiotensin-converting enzyme (ACE), ammonia, acetone, lactic acid, pyruvate, and renin specimens are temperature sensitive and should be placed in an ice bath immediately following collection; these samples also require transport in a chilled container. Bilirubin and erythrocyte protoporphyrin are very light sensitive; wrapping the tubes in aluminum foil decreases exposure to light and helps maintain the stability of the sample. It is advisable to contact the reference laboratory for detailed collection, handling, and submission protocols whenever there is a concern about a specific sample or test.

Troubleshooting technical problems associated with blood sample collection and handling

Hemolysis

Hemolysis can interfere with a number of laboratory test results; potassium and lactate dehydrogenase may be falsely elevated due to release of intracellular material; tests requiring analysis by spectrophotometry may be invalid due to interference. Hemolysis may be secondary to disease processes such as immune-mediated hemolytic anemia (IMHA), heavy metal toxicity (zinc), or parasitism (Babesia); improper collection or handling of blood samples is also commonly implicated in hemolysis (Protocol 47.10). A technique frequently used in emergency and critical care (ECC) settings involves venipuncture utilizing very small needles (25 gauge and smaller) and injecting the sample directly into hematocrit tubes for determination of PCV; this technique often results in hemolysis and may falsely lower the PCV. When hemolysis is noted, the sample should be redrawn using proper technique to minimize damage to RBCs.

Sample dilution

Blood samples may be inadvertently diluted during collection, which can result in erroneous results. Sample dilution is typically attributed to inadequate sample to

---

Protocol 47.10 Hemolysis troubleshooting checklist

Procedure
1. Choose an appropriate size needle and syringe or Vacutainer (Becton, Dickinson, Franklin Lakes, NJ) needle and tubes; avoid very small needles and large syringes.
2. Aspirate sample gently; avoid excessive negative pressure or pulsing.
3. Ensure that tourniquet use or vessel occlusion is limited to 2 minutes or less; 1 minute is preferred.
4. Avoid excessive isopropyl alcohol use; allow alcohol to dry prior to venipuncture.
5. Invert sample tubes following collection; allow serum samples to stand in a vertical position for 30 minutes to promote adequate clot formation prior to centrifugation.

Protocol 47.11 Collection of minimal samples for coagulation studies

Accurate determination of coagulation assays requires a 1:9 ratio of anticoagulant to blood; the following steps maintain that ratio with minimal sample volumes.

Procedure
1. Aspirate 0.1 mL of sodium citrate from a blue-top tube and inject it into a plain serum tube (red top).
2. Inject 0.9 mL of blood into the prepared tube.

---

anticoagulant ratio, inadequate discard volume during sample collection from a central line or arterial catheter, and aspiration of tissue fluids during venipuncture (relatively rare).

A common dilemma that arises in veterinary medicine is the need to collect sodium citrate samples from very small patients for coagulation assays. Commercially available sodium citrate collection tubes require either 1.8 or 2.7 mL of blood, which may be difficult to obtain from small or anemic patients. Coagulation testing demands a proper blood to anticoagulant ratio (Protocol 47.11) because dilute samples will not yield accurate results.

Platelet clumping

Platelets clumping is commonly encountered and may be due to prolonged collection times, delayed mixing of blood and anticoagulants, or other factors. It is acceptable to use blood from a sodium citrate tube for platelet counts when there is clumping in the EDTA sample; counts performed on sodium citrate samples should be multiplied by 1.1 to account for the dilutional differences between the tubes.

Delayed sample separation or analysis

Delays in separating or analyzing samples may have a significant negative effect on the quality of the specimen. Delayed analysis of arterial and venous blood gas samples may result in considerable changes in PaO_2, $PaCO_2$, and pH. Delayed centrifugation of serum and plasma samples allows prolonged contact with RBCs and often results in erroneous sample results including decreased glucose results and elevations in ammonia.

Troubleshooting patient problems associated with blood sampling

Information obtained from blood tests is often vital to the diagnostic process, and serial blood tests are frequently required to monitor a patient's condition and the efficacy of the treatment regimen. In some cases, obtaining blood samples can be problematic for the patient.

Iatrogenic anemia from frequent sampling

Frequent blood sampling, especially from small or anemic patients, can be associated with significant blood loss to a degree that is detrimental to the patient's condition. This is especially concerning in small patients, neonates, geriatric animals, and patients with anemia. There are several strategies to minimize blood loss in these patients:

1. Use Microtainer or other "mini" collection tubes to minimize sample volume requirements.
2. Use point-of-care testing equipment that requires minimal sample volumes instead of sending blood to reference laboratories that require larger sample volumes.
3. Use the push-pull or mixing method rather than the discard method when pulling blood samples from an IV catheter.

Hematoma formation

Hematomas (bruises) form when blood leaks from a vessel and pools under the skin. Hematomas may be minimized by holding direct pressure over a venipuncture site for at least 30 seconds and for a minimum of 5 minutes over an arterial puncture site. Pressure bandages may be placed over sampling sites on the limbs; these bandages need to be removed and the site should be carefully checked within 15 minutes of application. Patients requiring frequent sampling or with coagulopathies may benefit from a central catheter to allow administration of fluids and medications as well as to facilitate blood sampling.

Summary

- The person performing the venipuncture needs to be cognizant of safety concerns at all times.
- The quality of a blood sample and the accuracy of test results are dramatically affected by collection and handling techniques.
- Hemolysis is a significant issue that affects sample quality and can be minimized when proper techniques are utilized.
- Blood cultures require strict aseptic technique and specialized handling.

- The person performing venipuncture should assess each case individually and choose venipuncture sites and techniques best suited to that patient.
- Arterial and venous samples for blood gas analysis require special handling and must not be contaminated with room air.
- Risks to the patient including catheter-related infections and iatrogenic anemia can be significantly decreased by using aseptic techniques and minimizing the volume of blood drawn or discarded.

References

1. Anderson MEC, Montgomery J, Weese JS, Prescott JF. Infection Prevention and Control Best Practices for Small Animal Veterinary Clinics. Guelph, Ontario: Canadian Committee on Antibiotic Resistance; 2008.
2. Boyce JM, Pittet D. Healthcare Infection Control Practices Advisory Committee. Guideline for Hand Hygiene in Health-Care Settings: recommendations of the Healthcare Infection Control Practices Advisory Committee and the HICPA/SHEA/APIC/IDSA Hand Hygiene Task Force. Infect Control Hosp Epidemiol 2002;23(12 Suppl): S3–S40.
3. Becton, Dickinson and Company. *BD Vacutainer® Order of Draw for Multiple Tube Collections.* http://www.bd.com/vacutainer/pdfs/plus_plastic_tubes_wallchart_orderofdraw_VS5729.pdf (retrieved June 5, 2010).
4. Magee LS. Preanalytical variables in the chemistry laboratory. LabNotes 15(1). Franklin Lakes, NJ: Becton, Dickinson and Company; 2005.
5. Kennedy C, Angermuller S, King R, et al. A comparison of hemolysis rates using intravenous catheters versus venipuncture tubes for obtaining blood samples. J Emerg Nurs 1996;22:566–569.
6. Moureau NL. Drawing blood through a central venous catheter. Nursing 2004;34(2):28.
7. Schallom L, Bisch A. 2001. Blood sampling techniques for patients with arterial or venous catheters. Am Assoc Crit Care Nurs 2001;1(2). http://classic.aacn.org/aacn/practice.nsf/ad0ca3b3bdb4f33288256981006fa692/fd80e397d0ab6d5088256a4f007b00e3?OpenDocument.
8. Adlard K. Examining the push-pull method of blood sampling from central venous access devices. J Pediatr Oncol Nurs 2008;25(4):200–207.
9. Calvert CA, Wall M. Cardiovascular infections. In: Greene CE, ed. Infectious Diseases of the Dog and Cat. 3rd ed. St. Louis, MO: Saunders; 2006:847–849.
10. Hopper K, Rezende ML, Haskins SC. Assessment of the effect of dilution of blood samples with sodium heparin on blood gas, electrolyte, and lactate measurements in dogs. Am J Vet Res 2005;66(4):656–660.
11. Moses L, Curran A. Basic monitoring of the emergency and critical care patient. In: Battaglia AM, ed. Small Animal Emergency and Critical Care for Veterinary Technicians. St. Louis, MO: Saunders; 2007:15–18.
12. Becton, Dickinson and Company. Venous blood collection. *BD Vacutainer Blood and Urine Collecton—FAQs.* http://www.bd.com/vacutainer/faqs/ (retrieved May 27, 2010).

48

In-house hematologic evaluation

Karl E. Jandrey and Carine Laporte

Hematologic evaluation

Definition of hematologic evaluation

Hematologic evaluation is defined as the analysis of blood. In veterinary medicine, blood is analyzed by looking at seven parameters:

1. Hematocrit (HCT) and packed cell volume (PCV)
2. Total plasma or serum protein concentration (TP)
3. Hemoglobin concentration (Hgb)
4. Complete blood count (CBC), or blood cell and platelet concentrations per unit volume of blood
5. Erythrocyte (also called red blood cell or RBC) indices
6. Differential leukocyte (also called white blood cell or WBC) counts
7. Erythrocyte, leukocyte, and platelet morphology

Components of hematologic evaluation

The three main components of hematologic evaluation are:

1. **Blood sample collection, handling, and preservation.**
2. **Blood sample processing.** The processing of a blood sample varies based on the parameters of blood being measured and the hematologic procedures being performed, which may include a CBC, routine blood coagulation testing, and direct microscopic evaluation of the blood sample.
3. **Interpretation of results.** The results of a hematologic evaluation (Table 48.1) may aid in the diagnosis of pathologic conditions, help to tailor the

treatment regimen, and indirectly provide valuable information about the bone marrow.

Purpose of hematologic evaluation

Hematology plays a critical role in small animal veterinary medicine. Examination of blood samples can provide important information regarding two fundamental aspects of veterinary medicine:

1. **Diagnosis.** According to the *Manual of Canine and Feline Hematology and Transfusion Medicine,*[1] "Dogs and cats exhibit a wider range of hematologic pathology than other species so diagnostic hematology is very important in small animal medicine." Evaluation of blood parameters provides diagnostic information in three ways. First, hematologic evaluation may contribute to a more comprehensive understanding of the causative factors of a patient'sdisease state. This may occur, for example, with hematologic evidence of ongoing infection or inflammatory responses. Second, evaluation of blood may in itself constitute the primary basis for diagnosis, as is the case in certain leukemias. Finally, evaluation of blood can aid the veterinary practitioner to assess the severity of the patient's pathologic state.
2. **Treatment.** Evaluation of a patient's blood may direct a course of treatment. Hematology may provide a means to monitor the patient's response to treatment and allow the veterinarian to better tailor the treatment protocol to the patient's needs. For example, chemotherapeutic regimens for certain blood-related neoplastic conditions may be

Advanced Monitoring and Procedures for Small Animal Emergency and Critical Care, First Edition. Edited by Jamie M. Burkitt Creedon, Harold Davis.
© 2012 John Wiley & Sons, Inc. Published 2012 by John Wiley & Sons, Inc.

Table 48.1 Hematologic reference intervals for small animals

Parameter	Dog	Cat	Units
Plasma or serum protein	6.0–8.6	6.8–8.3	g/dL
Erythrocytes			
PCV/Hematocrit	40–55	30–50	%
Erythrocyte count	5.6–8.0	7.0–10.5	millions/L
Mean corpuscular volume (MCV)	65–75	42–53	fL
Mean corpuscular hemoglobin (MCH)	22–26	13–17	pg
Mean corpuscular hemoglobin concentration (MCHC)	33–36	30–33.5	g/dL
Reticulocyte count	7,000–65,000	7,000–60,000	%
Red blood cell distribution width (RDW)	11–14	14–18	%
Erythrocyte morphology	Biconcave disk, significant central pallor, 7.0 μm	Round cell, minimal central pallor, 5.8 μm	
Leukocytes			
Leukocyte count	6,000–13,000	4,500–14,000	per μL
Band neutrophils	Rare–300	Rare	per μL
Neutrophils	3,000–10,500	2,000–9,000	per μL
Lymphocytes	1,000–4,000	1,000–7,000	per μL
Monocytes	150–1,200	50–600	per μL
Eosinophils	0–1,500	150–1,100	per μL
Basophils	0–50	0–200	per μL
Platelets			
Platelet concentration ($\times 10^3$)	150–400	180–500	per μL
Mean platelet volume (MPV)	7–13	9–18	fL

Adapted from the University of California, Davis Veterinary Medical Teaching Hospital Clinical Laboratory.

modified based on the WBC count and the risk of myelosuppression.

There are a multitude of techniques by which blood may be evaluated, both in small animal clinics and in commercial laboratories. This chapter focuses on the logistics of in-house methods of hematologic evaluation, both manual and automated.

Advantages and disadvantages of in-house and commercial laboratory hematologic evaluation

Although all veterinary practices should have the capability to perform at least minimal manual blood evalu-

ation techniques such as blood smears, commercial veterinary reference laboratories also offer diagnostic hematologic evaluation services. The decision to perform blood analysis in house or to send the blood to an outside reference laboratory must be made with knowledge of the advantages and disadvantages of each option.

Advantages of in-house hematologic evaluation

The primary advantages of in-house evaluation are increased revenue to the practice and the immediacy of test result availability. Veterinary practices stand to benefit in productivity and revenue from maintaining as many diagnostic tests in house as can be accurately and cost effectively performed. In addition, the data provided from in-house tests are essential for urgent decision making for many patients. For example, in emergency patients, immediate access to the results of a hematologic evaluation may help direct lifesaving interventions. For these reasons, most emergency practices now have automated in-house CBC machines that accurately provide basic hematologic information regarding number, shape, size, and abnormalities of the various blood cell types. In-house microscopic evaluation of a blood smear can be used to provide additional hematologic information.

Disadvantages of in-house hematologic evaluation

Despite the increased revenue garnered from the performance of in-house blood evaluation, a small animal practice must consider cost efficiency to decide whether or not to perform blood evaluation in house. In-house diagnostic tests require technical time and expertise, both for the completion of tests and for the performance of quality control measures on the machines. Technicians must also be educated in the operation of these sensitive machines. Finally, the small animal clinic must consider the expense of maintenance, repair, and replacement of automated hematologic diagnostic machinery.

Advantages of commercial laboratory hematologic evaluation

Although there are advantages to in-house diagnostic laboratories in small animal practices, commercial laboratories can offer distinct advantages that make them a preferred option in some situations. This is particularly true for the less commonly performed hematologic evaluations. For example, commercial laboratories are able to acquire technology that smaller practices cannot afford or have sufficient demand to purchase. Furthermore, because a commercial laboratory analyzes samples from hundreds of practices, it will likely perform certain procedures at a higher frequency and with greater practical expertise than an individual practice. This expertise may then help ensure accuracy and guide interpretation of complex, discrepant, or species-specific results. For this reason, tests that are performed in a clinic less frequently than once weekly should be outsourced to a commercial laboratory that works with a larger volume of such cases.[2]

Disadvantages of commercial laboratory hematologic evaluation

Just as the advantages of in-house diagnostic testing include economic gain for the practice and rapid test results, less economic gain for the practice and a longer turnaround time for results can be disadvantageous when blood is sent for analysis at an outside laboratory. Another disadvantage is the possible damage to or leakage of the blood sample in transit. Care must be taken to properly package samples before shipment to minimize sample compromise. Finally, the technician or veterinarian must be aware that reference intervals vary between commercial laboratories. Therefore, the interpretation of normal or abnormal hematologic values must be made in light of the specific laboratory used.

In-house hematology laboratory equipment and safety

In-house laboratory equipment

The list in Box 48.1 refers to the minimal equipment required for an in-house hematologic laboratory.

In-house laboratory safety

All biologic materials, including blood, must be treated as potentially infectious. Certain bloodborne diseases may be zoonotic and easily transmissible both to humans and other animals, such as Leptospirosis in dogs. Therefore, all personnel should wear examination gloves when handling or transporting blood. In addition, due to the risk of accidental puncture, previously used needles should never be recapped but instead directly deposited into a designated sharps container. Spilled biologic material must be cleaned with 10% bleach solution and all waste materials properly disposed. A veterinarian or

---

Box 48.1 In-house laboratory equipment

- High-quality binocular microscope, preferably with plain achromatic (flat-field) lenses, a mechanical stage, a focusable substage condenser, and low dry, high dry, and oil immersion objectives
- Microhematocrit centrifuge capable of spinning tubes up to 12,000 rpm
- Standard centrifuge capable of spinning tubes up to 15 mL
- Refractometer
- Differential cell counter
- Hand tally counter
- Interval timer capable of recording elapsed time
- Hemocytometer
- Blood smear staining solutions
- In-house hematology analyzers
- Commercial test kits, such as enzyme-linked immunosorbent serologic assays (ELISAs)

senior technician should be consulted if any problems arise.

Blood

Blood composition

Whole blood is composed of three elements: plasma, blood cells, and platelets.

1. **Plasma.** Making up 55% of the blood's volume, plasma is itself composed of more than 90% water. The remaining 10% of plasma is made of electrolytes, proteins, fats, vitamins, and similar substances. Another way to describe plasma is as the portion of the blood composed of clotting factors plus **serum** (the fluid component of blood without clotting factors).

2. **Blood cells.** Blood cells and platelets make up the remaining 45% of the blood's volume. Blood cells include *erythrocytes* and *leukocytes*. There are many different types of leukocytes, and it is important to differentiate them in a complete hematologic evaluation (Table 48.2). Increased or decreased numbers of specific leukocytes may be strong diagnostic indicators of certain disease processes.

3. **Platelets.** Platelets (also called *thrombocytes*) are small anuclear cellular fragments derived from larger cells called *megakaryocytes* in the bone marrow. Along with erythrocytes and leukocytes,

Table 48.2 Blood cells

Cell	Diagram	Description	% Dog	% Cat	Size	Function
Erythrocyte		Biconcave disc		Cat 4.5 µm	Dog 7.0 µm	Carriage of oxygen
Lymphocyte (small)		Round with a large round purple nucleus which almost fills all the cell, with a pale blue rim of cytoplasm	12–30	20–55	8 µm	Immunity Production of antibodies
Lymphocyte (large)		Similar to small lymphocyte but more oval in shape of the lymphocytes	Variable, approximately 8%	Variable	12–14 µm	As above
Monocyte		Pleomorphic nucleus (slightly indented oval to horse shoe shaped with enlarged knob like ends. Blue staining cytoplasm which may contain vacuoles	3–10	1–4	20 µm	Chronic phagocyte
Neutrophil		Irregular lobed nucleus with pale bluish pink cytoplasm with diffuse indistinct pale granules	60–70	35–75	10–12 µm	Phagocyte
Immature, juvenile or band neutrophil		Nuclei horse shoe shaped and not as darkly staining as mature neutrophils	Variable, 0–3	Variable, 0–3		
Eosinophil		Bilobed or segmented nucleus. Numerous reddish pink granules that are rod-shaped in the cat, round in the dog	2–10	2–12	12–14 µm	Increased numbers in parasitic and allergic conditions
Basophil		Segmented or irregular shaped nucleus. Blue grey cytoplasm with dark, bluish granules	Very rare in both dog and cat	0–0.1	10–12 µm	Associated with the release of histamine and heparin

Colors as seen when smear stained with Romanowsky stains. Reprinted from Aspinall V, Complete Textbook of Veterinary Nursing, 2006, p. 696. Used with permission.

platelets are a major component of blood. They play an integral role in primary hemostasis, the repair of damaged vasculature, the inflammatory cascade, and wound healing.

Blood collection sample types

The success of a hematologic evaluation partially lies in the use of the appropriate blood collection sample type for the diagnostic test performed. For example, where some blood analyses require the presence of clotting proteins, these very proteins may constitute a diagnostic interference in other types of blood analyses. The three types of blood samples used in hematologic evaluation are whole blood, plasma, and serum.

1. **Whole blood** is composed of cellular elements (leukocytes, erythrocytes, and platelets) and plasma. Whole blood is collected by placing the appropriate amount of blood sample into a container with the proper anticoagulant (e.g., EDTA). The sample is then mixed by gently inverting or rolling the tube multiple times. Whole blood should not be refrigerated for delayed analysis because the cooling and rewarming processes may damage its cellular components.

2. **Plasma** is composed of serum and clotting factors and is the liquid portion of whole blood that does not include the cellular elements (as described earlier). Plasma is collected by sampling the appropriate amount of whole blood from the patient into a collection tube with the appropriate anticoagulant. The tube is then gently mixed similarly to whole blood. The closed tube is immediately centrifuged for 10 minutes at 2,000–3,000 rpm to separate the plasma from the cells, which will be found as a pellet at the bottom of the centrifuged tube. The plasma is separated from the cells by manual removal via pipette into a separately labeled tube. Care should be taken to avoid contamination of the plasma with the pelleted cells. The plasma may be refrigerated or frozen for delayed analysis.

3. **Serum** is defined as the liquid portion of whole blood that remains after a clot has formed. In other words, serum is plasma without clotting factors. Simple serum collection may be performed after blood is placed in a sample tube void of anticoagulant and allowed to sit undisturbed and clot. Without anticoagulant, a normal sample will clot in 5–15 minutes. Serum samples may also be acquired by the collection of whole blood into a sample tube void of anticoagulant that contains only a gel used to separate blood clots from serum once centrifuged.

An example of such a serum separator tube is the red-topped Vacutainer (Becton-Dickinson, Franklin Lakes, NJ) tube. Serum evaluation can be performed directly on the serum within the red-topped Vacutainer tube.

Anticoagulants

A variety of anticoagulants may be used in different hematologic procedures to either reversibly or irreversibly prevent the clotting of blood. Table 48.3 describes the most commonly used anticoagulants.

Methods of hematologic evaluation

As mentioned earlier, there are seven components to hematologic evaluation:

1. Hematocrit (HCT) and packed cell volume (PCV)
2. Total plasma or serum protein concentration (TP)
3. Hemoglobin concentration (Hgb)
4. Complete blood count (CBC)
5. Erythrocyte indices
6. Differential leukocyte counts
7. Erythrocyte, leukocyte, and platelet morphology

Although many blood analyses can be performed through direct microscopic evaluation by the technician, measurement of erythrocyte and leukocyte counts, hemoglobin concentration, and certain erythrocyte indices are fully automated in most laboratories and many practices. This section first discusses the techniques of CBC analysis and microscopic evaluation of blood films that are essential to overall hematologic evaluation in any small animal practice. It then examines the specific characteristics of hematologic evaluation in the context of the individual blood components.

Complete blood count analysis

A CBC is a technique used to evaluate the blood's cellular components through measurements of cell number, size, and maturity in a specific volume of blood. It consists of the analysis of four hematologic properties:

1. Erythrocyte and leukocyte counts (concentrations per unit blood volume)
2. PCV or HCT
3. Hemoglobin concentration
4. Erythrocyte indices

In addition, the CBC analysis is generally accompanied by tests that measure both the blood's platelet concentration and total plasma or serum protein

Table 48.3 Most commonly used anticoagulants

Anticoagulant	Mechanism of Action	Vacutainer Stopper Color	Test	Sources of Error
EDTA (1.8 mg/mL blood)	Irreversibly binds calcium, which is required for clotting to occur.	Lavender or purple.	Routine hematologic evaluation.	Morphologic changes may occur in stored EDTA anticoagulated samples: crenation, irregular cell membranes, and cytoplasmic vacuolation.
Sodium heparin (15 USP)	Reversibly prevents the conversion of prothrombin to thrombin by activating antithrombin.	Green.	Routine hematologic evaluation. Evaluation of avian blood.	A heparinized sample must be analyzed immediately because heparin: 1. Inhibits coagulation for only 8–12 hours 2. May cause the cells to clump. 3. Causes cells to stain poorly.
Sodium citrate (3.2%)	Reversibly binds calcium, which is required for clotting to occur.	Blue.	Coagulation profiles.	Not used in routine hematologic evaluation due to disruption of normal cell morphology. As a liquid anticoagulant, may also act as a diluent, thereby affecting such values as PCV.
No anticoagulant	Allows for the blood to clot naturally.	Red.	Used for serum biochemical analysis of blood (also called a "chemistry panel").	

concentration. A CBC may be performed manually or through the use of automated analyzers.

Manual CBC analysis

The manual CBC analysis is performed using a hemocytometer and Unopette system (Becton-Dickinson, Franklin Lakes, NJ). Because the technique differs slightly between each blood cell type, it is described later in the discussions of manual concentration evaluation for each blood cell type.

Automated CBC analysis

Automated CBC analyzers have the advantage of providing highly consistent, rapid, and accurate results. There are three methods by which automated CBC analyzers can evaluate cell concentrations: impedance analysis, quantitative buffy coat analysis, and laser flow cytometry.

Impedance analysis (coulter counter)

Impedance analysis is a technology based on the counting of cells in an electrolyte solution as the cells are drawn through an aperture. As they move through the

aperture, the cells displace a specific amount of electrolyte solution. Each displacement of solution is detected by an analyzer and counted as a cell. Impedance analysis is used by such automated CBC analyzers as VetScan HM2 Hematology System (Abaxis, Union City, CA), among others.

Although impedance analysis is a common and effective means of evaluating cell concentration, special considerations must be given to the fact that these instruments base their analyses on cell size. First, because normal cell sizes differ across species and the accepted normal variation in platelet size may differ between species, impedance analysis is species specific. Feline platelets, for example, have greater normal variation compared with dogs, presenting a potential diagnostic challenge with impedance analysis. Furthermore, cell size analysis can make the instruments prone to error under certain conditions. Clumps of platelets, for example, can present as the same size as leukocytes. In this situation, the cell counter may mistake these platelet clumps as leukocytes and the analysis may artifactually reflect increased leukocyte numbers that could mimic inflammatory states. Platelet clumping is particularly a problem in feline blood samples.

Quantitative buffy coat analysis

Quantitative buffy coat (QBC) analysis is a technique used to provide an *estimate* of cell count, rather than a true cell count, through analysis of cell densities within the buffy coat layer of a microhematocrit tube. QBC analysis involves the centrifugation of an EDTA anticoagulated blood sample in a commercially available stain-coated microhematocrit tube. Centrifugation of such a blood sample results in a clear delineation of layers corresponding with the different components of blood. The delineated layers of a blood sample in a microhematocrit tube are discussed in more detail later in this chapter with PCV/HCT determination. However, one such delineated layer, known as the "buffy coat," is composed of leukocytes and platelets. The buffy coat is distinctly separated into layers based on the density of the cells in QBC analysis. The granulocyte layer is the lowest of the buffy coat layers and composed of eosinophils, neutrophils, and basophils. Above this is found the agranulocyte layer, where lymphocytes and monocytes collect. The uppermost layer of the buffy coat contains platelets. In QBC analysis, the stained microhematocrit tube is placed in an optical scanning device that analyzes the degree of stain fluorescence in each cell layer. The analyzer provides a report with 12 hematologic values and a graph that provides information about cell numbers and the fluorescence of each cell layer. These 12 values include HCT, hemoglobin concentration, mean cell hemoglobin concentration, WBC concentration, granulocyte concentration and percentage, lymphocyte and monocyte concentration and percentage, fibrinogen concentration, and reticulocyte or nucleated red blood cell percentage (if present). In bovine and canine samples, eosinophil and neutrophil concentrations are also reported, where basophil concentration is included in the neutrophil concentration. This technology is used by analyzers such as QBC Vet Autoread (QBC Diagnostics, Port Mathilda, PA).

Special consideration must be given to the fact that QBC analyzers may not always correspond with the platelet counts from other automated analyses because the thickness of the cell layer above the lymphocyte and monocyte layer of the buffy coat is affected not only by platelet number but also by platelet size. As a result, total platelet concentration analyses may be artificially increased or decreased with increases or decreases in platelet size.

Laser flow cytometry

Laser flow cytometry is the third technique used by automated CBC count analyzers and is the most accurate of the three technologies. A focused laser beam is used to differentiate the relative size and density of the various cell types based on the refraction of light off of the cells. Although laser flow cytometers may be profoundly impacted by lipemia because lipid droplets may scatter light in a similar manner to platelets, this technology is rapid and has built-in quality control procedures. However, it is also the most expensive of the automated CBC analyzers and not commonly found in private practice.

It is important to note that although CBC analysis provides important information about the blood's cellular components, it cannot replace and must be accompanied by direct hematologic examination by the technician. A technician may directly examine a blood sample under a microscope to evaluate differential leukocyte concentrations, blood cell concentrations per unit volume of blood, and blood cell morphology. A microhematocrit tube can be used to evaluate total protein concentration. The combination of a CBC analysis (manual or automated) and direct microscopic and microhematocrit evaluation by the technician provides the complete hematologic evaluation.

Microscopic analysis of blood films

A *blood film* (or *peripheral blood smear*) is both a method of preserving a blood sample and a means of microscopic hematologic evaluation. Blood film evaluation is commonly used to analyze the blood's cellular components and their morphologies, detect the presence of blood parasites, and provide a rough estimation of platelet concentration. Therefore, blood film evaluation is an integral part of a comprehensive hematologic analysis. Many abnormalities (Box 48.2) are found on

---

Box 48.2 Abnormalities found on blood smear evaluation

- Abnormal numbers of immature erythrocytes (nucleated erythrocytes and reticulocytes)
- Abnormal numbers of immature leukocytes (lymphoblasts and band neutrophils)
- Toxic granulation of leukocytes
- Hypersegmentation of neutrophils
- Evidence of infectious agents (bacteria, extracellular hemoparasites, and intracellular inclusions from parasites or viruses)
- Platelet abnormalities (platelet clumps and macrothrombocytes)
- Abnormal numbers of basophils
- Neoplastic cells
- Heinz bodies (particularly in cats)

blood smears that are not reported by automated CBC analyzers.

Preparing a blood smear

Creating a proper blood smear requires technical expertise and practice (refer to Protocol 48.1).

There are many possible sources of error in blood smear preparation (Box 48.3) that may decrease diagnostic accuracy.

Staining a blood smear

The two main types of stains for peripheral blood smears are Romanowsky stains and Supra-vital stains.

Romanowsky stains

Romanowsky stains are mixtures of methylene blue, eosin, and other dyes that can be used to alter staining characteristics. Where the methylene blue component is used to stain blue the acidic cell structures such as the nucleus and RNA in the cytoplasm, the eosin component is used to stain red the more basic components such as hemoglobin. Romanowsky dyes are dissolved in methyl alcohol to act as a fixative. Examples of Romanowsky stains include Leishman stain and Giemsa stain. Although it is not technically a Romanowsky stain, the Diff-Quick stain functions similarly to the Romanowsky by using blue and orange dyes.[3] The Diff-Quick stain is commonly favored in many small animal practices for its ease, rapidity, and accuracy (see Protocol 48.2).

Romanowsky stains are used in four capacities. First, they can be used to detect changes in the size, shape, and staining of cells on a blood smear. Second, they can be used to perform differential WBC cell (leukocyte) counts. Third, they may be used to detect the presence of blood parasites such as *Mycoplasma haemofelis* and different *Babesia* species. Finally, Romanowsky stains may be used to make a rough estimate of the number of platelets in a blood sample.

Supra-vital stains

The second type of blood smear stain is the *supra-vital stain*. Because they highlight and stain the residual RNA of immature erythrocytes, supra-vital stains are used to detect Heinz bodies and perform reticulocyte counts. Examples of these stains include 1% new methylene blue (in citrate saline) and brilliant cresyl blue.

As with the production of the blood smear, errors made during the staining of the blood smear may result in inaccurate diagnostic conclusions. Sources of error may include failure to wash the stain off sufficiently, using stains at incorrect concentrations, staining over incorrect time periods, and using dirty, contaminated, or crystallized stains that may appear to represent hematologic infection.

Red blood cell (erythrocyte) evaluation

The evaluation of erythrocytes involves the analysis of six parameters:

1. PCV/HCT
2. Erythrocyte count
3. Reticulocyte count
4. Erythrocyte indices
5. Erythrocyte morphology

Packed cell volume/hematocrit

PCV and *hematocrit* are defined as the blood cell-to-fluid ratio. In other words, they represent the percentage of blood that is composed of RBC. However, whereas PCV is a *measured* value, HCT is a *calculated* value. See Equation 48.1 for the formula of PCV calculation. Although HCT usually corresponds to PCV values and the two terms are often used interchangeably, if the value of HCT does not correspond to that of the PCV, it is better to defer to the PCV value.

The measurement of PCV is most commonly performed by the microhematocrit method, which involves the use of capillary microhematocrit tubes that may be heparinized for use with fresh blood or void of contents for use with anticoagulated blood. The technique is among the most commonly performed and accurate in-house hematologic evaluations. Not only is the technique easily and rapidly performed, but the microhematocrit tube also requires only a small volume of blood (see Protocol 48.3).

PCV values can be determined from a microhematocrit tube using of a variety of methods, including scales on the centrifuge, handheld cards, or specialized microhematocrit readers. One popular tube reader is a plastic sheet called a Critocap chart (Oxford Labware/Sherwood Medical, St. Louis, MO). With this reader, the centrifuged microhematocrit tube is placed perpendicular to the chart lines with the clay-erythrocyte interface on the zero line. The tube is moved along the chart until the 100% line intersects the plasma–air interface in the center of the meniscus in the microhematocrit tube. The PCV is read as a percentage directly from the chart at the erythrocyte–buffy coat interface.

Other types of PCV readers allow the technician to determine the PCV by dividing the length of the column of erythrocytes by the total length of erythrocytes, buffy coat, and plasma. Multiplication of this value by 100 provides the PCV percentage.

Protocol 48.1 Blood smear preparation

Items Required
- Nitrile or latex gloves
- Grease-free microscope slide
- Pencil
- Blood sample anticoagulated with EDTA
- Capillary tube
- "Spreader": either the frosted edge of a second microscope slide or a slide coverslip
- 100% methyl alcohol (for delayed evaluation)
- Microscope with oil immersion lens
- Immersion oil

Important notes
- The following protocol has been written for a right-handed technician. For left-handed technicians, all reference to "right" and "left" in the protocol should be reversed.
- Nitrile or latex gloves should be worn throughout the entire procedure. Any biologic material from the patient, including blood, must be considered a possible source of zoonotic infection; thus direct contact with human skin or mucus membranes should be avoided. It is always advisable to make at least two smears from each blood sample in case the result obtained from one is not satisfactory. There will be one blood smear per microscope slide.

Procedure
1. Gather supplies
2. Label the underside or frosted edge of a grease-free microscope slide with a pencil to identify the slide. Labeling the wrong side or area of the microscope slide will result in the removal of the label during staining.
3. Place the microscope slide against a white background on the laboratory bench.
4. Draw a small sample of fresh blood or well-mixed EDTA blood into a capillary tube and place a small drop of blood on the right end of the slide about 1 cm from the edge. If the EDTA anticoagulated blood sample has been previously refrigerated, allow time for the sample to warm to room temperature and mix the sample thoroughly by inverting or rolling the collection tube before initiating the blood smear.
5. Create a "spreader" either by using a microscope coverslip or a second microscope slide. If the latter is performed, ensure that the edge of the spreader is smooth and does not have any chips or fractures that may cause irregular accumulations of blood along the edge of the spreader. The edge of the spreader should be narrower than the full width of the blood smear slide. This will prevent the spreader from pushing cells to the edge of the blood smear slide.
6. Hold the spreader in the right hand between the thumb and index finger with the cut (narrow) edge of the spreader facing downward.
7. Place the spreader in contact with the slide parallel to the short edge of the slide and a little to the left of the drop of blood. The angle of contact between the spreader and the slide is important and should be 20–30° to vertical. A more obtuse angle will cause a thicker smear, whereas a more acute angle will cause a thinner smear.
8. Pull the spreader to the right until it encounters the droplet of blood and allow the blood to run along the edge of the spreader.
9. After the blood has run the length of the spreader's edge, drag the spreader toward the opposite (left-hand) end of the slide with a steady uninterrupted motion. The blood along the spreader's edge will be drawn behind the spreader, creating a blood smear along the slide. The action of dragging rather than pushing the spreader in creating the smear is extremely important. Never place the spreader behind (to the right side of) the droplet of blood with the intent of *pushing* the blood across the slide because this will cause damage to the blood cells.
10. The ideal smear should cover about three-fourths of the length of the slide. It should be thick at one end and taper to a thin feathered edge at the other. The aim is to create a region on the slide where the cells are spaced far enough apart to be counted and differentiated.
11. Allow the smear to air dry in a horizontal position. Do not apply heat because it may distort the blood cells. Dried blood smears are fragile, so always handle with care.
12. If blood smear staining and evaluation will be delayed, fix the slide by submerging it in 100% methyl alcohol for 1 minute. This will enable a delay of staining for up to 3 days.
13. Blood smears should be examined under a microscope magnification of 10×, then 40×, and finally 100× with oil immersion.

Reproduced with permission from Aspinall V. *Complete Textbook of Veterinary Nursing.* Fig 31.7. London, UK: Butterworth-Heinemann; 2006:694.

Box 48.3 Sources of error in blood smear preparation

Blood Smear Appearance	Source of Error
Smear is too thick	• Droplet of blood was too large.
Smear is too thin	• Droplet of blood was too small.
Transverse alternating thick and thin bands across the smear	• Jerky hand motion, frequently due to hesitation while spreading.
Streaks throughout the entire length of the smear, particularly at the tail	• Irregular edge to the spreader. • Dried blood on the edge of a reused spreader. • Dust or particulate matter on the slide or in the blood.
Spots on the smear where blood is absent	• Grease or oil on the slide.
Very narrow, thick smear	• Smear was made before the blood had completely run along the spreading surface. • One surface of the spreader lifted during spreading.

Adapted with permission from Aspinall V. *The Complete Textbook of Veterinary Nursing*. London, UK: Butterworth-Heinemann; 2006:694–695.

Protocol 48.2 Diff-Quick staining of peripheral blood smears

Items Required
- Clean benchtop
- Previously prepared blood smear slide
- Staining set composed of fixative solution, stain solution I (methylene blue mixture), and stain solution II (eosin)
- Distilled water (to rinse the stained slide)

Procedure
1. Obtain a staining set composed of three solutions: fixative solution, stain solution I (methylene blue mixture), and stain solution II (eosin). The methylene blue solution is used to stain nuclei and certain organelles bluish purple, whereas the eosin solution stains hemoglobin and some leukocyte granules reddish orange.
2. Dip a previously prepared blood smear in the fixative solution five times, each for 1 second (total 5 seconds).
3. Allow the slide to drain.
4. Repeat the procedure for stain solution I (dip five times over a period of 5 seconds).
5. Allow the slide to drain.
6. Repeat dipping procedure with stain solution II.
7. Allow the slide to drain.
8. Rinse the slide with distilled water and allow it to dry in a horizontal position with the feathered edge pointed upward. This will allow the water to drip off the slide away from the smear.
9. Color intensity and degrees of shading can be varied according to the number of dips per solution/time in contact with the stain.

$$PCV = \frac{100 \times (\text{Length of the column of RBCs})}{(\text{Length of columns of RBCs} + \text{buffy coat} + \text{plasma})} \quad (48.1)$$

Interpretation of the information garnered from the microhematocrit method of PCV determination provides valuable insight into the patient's hematologic status (Box 48.4). A small animal practice may use the contents of the centrifuged microhematocrit tube not only to evaluate the patient's erythrocyte mass, but also to analyze the patient's plasma and gain a rough estimate of the leukocyte concentration.

Although the microhematocrit method of PCV determination has high precision, as with all laboratory diagnostics, one must consider potential sources of error. The major sources of error (Box 48.5) in PCV determination are generally associated with centrifugation.

Erythrocyte count

Similar to a PCV/hematocrit, the *erythrocyte count* measures the erythrocyte concentration of a sample of blood. In general, erythrocyte count (concentration) has no real advantage over PCV other than helping to deter-mine erythrocyte indices, discussed later in this chapter. Erythrocyte concentrations are reported as millions per microliter of blood ($n \times 10^6$ erythrocytes per microliter, or $n \times 10^{12}$ erythrocytes per liter in SI units). Normal values in the dog range from 5.6 to 8.0×10^{12} erythrocytes per liter of blood, whereas cat values range from 7.0 to 10.5×10^{12} erythrocytes per liter of blood. Erythrocyte count may be performed manually, through estimation based on the PCV value, or by using an automated counting device. Both the manual and automated methods require that the sample be diluted before the count.

Manual evaluation of erythrocyte count

The manual method for an erythrocyte count involves the use of the Unopette system and an improved

Protocol 48.3 PCV determination: microhematocrit method on anticoagulated blood

Items Required
- Anticoagulated blood
- Microhematocrit tube
- Sealant clay
- Microcentrifuge
- Microhematocrit chart

Procedure
1. Gather supplies.
2. Mix a sample of blood thoroughly with the appropriate anticoagulant.
3. Fill a microhematocrit tube by capillary action with the anticoagulated blood to 75% of the tube's capacity.
4. Wipe the outside of the tube clean and seal the unfilled end of the tube with sealant clay.
5. Place the tube in a microhematocrit centrifuge with the sealed end facing outward.
6. Balance the centrifuge with a second similarly filled microhematocrit tube placed directly across from the sample tube. This second microhematocrit tube can also be used as a backup in case the first tube breaks.
7. Spin the tubes in the centrifuge for 5 minutes at 10,000 rpm.
8. The resultant centrifuged microhematocrit tube will show delineated layers of blood cells. Red blood cells (erythrocytes) will concentrate at the bottom of the tube just above the sealant. If present, nucleated red blood cells will be found on top of the erythrocyte layer. Above this can be found the buffy coat, which will be light gray-cream in color and composed of WBCs (leukocytes) and platelets. Platelets will generally be found at the uppermost layer of the buffy coat and can occasionally be distinguished as having a slightly lighter cream color. Above the buffy coat layer will be found the plasma, or liquid, noncellular portion of the blood.
9. PCV values are determined based on the length of the erythrocyte layer in the microhematocrit tubes. Results are reported as percentages or liter per liter (L/L).

Box 48.4 Common abnormalities observed in PCV/HCT evaluation

- **Low PCV.** There are many causes for low PCV. However, the most common causes include anemia and artifact. For example, a patient's PCV will be artificially lowered both by iatrogenic hemolysis of the sample and by the use of a liquid anticoagulant.
- **High PCV.** High PCV may also be caused by a multitude of factors. Although a higher PCV may be normal in certain breeds of dogs, such as greyhounds, it can also indicate a pathologic state or physiologic response. Common causes of increased PCV include splenic contraction in dogs, relative hemoconcentration due to dehydration or hemorrhagic gastroenteritis, hyperadrenocorticism in dogs, hyperthyroidism in cats, and response to chronic hypoxic conditions, such as severe pulmonary disease, congenital right-to-left shunts, and high altitude. In rare cases, elevated PCV may indicate a bone marrow disorder known as polycythemia vera.
- **Abnormal plasma in the microhematocrit tube.** In a healthy fasted animal, the plasma at the top of the microhematocrit tube should be free of parasites and clear in color. However, plasma may differ in appearance depending on the health of the patient. For example, pink-colored plasma generally indicates hemolysis. This hemolysis may have occurred outside the body during sample collection or within the patient itself. A milky appearance likely indicates lipemia, or excessive fat in the plasma. This is a normal condition in nonfasted, postprandial animals; however, lipemia in fasted animals may indicate liver, pancreatic, or endocrine disease. Yellow or amber-colored plasma in the microhematocrit tube indicates the presence of excessive bilirubin, which can be associated with hemolytic diseases, liver dysfunction, or biliary tract obstruction. Heartworm positive animals may show *Microfilaria* that can be visualized at low power magnification (10×) as they move and displace the plasma at the buffy coat–plasma interface.
- **Abnormal plasma total protein concentration.** The plasma separated by the microhematocrit tube may also be evaluated for total protein concentration. Alterations in total plasma protein concentration may be due to a variety of causes ranging from dehydration to liver failure. The measurement of plasma total protein and the interpretation of values are discussed later in this chapter.
- **Abnormal width of the buffy coat.** An experienced technician will be able to note variations in the width of the buffy coat, reflecting increased or decreased WBC counts. Although this is a highly inaccurate method of leukocyte determination, it may raise the index of suspicion for a problem. Such suspicions should be confirmed through the appropriate manual or automated hematologic techniques.

Neubauer-ruled hemocytometer. The Unopette system consists of a calibrated coverglass, a disposable capillary pipette that holds a predetermined amount of blood, and a plastic reservoir chamber containing a premeasured volume of diluent and lysing agent. The Neubauer-ruled hemocytometer is a transparent glass chamber used for counting the number of cells per microliter of blood. This glass chamber is 0.1 mm deep with a well-defined space of known volume that holds a cell

Box 48.5 Sources of error in PCV determination associated with centrifugation

- **Polycythemia.** If a patient's PCV is greater than 50%, erythrocyte packing will not be as complete after 5 minutes of centrifugation as would be expected with a lower PCV. This may result in overestimation of the patient's erythrocyte concentration.
- **Anemia.** If a patient's PCV is less than 25%, erythrocyte packing may be tighter than expected and the analysis may show an exaggerated decrease in PCV. In this case, the animal would appear to be more anemic than it really is.
- **Overfilling the microhematocrit tube.** Overfilling the microhematocrit tube by more than 75% of its total length may reduce the rate of erythrocyte packing and may require increased centrifugation time for accurate determination of erythrocyte mass.

Adapted from the *BSAVA Manual of Canine and Feline Haematology and Transfusion Medicine,* edited by Michael Day, Andrew Mackin and Janet Littlewood, with the permission of BSAVA Publications. (c) BSAVA.

Protocol 48.4 Manual erythrocyte count using the Neubauer-ruled hemocytometer and Unopette system

Items Required
- Anticoagulated blood
- 10 µL Unopette pipette
- Reservoir containing 0.85% saline
- Hemocytometer and calibrated coverslip
- Lens cleaner and lens paper if needed
- Microscope (with 40× lens)
- Calculator

Procedure
1. Gather supplies.
2. Thoroughly mix the blood sample with the proper anticoagulant.
3. Fill the appropriate 10-µL Unopette pipette with blood by capillary action.
4. Wipe excess sample from the outside of the pipette, and transfer blood into the reservoir containing the diluent (0.85% saline).
5. Dilute the blood 1:200 to achieve the appropriate density of cells for counting with the diluent container. Thoroughly mix the blood and diluent by inversion.
6. Let the sample stand for the amount of time indicated by the Unopette instructions.
7. While allowing the sample to stand, make sure the hemocytometer and calibrated coverslip are clean and free of dirt or contaminant. If dirty, clean with lens cleaner and paper.
8. Resuspend the sample in order to deliver mixed representative sample to the hemocytometer.
9. Squeeze and discard three to four drops of the sample.
10. Immediately charge (fill) each side of the hemocytometer at the etched groove. Do not over- or underfill the hemocytometer because this can cause uneven distribution of cells and can contribute to an inaccurate erythrocyte count.
11. Place the hemocytometer on the microscope stage and lower the condenser of the microscope to improve contrast and thereby visualization of the cells.
12. Under 40× magnification, count the number of erythrocytes in the four corner squares of the hemocytometer. Cells that touch the lines between the two squares are considered within that square if they touch the top or the left line. Cells that touch the bottom or right-sided line are not counted within that square.
13. Perform the count in duplicate on different sides of the hemocytometer grid. Because erythrocytes are often tightly packed together, they may be difficult to enumerate; thus an agreement of 20% between the two counts is acceptable and considered "consistent."
14. If the two cell counts are consistent, average the two counts and multiply by the conversion factor 10,000 to get the erythrocyte count per liter of blood.

suspension beneath the microscope. This chamber volume is subdivided by two identical sets of fine grids known as Neubauer rulings. Each grid is divided into 9 large squares, and the 4 corner squares are further subdivided into 16 smaller squares. The central 1-mm square of the grid is further subdivided into 25 groups of 16 smaller squares (for a total of 400 small central squares). The area of each grid (Neubauer ruling) holds 0.9 µL of fluid. A technician may use this system to evaluate erythrocyte concentration of the sample by counting the number of erythrocytes in the four corner squares of the hemocytometer and multiplying by a conversion factor to get the total number of erythrocytes per liter of blood (see Protocol 48.4).

Although this system of manual erythrocyte counting may be useful in some circumstances, its disadvantages include low accuracy even with practice and the fact that it is very time consuming.

Estimation of erythrocyte count

In addition to the manual counting of erythrocytes, total erythrocyte counts may be estimated by dividing the PCV by 6. For example, if a patient comes into a clinic with a PCV of 42%, its erythrocyte count may be estimated to be somewhere around 7 million erythrocytes per microliter of blood.

$$\text{Erythrocyte Count} = \frac{\text{PCV}}{6}$$

Example: If PCV = 42%   (48.2)

then erythrocyte count = 42/6

$$= 7 \text{ million erythrocytes/}\mu\text{L}$$

Automated erythrocyte count

Automated determinations of erythrocyte count are performed by automated CBC machines. As mentioned earlier, these machines may use laser flow cytometry or impedance counters to detect and count erythrocytes in the blood sample. These automated counters require calibration for cell- and species-specific analysis.

Reticulocyte count

Reticulocytes are immature erythrocytes that have not yet lost their ribosomes to become fully developed erythrocytes. Although they have already extruded their nuclei, reticulocytes retain numerous organelles needed for hemoglobin production, such as ribosomes, mitochondria, and fragments of the Golgi apparatus. Reticulocytes have reduced oxygen-carrying capacity compared to mature erythrocytes, although they are capable of maturation to erythrocytes in the peripheral blood. A *reticulocyte count* is an expression of the percentage of immature erythrocytes in the peripheral blood. An increased number of peripheral reticulocytes indicates a regenerative anemia in all animals except horses, which do not release reticulocytes from the bone marrow (see Protocol 48.5).

Hemoglobin

Hemoglobin is a protein found in erythrocytes whose main function is to transport oxygen around the body. Hemoglobin is measured in grams per deciliter. Normal values range from 14–19 g/dL in dogs, and from 10–16 g/dL in cats.

Hemoglobin concentration may be estimated in a normal animal as a third of the PCV value. This ratio is based on a typical healthy small animal patient with an average erythrocyte size of 7 μm. Hemoglobin concentration is usually measured through automated instruments that rupture erythrocytes to release the hemoglobin from the cells. These analyzers then measure hemoglobin concentration by one of two methods. *Color-matching automated cell counters* compare the color of the lysed blood samples to specific hemoglobin concentrations. Because they provide information regarding

---

Protocol 48.5 Reticulocyte count

Items Required
- EDTA anticoagulated blood sample
- 1% new methylene blue solution
- Small test tube
- Microscope slide plus spreader (coverslip or a second microscope slide) to prepare a blood smear
- Wright stain (optional)
- Microscope with oil immersion lens (100×)
- Immersion oil
- Previously measured PCV value and erythrocyte concentration for the blood sample
- Calculator

Procedure
1. Gather supplies.
2. Mix a few drops of EDTA anticoagulated whole blood with an equal amount of 1% new methylene blue supra-vital stain in a test tube. New methylene blue will stain RNA blue and will thereby allow for visualization of intracellular ribosomal structures found in the reticulocytes in a blood sample.
3. Allow this mixture to stand for at least 10 minutes.
4. Prepare a blood smear using this mixture and allow to air dry in a horizontal position.
5. A Wright stain may be applied as a counterstain to color the red blood cells reddish and make aggregate granules stand out prominently in blue. This may make counting the reticulocytes easier.
6. Under an oil-immersion lens (100×), count the number of reticulocytes in an estimated total erythrocyte population of 1000. Feline blood samples will contain two types of reticulocytes: aggregate and punctate. Only aggregate reticulocytes should be considered in the reticulocyte count.
7. Calculate the percentage of reticulocytes in the blood sample by dividing the number of counted reticulocytes per 1000 erythrocytes by 10.

% Reticulocytes = No. of reticulocytes counted per 1000 RBCs/10

8. Correct this percentage for the degree of anemia present by multiplying the patient's PCV and dividing by the normal mean PCV (45% in the dog and 37% in the cat). A corrected reticulocyte count above 1% in dogs and above 0.4% in cats indicates regenerative anemia.
9. Absolute reticulocyte count may be calculated by multiplying the observed reticulocyte percentage by the erythrocyte count.

the concentration of only oxygenated hemoglobin, these color-matching automated cell counters are considered somewhat inaccurate. *Photometric hemoglobin analyzers* measure all forms of hemoglobin, regardless of oxygenation. Examples of automated analyzers are the various models of the HemoCue Whole Blood Hemoglobin System (HemoCue, Inc., Lake Forest, CA). HemoCue uses a specialized microcuvette to draw up a specific volume of whole blood via capillary action. When the cuvette containing the blood sample is placed in the HemoCue analyzer, hemoglobin concentration is displayed within 1 minute on the machine interface. This system uses dual wavelength photometers to account for lipemia, leukocytosis, and other sources of turbidity. For these reasons, and because it measures all hemoglobin types present, the photometric process is considered more accurate than color-matching technology.

Erythrocyte indices

The term *erythrocyte indices* refers to calculated or electronically derived values that describe the overall size of erythrocytes in a blood sample and the relative amount of hemoglobin within those erythrocytes. Erythrocyte indices include total erythrocyte numbers, hemoglobin concentration, and hematocrit of a blood sample.

They are used to describe four characteristics of erythrocytes:

1. **Mean corpuscular volume (MCV).** *Corpuscle* is an antiquated term for an erythrocyte. MCV indicates the average erythrocyte volume, which in turn is interpreted as denoting erythrocyte size. It is calculated from total erythrocyte count and hematocrit. Refer to Table 48.4 for the formula to calculate MCV. MCV is measured in femtoliters (fL, or 1×10^{-15} L).

2. **Mean corpuscular hemoglobin (MCH).** MCH refers to the mass of hemoglobin contained in the average erythrocyte. It is measured in picograms (pg, or 1×10^{-12} g) and is calculated using the formula found in Table 48.4. Because MCH is a value calculated from hemoglobin concentration and erythrocyte count rather than hematocrit, it is considered the least accurate of the erythrocyte indices.

3. **Mean corpuscular hemoglobin concentration (MCHC).** The MCHC is the average concentration of hemoglobin per erythrocyte and represents the relationship of the MCV to the MCH. It is expressed as a percentage and is calculated from hemoglobin concentration and hematocrit by the formula pro-

Table 48.4 Erythrocyte parameters

Parameters	Significance	Formula
Hematocrit	The percentage of total blood made of red blood cells (i.e., the erythrocyte mass).	$\text{Hematocrit} = \dfrac{(\text{RBC} \times \text{MCV})}{10}$
Mean cell volume (MCV)	The average size of the red blood cells.	$\text{MCV (fL)} = \dfrac{[\text{PCV (L/L)} \times 1000]}{\text{Total RBCs } (10^{12}/\text{L})}$
Mean corpuscular hemoglobin (MCH)	The weight of hemoglobin contained in an average red blood cell.	$\text{MCH (pg)} = \dfrac{\text{Hb concentration} \times 10}{\text{Total RBC count (number of millions)}}$
Mean corpuscular hemoglobin concentration (MCHC)	The average concentration of hemoglobin per red blood cell.	$\text{MCHC (g/dL)} = \dfrac{\text{Total Hb (g/dL)}}{\text{PCV (L/L)}}$
Reticulocyte count	The percentage of a red blood cell population that is reticulocytes.	Observed % of reticulocytes $= \dfrac{\text{No. of reticulocytes counted per 1000 RBCs}}{10}$ Corrected reticulocyte count $= \dfrac{\text{Observed \% of reticulocytes} \times \text{patient's PCV}}{\text{Normal mean PCV}}$ Absolute reticulocyte count (per µL blood) $=$ Observed % of reticulocytes $\times$ total RBC count

vided in Table 48.4. Because the RBC count is not involved in this formula, the results tend to be more standard and more easily reproducible.

4. **Red cell distribution width (RDW).** RDW is an electronic measurement of the variations in width of the RBCs. An increased RDW is called *anisocytosis* and reflects a variation in cell size above what is considered normal.

Morphologic evaluation of erythrocytes

Morphologic evaluation of erythrocytes is a critical component of any hematologic analysis and therefore an integral part of a complete blood smear evaluation. Morphology is evaluated through visual assessment of the cellular monolayer portion of the smear adjacent to the feathered edge seen with the 100× objective. A morphologic assessment of erythrocytes should include size, shape, color, inclusions, and other morphologic abnormalities.

Size

- *Normocytosis* refers to a state in which a cell is of the appropriate size for its particular species.
- *Anisocytosis* is defined as a variation in the size of RBC beyond what is normally anticipated for that particular species. One such variation in size may be microcytosis.
- *Microcytosis* is a smaller than normal erythrocyte, as measured by a decreased mean corpuscular volume (MCV).
- *Macrocytosis* is used to describe an erythrocyte that is larger than normal (has an increased MCV). This is usually a characteristic of juvenile erythrocytes, such as reticulocytes. Note that erythrocytes may swell when damaged or left at room temperature for 6–24 hours, resulting in an increased MCV (macrocytosis) as read by automated counters and an artifactually increased calculated hematocrit.

Shape

- *Normocytes* are cells with a normal appearance and shape. In canines, erythrocytes should be biconcave disks; in felines, they are rounder cells.
- *Poikilocytes* (poikilocytosis) are any abnormally shaped cell. This term requires further characterization:
  - *Schistocytes* are fragmented erythrocytes found in cases of vascular trauma, disseminated intravascular coagulation, or certain neoplasias.

  - *Acanthocytes* are erythrocytes with long irregular surface projections.
  - *Echinocytes* have regular surface projections (in contrast to acanthocytes).
  - *Spherocytes* are small dense erythrocytes with no area of central pallor, generally found in dogs as a result of autoimmune RBC destruction.
  - *Leptocytes* have an increased cell membrane surface relative to cell volume and appear as *target cells* or *codocytes*.
- *Crenated* erythrocytes are artifacts in which the erythrocytes look wrinkled due to an old sample or the addition of too much anticoagulant.

Color

- A *normochromic* erythrocyte is one in which there is a normal amount of hemoglobin present (normal MCHC).
- *Hypochromasia* describes an erythrocyte with less hemoglobin than normal. The result is an increased degree of central pallor and a decreased MCHC.
- *Hyperchromasia*, which represents an increased MCHC, is generally an artifact and may be associated with microcytosis.
- *Polychromasia* is found on a new methylene blue–stained blood smear and is characterized by the appearance of irregular areas of blue color within cells on the smear, intermingled with the normal orange-pink staining of mature erythrocytes. Because new methylene blue stains the reticulum of an immature red blood cell, polychromasia is associated with the presence of reticulocytes on a blood smear.

Inclusions

Many types of erythrocyte inclusions may be evaluated on a peripheral blood smear.

- *Nuclear remnants* may be observed with supra-vital stains as dark blue intracytoplasmic inclusions in reticulocytes.
- *Heinz bodies* can similarly be seen on supra-vital stains as round blue granular inclusions. Heinz bodies are the result of precipitation of denatured hemoglobin due to the action of drugs or infectious agents. They are found more commonly in feline than canine blood.
- *Howell-Jolly bodies* can be seen on Romanowsky stains as spherical blue-black granules near the periphery of the cell. These inclusions may indicate regenerative anemia in the feline or may remain as the result of splenectomy.

- *Basophilic stippling* may be observed as bluish granular bodies on the surface of an erythrocyte. Basophilic stippling is diagnostic for lead poisoning in small animals.

Morphologic abnormalities

- Parasites such as *Mycoplasma haemofelis*, *Babesia* species, *Cytauxzoon felis*, and the microfilariae of *Dirofilaria immitis* (heartworm) may be visualized on blood smear evaluation. *Microfilaria* are found near the feathered edge of a blood film and their length is approximately the width of an erythrocyte.
- *Rouleaux* refers to the stacking of erythrocytes so that they appear similar to a stack of coins. Although rouleaux is normal in equine blood and to a certain extent in feline blood, in small animals it is often an artifact as a result of slow spreading of a blood smear or an old sample.
- *Autoagglutination* is characterized by three-dimensional clumps of cells and is seen in immune-mediated hemolytic anemia.
- *Nucleated erythrocytes* may be observed on a blood smear in cases of regenerative anemia, lead poisoning, bone marrow disease, or extramedullary hematopoiesis. If this morphologic abnormality is noted, a correction factor must be used in the analysis of a total leukocyte count because the presence of nucleated erythrocytes may distort the automated count of similarly sized leukocytes (see Equation 48.3).

$$\text{Corrected total WBC count} = \frac{(\text{Total WBCs} \times 100)}{(100 + \text{nRBCs}/100 \text{ WBCs})}$$

$$(48.3)$$

Leukocyte evaluation

The evaluation of leukocytes involves the analysis of three parameters: (1) total leukocyte count, (2) differential leukocyte count, and (3) leukocyte morphology.

Total leukocyte count

Similar to erythrocyte count, *total leukocyte count* is a means of quantifying the concentration of WBCs in a certain volume of blood sample. It is assumed that the concentration of leukocytes in this volume is the same as that of the entire blood volume of the animal. Normal values for a dog range from 6 to 13 × 10^9 WBCs per liter of blood, whereas the cat ranges from 4.5 to 14.0 × 10^9 WBCs per liter of blood. As with erythrocytes, leukocytes may be counted manually or via automated analyzer.

Manual total leukocyte count

A manual total leukocyte count is performed using the Unopette system and a Neubauer hemocytometer in a similar manner to erythrocyte count. The major differences between the two types of cell count protocols include differing dilution factors (leukocytes require a dilution factor of 1:20 rather than the erythrocyte dilution of 1:200) and the fact that acetic acid must be used in the leukocyte protocol as a diluent to lyse erythrocytes and reduce interference with the count (see Protocol 48.6).

Automated total leukocyte count

Total counts of leukocytes in a volume of blood sample may be measured using impedance analysis, laser flow cytometry, and QBC analysis. Although automated leukocyte-counting systems are generally reliable, accurate, and provide rapid results, special considerations must be made when performing an automated cell count. Samples with large numbers of metarubricytes and rubricytes (nucleated red blood cells) artifactually elevate leukocyte counts because the counter mistakes the nucleated RBCs for leukocytes. The possible artifact of nucleated RBCs again illustrates the importance of direct microscopic evaluation of a stained peripheral blood smear in addition to any CBC. Correction factors are used if more than five nucleated red blood cells (nRBCs) are noted in a population of 100 leukocytes (see Equation 48.4).

Corrected leukocyte count

$$= \frac{100}{100 + (\text{nRBCs} \times \text{automated nucleated cell count})}$$

$$(48.4)$$

Differential leukocyte count

Whereas the total leukocyte count provides a description of the entire leukocyte population within a volume of blood sample, the purpose of the differential leukocyte count is to determine the relative proportions of different types of leukocytes in a blood sample. In such a way, it may provide insight into the health status of the patient. Differential cell counts may be performed manually or through automated analysis.

Manual differential leukocyte count

Differential leukocyte count is manually evaluated through microscopic examination of a stained peripheral blood smear. Traditionally, three stains have been

Protocol 48.6 Manual total leukocyte count using the Unopette and Neubauer hemocytometer system

Items Required
- Anticoagulated blood sample
- 20-µL Unopette pipette
- Reservoir containing 3% acetic acid diluent
- Hemocytometer and calibrated coverslip
- Lens cleaner and paper if needed
- Microscope with 100× lens
- Calculator

Procedure
1. Gather supplies.
2. Mix a blood sample with anticoagulant.
3. Using capillary action, fill the appropriate 20-µL Unopette pipette with the anticoagulated blood.
4. Wipe excess sample from the outside of the pipette and transfer blood into the reservoir containing the diluent (3% acetic acid).
5. Dilute the leukocytes by a factor of 1:20 to achieve the appropriate density of cells. Thoroughly mix the blood and diluent by inversion.
6. Let the sample stand for 10 minutes to allow complete lysis of erythrocytes.
7. Resuspend the sample to deliver a mixed, representative sample to the hemocytometer.
8. Ensure the hemocytometer and calibrated coverslip are clean and free of dirt or contaminants. Clean with lens cleaner and paper if needed.
9. Squeeze and discard three to four drops of the sample.
10. Immediately fill each side of the hemocytometer at the etched groove. As with total erythrocyte counts, do not over- or underfill the chamber because this may cause uneven distribution of cells and can lead to inaccurate cell counting.
11. Place the hemocytometer on the microscope stage and adjust the condenser for improved contrast.
12. Under a 100× microscope lens, count the number of cells in the nine large squares of the grid. The same rules as with erythrocytes apply for which cells are to be considered "inside" versus "outside" the counting squares.
13. Perform the count in duplicate on different sides of the hemocytometer grid. Because leukocytes are less tightly packed than erythrocytes, an agreement of 10% between the two counts is acceptable. If such an agreement is not achieved, clean the hemocytometer and repeat the cell count.
14. If the cell counts are consistent, average the two counts and multiply by 100% to calculate the total number of leukocytes per microliter of blood.

used to evaluate leukocytes: Wright stain, Wright-Giemsa stain, and Diff-Quick stain.

The two main techniques for analyzing these blood smears are described here. It is important to note, however, that despite different techniques of smear evaluation, in all cases the smear is first scanned at low power (using the 10× objective) to assess overall cell numbers and distribution, for platelet clumps, and potential blood parasites, such as *Microfilaria*.

1. **Analysis of the cell monolayer adjacent to the feathered edge of the smear.** The first technique of smear evaluation involves microscopic examination of the cell monolayer. The cell monolayer is an area where the cells are minimally overlapped and distributed the most evenly. In this method, a 10× objective is used to identify and assess the monolayer. Under oil immersion magnification, 100 leukocytes in the monolayer are then counted and the number of each leukocyte type recorded and converted to a percentage. The absolute value of each cell type can then be obtained by multiplying the total leukocyte cell count by the percentage of each cell type. If nucleated erythrocytes are observed, their numbers are tallied and reported per 100 leukocytes. As mentioned previously, this technique may be used to confirm accuracy of automated leukocyte analyses.

2. **Strip count technique.** In the strip count technique, rather than counting leukocytes along the monolayer, all leukocytes lying in one or more longitudinal strips running the complete length of the smear are identified and recorded in absolute numbers. When a minimum of 200 leukocytes have been observed, the differential cell count percentage is calculated for each type of leukocyte.

As described previously, manual hematologic evaluation such as the manual differential leukocyte count is an incredibly valuable technique, and the diagnostic value of a hematologic profile is seriously compromised when cell counts are interpreted without it. However, as with many manual methods of hematologic evaluation, manual differential leukocyte counts are time consuming and require expertise and practice to produce reliable results. Furthermore, the nonuniform distribution of leukocytes on a blood smear may contribute to inaccurate differential counts.

Automated differential leukocyte count

Automated counters for differential leukocyte counts use similar technologies to those instruments that evaluate total erythrocyte and leukocyte counts. As previously mentioned, sources of error must be considered in interpreting the results from automated cell counts. Sample damage, sample aging, platelet aggregation, and abnormalities in cell size may all cause the machines to analyze the cell counts of a blood sample erroneously.

Morphologic evaluation of leukocytes

Leukocyte morphology may provide valuable insight into the patient's disease state and severity of disease. Under normal conditions, a *neutrophil* in peripheral blood will be mature and contain an irregular, dark, and dense multilobulated nucleus. Its cytoplasm will be colorless to a pale pink, and it will be the most numerous leukocyte type. *Eosinophils* will also have a lobulated nucleus, but they will have red-orange granules in their cytoplasm. Eosinophils are generally less numerous in peripheral blood. *Basophils,* each of which has a lobulated nucleus and numerous dark purple granules in its cytoplasm, are rare in peripheral blood. Because differential and total leukocyte counts share information pertaining only to the *numbers* of leukocytes in the blood sample, evaluation of abnormal leukocyte morphology can provide unique evidence for a variety of disease conditions ranging from mild allergic responses to neoplasias and immune-mediated disease.

A great number of potential leukocyte variations may be observed upon morphologic evaluation. Some of the more common morphologic variations are discussed next.

Left shift

Left shift is used to describe an increase in the number of immature neutrophils in the peripheral blood due to increased bone marrow activity. Band neutrophils, metamyelocytes, and myelocytes are all types of immature neutrophils released under different left shift conditions. Left shift is usually indicative of an inflammatory condition, although it may also be seen due to abnormal leukocyte development in an inherited condition called Pelger-Huet anomaly. This anomaly has been reported in the Australian shepherd, as well as in such breeds as the American foxhound, basenji, Australian cattle dog, border collie, Boston terrier, cocker spaniel, German shepherd dog, Samoyed, and various coonhounds.

Toxic changes

Toxic changes refer to morphologic abnormalities in neutrophils due abnormal maturation. Although first observed in human patients with gram-negative sepsis and endotoxemia, the term *toxic change* is not necessarily associated with "toxemia." Most toxic changes reflect an asynchronous maturation between the nucleus and cytoplasm of the neutrophil. In the normal maturation of a neutrophil (called *granulocytopoiesis*), the nucleus lengthens and pinches in synchrony with the progressive loss of cytoplasmic basophilia and condensation of the chromatin. The normal mature segmented and late band neutrophil, therefore, has a white cytoplasm containing a fairly long nucleus and tightly condensed chromatin. Abnormal maturation (toxic changes) can be observed in any inflammatory condition severe enough to induce intense neutrophil production and thereby shorten maturation time in the bone marrow.

A number of toxic changes may be observed in peripheral leukocytes. Common toxic changes include the following:

- Improperly condensed chromatin and a basophilic cytoplasm due to abnormal retention of ribosomal RNA. This may be seen in segmented and band neutrophils in response to some bacterial or viral infection. This basophilia may be diffuse, focal, or streaked. Focal basophilic areas within the cytoplasm are known as Döhle bodies. *Döhle bodies* appear as coarse irregular gray to blue cytoplasmic inclusions and represent areas of retained ribosomal material and rough endoplasmic reticulum. However, it must be noted that Döhle bodies are common in feline neutrophils and not a significant abnormality in otherwise normally segmented neutrophils.
- Vacuolation is associated with lysosomal degranulation in inflammation, although it may also be artifactual due to prolonged exposure to anticoagulant.
- Toxic granulation refers to the appearance of numerous large granules that may be dark purple/red to black in color. Thought to be primary granules, toxic granules are unevenly spread throughout the cytoplasm of certain cells and can give the neutrophil a bluish appearance.

Hypersegmentation of neutrophils

A neutrophil is considered hypersegmented if its nucleus has five or more lobes. Hypersegmentation results from the aging of a neutrophil in the peripheral blood that accompanies abnormally prolonged circulation time. Glucocorticoid therapy is often associated with neutrophil hypersegmentation because neutrophils remain in circulation for an extended period in animals receiving these steroids. This effect on neutrophil circulation can also be observed with the endogenous release of glucocorticoids seen in chronic infection, Cushing disease, and stress. Hypersegmentation of neutrophils may also be observed in anemia.

Karyorrhexis, karyolysis, and karyopyknosis

Karyorrhexis, *karyolysis*, and *karyopyknosis* are terms used to describe nuclei that are fragmented, lysed, or condensed, respectively. In leukocytes, they represent artifact from inappropriate anticoagulant use.

Basket cells

Basket cells are degenerative leukocytes that have ruptured and appear as pale-staining amorphous bodies. Degenerative leukocytes may be due to artifact if the blood was held too long before making a smear, or they may indicate excessive cell fragility or leukemia.

Atypical lymphocytes

Atypical lymphocyte morphologic variations range from changes in color of the cytoplasm to changes in lymphocyte size, volume, and nuclear characteristics. These changes may indicate a variety of pathologic states, including neoplastic disease. *Reactive lymphocytes* contain a dark blue cytoplasm and dark irregular nuclei. Although they may be found in low numbers in health, increased percentages of reactive lymphocytes generally indicate chronic antigenic stimulation.

Parasites

Leukocyte parasites are best seen on a smear of the buffy coat on a microscope slide. Examples of these parasites include *Histoplasma* and *Ehrlichia*, an intracellular parasite of lymphocytes, monocytes, and neutrophils.

Platelet (thrombocyte) evaluation

Platelets may be evaluated via a *thrombogram,* a term used to refer to those portions of the CBC related to platelets (thrombocytes). The standard thrombogram includes analysis of: total platelet count, mean platelet volume (MPV) and size, platelet distribution width (PDW), platelet morphology, and thrombocrit (or plateletcrit). *Platelet distribution width* (PDW) is a reflection of platelet **anisocytosis** (size variation) as calculated from individual platelet volume. *Thrombocrit,* similar to hematocrit, measures the percentage of platelets in a given blood sample; however, this value is not often reported. Investigative research analyses more rarely may also include mean platelet component concentration and mean platelet component concentration distribution width. This section focuses on those parameters of platelets most commonly evaluated: total platelet count, mean platelet volume, and platelet morphology.

Total platelet count

Total platelet count, or platelet concentration, is defined as the number of platelets per unit volume of blood. Commonly accepted "adequate" values in small animals are 6–10 or more platelets per oil immersion field, where each single platelet corresponds to 10,000–15,000 platelets/µL circulating in the peripheral blood. However, the results of a total platelet count must be taken in light of the health of the patient. "Adequate" values of platelets are subjective terms that are only meaningful if the patient does not have occult or obvious bleeding. Accurate platelet concentrations may be determined with an automated analyzer, like a CBC machine, or by manual evaluation.

Manual platelet count

Platelets may be manually evaluated by two methods:

1. **Indirect platelet count** can be estimated via examination of a peripheral blood smear. Using this method, the number of platelets seen per 100 leukocytes is considered equivalent to the relative percentage of platelets. Simple multiplication of this percentage by the leukocyte cell count provides an estimation of the absolute number of thrombocytes per microliter of blood. Care must be taken in the interpretation of decreased platelet numbers if this platelet-counting method is used. Decreased numbers of counted platelets may truly reflect thrombocytopenia (an in vivo reduction in platelet numbers), or they may simply represent platelet aggregation on the blood film or tube of blood.

2. **Direct platelet count** is based on the same Neubauer hemocytometer and Unopette system used in manual erythrocyte and leukocyte counts. The procedure mimics that of manual leukocyte counting, with a few exceptions. First, the dilution factor is different, with platelets requiring a dilution of 1:100 rather than the leukocyte dilution of 1:20. Second, the diluent used for platelet counting differs from that of leukocytes and must be 1% ammonium oxalate to hydrolyze the erythrocytes while preserving the leukocytes and platelets. Finally, platelet counting must be performed after leukocyte counting because the platelets require a minimum of about 10 minutes to settle in the hemocytometer counting chamber. To perform the count, the platelets are examined under a 40× microscope lens and tallied in the 25 small squares located in the large center square of the grid. This number is then multiplied by 1000 to get the number of platelets per

microliter of blood. This technique is relatively labor intensive and has a much lower precision than the automated methods. However, it is important to perform a manual evaluation in cases of suspected platelet clumping or when many giant platelets are present (see Protocol 48.7).

Automated platelet count

Similar to erythrocytes and leukocytes, the platelet concentration may be measured by impedance counters, laser flow cytometers, and QBC analyzers. However, it is important to remember certain sources of artifact when reviewing these evaluations of platelet concentration. Refer to the section "Automated CBC Analysis" for sources of error.

Regardless of the system used, the automated platelet count should always be viewed with a certain level of suspicion and confirmed by manual estimation or direct count. Although an increased platelet count is unlikely to be a sampling or machine error and likely reflects a true thrombocytosis in the patient, a decreased automated platelet count may indicate either platelet clumping or a true thrombocytopenia.

Mean platelet volume

Mean platelet volume (MPV) is the average apparent volume of each individual platelet in the blood sample. The interpretation of MPV may be complicated for three reasons. First, reference ranges for MPV vary among analyzers and methods. Second, variables such as anticoagulants, sample storage temperature, and sample storage time may affect MPV values. Although these effects on MPV may be minimal, they should be considered when interpreting MPV, particularly in the upper and lower ranges of the reference limits. Finally, automated analyzers may provide inaccurate MPV evaluations. As discussed earlier, certain impedance analyzers may not be able to generate accurate MPV values in cases of severe thrombocytopenia. In addition, lipid droplets or cell fragments may be erroneously labeled as platelets by impedance analyzers and laser flow cytometers, contributing to a falsely elevated MPV analysis.[3] Despite sources of error and normal MPV variation in healthy animals of some species (particularly cats), accurate MPV values may be used to evaluate disease progression and severity.

Morphologic evaluation of platelets

A morphologic evaluation of platelets, similar to erythrocytes and leukocytes, can provide important informa-

---

Protocol 48.7 Manual platelet count using the Unopette and Neubauer hemocytometer system

Items Required
- Anticoagulated blood sample
- 20-μL Unopette pipette
- Reservoir containing 1% ammonium oxalate
- Hemocytometer and calibrated coverslip
- Lens cleaner and paper if needed
- Microscope with 100× objective
- Calculator

Procedure
1. Gather supplies.
2. Mix a blood sample with the appropriate anticoagulant.
3. Using capillary action, fill the appropriate 20-μL Unopette pipette with the anticoagulated blood.
4. Wipe excess sample from the outside of the pipette and transfer blood into the reservoir containing the diluent (1% ammonium oxalate).
5. Dilute the platelets by a factor of 1:100 to achieve the appropriate density of cells. Thoroughly mix the blood and diluent by inversion.
6. Let the sample stand for 10 minutes to allow complete lysis of erythrocytes.
7. Mix the sample and resuspend so that a consistent sample can be delivered to the hemocytometer.
8. Ensure the hemocytometer and calibrated coverslip are clean and free of dirt or contaminants. Clean with lens cleaner and paper if needed.
9. Squeeze three to four drops of the sample and discard.
10. Immediately fill each side of the hemocytometer at the etched groove. As with total erythrocyte counts, do not over- or underfill the chamber because this may cause uneven distribution of cells and can lead to inaccurate cell counting.
11. Place the hemocytometer on the microscope stage and adjust the condenser for improved contrast.
12. Under 40× magnification, count the number of platelets in the 25 small squares in the large center square of the grid. The same rules as with erythrocytes apply for which cells are to be considered "inside" versus "outside" the counting squares.
13. This number is then multiplied by 1000 to get the number of platelets per microliter of blood.

---

tion not reported in automated analyzers. Morphologic analysis should involve examination of platelet size, shape, and abnormal inclusions.

- **Size.** In health, platelets are generally uniform in size. With the exception of cats, which normally have greater platelet size variation, increased variation in platelet size may be taken to indicate changes in the patient's health status.

- **Shape.** In a healthy patient, nonactivated platelets should appear discoid. With the addition of anticoagulants, they may become more spherical. In cases of increased thrombopoiesis, however, these platelets may adopt a more elongated shape and acquire peripheral pseudopodia.
- **Inclusions.** Abnormal platelet inclusions are far less common than leukocytes or erythrocyte inclusions. However, granule inclusions are important to note in platelets because they serve as an indication of the activation status of the platelet. Whereas the granules of nonactivated platelets show on Wright staining to be small and pink to purple in color and surrounded by clear to pale blue cytoplasm, the granules of activated platelets will be more prominently centralized or completely absent if already secreted. Another type of platelet inclusion that may be noted on microscopic evaluation is caused by the parasite *Anaplasma platys*, whose morulae may be observed in certain platelets. However, the consistently low frequency of the parasite in the blood, combined with the induction of a cyclical thrombocytopenia the parasite (i.e., further decreases in the number of circulating platelets decreases the number of parasites in the blood), makes microscopic examination of *A. platys* an imprecise method of evaluation. Because of this, if *A. platys* infection is suspected, diagnosis must be confirmed by polymerase chain reaction (PCR) analysis.

Protocol 48.8 Measurement of plasma or serum total protein concentration with a refractometer

Items Required
- Previously centrifuged microhematocrit tube with blood sample
- Refractometer
- Overhead light source

Procedure
1. Gather supplies.
2. After centrifuging anticoagulated blood in a microhematocrit tube, break the tube just above the interface between the buffy coat and the plasma.
3. With the refractometer's cover plate closed, place the broken edge of the tube against the refractometer and allow the plasma to fill the space between the refractometer's cover plate and the glass surface by capillary action. Do not tap the sample out of the tube because this may scratch the glass surface of the refractometer.
4. Hold the refractometer horizontally and allow the overhead light to reach the top of the instrument.
5. Look through the viewfinder and focus the scale by turning the eyepiece.
6. The protein concentration will be read in grams per deciliter at the interface between the light and shaded areas. This reading may vary slightly between operators due to differences in interpretation of the location of this interface.
7. Clean the instrument with water and lens paper.

Total plasma or serum protein evaluation

Total protein evaluation, or protein concentration, is commonly performed in conjunction with PCV determination and most often analyzed with a handheld refractometer on blood serum or plasma. An example of a refractometer used in small animal clinics is the Reichert Rhino Vet360 refractometer (Reichert Analytical Instruments, Depew, NY). Measured in grams per deciliter, values for total protein in health range from around 6–8.6 g/dL for canines and felines (see Protocol 48.8).

Measured serum or plasma total protein concentration can be an important indicator of disease. When interpreted with increased or decreased PCV, protein concentration values may help elucidate certain pathologic conditions. However, as with all measured values, it is important to understand test limitations and sources of error. For instance, accurate plasma protein is difficult to determine in a lipemic blood sample because turbidity will cause the line of demarcation on the scale to become indistinct. Furthermore, in hemolysis, RBCs release hemoglobin. Because hemoglobin is itself a protein, hemoglobinemia will falsely increase plasma protein values. It is important to note that the yellow color of an icteric sample is *not* a source of error in evaluating blood total protein.

Specialized in-house analyzers: evaluation of hemostasis

In addition to the previously mentioned automated methods of hematologic evaluation, certain veterinary practices may also use more specialized in-house analyzers. This section focuses on the more common of these specialized in-house analyzers used to generate patient coagulation profiles in the assessment of hemostasis.

Hemostasis

Hemostasis is defined as the ability of the body's systems to maintain both blood fluidity and blood vessel integrity so as to preserve normal blood function.[4] It involves a highly complex interaction between blood cells, platelets, coagulation factors, fibrinolytic factors, and the endothelial cell lining of blood vessels with the ultimate goals of forming a cross-linked fibrin plug over areas of vascular damage and maintaining blood in a freely flowing state.

Coagulation profiles

In-house automated coagulation profile tests are designed to evaluate specific pathways within the hemostatic system. They may be used in small animal clinics when a bleeding disorder is suspected or as part of a standard presurgical screening protocol. Three hemostatic parameters commonly evaluated by these automatic analyzers are activated clotting time, prothrombin time, and activated partial thromboplastin time.

Activated clotting time

Activated clotting time (ACT) is a test performed to evaluate every clinically significant clotting factor except factor VII. ACT is a highly insensitive test in which abnormally increased activated clotting times indicate that the activity of one or more of these coagulation factors has been reduced by at least 95% (i.e., that the affected coagulation factors have at most only 5% of normal activity).

ACT may be evaluated manually after the collection of blood into a gray-top Vacutainer tube that contains diatomaceous earth. The time the sample takes to form a blood clot in the tube at 37°C with gentle rotation every 5–10 seconds is recorded as the ACT (see Protocol 48.9).

In addition to manual evaluation, automated analysis of ACT may be performed through the use of specialized coagulation analyzers in some practices. For example, an ACT cartridge may be inserted into the I-STAT System (Abbott Point of Care, Princeton, NJ) to provide laboratory-quality in-house analysis of ACT. The technology that underlies automated ACT analyses is different from the manual method and often includes internal quality control systems that are activated each time a sample is tested. With many of these analyzers, the internal quality system will suppress results if internal specifications are not met. The technology will also generally impose analyzer-specific blood collection requirements. It is important to consult the manufacturer's guidelines for automated analysis. For example, to use the I-STAT ACT cartridge, blood collection syringes or Vacutainer tubes must be made of plastic and devoid of anticoagulant. The device chosen for the initial transfer of the

---

Protocol 48.9 Manual act evaluation

Items Required
- Vacutainer tube with diatomaceous earth
- Blood sample
- Timer or any method of keeping time
- 37°C water bath or incubator

Procedure
1. Gather supplies.
2. Perform hand hygiene.
3. Perform venipuncture.
4. Collect 2 mL of blood directly into a gray-top Vacutainer tube that contains diatomaceous earth.
5. Begin a timer as soon as the blood enters the tube.
6. Gently invert the tube to mix its contents and place it in a 37°C incubator or water bath.
7. Rotate the tube gently every 5–10 seconds.
8. Examine the tube for clot formation at 60 seconds, and then every 5 seconds thereafter.
9. Record the time to blood clot formation. Normal time to clot is less than 120 seconds.

---

sample from the Vacutainer tube into the ACT cartridge must also be plastic. To collect blood into capillary tubes or to transfer directly from venipuncture for placement into the cartridge is not recommended by the manufacturer.

Prothrombin time/one-stage prothrombin time

Prothrombin time (PT), also known as one-stage prothrombin time (OSPT), is used to evaluate the extrinsic (i.e., Factor VII) and common coagulation pathways. PT is an insensitive test in which increases are only observed when the production, activity, or function of any of the coagulation factors is reduced by 70% or more. It, too, can be performed manually or through automated analyzers (see Protocol 48.10).

An example of an automated analyzer is the Coag Dx Analyzer produced by IDEXX (IDEXX Laboratories, Inc., Westbrook, ME). This machine analyzes both PT and PTT and can use fresh whole citrated blood. Reference ranges vary greatly between methods of automated PT analysis.

Activated partial thromboplastin time

Activated partial thromboplastin time (aPTT or PTT) is used to evaluate the intrinsic and common coagulation

Protocol 48.10 Manual prothrombin time

Items Required
- Citrate tube
- Sample of blood plasma
- Tissue thromboplastin reagent
- Timer or any method of keeping time

Procedure
1. Gather supplies.
2. Perform hand hygiene.
3. Perform venipuncture and place whole blood into sodium citrate for a ratio of 9:1.
4. Collect the plasma (i.e., the supernatant after centrifugation).
5. Add tissue thromboplastin reagent.
6. Add a reagent designed to recalcify the sample, thereby reversing sodium citrate's anticoagulant effects.
7. A clot should form in 6–20 seconds. A clot that takes longer than 20 seconds to form is considered to demonstrate a prolonged prothrombin time.

pathways. Its analysis most closely approximates that of ACT. Evaluation of PTT requires an automated coagulation analyzer. PTT is an insensitive test in which increases are only observed when the production, activity, or function of any of the coagulation factors is reduced by 70% or more.

In addition to these common parameters of coagulation, fibrinogen concentration may also be measured as a parameter of coagulation. Fibrinogen is produced by the liver and classified as an acute-phase protein, or a protein whose expression is upregulated during inflammation. Although fibrinogen determination is possible and may be diagnostically important, automated analysis of fibrinogen is complicated and not routinely available to in-house laboratories.[5]

General considerations and sources of error in hematologic evaluations

Spoiling of the samples

One of the most important considerations in a hematologic evaluation is the prevention of sample spoiling. The spoiling of a sample will completely invalidate the results of a diagnostic test. The resultant need to repeat venipuncture and collect a new sample of blood is not only time consuming, but it also causes increased discomfort to the patient. It is critical, therefore, not only to understand and anticipate causes of sample spoilage but also to be familiar with the means by which they may be prevented.

There are four major causes of sample spoiling in hematologic evaluation:

- **Clotting of the blood.** The clotting behavior of red blood cells is highly variable and based on the individual patient. Blood clotting may also result from poor mixing of the blood with the anticoagulant, or mixing of the blood sample with the incorrect anticoagulant.
- **Inappropriate filling of the sample tube (insufficient or excess).** Blood collection tubes are manufactured to contain a precise volume of anticoagulant to achieve a specific concentration in the blood sample given proper filling of the tube with the sample. If the collection tube is inappropriately filled with blood, the unintended ratio of blood to anticoagulant may artifactually change the characteristics of the blood sample. For example, insufficient filling of EDTA-containing tubes will lead to a relative excess of EDTA compared with the blood sample. This will lead to crenation (shrinkage) of the RBCs and iatrogenic, artifactual hemodilution.
- **Hemolysis of the blood sample.** RBCs are fragile and may be damaged by many factors in the process of blood collection. This is particularly a problem when measuring a patient's PCV because hemolysis will artifactually lower the PCV, invalidating the results.
- **Contamination of the blood sample.** Contaminants may include air dust, particles of skin, or elements from the operating personnel that inadvertently enter into the blood sample. Although it is unlikely that contaminants can be completely prevented, contamination from a blood sample can be minimized by adherence to proper blood collection protocols.

To avoid the invalidation of test results, a series of steps may be taken to prevent the spoiling of the blood samples. These methods of prevention may broadly be categorized as those focusing on blood collection and those focusing on sample preservation following the blood collection.

Blood collection

- **Perform venipuncture on a large central vein.** This will help to minimize damage to the fragile erythrocytes and decrease chance of venous collapse.
- **Avoid multiple venipuncture attempts.** Multiple traumas to the tissue will cause the release of tissue fluids that will induce blood clotting.

- **Avoid using a needle gauge that is too large or too small.** Smaller gauge needles decrease the damage to the erythrocytes by decreasing velocity and turbulence of blood flow, thereby minimizing hemolysis that may be induced by propulsion through a larger bore needle.[6] However, hemolysis may also occur with small-gauge needles due to the imposition of a large vacuum force on the blood and resultant shear stress on the RBCs.[7]
- **Use the smallest appropriate syringe size and avoid applying excess suction.** For example, if 1 mL of blood is required, a 2-mL syringe is sufficient. Small syringes are beneficial for two reasons. First, using a large syringe with a small-bore needle may cause hemolysis. An appropriate syringe size will decrease the risk of RBC rupture by decreasing the pressure imposed on the RBCs while the sample is drawn. No less importantly, larger syringes and suction pressures may increase the risk of collapsing the patient's vein. Avoid a forceful draw on the syringe plunger during blood collection with a needle and syringe.
- **Extract with a consistent suction pressure (vacuum).** This will decrease damage to the erythrocytes and thereby decrease probability of aggregation.
- **Remove the needle before transfer of blood from the syringe into the sample collection tube.** Ideally, blood should only pass through the needle once to reduce trauma to the erythrocytes. This will avoid causing the blood to pass through the needle twice under pressure (once going in and once coming back out of the syringe). For this reason, the stopper should ideally be removed from the tube and the needle removed from the syringe tip before blood is transferred directly into the tube. The stopper should then be replaced on the tube. In reality, however, blood samples are often transferred into the collection tube by insertion of the syringe needle through the rubber tube stopper and sometimes through forceful expulsion into the collection tube with the syringe plunger. In these cases, therefore, the needle is not removed from the syringe prior to transfer into the collection tube. To avoid hemolysis in these instances, the pressure applied to the syringe plunger must be slow to avoid any undue force on the erythrocytes.
- **Make sure the needle, syringe, and skin do not come into contact with water prior to venipuncture.** This will avoid any osmotic damage that could be inflicted on the fragile erythrocytes by water.
- **Upon transfer into the blood collection tube, do not shake the tube.** Instead, the tube should be gently rolled or inverted. Again, this functions to minimize trauma to the sensitive platelets and fragile erythrocytes.

Sample preservation

- **Examine sample immediately after collection.**
- **Store at the appropriate temperature.** Refrigeration at 4°C (about 39°F) is an important component of the storage of blood samples. Whereas erythrocytes will swell when left at room temperature for 6–24 hours, refrigerated erythrocytes will not undergo morphologic or physiologic alteration for 24 hours. However, it is important not to freeze the blood samples because the thawing process will damage both erythrocytes and platelets.
- **Avoid direct sunlight.**
- **Specific methods of preservation** may depend on the procedure to be performed on the blood sample. These methods may include the use of proper anticoagulants, the creation of a blood smear, or the preservation of whole blood (depending on the procedure to be performed).

Adapted with permission from Aspinall V. *The Complete Textbook of Veterinary Nursing.* London, UK: Butterworth-Heinemann; 2006:692.

Physiologic processes

Stress, fear, excitement, struggling, and restraint at the time of blood sampling may all play a role in altering hematologic characteristics, artifactually skewing diagnostic test results and potentially masking underlying disease processes. For example, during prolonged periods of stress, the patient will release glucocorticoids from its adrenal glands. This will ultimately induce a stress leukogram that can be noted on hematologic evaluation. Stress leukograms are characterized by a mature neutrophilia (increased concentration of mature neutrophils in the peripheral blood), monocytosis, lymphopenia, and eosinopenia. This increase in peripheral circulating neutrophils may in some cases be misinterpreted as the result of an inflammatory process. Furthermore, the release of epinephrine in an excited or struggling state may induce a *physiologic leukogram* in which a hematologic evaluation may again show mature neutrophilia, this time accompanied by a lymphocytosis, perhaps a thrombocytosis, and an increased PCV in dogs due to splenic contraction. This increase in PCV may be misinterpreted as relative hemoconcentration due to dehydration. To prevent errors in hematologic evaluation due to physiologic responses to the blood collection technique, the technician should choose to use large peripheral veins for easier and less stressful blood collection whenever possible. Manual compression of the spleen during restraint and lifting of the canine patient in particular may also induce splenic contraction, which may lead to an increase in the patient's PCV. The technician should use only the minimal amount of restraint necessary to immobilize an animal.

In addition to the technical aspects of blood collection technique, hematologic parameters may be altered by another physiologic process: digestion. In most cases, it is advisable to fast a patient prior to blood collection. As part of the normal digestion process, digested fat travels from the small intestine into the lymphatic circulation and thence to the peripheral circulation where it is deposited in adipose tissue for later use. Therefore, a postprandial blood sample in a healthy animal should be lipemic. Although this is a normal physiologic response to ingestion of fat, lipemia may induce hemolysis and impede accurate hematologic analysis.

Concurrent drug administration

Unless the purpose is to monitor treatment, blood should always be collected before pharmacologic treatment is administered. Different treatments may have biologic or dilution effects on sample or may influence test procedure. For example, sedatives and analgesics may mask disease processes by altering PCV and other hematologic parameters, and boluses of intravenous fluids may transiently dilute blood components.

Patient history

Patient history may play a significant role in the results of hematologic evaluation. Examples of significant factors include prior surgery, geographic origin, and recent vaccination history.

Improper blood collection and processing technique

Improper blood collection technique is a leading source of error in analysis of blood samples. For example, it is very important to avoid frequent blood collections from the same site on the patient. Not only will this cause the patient increased pain, trauma, and likelihood of hematoma formation, but it will also cause localized increases in platelet and leukocyte numbers.

In addition, as previously mentioned, proper technique for blood smear preparation is critical for a blood smear of diagnostic quality. Poor spreading technique will lead to blood smears that cannot be properly read or that contain damaged cells. Incorrect staining technique may likewise render a smear completely unreadable or invalid.

Inaccuracy of clinical instruments

Despite the many benefits of automated hematologic analysis, common instrumentation limitations may be significant sources of errors or diagnostic inaccuracies. First, an automated analysis will only be as good as the sample provided. Second, there are upper and lower limitations on the numbers of cells in a sample that an analyzer can accurately count. Third, automated analyzers are frequently limited in their ability to discriminate between cell types when cells are similar in appearance (size, weight, cytoplasmic inclusions, and nuclear components). Finally, automated systems are susceptible to certain interferences, such as *Microfilaria*, platelet and leukocyte aggregates, and microclots.[8]

To prevent these sources of error, quality control programs should be put in place. Effective quality control programs involve the following:

- **Regular maintenance of equipment and analysis of control materials.** It is important to note that "standards" should not be used in place of "controls." Whereas *standards* are nonbiologic materials used to calibrate the equipment, *controls* contain specific concentrations of blood components and are produced by the manufacturer for the purpose of equipment function evaluation. Equipment manufacturers provide guidelines as to how often these controls should be run. A small animal practice should chart and analyze control results regularly to help identify any changes in the performance of the equipment. In cases of aberrant test or control results, a second sample should be run. If the second sample produces similarly aberrant results, attempts should be made to evaluate the source of the error, whether from the instrument or the technicians' technique.
- **Instrument internal quality control programs.** Certain instruments may have internal quality control programs automatically performed with each blood sample to ensure accuracy.
- **Microscopic evaluation of stained blood smears.** Direct microscopic evaluation of all blood smears is invaluable to ensure accuracy and confirm cell identifications derived from machine analyzers.

References

1. Torrance A. Overview of haematologic diagnostic techniques. In: Day M, Mackin A, Littlewood J, eds. Manual of Canine and Feline Hematology and Transfusion Medicine. Gloucester, UK: British Small Animal Veterinary Association; 2000:1.
2. Tasker JB. The veterinary hospital laboratory. Vet Clin North Am 1976;6:523.
3. Stockham S, Scott M. Leukocytes. In: Stockham S, Scott M, eds. Fundamentals of Veterinary Clinical Pathology. 2nd ed. Ames, IA: Blackwell Publishing; 2008:61.

4. Day M, Mackin A, Littlewood J. Manual of Canine and Feline Hematology and Transfusion Medicine. Gloucester, UK: British Small Animal Veterinary Association; 2000:165.

5. Sirois M. Hematology and hemostasis. In: Sirois M, ed. Principles and Practice of Veterinary Technology. 2nd ed. St. Louis, MO: Mosby; 2004:224.

6. Moss G, Staunton C. Blood flow, needle size and hemolysis— examining an old wives' tale. N Engl J Med 1970;282(17):967.

7. Becton-Dickinson Web site. Blood and urine collection. http://www.bd.com/vacutainer/products (accessed June 2010).

8. Tighe M, Brown M. Urinalysis and hematology. In: Tighe MM, Brown M, eds. Mosby's Comprehensive Review for Veterinary Technicians. 3rd ed. St. Louis, MO: Mosby; 2008:50–51.

49

Electrolyte evaluation

Louisa J. Rahilly

Electrolytes are pivotal players in maintaining home-ostasis in the body. They have key roles in such physiologic functions as maintaining intracellular and extracellular fluid distribution; energy production and utilization; electrical conductivity and muscle contraction in cardiac, skeletal, and vascular smooth muscle; and clot formation. Many disease processes can cause electrolyte abnormalities including gastrointestinal disease; endocrine diseases such as diabetes, hyperadrenocorticism, hypoadrenocorticism, and thyroid disorders; renal and urinary disease; various neoplasms; sepsis; and skin disorders. Treatment interventions in critically ill animals can also precipitate electrolyte disorders or clinically significant shifts in electrolyte distribution and levels within the body. Appropriate treatment of electrolyte abnormalities may result in decreased morbidity and mortality. Many of the clinical signs of electrolyte abnormalities can be masked by or thought to be due to the underlying disease state. The role of the astute critical care technician is to monitor for potential sequelae of electrolyte abnormalities, appropriately obtain samples and use in-house analyzers, and alert the doctor to important changes noted on laboratory monitoring over the course of hospitalization.

Electrolyte concentrations in serum, plasma, or whole blood are ultimately the result of the combination of intake, excretion, shifts between the intracellular and extracellular space (note that we sample the extracellular space in the clinical setting), and artifactual influences *in vitro*.[1] Accurate measurement of electrolytes in the critical care setting is both necessary and challenging due to common artifacts such as dilution or binding with anticoagulants, sample exposure to air, and concurrent sample or patient abnormalities that spuriously alter electrolyte measurements. Electrolytes often need to be evaluated in the clinic using point-of-care (POC) analyzers because changes in electrolyte levels alter the treatment course on an hour-by-hour basis. Understanding the methodology and potential artifacts that may be caused by the POC analyzer in use is important, as some physiologic abnormalities, such as lipemia or hyperbilirubinemia, necessitate particular methodology and submission to a reference lab for accurate electrolyte measurement. This chapter introduces methods of electrolyte quantification and commonly used veterinary electrolyte analyzers, the physiologically significant electrolytes, disease states or treatments that may affect them, and recommendations on sample handling to ensure correct measurement and interpretation.

Methods of electrolyte quantification

The methods of electrolyte evaluation include flame photometry (FF), ion selective electrode assays (ISE), and enzymatic spectrophotometry (ES).[1,2] When serially evaluating a patient's electrolytes, values should always be measured with the same methodology and, ideally, the same analyzer because reference ranges and readings vary between the different methodologies and analyzers.[3–5] Flame photometry is typically only available in reference laboratories, making it impractical to use this methodology for POC analysis. FF was the gold standard for electrolyte analysis but has become obsolete due to both the logistics of utilization and inaccuracies in measurement with concurrent lipemia, hyperproteinemia, hemolysis, or hyperbilirubinemia.[1] Enzymatic

Advanced Monitoring and Procedures for Small Animal Emergency and Critical Care, First Edition. Edited by Jamie M. Burkitt Creedon, Harold Davis.
© 2012 John Wiley & Sons, Inc. Published 2012 by John Wiley & Sons, Inc.

spectrophotometry has clinical value in enabling electrolyte measurement utilizing in-house automated chemistry analyzers, but it has demonstrated the most interference in situations of hemolysis, hyperproteinemia, and lipemia.[2,6,7] Uremic samples with alterations in bicarbonate and potassium may also affect samples analyzed by ES.[7] Updated chemistry analyzers that use ES, such as the Catalyst DX chemistry analyzer (IDEXX, Westbrook, ME, operator's guide) and the Vetscan VS2 (Abaxis, Union City, CA) utilize filters to attempt to minimize the interference created by these abnormalities. One should interpret results in severely lipemic, icteric, hemolyzed, or hyperproteinemic samples carefully, however, and submit a paired sample to a reference laboratory that utilizes ISE to confirm in-house results.

Ion selective electrodes are now the method of choice and the reference method recommended by the Lab Medicine and Clinical Lab Standard Institute for the validation of POC analyzers.[2,3,7] The basic principle of ISE measurement is the comparison of an unknown value against a known value to compute the sample's electrolyte concentration (VetLyte electrolyte Analyzer, IDEXX Laboratories; Operator's Manual). Essentially, an ion sensitive membrane undergoes a reaction based on the electrical charge of the ion (electrolyte) causing a change in the specific ion-generated voltage. The analyzer then compares the change in voltage on the sample side of the membrane with a reference solution. An algorithm utilizing the measured voltages and a calibration curve derived from the ion concentration of known solutions is used to determine the electrolyte concentration within the sample (VetLyte electrolyte Analyzer, IDEXX Laboratories; Operator's Manual). Commonly used in-house veterinary analyzers that utilize ISE include the Vetscan i-STAT 1 (Abaxis), the Stat Profile Critical Care Xpress (Nova Biomedical, Waltham, MA), the VetLyte electrolyte analyzer (IDEXX Laboratories, Westbrook, ME), the VitalPath blood gas and electrolyte analyzer (Heska, Lovelane, CO), and the EasyLyte (Hemagen Diagnostics, Inc., Columbia, MD). Table 49.1 details each of these analyzers, which electrolytes they measure, and operator information.

Electrolytes vary with regard to the best sampling method and possible artifacts associated with measurement, the specifics of which are covered in the subsequent sections. Overall, however, electrolyte analysis should be performed on serum samples that are collected anaerobically.[3,4,8–11] Anaerobic conditions are most important for ionized calcium and magnesium analysis.[4,10–12] Whole blood, anticoagulated whole blood, and plasma can also be used, but one must consider various possible artifacts and the risk of clot formation prior to the completion of analysis when using whole blood. Careful attention to the timing of the sample collection and measurement is pivotal because various electrolyte concentrations can be affected by increased exposure time to platelets, exposure time to white blood cells, and alterations in protein binding associated with ongoing cellular metabolism (Vetscan i-STAT 1,user guide).[3,4,12]

Individual electrolytes

Table 49.2 details normal ranges and critical alert values for each of the physiologically significant electrolytes. It is important to remember, however, that these ranges should be used only as guidelines because each analyzer has its own manufacturer-determined reference intervals. A reference range specific to the analyzer used should be consulted when interpreting all electrolyte measurements. These ranges should be specific for sample type (i.e., plasma versus serum) and species within each analyzer.

Sodium

Sodium is the most abundant extracellular ion. It functions in determining the distribution of water throughout the body in the extracellular and intracellular compartments.[13–17] Disorders in sodium concentration are nearly always the result of changes in the volume of body water.[13,15,17] The sodium concentration should therefore be viewed as a reflection of relative free water in the body, rather than necessarily the amount of sodium in the body.[13,15–17] "Free water" is water that is free of sodium.

An increased sodium concentration is due to either the loss of body fluid containing relatively less sodium than plasma (hypotonic fluid), fluid containing no sodium (free water), or the ingestion or iatrogenic administration of relatively high-sodium substances.[13,15,16] Disease processes that can result in hypotonic fluid loss include gastrointestinal and renal disease, osmotic diuresis from hyperglycemia, ketonuria or mannitol administration, or postobstructive diuresis.[15] Lack of access to water and neurologic disease resulting in decreased water intake can also result in hypernatremia.[15,17] Animals with underlying metabolic disorders such as hyperadrenocorticism, hyperthyroidism, and hepatic disease have decreased urine concentrating abilities and are at risk of developing hypernatremia in the critical care setting if they have decreased water intake due to nausea or sedation.[15] Processes resulting in the loss of fluid that contains virtually no sodium (free water) include diabetes insipidus and panting.[15,17] Hyperaldosteronism, a rare disorder in dogs and cats,

Table 49.1 Common POC electrolyte analyzers used in veterinary medicine

Analyzer	Method	Electrolytes Measured (Reportable Range)	Sample Type Based on Manufacturer's Recommendations	Maintenance/Operator Tips
VetScan i-STAT 1 Abaxis	ISE	Na$^+$ (100–180 mmoL/L) K$^+$ (2.0–9.0 mmol/L) Cl$^-$ (65–140 mmol/L) iCa^{++} (0.25–2.50 mmol/L)	• Serum • WB • WB or plasma anticoagulated with balanced heparin	• Cartridges must be stored at 2–8°C and equilibrated to room temperature for 5 minutes prior to use • Once cartridges are equilibrated to room temperature they must not be returned to refrigerator and are good for 14 days. • Minimal maintenance
VetScan VS2 Analyzer Abaxis	ES	Na$^+$ (110–170 mmol/L) K$^+$ (1.5–8.5 mmol/L) iPhos (0–20 mg/dL)	• Serum • WB or plasma anticoagulated with lithium heparin	• Minimal maintenance • Self-calibrates with each sample
Stat Profile Critical Care Xpress Nova	ISE	Na$^+$ (blood 66–201 mmol/L; plasma 71–199 mmol/L) K$^+$ (blood 1.3–20.4 mmol/L; plasma 1.3–18.5 mmol/L) Cl$^-$ (blood 62–189 mmol/L; plasma 59–177 mmol/L) iCa^{++} (blood 0.3–4.7 mmol/L; plasma 0.7–4.4 mmol/L) iMg^{++} (blood 0.2–2.3 mmol/L; plasma 0.3–2.4 mmol/L)	• Serum • WB or plasma anticoagulated with lyophilized sodium or lithium heparin	• Automatic calibration • Sample inlet port should be cleaned when necessary with deionized water
Catalyst IDEXX	ES	Na$^+$ (85–180 mmol/L) K$^+$ (0.8–10 mmol/L) Cl$^-$ (50–160 mmol/L) iPhos (0.2–16.1 mg/dL) tMg^{++} (0.5–5.2 mg/dL 0.21–2.17 mmol/L)	• Serum • WB or plasma anticoagulated with lithium heparin	• Monthly quality control checks; internal and external cleaning
VetLyte IDEXX	ISE	Na$^+$ (40–205 mmol/L) K$^+$ (1.5–15 mmol/L) Cl$^-$ (50–200 mmol/L)	• Serum • WB or plasma anticoagulated with lithium heparin	• Daily and weekly cleaning recommended • Monthly cleaning involving cleaning the reference electrode • Electrodes should never be cleaned with abrasive cleaners such as alcohol or Amphyl
VitalPath Heska	ISE	Na$^+$ (20–250 mmol/L) K$^+$ (0.2–20.0 mmol/L) Cl$^-$ (20–250 mmol/L) iCa^{++} (0.1–4.0 mmol/L)	• Serum • WB or plasma anticoagulated with sodium or lithium heparin	• Automatic calibration
Easy-Lyte Hemagen	ISE	Na$^+$ (20–200 mmol/L) K$^+$ (0.2–40 mmol/L) Cl$^-$ (25–200 mmol/L)	• Serum • WB plasma anticoagulated with sodium or lithium heparin	• Automatic calibration • Minimal maintenance

FF, flame photometry; ES, enzymatic spectrophotometry; ISE, ion selective electrode; Na$^+$, sodium; K$^+$; potassium; Cl$^-$, chloride; iPhos, inorganic phosphate; iCa^{++}, ionized calcium; iMg^{++}, ionized magnesium; tMg^{++}, total magnesium; WB, whole blood.

Table 49.2 Reference ranges and alert values of each electrolyte[a]

Electrolyte	Normal Range Canine	Normal Range Feline	Critical Care Alert Values[b]	Common Artifacts
Na+	139–150 mmol/L	147–162 mmol/L	<120 mmol/L >170 mmol/L Change >1.0 mmol/L/h or >10 mmol/L/24 h	• Lipemia • Hemolysis • Hyperbilirubinemia • Hyperproteinemia • Sodium heparin
K+	3.4–4.9 mmol/L	2.9–4.2 mmol/L	<2.5 mmol/L >6.0 mmol/L	• Thrombocytosis • Leukocytosis • Potassium EDTA • Delay in serum or plasma separation
Cl−	106–127 mmol/L	112–129 mmol/L	<90 mmol/L	• Lipemia • Hemolysis • Hyperbilirubinemia • Hyperproteinemia • Sodium heparin
iPhos	2.5–6.0 mg/dL	2.4–8.2 mg/dL	<1.5 mg/dL	• Hemolysis • Citrate, oxalate and EDTA anticoagulation • Hyperlipidemia • Hyperbilirubinemia • Delay in serum or plasma separation
iCa++	1.12–1.40 mmol/L	1.20–1.32 mmol/L	<0.75 mmol/L > 2.0 mmol/L	• Aerobic sampling • Heparin dilution • Heparin binding • Delay in analysis
iMg++ tMg++	0.42–0.58 mmol/L 1.4–2.38 mg/dL	0.47–60 mmol/L 1.5–3.0 mg/dL		• Aerobic sampling • Heparin dilution • Heparin binding • Delay in analysis

[a]Catalyst DX chemistry analyzer (IDEXX Laboratories, Westbrook, ME), operator's guide, and Vetscan iSTAT 1 (Abaxis, Union City, CA), user guide.
[b]Critical care alert values refer to values that suggest impending severe physiologic compromise. Any value outside of the reference range is considered clinically significant, however.

results in increased sodium retention.[15,18] Dietary indiscretions can cause hypernatremia if the animal ingests excessive salt in the form of things such as table salt, sea water, homemade play dough, solid ice melts, or paintballs.[15] Iatrogenic causes of hypernatremia include the administration of high-sodium-containing solutions (sodium bicarbonate, hypertonic saline, and sodium phosphate enemas) and the administration of drugs that can affect the kidney's ability to concentrate urine (gentamicin, amphotericin B, methoxyflurane, and vinca alkaloids).[15,17] As evident by this extensive list of causes, many animals admitted to a veterinary intensive care unit are at risk of having or developing hypernatremia. Serial measurements to monitor for a rising sodium concentration are necessary to catch an animal trending toward hypernatremia before the clinical signs of hypernatremia develop, at which point irreversible neurologic damage may have occurred.

Hypernatremia results in cellular dehydration in the brain as water moves from the intracellular to the extracellular space.[16] The brain tissue shrinks, which can result in tearing of blood vessels and subarachnoid and intracerebral hemorrhage.[15,17] Clinical signs are related more to the rate of rise of sodium concentration than to the absolute concentration, and they include lethargy, nausea, depressed mentation, ataxia, and weakness.[15,16] Neurologic signs can progress to seizures, coma, and death.[15,16]

Decreased sodium concentrations are due to a relative gain of free water or hypotonic fluid within the extracellular space.[13] This may be due to a true increase in total body water or a decrease in total body water and sodium with sodium losses relatively exceeding water losses.[13,16] Measured hyponatremia may be due to an increase in osmotically active particles such as glucose or mannitol in the extracellular fluid causing a dilution of sodium molecules in the serum.[16] Gastrointestinal disease and severe burns can cause loss of both sodium and water with relatively more sodium loss, which results in hyponatremia.[16] Loss of sodium through the kidneys can occur with hypoadrenocorticism, diuretic administration, or sodium-wasting renal diseases.[16] Water retention and resultant hyponatremia can occur in cases of hypothyroidism with myxedema coma and water intoxication.[16,19] A pathophysiologic syndrome known as the syndrome of inappropriate antidiuretic hormone secretion (SIADH) has been described in humans and may be seen in veterinary patients. It is characterized by inappropriate release of antidiuretic hormone (ADH) resulting in the retention of free water.[13,16] This syndrome has been associated with certain neoplasms, pulmonary disease, central nervous system disease, perioperative patients, and certain drugs. There is documentation of SIADH in human patients associated with the administration of fentanyl, a drug used commonly in critically ill or injured veterinary patients.[20] Disease processes associated with decreased effective circulating volume such as hepatic disease and primary cardiac disease can cause hyponatremia as the thirst center is activated, increasing water consumption.[13,16]

Similar to hypernatremia, the severity of the clinical signs associated with hyponatremia depend on the rate of drop as well as the absolute sodium concentration.[16] Signs often do not occur unless the sodium concentration is <125 mmol/L.[16] Vomiting, ataxia, depression progressing to obtundation, seizures, and coma may occur as a result of cerebral edema as water moves into neurons.[19]

Treatment of sodium concentration abnormalities involves addressing the underlying cause and slowly returning the sodium concentration to normal with the administration of relatively hypertonic (in the case of hyponatremia) or hypotonic (in the case of hypernatremia) fluids. Table 49.3 details the sodium concentration of various electrolyte solutions that can be used to treat sodium abnormalities. Diuretic administration may be necessary to encourage sodium or water excretion.[13,15–17]

Table 49.3 Various fluid solutions and their sodium and potassium concentrations[47]

Fluid Type	Sodium Concentration (mEq/L)	Potassium Concentration (mEq/L)
5% dextrose in water	0	0
0.45% saline	77	0
2.5% dextrose in 0.45% saline	77	0
Lactated Ringer solution	130	4
Plasmalyte A	140	5
Normosol R	140	5
0.9% NaCl	154	0
Hetastarch	154	0
7.5% Hypertonic NaCl	1283	0

The fluid of choice depends on the rate of sodium drop and volume status of the patient. Cases of chronic sodium concentration abnormalities (>48 hours) should be treated with the goal to gradually correct the sodium concentration; acute cases can be addressed more aggressively.[16] Sodium concentration should not be changed >0.5–1 mEq/L/hour or 10 mEq/L over 24 hours.[15,16] Rapid adjustment of sodium concentration can result in neurologic sequelae. In the case of hyponatremia, neuronal dehydration resulting in a syndrome known as osmotic demyelination syndrome (ODS) or previously central pontine myelinolysis (CPM) can occur if the sodium concentration is raised too fast.[16,21] ODS is characterized by water moving out of brain cells during the correction of hyponatremia.[16,21] Signs of ODS can be delayed 1–6 days, and neuronal damage can be irreversible, making careful sodium monitoring vital because clinical signs may not immediately be apparent.[16] In the case of hypernatremia, rapid drops in sodium concentration can cause cerebral edema as extracellular water moves into neurons.[16] The signs of cerebral edema and rising intracranial pressure include depressed mentation, pupillary changes, thoracic limb rigidity, and seizures; the technician must monitor closely for these signs and pay close attention to serial sodium concentrations. Sodium concentration should be reassessed every 2–4 hours initially during the treatment of sodium derangements.[16]

Sodium concentration measurement

The reference standard for sodium measurement was traditionally flame photometry.[13] FF evaluates the entire volume of the sample, including both the aqueous and the nonaqueous phases.[13] Plasma is 93% water by volume, and sodium is present in the aqueous phase of plasma.[13] The distribution of sodium within only the aqueous portion of the sample results in a lower measured concentration of sodium in plasma than is truly present.[13] This difference is typically negligible, but in situations of hyperlipidemia and hyperproteinemia the nonaqueous portion of plasma increases.[13] When the nonaqueous portion of plasma is increased, the measured concentration of sodium will be significantly lower than the actual value, invalidating the results.[13] This artifact is known as pseudohyponatremia.[13] Ion selective electrodes measure sodium in water only, avoiding the artifact caused by increased lipid or protein in samples.[13,16] Enzymatic spectrophotometry can be used to measure sodium concentrations but can be inaccurate for hemolyzed, icteric, or hyperproteinemic samples and therefore should be used with caution in these circumstances.[2] Serum should be submitted to a reference laboratory that uses ISE for sodium and chloride concentration evaluation in icteric, lipidemic, or hyperproteinemic patients if the in-house electrolyte analyzer utilizes ES to verify the in-house results. Enzymatic spectrophotometry also has higher normal reference ranges for sodium concentration than FF or ISE, so one must use analyzer-specific reference ranges when interpreting results.[2]

Sodium heparin contains relatively high concentrations of sodium (160 mEq/L) and chloride (166 mEq/L) and can falsely elevate the measurement of both of these electrolytes when whole blood is anticoagulated with sodium heparin at concentrations >3.9%.[8] Therefore, if one uses sodium heparin to anticoagulate the sample prior to measurement of sodium or chloride concentrations, preparation of an "evacuated syringe" according to Hopper et al (see Protocol 49.1) or the purchase of commercially available syringes containing lyophilized 40 IU/mL heparin is necessary to avoid artifact.[8] One could also utilize lithium heparin for measurement of sodium or chloride concentrations.[8]

Chloride

Chloride is an extracellular ion that functions with sodium in maintaining water balance and has an important role in acid-base balance.[22] Chloride concentration often changes with sodium concentration, but certain situations can alter chloride concentration independent of changes in sodium. Hypochloremia can be caused by vomiting, gastrointestinal obstruction, metabolic alkalosis, and therapy with diuretics that block absorption of chloride in the kidneys (e.g., furosemide).[23,24] Hyperchloremia is often the result of loss of bicarbonate-rich, chloride-poor fluid in diarrhea and renal disease, and it

> **Protocol 49.1** Preparation of a heparinized syringe or "evacuated syringe" for blood sampling[8]
>
> **Items Required**
> 1. 3-mL syringe
> 2. 22-gauge needle attached to syringe
> 3. Liquid sodium heparin 1000 U/mL concentration
>
> **Procedure**
> 1. Aspirate 0.5 mL of heparin into the syringe.
> 2. Draw the plunger back to the 3-mL mark to coat the inner surface of the syringe.
> 3. Expel all of the air and heparin.
> 4. Draw 3 mL of air into syringe and expel it.
> 5. Repeat step 4 a total of three times.
> 6. Perform venipuncture.
>   - 7.8% with 0.5-mL sample: Inaccurate for all electrolyte measurements.
>   - 3.9% with 01.0-mL sample: Accurate for Na[+] and K[+] measurements.
>   - 2.0% with 2.0-mL sample: Accurate for iCa[++] measurements.
>   - 1.3% with 3.0-mL sample: Accurate for iCa[++] and iMg[++] measurements.

is associated with a metabolic acidosis.[24] Iatrogenic hyperchloremia can occur with the administration of bicarbonate-free fluids such as 0.9% NaCl.[24] To determine if the change in chloride concentration is due to an alteration in sodium, a formula was developed[22] (Eq. 49.1) that functions to determine the chloride concentration as high, low, or normal outside of the influences of free water.[22]

$$\text{Dog } Cl^- \text{ corrected} = Cl^- \times 146/Na^+$$
$$\text{Cat } Cl^- \text{ corrected} = Cl^- \times 156/Na^+ \tag{49.1}$$

The clinical signs of chloride derangements are typically associated with the underlying disease process or acid-base abnormality. The clinical sequelae of acidosis and alkalemia are addressed in Chapter 50, Acid-Base Evaluation. Treatment of chloride derangements involves addressing the underlying disorder and stopping any iatrogenic cause.

Chloride concentration measurement

Chloride measurement is similar to sodium in that it can be falsely lowered by lipemia and hyperproteinemia and elevated by the use of sodium heparin for anticoagulation.[2,8] Chloride concentration is more affected by dilution with sodium heparin than sodium concentration.[8] The sensitivity of chloride concentration measurements to sodium heparin anticoagulation is likely due to the high concentration (166 mmol/L) of chloride within sodium heparin. The concentration of chloride within sodium heparin is significantly higher than normal chloride concentrations and spuriously elevates the chloride measurement of the sample. Accurate chloride analysis should either be performed on serum or plasma or whole blood anticoagulated with lithium heparin. Red blood cells in venous blood carry more intracellular chloride than red blood cells in arterial blood, and the chloride concentration in venous blood is 3–4 mEq/L lower than arterial blood.[22] This variation is due to chloride shifting out of red blood cells in the presence of higher oxygen and lower carbon dioxide (generally the environment within arterial blood and room air relative to venous blood).[22,25] If a sample is exposed to room air and permitted to "arterialize," the chloride concentration measurement with be falsely elevated. Anaerobic sampling is therefore necessary when determining and interpreting chloride concentrations from venous blood.[22]

Potassium

Potassium is the most abundant cation in the body, but it is located primarily intracellularly, making measurement in whole blood, serum, or plasma an imperfect reflection of total body stores.[26] The large concentration gradient of potassium across cell membranes enables potassium to be a key player in the excitability and function of nerve and muscle cells, including those in cardiac and vascular smooth muscle.[26] Potassium concentration is a reflection of intake (primarily through nutrition); loss into the gastrointestinal tract (a factor exacerbated in animals with gastrointestinal disease); renal function, as the bulk of potassium is eliminated through the kidneys; and transcellular potassium shifts as occurs in some acid-base disorders and under the influence of insulin.[24,26]

Hyperkalemia can be caused by decreased renal excretion in acute renal failure, end-stage renal disease, or hypoadrenocorticism; urinary obstruction or intra-abdominal urine accumulation; and syndromes of massive cell death such as tumor lysis syndrome or rhabdomyolysis.[24,26] Drug therapy with angiotensin-converting enzyme inhibitors (e.g., benazepril and enalapril), nonsteroidal anti-inflammatory agents, β-blockers (e.g., atenolol), potassium itself, or potassium-sparing diuretics (e.g., spironolactone) has been shown to cause hyperkalemia in humans and may result in similar changes in small animal patients. Patients who are at higher risk are those prescribed a combination of these drugs and those with decreased renal delivery of

potassium as might be seen in dogs and cats with cardiac disease and dehydration.[26,27] A group of disease processes can cause concurrent hyperkalemia and hyponatremia with a decreased sodium-to-potassium ratio. This is the classic electrolyte picture with hypoadrenocorticism. A decreased sodium to potassium ratio can also be seen in dogs and cats with gastrointestinal disease, renal disease, pregnancy, body cavity effusions, and cardiac disease resulting in decreased effective circulating volume triggering free water retention and hyponatremia with concurrent decreased renal delivery of potassium for excretion resulting in hyperkalemia.[28,29]

Hyperkalemia can be life threatening as a result of the increased potassium concentration's effect on cardiac cell conduction and function.[24,26] Clinical signs include muscular weakness with progression to paralysis.[24,26] Cardiac toxicity is manifested by classic electrocardiogram (ECG) abnormalities including tall, tented T waves, a prolonged PR interval, loss of the P wave, bradycardia, and widening QRS complexes.[24,26] Ventricular tachycardia and fibrillation can occur.[24] In severe hyperkalemia the ECG progresses to a sine-wave pattern as the QRS complexes merge with the T wave. This latter rhythm is an indication of impending cardiac arrest, and rapid intervention is indicated.[26] Life-threatening hyperkalemia generally occurs at potassium concentrations >7.5 mEq/L,[24] but concurrent abnormalities such as hypovolemia, acidemia, hypocalcemia, and hyponatremia may exacerbate the condition and trigger rapid cardiac collapse at lower concentrations.[26] Treatment of hyperkalemia involves diuresis with intravenous fluid therapy, relieving urinary obstruction if present, cardiac protection with calcium gluconate or calcium chloride administration, and initiating intracellular movement of potassium with insulin, dextrose, β-agonists (e.g., terbutaline or albuterol) or bicarbonate therapy.[24,26,30,31] In refractory renal failure, hemodialysis or peritoneal dialysis is required to treat hyperkalemia.[24,26]

Low potassium concentration, or hypokalemia, is typically the result of excessive potassium loss through the gastrointestinal tract or through the kidneys due to renal disease or osmotic diuresis (e.g., hyperglycemia, ketonuria, postobstructive diuresis); hypokalemia can also result from intracellular potassium shifts in the face of metabolic alkalosis.[24,26] Hypokalemia is often confounded by decreased potassium ingestion in the face of nausea or anorexia.[24,26] Iatrogenic causes of hypokalemia include diuretics, steroids, β-agonists (e.g., terbutaline or albuterol) or insulin and dextrose therapy.[24] Hypomagnesemia can cause refractory hypokalemia in which the potassium concentration does not return to normal despite aggressive supplementation.[24] Hyperaldosteronism causes increased renal excretion of potassium and is a rare cause of severe hypokalemia in dogs and cats.[18,31]

Clinical signs of hypokalemia generally occur with serum potassium concentrations ≤2.5 mEq/L and include generalized weakness characterized classically by cervical ventriflexion that can progress to paralysis and respiratory difficulties, inability to concentrate urine, anorexia, vomiting, and decreased bowel motility.[24,26,32] Cardiac conduction abnormalities can occur and manifest on ECG by a depressed ST segment, decreased amplitude or inversion of the T wave, increased P wave amplitude, and prolonged PR and QRS intervals.[24] Multiple arrhythmias may also occur.[24,26] Treatment of hypokalemia involves potassium supplementation orally or parenterally, depending on the severity of hypokalemia and whether or not the patient is tolerant of enteral treatments.[24,26] Concurrent magnesium administration may be necessary to treat hypokalemia effectively.[24] Charts exist with recommended potassium supplementation based on degree of hypokalemia, but these should be viewed as a starting point. Rate of potassium administration depends on degree of total body depletion, renal and gastrointestinal losses of potassium, and rate of diuresis. Potassium concentration should be monitored at least once a day in patients on potassium supplementation and more frequently in animals with documented hypokalemia or pathophysiologic processes that may cause hypokalemia. Parenteral potassium supplementation should rarely exceed 0.5 mEq/kg/hour and should never exceed 1.0 mEq/kg/hour because rapid potassium administration can cause cardiac arrest.[24] The rate of potassium supplementation should be checked frequently, and fluids with potassium additives should not be administered rapidly as a bolus. Box 49.1 demonstrates how to determine the rate of potassium supplementation per kilogram based on the concentration of potassium in solution.

Potassium concentration measurement

Artifactually elevated potassium concentrations can be caused by anticoagulation with potassium EDTA as well as prolonged exposure to potassium-containing cells such as platelets and white blood cells.[28] Thrombocytosis and leukocytosis have been shown to cause pseudohyperkalemia.[9,28] Artifactual hyperkalemia can be seen in samples from Japanese breeds (e.g., Akita and Shiba Inu) due to leakage of potassium from these breeds' red blood cells.[9] Potassium concentrations are higher in serum than plasma due to release of potassium from cells during clotting.[9] Canine serum potassium concentrations are generally 0.35 mmol/L higher than canine plasma, and feline serum potassium was found to be

---

Box 49.1 Calculation of potassium supplementation (mEq/kg/h)

1. Determine the amount of potassium in the solution by adding the amount of supplemented potassium to the amount already present in the fluid (see Table 49.3).
2. Divide the total amount of potassium by the total volume of the fluid to determine the concentration of potassium in solution.
3. Determine the total amount of potassium being administered per hour by multiplying the amount of potassium per milliliter by the fluid rate of the patient in mL/h.
4. Determine the rate of administration in mEq/kg/h by dividing the amount of potassium per hour by the weight of the patient in kilograms.

Case example: A 10-kg Boston terrier being treated with lactated Ringer solution with 40 mEq/L of potassium added at a rate of 40 mL/h.

1. Total amount of potassium in solution:
   40 mEq (supplemented) + 4 mEq (already present in fluid) = 44 mEq
2. Concentration of potassium in solution:
   44 mEq (total amount of potassium) ÷ 1000 mL (total volume) = 0.044 mEq/mL
3. Amount of potassium administered per hour:
   0.044 mEq/mL × 40 mL/h = 1.76 mEq/h
4. Rate of administration:
   1.76 mEq/h ÷ 10 kg = 0.18 mEq/kg/h

0.47 mmol/L higher than feline plasma.[9] This degree of variation between serum and plasma samples necessitates consideration of the sample type used to create the reference interval on the analyzer being used.[9] Serial samples on the same patient should always be run using the same type of sample. Although the changes caused by anticoagulation with potassium EDTA or potassium leakage from cells are typically minimal, they may result in pseudohyperkalemia or pseudo normokalemia if the patient's actual value is at the high end of normal or just below the reference range, respectively.[9] Ideally, potassium samples should be run on whole blood, heparin-anticoagulated whole blood, or plasma rapidly separated from the cell pellet to minimize length of exposure to potassium-containing cells.[9]

Hemolysis and elevated total protein concentration appear to have less of an effect on potassium measurement than on sodium and chloride measurements, although analysis with ES showed more variation in potassium measured in a hemolyzed sample than either FF or ISE.[2] Like sodium and chloride, however, values obtained via ES are generally higher than those obtained via FF or ISE.[2] Because ES potassium concentration measurement can show more variation than other methods, plasma potassium levels should be submitted for ISE analysis to a reference laboratory in patients with severe hemolysis or hyperbilirubinemia if the available POC analyzer utilizes ES.

Samples anticoagulated with heparin can cause dilution and artifactual lowering of potassium concentrations.[8] Syringes should be prepared for blood sampling utilizing the "evacuated syringe" technique (see Protocol 49.1).[8] Use of a commercially available syringe coated with lyophilized 40 IU/mL heparin is also an option to avoid dilutional artifact.[8]

Phosphorus

Phosphate is a vital intracellular ion in many physiologic processes including maintenance of cell membrane integrity, enzyme activation and deactivation, acid-base balance, clot formation, and energy production and use.[33,34] Most of the phosphorus in the body is within the mineralized bone matrix with the remainder mostly intracellular.[33,34] Only a small portion (<1%) is present in the extracellular fluid.[33,34] Only a third of total plasma phosphorus, in the form of inorganic phosphate, is measured by chemistry analyzers.[34] Similar to potassium, changes in total body stores of phosphorus are not necessarily reflected in blood phosphate levels.[33,34] An elevated measured phosphorus concentration may occur in situations of normal or low total body phosphorus stores.[33] Transcellular shifts contribute to many of the alterations seen in phosphate concentrations measured in critically ill patients.[33,34]

Hypophosphatemia can be due to a number of disease processes as well as secondary to treatment of various disease states. It can be seen in patients with decreased intestinal absorption, increased renal losses, hypomagnesemia, rapid tissue regeneration (i.e., liver regeneration after an episode of acute hepatic failure), head trauma, hypothermia, and shifting of phosphorus into cells with respiratory alkalosis, metabolic acidosis, or insulin or dextrose administration (particularly in diabetic ketoacidosis).[33,34] Respiratory alkalosis with associated hypophosphatemia can be seen in critically ill patients who are hyperventilating as a result of pain, anxiety, fever, or seizures.[33] Treatment of patients with phosphate-binding antacids (e.g., aluminum hydroxide) or aggressive diuresis in the face of decreased intake can result in hypophosphatemia.[34]

Clinical signs generally do not occur unless hypophosphatemia is severe.[33,34] The most significant clinical sequelae of hypophosphatemia are decreased delivery of oxygen to the tissues due to an increased affinity of hemoglobin for oxygen, impaired white blood cell function, and the development of hemolytic anemia as a result of altered integrity of the red blood cell membrane.[33,34] Decreased oxygen delivery to tissues may cause subtle clinical signs, but severe cases may demonstrate neuromuscular depression first noted with diaphragmatic weakness and possibly progressive neurologic signs.[33] Other signs of hypophosphatemia such as ileus, anorexia, and vomiting are often thought to part of the underlying disease.[33] Hemolysis in dogs has not been documented until phosphorus concentrations are <0.5 mg/dL, but cats appear to be more sensitive and have been shown to hemolyze at 1 mg/dL.[33] A decreased hematocrit may take 24–48 hours to become apparent following hemolysis triggered by hypophosphatemia.[33,34] Treatment of hypophosphatemia involves managing the underlying condition, addressing any acid-base abnormality contributing to transcellular shifts, and administering phosphorus supplementation either enterally or parenterally in more severely affected or nauseated animals.[33] It is recommended to treat phosphorus concentrations <3 mg/dL.[33] Parenterally administered potassium phosphate should be diluted before use because it is hypertonic and can cause tissue irritation.[33] It should be administered in calcium-free fluids (0.9% saline or 5% dextrose in water) to prevent precipitation of calcium salts.[33] Similar to other electrolytes, the dose depends on the rate of phosphorus loss and the underlying cause of hypophosphatemia. Recommended doses of parenteral phosphorus range from 0.01 to 0.06 mmol/kg/hour.[33,34] Phosphorus concentration should be monitored every 3–6 hours to ensure appropriate supplementation.[33] Sodium, potassium, and ionized calcium concentrations should also be closely monitored while patients receive phosphorus therapy because sodium or potassium phosphate can cause elevations in these electrolytes, and calcium concentration can drop due to binding of calcium to phosphorus.[33]

Hyperphosphatemia is generally caused by decreased urinary excretion of phosphorus due to renal disease or urinary obstruction; increased phosphorus release during cell death (e.g., tumor lysis syndrome); hypoparathyroidism; or iatrogenically through the administration of phosphate-containing enemas.[34] Phosphate concentration is normally higher in dogs up to 1 year of age due to rapid bone turnover; therefore, adult dog reference intervals usually underestimate the normal growing dog's phosphorous concentration.[34] Toxicities with vitamin D–containing rodenticides, anti-psoriasis creams (e.g., calcipotriol and calcipotriene), or zinc phosphide (a pesticide used in gopher bait) can cause serious and potentially fatal elevations in phosphorus.[34]

Clinical signs of hyperphosphatemia include weakness, tetany, seizures, tachycardia, and torsades de pointes, a potentially fatal cardiac dysrhythmia.[34] Initial treatment should directly address severe sequelae of hyperphosphatemia such as seizures and torsades de pointes. Following stabilization, therapy to lower phosphorus concentrations includes diuresis with crystalloid therapy and potentially dextrose administration to drive phosphorus into cells.[34]

Phosphate concentration measurement

Phosphate should be measured on serum or heparinized plasma using enzymatic spectrophotometry or flame photometry.[33,35] Citrate, oxalate, and EDTA can interfere with the enzymatic assays and should therefore not be used.[33] Hemolysis of the sample causes artifactual hyperphosphatemia as inorganic phosphate is released from red blood cells and quantified along with the serum fraction. Similar to potassium, serum or plasma should be separated from cells within 1 hour of sampling to prevent leakage of cellular phosphorus into the sample.[33] Hyperlipidemia and hyperbilirubinemia may falsely decrease the phosphate concentration due to interference with colorimetric determination.

Calcium

Like phosphorus, most of the body's calcium is stored in bone with <1% readily available in plasma. Calcium exists in three forms in plasma or serum: ionized or "free" calcium (iCa^{++}), complexed or chelated calcium bound to other substances such as phosphate and sulfate, and protein-bound calcium.[11] Ionized calcium is the biologically active form of calcium and has a role in many physiologic functions including intra- and extracellular messaging, cardiac conduction, and muscle contraction.[36]

The most common cause of hypercalcemia in veterinary patients is neoplasia, specifically lymphoma.[14,36] Other neoplasms can cause hypercalcemia as well.[14,36] Other causes of hypercalcemia include renal failure, hyperparathyroidism, hypoadrenocorticism, and systemic pyogranulomatous disease.[14,36] Toxicities that can result in hypercalcemia include vitamin D rodenticides, anti-psoriasis creams (e.g., calcipotriol, calcipotriene), and day-blooming Jessamine ingestion.[14]

Hypercalcemia results in nausea, anorexia, abdominal pain, constipation, polyuria and polydipsia, and soft tissue mineralization.[14] It is treated with promotion of calciuresis by intravenous fluid therapy, furosemide and glucocorticoids, treatment of the underlying cause, and medications to inhibit bone resorption (e.g., calcitonin and bisphosphonates).[14]

Hypocalcemia is common in critically ill humans and has been documented in hospitalized dogs and cats.[37,38] It can occur in many disease states such as renal failure, diabetic ketoacidosis, pancreatitis, eclampsia, malabsorptive syndromes, feline lower urinary tract obstruction, ethylene glycol toxicity, tumor lysis syndrome, hypomagnesemia, and sepsis.[39] The systemic inflammatory response syndrome in a number of disease states including neoplasia, trauma, and gastrointestinal disease seems to be linked to hypocalcemia.[38] Iatrogenic causes of hypocalcemia include parathyroidectomy, phosphate enema, sodium bicarbonate, and furosemide. Multiple blood transfusions can cause hypocalcemia because the anticoagulant in the blood products chelates calcium.[39]

Clinical sequelae of hypocalcemia include restlessness or excitation, facial rubbing, muscle tremors, tetany, seizures, tachycardia, hyperthermia, and cardiopulmonary arrest.[39] Hypotension has been documented in human patients.[39] ECG changes include a prolonged QT interval.[39] Symptomatic hypocalcemia is life threatening and should be treated. Emergent treatment involves intravenous administration of 10% calcium gluconate at a dose of 1.0–1.5 mL/kg over 20–30 minutes with continuous ECG monitoring to watch for bradycardia.[14] If bradycardia occurs, the infusion should be discontinued until a normal heart rate returns.[14] Severe cases may require a constant rate infusion of 10% calcium gluconate (5–10 mL/kg over 24 hours) or repeated doses every 6–8 hours.[14] Calcium solutions should not be added to bicarbonate-containing solutions because calcium carbonate can precipitate.[14] Careful monitoring of ionized calcium levels to watch for overcorrection and repeated patient assessment for the clinical signs of hypercalcemia or relapsing hypocalcemia are necessary.[14]

Calcium concentration measurement

Calcium can be measured as either total calcium (tCa, a reflection of all three forms in plasma) or iCa^{++}. Total calcium can be affected by protein concentration, as a portion of total calcium is protein bound. Historically, formulas were created to correct total calcium for the influence of hypoalbuminemia as a clinically appropriate way to assess calcium.[11,37] These formulas have since been shown to cause spurious interpretation of calcium levels in the face of hypoproteinemia.[11,37] Total calcium measurements correlate poorly with ionized calcium in situations of renal insufficiency and acid-base imbalance.[4,12] Total calcium measurement can also be spuriously affected by hemolysis, hyperbilirubinemia, and lipemia.[11] Ionized calcium assessed by ISE, which minimizes interference by other ions, protein, hemolysis, and lipemia, is considered the most accurate and clinically appropriate measurement of calcium.[11,37]

Measurement of ionized calcium must be carefully planned and performed due to potential artifact associated with exposure to air, the anticoagulant used, hemodilution with the anticoagulant, and alterations in ionized calcium with prolonged handling time. Calcium can be measured in whole blood, plasma, or serum, but reference ranges for each sample type may vary slightly depending on the analyzer used.

Ionized calcium concentration is affected by pH because hydrogen ions compete with iCa^{++} for binding sites on albumin and displace ionized calcium from the protein.[10,11] Acidemia, therefore, is associated with an elevated ionized calcium concentration. Exposure of the sample to air decreases the sample's carbon dioxide tension, raising its pH and falsely lowering the ionized calcium concentration.[3,4,11,12] The change in ionized calcium with exposure to air appears to be about 7.2% and will only cause spurious results if a patient has a mildly elevated or low end of normal calcium concentration.[10] It has been found that there is acceptable correlation between iCa concentration measurements sampled anaerobically and those measured aerobically with correction to a pH of 7.4.[11] Automatic correction utilizing formulas based on the predictable linear change in ionized calcium with changes in pH are available with some POC analyzers.[4,8,11] One must be very careful in veterinary medicine, however, because most POC analyzers are using an algorithm to correct the iCa to a pH of 7.4 based on human data that are not validated in dogs and cats.[4,8,11] If an analyzer has an algorithm for iCa correction to a pH of 7.4 that has been validated in dogs and cats, corrected aerobic measurements can be considered accurate. In most cases, however, this is not the case, and these authors recommend strictly anaerobic sampling for measurement of iCa concentrations.

Anaerobic blood sampling is best performed utilizing Vacutainer tubes (Becton Dickinson, Franklin Lakes, NJ). Silicone serum separator tubes should be avoided because the silicone releases calcium and falsely increases the ionized calcium value.[11] Once the blood is clotted, the sample is centrifuged for serum separation. Serum can be removed from the tube using a spinal needle attached to a non-air-containing syringe through the red-top stopper without exposing the sample to air.[11] Anaerobic sampling can also be achieved through the use of a sampling line (a central venous catheter or arterial catheter). Anaerobic sampling from a sampling line involves letting the syringe fill with arterial pressure if utilizing an arterial line and gentle negative pressure avoiding air bubbles or air spaces from a venous sampling line (Vetscan i-STAT 1, user guide). A rubber stopper can be placed on the needle if the sample cannot be placed directly into the cartridge or analyzer.

Calcium concentration also changes with time after a sample has been collected as cells undergo metabolism and produce lactic acid, which drops the pH in the sample.[3] Various studies have demonstrated slightly different results regarding the length of time an ionized calcium sample is stable at varying temperatures, but conservative collective interpretation of these studies indicates that if a sample is not analyzed within 8 hours of collection it should be refrigerated (4°C) for up to 48 hours or frozen at −20°C for up to 1 week.[3,4,12]

Sodium and lithium heparin bind or chelate calcium, which causes ionized calcium to drop.[3,8,11] Zinc heparin displaces calcium from binding sites and causes ionized concentrations to increase.[11] Oxalate, citrate, and EDTA also bind calcium. Therefore, none of these anticoagulants should be used when collecting a sample for measurement of ionized calcium concentration.[11] It has been shown that 40 IU/mL of dry coated lithium heparin syringes or 30 IU/mL self- prepped liquid sodium heparin syringes do not cause significant dilution or binding of ionized calcium.[3] One study recommended using ≤15 IU/mL of heparin or less to assess ionized calcium or magnesium accurately.[8]

Ionized calcium concentrations are lower in plasma than in whole blood or serum.[4,12] This may be due to increased exposure time to heparin, causing increased calcium binding to heparin.[4,12] These authors recommend utilizing either non-anticoagulated whole blood or low concentration (≤30 IU/mL) heparin anticoagulated whole blood for measurement of ionized calcium concentrations. Samples must be run relatively quickly after they are obtained to avoid premature clotting or prolonged exposure to heparin. One can use whole blood to measure calcium concentration utilizing the Vetscan i-STAT 1 analyzer to avoid error caused by anticoagulant, but efficient sampling and running are necessary to avoid clotting of the sample. Most other POC analyzers that measure ionized calcium require anticoagulation (Table 49.1), and low concentration (≤30 IU/mL) heparin should be used. Animals with hypercoagulable states and cats are more likely to clot prematurely (Vetscan i-STAT 1, user guide). Samples obtained from animals with a known or suspected hypercoagulable state should be anticoagulated with a low (≤30 IU/mL) concentration of heparin.

Magnesium

Magnesium is a predominantly intracellular ion distributed mostly in bone and muscle. Similar to calcium and phosphorus, approximately 1% exists in plasma and interstitial body fluid.[40] The plasma component has three portions: ionized (iMg^{++}), protein bound, and complexed to molecules such as phosphate and bicarbonate.[40] Ionized magnesium is the active form.[40] Magnesium functions mainly in the production and use of energy, maintenance of the sodium-potassium gradient across cell membranes, regulation of intracellular calcium, and muscle and cardiac contraction.[40]

Hypomagnesemia is a common condition in critically ill humans, dogs, and cats.[40–42] It is linked to a number of other electrolyte disorders including hypokalemia, hypocalcemia, hypophosphatemia, and hyponatremia.[40] Causes of hypomagnesemia include increased gastrointestinal losses, decreased intake or malabsorption, acute pancreatitis, renal disease, diabetic ketoacidosis, hyperthyroidism, hyperparathyroidism, sepsis, hypothermia, and massive blood transfusion.[40] Iatrogenic causes of hypomagnesemia include insulin administration causing intracellular shifts and increased renal losses of magnesium due to the administration of furosemide and osmotic agents such as mannitol.[24,40]

Clinical sequelae of hypomagnesemia include cardiac arrhythmias, anemia, neuromuscular weakness that can manifest as dysphasia or dyspnea if esophageal or respiratory muscles are affected, muscle twitching, ataxia, seizures, coma, refractory hypokalemia, and hypocalcemia.[24,40] ECG changes include prolonged PR interval, widened QRS complex, depressed ST segment, and a tented T wave.[40] Multiple arrhythmias can occur, one of which is torsades de pointes.[40] Treatment of hypomagnesemia involves the parenteral administration of magnesium sulfate at a rate determined by the degree of depletion and the estimated rate of ongoing losses (dose range: 0.3–1.0 mEq/kg/day).[24,40] Magnesium supplementation can cause burning at the catheter site, cutaneous vasodilation, and hypotension.[40] Iatrogenic overdose of magnesium can cause vomiting, hypotension, bradycardia, flaccid paralysis, and severe mental obtundation.[43] Intravenous calcium gluconate counteracts the physiologic effects of magnesium and can be used along with 0.9% saline diuresis to reverse these complications.[43]

Hypermagnesemia appears to be less common than hypomagnesemia.[40–42] It is most commonly caused by decreased renal clearance due to renal disease but can also be seen with some endocrinopathies such as diabetic ketoacidosis, hypoadrenocorticism, and thyroid disorders.[24,40] Hypermagnesemia can be caused iatrogenically through multiple doses of magnesium-containing cathartics or overdosing parenteral magnesium formulations.[24,40,43]

As noted in the description of magnesium overdose, hypermagnesemia can cause obtundation, weakness, and hypotension.[24,40] ECG changes include a prolonged PR interval and widened QRS complexes.[40] Severe hypermagnesemia can cause respiratory depression to apnea, coma, and cardiac arrest.[40] Therapy for hypermagnesemia includes diuresis with fluid therapy and potentially furosemide.[24,40] Calcium gluconate therapy should be used in severe cases if severe obtundation, respiratory depression, hemodynamic instability, or arrhythmias are present.[24,40]

Magnesium concentration measurement

Because magnesium is primarily intracellular, it is still unclear which clinical magnesium sample best reflects total body stores.[44] Clinicopathologic options for magnesium concentration quantification include ionized magnesium, total serum or plasma magnesium, intracellular quantification of magnesium, and magnesium clearance tests whereby a quantity of magnesium is administered and the percentage excreted is thought to reflect the total body stores. A study evaluating intracellular versus total serum magnesium in dogs with gastric dilatation and volvulus demonstrated no correlation between the two sampling methods.[45] Because ionized magnesium is the biologically active form, and total magnesium concentration is influenced by factors similar to those that affect total calcium concentration (protein concentration, renal function, and acid-base balance), ionized magnesium concentration is theoretically the POC analyte of choice.[3,4,46] Ion selective electrode assay is the method of choice for determining magnesium concentration because there is less interference caused by icterus, lipemia, and hemolysis.[37]

Sample handling and causes of artifact are very similar for ionized magnesium as they are for ionized calcium. Aerobic sampling causes artifactual decreases in iMg^{++} due to an increased pH and increased protein binding.[4] Both lithium and zinc heparin formulations can interfere with the magnesium electrode and cause falsely elevated iMg^{++} concentrations.[4,12] Serum values of iMg^{++} may be higher than for whole blood or plasma due to possible release of magnesium from platelets during clotting. Despite this, anaerobically obtained serum samples are considered the most accurate for determination of magnesium and calcium concentrations due to lack of dilution, binding, or interference from anticoagulant. Sample storage for measurement of magnesium is similar to that for calcium: Ionized magnesium concentration should be analyzed within 8 hours if kept at room temperature (22°C), within 24 hours if kept at 4°C, and within 1 week if stored at −22°C.[4] Ionized magnesium concentration dropped with time if samples were held too long or were stored inappropriately. Feline samples were found to be stable for 24 hours at 22°C, 72 hours at 4°C, and 4 weeks at −20°C.[46]

References

1. Stockham SL, Scott MA. Monovalent electrolytes and osmolality. In: Stockham SL, Scott MA, eds. Fundamentals of Veterinary Clinical Pathology. Ames, IA: Iowa State Press; 2002: 340–349.

2. Bernardini D, Gerardi G, Contiero B, et al. Interference of hemolysis and hyperproteinemia on sodium, potassium, and chloride measurements in canine serum samples. Vet Res Comm 2009;33(Suppl 1):S173–S176.

3. Tappin S, Rizz F, Dodkin S, et al. Measurement of ionized calcium in canine blood samples collected in prefilled and self-filled heparinized syringes using the i-STAT point-of-care analyzer. Vet Clin Pathol 2008;37(1):66–72.

4. Unterer S, Lutz H, Gerber B, et al. Evaluation of an electrolyte analyzer for measurement of ionized calcium and magnesium concentrations in blood, plasma, and serum of dogs. Am J Vet Res 2004;65(2):183–187.

5. Hristova EN, Cecco S, Niemela JE, et al. Analyzer-dependent differences in results for ionized calcium, ionized magnesium, sodium and pH. Clin Chem 1995;41(11):1649–1653.

6. van Pelt J. Letter to the editor: Enzymatic determination of sodium, potassium and chloride in serum compared with determinations by flame photometry, coulometry and ion-selective electrodes. Clin Chem 1994;40(5):846–847.

7. Hübl W, Wejbora R, Shafti-Keramat I, et al. Enzymatic determination of sodium, potassium, and chloride in abnormal (hemolyzed, icteric, lipemic, paraproteinemic, or uremic) serum samples compared with indirect determination with ion-selective electrodes. Clin Chem 1994;40(8):1528–1531.

8. Hopper K, Rezende ML, Haskins SC. Assessment of the effect of dilution of blood samples with sodium heparin on blood gas, electrolyte, and lactate measurements in dogs. Am J Vet Res 2005;65(4):656–660.

9. Gunn-Moore DA, Reed N, Simpson KE, et al. Effect of sample type, and timing of assay, on feline blood potassium concentration. J Feline Med Surg 2006;8:192–196.

10. Brennan SF, O'Donovan J, Mooney CT. Changes in canine ionized calcium under three storage conditions. J Small Animal Pract 2006;47:383–386.

11. Schenck PA and Chew DJ. Calcium: total or ionized? Vet Clin Small Anim 2008;38:497–502.

12. Unterer S, Gerber B, Glaus TM, et al. Evaluation of an electrolyte analyzer for measurement of concentrations of ionized calcium and magnesium in cats. Vet Res Comm 2005;29: 647–659.

13. Marino PL, Sutin KM. The ICU Book. 3rd ed. Philadelphia, PA: Lippincott Williams and Wilkins; 2007:595–609.

14. Schaer M. Therapeutic approach to electrolyte emergencies. Vet Clin Small Anim 2008;38:513–533.

15. Goldkamp C, Schaer M. Hypernatremia in dogs. Compend Contin Educ Pract Vet 2007;29(3):148–160.

16. Lin M, Liu SJ, Lim IT. Disorders of water imbalance. Emerg Med Clin North Am 2005;23:749–770.

17. Temo K, Rudloff E, Lichtenberger M, et al. Hypernatremia in critically ill cats: pathophysiology. Compend Contin Educ Pract Vet 2004;26(6):422–433.

18. Ash, RA, Harvey AM, Tasker S. Primary hyperaldosteronism in the cat: a series of 13 cases. J Feline Med Surg 2005;7:173–182.

19. Toll J, Barr SC, Hickford FH. Acute water intoxication in a dog. J Vet Emerg Crit Care 1999;9(1):19–22.

20. Kokko H, Hall PD, Afrin LB. Fentanyl associated syndrome of inappropriate antidiuretic hormone secretion. Pharmacotherapy 2002;22(9):1188–1192.

21. Churcher RK, Watson ADJ, Eaton A. Suspected myelinosis following rapid correction of hyponatremia in a dog. J Am Anim Hosp Assoc 1999;35:493–497.

22. de Morais HAS. Chloride ion in small animal practice: the forgotten ion. J Vet Emerg Crit Care 1992;2(1):11–24.

23. Boag AK, Coe RJ, Martinez TA, et al. Acid-base and electrolyte abnormalities in dogs with gastrointestinal foreign bodies. J Vet Intern Med 2005;19:816–821.

24. Schaer M. Disorders of serum potassium, sodium, magnesium and chloride. J Vet Emerg Crit Care 1999;9(4):209–217.

25. West JB. Gas transport by the blood. In: West JB, ed. Respiratory Physiology: The Essential. 7th ed. Baltimore, PA: Lippincott Williams & Wilkins; 2005:75–92.

26. Alfonzo AVM, Isles C, Geddes C. Potassium disorders—clinical spectrum and emergency management. Resuscitation 2006;70: 10–25.

27. Nielsen L, Bell R, Zoia A, et al. Low ratios of sodium to potassium in the serum of 238 dogs. Vet Record 2008;162: 431–435.

28. Bell R, Mellor DJ, Ramsey I, et al. Decreased sodium: potassium ratios in cats: 49 cases. Vet Clin Pathol 2005;34(20): 110–114.

29. Bissett SA, Lamb M, Ward CR. Hyponatremia and hyperkalemia associated with peritoneal effusion in four cats. J Am Vet Med Assoc 2001;218(10):1590–1592.

30. Carvalhanna V, Burry L, Lapinsky SE. Management of severe hyperkalemia without hemodialysis: case report and literature review. J Crit Care 2006;21:316–321.

31. Sowinski KM, Cronin D, Mueller BA, et al. Subcutaneous terbutaline use in CKD to reduce potassium concentrations. Am J Kidney Dis 2005;45(6):1040–1045.

32. Haldane S, Graves TK, Bateman S, et al. Profound hypokalemia causing respiratory failure in a cat with hyperaldosteronism. J Vet Emerg Crit Care 2007;17(2):202–207.

33. Visser't Hooft K, Drobatz KJ, Ward CR. Hypophosphatemia. Compend Contin Educ Pract Vet 2005;27(12):900–910.

34. Schropp DM, Kovacic J. Phosphorus and phosphate metabolism in veterinary patients. J Vet Emerg Crit Care 2007;17(2): 127–134.

35. Melton LA, Tracy ML, Moller G. Screening trace elements and electrolytes in serum by inductively-coupled plasma emission spectrometry. Clin Chem 1990;36:247–250.

36. Messinger JS, Windham WR, Ward CR. Ionized hypercalcemia in dogs: a retrospective study of 109 cases (1998–2003). J Vet Intern Med 2009;23:514–519.

37. Sharp CR, Kerl ME, Mann FA. A comparison of total calcium, corrected calcium, and ionized calcium concentrations as indicators of calcium homeostasis among hypoalbuminemic dogs requiring intensive care. J Vet Emerg Crit Care 2009;19(6): 571–578.

38. Holowaychuk MK, Hansen BD, DeFrancesco TC, et al. Ionized hypocalcemia in critically ill dogs. J Vet Intern Med 2009;23: 509–513.

39. Holowaychuk MK, Marin LG. Review of hypocalcemia in septic patients. J Vet Emerg Crit Care 2007;17(4):348–358.

40. Martin LG, Wingfield WE, Van Pelt DR, Hackett TB. Magnesium in the 1990's: implications for veterinary critical care. J Vet Emerg Crit Care 1993;3(2):105–114.

41. Martin LG, Matteson VL, Wingfield WE, et al. Abnormalities of serum magnesium in critically ill dogs: incidence and implications. J Vet Emerg Crit Care 1994;4(1):15–20.

42. Toll J, Erb H, Birnbaum N, et al. Prevalence and incidence of serum magnesium abnormalities in hospitalized cats. J Vet Intern Med 2002;16:217–221.

43. Jackson CB, Drobatz KJ. Iatrogenic magnesium overdose: 2 case reports. J Vet Emerg Crit Care 2004;14(2):115–123.

44. Bateman S. Editorial: Cats and magnesium—another species to consider. J Vet Intern Med 2002;16:215–216.

45. Bebchuk TN, Hauptman JG, Braselton WE, et al. Intracellular magnesium concentrations in dogs with gastric dilatation-volvulus. Am J Vet Res 2000;61(11):1415–1417.

46. Gilroy CV, Burton SA, Horney BS, MacKenzie AL. Validation of the Nova CRT8 for the measurement of ionized magnesium in feline serum. Vet Clin Path 2005;34(2):124–131.

47. Driessen B, Brainard B. Fluid therapy for the traumatized patient. J Vet Emerg Crit Care 2006;16(4):276–299.

50

Acid-base evaluation

Steve C. Haskins

Overview of acid-base interpretation

Acid-base evaluation should be performed in any patient with a serious metabolic disturbance (Box 50.1). In these patients, the magnitude of acid-base derangement is difficult to ascertain by clinical signs alone, and the measurement of acid-base status is an important component of the initial assessment and ongoing patient monitoring.

The pH is a unitless expression of the hydrogen ion concentration. Normal plasma pH is about 7.40 ± 0.5 units. Values <7.35 represent an acidemia, whereas values >7.45 represent an alkalemia. Aberrations of pH are due to either respiratory or metabolic disturbances. The respiratory contribution to the acid-base disturbance is defined by arterial PCO_2. Normal $PaCO_2$ is about $40 \pm 5\,mm\,Hg$ (cats may be slightly lower) (Table 50.1). Values <35 mm Hg represent a respiratory alkalosis; values >45 mm Hg represent a respiratory acidosis. The metabolic component is best represented by the base deficit/excess calculation (SBE or BE_{ecf}) on analyzer printouts. Surrogate markers for BD/E include plasma standard bicarbonate concentration, bicarbonate concentration, and total carbon dioxide. The BD/E ranges between 0 and $-4\,mEq/L$ in dogs (cats may be slightly lower); normal plasma bicarbonate concentration ranges between 20 and 24 mEq/L, and total carbon dioxide concentration between 21 and 25 mEq/L (cats may be slightly lower). BD/E values more negative than the normal range or values below the normal range for any of the surrogate markers represent a metabolic acidosis; BD/E values more positive than the normal range or values above the normal range for any of the surrogate markers represent a metabolic alkalosis.

Sampling and storage of blood for acid-base measurement

Normal acid-base values are referenced to arterial blood, which should be used when evaluating the ability of the lung to oxygenate the blood (see Chapter 22, Blood Gas Analysis, for more information). For acid-base measurements, venous blood can generally be used. Venous pH tends to be 0.03–0.05 units lower, PCO_2 3–5 mm Hg higher, bicarbonate 1–2 mEq/L higher, and base deficit 1 mEq/L lower than arterial blood.[4,7] Unfortunately, certain common events in critically ill animals can increase the disparity between arterial and venous blood values: sluggish peripheral blood flow[8] and cardiac arrest,[9] and impaired carbon dioxide carriage (anemia,[10] administration of carbonic anhydrase inhibitor) increase PCO_2 and decrease pH in venous blood compared with arterial blood.

The technique for collecting a blood sample for pH and blood gas analysis is outlined in Protocol 50.1. Dilution of the blood sample by anticoagulant should be minimized. Heparin solution has a pH of about 6.66 and a PCO_2 of about 5 mm Hg.[11] The dead space of a 3-mL syringe and needle is about 0.094 mL,[11] which represents a 9.4% dilution of a 1 mL blood sample and a 3.1% dilution of a 3 mL blood sample. After drawing liquid heparin into the syringe, evacuate as much of it as possible; there will still be sufficient heparin remaining to anticoagulate the blood sample.

Advanced Monitoring and Procedures for Small Animal Emergency and Critical Care, First Edition. Edited by Jamie M. Burkitt Creedon, Harold Davis.
© 2012 John Wiley & Sons, Inc. Published 2012 by John Wiley & Sons, Inc.

Box 50.1 Interpretation of acid-base measurements

	Parameter (normal range for dogs)	Acidosis	Alkalosis
Overall hydrogen ion concentration	pH (7.35–7.45)	Below normal	Above normal
Respiratory contribution	$PaCO_2$ (35–45 mm Hg)	Above normal	Below normal
Metabolic contribution	Base deficit/excess (0 to −4 mEq/L) Standard bicarbonate (20–24 mEq/L) Bicarbonate (20–24 mEq/L) Total carbon dioxide (21–25 mEq/L)	More negative Below normal	More positive Above normal

Table 50.1 Arterial acid-base values for normal individuals

	Human[1]	Dog[2–4]	Cat[3,5,6]
pH	7.40 (7.35–7.45)	7.39 (7.35–7.43)	7.39 (7.33–7.45)
$PaCO_2$, mm Hg	40 (35–45)	37 (31–43)	32 (26–38)
Base deficit, mEq/L	0 (−2 to +2)	−2 (+1 to −5)	−6 (−3 to −9)
Bicarbonate concentration, mEq/L	24 (22–26)	22 (19–25)	18 (15–21)

Blood should be collected anaerobically. Exposure to small air bubbles allows equilibration of gases between the blood and the air, which has a PCO_2 of about 0.275 mm Hg and a PO_2 of about 160 mm Hg. Air mixing will lower the partial pressure of carbon dioxide, which will change the pH.

The sample should be analyzed as soon as possible after collection to minimize *in vitro* changes due to metabolism and diffusion of gases into and through the plastic wall of the syringe. Although this is particularly important for PO_2 measurements, it is also somewhat true for PCO_2 and pH. *In vitro* metabolism by nucleated cells increases the PCO_2. Diffusion of carbon dioxide into and through the walls of the plastic container decreases the PCO_2. If the time to analysis is greater than about 10 minutes, the blood sample should be stored in ice water.[12] Ice water storage for as long as 6 hours has been reported to result in very little change in PCO_2 and pH values.[13] Samples can be stored in screw-top or vacuum heparin collection tubes for at least 30 minutes with minimal changes in measured values.[14] Repeated measurements from the same syringe or container will result in changed values due to the repeated exposure of the blood sample to room air.[14]

If air is accidentally drawn into the analyzer during sample aspiration/insertion, pH and PCO_2 values may be erroneous. Measurements marked with error codes on the analyzer printout should be repeated. Measurements that seem unbelievable should not be believed and should be repeated.

Blood gases are measured at the temperature of the blood gas analyzer water bath, which is usually set at 37°C. When the animal's body temperature is lower than the water bath, the PO_2 and PCO_2 will increase and the pH will decrease when the blood sample is warmed to 37°C for analysis. The patient's temperature should always be input at the time of sample analysis so that the analyzer can calculate and report the values corrected to the patient's body temperature in addition to those measured at 37°C (the magnitude of temperature-induced changes can be readily observed). If one wants to know the values in the patient at the time of sampling, the temperature-corrected values should be used. This may be important if one is tracking blood gas and acid-base changes over time, which is also associated with changing body temperature. Published normal reference values were established for normothermic patients, however, and perhaps characterization of acid-base

Protocol 50.1 Protocol for collecting a blood sample for pH and blood gas analysis

Items Required
- Use either a commercial blood gas syringe with dry anticoagulant or prepare a sampling syringe by drawing an aliquot of liquid heparin solution into it and then blowing as much of the liquid heparin out of the dead space of the syringe as possible.
- If blood is to be taken from a catheter: (1) use a separate syringe with about 1 mL of heparinized saline to scavenge fluid and blood from the catheter prior to sample collection; (2) use a separate syringe with about 3 mL of heparinized saline to flush the catheter after the scavenged fluid and blood has been returned to the patient.

Procedure
Blood taken via direct vessels puncture:
1. Gather supplies.
2. Perform hand hygiene.
3. Clip the hair and aseptically prepare the skin over the intended puncture site.
4. Aseptically puncture the vessels and anaerobically obtain at least a 1 mL blood sample.

Blood taken from a catheter:
1. Scrub the injection port with antiseptic solution. The fluid infusion must be stopped.
2. Remove at least 3 mL of fluid and blood from the catheter so you can obtain a pure blood sample.
3. Take at least a 1 mL blood sample.
4. Return the scavenged fluid and blood to the patient.
5. Flush the catheter with heparinized saline.

Storage and analysis:
1. Analyze the samples immediately.
2. If the sample cannot be analyzed within 10 minutes, store it in ice water.
3. Mix the sample prior to analysis by vigorously rolling the syringe between your hands.
4. Insert the blood anaerobically into the analyzer as per the manufacturer's guidelines.
5. Input the patient's identification and temperature.

status and therapeutic decisions should be based on the values as measured at 37°C.

Hydrogen ion concentration

Hydrogen ions are highly reactive with anionic regions of macromolecules like proteins. This interaction changes charge distribution within the protein resulting in a change in conformation and function of the protein.

Changing the catalytic activity of protein enzymes alters many physiologic cell functions such as mentation, hemoglobin affinity for oxygen, myocardial contractility and other skeletal muscle function, vasomotor tone and other smooth muscle function, coagulation, inflammation, digestion, hepatic metabolism, and renal excretion. Enzyme systems are most active within a narrow pH range and become inactive when the hydrogen ion concentration varies too far from normal. All aspects of cell function depend on a fairly normal hydrogen ion concentration.

The pH is a convenient negative logarithmic expression of the hydrogen ion concentration (or, more specifically, activity) that compresses a very wide range of hydrogen ion activities into a scale that is much easier to use (Appendix 50.1). The logarithmic pH scale is also useful clinically because the physiologic effects of changes in pH is more linearly related to pH than it is to hydrogen ion concentration (i.e., a pH decrease of 0.2 units would be similarly disruptive to cellular function as would an increase of 0.2 units even though the corresponding change in hydrogen ion concentration is dramatically different).

The pH is the net balance of all of the acids (hydrogen ion donors) and all of the bases (hydrogen ion acceptors) in the body at any point in time. Hydrogen ion concentration depends on the balance between intake and elimination of acids and bases. Buffers are acid-base pairs that cushion the effect on pH of a given acid or base load; they do not change the direction of change, just minimize the magnitude of change (Appendix 50.2). The pH is regulated by a respiratory component (carbonic acid) and a metabolic component (all of the other acids and bases).

The respiratory component of the acid-base balance

Carbonic acid (H_2CO_3) is in a two-way equilibrium with carbon dioxide and water, and with hydrogen and bicarbonate:

$$CO_2 + H_2O \leftrightarrow H_2CO_3 \leftrightarrow H^+ + HCO_3^- \qquad (50.1)$$

Each reaction obeys the law of mass action.* The left-hand reaction is between carbon dioxide and water, and carbonic acid. This reaction is greatly accelerated by

---

*All reactions have a proportional equilibrium (which depends on temperature and the environmental pH relative to the pK of the reaction). When reactant is added to one side of an equilibrium, some of it will move to other side so as to reestablish the proportional equilibrium.

carbonic anhydrase (located in red blood cells, renal tubular epithelial cells, and intestinal epithelial cells where rapid fluxes are important). When carbon dioxide increases, some of the CO_2 will combine with H_2O to form H_2CO_3. When H_2CO_3 increases, it will dissociate into hydrogen and bicarbonate in a 1:1 ratio. This is very acidifying because the normal H^+:HCO_3^- ratio (at 7.4) is about 0.00000167:1.

The respiratory contribution to the acid-base balance is defined by the $PaCO_2$. The medullary respiratory centers regulate $PaCO_2$ by adjusting alveolar minute ventilation. $PaCO_2$ is the marker of alveolar ventilation and of the respiratory contribution to the pH. Carbon dioxide production does not vary enough in comparison with how much ventilation can change (except in malignant hyperthermia) to be a material player in determining $PaCO_2$.

Surrogate markers of PaCO₂: venous PCO₂ (PvCO₂) and end-tidal PCO₂ (PetCO₂)

When arterial blood is not available, venous blood may be used for PCO_2 measurements. $PvCO_2$ values are normally 3–5 mm Hg higher than $PaCO_2$ (due to tissue metabolic CO_2 production). The arterial-venous gradient is not a fixed value, however, and it can increase in common disease states such as hypovolemia and anemia. $PvCO_2$ is actually a marker of tissue PCO_2, which in turn is the balance between $PaCO_2$, metabolic CO_2 production, and tissue perfusion. Changes in $PvCO_2$ will lag behind changes in $PaCO_2$ in transition states (e.g., acute hyperventilation following prolonged hypoventilation).

When a blood gas analyzer is not available, $PetCO_2$ may be used as a surrogate marker of $PaCO_2$. Normally $PetCO_2$ is only about 3–5 mm Hg below $PaCO_2$ (due to lung regions with high ventilation to perfusion ratios). $PetCO_2$ values are disproportionately lower than $PaCO_2$ when there is increased alveolar dead space ventilation (hypovolemia, pulmonary thromboembolism, or PPV with large tidal volumes) and tachypnea when there is mixing of anatomic dead space gases and functional alveolar space gases. See Chapter 26, Capnography, for more information about $PetCO_2$.

Respiratory acidosis

The causes of respiratory acidosis are cited in Box 50.2. $PaCO_2$ values >45 mm Hg define hypoventilation and respiratory acidosis; $PaCO_2$ >60 mm Hg may warrant treatment. Without supplemental oxygen therapy, this magnitude of hypoventilation is likely to be associated with hypoxemia. Without metabolic compensation, this magnitude of respiratory acidosis may be associated with a pH < 7.2. Hypercapnia causes cerebral vasodila-

---

> **Box 50.2** Cause of respiratory acidosis/alkalosis
>
> Respiratory acidosis (hypercapnia)
> - Hypoventilation
> - Neuromuscular disease
> - Airway obstruction
> - Open pneumothorax or flail chest
> - Anterior displacement of the diaphragm by abdominal space filling disorders
> - Pleural space filling disorders
> - Pulmonary parenchymal disease (late)
> - Compensation for metabolic alkalosis
> - Carbohydrate-rich IV feeding solutions in debilitated patients
> - Bicarbonate therapy in patients with respiratory compromise
> - Rebreathing of just exhaled alveolar gases due to mechanical dead space
> - Malignant hyperthermia
>
> Respiratory alkalosis
> - Hypotension
> - Fever and heat-induced illness
> - Systemic inflammatory response and sepsis
> - Excitement and exercise
> - Pain
> - Pulmonary thromboembolism
> - Pulmonary parenchymal disease (early)
> - Inappropriate ventilator settings
> - Compensation for metabolic acidosis

---

tion, which increases cerebral blood flow that may be harmful in patients with intracranial disease. With proper support and time for compensation, and in patients without intracranial disease, considerably higher PCO_2 values may be permissible without apparent harm to the patient.

The first treatment for hypercapnia is effective treatment for the underlying disease process that is causing the hypoventilation (relief or bypass of airway obstructions, removal of pleural filling disorders, etc.). The symptomatic therapy for hypoventilation is positive pressure ventilation until such time as effective treatment of the underlying disease can be implemented. The general guidelines for positive pressure ventilation of animals with relatively normal lungs are outlined in Box 50.3: (1) peak proximal airway pressure: 10–15 cm H_2O; (2) tidal volume: 10–15 mL/kg; (3) inspiratory time: about 1 second (just long enough to achieve a full tidal volume); (4) ventilatory rate: 10–15 times per minute; (5) minute ventilation: 150–250 mL/kg/minute. Diseased lungs are stiffer (less compliant) than normal lungs, and ventilator settings (except tidal volume) will

Box 50.3 Guidelines for positive pressure ventilation

Normal lungs
- Proximal airway pressure 10–15 cm H_2O
- Tidal volume 10–15 mL/kg
- Breathing rate 10–15 breaths/minute
- Inspiratory time 0.5–1 second
- Minute ventilation 150–250 mL/kg/minute

Diseased lungs
- Higher airway pressures (>15 cm H_2O) and breathing rates (>15/minute) as necessary but with smaller tidal volumes (<10 mL/kg)

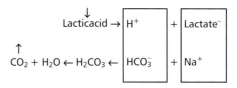

Figure 50.1 Lactic acid buffering by the carbonic acid-bicarbonate buffer system: the increased hydrogen combines with bicarbonate to form carbonic acid. The decrease in bicarbonate concentration approximately equals the increase in lactate concentration.

probably need to be higher than those for normal lungs. The primary ways to improve ventilation are to increase respiratory rate or proximal airway pressure. Tidal volumes should not be increased above normal when there is diffuse lung disease because this predisposes to ventilator-induced lung damage.[15] Inspired oxygen, end-expiratory pressure, and inspiratory time are alterable parameters that primarily affect oxygenation and may have little on PCO_2. Make sure there is patient synchrony and that other untoward events (hyperthermia, pneumothorax) are not present. See Chapter 27, Mechanical Ventilation, for more information regarding positive pressure ventilation.

Respiratory alkalosis

The causes of respiratory alkalosis are listed in Box 50.2. $PaCO_2$ values <35 mm Hg define hyperventilation and respiratory alkalosis; $PaCO_2$ <20 mm Hg may warrant treatment. This magnitude of hypocapnia may be associated with cerebral vasoconstriction and cerebral hypoxia. Without metabolic compensation, a $PaCO_2$ <20 mm Hg may be associated with a pH >7.6. The muscular effort necessary to maintain the hyperventilation may be associated with disproportionately high oxygen consumption. The first and only treatment for hypocapnia is effective treatment for the underlying disease process that is causing the hyperventilation.

The metabolic component of the acid-base balance

In contrast to the respiratory component, the metabolic component includes many acids and has many markers. This complexity has spawned a number of different ways by which its contribution to the acid-base balance can be characterized.

Overview of markers of the metabolic component

Bicarbonate

Plasma bicarbonate concentration is the time-honored overview marker of the metabolic contribution to acid-base balance. Bicarbonate is intimately associated with hydrogen in the carbonic acid equilibration equation and in the carbonic acid–bicarbonate buffer system (Eq. 50.1). The hydrogen ion of any added acid will bind with bicarbonate to form carbonic acid, which dissociates to carbon dioxide and water; the carbon dioxide is eliminated by alveolar ventilation (Fig. 50.1). Because it is ventilated to the atmosphere, carbon dioxide does not pile up on the left side of the carbonic acid equilibration; this allows bicarbonate buffering of additional lactic acid. Because the carbonic acid–bicarbonate buffer system is open ended, it is quantitatively the most powerful buffer system in the body. The binding of bicarbonate by the hydrogen of any acid will decrease the plasma bicarbonate concentration, which then can be used as a marker of the magnitude of the acidosis.

In a pH and blood gas analyzer, pH and PCO_2 are measured and bicarbonate concentration is calculated via the Henderson-Hesselbach equilibration:

$$pH = -\log(HCO_3 / H_2CO_3) \qquad (50.2)$$

There will be no error in the bicarbonate calculation; there can be only one bicarbonate concentration for the measured pH and PCO_2 values. If there were errors in sampling, storage, or measurement, there may, however, be unrepresentative pH or PCO_2 measurements that would, in turn, lead to incorrect bicarbonate concentration calculation.

Dogs normally have a bicarbonate concentration in the range of 20–24 mEq/L; cats are slightly lower (16–20 mEq/L) (Table 50.1). Values below these respective ranges represent hypobicarbonatemia and serve as a marker of metabolic acidosis; values above these ranges represent hyperbicarbonatemia and mark a metabolic alkalosis.

Standard bicarbonate

Carbon dioxide and bicarbonate are both part of the carbonic acid–bicarbonate equilibration equation. A primary change in bicarbonate *does not* cause a change in arterial PCO_2 *in vivo* because $PaCO_2$ is monitored and controlled by medullary chemoreceptors. Changes in PCO_2 *do*, however, cause small changes in plasma bicarbonate concentration (approximately 0.15 mEq/L per mm Hg decrease in PCO_2 below 40 and 0.075 mEq/L per mm Hg increase in PCO_2 above 40).[16] Standard bicarbonate is a mathematically adjusted bicarbonate concentration (to a PCO_2 of 40 mm Hg) to eliminate the effect of changes in PCO_2 on bicarbonate concentration.

If both standard bicarbonate and an (undesignated) bicarbonate concentration are available on the printout from the analyzer, the standard bicarbonate would be the more accurate representation of the metabolic contribution to the acid-base balance.

Total carbon dioxide concentration

A blood gas analyzer is not always available to measure pH and PCO_2. Total CO_2 concentration can be easily measured and is a common component of commercial chemistry panels. Carbon dioxide exists in many forms in the plasma, almost all of which is as bicarbonate anion. Very small amounts exist in the form of carbonic acid, dissolved CO_2, and as carbamino groups on various proteins. Total CO_2 concentration is only about 1 mEq/L above bicarbonate concentration, and total CO_2 concentration can be interpreted as if it were bicarbonate concentration. Total CO_2 has nothing to do with the partial pressure of CO_2, and total CO_2 should not be considered to be a surrogate marker of PCO_2.

Base deficit/excess

The carbonic acid–bicarbonate buffer system is not the only buffer in blood; hemoglobin protein, plasma protein, and phosphate buffers also absorb hydrogen ion and also act to cushion the impact of a given load of acid on pH (there are also intracellular and bone buffers).

The quantitative impact of all of the buffer systems in whole blood has been determined by titrational experiments and is termed base deficit (a deficit of base indicates the presence of a metabolic acidosis) or base excess (an excess of base indicates a metabolic alkalosis). Base deficit/excess values are usually considered to be the most accurate index of the metabolic contribution to

acid-base balance. Alignment nomograms were originally developed to hand-determine the base deficit/excess and bicarbonate and total CO_2 concentrations from the measured pH and PCO_2.[16] Nowadays these values are calculated by the blood gas analyzer and are displayed and printed out for the user. Acronyms for base deficit/excess include SBE and BE_{ECF}.*

The normal base deficit/excess ranges between 0 and −4 mEq/L for the dog and between −4 and −8 mEq/L for the cat (Table 50.1); more negative values mark a deficit of base and a metabolic acidosis; more positive values mark an excess of base and a metabolic alkalosis.

Anion gap

The anion gap is usually calculated by the following equation:

$$Na + K - Cl - HCO_3 \qquad (50.3)$$

There can be no anion gap in reality (the number of cations always equals the number of anions), but not all of them are routinely measured. In this calculation, $Na + K$ normally exceeds $Cl + HCO_3$ by 15 to 20 mEq/L.[†] Normally the negative charges on albumin comprise most of this apparent gap. Phosphorous and lactate make up a small portion of the gap in the normal animal, but this can increase in disease states.

An increase in anion gap is usually considered to mark the presence of an accumulation of unmeasured anions, most of which represent anions of organic acids such as lactic acid, ketoacids, phosphoric and sulfuric acids, or acid intoxicants such as glycolic acid from ethylene glycol, salicylic acid from salicylate, formic acid from methanol, or various acidic amino acids from rhabdomyolysis).

Hyperalbuminemia can also cause an increase in anion gap associated with a metabolic acidosis. Metabolic acidosis can also be caused by renal and gastrointestinal bicarbonate losses or hydrogen retention, without an increase in anion gap.

The anion gap calculation (with the standard formula) is difficult to interpret and rarely adds meaningful infor-

---

* SBE: standard base excess; the word *standard* implies the use of the *in vivo* buffer curve. BE_{ECF}: the "ECF" implies the use of the *in vivo* buffer curve. In both terminologies the term *negative base excess* is used instead of the term *base deficit*. The original experiments were done with blood in test tubes and constitute an *in vitro* buffer curve. The *in vivo* buffer curve, which incorporates the effects of dilution and buffering by the interstitial fluid compartment, is flatter than the *in vitro* buffer curve (less change in pH per change in bicarbonate or base deficit/excess).

† Sometimes potassium is eliminated from the calculation; normal values would then range between 10 and 15 mEq/L.

mation to the patient assessment. First, by the time one has the measurements needed to calculate the anion gap, there is usually enough information (historical, physical, or laboratory) with which to define the nature of the metabolic acidosis. If a patient has metabolic acidosis and signs of poor tissue perfusion, the odds-on bet would be a lactic acidosis; if a patient has metabolic acidosis and urine ketones, a ketoacidosis; a metabolic acidosis and uremia, a phosphoric acidosis, and so on.

Second, animals rarely have a pure acidosis from a singular source; most acid-base derangements represent a variable combination of acidotic and alkalotic processes that culminate in the measured acid-base abnormality. This may have the net effect of increasing or decreasing the calculated anion gap, or processes may cancel one another out so as to result in a normal anion gap calculation (e.g., hypoproteinemia and lactic acidosis). An increased anion gap surely marks the presence of unmeasured anions, the acids of which are possibly contributing to the metabolic acidosis. A normal value may be normal or may represent multiple off-setting acid-base derangements. A decreased value surely marks a hypoproteinemia.

The expanded anion gap

Albumin, phosphorous, and lactate are commonly measured, and their contributions to the anion gap can be easily calculated (Box 50.4):

$$Na + K + Ca\ effect + Mg\ effect - Cl - HCO_3 -$$
$$lactate - albumin\ effect - phosphate\ effect \quad (50.4)$$

The expanded anion gap accounts for many of the usually unmeasured anions; normal values for the expanded anion gap range between 0 and 4 mEq/L. This residual anion gap is composed of the remaining unmeasured anions such as sulfates, ketones, and various amino acids. The expanded anion gap formula moves many of the relevant players in the anion gap calculation from an unknown to a known category, which allows for a more comprehensive evaluation of the acid-base status.

Strong ion difference

Strong ion difference (SID) is the difference between the strongly dissociated cations and the strongly dissociated anions; however the usual formula is much abbreviated:

$$Na + K - Cl \quad (50.5)$$

> **Box 50.4** Calculating the expanded anion gap
>
> $$AG_{expanded} = Na + K + Ca\ effect + Mg\ effect - Cl -$$
> $$HCO_3 - lactate - albumin\ effect - phosphate\ effect$$
>
> For Na, K, Cl, HCO_3, and lactate, use the measured value (mEq or mM/L).
>
> Calcium effect = ionized calcium mM/L $\times 2$
> $\qquad$ = mEq/L (ionized calcium may be
> $\qquad\qquad$ estimated as half of total calcium)
> $\qquad\qquad$ (mg/dL $\times 0.3 \approx$ mM/L)
>
> Magnesium effect
> $\quad$ = ionized magnesium mM/L $\times 2$
> $\quad$ = mEq/L (ionized magnesium may be
> $\qquad$ estimated as half of total magnesium)
> $\qquad$ (mg/dL $\times 0.45 \approx$ mM/L)
>
> Albumin effect = albumin g/dL $\times 3.7$ (g/L $\times 0.37$)
>
> Phosphate effect =
> $\quad$ phosphorous mg/dL $\times 0.58$ (mM/L $\times 1.8$)

The only difference between this SID formula and the traditional anion gap formula is the absence of HCO_3. In this context one might anticipate that the criticisms of anion gap would also apply to SID. It has been proposed that a decrease in SID can be used as a marker of metabolic acidosis and an increase in SID as a marker of metabolic alkalosis.[17–19] When the decrease in SID is due to a decrease in bicarbonate, it is indeed associated with a metabolic acidosis. However, hypoalbuminemia also decreases SID, and this would be associated with a metabolic alkalosis (see "Albumin" below). Increases in anions of salts (such as sodium lactate or sodium acetate) increase both anion gap and SID calculations, but they have no effect per se on acid-base balance. In the end, SID, like anion gap, provides a broad categorization of underlying events and is difficult to interpret without any further information. Broad categorical descriptions of acid-base balance are of limited use and one might be better served to evaluate the specific contributors insofar as possible (see "Markers of Specific Contributors to the Metabolic Component" below).

A$_{TOT}$

Strong ion difference describes an apparent gap between commonly measured strongly dissociated cations and anions (SID$_{apparent}$). This gap is composed of the anions of weakly dissociated acids: albumin and phosphate (A$_{TOT}$). A$_{TOT}$ (the albumin effect and the phosphate effect), as calculated for the expanded anion gap formula (Box 50.4). An increase in A$_{TOT}$ caused by hyperphosphatemia (see "Phosphorous Effect" below) or hyperalbuminemia (see "Albumin Effect" below) would be associated with a metabolic acidosis, and *vice versa*. A$_{TOT}$ is another grouping assessment, and one might be better served to evaluate the specific contributors insofar as possible (see "Markers of Specific Contributors to the Metabolic Component" below).

The remaining important weakly dissociated acid is carbonic acid; the conjugate anion is bicarbonate. A$_{TOT}$ and HCO$_3$ comprise SID$_{effective}$. SID$_{apparent}$ and SID$_{effective}$ generally have a similar value because the former is an assessment of the stuff around the gap and the latter is an assessment of the stuff of the gap itself.*

The Stewart approach to acid-base balance

The Stewart approach to acid-base balance is a much discussed so-called new approach to acid-base interpretation. Stewart was a chemist who described acid-base balance from a chemical (not a clinical) point of view.[20] The Stewart approach is similar to the whole blood buffer base concept proposed by Singer and Hastings in 1948.[21] Because all cations and anions are always balanced, one can describe acid-base balance from several different perspectives. Stewart chose to solve his equations for bicarbonate as the dependent variable (i.e., bicarbonate concentration can be calculated from the concentration of all of the other cations and anions). Perhaps this is justified from the perspective that bicarbonate is a tricky anion to predict; it is involved with hydrogen in many other buffer systems and can disappear or reappear in the name of carbon dioxide. Stewart could just as well have solved his equations for any other cation or anion. There is nothing incorrect about Stewart's observations and calculations; however, one must take care not to misapply Stewart's proposals in the clinical management of patients.

According to the Stewart approach, the three causes of acid-base disturbances are changes in PCO$_2$, changes in SID$_{apparent}$, and changes in A$_{TOT}$. Bicarbonate has been relegated to "dependent" ion status, and as such it cannot primarily affect acid-base balance; it can only be affected by changes in the other parameters. This approach divides the very large metabolic component of the traditional approach (base deficit/excess or bicarbonate) into two (still fairly large) subgroups. The problems inherent in associating a specific directional change in SID$_{apparent}$ were discussed earlier and, again, one might be better served to evaluate the specific individual contributors to SID$_{apparent}$ and A$_{TOT}$ (see "Markers of Specific Contributors to the Metabolic Component" below).

The value of the Stewart approach might be in its ability to suggest directional acid-base changes when pH and PCO$_2$ measurements are not available. The Fencl-Leith quantitative expansion of the Stewart approach might be useful to help define individual contributions to the overall base deficit/excess[22,23] (see Box 50.5). It seems that it should not so much be a debate of whether to use the traditional approach or the Stewart approach to acid-base interpretation as it is a discussion of how to use them both together to best define the patient's condition at the time of measurement.

Markers of specific contributors to the metabolic component

Lactate

Blood lactate concentration can now be measured by many commercial analyzers. In lactic acidosis, lactate accumulates in the plasma as the hydrogen ion is buffered by bicarbonate; the magnitude of the lactate increase is similar to the decrease in bicarbonate (if there were no other influences on the bicarbonate concentration). The lactate concentration can be used as a marker of the quantity of lactic acid that has been added to the extracellular fluid (ECF). Each 1 mEq or mM/L increase in lactate would have a 1 mEq/L base deficit effect. Normal animals generally have a lactate concentration below 1 mEq/L; the normal range is often considered to extend up to 2 mEq/L.

It is not the lactate anion that causes the acidosis; it is the hydrogen that came with it. Sodium lactate (such as in lactated Ringer or Hartmann solution) is a salt, not an acid, and will have no impact, per se, on acid-base balance (see "The Acid-Base Impact of Crystalloid Sodium Solutions" in Appendix 50.3). If a blood sample is contaminated with sodium lactate, the measured lactate may be very high but will not be associated with an acidifying effect.

Ketones

Acetoacetate can be measured in the urine by nitroprusside reaction on most urine reagent strips. This color-

---

*SID$_{apparent}$ and SID$_{effective}$ essentially calculate the same thing; SID$_{apparent}$ calculates the stuff around the gap (you can tell how big the hole is by what is missing; you measure it indirectly), whereas SID$_{effective}$ calculates the stuff in the gap (you can tell how big the hole is by measuring it directly).

Box 50.5 Quantitative assessment of the metabolic contributions to acid-base balance

Overall equation: Base deficit / excess

   = −lactate − ketones ± phosphorous effect

    ± albumin effect ± water effect

    ± chloride-bicarbonate effect

    ± unmeasured effect

Lactate: enter measured lactate (mM/L)
Ketone: enter measured ketones (mM/L)
Phosphorous effect:

Change in phosphorous (in mg/dL) from normal
(4 mg/dL)×0.58 = phosphorous effect (mEq/L)

                      (Equation 50.6)

Change in phosphorous (in mM/L) from normal
(1.3 mM/L)×1.8 = phosphorous effect (mEq/L)

                      (Equation 50.7)

Albumin effect:

1 g/dL (10 g/L) change in albumin concentration
(from normal)×3.7 mEq/L of BD/E effect

                      (Equation 50.8)

Water effect:

$(Na_{measured} − Na_{normal})×0.25$ (Equation 50.9)

Na_{normal} = 145 mEq/L (mM/L) in the dog and 155 in the cat.
Chloride-bicarbonate effect:
  Adjusted chloride concentration:
  Normal [Cl⁻] (145 for dog; 155 for cat)
  ± change in [Na⁺] × 0.75
Chloride-bicarbonate effect:
  Adjusted − measured chloride concentration
Unmeasureds effect: Base deficit/excess − all of above

---

indexed assessment is semiquantitative. Acetoacetate represents a much lower proportion of the ketoacids compared with β-hydroxybutyrate in ketoacidosis. Plasma β-hydroxybutyric acid can be measured in the laboratory or with handheld instrumentation by measuring the NAD⁺:NADH ratio, a reduction/oxidation reaction. The units of measure are mM/L that have a 1:1 relationship with the mEq/L contribution to the acid base balance. Plasma ketones are normally zero.

Phosphate

Plasma inorganic phosphate is commonly measured and reported as elemental phosphorous in mg/dL or mM/L in serum chemistry testing profiles. Plasma phosphate anion is also associated with other plasma cations such as sodium, potassium, calcium, magnesium, and, of importance to the present discussion, with hydrogen as phosphoric acid. Phosphoric acid (H_3PO_4) could potentially exist as H_3PO_4, $H_2PO_4^{1-}$, HPO_4^{2-}, or PO_4^{3-}, depending on the pH of the fluid. At a pH of 7.4, approximately 90% of phosphoric acid exists as HPO_4^{2-} and 10% exists as $H_2PO_4^{1-}$.

The hyperphosphatemia of renal disease is associated with a phosphoric acidosis. A coexistent sulfuric acidosis (another end product of protein metabolism) would be expected but is not measured. The magnitude of the phosphoric acidosis contribution to the metabolic component can be calculated.*

Change in phosphorous (in milligrams per deciliter)
    from normal (4 mg/dL)×0.58 =
    phosphorous effect (mEq/L)

                      (50.6)

Change in phosphorous (in mM/L)
    from normal (1.3 mM/L)×1.8 =   (50.7)
    phosphorous effect (mEq/L)

Albumin

Albumin is a multivalent anion associated with many plasma cations: sodium, potassium, calcium, magnesium, and, of concern to this discussion, hydrogen. Hypoalbuminemia is associated with a decrease in the "H-Alb acid," resulting in a metabolic alkalosis, whereas hyperalbuminemia is associated with an acidosis. Changes in globulin have little effect on acid base balance.[24] The impact of changes in albumin concentration on acid-base balance can be calculated:

1 g/dL (10 g/L) change in albumin concentration
   ×3.7 mEq/L of BD/E effect

                      (50.8)

An increase in albumin has an acidifying effect; a decrease has an alkalinizing effect.

---

*To convert from mg/dL to mM/L: mg/dL × 1 mM/31 mg × 10 dL/L (= phosphorous in mg/dL × 0.323). To convert mM/L to mEq/L: phosphorous in mM/L × 1.8 (90% HPO_4^{2-}; 10% $H_2PO_4^{1-}$).

Water

Water dissociates to a small extent, in a temperature-dependent manner, into H^+ and OH^-. Water has a pK of 7.00 at room temperature and a pK of 6.80 at body temperature. Compared with the body at a pH near 7.40, water is acidic. This acidic effect is magnified *in vivo* because once the water is equilibrated with existing levels of carbon dioxide it has considerable titratable acidity.[25]

The concentration of free water is not measured, but the consequence of changes in the concentration of free water (i.e., the sodium concentration) is commonly measured. Changes in sodium concentration are used to calculate the free water effect. Changes in sodium, per se, do not have an impact on acid-base balance; it is not the sodium, it is the water, even though it is sometimes referred to as the "sodium effect." The acid-base effect of changes in water concentration is calculated as follows:

$$(Na_{measured} - Na_{normal}) \times 0.25 \qquad (50.9)$$

Na_{normal} is often considered to be 145 mEq/L (mM/L) in the dog and 155 in the cat. An increase in free water (marked by a decrease in sodium concentration) has an acidifying effect; a decrease has an alkalinizing effect.

Chloride-bicarbonate effect

This category is sometimes referred to as the "chloride effect," suggesting it is the chloride that has the effect. Terminology like "hyperchloremic metabolic acidosis and hypochloremic metabolic alkalosis" further this concept. But changes in chloride concentration, per se, do not have an impact on acid-base balance. As noted earlier, bicarbonate is a rather complex anion that is influenced by several buffer systems and respiratory handling of carbon dioxide; bicarbonate concentration is difficult to predict. Many processes in the body, however, involve the reciprocal handling of chloride and bicarbonate (i.e., when one is lost, the other is retained, and vice versa). In this manner, changes in chloride concentration can be used as a marker for the change in bicarbonate concentration that would have occurred (equal and opposite) had there been no other influences operating on the bicarbonate concentration.

Like sodium, chloride is affected by changes in water concentration. Because the effect of changes in water concentration have already been considered, effect on chloride concentration must now be eliminated from consideration. This is done by calculating an "adjusted chloride concentration" reference value:

$$Normal\ chloride\ concentration\ (110\ mEq/L\ [mM/L]$$
$$in\ dog;\ 120\ in\ cat) \pm (change\ in\ sodium$$
$$concentration \times 0.75^*)$$

$$(50.10)$$

A higher than anticipated measured chloride concentration marks a proportional base deficit effect (a metabolic acidosis); a lower than anticipated measured chloride concentration marks a base excess effect.

Metabolic acidosis

The causes of metabolic acidosis are listed in Box 50.6. The treatment of metabolic acidosis should be primarily aimed at correction of the underlying disease process and should be the only therapy necessary if the metabolic acidosis and the pH disturbance is mild to moderate and the underlying disease is readily treatable. If, however, the metabolic acidosis is severe (base deficit >10 mEq/L; bicarbonate concentration <14 mEq/L; pH <7.2) and the underlying disease is difficult to treat, symptomatic alkalinization therapy may be indicated. Sodium bicarbonate is the most common agent used to treat metabolic acidosis. Guidelines for the calculation of bicarbonate dosage are detailed in Protocol 50.2. Sodium bicarbonate may be associated with a number of problems when used in a cavalier manner; these problems and their avoidance are detailed in Box 50.7.

Metabolic alkalosis

The causes of metabolic alkalosis are listed in Box 50.6. Most cases of metabolic alkalosis encountered clinically are either mild (do not need symptomatic treatment) or iatrogenic. The treatment of metabolic alkalosis relies on effective treatment of the underlying disease process. On the rare occasion that acidifying therapy is warranted, a dilute solution of hydrochloric acid, lactic acid, or acetic acid could be administered. Saline, acetazolamide, potassium-sparing diuretics (spironolactone, amiloride, and triamterene) and ammonium chloride are also acidifying therapies. Coexistent electrolyte abnormalities such as hypochloremia and hypokalemia potentiate metabolic alkalosis and should be treated.

---

*The normal sodium-to-chloride ratio is about 4:3 (150:110). For each 4-unit change in sodium, there should be a 3-unit change in chloride in the same direction (example: a decrease in sodium from 150 to 122 (a decrease of 28) would be associated with a proportional decrease in chloride concentration to 89 ($-28 \times \frac{3}{4} = -21$; $110 - 21 = 89$).

Box 50.6 Causes of metabolic acidosis and alkalosis

Metabolic acidosis
  Without anion gap:
- Gastrointestinal losses of bicarbonate (diarrhea, vomiting with reflux from the duodenum)
- Renal loss of bicarbonate (proximal tubular acidosis, carbonic anhydrase inhibitors)
- Renal hydrogen retention (distal tubular acidosis, hypomineralocorticism)
- Intravenous nutrition
- Large-volume saline administration
- Free water administration
- Compensation for respiratory alkalosis
- Ammonium chloride administration
  With anion gap:
- Lactic and pyruvic acidosis
- Ketoacidosis (insulin deficiency, acute starvation)
- Phosphate and sulphate acidosis (oliguric renal disease)
- Ethylene glycol intoxication
- Methanol intoxication
- Salicylate poisoning
- Rhabdomyolysis
  Metabolic alkalosis
- Gastric losses of hydrogen ion (vomiting due to a pyloric obstruction, gastric suctioning)
- Furosemide administration
- Hypermineralocorticism
- Organic anion (lactate, acetate, gluconate, citrate or ketone) metabolism
- Carbenicillin and other penicillin derivatives
- Free water deficit
- Alkalinization therapy
- Compensation for respiratory acidosis
- Hypochloremia
- Hypokalemia

Expected compensation for a primary abnormality

When a primary change occurs in either the respiratory or the metabolic component, the other component should change in a direction so as to return pH toward normal (i.e., a primary metabolic acidosis should be compensated by a respiratory alkalosis). The general concept is that compensatory mechanisms do not over-compensate. Therefore, the component that varies in the same direction as the pH is probably the primary abnormality, whereas the component that varies in a direction opposite to that of pH is probably the secondary, compensatory abnormality. This is not always a safe assumption because many acid-base disturbances in critically ill

Protocol 50.2 How to calculate and administer a dose of bicarbonate

Procedure
1. Pick a conservative base deficit or bicarbonate concentration treatment goal (such as a base deficit of -5 mEq/L [mM/L] for the dog [-8 for the cat] or a bicarbonate concentration of 18 mEq/L [mM/L] for the dog [15 for the cat]).
2. Determine the difference between the measured and the goal value.
3. Multiply this difference times the estimated extracellular fluid space (0.3 × kg body weight).
4. Administer slowly over a minimum of about 30 minutes.
   - A single undiluted dose of sodium bicarbonate can be administered intravenously.
   - Undiluted solutions (1 mEq or mM/L) have an osmolality of 2000 mOsm/kg, which will cause phlebitis with extended infusions and a sodium concentration of 1000 mEq or mM/L, which can cause hypernatremia with large infusions.
   - Sodium bicarbonate can be administered with other fluids.
   - However, it will bind divalent cations (calcium and magnesium) as carbonates.

Box 50.7 Dangers of sodium bicarbonate administration and their avoidance

  Excessive alkalinization of the patient: calculate dosages carefully; monitor acid-base balance.
  Excessive alkalinization of the vascular fluid compartment: administer calculated dose over at least 30 minutes.
  Hypotension, restlessness, nausea and vomiting, collapse, and death: administer calculated dose over at least 30 minutes.
  Hypokalemia: administer carefully and with concurrent potassium in hypokalemic patients; monitor potassium concentration.
  Hypo(ionized)calcemia: administer carefully and with concurrent calcium in hypocalcemic patients; monitor ionized calcium.
  Hypercapnia: administer carefully and with carbon dioxide monitoring in patients with ventilator compromise and with ventilator support in patients that develop hypercapnia.
  "Paradoxical" intracellular acidosis: avoid hypercapnia.
  Phlebitis with continuous infusions: dilute with other fluids (a 1:3 dilution with a sodium-free solution such as 5% dextrose in water will decrease the osmolality to 500 mOsm/kg).
  Hypernatremia with large infusions: monitor sodium with repeated dosages of sodium bicarbonate, dilute with distilled water (usually as 5% dextrose in water) as necessary (a 1:3 dilution with a sodium-free solution such as 5% dextrose in water will decrease the sodium concentration to 250 mEq or mM/L).

Table 50.2 Expected magnitude of compensation for a primary abnormality[6]

Primary Event	Expected Compensation
Metabolic acidosis	$\downarrow$ PaCO$_2$ of 0.7 mm Hg per 1 mEq/L $\downarrow$ HCO$_3$
Metabolic alkalosis	$\uparrow$ PaCO$_2$ of 0.7 mm Hg per 1 mEq/L $\uparrow$ HCO$_3$
Respiratory acidosis	$\uparrow$ 0.15 to 0.35* mEq/L HCO$_3$ per 1 mm Hg $\uparrow$ PaCO$_2$
Respiratory alkalosis	$\downarrow$ 0.25 to 0.55* mEq/L HCO$_3$ per 1 mm Hg $\downarrow$ PaCO$_2$

patients are multifactorial and what might otherwise appear to be a "secondary, compensatory" component may well be driven by one or several primary abnormalities. Calculating expected magnitudes of compensation is an attempt to determine whether or not there may be a coexistent problem within the compensatory component. In humans and dogs, but not cats, normal ranges of expected compensation have been established (Table 50.2).

The clinical relevance of calculating expected magnitudes of compensation is limited because the assumptions inherent in the calculation may not be true for the patient. Compensation assumes a stable primary component for a sufficient period of time to allow full compensation. Although this may be true in some chronic medical conditions, it is unlikely a valid assumption in acute critical illnesses. So levels of compensation that do not fall within the predicted range do not prove a problem with the compensatory component nor the presence of co-driving disease. Similarly levels of compensation within the predicted range do not prove the competence of compensation or the absence of coexistent disease. Critically ill patients often have multiple problems causing their acid-base derangement; a full list of differentials should be considered for each identified abnormality.

Appendix 50.1

The correlation between hydrogen ion concentration (activity) and pH

[H$^+$] (nM/L)[a]	[H$^+$] mEq or mM/L[b]	pH (units)[c]	
0.0001	0.000,000,000,1	14.0	
10	0.000,010	8.0	Upper pH limit of survivability
26	0.000,026	7.6	Upper treatable pH level
40	0.000,040	7.4	Normal
63	0.000,063	7.2	Lower treatable pH level
100	0.000,100	7.0	
160	0.000,160	6.8	Lower pH limit of survivability
1,000,000,000 (1 M)	1,000	1.0	

[a]Nanomoles are the traditional unit used to express the small concentrations of hydrogen ion in the mammalian body at normal pH; 1 nanomole = 0.000,000,001 moles (1×10^{-9}).
[b][H$^+$] expressed in units similar to other common electrolytes (mEq/L or mM/L) to illustrate that hydrogen concentrations are very low in comparison.
[c]Corresponding pH values to illustrate that the pH scale logarithmically compresses a very wide range of hydrogen ion concentrations into numbers that are much easier to use.

Appendix 50.2 Buffers

Buffers are acid-base pairs with pK values near 7.4. The pK is the pH at which an acid or base is 50% undissociated and 50% dissociated. A buffer functions to absorb added acids or bases so as to diminish their impact on pH. Buffers combine with acids and bases so as to eliminate much of their influence on pH. The primary buffer systems are carbonic acid–bicarbonate (pK 6.1), phosphoric acid–phosphate ($H_2PO_4^-$ – HPO_4^{2-})(pK 6.8), and various proteins (hemoglobin, albumin, intracellular) (HPr – Pr$^-$) (pK 5.5–8.5). Compounds with pK values more than about 2 pH units away from 7.4 are too highly dissociated at normal-range body pH to function as effective buffers. HCl (pK 1.0), lactic acid (pK 3.5), hydroxybutyric acid (pK 4.7), acetoacetic acid (pK

3.6), phosphoric acid ($H_3PO_4 - H_2PO_4^-$) (pK 2.0) are totally dissociated acids at body pH; the anionic dissociated component will not bind hydrogen and cannot act as a buffer. These substances should be considered strong acids.

Appendix 50.3 The acid-base impact of crystalloid sodium solutions

Granular sodium chloride, sodium lactate, sodium acetate, sodium gluconate, and sodium citrate have no acid-base impact when added to whole blood *in vitro*. Sodium and the respective anion increase in proportion to the amount added and SID changes (decreases with sodium chloride; increases with sodium lactate, acetate, gluconate, and citrate), but pH does not change. The same would be true *in vivo* if the organic anions (lactate, acetate, gluconate, and citrate) were not metabolized.

The addition of distilled water to whole blood has an acidifying effect by two mechanisms. First, distilled water at body temperature has a pH of about 6.8 and is therefore acid when compared with plasma at a pH of 7.4. Water itself has very little titratable acidity (0.2 mM/L)[25], which means that its addition would have little quantitative effect on acid-base balance. But when water is equilibrated to a PCO_2 of 40 mm Hg, the carbonic acid–bicarbonate buffer system is "activated," the pH decreases to between 4.9 and 5.6, and the titratable acidity increases to 24 mM/L.[25]

Second, the water dilutes the bicarbonate concentration (to a proportionately greater extent than it does the hydrogen concentration) causing carbonic acid to dissociate, which adds more hydrogen ions to the milieu.

When sodium chloride, sodium lactate, sodium acetate, sodium gluconate, and sodium citrate *solutions* are added to whole blood *in vitro*, they will have a mild acidifying effect similar to that of adding the same amount of distilled water. It is the water, not the electrolytes, that causes the initial acidifying effect. The same thing occurs when these solutions are initially administered to patients (before the anions are not metabolized). With saline, the chloride is not metabolized, but the bicarbonate is diluted and a mild metabolic acidosis would occur until the animal compensated.

The organic anions of the remaining sodium solutions are metabolized. As they are metabolized, an equal number of hydrogen ions are also removed. As the hydrogen ions are removed from the plasma, additional carbonic acid dissociates and bicarbonate is generated. These organic anions are not *metabolized to bicarbonate*; they are *replaced by* bicarbonate (via new carbonic acid dissociation). So the metabolism of these organic anions

has an alkalinizing effect and the magnitude of the alkalinization depends on their relative concentration in the crystalloid compared with that of bicarbonate in plasma. In lactated Ringer and Hartmann solutions, where the lactate concentration is about the same as plasma, there will be minimal net effect on acid-base. In Normosol R and Plasmalyte 148, where the acetate plus gluconate concentrations far exceed plasma bicarbonate, there will be a net alkalinizing effect.

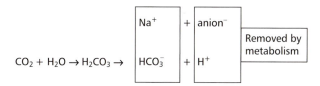

Metabolism of the organic anion and an accompanying hydrogen causes dissociation of additional carbonic acid and the generation of "new" bicarbonate.

Whether a patient actually develops the predicted acidosis or alkalosis associated with the administration of these fluids depends on variables such as volume and rate of administration, time of sampling compared with the time of administration, and the animal's ability to maintain acid-base homeostasis.

References

1. Martin L. All You Really Need to Know to Interpret Arterial Blood Gases. 2nd ed. Philadelphia: Lippincott Williams & Wilkins, 1999.
2. Lawler DF, Kealy RD, Ballam JM, Monti KL. Influence of fasting on canine arterial and venous blood gas and acid-base measurements. J Vet Emerg Crit Care 1992;2:80–84.
3. DiBartola SP. Fluid, Electrolyte, and Acid-base Disorders in Small Animal Practice. 3rd ed. Philadelphia: WB Saunders, 2006.
4. Haskins SC, Pascoe PJ, Ilkiw JE, Fudge J, Hopper K, Aldrich A. Reference cardiopulmonary values in normal dogs. Comp Med 2005;55:156–161.
5. Herbert DA, Michell RA. Blood gas tensions and acid-base balance in awake cats. J Appl Physiol 1971;30:434–436.
6. Middleton DJ, Ilkiw JE, Watson ADJ. Arterial and venous blood gas tensions in clinically healthy cats. Am J Vet Res 1981;42:1609–1611.
7. Ilkiw JE, Rose RJ, Martin ICE. A comparison of simultaneously collected arterial, mixed venous, jugular venous and cephalic venous blood samples in the assessment of blood gas and acid-base status in dogs. J Vet Int Med 1991;5:294.
8. Haskins SC, Pascoe PJ, Ilkiw JE, Fudge J, Hopper K, Aldrich A. The effect of moderate hypovolemia on cardiopulmonary function in dogs. J Vet Emerg Crit Care 2005;15:100–109.
9. Weil MH, Rackow EC, Trevino R, et al. Difference in acid-base state between venous and arterial blood during cardiopulmonary resuscitation. N Engl J Med 1986;315:153–156.
10. Kawashima Y, Yamamoto Z, Manabe H. Safe limits of hemodilution in cardiopulmonary bypass. Surgery 1974;76:391–396.

11. Hopper K, Rezende ML, Haskins SC. Assessment of the effect of dilution of blood samples with sodium heparin on blood gas, electrolyte, and lactate measurements in dogs. Am J Vet Res 2005;65:656–660.

12. Burnett RW, Covington AK, Fogh-Andersen N, et al. Approved IFCC recommendations on whole blood sampling, transport and storage for simultaneous determination of pH, blood gases and electrolytes. Eur J Clin Chem Clin Biochem 1995;33:247–253.

13. Rezende ML, Haskins SC, Hopper K. The effects of ice-water storage on blood gas and acid-base measurements. J Vet Emerg Crit Care 2007;17:67–71.

14. Ritchey MT, McGrath CJ, Portillo E, Scott M, Claypool L. Effect of sample handling on venous PCO_2, pH, bicarbonate, and base excess measured with a point-of-care analyzer. J Vet Emerg Crit Care 2004;14:253–258.

15. Ventilation with lower tidal volumes as compared with traditional tidal volumes for acute lung injury and the acute respiratory distress syndrome. The Acute Respiratory Distress Syndrome Network. N Engl J Med 2000;342:1301–1308.

16. Siggaard-Andersen O. Blood acid-base alignment. Scand J Lab Clin Invest 1963;13:211–217.

17. Kellum JA. Determinants of blood pH health and disease. Crit Care 2000;4:6–14.

18. Corey HE. Stewart and beyond: new models of acid-base balance. Kidney Int 2003;64:777–787.

19. Autran deMorais HS, Constable PD. Strong ion approach to acid-base disorders. In: DiBartola SP, ed. Fluid, Electrolyte, and Acid-base Disorders in Small Animal Practice. 3rd ed. Philadelphia: WB Saunders, 2006:chapter 13.

20. Stewart PA. Modern quantitative acid-base chemistry. Can J Physiol Pharmacol 1983;61:1444–1461.

21. Singer RB, Hastings AB. Improved clinical method for estimation of disturbances of acid-base balance of human blood. Medicine 1948;27:223–242.

22. Hopper K, Haskins SC. A case-base review of a simplified quantitative approach to acid-base analysis. J Vet Emerg Crit Care 2008;18:467–476.

23. Kurtz I, Kraut J, Ornekian V, Nguyen MK. Acid-base analysis: a critique of the Stewart and bicarbonate-centered approaches. Am J Physiol Renal Physiol 2008;294:F1009–F1031.

24. Figge J, Mydosh T, Fencl L. Serum proteins and acid-base equilibria: a follow-up. J Lab Clin Med 1992;120:713–719.

25. Gaudry PL, Duffy C, Bookallil MJ. The pH and titratable acidity of intravenous infusion solutions. Anaesth Intensive Care 1972;1: 41–44.

51

Osmolality and colloid osmotic pressure

Elke Rudloff and Angel Rivera

Water is the most essential nutrient of the body. Within the vessel, water is the transport medium that delivers oxygen, solutes, and hormones to the interstitium while removing waste products for breakdown and excretion. Within the interstitial space, water is the vehicle that moves these substances between the capillary and the cell. Within the cell, water provides a medium for organelles and for cell membrane expansion. Water also provides a means to dissipate heat through evaporation.

Identifying water imbalance in the critically ill animal can be one of the most important challenges of patient management. Qualitative information of a patient's water needs is obtained through evaluation of physical parameters of perfusion and hydration.[1] Quantitative information can be obtained with laboratory evaluation of osmolality as well as colloid osmotic pressure (COP). This chapter focuses on the basic concepts behind the role of osmolality and COP in the movement of water in the body, as well as understanding, measuring, and interpreting osmolality and COP.

Physiology of water movement: osmolality

An *osmole* is a unit term used to describe a particle; 1 osmole is equivalent to 1 g molecular weight (1 mol; 6.02×10^{23} particles) of any nondissociable substance, regardless of the substance's composition, charge, size, or weight.[2] Osmoles are often expressed in terms of *milliosmoles* (1 osmole = 1000 milliosmoles). *Osmolarity* describes the total concentration of all solutes dissolved in water and is expressed as milliosmoles/L. *Osmolality* describes the total concentration of all solutes dissolved in solution when expressed as milliosmoles/kg (mOsm).

Because 1 L of water weighs just about 1 kg, the terms *osmolarity* and *osmolality* tend to be used interchangeably when discussing body water, except when significant hyperlipidemia exists.

Water moves freely across nearly all membranes, separating the intravascular, interstitial, and intracellular compartments in the body. The two important factors that affect the movement of water across the membranes are (1) the difference in the concentration of water molecules (in relation to solutes or *osmoles*, as above) on one side of the membrane compared with the other, and (2) the difference in the hydraulic pressure on one side of the membrane compared with the other.

As an uncharged molecule, water's movement is governed passively by its chemical gradient, also called its concentration gradient, across a membrane: Water molecules will move from areas of higher water concentration to areas of lower water concentration. The pressure that leads to the passive movement (also called *diffusion*) of water along its concentration gradient is called *osmotic pressure*. Areas of high osmotic pressure have relatively low water concentration in relation to solute, whereas areas of low osmotic pressure have relatively high water concentration in relation to solute. Osmotic pressure is therefore a chemical pressure generated by the particles (solutes) dissolved in water that tends to hold water on the particles' side of a semipermeable membrane.

Hydraulic pressure in the capillary is physical pressure generated primarily by the combination of cardiac output and the pressure of the fluid in the venular network exiting the end of the capillary. Hydraulic pressure in the interstitium is created by the interaction of collagen fibrils, fibroblasts, and the lymphatics, which

Advanced Monitoring and Procedures for Small Animal Emergency and Critical Care, First Edition. Edited by Jamie M. Burkitt Creedon, Harold Davis.
© 2012 John Wiley & Sons, Inc. Published 2012 by John Wiley & Sons, Inc.

are dynamic. By expanding, contracting, and pumping, they can affect interstitial hydraulic pressure, and in health they maintain a negative interstitial hydraulic pressure. Water is in equilibrium across a membrane when the net driving force for water movement is zero. In other words, at equilibrium, water does not move across a membrane because the osmotic pressure gradient is equal to the hydrostatic pressure gradient across that membrane.

The primary solutes that produce osmotic pressure in the extracellular (intravascular and interstitial) compartment of dogs, cats, and humans are the most plentiful dissolved substances: sodium, chloride, glucose, and urea.[2,3] The primary solutes that produce intracellular osmotic pressure are potassium and magnesium because they are the most plentiful dissolved intracellular molecules.[2,3] Effective osmolality (also called *tonicity*) is generated by solutes that are unable to pass between the intracellular and extracellular compartments. Because they do not freely cross the cellular membrane, they can affect water movement. When there is a difference in tonicity between the intracellular and extracellular compartments (i.e., an osmolar gradient), water will freely move from the compartment with fewer solutes to the compartment with more solutes until the osmolality (concentration of solutes) is equal between compartments. This process is called *osmosis* (Fig. 51.1).

Like water, urea is able to pass across most mammalian membranes without energy and is therefore considered an *ineffective osmole* except under rare conditions. Urea can act as an effective osmole when changes in urea concentration occur more rapidly than equilibrium occurs across the cell membrane, such as urea extraction during dialysis or intravenous infusions of urea.

Changes in plasma osmolality affect water movement between the intracellular and extracellular compartments. Rapid increases in plasma osmolality will cause water to move from the cells and interstitium into the intravascular space, and dehydrate the cells and interstitium. This is the principle by which mannitol works in patients with cerebral edema.

Isotonic solutions that contain added dextrose and parenteral nutrition are hyperosmolar compared with normal plasma. Their infusion in peripheral veins can create a local osmolar gradient causing water to move out of the endothelial cell and into the plasma, leading to endothelial cell dehydration and damage at the site of injection and localized pain and tissue swelling. In contrast, when large volumes of 5% dextrose in water are rapidly infused, the dextrose is quickly metabolized and the remaining hypotonic water will decrease plasma serum osmolality, resulting in water moving from the intravascular space into the interstitium and cells, causing interstitial edema and cell swelling.

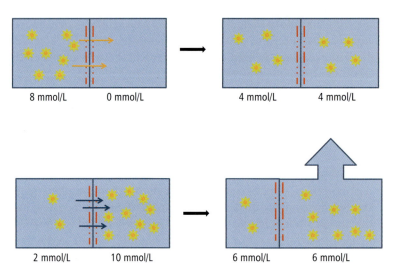

8 mmol/L   0 mmol/L   4 mmol/L   4 mmol/L

2 mmol/L   10 mmol/L   6 mmol/L   6 mmol/L

Figure 51.1 Osmotic forces across a semipermeable membrane. The top figure demonstrates that when more solutes (star-shaped dots) exist on one side of a semipermeable membrane (dashed lines) and the membrane is permeable to those solutes, solute particles will diffuse across the membrane until they are in equal concentration on either side of the membrane. Permeable solutes are thus considered ineffective osmoles because their presence on one side of the membrane (or the other) does not cause water to move across the membrane; the solutes move instead.

The bottom figure demonstrates that when more solutes exist on one side of a semipermeable membrane and the membrane is *not* permeable to those solutes, *water* will move across the membrane until the solutes are in equal concentration; this movement is caused by *osmotic pressure*. When the impermeable solutes that generate the osmotic pressure are colloid particles, then the pressure generated is called *colloid osmotic pressure*.

The brain is most susceptible to rapid changes in plasma osmolality (>30–35 mOsm), and damage caused by rapid swelling or shrinking of neurons can result in altered mentation, seizures, and intracranial bleeding.[4] The brain is encased in the skull, so that any type of increase in brain volume from neuronal swelling will compress and damage functional neurons and brain vessels. However, when plasma osmolality increases slowly, brain cells produce idiogenic osmoles (e.g., amino acids, glutamine, inositol) that prevent the development of a transcellular osmotic gradient and maintain intracellular water content.[4]

When a patient is hyperosmolar (e.g., a diabetic cat with hyperglycemia and ketosis), special attention should be given to the type and rate of fluids infused. It would be highly detrimental to infuse large volumes of hypotonic fluids (e.g., lactated Ringer solution or half-strength solutions) because a large osmotic gradient could result in a rapid shift of water into brain cells. To prevent rapid osmotic shifts during fluid administration, isotonic fluids with a more normal osmolality (e.g., Normosol-R) are used, or fluids can be modified by mixing with concentrated sodium and chloride and increasing the osmolality closer to the patient's osmolality, so that they produce less of an osmotic gradient.

Physiology of water movement: colloid osmotic pressure

The capillary endothelial membrane is freely permeable to small solutes as well as water, allowing a passive exchange of most small solutes between the intravascular and interstitial compartments (Fig. 51.2). The sum of all forces that affect water movement are summarized

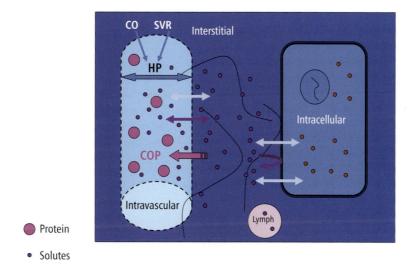

● Protein

• Solutes

Figure 51.2 Relationship of forces governing water movement between the fluid compartments. Total body water is distributed between two major body compartments: the intracellular space and the extracellular space. The extracellular compartment is further divided into the interstitial space and intravascular space. The cell membrane is freely permeable to solute-free water (white arrows), which moves in and out of the cell as a result of osmolar gradients established between the intracellular and interstitial fluid compartments. The concentration gradient of solutes on either side of a membrane dictates how water will move by osmosis across the cell membrane. Changes in the intracellular concentration affect the osmolar gradient and depend on the molecules' ability to move through the cell membrane by active membrane pumps and restricted channels.

The capillary membrane is permeable to water and small solutes, and it is relatively impermeable to blood cells and large molecules such as proteins. The most abundant small solutes in the extracellular fluid are sodium, glucose, chloride, bicarbonate, and urea, which are equally distributed across the vascular membrane. Plasma water is the vehicle transporting oxygen and solutes to the capillary.

Starling's forces dictate water movement and retention in the extracellular space. The capillary hydrostatic pressure (HP) is produced by the forces generated by cardiac output (CO) and systemic vascular resistance (SVR). The intravascular colloid osmotic pressure (COP) opposes the HP, retaining water in the vessel. The vascular membrane creates a barrier that under normal conditions prevents the movement of large molecules, primarily proteins, out of the vessels. Under normal conditions, the concentration of proteins is greater in the blood vessel than in the interstitium, promoting water retention within the capillary. Lymphatic vessels are within the interstitial matrix and carry excess fluid, proteins, and solutes from the interstitium back to the circulation.

in the Starling equation.[5] One major force that opposes hydrostatic pressure across the vascular membrane and thus prevents great movements of water out of the vessel and into the interstitium is plasma *colloid osmotic pressure* (COP).[3,5] COP is generated by the presence of large molecules (primarily proteins) that do not readily move across the capillary membrane, creating an osmotic effect (Fig. 51.1) As it pertains to proteins, synonyms of COP include *protein osmotic pressure* and *oncotic pressure*. Albumin is the most abundant protein in the plasma, and when present in normal concentration, it produces approximately 75% of the total intravascular COP. Other proteins such as fibrinogen and globulins contribute the remaining 25%. The albumin molecule expresses a negative charge that attracts positively charged sodium ions, increasing the water attraction of albumin. This additional water-holding effect is called the *Gibbs-Donnan effect* and increases the COP by approximately 20%. When there is a break in the endothelial barrier or the capillary membrane becomes more permeable during inflammatory states, protein molecules can pass from the intravascular compartment into the interstitial compartment causing a decrease in plasma COP and an increase in interstitial COP. When plasma COP is significantly reduced, intravascular water retention is reduced. This can result in hypovolemia, interstitial edema, and fluid losses into body cavities (e.g., pleural space, abdominal cavity, gastrointestinal tract) (Fig. 51.3). Hypovolemia reduces oxygen delivery to the tissues. Significant interstitial edema of the tissues

inhibits transport of metabolic substances to and from the cell. Significant leakage of fluid into the lung interstitium, pleural space, and abdominal cavity may affect oxygenation, ventilation, and increase the work of breathing.

Synthetic colloid fluids (e.g., hydroxyethyl starch) and Oxyglobin (Biopure, Cambridge, MA) contain large molecules that generate COP. When the molecules are larger than the interendothelial pore size, they can maintain intravascular COP during states of hypoproteinemia and increased capillary permeability. Synthetic colloid fluids are commonly used to resuscitate and maintain intravascular volume in critical patients with hypovolemic shock and with diseases causing a systemic inflammatory response (e.g., pancreatitis, severe gastroenteritis, pneumonia).

Frequent monitoring of both the patient as well as laboratory monitoring of osmolality and COP can provide the veterinary team with information on a patient's needs and response to specific therapy affecting fluid balance. Clinical monitoring of a patient's water balance is addressed elsewhere (see Chapter 49, Serum Electrolyte Evaluation).

Calculating plasma osmolality

Osmolality can be *calculated* by knowing a patient's blood urea nitrogen (BUN), glucose, and sodium (Na) levels. Four equations are reported to be used in the calculation of osmolality.[6] The two that correlate

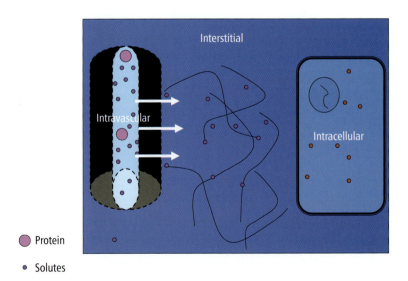

Protein

Solutes

Figure 51.3 Decreased intravascular colloid osmotic pressure. Decreased intravascular colloid osmotic pressure results in movement of intravascular water into the interstitium, which can lead to reduced blood flow through the capillary, interstitial edema, and decreased tissue oxygen delivery.

most accurately to measured plasma osmolality are as follows:

$$\text{Osmolality (mOsm)} = 2(\text{Na} + \text{K})(\text{mEq/L})$$
$$+ \text{Glucose (mg/dL)}/2.8$$
$$+ \text{BUN (mg/dL)}/18$$

$$\text{Osmolality (mOsm)} = [1.86(\text{Na} + \text{K})(\text{mEq/L})$$
$$+ \text{Glucose (mg/dL)}/2.8$$
$$+ \text{BUN (mg/dL)}/18] \div 0.93$$

The units 18 and 2.8 convert the mg/dL of BUN and glucose to milliosmoles.[2] In the second equation, the 1.86 accounts for the incomplete dissociation of the salts, and the 0.93 accounts for the body percentage of water when measuring whole blood.[7,8] An increase or decrease in *calculated* osmolality is caused by an increase or decrease in sodium, glucose, or BUN. Other, potentially toxic, substances will increase osmolality, but the only way to detect them is by *measuring* osmolality using an osmometer. In contrast to *calculating* milliosmoles, an osmometer *measures* not only the normal solutes (BUN, glucose, Na) but also other small solutes. There is a normal 10 mOsm difference between the calculated and measured milliosmoles (*osmolar gap*).[6] If the osmolar gap is significantly increased, toxins should be investigated for (Table 51.1).

Measuring plasma osmolality

A variety of osmometers are available for clinical laboratory monitoring. Some measure osmolality using a freezing-point depression method (Fig. 51.4), and others use room-temperature controls and vapor-point depres-

sion (Fig. 51.5). The freezing point depression determination of osmolality compares the freezing point of solute-free water and the freezing point of the sample. Water has a freezing point of 0°C, and a solution with saline concentration of 1 mOsm/kg has a freezing point

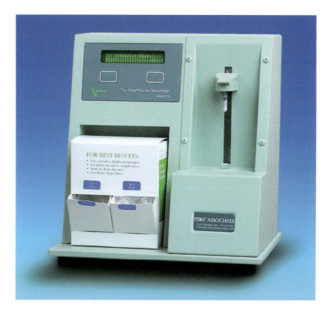

Figure 51.4 Fiske 210 freezing-point depression osmometer (Cardinal Health). Osmotically active substances decrease the freezing point, and the freezing point depression difference is translated by a thermistor into measured milliosmoles. This type of osmometer is the most commonly encountered in veterinary medicine because it can detect consumed alcohol-based toxins such as ethylene glycol.

Table 51.1 Substances that increase osmolar gap

Acetone
Ethylene glycol
Ethanol
Ether
Glycerol
Inositol
Isopropyl alcohol
Ketones
Lactate
Mannitol
Methanol
Paraldehyde
Sorbitol
Uremia

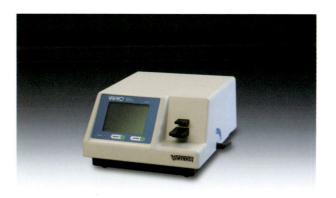

Figure 51.5 VAPRP 5520 vapor pressure osmometer (Wescor, Logan, UT). Sample volumes of 10 μL are typically used, but the osmometer allows for testing of sample volumes as small as 2 μL. Results are available in 20 seconds and expressed as mmol/kg. The osmometer is able to store up to 32 sample results and can be easily connected to a printer or computer to download data. The instrument needs to be calibrated and has control solutions for high, normal, and low osmolality.

of −1.858 °C. Osmotically active substances decrease the freezing point, and the freezing point depression difference is translated by a thermistor into measured milliosmoles.

A vapor-point depression osmometer analyzes the vapor pressure of an osmotically active solution: the lower the vapor pressure, the higher the osmolality of a solution. A sample of solution is pipetted onto a small solute-free paper disk that is inserted into the sample chamber that contains a thermocouple hygrometer. The temperature of the sample and the temperature of the chamber equilibrate. An electrical current is passed through the thermocouple, cooling it to a temperature below dew point. Water condenses from air in the chamber to form microscopic droplets on the surface of the thermocouple. When the temperature of the thermocouple reaches the dew point, condensation ceases, causing the thermocouple temperature to stabilize.

In contrast to freezing-point depression osmometers, vapor-point depression osmometers are not affected by artifacts caused by increased viscosity of a solution, suspended particles, or other conditions. However, because vapor-point depression osmometers require larger sample volumes and do not detect alcohols such as ethylene glycol, they are used less frequently in clinical medicine. Freezing point depression osmometers can detect not only nonvolatile particles but also commonly encountered toxic volatile alcohols that can increase the osmolar gap. The Advanced Micro Osmometer Model 3300 (Advanced Instruments, Inc., Norwood, MA), a freezing point depression osmometer, has been validated for measuring plasma and whole blood samples in normal dogs.[6]

Osmometers can test a variety of fluid and tissue samples, and plasma, serum, blood, and urine are the most commonly tested samples in veterinary medicine. Serum osmolality can be compared with urine osmolality to evaluate for the cause of water imbalances. As the serum osmolality rises, the urine osmolality should also rise. The normal kidney will reabsorb water from the renal tubules in the hyperosmotic patient and concentrate the urine. When there is an excess of water in the body, normal kidney function dilutes the urine, eliminating extra body water. Normal serum osmolality ranges from 290 to 310 mOsm in the dog and from 290 to 330 mOsm in the cat.[9] Whole blood osmolality is a little higher than plasma osmolality.[6] Normal urine osmolality can range between 161 and 2830 mOsm in dogs.[10] The urine osmolality will increase when water intake is withheld as long as kidney function is normal. Each individual laboratory should establish the normal reference range in each species for its osmometer.

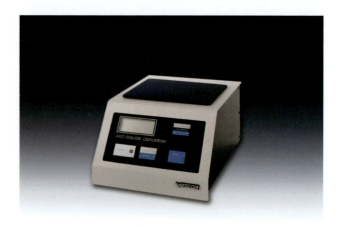

Figure 51.6   Model 4420 Colloid osmometer (Wescor). Heparinized whole blood, plasma, and serum can be analyzed. Sample volume requirements are normally 350 μL; however, special procedures allow for measurements of sample volume as low as 125 μL. The osmometer requires frequent calibration with high (25 mm Hg), low (15 mm Hg), and normal (20 mm Hg) reference solutions. The membrane requires periodic changing, and saline solution is regularly infused to prevent the membrane from drying out.

Measuring colloid osmotic pressure

Colloid osmotic pressure cannot be accurately predicted and must be directly measured using a colloid osmometer (Figs. 51.6 and 51.7). The colloid osmometer uses a semipermeable membrane to simulate the role of the natural vascular membrane in the establishment of colloid osmotic pressure responsible for water flow between interstitial fluid and blood. The effects of both natural and synthetic colloid molecules are measured by colloid osmometers. The normal values reported for plasma COP range from 14 to 27 mm Hg in the dog and 21 to 34 mm Hg in the cat.[10–13] Whole blood COP is reported to be 19.95 ± 2.1 mm Hg in the dog, and 24.7 ± 3.7 mm Hg in the cat.[14] When whole blood is being measured, the sample should be collected with lyophilized heparin. Each individual laboratory will establish the normal reference range in each species for its colloid osmometer.

Severe hemolysis (with release of hemoglobin into plasma), as well as severe hypergammaglobulinemia (caused by multiple myeloma or feline infectious peritonitis) and hyperalbuminemia (associated with hepatocellular carcinoma), can increase COP. A decrease in COP can indicate dilution of the blood or a deficiency in intravascular albumin molecules (Table 51.2).

In summary, the osmolality and COP play an important role in water homeostasis of our patients. Veterinary

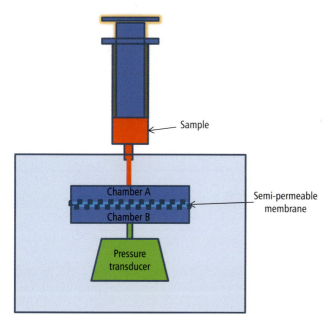

Figure 51.7 Principles of the colloid osmometer. The sample is injected into Chamber A and allowed to equilibrate with the reference Chamber B, which contains 0.9% sodium chloride. The artificial membrane does not allow molecules >30,000 Da to pass. The colloid osmotic pressure of the sample causes water and small solutes to move from Chamber B to Chamber A, causing a reduction in pressure in Chamber B. The negative pressure produced is measured by the pressure transducer and equals the COP of the sample in Chamber A. The results are displayed in mm Hg, cm H_2O, or kilopascals (kPa).

Table 51.2 Causes of hypoalbuminemia

Decreased production (liver failure)
Portosystemic shunt
Chronic active hepatitis
Acute hepatotoxicity
Increased loss
    Protein-losing glomerulonephropathy
    Protein-losing enteritis
    Systemic inflammatory response syndrome
    Acute allergic reaction

technicians who understand the physiology and monitoring of osmolality and COP, and how it relates to abnormal water balance, will have a greater ability to anticipate and prevent morbidity in their patients.

References

1. Tonozzi C, Kirby R, Rudloff E. Perfusion versus hydration: impact on the fluid therapy plan. Compend Contin Educ Vet 2009;31(12):E1–E14.
2. Wellman ML, DiBartola S, Kohn CW. Applied physiology of body fluids in dogs and cats. In: DiBartola S, ed. Fluid, Electrolyte and Acid-Base Disorders in Small Animal Practice. St. Louis, MO: Saunders-Elsevier; 2006:3–25.
3. Aronson PS, Boron WF, Boulpaep EL. Physiology of membranes. In: Boron WF, ed. Medical Physiology: A Cellular and Molecular Approach. Philadelphia, PA: Elsevier-Saunders; 2005:50–86.
4. Lien YHH, Shapiro JI, Chan L. Effects of hypernatremia on organic brain osmoles. J Clin Invest 1990;85:1427–1435.
5. Starling EH. On the absorption of fluids from the convective tissue spaces. J Physio (Lond) 1896;19:312–326.
6. Barr JW, Pesillo-Crosby SA. Use of the advanced micro-osmometer model 3300 for determination of a normal osmolality and evaluation of different formulas for calculated osmolarity and osmole gap in adult dogs. J Veterinary Emerg Crit Care 2008;18:270–276.
7. Dorwart WV, Chalmers L. Comparison of methods for calculating serum osmolality from chemical concentrations, and the prognostic value of such calculations. Clin Chem 1975;21(2):190–194.
8. McQuillen KK, Anderson AC. Osmol gaps in the pediatric population. Acad Emerg Med 1999;6(1):27–30.
9. DiBartola S. Disorders of sodium and water: hypernatremia and hyponatremia. In: DiBartola S, ed. Fluid, Electrolyte and Acid-Base Disorders in Small Animal Practice. St. Louis. MO: Saunders-Elsevier; 2006:47–79.
10. van Vonderen IK, Kooistra HS, Rijnberk A. Intra- and interindividual variation in urine osmolality and urine specific gravity in healthy pet dogs of various ages. J Vet Intern Med 1997;11:30–35.
11. Smiley LE, Garvey MS. The use of hetastarch as adjunct therapy in 26 dogs with hypoalbuminemia. A phase two clinical trial. J Vet Intern Med 1994;8(3):195–202.
12. Thomas LA, Brown SA. Relationship between colloid osmotic pressure and plasma protein concentration in cattle, horses, dogs and cats. Am J Vet Res 1992;53:2241–2243.
13. Rudloff E, Kirby R. Colloid osmometry. Clin Tech Small Anim Pract 2000;15(3):119–125.
14. Culp AM, Clay ME, Baylor IA, King LG. Colloid osmotic pressure and total solids measurements in normal dogs and cats [abstract]. Proc 4th Int Vet Emerg Crit Care Symp 1995:705.

52

Cytology

Rebecca J. Greer and Timothy Koors

Cytology can be defined as the study of the microscopic appearance of cells, especially for the diagnosis of abnormalities and malignancies.[1] Microscopic examination of tissue aspirates and fluid is a valuable tool for the emergency clinician and technician. Cytology can provide the clinician with a quick diagnosis, help guide treatment, and provide information about prognosis. Most samples for cytology are obtained by fine-needle aspiration; other techniques such as impression smears are also utilized. This technique is fairly benign in most cases, which makes cytology a useful tool in critically ill patients that may not tolerate more invasive procedures or general anesthesia. A high-quality sample is necessary for accurate interpretation. Several factors can affect the diagnostic quality of a sample, including sample collection technique, sample preparation, slide staining, and the microscope. Scanning and evaluation of the slide also play an important role in diagnosis. This chapter discusses some of the common situations encountered by the emergency clinician and technician where cytology is useful. It also details the equipment required and preparation necessary to obtain the most information from cytology samples.

Indications

There are many indications for evaluating cytology in emergency practice (Box 52.1). The following is a description of some of the more common indications.

Effusion analysis

Fluid accumulation in body cavities is a presenting complaint frequently encountered in the emergency setting.

Normal dogs and cats have very little fluid in the pleural, peritoneal, and pericardial spaces. Accumulation of fluid in these potential spaces is pathologic and can be caused by a variety of disease processes. Collection of this fluid can be both therapeutic and diagnostic See Chapter 14, Pericardiocentesis; Chapter 30, Pleural Space Drainage; and Chapter 35, Peritoneal Evaluation, for more information regarding sample collection from these spaces. Samples should be evaluated for the presence of cells (red blood cells [RBCs], white blood cells [WBCs], neoplastic cells, etc.) and infectious organisms (bacteria and fungi).

Effusions are separated into three classifications (Table 52.1) based on protein and cellular content,[2] although there is some overlap between the classes. Transudates have a low protein concentration (<2.5 g/dL) and cellular content (<1000/μL).[2] Transudates are colorless and clear, and they typically occur due to increased vascular hydrostatic pressure or decreased plasma colloidal osmotic pressure. Common causes of transudates include hypoalbuminemia, portal hypertension, portosystemic shunt, and right-sided congestive heart failure.[2]

The second class of effusions is exudates. Exudates are characterized by high protein concentration (>3.0 g/dL) and high cellularity (>7000/μL).[2] Exudates can be subclassified as septic or nonseptic. Septic exudates result from infectious causes (bacterial, viral, protozoal, fungal); nonseptic exudates are a result of sterile inflammation (as is often seen in pancreatitis, for instance) or neoplasia. Fluid that accumulates in the body cavity due to feline infectious peritonitis (FIP) is a unique example of a septic exudate. In FIP the cell count may be less than a typical exudate (<7000/μL), but the

Advanced Monitoring and Procedures for Small Animal Emergency and Critical Care, First Edition. Edited by Jamie M. Burkitt Creedon, Harold Davis.
© 2012 John Wiley & Sons, Inc. Published 2012 by John Wiley & Sons, Inc.

Box 52.1 Indications for cytology

1. Effusions
   a. Pleural
   b. Pericardial
   c. Peritoneal
   d. Joint
2. Lymphadenopathies
3. Masses
4. Dermatitis
   a. Ears

protein concentration in the fluid is generally very high (>4.5 g/dL). Thus the high protein concentration is what classifies the FIP fluid as an exudate. On cytologic examination of FIP fluid there is usually granulated pink material in the slide background due to precipitated protein.[2]

The third class of effusions is modified transudates. As the name suggests, modified transudates are a hybrid between pure transudates and exudates. They result from the addition of protein and cells to a pure transudate. The protein concentration is typically at least 2.5 g/dL and can be as high as 7.5 g/dL.[2] The cell count is usually between 1000 and 7000/μL.[2] Modified transu-

dates result from leakage of fluid from the lymphatics or blood vessels due to increased hydrostatic pressure or increased vessel permeability. Modified transudates are the most common effusions in dogs and cats. Hemorrhagic and chylous effusions fall into this category.

Pericardial effusions

The etiology of pericardial effusions can be difficult to determine cytologically. These effusions can be pure transudates, modified transudates, or exudates; however, the majority are modified transudates (hemorrhagic). Many pericardial effusions are idiopathic; no underlying etiology can be identified. When an etiology is identified, the most common is neoplasia.[3] The common neoplasms that cause pericardial effusion in dogs are hemangiosarcoma and chemodectoma, neither of which tends to exfoliate cells, which prevents an etiology from being found with cytology. Mesothelioma cells do exfoliate, but it can be difficult to distinguish the mesothelioma cells from reactive nonneoplastic cell. The preceding discussion explains why it can be challenging to make a diagnosis of neoplasia using cytologic evaluation of pericardial effusion, even when neoplasia is the underlying etiology. Cytology can be useful in diagnosing infectious etiologies of pericardial effusion, especially if organisms can be identified.[3]

Table 52.1 Evaluation of Effusions

Effusion	Cell Count	Total Protein	Causes
Transudate	<1000 cells/μL	<2.5 g/dL	Hypoalbuminemia Right heart failure Portal hypertension
Modified transudate	1000–7000 cells/μL	2.5–7.5 g/dL	*Most common:* Heart failure Neoplasia Inflammation Chylous Hemorrhagic
Exudate	>7000 cells/μL	>3 g/dL	
Septic exudate	Visualize infectious organism(s)		Bacterial Viral Protozoal Fungal
Nonseptic exudate	No infectious organism(s) seen		Inflammation Pancreatitis Peritonitis Neoplasia

Joint effusions

Animals may also present with swollen, painful joints. If joint effusion is present, cytology may help to make a diagnosis and therefore to guide treatment. Cytology is generally the most important evaluation to perform on joint effusions, so if only a small sample can be obtained, cytology should be prioritized over total protein concentration or cell counts. Normal synovial fluid is grossly viscous and has a low protein concentration (<2.5 g/dL) and cell count (<3000/μL).[2] There is very little fluid present in healthy joints. Pathologic joint effusions can be septic or nonseptic. Septic arthritis is usually caused by a bacterial or fungal infection and usually localized to one joint, although multiple joints can be affected. Infection can be caused by hematogenous spread or by direct inoculation. The cell count in septic arthritis is typically very high (5000–10,000/μL), with neutrophils as the predominant cell.[2] Generally, the neutrophils present are degenerate. Neutrophil degeneration may not always be apparent and organisms may not be identified in septic arthritides. If enough fluid can be obtained, a culture should also be performed. Joint fluid in nonseptic arthritis has an increased cell count (1000–10,000/μL) but not usually as high as seen with septic arthritis.[2] The neutrophils present are nondegenerate, and no infectious organisms are present. Causes of nonseptic arthritis include ehrlichiosis, Lyme disease, drug mediated, immune mediated, and systemic lupus erythematosus. Nonseptic arthritis can also be secondary to neoplasia or infection in distant areas of the body. Neoplastic cells may be present in cases of synovial cell sarcoma, but histopathology is generally required to differentiate between reactive synovial cells and neoplasia. Trauma or coagulopathies may also cause joint effusion. In this case the fluid resembles peripheral blood.[2]

Lymph node evaluation

Lymphadenomegaly may be noted by owners, or it may be found on physical examination. Lymph nodes may be enlarged due to a primary problem within the nodes themselves or in response to disease elsewhere in the body. The prescapular and popliteal nodes are the sites of choice to aspirate when generalized lymphadenomegaly is present. The submandibular lymph nodes are not the best diagnostic nodes because they often have a strong inflammatory component secondary to draining the mouth that can mask other diseases. The size of the nodes should also be considered. Very large lymph nodes tend to have necrotic centers, which makes diagnosis difficult. Therefore, it is advisable to sample slightly or moderately enlarged nodes if possible.[2] Common conditions that cause lymphadenomegaly include lymphoma,

metastatic neoplasia, infection (bacterial, fungal, rickettsial), inflammation, and immune mediated.

Mass evaluation

Masses are commonly found on and in small animals. Intra-abdominal and intrathoracic masses are generally aspirated with ultrasound guidance. The sample is then evaluated to help determine if the mass is neoplastic, inflammatory, or benign. Dermal or subcutaneous masses are generally only evaluated in the emergency setting if there is concern that they are related to significant disease pertinent to the current visit. Examples of skin/subcutaneous masses related to systemic disease include mast cell tumors, cutaneous lymphoma, and blastomycosis.

Skin and ears

Dermatologic diagnoses are not typically intensely pursued in the emergency setting; however, there are certain urgent care situations when cytology of the skin and external ear canals can be beneficial. It is not uncommon for an animal to present to the emergency clinic with severe skin lesions, itchy skin, or ear disease. Cytology is beneficial in making a correct diagnosis and therefore selecting appropriate initial treatment. Excessive amounts of bacteria may require systemic antibiotics. Severely pruritic animals require skin scraping with cytologic evaluation to look for evidence of mites. Animals with signs of ear disease require ear cytology to determine if topical treatment alone will be adequate or if systemic treatment is necessary. Furthermore, cytologic examination of skin lesions may give a diagnosis in debilitated animals not stable enough for more invasive diagnostic tests or general anesthesia. For example, patients with debilitating systemic blastomycosis may have skin lesions that allow for rapid noninvasive cytologic diagnosis of the systemic problem.

Equipment

A compound binocular microscope with a set of high-quality objectives is required for diagnostic cytologic examination. The microscope should have a light source with a substage condenser to provide optimal contrast and eliminate artifact. Most microscopes have four standard objectives: 4×, 10×, 40×, and 100× oil immersion. A good quality microscope is essential.

The microscope must be adjusted before each use to allow the best image. First the oculars should be adjusted for the width of the examiner's eyes. Each ocular can be individually focused to account for differences in the focusing abilities of the viewer's eyes. Once an image is

Protocol 52.1 Adjusting the microscope

Items Required
- Microscope
- Specimen slides

Procedure
1. Place the slide on the stage; secure slide in place with the stage clips.
2. Move the 4× or 10× objective into use. Adjust the coarse focus knob to move the slide up as close as possible to the objective, taking care not to bump the slide into the lens. Using the 4× or 10× it should not be possible to touch the slide to the objective.
3. Illuminate a stained area of the slide.
4. While looking through the ocular lenses, slowly adjust the coarse focus knob (moving the specimen away from the objective) until the specimen is visible.
5. Change to the fine focus knob and bring the image into sharper view.
6. Adjust the individual oculars for the best focus.
7. Adjust the condenser lens and/or light source so the illumination is optimal.
8. Readjust the fine focus knob as needed to improve the image.
9. Move to higher objectives without changing the focus from the previous objective. Use the fine focus knob to bring the image into sharp focus.

Protocol 52.2 Kohler illumination

Items Required
- Microscope
- Specimen slides

Procedure
1. Bring image into focus (see Protocol 52.1).
2. Completely close diaphragm.
3. Raise or lower condenser until circle of light is in sharp focus.
4. Center light in the field of view.
5. Open diaphragm until only the field of view is present (i.e., circle of light just outside field of view).
6. Open or close condenser aperture to allow best contrast.

Box 52.2 Microscope maintenance

1. Wipe 100× with lens paper with every use.
2. Wipe objectives, oculars, and stage once daily.
3. Clean lenses with cleansing solution weekly.
4. Perform regular service as recommended by manufacturer.

path that light takes from the light source to the viewer's eye and will help eliminate scatter. The sample must first be in focus, following the nine steps listed in Protocol 52.1 for focusing. The diaphragm is then closed all the way resulting in a blurry area of light in the field. Using the condenser knob, raise or lower the condenser until the circle of light is in sharp focus. Then use the condenser placement screws to center the light circle in the field of view. Open the diaphragm until only the field of view is illuminated, meaning the circle of light is just outside the field of view. Open or close the condenser aperture to allow the best contrast.[4,5]

If the image is difficult to get into focus, the lenses may need to be cleaned or the light source adjusted. Opening or closing the aperture and/or adjusting the strength of the light source may help.

Maintenance of the microscope (Box 52.2) includes weekly cleaning of the objective and ocular lenses with a lens cleansing solution. Use the recommended solution for the particular microscope but not alcohol or water because standard immersion oil is not dissolved by these substances.[6] The lens is then wiped with lens paper that has the appropriate solution applied to the paper and wiped in a circular motion. Lens paper is the only material that should be used to actually wipe the lenses because other paper or materials may scratch the lens surface. The ocular pieces can be removed from the eyepiece tube and wiped down, but do not attempt to take the actual lenses apart. The objectives should be wiped with plain lens paper at least once a day and the high power oil objective (100×) should have the oil removed with plain lens paper every time it is used. If the microscope is not properly maintained, the lenses will become damaged and a clear, focused image will not be obtained. The stage should be wiped as needed. This area of the microscope can be cleaned with ordinary cleansing materials; oil spills and water will cause the slides to stick to the stage preventing appropriate movement. The owner's manual of each microscope lists specific solutions and cleaning recommendations for that microscope. The microscope should be serviced regularly as recommended by the manufacturer.

visible, a combination of adjustments will be made to achieve the best focus. Protocol 52.1 lists the general sequence of events.

For the best images, the Kohler method of illumination (Protocol 52.2) should be used and readjusted every time an objective is changed. This method deals with the

---

Box 52.3 Other equipment

1. Glass slides, preferably frosted on one end
2. Coverslips: glass or plastic
3. Needles: 21–25 gauge
4. Syringes: 3–20 cc
5. Serum tubes
6. EDTA tubes
7. Centrifuge
8. Stains: Romanowsky type
9. Pencil

The other supplies needed are inexpensive and readily available. These supplies include the following: glass slides with a frosted end, glass or plastic coverslips, needles (21–25 gauge), syringes (3–20 cc), serum tubes, EDTA tubes, centrifuge for spinning down samples, stains, and a pencil (Box 52.3).

Slide preparation

Slide preparation varies by the type of sample to be analyzed (i.e., tissue vs. fluid).

Fluid

Examination can be performed on fluid directly, or samples can be centrifuged to concentrate cells. Slides from fluid samples are prepared in the same way as a blood smear. A small drop is placed near the frosted end of the slide. A second slide is backed into the sample with the acute angle toward the operator (frosted end of the slide). The second slide is then drawn away from the operator. The speed at which the slide is moved depends on the viscosity of the fluid.[2] Thinner samples should be spread faster than more viscous samples to ensure even distribution over the slide. All fluid applied to the slide originally should remain on the slide. Care should be taken not to allow excess fluid to be drawn off the end of the slide. Neoplastic cells tend to clump and stick to the spreader slide. If excess fluid is removed with the spreader slide and discarded, valuable diagnostic material may be lost. If excess fluid is a problem, the spreader slide can be stopped before it reaches the end of the specimen slide. Excess fluid on the spreader slide can then be transferred to another slide. An alternative is to allow the excess fluid to run back on itself for a short distance. With this procedure the thin part of the specimen can be used to estimate cell numbers while the area of excess fluid can be evaluated for abnormal cells or infectious organisms.

Samples can be centrifuged to concentrate fluids of low cellularity. After centrifuging for 5 minutes, the pellet is resuspended in 1–2 drops of supernatant. This solution is then prepared as previously described. Micro-hematocrit tubes can be used if there is a small volume of fluid. The same is then spun just like a packed cell volume (PCV). The buffy coat or cellular layer is then applied to a slide.[2] The slide is prepared utilizing the squash technique described later.

Tissue

Slides with tissue samples can be obtained in several different ways. Fine-needle aspiration is a common method to obtain samples.[2] Once the tissue sample has been obtained, the needle is removed from the syringe. A syringe with air is attached to the needle. The sample is then blown onto the slide using the air in the syringe. This process may be repeated a few times to ensure complete transfer of sample material to a slide (Fig. 52.1A and B). Once the sample material is on a slide, a compression (squash) preparation can be made.

Squash preparation

A squash preparation is accomplished by placing a sample on the slide and then placing a second glass slide over the sample at a right angle to the specimen slide. The sample is gently but firmly compressed. Generally the only pressure for compression is the weight of the second slide. The second slide is then drawn away from the frosted end of the specimen slide. This process should be performed with a smooth and continuous motion.[2] Care should be taken especially with lymph node aspirates because lymphoma cells rupture easily.[7] The resulting specimen should be oblong in shape and have a cellular monolayer at the end (see Fig. 52.1C and D).

Impression smear

Slides can also be prepared by making an impression smear. This technique can be used for skin or excised tissue. With excised tissue, the cut surface is blotted with a paper towel to remove blood or other fluids. The tissue is then gently pressed or touched against a slide at several different places. The tissue should lightly stick to the slide. A clean slide can also be pressed against skin to obtain skin cytology. A variation of the slide to skin technique utilizes a clear adhesive tape preparation. A piece of transparent acetate tape is used. The adhesive side of the tape is pressed against the area of interest, being sure to leave uncompromised adhesive on each side for affixing to the slide. The sample area is placed on the middle of a glass slide and the tape edges used to

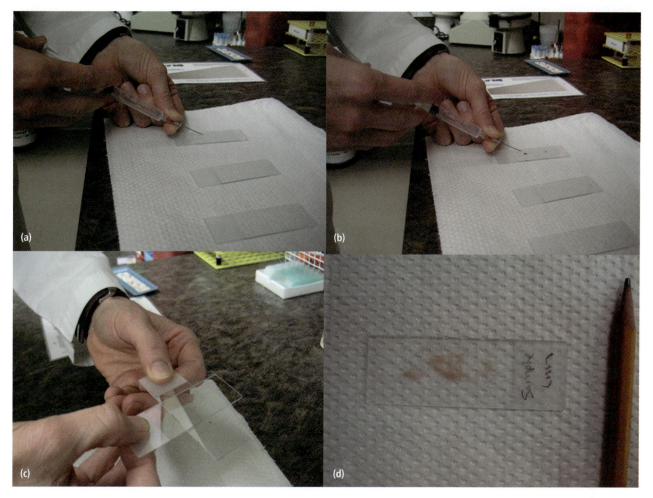

Figure 52.1 Preparing squash sample from an aspirate. (a) Aligning the needle above the slide; needle aspiration has been performed and sample is in the needle. (b) The sample was blown out of the needle using the air in the syringe. This results in a small amount of sample on the slide. (c) A second, clean slide is aligned over the slide with the sample, the weight of the slide is used to squash the sample, and then the top (second) slide is drawn off the end of the sample slide. (d) Finished squash sample, unstained.

affix the tape to the slide. The slide with adhered tape can then be stained. If using the Diff-Quik solution, the fixative step is skipped because it will dissolve the adhesive, and the slide is dipped into the stains and rinsed in standard fashion. An alternative staining method is to place a single drop of stain on the slide and then affix the tape with the sample section in the stain. In this method, the stain is not rinsed off but the tape, drop of stain, slide combination is directly viewed with the microscope.[8] The tape method of obtaining samples is especially useful for the paws and around the nose.[2]

After the sample is obtained and placed on a slide, the slide should be labeled with patient identification and type of sample. A pencil will write easily on the frosted end and remain visible even after staining. Marks made by pens and permanent markers will rinse off during the staining process.

Staining

Many different stains are available for staining cytology samples. The most commonly used in veterinary medicine are the Romanowsky-type stains.[9] Romanowsky-type stains include Wright, Giemsa, and Jenner stains. Romanowsky-type stains are defined by the use of a combination of eosin and methylene blue. Characteristically these stains color a cell's nucleus purple and its cytoplasm blue or pink.[10] A proprietary example is the Diff-Quik stain (Andwin Scientific, Tryon, NC). The Diff-Quik brand (Fig. 52.2) is one of the most commonly used Romanowsky-type stains due to the quick results and ease of use. Staining times with Diff-Quik vary depending on the thickness of the sample. Thick samples may require as much as 60–120 seconds in each solution. A general guide for staining with Diff-Quik

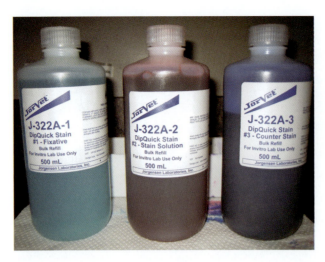

Figure 52.2 Bulk DipQuick, another proprietary version of Diff-Quik stain.

Protocol 52.3 General guidelines for Diff-Quik stain

Items Required
- Diff-Quick stains
- Specimen slides

Procedure
1. 60–120 seconds in fixative
2. 30–60 seconds in solution 1
3. 5–60 seconds in solution 2
4. 15- to 30-second rinse in cold water
5. Air dry or blot
   Times will vary depending on thickness of sample (longer for thicker samples)

---

solutions is as follows (Protocol 52.3): 60–120 seconds in fixative, 30–60 seconds in solution 1, and 5–60 seconds in solution 2. The slide should then be rinsed with cold water for 15–20 seconds to remove any stain precipitate and then allowed to air dry in a nearly vertical position.[2] If time is of the essence, the samples could be dried by blotting with bibulous paper or a hair dryer on low. Common errors in staining are discussed later.

New methylene blue is another valuable stain to have in the emergency practice because it stains nuclei, bacteria, fungi, platelets, and mast cell granules.[9] Diff-Quik solutions may not always stain mast cell granules adequately; therefore a new methylene blue stain may help distinguish the cells in low-granule mast cell tumors. New methylene blue stain can also be used in cases with anemia to look for reticulocytes. New methylene blue is more labor intensive than Diff-Quik because it requires

preparing the solution and proper disposal of formalin. To prepare the solution, new methylene blue is mixed with 0.9% saline and formalin. The solution is passed through filter paper before using to remove precipitates. The stain should be replaced and filtered weekly.[2] A drop of the prepared solution is then placed on a slide, and a coverslip is placed on top. The slide should be examined immediately because the stain evaporates quickly.

Slide scanning and evaluation

Slides should be examined first with 4× or 10× to evaluate overall sample quality and staining. Slides that are too lightly stained can be re-stained to improve quality. The slide is then scanned at 10× to find the area of the slide that will be of highest diagnostic yield. The slide should be scanned in a consistent manner to be sure the entire slide is evaluated. Starting at one corner of the slide, a back and forth pattern is used until the entire slide has been evaluated. Large objects such as parasites and some fungal elements may be seen at this low power. Once the initial evaluation is performed, a more detailed study is made. The best area to examine is the area where the cells are in a monolayer. The 40× objective is used to obtain an overview of the cell population. At this magnification it is possible to compare cell sizes and determine the proportions of different cell types. This power should provide enough detail to make a presumptive diagnosis if there is not enough time to thoroughly examine the slide in the emergency setting. To further improve resolution, a drop of immersion oil is applied directly to the stained surface (or on top of the coverslip if one is in place), and the slide is reexamined with the 100× oil immersion objective. Take care not to touch immersion oil to *any* objective other than the oil immersion (generally 100×) because this is the only objective that is sealed and designed for oil use.[11] This objective shows greater detail of individual cells (Protocol 52.4). Nuclear structures and cytoplasmic granules can be seen at this magnification. Cellular inclusions may also be seen at this magnification.[2]

Troubleshooting

Making a diagnosis from cytology can be very rewarding. However, there are some pitfalls that can make examining slides frustrating. Here is a list of commonly encountered problems and their solutions.

Nondiagnostic samples

Obtaining nondiagnostic samples can be frustrating, especially in an emergency situation. One of the

Protocol 52.4 Slide scanning and evaluation

Items Required
- Microscope
- Immersion oil
- Specimen slides

Procedure
1. Systematic scan at low power (4× or 10×).
   a. Use back-and-forth technique.
   b. Evaluate staining technique.
   c. Identify monolayer.
   d. Look for large organisms (fungus or parasites).
2. Increase magnification (40×).
   a. Evaluate cellular structure.
3. Increase magnification (100×).
   a. Place drop of immersion oil on slide.
   b. Evaluate for more detailed cellular structure.

most common causes for nondiagnostic samples is hemodilution. This phenomenon occurs commonly when aspirating vascular organs such as the spleen. If a large amount of blood is aspirated, it can be smeared like a blood film to look for diagnostic cells. The best way to avoid blood contamination in vascular organs is to use a fine-needle biopsy approach without aspiration, also called a fenestration approach.[7] A needle (alone or attached to a syringe) is directed into the area of interest. Multiple fenestrations are made in the tissue without applying negative pressure to the syringe. The needle is then attached to a syringe with air, or if already attached to a syringe, the air is used to blow the sample out and it is prepared as a squash. If using the aspiration technique in a tissue where peripheral blood contamination is expected to be a problem, release the negative pressure on the syringe before removing the needle from the tissue. This precaution will prevent blood from being drawn into the syringe as the needle is removed. It will also prevent the sample from being sucked into the barrel of the syringe when the pressure in the syringe equilibrates with room air.[7]

Nondiagnostic samples are also obtained if the material on the slide is too thick or if there is poor separation of cells. A common mistake is to place too much material on a slide. It is then impossible to obtain a monolayer of cells with a squash preparation. This problem can be avoided by making sure only a small amount of sample is applied to a slide.[2] Multiple slides can be made from a single fine-needle aspiration. It takes practice to know the right amount of material to apply to a slide.

Fractured cells and naked nuclei also make diagnosis difficult. Certain neoplastic cells are fragile and break when preparing the sample. One step to help avoid this problem is to not apply excessive vacuum when aspirating the sample. In general, 0.5–1 cc of vacuum is all that is needed. Overzealous compression of the sample during squash preparation can also fracture cells.[2] Care should be taken when preparing slides, especially of enlarged lymph nodes because lymphoma cells rupture easily.

Staining

Most errors that occur with staining are due to inadequate time in the solutions or use of old solutions. Slides may appear dull or washed out. In most cases the problem can be remedied by replacing the slide into one or all of the staining solutions. Staining times vary depending on the kind of material being stained. In general, thicker cellular material requires more contact time than thinner, less cellular material. Stain precipitates may be present on the slide if it has not been rinsed adequately.[9] The same problems can be seen if the staining solutions are not maintained properly. Manufacturer recommendations should be followed regarding maintenance and changing or replacement of the solutions and their containers.

Prolonged contact time in the stain may also result in problems. When using the Romanowsky-type stains, slides may appear too pink or too blue. It is important to use the same brand of stain consistently to obtain a feel for the appropriate length of time to stain different material.[9]

If technique is followed properly, and the slide is still not stained appropriately, there may be a problem with the stain itself. This problem usually occurs as the stain deteriorates with age.[9] The stain should be replaced with fresh solution when this occurs (Protocol 52.5). Aggregates of stain precipitate can form and give the false appearance of cocci bacteria or inclusion bodies. False results can have life-threatening consequences in an emergency situation. For example, if these cocci-appearing aggregates are seen in a sample of abdominal fluid from a critically ill patient, that patient may be taken for an abdominal exploration resulting in an unstable patient undergoing a risky and unnecessary procedure. This problem can be avoided by changing the stain regularly. The timeframe varies from clinic to clinic depending on the number of slides stained and the type of stain used. Manufacturer recommendations should be followed regarding how often to change the solutions. It is good practice to have separate stains for clean (blood, aspirates, fluid) and dirty (skin, fecal, abscess)

Protocol 52.5 Troubleshooting

Procedure
Nondiagnostic sample:
1. Retake sample.
   a. Decrease force of aspiration.
   b. Use needle biopsy technique.
Staining:
1. Too lightly stained:
   a. Re-stain.
   b. Replace old stain solution.
2. Stain granules:
   a. Rinse slide thoroughly.
   b. Re-stain new sample in fresh stain.

samples. Bacteria from dirty samples can contaminate the stain, resulting in bacteria on the slide of a sample that did not truly contain bacteria. If only one staining station is available, the stain should be changed immediately if has come in contact with infectious organisms or debris.

Conclusion

Cytology is an important tool for the emergency clinician. A diagnosis made by in-house cytology can prevent a delay in definitive treatment. A quick diagnosis benefits the patient and the owner. If a diagnosis cannot be made in the clinic, samples should be submitted to a diagnostic laboratory for analysis. Good sample collection technique and sample preparation will ensure that the pathologist has the best chance of making a diagnosis. There are some instances where cytology will not provide an answer. In these instances, biopsies should be taken after the patient has been stabilized.

Summary

- Indications for cytology
  - Presence of effusions
  - Lymphadenopathy
  - Masses
  - Dermatologic problems
- Equipment required
  - Microscope
  - Microscope slides
  - Coverslips
  - Needles (21–25 guage)
  - Syringes (3–12 cc)
  - Stains
    - Romanowsky type
    - New methylene blue
  - Pencil
- Microscope use
  - Place the slide on the stage; secure slide in place with the stage clips.
  - Move the 4× or 10× objective into use. Adjust the coarse focus knob to move the slide up as close as possible to the objective, taking care not to bump the slide into the lens. Using the 4× or 10×, it should not be possible to touch the slide to the objective.
  - Illuminate a stained area of the slide.
  - While looking through the ocular lenses, slowly adjust the coarse focus knob (moving the specimen away from the objective) until the specimen is visible.
  - Change to the fine focus knob and bring the image into a sharper view.
  - Adjust the individual oculars for the best focus.
  - Adjust the condenser lens and/or light source so the illumination is optimal.
  - Readjust the fine focus knob as needed to improve the image.
  - Move to higher objectives without changing the focus from the previous objective. Use the fine focus knob to bring the image into sharp focus.
- Microscope maintenance
  - Daily lens wiping with lens paper
  - Weekly lens cleaning with a recommended cleaning solution
  - Routine service
- Slide preparation
  - Fluids
    - Make a smear
  - Aspirates
    - Squash preparation
- Staining
  - Romanowsky type
    - Adequate time in each solution
    - Rinse well
- Slide scanning and evaluation
  - Systematic scan at low power
    - Evaluate staining technique
    - Identify monolayer
  - Increase magnification
    - Evaluate cellular structure
    - Look for organisms
- Troubleshooting
  - Nondiagnostic sample
    - Retake sample
    - Decrease force of aspiration
    - Try needle biopsy rather than aspiration

- Staining
  - Too lightly stained
    - Re-stain
    - Replace old stain solutions
  - Stain granules
    - Rinse slide thoroughly

References

1. Dictionary.com. Definition of cytology.
2. Raskin RE, Meyer DJ. Atlas of Canine and Feline Cytology. Philadelphia, PA: Saunders; 2001.
3. Rush JE, Shaw SP. Canine pericardial effusion: diagnosis, treatment, and prognosis. Compend Cont Educ Pract Vet 2007;29: 405–411.
4. BerkelyTutorialonline. Kohler Illumination: http://microscopy.berkeley.edu/courses/TLM/condenser/kohler.html.
5. Oldfield R. Light Microscopy an Illustrated Guide. Aylesbury, UK: Wolf Publishing; 1994.
6. MicroscopeWorld.com. Microscope Maintenance http://www.microscopeworld.com/MSWorld/microscope_maintenance.aspx, 2010.
7. LeBlanc CJ, Head LL, Fry MM. Comparison of aspiration and nonaspiration techniques for obtaining cytologic samples from the canine and feline spleen. Vet Clin Pathol 2009;38: 242–246.
8. Rosenkrantz W. Cutaneous cytology: a quick review of an indispensable test. Vet Med 2008. Available at: http://veterinarymedicine.dvm360.com/vetmed/Medicine/ArticleStandard/Article/detail/522835.
9. Jorundsson E, Lumsden JH, Jacobs RM. Rapid staining techniques in cytopathology: a review and comparison of modified protocols for hematoxylin and eosin, Papanicolaou and Romanowsky stains. Vet Clin Pathol 1999;28:100–108.
10. Turgeon ML. Clinical Hematology: Theory and Procedures. 4th ed. Baltimore, MD: Lippincott Williams & Wilkens; 2005.
11. Fankhauser DB. Immersion oil microscopy. http://biology.clc.uc.edu/fankhauser/labs/microscope/Oil_Immersion.htm, 2001.

53

Blood typing and cross-matching

Nicole M. Weinstein and Carolyn A. Sink

Knowledge of blood types, necessary equipment, blood type and crossmatch test procedures, and test interpretation are paramount in effective and safe transfusion medicine. A blood type and, in some instances, a crossmatch test should be performed prior to packed RBC (pRBC) or whole blood (WB) transfusions in dogs and cats. The benefits of blood transfusion are numerous and can be maximized with safe transfusion and blood banking practices. Although some complications of transfusion cannot be predicted or even prevented, determination of patient and blood donor blood compatibility can minimize the risk of a hemolytic transfusion reaction. The veterinary care worker should understand dog and cat blood typing and the basics of crossmatching before the bleeding or anemic patient arrives at the clinic.

Agglutination, hemagglutination, and autoagglutination

To interpret information and tests discussed in this chapter, one must first understand some terminology pertaining to red blood cells (RBCs). The general term used to describe the visible clumping together of RBCs is *agglutination* or *hemagglutination*. RBCs agglutinate when antibodies present in plasma adhere to substances (antigens) on the surfaces of neighboring RBCs, thus linking and binding these neighboring RBCs together into clumps that can be visualized *in vitro*. Generally, hemagglutination occurs because prospective transfusion recipient plasma contains antibodies to prospective donor RBCs. Animals do not normally produce antibodies to their own RBCs. The term *autoagglutination*

is used to describe specifically hemagglutination of a patient's own RBCs to each other due to the production of antibodies to one's own RBCs. Both canine and feline patients can develop these RBC "autoantibodies," which can result in RBC destruction and immune-mediated hemolytic anemia. Because hemagglutination is used as the "positive" (i.e., reactive) end point of both blood typing and crossmatch tests, autoagglutination could lead to a false reactive interpretation of the test. Blood typing and crossmatch procedures include a step to evaluate for the presence of autoagglutination (Protocols 53.1–53.4). If autoagglutination is determined to be present, patient RBCs should be washed (Protocol 53.5) prior to performing the blood typing or crossmatch procedure.

Canine blood types

Blood types are antigens present on the surface of the RBC membrane and are species specific. Several blood group systems have been documented in dogs, but significance, antigenicity, and ability to test for these different groups is highly variable. The dog erythrocyte antigen system (DEA), in which a number denotes the blood type, is the traditional schema used.[1–4] DEA 1.1 is considered the most clinically relevant because of its potential to cause a hemolytic transfusion reaction.[5–7] In-clinic tests are available for DEA 1.1 typing.

A dog can be positive or negative for a specific blood type. Using DEA 1.1 as an example, RBCs from a single dog can either display the 1.1 antigen, denoted DEA 1.1 positive, or not display it, denoted DEA 1.1 negative. Several other blood groups are described in dogs, but

Advanced Monitoring and Procedures for Small Animal Emergency and Critical Care, First Edition. Edited by Jamie M. Burkitt Creedon, Harold Davis.
© 2012 John Wiley & Sons, Inc. Published 2012 by John Wiley & Sons, Inc.

Protocol 53.1 Canine (DEA 1.1) blood type: DMS card

Items Required
- Whole blood (in EDTA)
- Autoagglutination saline screen card (provided in kit)
- Pipette (provided in kit)
- Wooden stirrer (provided in kit)
- Diluent (provided in kit)
- Rapid-Vet H (Canine 1.1) card (provided in kit)

Procedure
Autoagglutination saline screen
1. Apply one drop of diluent and canine whole blood (in EDTA) to well.
2. Mix thoroughly with provided wooden stick for 10 seconds.
3. Rock card to a slight angle looking for agglutination.
   - If negative, proceed to DEA 1.1 typing.
   - If positive, see text.

Procedure
1. Apply one drop of diluent into each well.
2. Apply one drop of canine whole blood (in EDTA) into each well (patient, positive control, negative control).
3. Mix each test thoroughly with a wood stick for 10 seconds; use a separate stick or stick end for each well so not to cross-contaminate.
4. Rock the card for 1 minute; observe for agglutination.

Interpretation

DEA 1.1 Positive	Hemagglutination in Patient Test Well
DEA 1.1 Negative	No hemagglutination in Patient Test well
DEA 1.1 Positive Control	Hemagglutination should be seen
DEA 1.1 Negative Control	No hemagglutination should be seen

Protocol 53.2 Feline (AB) card blood type

Items Required
- Whole blood (in EDTA)
- Rapid Vet H (Feline A, B, AB) blood typing card (provided in kit)
- Pipette (provided in kit)
- Wooden stirrer (provided in kit)
- Diluent (provided in kit)

Procedure
1. Apply one drop of diluent and feline whole blood (in EDTA) to well marked Auto-Agglutination Saline Screen.
2. Mix thoroughly with wooden stick for 10 seconds.
3. Rock card to a slight angle looking for agglutination.
   - If negative, proceed to number 4.
   - If positive, see text.
4. Apply one drop of diluent into each of the two remaining wells labeled Patient Test.
5. Apply one drop of feline whole blood (in EDTA) into each of the wells.
6. Using a new wooden stick stirrer, press firmly downward so to spread and mix the material within the entirety of the well.
7. Repeat with the other well using a *new* wooden stirrer.
8. Add a *second* drop of diluent to the well labeled type A.

   Do not stir the fluid in this well a second time.

9. Rock the card for 1 minute or less until hemagglutination has occurred in one of the Patient Test wells. Take care not to cross-contaminate the samples within the wells.

Interpretation

Blood type A	Strong hemagglutination in well labeled type A.
Blood type B	Strong hemagglutination in well labeled type B.
Blood type AB	Strong hemagglutination in wells labeled type A and type B.

typing reagents are available for only a handful, including DEA 3, 4, 5, 7, and, more recently, the *Dal* blood type.[1–4,8,9] Testing for these other blood groups is typically performed only by some commercial blood banks or academic veterinary hospitals.[5,10]

Little is known about the potential functions these antigens serve or their biochemical makeup in dogs, but their potential antigenicity has been well described.[5–9,11] In dogs, naturally occurring alloantibodies (antibodies formed against a RBC antigen the recipient *lacks*, i.e., non-self antigen) are seen infrequently and are not considered clinically relevant.[12] Transfusion of a RBC-containing product, either packed pRBCs or WB, can cause a dog to produce alloantibodies to the non-self RBC antigen(s) present in the transfused product. For example, a DEA 1.1 negative patient who receives donor DEA 1.1 positive RBCs will produce anti-DEA 1.1 alloantibodies against the DEA 1.1 antigen. This is true for other DEA types as well. Alloantibodies are typically formed in as few as 4 days to as long as months, following exposure to the novel antigen.[3,4,6,7] Identification of these alloantibodies is accomplished with a crossmatch

Protocol 53.3 Feline AB slide typing

Items Required
- Whole blood (in EDTA)
- Three glass slides
- Plastic pipettes (four minimum)
- Serum or plasma from a type B cat (Anti-A reagent; see text)
- *Triticum vulgaris* lectin solution (Anti-B reagent; see text)
- Buffered saline

Procedure
1. Label the three slides A, B, and C.
2. To slide A, add 2 drops of anti-A reagent (B cat serum or plasma).
3. To slide B, add 2 drops of anti-B reagent.
4. To slide C, add 2 drops of PBS or buffered saline.
5. Add 1 drop of patient whole blood to each of the three slides without contacting the liquid on the slide.
6. Gently rock each slide and observe for hemagglutination.

Interpretation

Type A:	Hemagglutination on slide labeled A
Type B:	Hemagglutination on slide labeled B
Type AB:	Hemagglutination on slides labeled A and B
Autoagglutination	Hemagglutination on slide labeled C. This indicates red blood cells need to be washed (Protocol 53.5).

test. Where blood typing identifies specific antigens on the RBC surface (i.e., DEA 1.1 positive or negative), a crossmatch test detects these alloantibodies against RBC antigen(s) present in the plasma or serum. Alloantibodies may result in destruction of the donor RBCs and a shortened lifespan for the transfused RBCs. A second exposure to the DEA 1.1 antigen (i.e., in the form of a pRBC or WB transfusion) would result in more rapid production of additional anti-DEA 1.1 alloantibodies with destruction of RBCs.[3–7] It was once believed that previous pregnancy in female dogs could result in significant production of red cell alloantibodies; this has been shown not to be the case.[13]

DEA 1.1 is considered the most antigenic canine RBC antigen (i.e., the most capable of provoking an immunologic response from the recipient), so potential canine donors or transfusion recipients should be blood typed to determine whether they are DEA 1.1 positive or negative. In-clinic blood typing methods for DEA 1.1 exist that allow for blood type–specific transfusions. If recipi-

ent blood type cannot be determined, DEA 1.1 negative whole blood or packed red blood cells should be administered. A pretransfusion recipient blood sample should be drawn. The sample can be used for later DEA 1.1 blood typing; transfused RBCs could potentially alter test results if a significant volume of blood is transfused and the donor and recipient are of different DEA 1.1 blood types. In the event of a hemolytic transfusion reaction, collection of a pretransfusion recipient blood sample may also be useful for retrospectively evaluating pretransfusion recipient–donor compatibility. This is typically reserved for cases where a pretransfusion crossmatch test was not performed.

DEA 1.1 blood typing

Two in-clinic tests are available for canine blood typing.

DMS card test for DEA 1.1

A blood typing card test, RapidVet-H (Canine DEA 1.1) (DMS Laboratories, Inc., Flemington, NJ) is available for in-hospital blood typing of dogs. The DMS card identifies dog blood as either DEA 1.1 positive or negative. Canine RBCs that display DEA 1.1 surface antigen react with a lyophilized murine monoclonal antibody on the test card; RBCs lacking the surface antigen will not react. The observation of strong hemagglutination (Fig. 53.1). DEA 1.1 positive blood type indicates the blood sample, and thus the dog being tested is DEA 1.1 positive. Autoagglutination due to RBC autoantibody in diseases such as immune-mediated hemolytic anemia (IMHA) must be ruled out prior to performing the test. Because hemagglutination is the positive end point of the card blood typing test, as described earlier, hemagglutination due to autoagglutination could not be distinguished from hemagglutination from a DEA 1.1 positive blood sample. A DEA 1.1 negative dog with autoagglutination could be misclassified as DEA 1.1 positive. A separate card, provided by the manufacturer, serves as the autoagglutination screen. Autoagglutination saline screen provides three separate wells for testing. The card can be cut so different patients can be tested, minimizing waste. The presence of autoagglutination in a potential recipient's sample would warrant washing of the recipient's RBCs prior to repeating the test (Protocol 53.5). Given the subjectivity of hemagglutination grading as well as the potential for an adverse transfusion outcome, the use of DEA 1.1 negative donor blood may be a better option in patients with autoagglutination.

The benefits of the DMS card method for canine blood typing include rapid turnaround (<2 minutes) as well as reliable results. Test kits can be purchased

Protocol 53.4 Tube crossmatch procedure

Items Required
- Patient whole blood (in EDTA) with or without patient serum
- Donor whole blood (can be from segment; segments are sections of blood-filled plastic tubing coming from the blood collection bag)
- Centrifuge (capable of 1000 × g or 3400 rpm)
- Disposable pipettes
- 3–5× magnification lens (optional)
- Normal or buffered saline
- Optional: Microscope, microscope slides, coverslips

Preparation of a 3%–5% red cell suspension for patient and blood donor(s)
1. Label a 12 × 75 mm tube with recipient or donor identification (ID).
2. Pipette approximately 2 drops of whole blood (or 1 drop of packed red blood cells) into tube.
3. Fill tube approximately three-quarters full with buffered or normal saline. Mix thoroughly.
4. Centrifuge (1000 × g or 3400 rpm) for 60 seconds.
5. Aspirate or decant the supernatant saline from the red blood cells.
6. Repeat steps 3–5 two additional times.
7. After the last wash, decant the supernatant and centrifuge the red cells for 15 additional seconds to prepare a packed cell button.
8. Fill the tube approximately three-quarters full (4 mL) with buffered or normal saline. Mix thoroughly. The red cell suspension should have the appearance of red Kool-Aid.

Tube Preparation
Major crossmatch
1. Label a test tube with donor ID and word *Major*.
2. Add 2 drops of patient serum or plasma.
3. Add 1 drop of donor RBC suspension.

Minor Crossmatch
1. Label a test tube with donor ID and word *Minor*.
2. Add 2 drops of donor serum or plasma.
3. Add 1 drop of patient RBC suspension.

Recipient Autocontrol
1. Label a test tube with patient ID and *Patient AC*.
2. Add 2 drops of patient serum or plasma.
3. Add 1 drop of patient RBC suspension.

Donor Autocontrol
1. Label a test tube with donor ID and *Donor AC*.
2. Add 2 drops of donor serum or plasma.
3. Add 1 drop of patient RBC suspension.

Incubation and Centrifugation
1. Shake each tube gently to mix the contents within.
2. Cover each tube or the entire group with plastic or Parafilm to prevent condensation from entering any of the tubes.
3. Incubate all tubes at 37° C for 15 minutes.
4. Centrifuge (1000 × g or 3400 rpm) the tubes for 15 seconds.
5. Read each tube and grade according to the chart below. Reactions should be read in a well-lit area, preferably with a white background to maximize visualization. A 3 × 5 magnification lens can be used, if needed.

Grading
1. Remove one tube from the centrifuge at a time, taking care not to dislodge the red cell button.
2. Note the color of the supernatant. Free hemoglobin (red-tinged supernatant) greater than the amount in the original blood sample denotes hemolysis. Hemolysis is considered a *positive* reaction.

(Continued)

3.   While viewing the tube and red cell button, gently shake the tube back and forth to dislodge the red cell button.
4.   Observe the manner in which the red cells leave the button.
5.   Microscopic evaluation (optional): For samples lacking obvious macroscopic (visual to the naked eye) hemagglutination, a drop of the resuspended RBC-plasma mixture is placed on a microscope slide followed by a coverslip and evaluated at ×40.

Grade the reaction based on the following criteria:

Result	Description
Negative	No hemagglutination
Negative	Rouleaux* (see below)
Positive	Hemolysis
Positive microscopic	Negative macroscopic
	Red cell aggregates (look like clusters of grapes rather than stacks of coins)
Weak positive	Minimal hemagglutination
1+	Small red cell aggregates
2+	Small and large red cell aggregates
3+	Many large red cell aggregates
4+	One solid button of red cells

*Suspected rouleaux ("stacked coin" appearance) must be confirmed by saline replacement as follows:

1.   Recentrifuge the tube containing suspected rouleaux.
2.   Remove the residual serum/plasma.
3.   Resuspend the cells using 2 drops of normal saline.
4.   Centrifuge for 15 seconds.
5.   Read and grade reaction as above. If hemagglutination persists, it suggests true incompatibility. If hemagglutination resolves, it confirms rouleaux.

Note: True red cell antigen-alloantibody reactions will not disperse with the addition of saline.

Tube/test	Result	Interpretation
Recipient Autocontrol	Positive	Patient has formed autoantibodies against self RBCs; these autoantibodies may also cause hemagglutination of donor RBCs in vitro and/or in vivo. Recommend finding a compatible donor or the "least incompatible" donor (hemagglutination in major is less than in autocontrol).
Recipient Autocontrol	Negative	No detectable autoantibodies.
Major (Recipient)	Positive	Recipient of intended whole blood or pRBCs has alloantibodies against an antigen(s) on the donor RBC surface. *Do not use this donor's red blood cells.*
Major (Recipient)	Negative	Recipient of intended whole blood or pRBCs is compatible with donor RBCs.
Minor (Recipient)	Positive	Donor has alloantibodies against patient RBCs. <ul><li>Donor screening should exclude donors who have previously received blood products so to decrease the risk of alloantibody production.</li><li>This could reflect an AB blood type incompatibility in a cat if not properly blood typed prior to crossmatch testing.</li><li>In cats, the presence of non-AB blood type alloantibodies may result in a positive minor crossmatch.</li></ul>
Minor (Recipient)	Negative	Donor plasma does not contain detectable alloantibodies to recipient RBCs.
Rouleaux	Present	Hemagglutination that disperses following saline replacement suggests an increase in plasma proteins is causing red blood cells to loosely aggregate. This is not thought to be of clinical relevance in transfusion of red blood cells.

Protocol 53.5 Washing of red blood cells

Items Required
- Whole blood (in EDTA)
- Centrifuge
- Saline
- Pipette(s)

Procedure
1. Pipette approximately 2 drops of whole blood or packed red blood cells into 12 × 75 mm tube.
2. Fill tube approximately three-quarters full with buffered or normal saline. Mix thoroughly.
3. Centrifuge (1000 × g or 3400 rpm) for 60–90 seconds.
4. Aspirate or decant the supernatant saline from the red blood cells.
5. Repeat steps 2–4 two additional times.
6. After the last wash, decant the supernatant and centrifuge the red cells for 15 additional seconds to prepare a packed cell button.

individually or in larger numbers. Severely anemic samples, those with a packed cell volume (PCV) of 15% or less could cause a false-negative result (i.e., weak or absent hemagglutination in a DEA 1.1 positive sample. This, however, provides relatively minimal risk to the

patient that is DEA 1.1 positive and who can safely receive DEA 1.1 positive or DEA 1.1 negative blood; if mistyped as DEA 1.1 negative, DEA 1.1 negative blood would be given. A sample of whole blood can be concentrated by removing some plasma to mimic a more normal PCV so to blood type the patient accurately.

Quick Test DEA 1.1

A second in-clinic DEA 1.1 blood type test is also available. The Quick Test DEA 1.1 (Alvedia, Lyon, France) is an immunochromatographic cartridge system for DEA 1.1 typing. It uses a membrane containing a monoclonal antibody to the DEA 1.1 antigen; capillary action, under the influence of a buffer, results in migration of the erythrocytes on the membrane. Red cells positive for DEA 1.1 will be retained resulting in a red band in the middle of the membrane. DEA 1.1 negative RBCs are not retained in the membrane; thus no red band appears. An internal control for the test is manifestation of a red band (Fig. 53.2).

Proposed advantages of this Quick Test include fast turnaround (<2 minutes) and the ability to perform a blood type test even in samples exhibiting autoagglutination.[14] The Quick Test cartridge traps agglutinated RBCs at the start of the test so that only nonagglutinated cells migrate through the membrane and participate in testing. Even anemic samples can be blood typed; removal of some plasma to approximately a more normal PCV is still an option as in the DMS card typing procedures.

The Quick Test (Alvedia) and the RapidVet-H DEA 1.1 (DMS Laboratories) blood typing card were recently

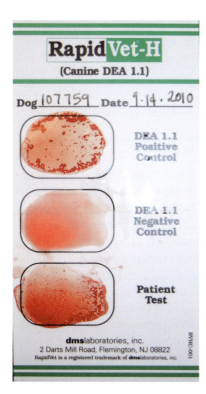

Figure 53.1 The observation of strong hemagglutination DEA 1.1 positive blood type indicates the blood sample, and thus the dog being tested is DEA 1.1 positive.

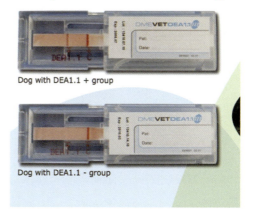

Figure 53.2 Quick Test DEA 1.1 positive and negative. Examples of dogs with DEA 1.1 positive (top) and a DEA 1.1 negative (bottom) blood are shown.

evaluated and compared with other methods typically reserved for larger clinical laboratory settings.[14] In this comparison, the accuracy of the quick test was 93%, slightly better than the DMS typing card. The Quick Test resulted in a few false negatives (DEA 1.1 positive dogs typed incorrectly as 1.1 negative); this occurred primarily in samples demonstrating autoagglutination, possibly from trapping of the majority of erythrocytes. The DMS card displayed both a few false-positive results and false-negative results. Overall, the study revealed good agreement when performed by experienced personnel between the various tests when judged against the laboratory technology. Ease of interpretation was considered superior with the Quick Test DEA 1.1 (Alvedia).

Feline blood types

The AB blood group system, the most widely recognized blood group system in cats, includes blood types A, B, and AB. Although similar in name, these are unrelated to the human ABO blood types. Blood type prevalence varies both by geographic location and between cat breeds (Table 53.1).[15]

In the United States, feline blood type A is the most common with fewer numbers of type B cats; type AB cats are uncommon, occurring only within the relatively small population of cats that exhibit the B type.[15,16] Greater percentages of type B cats are seen on the West Coast compared with the East Coast of the United States, and relatively higher proportions of type B cats are present in other countries.[15,16]

Feline blood type A or B is determined by the presence of certain RBC membrane glycolipids; type AB contains a mixture of both types.[17-20] Unlike dogs, by 1–2 months of age, cats produce alloantibodies against RBC antigens they lack without prior sensitization from a blood transfusion.[21] Because blood transfusion is not required for the production of these antibodies, they are referred to as "naturally occurring" alloantibodies. The presence of these naturally occurring alloantibodies necessitates blood typing prior to all blood transfusions in cats. High levels of strong antibodies capable of both hemolysis and hemagglutination of type A RBCs are produced by type B cats.[21] As little as 1 mL of type A blood transfused into a type B cat can result in death.[21-23] Type A cats also produce anti-B alloantibodies, which are present in varying levels and are of various strengths depending on the cat.[21,23] Type AB cats do not produce anti-A or anti-B alloantibodies because they recognize both antigens as "self."[18]

There are other indications for blood typing in cats in addition to blood transfusion. Neonatal isoerythrolysis results from type A or type AB kittens ingesting the colostrum from a type B queen. The kittens, following colostrum ingestion, absorb strong anti-A antibodies; these anti-A antibodies result in hemolysis, severe anemia, and potentially death in blood type A and blood type AB kittens.[24-26] Type B kittens are unaffected. AB blood type determination of queens is advised, especially in breeds with a relatively high proportion of type B cats.

AB blood typing

In-house feline AB blood typing is possible using either a slide test (Protocol 53.3) or using a commercial blood typing kit. Necessary reagents for the slide test include serum from a type B cat, used as the anti-A solution, and a prepared solution of *Triticum vulgaris* lectin (Sigma Chemical Co., Product L9640, St. Louis, MO), used as the anti-B solution.[17,19,27] *Triticum vulgaris*, a wheat germ lectin, when prepared at a specific concentration, preferentially causes agglutination of type B feline RBCs. A stock solution is prepared: 25 mg of lyophilized *Triticum vulgaris* lectin powder is resuspended in 12.5 mL of 0.9% saline and kept frozen. To prepare the slide solution, 32 µL of stock solution is added to 968 µL of 0.9% saline resulting in a concentration of 64 µg/mL. The prepared slide solution can be divided into aliquots; one aliquot is kept at 4°C for testing purposes. Others can be thawed

Table 53.1 Frequencies of type A and B cats in the United States[15,16]

Breed	Type A	Type B	Breed	Type A	Type B
Abyssinian	84%	16%	Maine Coon	97%	3%
American Shorthair	100%	0%	Norwegian Forest	93%	7%
Birman	82%	18%	Oriental Shorthair	100%	0%
British Shorthair	64%	36%	Persian	86%	14%
Burmese	100%	0%	Scottish Fold	81%	19%
Cornish Rex	67%	33%	Siamese	100%	0%
Devon Rex	59%	41%	Somali	82%	18%
Exotic Shorthair	73%	27%	Sphinx	83%	17%
Himalayan	94%	6%	Tonkinese	100%	0%
Japanese Bobtail	84%	16%	Turkish Angora	50%	50%

as needed.[19,27] The slide test allows for rapid determination of blood type as long as all reagents are readily available; it also evaluates for autoagglutination.

Two commercial blood type kits are available for AB blood group typing: the RapidVet-H Feline (DMS Laboratories) and the Quick Test A + B (Alvedia).

RapidVet-H (Feline)

The RapidVet-H Feline (DMS Laboratories) blood typing card is used for determination of blood types A, B, or AB in cats. It contains three wells: a control well, an anti-A well, and an anti-B well. The presence of autoagglutination is determined in the control well prior to determination of blood type. The anti-A well, used to identify type A red cells, contains lyophilized murine monoclonal antibody against the A-antigen. The anti-B well, used to identify type B erythrocytes, contains the *Triticum vulgaris* lectin. Hemagglutination in a well indicates the cat's red blood cells display that RBC antigen; that is, hemagglutination in the anti-A well indicates the cat's red blood cells displays blood type A.

The presence of autoagglutination would require washing of red cells prior to testing or confirmation with another blood type method (Protocol 53.5).

Quick Test A + B (Feline)

Similar to the typing system for dogs, the Quick Test is an immunochromatographic cartridge system. Monoclonal antibodies specific to red cell antigens A and B are present in the membrane. Red blood cells migrate on the membrane under the influence of a buffer and capillary action. The anti-A and anti-B antibodies present in the membrane will bind the corresponding red blood cells, resulting in a red band under the corresponding letter A or B on the kit. Type AB red cells would result in two lines. A control band present in the membrane and denoted with a 'C' must appear to ensure a successful test.

The RapidVet-H Test Feline (DMS Laboratories) and the Quick Test A + B (Alvedia) were recently compared to each other and to other test methodologies for AB blood determination.[28]

Both the Quick Test and the DMS card misidentified some cats, but both tests generally provided accurate typing results.[28] The ease of interpretation of the Quick Test was seen as an advantage. Type AB cats posed a greater challenge in definitive determination of blood type.

Crossmatch testing

The crossmatch test is performed to determine blood component compatibility between blood donor and recipient with the primary objective of selecting donor units that will provide the maximum benefit (and the minimum harm) to the patient. Major and minor crossmatch tests are performed *in vitro*; crossmatch-compatible blood products are selected in an effort to prolong RBC lifespan and efficacy *in vivo*.

Typically, a crossmatch test is performed between the intended recipient and potential donor(s) when the patient has received blood in the past, roughly >4 days prior. An unknown transfusion history is another indication for compatibility testing. There is some debate regarding when to crossmatch and which patients to crossmatch. Most would agree, given the absence of significant naturally occurring alloantibodies in dogs, a crossmatch test is only indicated when a canine patient has been previously transfused. The distinction is less obvious for cats. It has been demonstrated that some cats have naturally occurring alloantibodies *outside the AB blood group designations.*[29] Despite AB compatibility, plasma from these cats causes hemagglutination of red blood cells; this indicates a non-AB alloantibody has been formed against a RBC antigen other than blood type A or B. The *Mik* red cell antigen has been described in three unrelated feline blood donors that were all type A and had never received a blood transfusion.[29] Inadvertent transfusion of *Mik*-positive RBCs into a *Mik*-negative recipient resulted in an acute hemolytic transfusion reaction, demonstrating the clinical relevance of non-AB red cell antigens and alloantibodies. Other non-AB, non-*Mik* red cell antigens are also suggested by incompatible crossmatch results.[30,31] Overall, naturally occurring, non-AB alloantibodies occur in a relatively small proportion of cats; therefore, crossmatch testing of all cats prior to transfusion may be unnecessary.

Crossmatch testing cannot prevent all hemolytic transfusion reactions or prevent decreased red blood cell survival in recipients that produce alloantibodies following transfusion. Even with blood type specific blood, the potential exists for acute or delayed hemolytic transfusions. For additional information about monitoring patients for transfusion reactions, see Chapter 59, Administration of Biologic Products.

Crossmatch tests are more time consuming and more technically challenging than blood typing procedures, especially given commercially available blood typing kits. Also, lack of standardization of the crossmatch test procedures and test result interpretation complicates matters.[32] The tube crossmatch has been considered the gold standard for years in human blood banking; in many blood banks, however, it has been replaced with a gel column technology. Whereas the tube crossmatch requires a minimum amount of equipment, gel column crossmatch requires specialized equipment and specially prepared gel column test cards; it is typically reserved for larger clinical laboratories and commercial blood banks.[10] Crossmatch test procedures for in-clinic crossmatch testing include the tube crossmatch and a commercially available RapidVet-H Crossmatch Test Kit (DMS Laboratories), which is a modified gel test (see Protocol 53.4).

Although the tube crossmatch includes many steps and some basic laboratory skills, it is relatively straightforward. The crossmatch test includes, for each potential blood donor, both a major and minor crossmatch. For the major crossmatch, recipient plasma or serum is incubated with donor RBCs in a 3%–5% suspension with saline; this is the most important reaction along with the recipient autocontrol. The major crossmatch tests for alloantibodies in recipient plasma or serum against a potential blood donor; hemagglutination or hemolysis indicates a positive reaction and incompatibility between the two. The recipient autocontrol allows for evaluation of autoantibody, similar to the purpose of an autoagglutination screen in blood typing; it utilizes recipient plasma or serum and recipient RBC suspension. A negative or compatible result is expected for the minor crossmatch where recipient RBC suspension and donor plasma or serum is incubated. The ideal blood donor should have no history of prior RBC or plasma transfusions; the formation of alloantibodies is very unlikely in a dog that has never received a transfusion. This is also true in cats for the most part, but a non-AB blood group alloantibody is a possibility in cats that have never been transfused. In addition to understanding the terminology of crossmatch tests, two of the biggest challenges are preparing an appropriate RBC suspension and grading of the reactions. Protocol 53.4 describes preparation of a RBC suspension. Many describe the appropriate color similar to the appearance of red Kool-Aid (Fig. 53.3). For reaction grading, gentle resuspension of the red cell button is key with continued observation; vigorous shaking could result in the observer missing the reaction (i.e., a false negative). A lack of RBC agglutinates is considered a negative or compatible reaction. Macroscopic hemagglutination, which is visible to the naked eye, is graded according to the provided chart in the protocol (Fig. 53.4). A 2+ incompatible reaction is occurring in the tube on the left and the tube on the right (patient autocontrol) reveals no hemagglutination. In Figures 53.5 and 53.6, a 3+ and 4+ hemagglutination incompatible reaction are present, respectively indicating incompatibility between blood donor and recipient. In both images, the tube on the left shows no hemagglutination. If no macroscopic agglutination is observed, some recommend evaluation

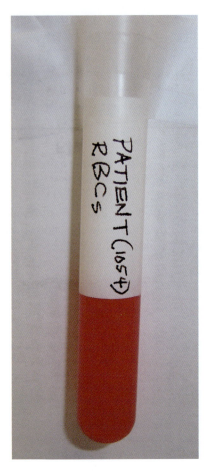

Figure 53.3 Appropriate RBC suspension color.

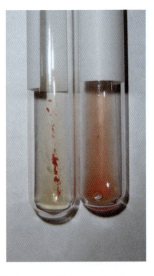

Figure 53.4 A 2+ incompatible reaction is occurring in the tube on the left and the tube on the right (patient autocontrol) reveals no hemagglutination.

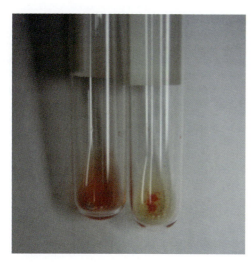

Figure 53.5 3+ incompatible reaction in tube on right. Patient autocontrol (tube on left) is negative.

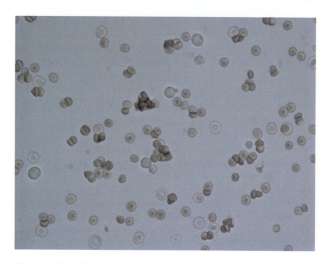

Figure 53.7 Positive microscopic hemagglutination, 40×.

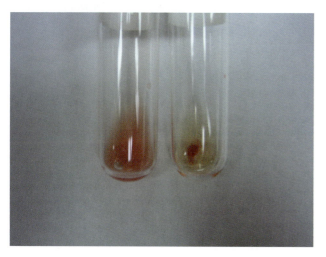

Figure 53.6 4+ incompatible reaction in tube on right. Patient autocontrol (tube on left) is negative.

microscopically; a drop of the resuspended mixture is evaluated at ×40 and graded as positive or negative. Aggregates or grape-like clusters of RBCs are considered an incompatible reaction (Fig. 53.7). The tube cross-match procedure does require practice and takes some skill in accurate interpretation.

The RapidVet-H Companion Animal Crossmatch Test Kit Major is available from DMS Laboratories. The provided kit comes with a thorough set of instructions as well as centrifuge specifications because the final step of the gel requires a certain type of centrifuge. It offers a more standardized approach for both the procedure itself and the interpretation step. Visit the DMS website for the complete instructions and information regarding this methodology.[33]

Familiarity with both blood typing and crossmatch testing are essential to the practice of veterinary transfusion medicine. Knowledge of blood types in both cats and dogs allows for informed donor selection and screening and decreases the risk of a hemolytic transfusion reaction in an intended recipient. Commercially available blood typing tests are available for both dogs and cats; they can be performed in a veterinary clinic, offer fast turnaround, and are relatively simple to use. In some situations when recipients have a prior transfusion history, a crossmatch test is indicated. Although commercial blood typing tests allow for determination of AB blood type and DEA 1.1 blood type in cats and dogs, respectively, a recipient can produce alloantibodies to other RBC antigens following a blood transfusion. A crossmatch test is needed, prior to subsequent transfusions, to test for these alloantibodies. Crossmatch test protocols are more time consuming and less standardized than blood types but are equally necessary in some patients.

References

1. Vriesendorp HM, Albert ED, Templeton JW, et al. Joint report of the Second International Workshop on Canine Immunogenetics. Transplant Proc 1976;8:289–314.
2. Vriesendorp HM, Westbroek DL, D'Amaro J, et al. Joint report of 1st International Workshop on Canine Immunogenetics. Tissue Antigens 1973;3:145–163.
3. Swisher SN, Young LE. The blood group system of dogs. Physiol Rev 1961;41:295–314.
4. Swisher SN, Bull R, Bowdler J. Canine erythrocyte antigens. Tissue Antigens 1973;3:164–165.
5. Giger U, Gelens CJ, Callan MB, et al. An acute hemolytic transfusion reaction caused by dog erythrocyte antigen 1.1 incompatibility in a previously sensitized dog. J Am Vet Med Assoc 1995;206:1358–1362.

6. Young LE, Ervin DM, Yuile CL. Hemolytic reactions produced in dogs by transfusion of incompatible dog blood and plasma; serologic and hematologic aspects. Blood 1949;4:1218–1231.

7. Young LE, Yuile CL, et al. Observations on hemolytic reactions produced in dogs by transfusion of incompatible dog blood. J Clin Invest 1948;27:563.

8. Blais MC, Berman L, Oakley DA, et al. Canine *Dal* blood type: a red cell antigen lacking in some Dalmatians. J Vet Intern Med 2007;21:281–286.

9. Callan MB, Jones LT, Giger U. Hemolytic transfusion reactions in a dog with an alloantibody to a common antigen. J Vet Intern Med 1995;9:277–279.

10. Kessler RJ, Reese J, Chang D, et al. Dog erythrocyte antigens 1.1, 1.2, 3, 4, 7, and Dal blood typing and cross-matching by gel column technique. Vet Clin Pathol 2010;39:306–316.

11. Melzer KJ, Wardrop KJ, Hale AS, et al. A hemolytic transfusion reaction due to DEA 4 alloantibodies in a dog. J Vet Intern Med 2003;17:931–933.

12. Hale AS. Canine blood groups and their importance in veterinary transfusion medicine. Vet Clin North Am Small Anim Pract 1995;25:1323–1332.

13. Blais MC, Rozanski EA, Hale AS, et al. Lack of evidence of pregnancy-induced alloantibodies in dogs. J Vet Intern Med 2009;23:462–465.

14. Seth M, Winzelberg S, Jackson KJ, et al. Comparison of gel column, card and cartridge techniques for DEA 1.1 blood typing of dogs (abstr). J Vet Intern Med 2008;22(3):775.

15. Giger U, Kilrain CG, Filippich LJ, et al. Frequencies of feline blood groups in the United States. J Am Vet Med Assoc 1989;195:1230–1232.

16. Giger U, Bucheler J, Patterson DF. Frequency and inheritance of A and B blood types in feline breeds of the United States. J Hered 1991;82:15–20.

17. Andrews GA CP, Smith JE, Rich L. N-glycolylneuraminic acid and N-acetylneuraminic acid define feline blood group A and B antigens. Blood 1992;79:7.

18. Auer L, Bell K. The AB blood group system of cats. Anim Blood Groups Biochem Genet 1981;12:11.

19. Griot-Wenk M, Pahlsson P, Chisholm-Chait A, et al. Biochemical characterization of the feline AB blood group system. Anim Genet 1993;24:401–407.

20. Griot-Wenk ME, Callan MB, Casal ML, et al. Blood type AB in the feline AB blood group system. Am J Vet Res 1996;57:1438–1442.

21. Bucheler J, Giger U. Alloantibodies against A and B blood types in cats. Vet Immunol Immunopathol 1993;38:283–295.

22. Giger U, Akol KG. Acute hemolytic transfusion reaction in an Abyssinian cat with blood type B. J Vet Intern Med 1990;4:315–316.

23. Giger U, Bucheler J. Transfusion of type-A and type-B blood to cats. J Am Vet Med Assoc 1991;198:411–418.

24. Bucheler J. Fading kitten syndrome and neonatal isoerythrolysis. Vet Clin North Am Small Anim Pract 1999;29:853–870, v.

25. Casal ML, Jezyk PF, Giger U. Transfer of colostral antibodies from queens to their kittens. Am J Vet Res 1996;57:1653–1658.

26. Giger U, Casal ML. Feline colostrum—friend or foe: maternal antibodies in queens and kittens. J Reprod Fertil Suppl 1997;51:313–316.

27. Butler MAG, Smith JE. Reactivity of lectins with feline erythrocytes. CompHaematol Int 1991;1:217–219.

28. Seth M, Jackson KJ, Giger U. Comparison of gel column, card, cartridge, slide and tube techniques for AB blood typing of cats [abstract]. J Vet Intern Med 2008;22(3):741.

29. Weinstein NM, Blais MC, Harris K, et al. A newly recognized blood group in domestic shorthair cats: the *Mik* red cell antigen. J Vet Intern Med 2007;21:287–292.

30. Weingart C, Giger U, Kohn B. Whole blood transfusions in 91 cats: a clinical evaluation. J Feline Med Surg 2004;6:139–148.

31. Henson MS, Kristensen AT, Armstrong PJ, et al. Feline blood component therapy: Retrospective study of 246 transfusions. American College of Veterinary Internal Medicine, 12th Congress, San Francisco, CA, 1994.

32. Scott M, et al. Standard crossmatching protocol. Association for Veterinary Hematology and Transfusion Medicine, American College of Veterinary Internal Medicine, 21st Congress, Charlotte, NC; 2003.

33. RapidVet-H Companion Animal Crossmatch Test Kit Major. http://www.rapidvet.com/xmatch.htm (accessed December 12, 2010).

SECTION VIII

Infection control

54

Minimizing nosocomial infection

Amanda K. Boag and Katherine Jayne Howie

Nosocomial infections are infections that develop more than 48 hours after a patient has been hospitalized or that occur in a patient who has been hospitalized in the 2 weeks prior to the current admission.[1] The term healthcare- (or hospital-)associated infection (HAI) is now being recommended to describe infections associated with healthcare delivery in any setting.[2] This reflects the difficulty in determining with certainty where the pathogen was acquired in many patients; the terms may be used interchangeably. As nosocomial infections are by definition acquired in a healthcare setting, the veterinary team and especially technicians who spend most time interacting with the patient have a very important role to play in minimizing their occurrence.

Nosocomial infections have been a major problem in human healthcare for many years. Latest figures from the Centers for Disease Control and Prevention (CDC) suggest HAI occur in 1.7 million human patients a year with an annual cost of more than $30 billion. They are responsible for approximately 99,000 deaths annually, making HAI one of the top 10 leading causes of death in the United States.[3] Both in the United States and Europe, HAI have been found to occur with the greatest frequency in patients in the intensive care unit (ICU).[4] The incidence of nosocomial infections in the field of small animal veterinary medicine is not known but appears to be increasing.[5,6]

It is thought that factors associated with an increased risk of acquiring a nosocomial infection in human hospitals are also likely to be associated with increased risk in veterinary patients. In particular these include the more intensive treatment of critically ill animals with increasing use of invasive devices such as urinary and intravenous (IV) catheters, increased duration of hospitalization, increase in intensive care techniques such as mechanical ventilation, and the wider use of antimicrobial and immunosuppressive drugs.[7-8] A high veterinary technician-to-patient ratio is also a risk factor in some studies.[9] Importantly, many of the bacteria that cause nosocomial infection are normal commensal organisms that may be found on the skin/mucosa or in the gastrointestinal tract of normal healthy dogs and cats. These healthy animals are described as being colonized. Although the relationship between colonization and subsequent infection is complex, patients entering an ICU with prior colonization may be at higher risk of subsequent infection and may act as reservoirs for other noncolonized patients.[10,11]

Nosocomial infections may complicate the course of both medical and surgical diseases. They may range from mild superficial skin infections to infection causing sepsis and septic shock. In human medicine, common nosocomial infection sites include blood stream infections (previously known as septicemia), urinary tract infections, surgical wound infections, infectious diarrhea, and pneumonia. This would seem to be similar in veterinary medicine, although nosocomial pneumonia appears anecdotally to be less common. This may reflect the fact that relatively few veterinary patients undergo long-term mechanical ventilation.

Although many bacterial species can cause nosocomial infections, including some that are easy to treat, a proportion of nosocomial infections are caused by bacteria that are resistant to multiple antibiotics. These bacteria are of

Advanced Monitoring and Procedures for Small Animal Emergency and Critical Care, First Edition. Edited by Jamie M. Burkitt Creedon, Harold Davis.
© 2012 John Wiley & Sons, Inc. Published 2012 by John Wiley & Sons, Inc.

particular concern as they are often difficult and expensive to treat. Moreover, they may represent a zoonotic risk to veterinary staff attending infected patients as well as being a risk to other patients in the ICU.

Bacteria causing nosocomial infection

Nosocomial infections may be caused by a large number of bacterial species. Much of the published information focuses on infection with specific multidrug-resistant bacteria (as described below), and infections caused by these pathogens can be particularly challenging to treat. However, these infections remain relatively rare in clinical veterinary medicine. In the authors' experience, these bacteria are the cause of a small but significant proportion of veterinary HAI.

Methicillin-resistant Staphylococcus aureus (MRSA)

MRSA is one of the most significant bacteria causing nosocomial infection in human medicine and has been identified with increasing frequency in veterinary patients since it was first reported in 1999.[12] Staphylococci are gram-positive cocci that are a common commensal of mucosa and skin and do not typically cause disease in healthy individuals. In unwell humans and animals, they can cause a wide range of infections including postoperative wound infections, infection of implants, infections associated with catheters, endocarditis, and sepsis. The antimicrobial methicillin was first used in human clinical practice in 1959, and the first human case of MRSA infection was identified in 1961.[13] Although methicillin is no longer used clinically, the majority of MRSA strains are also resistant to most other commonly used antibiotics, making infections hard to treat once they have occurred. Genetic analysis of MRSA isolates show that new strains have arisen on only a very small number of occasions; most infections are caused therefore by transmission of the bacteria from one individual to another. Moreover, the majority of MRSA strains isolated from small animal veterinary patients are identical to human hospital-acquired strains, and it is highly likely that humans are ultimately the source. Veterinary staff (including technicians) may be at higher risk of colonization with MRSA than the general human population with colonization rates of approximately 10% being reported in several studies.[14–15] Veterinary patients may also become colonized with MRSA, although the frequency and duration of colonization is unknown. There is also good evidence that MRSA can be passed between pet animals and owners with the possibility for zoonotic infections.[16–17] The

problem of MRSA is evolving in the human field with recent identification of new strains of community acquired MRSA with increased ability to cause disease and new hospital strains with even more marked antimicrobial resistance, including to the drug vancomycin.[18] To date, these strains have not been identified in veterinary patients.

Methicillin-resistant *S. pseudintermedius* (previously known as *S. intermedius)* has been reported recently as causing disease in canine and feline patients[19,20]; the emergence of resistant *S. pseudintermedius* is potentially a greater concern to veterinary patients as it is the principle staphylococcal species colonizing healthy dogs.

Extended spectrum beta-lactamase Escherichia coli (ESBL E. coli)

E. coli is a gram-negative bacteria that is a commensal of the gastrointestinal tract. Multidrug-resistant *E. coli* (including ESBL *E. coli*) is emerging as a significant public health concern in human medicine. Reports of ESBL *E. coli* causing clinical disease in veterinary patients are limited[21–22]; however, it may be under-reported as veterinary microbiology laboratories rarely identify them specifically. Cultures of fecal samples from healthy dogs and pet therapy dogs have identified colonization by ESBL *E. coli*.[23–24] As with other bacteria this is likely to represent a risk factor for subsequent infection. *E. coli* is commonly implicated in nosocomial infections, especially urinary tract infections, and a recent publication reported that 67% of bacteria isolated from IV catheter tip cultures were coliform bacteria.[25] Prolonged ICU stay has also been shown to be associated with increasing proportions of resistant *E. coli* isolates from rectal swabs in veterinary patients.[26] ESBL *E. coli* is of particular concern as they are resistant to many different antibiotics including the third-generation cephalosporins, limiting the choice of therapy for these pathogens to carbapenems (e.g., imipenem) and occasionally aminoglycosides.

Vancomycin-resistant enterococcus

Vancomycin-resistant enterococcus (VRE) is another multidrug-resistant bacterium that can cause nosocomial infection. To date, there have been very few cases of clinical infection reported in veterinary medicine,[27–28] but it has been found to colonize a small proportion of healthy dogs in both Europe and the United States.[29] Enterococci form part of the normal human and animal gut flora. They are gram-positive cocci with *E. faecium* and *E. faecalis* being the most frequent isolates. *E. faecium* is generally more resistant than *E. faecalis*. VRE was first identified in human hospitals in the United

States in the 1980s. There is little clinical experience with it in small animal patients, but treatment is likely to be very challenging as VRE is generally resistant to all antibiotics. In some cases (e.g., urinary tract infection), the animal may manage to clear the infection itself if the underlying cause/predisposing factors for the infection can be resolved.

Transmission of infection and colonization

The majority of bacteria that cause nosocomial infection exist as commensal organisms in healthy individuals as well as pathogenic organisms. It is well recognized that the hands of healthcare workers represent the main mode of transmission of these bacteria between patients with the main reservoir being other infected or colonized patients or colonized healthcare workers.[30] The percentage of veterinary staff and animals entering our clinics that are colonized is unknown; however, it is safe to say that it is not zero. All strategies to minimize nosocomial infection must recognize this fact.

Contamination of the environment may also play a role in infection with veterinary staff picking up bacteria from environmental surfaces and transferring them to patients. Survival of bacteria in the environment varies with bacterial species, but it is known that MRSA can survive in conditions similar to those found in the hospital environment for long periods of time (days) and that thorough cleaning of the environment is necessary to control outbreaks of MRSA.[31]

Airborne transmission is thought to be much less important for the majority of nosocomial infections. It is possible that veterinary staff could become colonized by inhaling MRSA and can then transmit the infection to other patients.

Control strategies for nosocomial infection

Considering the potential for nosocomial infection to cause increased morbidity and mortality, infection control measures and prevention strategies are a key part of the management of nosocomial infections. Technician and nursing staff have a vitally important role to play in this. Evidence-based information specifying the importance of different control measures does not currently exist in the veterinary literature; however, there is a wealth of information from the human field including several guidelines focused on control of particular bacteria.[32,33] A major challenge with interpreting published reports is that the majority of studies of successful control involve implementation of multiple interventions concurrently, making it difficult to compare the efficacy and importance of each individual intervention.

Many of the principles employed will be of benefit in the control of all nosocomial infections. When designing a strategy for your clinic to minimize nosocomial infection, the following should all be considered:

- Hand hygiene
- Environmental hygiene
- Barrier nursing technique and isolation
  - Including identification of at-risk patients
- Antimicrobial stewardship

Hand hygiene

Diligent hand hygiene is arguably the single most important measure used in the control of nosocomial infection.[34] Although the need and technique for surgical scrubbing is well recognized, techniques for hand hygiene outside the surgical suite are often overlooked, and experience suggests that hand hygiene is often a neglected priority in day-to-day veterinary practice. As people become increasingly concerned about and educated in the need for good hygiene practices to reduce the risk of hospital-acquired infections in human health care, they also expect the same high standards to be applied to their animals.

The importance of good hand hygiene has been recognized for over 150 years. A Hungarian obstetrician working in Vienna named Ignaz Semmelweis first suggested it was important in 1847. He noted that puerperal fever was more common on a maternity ward staffed by medical students and doctors than one staffed by midwives. The medical students and doctors worked in other areas of the hospital including the morgue, whereas the midwives did not. Semmelweis introduced a policy of requiring all medical students and doctors to wash their hands before entering the maternity ward. Although very unpopular with the doctors, the infection and mortality rate in Semmelweis's hospital dropped dramatically, from ~20% to around 1%-2% when handwashing was introduced. Unfortunately, the importance of Semmelweis's discovery was not widely recognized until after his death.

Hand hygiene can be performed in a number of ways, including

- Hand washing with plain soap and water
- Antiseptic hand washing
- Using alcohol-based hand rubs
- Surgical hand hygiene/antisepsis

The aim of all hand hygiene procedures is to reduce the number of potentially pathogenic bacteria on the hands.

There are two major groups of microorganisms found on skin, which are the following.

- **Transient (contaminating) flora.** This refers to bacteria that do not usually live on the skin but may be found on the skin for short periods of time. Typically, these bacteria are acquired onto the hands following contact with the environment, other patients/people, or colonized sites on the same person (e.g., nose). Most nosocomial infections are caused by transient flora, which can be easily removed by hand washing.
- **Resident (colonizing) flora.** This refers to bacteria that live on healthy skin. They are not normally pathogenic and help protect the skin from invasion by pathogenic species. Rarely, however, they can cause infection, usually following surgery or other invasive procedures. They are difficult to remove completely, but their numbers are minimized by a surgical hand scrub.

Hand washing alone will remove dirt and a proportion of loose transient bacteria. An antiseptic hand wash or use of an alcohol hand rub combines hand washing with an antiseptic solution. Both transient and resident micro-organisms will be killed. Furthermore, the multiplication of resident flora is also temporarily reduced if the antiseptic has persistent or residual activity. Surgical hand hygiene describes the conventional presurgical scrub procedure. This takes longer to perform than a simple antiseptic hand wash but leads to a greater reduction in resident flora. When nursing critical care patients, an antiseptic hand wash or use of an alcohol hand rub represents the most appropriate form of hand hygiene in the majority of situations.

There are a number of antiseptic products used for hand hygiene in veterinary practice. The most commonly used solutions are chlorhexidine, iodophors (e.g., povidone-iodine), and triclosan. They are all acceptable, although the iodophors in particular do not work well in the presence of organic matter; thus a thorough hand wash with soap and water must be done first.

How to perform a hygienic hand wash

Although it sounds simple, numerous studies have shown that hand washing is rarely performed correctly. To be effective, all surfaces of the hand and wrist must be washed. If using an antiseptic, it must also be in contact with the skin for a suitable period of time according to the manufacturer's instructions, which for a chlorhexidine-based solution, for example, is typically 1 minute. The most effective way to ensure all parts of the hand are cleaned is to follow a staged hand wash protocol (see Protocol 54.1), illustrated in Figure 54.1.

When a protocol is not followed routinely, hand washing is often inadequately performed with some areas of the hands not cleaned properly. The efficacy

---

Protocol 54.1 How to perform an antiseptic hand wash

Use free-flowing water at a temperature suitable for thorough wetting and rinsing of hands.
1. Wet hands thoroughly and apply the antiseptic solution
2. Rub hands together palm to palm
3. Rub right palm over back of left hand and vice versa
4. Rub hands together palm to palm with fingers interlaced
5. Bend and interlock fingers (as if holding hands with yourself)
6. Clean thumbs by grasping right thumb in left palm and vice versa
7. Use fingers of right hand to rub left palm focusing on base of left fingers and vice versa
8. Use left hand to rub right wrist and vice versa (optional)

- **Faucets** should be turned off using a no-touch technique.
- Hands should be dried using paper toweling.
- Paper toweling should be disposed of in a foot-operated pedal bin.
- The whole process should take around one minute.

---

of a hand-washing protocol can be tested using hand creams that fluoresce under UV light if not properly washed off (e.g., www.glitterbug.com, www.germjuice.com).

Hand rubs

Complete and diligent hand washing takes a real amount of time to perform, and in a busy critical care environment it can be difficult to achieve on all the occasions in which it is required. Alcoholic hand rubs are an alternative to antiseptic hand washing that can be used provided the hands are not grossly dirty; that is, hands must be free of visible dirt, blood, or other proteinaceous material or body fluids. Recent recommendations in the human field suggest use of an alcohol-based hand rub is the preferred means for hand hygiene in most clinical situations.[35,36] Alcohol hand rubs usually contain a combination of an alcohol (typically 60%-95% ethanol or isopropanol), an antiseptic agent such as chlorhexidine, and an emollient. Both liquid and gel formulations are available and can be bought as wall dispensers or small bottles. The rub is applied to all parts of the hands (using a protocol similar to that used for antiseptic hand washing) for 15–20 seconds and the hands are allowed to air dry. Their use may be encouraged by wearing the small bottles on clinical clothing and/or by placing them strategically on kennel doors (see Fig. 54.2).

The advantages of alcohol-based hand rubs compared with antiseptic hand washing include a reduction in the

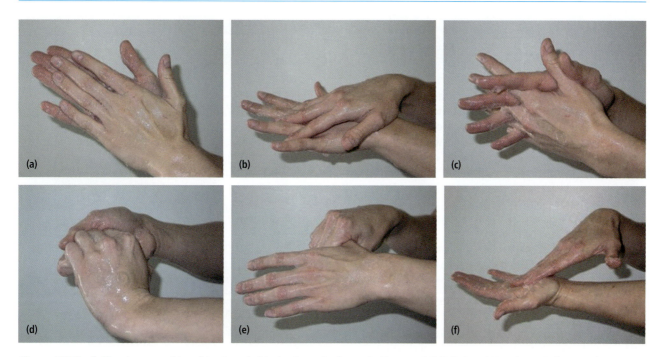

Figure 54.1a–f The six steps of hand hygiene (with thanks to Professor S. Gregory, MRCVS, Royal Veterinary College, UK).

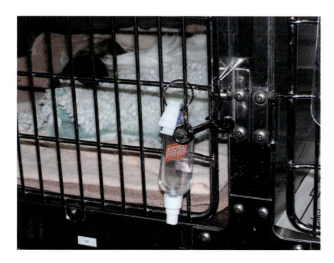

Figure 54.2 An alcohol hand rub placed on a kennel door.

time taken to complete effective hand hygiene, more rapid action, and less skin irritation. Alcohol-based hand rubs also do not require the presence of a sink or hand-drying facilities. All of these factors have been demonstrated to improve hand hygiene compliance in human medicine.[37,38]

Regardless of the technique chosen, it is important that fingernails are kept short and clean and any cuts or abrasions are covered with waterproof dressings. Artificial nails should not be used.[39,40] All jewelry (other than a plain wedding band) and wristwatches should be removed, and sleeves should be short.

Timing of hand hygiene and use of gloves

There are many occasions on which hand hygiene should occur (see Box 54.1).[41] For basic care procedures such as physical examination, correct use of an alcohol hand rub or diligent washing with soap and water using a routine process (see Protocol 54.1) is sufficient. Soap and water should always be used if the hands are visibly soiled and after the healthcare worker performs any personal hygiene procedures such as visiting the bathroom. An alcohol hand rub *or* an antiseptic hand wash should be performed before touching wounds or performing invasive procedures and after dealing with infected or contaminated patients or tissues. Use of gloves can reduce the bacterial contamination of hands as well as acting as barrier protection during contact with body fluids. Gloves do not, however, provide complete protection against hand contamination; this may occur via small defects in the glove or via contamination of the hands during glove application and removal. Gloves should be worn whenever it can be reasonably anticipated that there will be contact with potentially infectious material or nonintact skin. Gloves should be removed after each

Box 54.1 Hand hygiene guidelines

Hand hygiene should be carried out
- Before and after touching or examining the patient*
- Before and after touching any invasive devices such as intravenous catheters and urinary catheters*
- After contact with any body fluids or excretions, mucosal surfaces, nonintact skin, or wound dressings*
- If moving from a contaminated/infected body site to another body site of the same patient*
- After contact with inanimate objects in the immediate vicinity of the patient
- Before handling medication or preparing food
- When arriving and leaving work
- Before and after performing any personal hygiene procedures such as visiting the bathroom or blowing the nose
- Before and after eating
- Before and after removing gloves

*Glove use should be considered if there is a high risk that the hands may come into contact with potentially infectious material or nonintact skin.

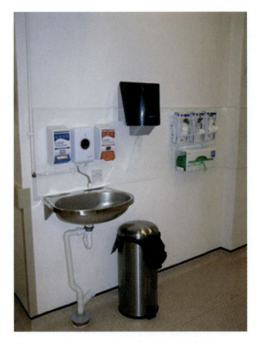

Figure 54.3 An appropriate area for hand washing in a veterinary clinic.

procedure and if moving from a contaminated to another body site on the same patient. Hands should always be washed after removing gloves, and glove use should *not* reduce the frequency of hand washing. If hands are known to have become heavily contaminated with infected fluids during patient treatment, a full surgical scrub may be performed.

Despite the fact that it is acknowledged that hand washing is the single most important means of preventing nosocomial infections, there are major problems regarding compliance. Numerous studies in human hospitals show that many hospital care workers fail to perform hand hygiene at appropriate times.[42,43] Studies of poor compliance in human hospitals reveal that there are many factors associated with poor hand hygiene compliance, including being a doctor or nursing assistant (as opposed to a nurse), being male, working in a critical care environment, a high intensity of patient care, wearing gloves and gowns, undertaking activities with a high risk of cross-transmission, being too busy and failing to think about it, lack of easy availability of facilities such as sinks, and skin irritation with frequent washing.[42] A lack of knowledge is also often highlighted with some reports of skepticism about the effectiveness of hand hygiene and lack of knowledge of hospital protocols.[42] Additional perceived barriers include lack of role models[44] and low institutional

priority with lack of administrative sanctions for noncompliers.[45]

Methods to improve hand hygiene compliance include education and teaching with constant reinforcement within the workplace, getting senior staff to set a good example, and making sure the staff-to-patient ratio is favorable. The introduction of conveniently placed alcohol hand rubs, removing the need to hand wash after every patient contact and allowing opportunities for hand hygiene remote from washing facilities, also facilitates compliance. Good hand hygiene is vitally important and should be adopted by all those working in clinical veterinary medicine (see Fig. 54.3). It is easy to perform, and if done well will result in a minimization of risk of nosocomial infection. Technicians have a large role to play both in ensuring they themselves comply and in reminding the rest of the veterinary team as to its importance.

Environmental cleaning

Although the principle route of infection for most nosocomial infections involves transmission of bacteria from one infected or colonized person or patient to another on healthcare workers' hands, the role of the environment should not be ignored. The environment may act as a source for contamination of healthcare worker's hands. Many of the bacteria that cause nosocomial infection can survive in the environment for prolonged periods of time.

Although specific responsibility for environmental cleaning may reside with one group of staff, all staff should take some degree of responsibility for maintaining a clean clinical environment, and the policy of "clean as you go" should be adopted. This also applies to senior staff, who should set an example of good practice. Positive feedback is also extremely important, and the value of performing a cleaning task well should never be overlooked. All clinics should have a clear cleaning schedule with checks to ensure regular cleaning is being performed.

Floors and all surfaces should be cleaned at least once daily. Floors should be constructed of nonporous, nonslip materials, and ideally the junction between floor and wall should be curved to facilitate cleaning. Gross debris should be swept or vacuumed up and the floors cleaned with a disinfectant that is ideally virucidal, bacteriocidal, mycocidal, nonirritant, noncorrosive, and nonstaining (see Chapter 56, Antiseptics, Disinfectants, and Sterilization, for more information). Disinfectants should be used according to the manufacturer's instructions; although there is a limited evidence, it is recommended that their use should be rotated on a regular schedule to prevent resistance.[46] Mops should be kept clean and replaced on a regular basis. Mop buckets should be emptied and rinsed after each use and should also undergo regular full bucket disinfection. Floors should be deep cleaned on a regular basis with the frequency dependent on use and soiling.

Examination and operating tables should be disinfected after each use, using a suitable disinfectant with properties similar to those used on the floor. As most disinfectants are not effective in the presence of organic matter, any gross contamination should be removed using soap and water first.

Work surfaces in clinical areas and kennels should be constructed of material that can be thoroughly cleaned and is impervious to disinfectant. Seams should be sealed to prevent accumulation of contaminated material, and junctions should be rounded to facilitate cleaning. They should be regularly disinfected at least twice daily but more regularly if they become soiled. If soiling is heavy, they may need to be cleaned more than once before the area is reused; the use of more than one disinfectant can be considered for synergistic effects. Similarly to patients with any infection, movement of patients between kennels should be minimized. Sinks and showers must be kept clean, and in hard water areas lime scale should be controlled and soap scum removed daily with a scouring preparation. Areas not immediately visible, for example, the tops of kennels, should not be forgotten, and the cleaning schedule should include a frequent (e.g., weekly) general cleaning and inspection of these areas.

Garbage bins used for clinical waste should be covered and the cover should be foot-operated and not allowed to overflow. Soap, antiseptics, and paper towels should be replenished daily and fresh supplies stored for easy access if supplies run out. Animal bedding should be cleaned of gross soiling and then washed using a hot cycle (60°C, 140°F) with a biological washing powder. Drying in a hot tumble dryer is recommended. If the bedding has been exposed to an animal with a known infectious disease, it may need to be soaked in a suitable disinfectant for a period of time before laundering. If heavily soiled, it may be disposed of or washed and then autoclaved before returning to use. Feeding bowls should also be made of a material that can be disinfected. The use of disposable (cardboard) feeding bowls should be considered for patients with any infectious condition, including nosocomial disease.

Recently, there has been a focus on the concept of "high hand touch areas." This refers to areas very close to the patient that are often touched just before or after a patient contact.[47] Examples include infusion pumps, kennel doors, and monitoring equipment. Door handles, medical records, computers, and telephones are also considered to be high hand touch regions. These areas, although usually superficially clean, may be at greatest risk of becoming contaminated with bacteria due to their proximity to the patient and the high frequency with which staff touch them. They should be cleaned more regularly than other sites; some authorities recommend 4× daily wiping with soapy water. Medical equipment used for physical examination (e.g., stethoscopes, thermometers) may also be considered in the same way. Hand rubs should also be readily available near these sites.

Barrier nursing and isolation

All practices should have facilities and policies for isolation and barrier nursing. These facilities may be used for animals with a known infectious disease but also on occasion for patients with a known risk of contracting an infectious disease, for example, unvaccinated or immunosuppressed animals. Barrier nursing may also be used for patients in which there is a high index of suspicion for a nosocomial infection prior to receipt of microbiological culture results, for example, those with chronic nonhealing wounds that have received multiple courses of antibiotics. Evidence to support strict isolation as opposed to enforcement of strict barrier nursing procedures or cohort nursing is lacking in many human studies.[48,49]

True isolation facilities are completely self-contained areas that do not share an air space with other animal accommodation. As the facility must be completely self-contained, it must have its own equipment for feeding, nursing, and cleaning, including hot and cold water, medical supplies, and an examination table. Not all practices have an area that fulfills all these requirements, and guidelines must be adapted for the local situation.

For animals where strict isolation is not required, barrier nursing may be more appropriate. This may include patients where an increased level of vigilance is appropriate to protect the animal from infection or where the animal has a known infection but is considered a low contagious risk. Barrier nursing may be provided within a separate ward or a partitioned area of an existing ward. It should be remembered that animals that are isolated are inevitably barrier-nursed; however, not all animals that are barrier-nursed are effectively isolated.

Regardless, each animal being isolated or barrier-nursed should have dedicated equipment. Any equipment can act as a fomite and facilitate transmission to other patients.[50] The isolation or barrier-nursing area should have dedicated leads or leashes, thermometers, and stethoscopes. As far as possible equipment including bedding and feeding bowls used in this area should be disposable, and robust cleaning protocols should be in place for any equipment that will be used subsequently with other patients. If bedding is to be reused, it should be clearly identifiable as belonging to the isolation area; for example, it may be a color different from that used in the rest of the clinic. The location of the medical record should also be considered; if paper records are used, they should not then be carried to other sites in the clinic. Dedicated pens should be used.

Isolated patients should not have contact with other patients. If canine patients are allowed outside, it should be to an area that is not frequented by other canine patients. Procedures such as radiography or ultrasound that must be carried out in other areas of the clinic should be scheduled for the end of the day, and all staff involved should be alerted as to the nature of the patient's disease. These areas should be thoroughly cleaned after use.

Staffing of isolation areas will depend on the size of the clinic. Ideally, one technician should be allocated to this area and this technician should have minimal responsibilities in other animal areas, especially with any high-risk patients. Protective clothing (disposable overalls and/or aprons, rubber boots or shoe covers, disposable gloves, masks, and caps) should be worn when entering the area and must be removed on exit (see Fig. 54.4). For true isolation areas, a foot bath containing an

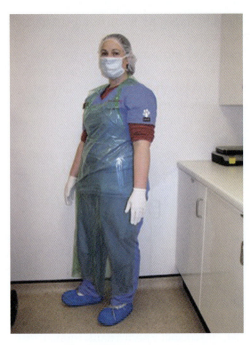

Figure 54.4 Clothing appropriate for use in an isolation area or when barrier nursing a patient.

appropriate disinfectant should be available on entry and exit of the area. Personal and environmental hygiene must be strict and all waste must be disposed of safely. Staff and owners should be apprised of any possible zoonotic risks, and owners should be allowed to enter only in exceptional circumstances. If owners are allowed to visit, they should observe the same hygiene and clothing precautions as staff members. Notices should be placed at the entrance of the isolation area or around the barrier nursing area clearly stating what measures must be instituted on entry (see Protocol 54.2). The veterinarian in charge of the case should consider carefully when to examine the patient dependent on his or her other patients and daily tasks; generally, examining the patient at the end of the working day reduces the risk of transmission to other patients.

The cost of isolating or barrier nursing patients is high in terms of both consumables and staffing, and therefore additional fees should be set and owners apprised of this. Owners should also be warned that highly intensive monitoring and treatment, which may otherwise be available, may not be possible to deliver in the isolation unit.

In some instances, it may be preferable or necessary to treat a patient with a nosocomial infection as an outpatient. Many patients with nosocomial infections are clinically well and with appropriate owner information and consent may be managed at home. It is vital that the

Protocol 54.2 Suggested rules for use with a barrier nursed/isolated patient

Rules for isolation area
1. Only designated personnel should enter the isolation unit; visitors are permitted only with the express permission of the attending clinician and must be accompanied at all times.
2. Protective clothing should be worn when entering the area and should include:
   - Disposable plastic apron or gown
   - Plastic overshoes
   - Disposable gloves
   - Caps and masks
3. All protective clothing should be removed and disposed of on exiting the isolation area.
4. Hands should be cleaned (antiseptic hand wash) both before entering and on leaving the isolation area.
5. All patients in the isolation area should be allocated a lead/leash, stethoscope, feeding utensils, litter tray (if appropriate), and thermometer for their sole use. These should be kept together in a plastic box and sterilized/disinfected between patients.
6. Medications must not be removed from the isolation area.
7. All clinical waste should be disposed of in the garbage bin within the isolation area and the bag should be sealed and double-bagged before removal from the area.
8. Disposable bedding should be used.
9. The isolation area must be thoroughly cleaned once the patient has been discharged.

owners are educated as to zoonotic risks and that if there are any concerns that humans in the animal's environment are at risk, advice should be sought from medical professionals as to whether management at home is appropriate from the human health perspective. If patients are dealt with on an outpatient basis, it is essential that they are clearly identifiable on revisits. Owners should be educated to wait outside the clinic until their appointment time to reduce the risk of transmission to other patients in the waiting room. As far as possible, revisits should be scheduled for the end of the day to allow thorough cleaning of the consult room following the visit.

Antimicrobial stewardship

Antimicrobials are commonly prescribed drugs and are often used on an empirical basis, especially while awaiting microbiological culture results. In human medicine approximately one third of hospitalized patients receive antimicrobial therapy at some point in their hospital stay, and a significant proportion of this use is unnecessary or inappropriate.[51,52] Moreover, studies have shown that inappropriate antibiotic use is associated with higher mortality, which is not necessarily reversed if the antibiotic is changed once culture results are known.[53,54] Although this information does not exist for the veterinary field, it seems likely that the figures are similar. The use of most common antimicrobials is rarely associated with adverse effects for that individual patient; most of the commonly prescribed drugs have a high therapeutic index and it is easy to feel that by prescribing an antibi-

otic we "may be doing some good and are unlikely to be doing harm" to the individual patient. However, viewed on a population basis and considering the rise of antimicrobial resistance, this thinking should be carefully questioned.

Antibiotic therapy may contribute to an increase in antibiotic resistance in a number of ways:

1. Some bacteria contain genes encoding inducible resistance; the presence of certain antimicrobials may induce synthesis of enzymes that inactivate that drug and potentially other drugs as well.
2. More importantly, the use of antimicrobials (especially broad-spectrum antimicrobials) alters selection pressures. Any commensal or colonizing microbes that display mechanisms of resistance will enjoy a selective advantage. New mechanisms of resistance arise rarely, but the use of antimicrobials encourages the dissemination of pre-existing resistant strains. The clustering of multiple resistance genes on plasmids and other genetic elements makes the problem especially challenging, as exposure to one antimicrobial may coselect for bacteria that are resistant to several unrelated agents.[55]

For most important nosocomial infections (i.e., MRSA, VRE, and ESBL *E. coli*), prior colonization of the skin, mucosa, or gastrointestinal tract with that bacteria results in a much-increased risk of nosocomial infection with the multidrug-resistant strain.[56,57]

Numerous studies in human medicine suggest that prior use of antimicrobials is a major risk factor for a multidrug-resistant infection. Certain classes of antimicrobials appear to be particularly associated with subsequent development of resistant infections. For MRSA and ESBL *E. coli* prior use of fluoroquinolones and cephalosporins (especially third-generation cephalosporins) have been consistently identified as a risk factor in various groups of patients.[58,59] For VRE, third-generation cephalosporins and antibiotics with potent anti-anaerobic activity have been implicated.[60] Other studies have shown a reduction in rates of drug-resistant infections when use of antimicrobials has been controlled or restricted.[61–62] The data are sometimes difficult to interpret, as most studies are done in human hospitals in the face of increasing infection rates where multiple control strategies are implemented concurrently. However, it is widely accepted that rational antimicrobial use is an important step in helping reduce resistant infection rates. Of the drug classes most commonly identified in human medicine that are associated with increased rates of resistant infections, both the fluoroquinolones and cephalosporins are frequently used in small animal medicine. The evidence available in the small animal veterinary field regarding the role of antimicrobial use is less strong. One study documented changes in fecal flora in dogs hospitalized in a veterinary ICU and showed that the proportion of dogs colonized with resistant bacteria increased with duration of hospitalization regardless of antimicrobial use. Dogs that were treated with enrofloxacin were 25.6 times more likely to be colonized by a resistant strain.[63] Other studies of the bacteria causing urinary tract infection in dogs have shown increasing levels of resistance.[64,65]

Thus it is clear that to minimize the risk of nosocomial infection, the use of antimicrobials should always be considered carefully. Although technicians are not responsible for prescribing drugs, it is reasonable to question doctors on their decision making. It is also important that when antimicrobials are prescribed they are used at an appropriate dose and given at the correct time intervals.[66] Following up on culture results with adjustment of antimicrobial therapy, if necessary, is also vitally important.

Role of screening for pathogenic bacteria

Screening involves taking microbiological samples from the environment, patients, or staff to look for the presence of multidrug-resistant bacteria.

Environmental screening to ensure that cleaning has been effective may be a useful technique to support measures to minimize nosocomial infection. Interpretation

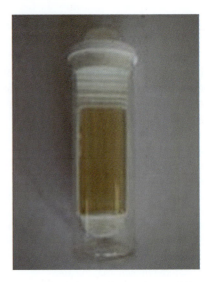

Figure 54.5 Agar dipslide, which may be used for quantitative screening of environmental cleanliness.

of environmental screening results must be undertaken carefully and with knowledge of the screening methodology used. It is not reasonable to expect a hospital environment to be sterile, and assessment of the amount of bacteria present may be as important as whether they are present at all. Quantitative assessment of microbiological load at high hand touch sites may be carried out using agar-impregnated slides (see Fig. 54.5) with the agar used chosen to reflect the microbe of interest.[55]

Screening of patients prior to hospital admission has been used in human medicine as a control strategy for certain microbes, notably MRSA. Some European countries (e.g., Denmark, Holland) have very low MRSA infection rates largely because they have a comprehensive screening program for both patients and staff.[67] Patients are screened before admission for elective procedures, and if found to be positive for MRSA, the procedure is delayed until the person is decolonized. Although this technique has worked very well for minimizing nosocomial infection with MRSA in these areas, it relies on a well-controlled and well-funded public health system and is therefore not currently applicable to veterinary medicine.[68] It also minimizes the risk of infection only with the bacteria that is being screened for rather than reducing the global infection risk.

Screening of staff may also be discussed but has many challenges associated with it. As with patient screening, it minimizes risk associated only with a single bacterial species. Furthermore, identifying that a member of staff is colonized does not necessarily mean that the person is a source of infection; if the basic measures of good hand hygiene and appropriate barrier nursing as described above are carried out, then a colonized staff member should pose minimal risk. Screening of staff is recommended only in the face of an outbreak, and advice should be sought from human healthcare professionals and infectious disease specialists prior to embarking on this process.

Summary

Nosocomial infections can cause significant morbidity and mortality and can lead to increased expense and stress for owners. It is likely that as critical care continues to develop within veterinary medicine and we treat increasing numbers of high risk patients, nosocomial infections will become more common. Moreover, many of these infections may be with multidrug-resistant organisms, and the age of relying on ever more powerful antibiotics seems to be drawing to a close. To minimize the risk of nosocomial infection, it is vitally important that we utilize multiple infection-control strategies based on an understanding of the epidemiology and transmission of these microbes. Diligent hand washing, good environmental cleaning, and appropriate barrier nursing and isolation are all key parts of an infection control strategy where technicians have a very large role to play.

References

1. Crowe MJ, Cooke EM. Review of case definitions for nosocomial infection—towards a consensus. J Hosp Infect 1998;39:3–11.
2. Siegel JD, Rhinehart E, Jackson M, et al. Guidelines for isolation precautions: preventing transmission of infectious agents in healthcare settings. 2007. Available at: http://www.cdc.gov/hicpac/2007IP/2007isolationPrecautions.html2007. Accessed July 2, 2010.
3. Centers for Disease Control and Prevention website. Available at http://www.cdc.gov/hai/index.html. Accessed July 2, 2010.
4. Hildron AI, Edwards JR, Patel J, et al. Antimicrobial-resistant pathogens associated with healthcare-associated infections: annual summary of data reported to the National Healthcare Safety Network at the Centers for Disease Control and Prevention 2006–2007. Infect Cont Hosp Epidem 2008;29:996–1011.
5. Rich M, Roberts L. MRSA in companion animals. Vet Rec 2006;159:535–536.
6. Ogeer-Gyles J, Mathews KA, Boerlin P. Nosocomial infections and antimicrobial resistance in critical care medicine. J Vet Emerg Crit Care 2006;16:1–18.
7. Warren DK, Kollef MH, Seiler SM, et al. The epidemiology of vancomycin-resistant Enterococcus in a medical intensive care unit. Infect Control Hosp Epidemiol 2003;24:238–241.
8. Oztoprak N, Cevik M, Akinci E, et al. Risk factors for ICU-acquired methicillin-resistant Staphylococcus aureus infections. Am J Infect Control 2006;34:1–5.
9. Stone PW, Pogorzelska M, Kunches L, et al. Hospital staffing and healthcare associated infections: a systematic review of the literature. Clin Infect Dis 2008;47:937–944.
10. Safdar N, Bradley E. The risk of infection after nasal colonization with Staphylococcus aureus. Am J Med 2008;121:310–315.
11. Linden PK. Enterococci: resistance update and treatment options. In: Owens RC Jr, Lautenbach E, eds. Antimicrobial Resistance: Problem Pathogens and Clinical Countermeasures, Informa Healthcare, New York, 2008:89–110.
12. Tomlin J, Pead MJ, Lloyd DH, et al. Methicillin-resistant Staphylococcus aureus infections in 11 dogs. Vet Rec 1999;144:60–64.
13. Jevons PE "Celbenin"-resistant staphylococci. BMJ 1961;1:124–125.
14. Loeffler A, Boag AK, Sung J, et al. Prevalence of methicillin-resistant Staphylococcus aureus among staff and pets in a small animal referral hospital in the UK. J Antimicrob Chemother 2005;56:692–697.
15. Anderson ME, Lefebvre SL, Weese JS. Evaluation of prevalence and risk factors for methicillin-resistant Staphylococcus aureus colonization in veterinary personnel attending an international equine veterinary conference. Vet Microbiol 2008;129:410–417. staphylococci in companion animals. Emerg Infect Dis 2005;11:1942–1944.
16. Anderson ME, Lefebvre SL, Weese JS. Evaluation of prevalence and risk factors for methicillin-resistant Staphylococcus aureus colonization.
17. Strommenger B, Kehrenberg C, Kettlitz C, et al. Molecular characterization of methicillin-resistant Staphylococcus aureus strains from pet animals and their relationship to human isolates. J Antimicrob Chemother 2006;57:461–465.
18. Gonzalez BE, Rueda AM, Shelburne SA 3rd, et al. Community-associated strains of methicillin-resistant Staphylococccus aureus as the cause of healthcare-associated infection. Infect Control Hosp Epidemiol 2006;27:1051–1056.
19. Sasaki T, Kikuchi K, Tanaka Y, et al. Methicillin-resistant Staphylococcus pseudintermedius in a veterinary teaching hospital. J Clin Microbiol 2007;45:1118–1125.
20. Loeffler A, Linek M, Moodley A, et al. First report of multiresistant, mecA-positive Staphylococcus intermedius in Europe: 12 cases from a veterinary dermatology referral clinic in Germany. Vet Dermatol 2007;18:412–421.
21. Sanchez S, McCrackin Stevenson MA, Hudson CR, et al. Characterization of multidrug-resistant Escherichia coli isolates associated with nosocomial infections in dogs. J Clin Microbiol 2002;40:3586–3595.
22. Sidjabat HE, Townsend KM, Hanson ND, et al. Identification of bla(CMY-7) and associated plasmid-mediated resistance genes in multidrug-resistant Escherichia coli isolated from dogs at a veterinary teaching hospital in Australia. J Antimicrob Chemother 2006;57:840–848.
23. Costa D, Poeta P, Brinas L, et al. Detection of CTX-M-1 and TEM-52 beta-lactamases in Escherichia coli strains from healthy pets in Portugal. J Antimicrob Chemother 2004;54:960–961.
24. Sidjabat HE, Townsend KM, Lorentzen M, et al. Emergence and spread of two distinct clonal groups of multidrug-resistant Escherichia coli in a veterinary teaching hospital in Australia. J Med Microbiol 2006;55:1125–1134.
25. Marsh-Ng ML, Burney DP, Garcia J. Surveillance of infections associated with intravenous catheters in dogs and cats in an intensive care unit. J Am Anim Hosp Assoc 2007;43:13–20.
26. Ogeer-Gyles J, Mathews KA, Sears W, et al. Development of antimicrobial drug resistance in rectal Escherichia coli isolates from dogs hospitalized in an intensive care unit. J Am Vet Med Assoc 2006;229:694–699.

27. Boerlin P, Eugster S, Gaschen F, et al. Transmission of opportunistic pathogens in a veterinary teaching hospital. Vet Microbiol 2001;82:347–359.

28. Pressel MA, Fox LE, Apley MD, et al. Vancomycin for multi-drug resistant *Enterococcus faecium* cholangiohepatitis in a cat. J Fel Med Surg 2005;7:317–321.

29. Herrero IA. Dogs should be included in surveillance programs for vancomycin-resistant enterococci. J Clin Microbiol 2004;42:1384–1385.

30. Boyce JM, Pittet D. Guidelines for hand hygiene in health care settings: recommendations of the healthcare infection control practices advisory committee and the HICPAC/SHEA/APIC/IDSA Hand Hygiene Task Force. Infect Control Hosp Epidemiol 2002;23:1–48.

31. Wagenvoort JHT, Sliuijsmans W, Penders RJR. Better environmental survival of outbreak vs. sporadic MRSA isolates. J Hosp Infec 2000;45:231–234.

32. Muto CA, Jernigan JA, Ostrowsky BE, et al. SHEA Guideline for preventing nosocomial transmission of multidrug-resistant strains of *Staphylococcus aureus* and *Enterococcus*. Infect Control Hosp Epidemiol 2003;24:362–386.

33. Coia JE, Duckworth GJ, Edwards DI, et al. Guidelines for the control and prevention of meticillin-resistant *Staphylococcus aureus* (MRSA) in healthcare facilities. J Hosp Infect 2006;63:S1–S44.

34. Boyce JM, Pittet D. Guidelines for hand hygiene in health care settings: recommendations of the healthcare infection control practices advisory committee and the HICPAC/SHEA/APIC/IDSA Hand Hygiene Task Force. Infect Control Hosp Epidemiol 2002;23:1–48.

35. Pittet D, Allegranzi B, Boyce J, et al. The World Health Organization guidelines on hand hygiene in health care and their consensus recommendations. Infect Control Hosp Epidemiol 2009;30:611–622.

36. Picheansathian W. A systematic review of the effectiveness of alcohol-based solutions for hand hygiene. Int J Nurs Pract 2004;10:3–9.

37. Larson EL, Aiello AE, Bastyr J, et al. Assessment of hand hygiene regimens for intensive care unit personnel. Crit Care Med 2001;29:944–951.

38. Maury E, Alzieu M, Baudel JL, et al. Availability of an alcohol solution can improve hand disinfection compliance in an intensive care unit. Am J Respir Crit Care Med 2000;162:324–327.

39. McNeil SA, Foster CL, Hedderwick SA, Kauffman CA. Effect of hand cleansing with antimicrobial soap or alcohol-based gel on microbial colonization of artificial fingernails worn by health care workers. Clin Infect Dis 2001;32:367–372.

40. Gordin FM, Schultz ME, Huber R, et al. A cluster of hemodialysis-related bacteremia linked to artificial fingernails. Infect Control Hosp Epidemiol 2007;28:743–744.

41. Sax H, Allegranzi B, Uckay I, et al. "My five moments for hand hygiene": a user-centred design approach to understand, train, monitor and report hand hygiene. J Hosp Infect 2007;67:9–21.

42. Erasmus V, Daha, TJ, Brug H, et al. Systematic review of studies on compliance with hand hygiene guidelines in hospital care. Infect Control Hosp Epidemiol 2010;31:283–294.

43. Pittet D, Mourouga P, Perneger TV. Compliance with handwashing in a teaching hospital. Ann Intern Med 1999;130:125–130.

44. Pessoa-Silva CL, Posfay-Barbe K Pfister R, et al. Attitudes and perceptions towards hand hygiene among healthcare workers caring for critically ill neonates. Infect Control Hosp Epidemiol 2005;26:305–311.

45. Pittet D. Improving compliance with hand hygiene in hospitals. Infect Control Hosp Epidemiol 2000;21:381–386.

46. Murtough SM, Hiom SJ, Palmer M, Russell AD. A survey of rotational use of biocides in hospital pharmacy aseptic units. J Hosp Infect 2002;50:228–231.

47. Dancer SJ. How do we assess hospital cleaning? A proposal for microbiological standards for surface hygiene in hospitals. J Hosp Infect 2004;56:10–15.

48. Cooper BS, Stone SP, Kibbler CC, et al. Isolation measures in the hospital management of methicillin resistant *Staphylococcus aureus* (MRSA): systematic review of the literature. BMJ 2004;329:533–540.

49. Cepeda JA, Whitehouse T, Cooper B, et al. Isolation of patients in single rooms or cohorts to reduce spread of MRSA in intensive care units: prospective two-centre study. The Lancet 2005;365:295–304.

50. Siegel JD, Rhinehart E, Jackson M, et al. Guidelines for isolation precautions: preventing transmission of infectious agents in Healthcare settings. 2007. Available at: http://www.cdc.gov/ncidod/dhqp/gl_isolation.html.

51. Erbay A, Colpan A, Bodur, et al. Evaluation of antibiotic use in a hospital with an antibiotic restriction policy. Int J Antimicrob Agents 2003;21:308–312.

52. Hecker MT, Aron DC, Patel MP, et al. Unnecessary use of antimicrobials in hospitalised patients: current patterns of misuse with an emphasis on the anti-anaerobic spectrum of activity. Arch Intern Med 2003;163:972–978.

53. Kollef MH. Inadequate antimicrobial treatment: an important determinant of outcome for hospitalized patients. Clin Infect Dis 2000;31 Suppl 4:S131-S138.

54. Kollef MH, Sherman G, Ward S, et al. Inadequate antimicrobial treatment of infections: a risk factor for hospital mortality among critically ill patients. Chest 1999;115:462–474.

55. Ogeer-Gyles JS, Mathews KA, Boerlin P. Nosocomial infections and antimictobial resistacne in critical care medicine. J Vet Emerg Crit Care 2006;16:1–18.

56. Mest DR, Wong DH, Shimoda KJ, et al. Nasal colonization with methicillin-resistant *Staphylococcus aureus* on admission to the surgical intensive care unit increases the risk of infection. Anesth Analg 1994;78:644–650.

57. Tornieporth NG, Roberts RB, Hafner JJ, et al. Risk factors associated with vancomycin-resistant *Enterococcus faceium* infection or colonization in 145 matched case and control patients. Clin Infect Dis 1996;23:767–772.

58. Zinn CS, Westh H, Rosdahl VT. An international multicenter study of antimicrobial resistance and typing of hospital *Staphylococcus aureus* isolates from 21 laboratories in 19 countries or states. Microb Drug Resist 2004;10:160–168.

59. Lepelletier D, Caroff N, Riochet D, et al. Risk-factors for gastrointestinal colonisation with resistant Enterobacteriaceae among hospitalised patients: a prospective study. Clin Microbiol Infect 2006;12:974–979.

60. Linden PK. Enterococci: resistance update and treatment options. In: Antimicrobial Resistance Problem Pathogens and Clinical Countermeasures Eds. Owens RC, Lautenbach E. Informa Healthcare USA, 2008:89–110.

61. Gross R, Morgan AS, Kinky DE, et al. Impact of a hospital-based antimicrobial program on clinical and economic outcomes. Clin Infect Dis 2001;33:289–295.

62. Davey P, Brown E, Fenelon L, et al. Interventions to improve antibiotic prescribing practices for hospital inpatients. The Cochrane Library 2, 2008.

63. Ogeer-Gyles J, Mathews KA, Sears W, et al. Development of antimicrobial drug resistance in rectal *Escherichia coli* isolates from dogs hospitalized in an intensive care unit. J Am Vet Med Assoc 2006;229:694–699.

64. Ball KR, Rubin JE, Chirino-Trejo M, et al. Antimicrobial resistance and prevalence of canine uropathogens at the Western College of Veterinary Medicine Veterinary Teaching Hospital, 2002–2007. Can Vet J 2008;49:985–990.

65. Cohn LA, Gary AT, Fales WH, et al. Trends in fluoroquinolone resistance of bacteria isolated from canine urinary tracts. J Vet Diagn Invest 2003;15:338–343.

66. MacKellar QA, Sanchez Bruni SF, Jones DG. Pharmacokinetic/pharmacodynamic relationships of antimicrobial drugs used in veterinary medicine. J Vet Pharmacol Therap 2004;27:503–514.

67. Wertheim HF, Vos MC, Boelens HA, et al. Low prevalence of methicillin resistant *Staphylococcus aureus* (MRSA) at hospital admission in the Netherlands: the value of search and destroy and restrictive antibiotic use. J Hosp Infect 2004;56:321–325.

68. Sturenberg E. Rapid detection of methicillin resistant *Staphylococcus aureus* directly from clinical samples: methods, effectiveness and cost considerations. Ger Med Sci 2009;7:1–19.

55

Care of indwelling device insertion sites

Elana Moss Benasutti

Most indwelling devices used in the emergency room and intensive care unit are necessary because they aid in the provision of life-saving care, but their use is not without complication. These devices circumvent the patient's innate immune system and often create a direct pathway between the external environment and the sterile environment of the body. Bacteria and other microorganisms can travel along these devices, which can lead to infection. For example, any device that passes through the skin compromises the integrity of the skin's protective barrier and allows external microorganisms to gain access to interior sites. Any device that enters the body through a natural opening disables that opening's natural mechanism for keeping pathogens out; urinary catheters, for example, abolish the one-way flushing mechanism that usually helps prevent retrograde bacterial invasion. Indeed, infection is the one risk that all indwelling devices share. Noninfectious device complications include device dislodgement, device lumen occlusion, patient injury (e.g., vascular occlusion or thrombosis in the case of vascular catheters), or loss of device function for another reason.

A device-associated infection threatens the patient's status in two ways: (1) the infection's effects may be systemic (i.e., **sepsis**, the systemic response to infection), which can put the patient's life at risk, and (2) even if the infection is localized with no systemic effects, the device itself may be lost. The device may need to be removed to prevent infection spread, or it may become displaced due to breakdown of local tissue, allowing it to slip. Either way, its loss can have dire consequences for the patient. For example, a lost thorocostomy tube may jeopardize a patient's ability to breathe and may require a high-risk general anesthetic procedure for

replacement. The loss of even a simple venous catheter can make patient treatment quite challenging.

Hospitalized patients are susceptible to **nosocomial (hospital-acquired) infection**, and it appears that each additional indwelling device further increases the risk.[1] The medical professionals handling the patient and its indwelling devices play a significant role in the spread of pathogens and thus in the likelihood of hospital-acquired infection.[2] Nosocomial infections increase morbidity and mortality, lengthen hospital stays, and add cost to patient care. In veterinary medicine, increased morbidity or cost can lead to euthanasia, as most owners have a finite amount of money to spend.

Attention to strict aseptic technique in the placement, handling, and maintenance of indwelling devices decreases the risk of infection significantly.[3] The existence of set protocols for the placement, handling, and maintenance of indwelling devices and strict adherence to these protocols significantly decreases the incidence of nosocomial infection. Included in these protocols should be a good system of hand hygiene, as it has been shown that many nosocomial infections come from the hands of the healthcare worker.[4] Because all devices circumvent the patient's innate immunity, because modes of microorganism transmission are similar regardless of device or site, and because all devices can malfunction, most device insertion sites require the same basic care.

Device insertion site infection

Local device insertion site infections can occur without causing systemic problems, and device-associated systemic sepsis can occur without an insertion site

Advanced Monitoring and Procedures for Small Animal Emergency and Critical Care, First Edition. Edited by Jamie M. Burkitt Creedon, Harold Davis.
© 2012 John Wiley & Sons, Inc. Published 2012 by John Wiley & Sons, Inc.

infection. Therefore, when a site infection occurs, the doctor must decide whether to remove the device or leave it in place. Risks and benefits must be considered, and close monitoring of rectal temperature, blood pressure, complete blood count (CBC), and blood glucose concentration may aid in decision making. If the infection appears to be localized, it is sometimes best to leave the device in. For instance, in the author's experience, localized feeding tube insertion site infections are often treated successfully with diligent, daily site cleaning with a 2% chlorhexidine (CHX) gluconate scrub; thorough site drying before bandaging; and sometimes systemic antibiotic therapy. Minor infection related to a human pediatric patient's central venous catheter is sometimes managed with diligent site care and systemic antibiotics for up to three days, after which time the device is usually removed if the infection persists,[1] though the Centers for Disease Control (CDC) recommend removal of vascular catheters if there is evidence of phlebitis or purulence.[5]

Hand hygiene

Good hand hygiene is an essential aspect of nosocomial infection prevention.[6] Without adequate hand hygiene practices, other indwelling device site care practices are likely in vain. The CDC has extensive recommendations for how and when to perform hand hygiene measures,[6] which are detailed in Chapter 54, Minimizing Nosocomial Infection. A hygienic handwashing protocol is available in Protocol 54.1.

General care of insertion sites

Insertion site care varies somewhat by patient and device, but some principles generally hold true across the board.

Bandaging

Insertion sites that penetrate the skin (excepting tracheostomy sites) should be kept covered with a sterile, nonadherent pad, or a sterile, self-adherent bandage, and wrapped with gauze. Cast padding may be placed over the gauze to help secure it, and an outer, water-resistant wrap may be applied as a final barrier. This general bandage will work in many situations, but isn't appropriate for all devices. More specific wraps will be described later in the chapter.

Handling

As stated above, good hand hygiene is paramount in the basic care of indwelling devices. After proper hand hygiene is performed, clean examination gloves should be worn before handling any device or insertion site. Sterile gloves may be indicated in some instances, such as when handling the inner cannula of a tracheostomy tube (see Chapter 24, Temporary Tracheostomy).

Maintenance

Most sites should be unwrapped, evaluated, and rewrapped regularly, at least once daily. The insertion site should appear clean with no redness, swelling, oozing fluid, or other signs of inflammation. The area should not feel excessively warm and should not be unduly painful to the patient. If the device is sutured in place, the sutures should be assessed for functionality and suture sites evaluated for inflammation. The device should be securely in place with no signs of slippage or migration. When a device is inserted, a note should be made on the treatment sheet as to the device's size, functionality (e.g., for an intravenous [IV] catheter, does it flush? does it aspirate?), and placement depth. Some devices have depth markers on them that can be used as a reference when performing daily evaluation. If there are no markers, the length of the device extending from the body can be measured and a note made in the treatment sheet.

If the site shows any signs of inflammation or infection, it should be scrubbed with a 2% tincture of CHX preparation, the CHX should be left on the site, and the site should be allowed to air dry before rewrapping.[5] A doctor should be notified of the inflammatory change and the patient should be checked for signs of systemic infection. Similarly, any migration from the original position or altered functionality should be reported to the clinician. Device removal should be at clinician discretion. Insertion sites should be kept clean and dry.

Care of associated lines and connections

As long as they are clean and no complications are present, disposable lines or connections used with the indwelling devices (fluid lines, stopcocks) can remain in place for 72–96 hours;[5] however, they should be changed immediately when dirty, or whenever contaminated with body fluids or feces. Injection ports may be preferable to stopcocks.[4] All ports should be swabbed with 70% alcohol or an iodophor (e.g., povidone-iodine) prior to being punctured with a sterile needle, and when stopcocks are used, they should be capped aseptically when not in use.[5] Each port to a device increases the chance for site or bloodstream (vascular catheters) infection, so port number should be kept to a minimum.

Care of specific insertion sites

Peripheral venous and arterial catheters

Venous access is required in most acutely or critically ill patients for administration of IV fluids and medications. Many critically ill patients require multiple simultaneous constant rate infusions, which often requires multiple venous catheter ports. Arterial catheters are indicated for direct blood pressure monitoring or frequent sampling of arterial blood. Because vascular access plays a dominant role in quality veterinary care, the proper care of venous and arterial catheters is a top priority of good nursing.

Many catheter-related infections begin with the placement of the catheter. Pathogen migration from the insertion site into the cutaneous catheter tract is the main cause of infection in peripheral catheters.[5] Contamination of the catheter hub is often the source of central venous catheter (CVC) infections.[5] Systemic antibiotics should not be administered routinely before insertion or during the use of intravascular catheters for the purpose of preventing catheter-associated infection.[5]

Catheter materials

Choosing the appropriate catheter type is important in the prevention of catheter-related infections. According to the CDC, catheters made of Teflon® or polyurethane are preferred over those made of polyvinyl chloride or polyethylene, to help reduce the incidence of infection.[5] Also, catheter diameter has been shown to be significant in the formation of thrombi. To decrease the chance of venous thrombosis, the smallest catheter diameter required to meet needs should be used.[7]

Site preparation for peripheral IV and arterial catheters

The proposed insertion site should be completely clean and should be free of local trauma and infection. The region is clipped of fur as close to the skin as possible with a clean blade. When possible, a margin of 1.5–2 inches (5 cm) of fur should be removed on all sides of the proposed puncture site.[8]

A healthy venous or arterial catheter site starts with proper aseptic placement. After performing appropriate hand hygiene (see Chapter 54, Minimizing Nosocomial Infection, and Protocol 54.1), clean gloves should be donned and the proposed insertion site scrubbed. The scrub should not be too vigorous, as damage to the skin invites infection.

There is not currently a single, definitive recommendation for catheter insertion site preparation.[5] A 30-second scrub with 2% CHX may be the most effective at preventing catheter related infections; a 10% povidone iodine scrub for 2 minutes is also acceptable.[4,5] While 70% isopropyl alcohol is an effective antimicrobial for the skin, it should not be used on sensitive or delicate skin, as it drying and therefore can be damaging to such skin; sterile water can be used instead as a damp wipe/rinse for the scrub solution.[4] Additionally, alcohol inactivates povidone-iodine, so alternating these two antiseptics for site preparation is not recommended (see Chapter 56, Antiseptics, Disinfectants, and Sterilization). See Protocol 55.1 for instructions on vascular device insertion site preparation.

After preparing the site, gloves are removed, hand hygiene again performed, and clean gloves donned prior to catheter placement (sterile gloves for arterial catheterization). Instruction on catheter placement is found in Chapter 4, Catheterization of the Venous Compartment, and Chapter 5, Arterial Puncture and Catheterization.

Protocol 55.1 Site preparation for peripheral IV and arterial catheters

Items Required
- Clippers with clean blade
- Examination gloves
- Skin scrub
  2% CHX scrub (preferred)
  10% povidone-iodine scrub (acceptable)
- Skin rinse
  70% isopropyl alcohol
  Sterile water (for sensitive or delicate skin)

Procedure
1. Collect necessary supplies.
2. Clip fur with a radius of 2 inches (5 cm) from proposed insertion site. Clip fur as close to the skin as possible.
3. Perform hand hygiene and don clean examination gloves.
4. Perform a gentle 30-second scrub with 2% CHX, or a gentle 1-minute scrub if using 10% povidone-iodine. Do not scrub so vigorously that skin is damaged.
5. Rinse the skin with 70% isopropyl alcohol if using CHX and the skin is not overly delicate or damaged. Rinse the skin with sterile water if using povidone-iodine or the skin is delicate or damaged.
6. Remove gloves, perform hand hygiene, and don clean gloves appropriate to the task prior to catheter insertion.

Dressing

The catheter insertion site should be covered with sterile gauze or sterile, transparent, adhesive dressing.[5] The site may then be dressed with clean gauze or cotton cast padding, as listed above in general recommendations. Topical antibiotic ointment or cream should not be applied to the catheter insertion site due to its tendency to promote fungal growth and encourage bacterial resistance.[5] It is unclear whether flushing catheters with heparinized saline is more effective at preventing catheter failure than flushing with plain 0.9% NaCl.

The catheter should be protected so that the animal does not chew or lick the area. Many commercial products are available to limit animal access to vascular catheters, including Elizabethan collars, no bite collars, catheter guards, various wrapping materials, and noxious-tasting, antilick sprays.

Care and maintenance of peripheral vascular catheter insertion sites

A peripheral catheter should be evaluated at least every 2 hours.[9] The wrap should be snug, clean, and dry. Loose or soiled dressings should be changed immediately, and if the dressing is soiled or wet to the level of the catheter insertion site, the clinician should be notified. During the dressing change, the site should be cleaned with 2% CHX scrub; allowed to air dry or dried with sterile gauze; and rewrapped with new, clean dressings. The vessel above the site should not be hard or "ropey" on palpation, the skin above the site should not be excessively warm, there should be no edema proximal or distal to the catheter, and there should be no bandage strike-through or oozing at the site. If any of these abnormalities are noted, the clinician should be notified and a dressing or catheter change considered.

There are not clear guidelines as to how often a vascular insertion site should be directly evaluated.[5] Standard veterinary practice is to unwrap and evaluate, and dress vascular catheter insertion sites with clean, new materials once daily.[9] There should be no redness or swelling at the site. The site should be clean and dry with no leaking blood or fluid. Such abnormalities should be brought to the clinician's attention; the CDC recommends removal of temporary vascular catheters with evidence of phlebitis or infection.[5]

Proper hand hygiene (washing or alcohol-based hand rub) should be performed prior to any contact with a catheter or its insertion site, and clean gloves should be worn every time the catheter is accessed (see Chapter 54, Minimizing Nosocomial Infection, and Protocol 54.1). The catheter should be handled gently. Irritation of the vessel caused by catheter handling increases the risk for phlebitis. When accessing the catheter, be aware of the anatomy of the vessel and try to avoid bending the catheter against the vessel's direction. Take care not to dislodge the catheter when accessing it. Always hold the catheter by the hub with one hand (properly cleaned and gloved) while accessing it with the other hand so as not to dislodge the catheter or its connections during manipulations.

Any vascular catheter that is no longer essential should be removed immediately. In human adults, it is recommended that peripheral venous catheters be replaced every 72–96 hours to help prevent phlebitis; however, it is recommended to leave uncomplicated catheters in place in children until they are no longer essential.[5] Thus, although the most common veterinary practice is to replace peripheral venous catheters every 72 hours, it is unclear whether this routine replacement is required. The CDC does not recommend the routine replacement of arterial or central venous catheters unless catheter-associated complications arise.[5]

Possible complications of indwelling vascular catheters

Despite the best care, complications can still arise. Localized infection at the site, bloodstream infection or sepsis, phlebitis, thrombosis, and edema are all potential consequences of intravascular catheters. The severity of these complications ranges from mild to life threatening. See Table 55.1 regarding some common complications of vascular catheters.

Catheter, line, or dressing damage or dislodgement

In the event of catheter, line, or dressing complication, unwrap the catheter. If the catheter or insertion site is wet or dirty, clean site with a 2% solution of CHX scrub and allow the site to air dry before being rewrapped.[5] If air drying is impossible, dry the insertion site with sterile gauze prior to rewrapping. Do not rewrap a wet site, as this encourages the growth of pathogens. Before rewrapping, make sure the catheter is at the proper angle in relation to the vessel.

Flush and attempt to aspirate blood back from the catheter while it is unwrapped to ascertain that the catheter is still in the vessel. If no blood appears after aspiration, place clean, gloved fingers above the insertion site while injecting saline; if the catheter is still in the vessel one can sometimes feel a "jet" or "stream" of fluid as it flows up the vessel (particularly in a vein). If no intravascular fluid stream is palpable, watch this area closely while flushing. If the catheter tip is in the subcutaneous space, fluid will accumulate subcutaneously. Whenever flushing a catheter (wherever its tip may be),

Table 55.1 Signs of and appropriate actions for phlebitis and thrombosis of vascular catheter insertion sites

Condition	Signs	Action
Phlebitis	• Redness around site • Heat • Swelling • Pain on palpation of site or upon catheter flushing	• Inform clinician • Catheter should be removed • If clinician elects to leave catheter in place, clean site with 2% CHX, allow to dry, and redress with new, clean materials
Thrombosis	• Pain on palpation of site or upon catheter flushing • Vessel feels hard or "ropey" • Vessel appears distended without being occluded • Edema above or below site • Catheter becomes difficult to flush or aspirate	

consider the size of the animal, the prescribed fluid rate, and the animal's ability to handle volume (and heparin if flushing with heparinized saline). This is especially important when working with very small animals such as toy breeds, neonates, and small mammals such as ferrets.

If unable to ascertain whether an IV catheter is in the vessel, but the clinician is reluctant to remove the catheter, it should only be used to infuse plain fluids. Infuse slowly while observing closely for leaking or the subcutaneous accumulation of fluids. If fluids accumulate subcutaneously, the catheter must be removed.

The insertion site of an intact vascular catheter should be redressed with new materials as previously mentioned, and protected from animal-induced damage by using an Elizabethan collar or by wrapping more extensively and applying a commercial antilick product. Commercial plastic catheter guards are also available. Secure the fluid line in such a way as to minimize pulling on the catheter itself, as trauma to the vessel leads to phlebitis and thrombosis.

Edema distal to the catheter insertion

Swelling distal to the catheter wrap usually indicates that the wrap is too tight. This swelling should be "cool" and should pit with pressure from a finger. In such cases, remove the bandage, rewrap the site more loosely with new bandage materials, and monitor. Evaluate the patient's other limbs and its skin turgor for evidence of generalized edema, which could indicate a compromise in the patient's vascular retention status due to low colloid osmotic pressure (COP; see Chapter 51, Osmolality and Colloid Osmotic Pressure, for more details). If distal swelling persists despite a loosened bandage,

inform the clinician, who may elect to replace the catheter or continue to monitor the situation.

If the swelling distal to the catheter is warm, the skin is reddened, the limb seems painful, or the swelling does not pit with pressure from a finger, it may be due to phlebitis or infection. The clinician should always be notified in such cases, and the catheter will likely need to be removed.

Swelling above (or both above and below) the insertion site

Swelling above the insertion site often indicates phlebitis or thrombosis of the vessel. The site should be unwrapped and evaluated. If no signs other than edema are present, consider the patient's vascular fluid retention status as above. However, if redness, heat, or pain is noted, phlebitis or thrombosis may be present. Signs are described in Table 55.1.

Phlebitis is inflammation of the vessel. If phlebitis is present, the catheter should ideally be removed. If vascular access is limited and the catheter is still needed, the catheter should be flushed while unwrapped to make sure there is no leakage at the site. If the site leaks when flushed the catheter must be removed. If there is no leakage at the site the doctor should evaluate the patient and the site. If the phlebitis is minor and no signs of systemic inflammation are present, the clinician may elect to leave the catheter in place. At a minimum, the site should be cleaned with 2% CHX scrub, air dried or dried with sterile gauze, and rewrapped. If phlebitis has been found, the wrapped site should be checked every 2 hours, unwrapped and evaluated every 6–12 hours, and the patient monitored closely for signs of systemic inflammation. If infectious phlebitis is suspected, systemic antibiotics are sometimes used. If there are no signs of improvement in the phlebitis within 1–3 days, or if systemic inflammatory signs have evolved and are believed secondary to the catheter, the catheter must be removed. Blood cultures may be taken aseptically, one from the infected catheter, and at least one from a different site, to help confirm and diagnose a catheter-related infection.

Vessel thrombosis occurs with thrombus formation at the tip of or along the outer length of the catheter. A thrombosed vessel can be painful and increases the chance of pulmonary embolism. As with phlebitis, ideally the catheter would be removed, but sometimes that is not possible. Thrombosis varies in severity and common sense must be used when deciding when to leave or remove a catheter. The location and degree of edema should be considered. For instance, swelling only near the insertion site might warrant less drastic action than swelling that involves a large portion of a limb, and more severe edema may warrant catheter removal more often than milder edema. The degree of hardness or "ropiness" of the vessel should also be considered. Is it mild or severe, and how much of the length of the vessel is affected? Once the vessel begins to harden, a catheter may be left in for a short period of time (usually 12–24 hours) before the condition worsens and the catheter needs to be pulled or ceases to function (leaking at site, no longer patent). If leaving a catheter in place, one may consider massaging and wrapping the limb to inhibit fluid retention.

Redness, heat, swelling, pain, or purulence at the catheter insertion site

Taken together, redness, heat, swelling, and pain are signs of inflammation or infection. The patient's temperature and other vital parameters should be assessed and reported to the clinician as soon as possible. The catheter should be removed as soon as possible.[5] If the doctor decides to leave the catheter in place, the site and the patient should be monitored closely and cared for in the same manner as for phlebitis, detailed above.

Oozing at the catheter insertion site

Ascertain whether the tissue itself is oozing, or if fluids being placed into the catheter are leaking out at the site. This is done by unwrapping the catheter and flushing it with sterile saline. Watch the insertion site closely for leakage while flushing the catheter. Tissue oozing may indicate infection and should be treated as such (see above). If fluids administered are leaking, the catheter should be removed.

Central venous catheter and peripherally inserted central catheter insertion sites

Insertion

CVCs and peripherally inserted central catheter (PICC) lines travel to the vena cava, and because they can dwell much longer (>1 month) than peripheral catheters, the CDC recommends they be placed with a more stringent aseptic technique than is necessary for peripheral venous catheters.[5] The catheter with the fewest required ports should be inserted. During CVC or PICC insertion, the operator should don a full sterile gown, sterile gloves, cap, and mask, and a large sterile drape should be used to create a sterile field. Skin insertion site preparation is the same as for peripheral venous and arterial catheters, though a very wide margin of fur should be clipped in such cases. Dressing recommendations are the same as for peripheral vascular catheters.

Maintenance

A central catheter should be maintained in much the same manner as a peripheral catheter. Length of dwell time has been found to be a significant risk factor for catheter-related infection. Since these catheters are accessed frequently and are expected to dwell for extended periods of time, good hand hygiene and donning clean gloves when handling these catheters are imperative. The catheter should be unwrapped and the site evaluated at least every 48 hours if wrapped in gauze, and at least every 7 days if covered with transparent, adhesive dressing.[5] The site should be checked for any redness, swelling, leakage of administered fluids, or oozing of the tissue at the site. The area around the insertion site should be gently palpated for any signs of pain or hardening of the vessel. The area should also be checked for excessive warmth. If any of these signs are present, the doctor should be notified and the situation addressed. Catheters with associated inflammation should be removed.[5]

There is not currently a single, definitive recommendation for central catheter insertion site care.[5] Standard veterinary practice is generally that central line insertion sites be cared for in a manner similar to peripheral catheter insertion sites. Generally, sites are cleaned every time they are directly evaluated with a 2% solution of CHX scrub, and allowed to air dry or are dried with sterile gauze, then dressed again with new materials. Direct site evaluation, cleansing, and redressing should also be done any time the area is soiled or the site becomes exposed. The CDC does not recommend the routine application of povidone iodine or triple antibiotic ointment to the site, as the moisture encourages the growth of pathogens. The CDC does approve the use of sponges impregnated with CHX at the CVC insertion site.[5]

Intraosseous catheter insertion sites

The intraosseous (IO) catheter is the epitome of the life-saving device because of the ease and speed with which the catheter can be placed in hypovolemic and neonatal patients. Resuscitative fluids, blood products, and most any drug that can be administered intravenously can be administered intraosseously. As with all indwelling devices, IO catheters have a few risks. Complications such as infection (such as osteomyelitis) can usually be avoided by proper aseptic placement and proper care of the site and catheter once placed.

Insertion

IO catheter insertion site preparation is the same as for peripheral venous and arterial catheters. Once placed, the catheter should be secured by wrapping a tape butterfly around the hub and suturing the butterfly to the skin or periosteum. Some IO catheters come with their own permanent butterflies. If desired, the sutures may be glued to the patient with a cyanoacrylate glue. The manufacturer of the catheter should be consulted for compatibility. If possible, the secured catheter should be protected by an outer bandage. For more detail on placing and securing an IO catheter, see Chapter 4, Catheterization of the Venous Compartment.

Maintenance

IO catheters usually dwell for only a short period (3–4 hours), until vascular access is achieved. If left in for an extended period, they should be maintained in much the same manner as an IV catheter. Hand hygiene should be performed and clean examination gloves worn every time the catheter is handled. Standard practice is to flush the IO catheter with a small amount of heparinized or plain saline every 6 hours. Rewrapping an IO catheter is not always feasible. There may be cases in which the patient is too small, too young, or too critical to make routine rewrapping possible. Once again, common sense must be used to decide what is best for the patient. An IO catheter should be left in for no longer than 96 hours.

Complications of IO catheters
Fluid extravasation

Extravasation of fluid may be the most common complication of IO catheters. This usually occurs when the needle is misplaced upon insertion, either because the catheter does not penetrate fully through the cortex and into the medullary cavity or because it has passed out of the bone's medulla and through the far cortex, into the muscle. Fluid extravasation can also occur when the patient moves excessively after proper placement of the IO catheter. When hypertonic fluids or caustic medications extravasate, muscle necrosis can occur.

There are a few ways to confirm an IO catheter's position. When the IO catheter is properly positioned, it should flush easily with little resistance. Radiographic imaging shows the catheter's placement as well. If administered drugs or fluids leak at the site, one should suspect the catheter is not properly seated, and it should be removed. Replacing the IO catheter in the same site is not recommended, as fluid may escape from the hole left from the first catheter. For the same reason, it is not recommended to make more than one attempt at the same site when placing the IO catheter.

Compartment syndrome

Compartment syndrome occurs when fluids extravasate from an IO site for an extended period of time. When a large amount of fluid leaks into the muscle, a pocket is formed within the muscle, which can cause muscle necrosis. It is recommended that there be no repeated attempts in the same bone if the first IO catheterization fails. Another site should be chosen, as fluid will sometimes leak from the hole made on the first attempt. The best way to minimize serious harm to the patient from compartment syndrome is to monitor the catheter site and associated limb closely.

Infection and osteomyelitis

Localized site infection or osteomyelitis occurs rarely, particularly if the IO catheter is removed after only a few hours' time. Infection most often occurs when proper aseptic technique was not followed on insertion. The IO catheter should be removed if signs of infection are present; systemic antibiotics are usually indicated.

Thoracostomy tube insertion site maintenance

Great care must be taken to keep the insertion site of a thoracostomy tube healthy. Having to remove a tube due to infection, or having the tube migrate out of the pleural space due to breakdown of the tissue at the site due to infection, can greatly compromise the patient. Also, care must be taken not to introduce bacteria into the pleural space.

Prior to contacting the thoracostomy tube or insertion site, hands should be cleaned using good hand hygiene practice as recommended by the CDC and described in Chapter 54. Clean examination gloves should worn any time the site or tube system is handled. The insertion site should be kept clean and dressed. Though specific, evidence-based recommendations are unavailable, the site should probably be unwrapped, evaluated, and redressed at least as often as a vascular catheter insertion site, so probably at least every 24 hours if no obvious complications are present. The site should be covered with a sterile, nonadherent pad before bandaging. Self-adherent, transparent bandages can be used in place of the nonadherent pad and are preferable in smaller animals where a bulky wrap would be uncomfortable. A body stockinette can be placed to further cover the site, and the tube itself can then be fastened to the stockinette with tape and suture, or plastic clamps.

It can be very challenging to keep a thoracostomy tube site properly bandaged. Large breed dogs are especially difficult due to their body conformation. It may help to criss-cross the bandage across the dog's chest. But when a patient is mobile, all attempts at keeping the site covered sometimes fail. One solution is to cover the site with a sterile, self-adherent bandage. A clean T-shirt is then put on the dog and tied to a close on top of the dog's back. A hole is cut in the shirt and the thoracostomy tube is passed through the hole and clamped to the T-shirt. This method works well to keep the site covered and also helps to stabilize the tube from excessive movement. This would not be suitable for a dog attached to a continuous suction device, in which case a more stabilizing wrap is needed.

Any animal with a thoracostomy tube requires constant monitoring and an Elizabethan collar. No matter how closely watched, some animals still manage to remove their tubes and sometimes tubes can migrate out of the thorax and into the subcutaneous space just through the movement of the animal's body. Thus, respiratory rate and effort should be watched closely and the chest ausculted frequently (every 2–4 hours). Care should be taken to ensure that the tube is not accidentally pulled upon, as this can cause inflammation of the pleura and the insertion site.

Nephrostomy tube insertion site maintenance

The collecting tip of a nephrostomy tube is placed within the renal pelvis and the tube travels through the body wall with its egress end outside the skin. The draining end of the tube is outside of the animal, attached to a sterile, closed urinary collection system. Keeping the insertion site clean helps to decrease pathogen introduction into the retroperitoneal space and the kidney. The bandaged tube should be evaluated every 2 hours, checking for any wetness and making sure that the bandage and tube are still wrapped in the proper position. At the author's institution, the site is unwrapped and evaluated every 8–12 hours.

Whereas most indwelling devices are situated in a fairly large space such as the pleural space, or a lumen as with a central line or a feeding tube, the nephrostomy tube is placed inside a tiny space within a delicate organ. Therefore it is vital that there be no tugging or pulling of the tube by handlers or the animal. The tubes are usually long enough to allow them to be curled several times before being wrapped closely to the body. A "butterfly" can be made of tape wrapped around the tube and then sutured to a stockinette, which is worn by the patient, or, if the surgeon chooses, sutured directly to the patient. Most cats and small dogs seem to prefer the stockinette to a bandage wrap. A sterile, transparent, self-adherent bandage works well over the site. The stockinette provides a clean covering and takes the brunt of any pulling that may occur. Enough slack must be left in the tube so that when the stockinette is pulled, it does not affect the site. If a bandage wrap is used the excess tubing can be curled and incorporated in the wrap so any tugging will not affect the tube site. An Elizabethan collar should be used and the animal watched closely.

In addition to monitoring the site for signs of infection, the nephrostomy tube site should be watched for leakage. While this could imply infection, it could also indicate retroperitoneal urine leakage. If effusion is noted from the insertion site, a doctor should be alerted immediately so that uroabdomen can be ruled out.

Another complication of the nephrostomy tube is the tube becoming clogged with stones or debris. Once approved by the doctor on the case, gentle aspiration and retropulsion can be attempted. If this is not successful, imaging may be necessary to determine the cause of the occlusion, and tube removal may be necessary.

Surgical drain insertion site maintenance
Jackson Pratt drain insertion sites

The Jackson Pratt (JP) drain is typically placed in the abdomen to drain peritoneal effusion postoperatively. It is also used to drain effusion from the subcutaneous space postoperatively in cases where excessive fluid buildup is expected. The drain consists of a surgical drainage tube placed inside the body, which attaches to thin rubber tubing that passes through the body wall to the outside and is then attached to a rubber squeeze bulb. When squeezed and then closed, the bulb creates suction, which draws fluid into the bulb where it is collected.

The insertion site of the JP drain should be kept clean, dry, and covered. The site should be covered with a nonadherent pad or a sterile, self-adherent bandage and then wrapped. The bandaged site should be checked every 2 hours, and the bandage should be dry. At the author's institution, the site is unwrapped and evaluated every 8–12 hours.

Insertion sites into the cranial abdomen are fairly easy to keep covered. Insertion sites into the inguinal area are very difficult. The variations in the size and shape of the many breeds of dog make it necessary to be creative with the bandage material. Usually it is necessary to rewrap these sites often, as bandages seem to slide off of them easily. Also, the bandage may sometimes become soiled with urine or feces, which can wick up towards the insertion site. If the urine or feces would not come into contact with the insertion site without the wrap acting as a wick, it may be better to forgo the wrap and just use a sterile, self-adherent bandage.

The tubing of the JP drain is long, and can be curled and then wrapped into the bandage material, with slack enough between the site and the wrapped portion of tubing that the weight of the bulb will not pull on the site. The bulb itself can also be taped to the bandage. In cases where the site is only covered with a sterile, self-adherent bandage, a clean t-shirt can be worn by the patient, brought to the top of the back and tied. The drain is passed through a hole cut in the shirt and attached to the shirt with a plastic clamp. A stockinette can be used in place of the t-shirt in smaller animals.

The drain insertion site should be monitored for infection, and treated accordingly, as stated earlier in this chapter. When a site is inflamed, it may allow the effusion to leak out at the site. If the drain is to be left in, some sterile gauze sponges should be added to the wrap to absorb the fluid. In cases where it is not physically possible to keep a bandage on, such as the inguinal area, care should be taken to keep the site and area around the site as clean and dry as possible. Fluid should be gently and aseptically wiped from the site, taking care to wipe in motions away from the site and not towards it. A 2% solution of CHX scrub should be used to clean the area. The area should be allowed to air dry if possible or be dried with sterile gauze. If the animal is recumbent, the limbs can be propped apart with clean towels to aid in keeping the area dry. Also if the animal is recumbent, sterile gauze can be placed around the site without an outer wrap. Of course, good hand hygiene as stated earlier in this chapter should be used any time the site or the drain itself is handled, and clean examination gloves worn.

Care should be taken to ensure that the tubing does not become kinked, preventing suction. The bulb should be kept empty of air and fluid to ensure adequate suction. Fluid should be emptied from the drain as often as needed, and fluid volumes recorded in the patient treatment sheet.

Penrose drain insertion sites

The Penrose drain is a passive drain. It consists of a simple rubber tube placed in a wound or incision to drain fluid from the site out of the animal. This helps to prevent infection, and also aids in patient comfort.

The Penrose drain site is a messy site, with fluid draining out freely and being caught only by any bandage material. If present, the external bandage should be checked every 2 hours for strikethrough. When strikethrough is present the bandage should be removed and the site examined, cleaned with a 2% solution of CHX, dried with sterile gauze, and redressed. At the author's institution, if there is no strikethrough present, the site is examined, cleaned, and rebandaged every 8 hours.

Care should be taken to prevent the animal licking or chewing the drain or site. This is best achieved with an Elizabethan collar.

Feeding tube insertion sites

Nasoesophageal and nasogastric tube insertion sites

Nasoesophageal (NE) tubes enter the nares and terminate in the esophagus; nasogastric (NG) tubes terminate in the stomach. The tube is generally secured with a sutured or stapled tape "butterfly" just caudal to the nostril and then again into the cheek of the animal. The nostril housing the tube should be monitored for signs of inflammation or infection such as pain or exudate, and treated accordingly.

There is significant risk of the tube leaving the esophagus and entering the trachea. The tube should be measured and a note made in the record as to how much tubing is external. Every time the tube is used, external placement should be checked. The sutures should all be in place and the tube seated securely with no slippage visible. The tube should be aspirated and negative pressure achieved if the tube is in the esophagus; negative pressure or gastric fluid if the tube is in the stomach. If gas is aspirated, a radiograph should be taken to check tube placement before anything is instilled into the tube. Animals with NE or NG tubes should always wear an Elizabethan collar.

Esophagostomy, percutaneous endoscopically placed gastric, and jejunostomy tube insertion sites

The insertion sites of these devices should be evaluated at least once daily. The site should be covered with a sterile nonadhering pad or a sterile, self-adherent bandage, and wrapped with clean, soft, bandage material. The animal should always wear an Elizabethan collar and the wrap should be substantial enough to protect the site and tube in the event that the animal escapes or evades the collar. Esophagostomy tubes are especially vulnerable to clawing.

In addition to monitoring for infection, it is imperative that the device's proper placement is evaluated, as much as can be determined from the insertion site. Feeding tubes can migrate due to breakdown of the site, or due to tugging or pulling by the animal. If displaced, food may end up in the airways, the peritoneal cavity, or the subcutaneous space. It is impossible to ascertain whether the device is placed properly just from evaluation of the insertion site, but a healthy insertion site gives confidence to that assumption. All feeding tubes should be checked for negative pressure or reflux to ensure proper placement prior to feeding through the tube. The tube should be marked in some way so that tube migration can be assessed. The site should also be checked for leakage of food or other fluid. If any food or fluid leaks from the site the feeding should be stopped immediately and a doctor notified.

These types of feeding tubes generally remain functional for extended periods of time (up to months), and can be maintained and used by the owner at home if they are properly educated in the care of the tube. Because of the length of time that the tube remains in the patient, a moist dermatitis sometimes develops. If the tube and sutures are all securely in place it may help to leave the site unwrapped for 15–20 minutes after each cleaning and drying. The animal should be held during this time to ensure that it does not rip out the tube.

In the author's experience, minor infections of enteral feeding tube insertion sites can often be successfully treated by frequent (2–3 times a day) cleaning and rewrapping. Systemic antibiotic therapy may be considered. These patients should be closely monitored by a doctor.

An infected, soiled, or exposed site should be cleaned with a 2% CHX solution, allowed to air dry or dried with sterile gauze, and rewrapped with new, clean material. If the tissue at the site is oozing, sterile gauze can be placed over the site to absorb the fluid. It is important to keep the site as dry as possible. If the site is red and inflamed, but not oozing fluid or overly moist, povidone iodine may be helpful in eliminating the infection. In general, it is not recommended to use iodine or triple antibiotic ointment on these sites, as the excess moisture promotes the growth of certain pathogens.

Epidural catheter insertion sites

Epidural catheters are often placed in cases in which pain management is expected to be difficult. These catheters must be placed aseptically and maintained with stringent aseptic technique. After placement, povidone iodine can be applied to the area around the site with sterile iodine-soaked swabs. Sterile gauze sponges can be placed under the injection cap, both to aid in keeping the catheter laying evenly along the animal's back, and to absorb any leaking fluid. The site should be covered with a clear, sterile, self-adherent bandage. It is not recommended to unwrap an epidural catheter, so the clear bandage allows a periodic visual site check every few hours. It is not unusual to note clear fluid leaking from the site. This is one reason to place sterile, gauze sponges beneath the epidural catheter. If any colored fluid, swelling, or other signs of inflammation are seen, a doctor should evaluate the site immediately. If any sign of infection is seen, the catheter should be removed.

To avoid introducing bacteria into the epidural space, the injection cap to the catheter should be scrubbed with a 2% solution of CHX and a gauze sponge soaked in 2% CHX placed over it for a full 3 minutes prior to being punctured with a sterile needle. Proper hand hygiene should be performed as stated above, and sterile gloves must be worn when utilizing this device.

Extreme care should be taken to not displace the catheter. Although rare, epidural hematomas, epidural abscesses, and arachnoiditis are possible complications. There is a limit to the volume that can be injected into an epidural catheter. The doctor's orders should be specific as to that amount.

Summary

The importance of properly caring for the insertion sites of indwelling devices cannot be overstated. Most insertion sites will remain healthy and the device functional for as long as needed if well maintained. Paying close attention to the site can greatly reduce the incidence of infection and other possible complications.

References

1. de Jonge RC, Polderman KH, Gemke RJ. Central venous catheter use in the pediatric patient: mechanical and infectious complications. Pediatr Crit Care Med 2005;6(3):329–39.

2. Eggimann P, Pittet D. Infection control in the ICU. Chest 2001;120:2059–93.

3. Strong S, Mukai L. A new quality approach to reducing vascular access infections. Nephrol Nurs J 2010;37(5):547–50.

4. Nosocomial infections in the newborn intensive care unit: catheter related practices. Available at: www.medscape.com/medscapetoday. Accessed January 2011.

5. Centers for Disease Control and Prevention website. Guidelines for the prevention of intravenous catheter related infections. Available at: www.cdc.gov/mmwr/PDF/rr/rr5116.pdf. Accessed January 2011.

6. Centers for Disease Control and Prevention website. Guideline for hand hygiene in health care settings. Available at: www.cdc.gov/mmwr/PDF/rr/rr5116.pdf. Accessed January 2011.

7. Grove JR, Pevec WC. Venous thrombosis related to peripherally inserted central catheters. JVIR 2000;11:837–40.

8. Busch SJ. Small Animal Surgical Nursing: Skills and Concepts. Elsevier/Mosby, 2006:23.

9. Battaglia AM. Patient's lifeline: intravenous catheter. In: Battaglia AM, ed. Small Animal Emergency and Critical Care for Veterinary Technicians, 2nd edition. Saunders, Elsevier, 2007:47.

56

Antiseptics, disinfectants, and sterilization

Jennifer Devey and Connie M. Schmidt

Antisepsis is defined as the destruction or inhibition of the growth of microorganisms through the use of antiseptics with the end goal of preventing infection. An **antiseptic** is a chemical agent or substance that kills or prevents growth of microorganisms on living tissue through topical application. This is as opposed to a **disinfectant**, which has the same role but is used on inanimate objects. Antiseptics and disinfectants are not expected to kill spores whereas **sterilization** is, although some disinfectants are sporicidal if left in contact with the surface for an extended period of time. Antiseptics and disinfectants typically have a broad spectrum of activity as compared with antibiotics, which target a specific bacterial population.

Disinfectants and antiseptics must remain in direct contact with the surface of the inanimate object or the tissue, respectively, for a certain length of time in order to be effective. This **contact time** must be continuous and varies with each chemical. For example, a surgical preparation of 2 minutes means 2 minutes of continuous contact time of the antiseptic with the skin. Disinfectants and antiseptics have variable **residual activity**, or activity that remains after the initial contact time. Contact times and residual activities of different chemicals will be described below.

The term **aseptic technique** is used to describe all of the precautions taken to prevent contamination and ultimately infection during medical and surgical procedures. Aseptic technique should be used for all surgical procedures and all procedures where contact is being established between the inner and outer surfaces of the body. Aseptic technique requires the appropriate use of antiseptics as well as appropriate personnel preparation and sterile instruments, suture, fluids, tubes, catheters, bandaging material, and so on. While the use of caps, masks, sterile gowns, and gloves helps minimize surgical infection, it has been shown that skin disinfection plays a more important role, thus the importance of skin decontamination cannot be overemphasized.

Aseptic technique during placement of catheters and tubes is essential as is aseptic management while they are in use. Infections secondary to tubes and catheters can occur from direct contamination from hospital surfaces, hospital equipment, or from the hands of hospital personnel. Infections can also result from introduction of the patient's own flora during the time of insertion, subsequent migration of microorganisms (either from the environment or contamination from the patient's urine or feces) along or through the catheter or tube, secondary to contamination of catheter hubs or infusion of contaminated fluid. The goal is to minimize all of these factors as much as possible, particularly the factors that are more easily controlled.

Hospital surface disinfection is paramount in preventing the spread of infectious disease, as many bacteria, fungi, and viruses can persist in the hospital environment for extended periods of time. Unenveloped viruses like parvovirus and microorganisms that sporulate can pose a particular challenge, and surface disinfection products and techniques must be applied properly to be effective. Proper instrument sterilization is crucial to help prevent infections associated with procedures that involve introduction of devices into body parts usually protected from the outside environment.

This chapter focuses on the rationales behind and different properties of antiseptics, disinfectants, and

Advanced Monitoring and Procedures for Small Animal Emergency and Critical Care, First Edition. Edited by Jamie M. Burkitt Creedon, Harold Davis.
© 2012 John Wiley & Sons, Inc. Published 2012 by John Wiley & Sons, Inc.

sterilization. Proper selection and use of these chemicals and methods are crucial to the prevention of **nosocomial (hospital-acquired) infection**, whether the patient is undergoing a surgical procedure, has an indwelling device, is being mechanically ventilated, or is simply hospitalized. See Chapter 54, Minimizing Nosocomial Infection, for an expanded discussion of other precautions against hospital-acquired infection.

Sterilization

Sterilization is defined as the use of a physical or chemical process to kill all microorganisms including bacteria, viruses, fungi, mycobacteria, protozoa, and spores. The two most commonly used methods of sterilization are autoclaving and gas sterilization. Autoclaving uses pressurized steam, which causes denaturation and coagulation of microorganism proteins. Gas sterilization is performed with ethylene oxide. It works by destroying the organisms through alkylation of deoxyribonucleic acid. Most items that cannot be autoclaved such as plastics and endoscopes can be safely gas sterilized.

Each method of sterilization requires that the item be packaged in a specific manner to permit penetration of the steam or gas. The exception to this is "flash" sterilization. If an instrument is needed on an emergency basis it can be sterilized in an open, unwrapped tray very quickly. Flash sterilization is not recommended for devices that are going to be implanted. All packs to be sterilized, whether by autoclaving or gas, should contain appropriate indicator strips that turn a specific color once the contents have been appropriately sterilized. Autoclaved sterile packs should not be placed into storage until they are completely dry. Gas sterilized items must be allowed to vent for an appropriate length of time per the manufacturer's instructions. Sterile packs should be stored in closed cabinets.

Sterile items should not be used if the packaging is damaged in any fashion. Instruments must be packaged in such a manner that sterility is not broken as the wrap is opened. The size of the sterile field that is prepared, whether for an exploratory celiotomy or placement of a central venous catheter, should be large enough to ensure that instruments and devices do not become contaminated during the procedure. Indicators should always be checked to ensure sterility has been achieved prior to use of the pack contents.

Glutaraldehyde

Glutaraldehyde is used to **"cold sterilize"** instruments. It is the chemical used in cold sterile trays used in most veterinary hospitals. Glutaraldehyde is considered a chemical sterilant since it has a broad spectrum of activity including being sporicidal. It acts by alkylating microorganism proteins. To ensure it is sporicidal the solution must be made alkaline. Unfortunately this leads to a steady loss of activity, which makes the glutaraldehyde solution ineffective after a maximum of 30 days. The shelf life varies depending on the formulation; therefore, manufacturer's guidelines must be followed. In a 2% glutaraldehyde solution, most bacteria are killed within 2 minutes of contact; fungi, virus, and mycobacteria within 10 minutes; and spores within 3 hours. It is noncorrosive and most objects that can be submerged in water may be safely sterilized using glutaraldehyde. Like all chemical disinfectants it is toxic to cells and irritating to skin, membranes, and airways, so all materials sterilized with glutaraldehyde must be rinsed thoroughly immediately prior to use.

Disinfectants and antiseptics

A disinfectant is a chemical agent or substance that kills or prevents growth of microorganisms on inanimate objects through topical application. In contrast, an antiseptic is an agent applied topically to living tissue. Many of the antiseptic agents discussed below can be used as disinfectants. A disinfectant is usually of a higher concentration than one can use safely on skin and tissues; therefore, most disinfectants cannot be used as antiseptics. Some disinfectants should be diluted prior to use. Those that require dilution should always be diluted according to the manufacturer's instructions.

An antiseptic is a chemical agent or substance that kills or prevents growth of microorganisms on living tissue through topical application. A variety of different antiseptics are available in veterinary medicine. Each has advantages and disadvantages, and none is effective against all organisms (see Table 56.1). Commonly used antiseptics include acids, alcohols, halogen-releasing agents, oxidizing agents, phenols, quaternary ammonium compounds, silver, and honey. A discussion of all antiseptics is beyond the scope of this chapter and the reader is referred to other sources for more detailed information (see Recommended Reading at the chapter's end).

Many antiseptics are available as aqueous solutions; some are also available as scrubs, which are detergents or soaps. The presence of detergent or soap in wounds may also potentiate wound infection. Detergents and soaps are irritating and cytotoxic, and thus should only be used on intact skin, and should never contact mucous membranes or subcutaneous tissues. Product labels must always be consulted for proper mixing and diluting instructions. Over- or under-diluting the product can

Table 56.1 Commonly Used Antiseptics

Antiseptic	Spectrum of Activity	Ineffective Activity	Residual Activity	Decreased Effectiveness
Alcohol	Bacteria, unenveloped viruses, some fungi, mycobacteria	Variable enveloped viruses, no spores	None	Organic material
Chlorhexidine solution	Gram-positive bacteria, some gram-negative bacteria, unenveloped viruses, fungi, mold, yeast	Variable gram-negative bacteria, variable enveloped viruses, no mycobacteria, no spores	4–6 hours, occasionally up to 2 days	Organic material
Povidone-iodine	Bacteria, enveloped viruses, fungi, yeast, mycobacteria	Variable enveloped viruses, no spores	Up to 4–6 hours	Organic material, alcohol

result in poor efficacy or exacerbation of skin irritation and toxicity, respectively.

Acids

Boric acid and acetic acid are the most commonly used **acid antiseptics** and are typically used in wounds at concentrations of 0.25 to 0.5%. They primarily act by disrupting cell membranes and are effective against bacteria (especially urea splitting organisms such as *Pseudomonas aeruginosa*), yeast, and fungi. At a pH of approximately 3.6, acids are bacteriostatic, and at a pH of approximately 3 they are bactericidal; therefore, the pH of the product being used should be confirmed. They are toxic to fibroblasts but these acids' impact on wound healing is unknown.

Alcohol

Alcohol is used both as an antiseptic and a disinfectant. It denatures proteins and disrupts metabolic function, causing precipitation of cell proteins and cell lysis. It also helps solubilize fats and may enhance the effectiveness of some antiseptics. It is effective against gram-positive and gram-negative bacteria, mycobacteria, some fungi, and some enveloped viruses; however, it has variable effectiveness against enveloped viruses and is not effective against Lyssaviridae (rabies virus). It is ineffective against bacterial spores. Unlike other commonly used antiseptics it has no residual effect because it rapidly evaporates. The presence of organic material such as blood or mucus also decreases its effectiveness. Ethyl and 70% isopropyl alcohol are the most effective forms. Within 2 minutes 90% kill is expected although effective kill of many bacteria occurs within 10 seconds of sustained exposure. As a general rule, extended exposure is needed and a cursory swipe with an alcohol-soaked swab on an animal's skin does little to disinfect the skin

site. Alcohol is cytotoxic and neurotoxic when applied to open wounds.

Chlorhexidine

Chlorhexidine is a bisguanide and the most commonly used **bisguanide antiseptic** in veterinary medicine. Bisguanides work by binding with proteins in the cell wall thus disrupting the cell wall, which causes leakage of cell contents. Bisguanides also precipitate cell proteins that are released during this process. Chlorhexidine has a spectrum of activity against most gram-positive and some gram-negative bacteria (including *Escherichia coli* and *Pseudomonas aeruginosa*), although it has somewhat variable activity against many gram-negative bacteria. It is effective against mold, yeast, and many viruses although it has variable activity against enveloped viruses and is not considered effective against Lyssaviridae (rabies virus). It is ineffective against bacterial spores and mycobacteria. It is suggested that there is an approximately 90% kill within 30 seconds of contact time. Although a preparation time of 5 to 7 minutes is recommended it is possible that two 30 second preps are sufficient. Since chlorhexidine binds to keratin, contact time may be less of an issue than with some other antiseptics. Chlorhexidine is considered to provide equally effective skin decontamination as povidone-iodine, but it has a longer residual effect than povidone-iodine of up to 2 days. When used as a wound lavage it has an immediate antimicrobial effect with a lasting residual effect. Chlorhexidine is generally not negatively impacted by the presence of alcohol, soaps, or lavage fluids, but the presence of moderate amounts of blood or organic matter can interfere with its effectiveness. Also, chlorhexidine's activity is pH dependent, being more soluble and thus more effective at lower pH.

Chlorhexidine is toxic to eyes and should never come in direct contact with them. It should not be used in the

Protocol 56.1 Formulating a 0.05% Chlorhexidine Solution

Items Required
- Chlorhexidine stock solution
- Water: deionized, distilled, or tap water

Procedure
If stock chlorhexidine solution is 4%
- To make 250 mL total volume, add 3.1 mL of 4% solution to 247 mL of water.
- To make 500 mL total volume, add 6.2 mL of 4% solution to 494 mL of water.

If stock chlorhexidine solution is 2%
- To make 250 mL total volume, add 6.2 mL of 2% solution to 244 mL of water.
- To make 500 mL total volume, add 12.5 mL of 2% solution to 488 mL of water.

Solution will be stable for 1 week if tap water is used.
 Solution will be stable for 6 weeks if distilled or deionized water is used.

ear if there is any concern that the tympanic membrane is not intact. It has a lower incidence of causing allergic reactions and skin irritation, and is less cytotoxic than iodine-based solutions; however, prolonged skin contact with concentrations of greater than 0.5% may be harmful and may impair fibroblast activity.

Currently solutions of 0.05% are recommended for wound lavage. This concentration can be prepared by diluting 1 part of a 2% stock solution with 40 parts of water (see Protocol 56.1). At this concentration chlorhexidine has been shown to help promote wound healing. If stock solution is diluted with tap water it is considered stable for 1 week. If it is diluted with distilled or deionized water it is considered stable for 6 weeks. A 1% ointment is useful for treatment of external wounds.

Halogen-releasing agents

Iodophors

Povidone-iodine is the most commonly used **iodophor** in veterinary medicine and is usually used as a scrub or solution commonly known as Betadine® (Purdue Frederick Company, Stamford, CT), which is a 10% povidone-iodine formulation. **Cadexomer iodine** is available as an ointment or dressing. Iodophors contain polymerized iodine so the free iodine is slowly released with the goal of minimizing tissue irritation and enhancing the delivery of iodine to the tissues. The iodine penetrates the cell wall where it causes oxidation of the intracellular contents and replaces microbial contents

with iodine. It has a broad spectrum of activity against vegetative gram-positive and gram-negative bacteria, fungi, enveloped viruses, yeast, and mycobacteria. It is considered ineffective against bacterial spores and unenveloped viruses. Approximately 90% kill is expected within 30 seconds of contact time although a minimum of 2 minutes of contact time is advised and a 5 to 7 minute scrub time is recommended. Povidone-iodine has a very rapid onset of activity and up to 4 to 6 hours of residual activity. It is inactivated by the presence of blood, plasma, and organic material so the presence of any of these rapidly diminishes the residual bactericidal activity. Iodophors are also affected by pH and temperature as well as the presence of alcohol and detergent. Alternating povidone-iodine with alcohol may actually decrease the effectiveness of the iodine by decreasing the contact time of the povidone-iodine with the skin. In addition, the presence of alcohol may interfere with the effectiveness of the povidone-iodine. The practice of alternating the povidone-iodine prep with alcohol is not advised. Although the presence of alcohol may decrease the effectiveness of povidone-iodine, alcohol-based iodophors have been shown to be more effective at decreasing central venous catheter colonization when compared with aqueous solutions.

Stock solution of povidone-iodine is usually 10%. Dilution of 1 part stock solution and 9 parts water creates the commonly used 1% solution (see Protocol 56.2). Either water or an electrolyte solution can be used to dilute the stock solution. Dilution both increases the bactericidal activity and decreases the cytotoxicity, although even at concentrations of 0.5% povidone-iodine can impair tissue fibroblast proliferation. At concentrations greater that 0.05% povidone-iodine can impair lymphocyte blastogenesis and granulocyte and monocyte viability and migration. Given that the most commonly used solution in practice is 1% it should be

Protocol 56.2 Formulating 1% Povidone-Iodine Solution

Items Required
- Povidone-iodine stock solution
- Water or electrolyte solution

Procedure
Stock povidone-iodine solution is 10%
- To make 250 mL total volume, add 25 mL of 10% solution to 225 mL of water.
- To make 500 mL total volume, add 50 mL of 10% solution to 450 mL of water.
Solution can be made using water or an electrolyte solution.

kept in mind that at this concentration there may be negative side effects. These side effects do not appear to be clinically relevant in most patients. It may be clinically relevant in some patients such as those with chronic wounds requiring repeated contact or those with underlying conditions predisposing them to delayed wound healing. Iodophors are more irritating to skin than bisguanides and can cause contact dermatitis and pruritus at concentrations as low as 0.1%.

Tincture of iodine is a commercially available solution of 2% iodine in 50% ethyl alcohol and is intended for use on intact skin only.

Iodophors should not be used on silicone.

Sodium hypochlorite

Sodium hypochlorite (household **bleach**) is an alkali that when mixed with an acid releases free chloride and oxygen. The chloride combines with water to form hypochlorous acid. It oxidizes and inactivates bacterial membranes and cytoplasmic enzyme systems, kills bacteria, and liquefies necrotic tissue. It has a broad spectrum of activity against gram-positive and gram-negative bacteria, mycobacteria, spores, fungi, enveloped and unenveloped viruses, and protozoa except for *Cryptosporidium*. It is also effective against biofilms. It has diminished activity in the presence of organic material and cationic detergents. It is corrosive and cytotoxic with a detrimental impact on neutrophils, fibroblasts, and endothelial cells at higher concentrations. For wound antisepsis it is used as a 0.5% solution (commonly called **Dakin's solution**) which is made by diluting 1 part regular laundry bleach with 9 parts water. (see Protocol 56.3). Although some rapid kill occurs, approximately 10 minutes of contact time ensures destruction of most microorganisms. It is unstable in solution and deteriorates rapidly, a process that is hastened with exposure to metal, high temperatures, light, and acid. Because of this instability the solution should be made

up immediately prior to use and any remaining solution should be discarded.

Honey

Honey has been used to treat wounds for over 4000 years. Its antiseptic properties are a result of its hyperosmolality, acidity, and ability to generate hydrogen peroxide; however, the concentration of hydrogen peroxide that is generated is 1,000 times less than that in 3% hydrogen peroxide. The phytochemical components, as well as the low pH of honey (approximately 3.6), also increase its antiseptic properties. It has a broad spectrum of activity against gram-positive and gram-negative bacteria as well as yeast.

Oxidizing agents

Hydrogen peroxide (H_2O_2) is a commonly used, foaming wound irrigant that dislodges bacteria and debris by effervescence. It releases oxygen, which causes lipid peroxidation of cell walls. At the high concentrations commonly found in disinfectants it is effective against vegetative gram-positive bacteria, gram-negative bacteria, mycobacteria, fungi, enveloped and unenveloped viruses, and protozoa; is variably effective against fungi; and is a good sporicide. Significant tissue damage can occur at concentrations of greater than 3%. At the 3% concentration used in antiseptic solutions, it is likely only effective against gram-positive bacteria, unless the bacteria contain catalase, in which case it is rendered ineffective. Its duration of effect is short-lived since it is not absorbed and has no residual activity.

Phenols

Phenols are effective antiseptics with a variable spectrum of activity that depends on the formulation. Phenols act primarily by binding cell membranes with subsequent disruption of the cell wall and leakage of intracellular contents, followed by binding with and precipitating the proteins that are released from the cell. Phenol (**carbolic acid**) has a broad spectrum of activity against gram-positive and gram-negative bacteria at a 0.1 to 1% concentration, and mycobacteria and fungi at a 1 to 2% concentration. It has variable activity against enveloped viruses, is ineffective against spores except at very high concentrations (5%), and has questionable activity against protozoa. At concentrations greater than 0.5% it has local anesthetic properties. Because phenol is highly toxic to tissues, it is not used commonly except at low concentrations (0.5%). It is highly corrosive and extended exposure can cause neurotoxicity.

Hexachlorophene has a broad spectrum of activity against gram-positive organisms. It is inactivated by

---

Protocol 56.3 Formulating 0.5% Sodium Hypochlorite (Dakin's) Solution

Items Required
- Household bleach
- Water

Procedure
- To make 250 mL total volume, add 25 mL of household bleach to 225 mL of water.
  Use immediately and discard unused solution.

alcohol. It is primarily incorporated into hand-washing soaps where repeated use leads to buildup of a residue on the skin that prolongs its bacteriostatic action. Washing hands with any other soap removes this residue. Severe neurotoxicity can occur with prolonged contact to high concentrations.

Chloroxylenol is a manmade phenolic compound that is minimally affected by the presence of organic debris. It works by inactivating enzyme systems and disrupting cell walls. It has a broad spectrum of activity against gram-positive bacteria and some gram-negative bacteria.

Quaternary ammoniums

Quaternary ammonium compounds are **cationic surfactants**, also known as **detergents**, that act by disrupting cell membranes, denaturing proteins, and inactivating enzyme systems. They are very effective against gram-positive bacteria and enveloped viruses but have variable effectiveness against gram-negative bacteria, fungi, and protozoa. They are mycobacteriostatic and sporostatic. They are ineffective against unenveloped viruses. They are inactivated by hard water, soaps and detergents, cotton, iodine, rubber, and organic material; this list should be considered when applying quaternary ammonium compounds. These compounds are corrosive at higher concentrations, are irritating to membranes, and can cause dermatitis after repeated use. However, the quaternary ammonium compound benzethonium, at 0.1 to 0.2%, is a safe and effective topical antiseptic.

Silver

Silver compounds have been used for many years as topical antiseptics, predominantly in burn patients. Silver ions act primarily by binding with thiol groups, which precipitates proteins and impairs the metabolic activities of cells. Silver is most commonly used in veterinary medicine as **silver sulfadiazine,** which is a 1% cream composed of two antibacterial agents. It has a broad spectrum of activity against gram-positive and gram-negative bacteria as well as yeast.

Handwashing

Handwashing plays a vital role in preventing infection. The importance of adequate hand washing in preventing infection was first noted by Oliver Wendell Holmes in 1843 and Ignaz Semmelweiss in 1846. Despite this knowledge and continued confirmation that infection is often transmitted by health care workers' hands, compliance rates remain poor. Even when handwashing occurs, often not all surfaces of the hands come in contact with the soap or antiseptic.

Medical staff should wash their hands before coming on duty, before and after direct or indirect contact with patients, before and after performing any bodily function such as nose blowing or using the restroom, before preparing or serving food, before preparing and administering medication, after direct or indirect contact with a patient's excretions, secretions, or blood, and after completing a shift.

Regular soap is not recommended for use in the surgical or intensive care unit setting. The primary action of soap is the mechanical removal of viable transient microorganisms. Regular soap should be used if gross contamination is present, and then always followed with the use of an antiseptic. If gross contamination is not present then this step can be skipped. Good hand hygiene can be achieved by using a waterless alcohol-based product or an antibacterial soap and water with adequate rinsing (i.e., any hand washing product with antimicrobial agents). An alcohol-based hand rub should be applied and the hands should be vigorously rubbed for at least 15 seconds. If an antimicrobial soap is being used, hands should be washed for at least 30 seconds.

Multiuse cloth hand towels should be avoided. Artificial nails and nails longer than 0.25 inches have been associated with an increased likelihood of infection. Please see Chapter 54, Minimizing Nosocomial Infection, for an in-depth discussion of hand hygiene and for a handwashing protocol.

Surgical scrubbing: personnel

All jewelry should be removed. Gross contamination should be removed using soap and water. Debris should be removed from under the nails using a nail pick under running water. Arms and forearms should be scrubbed starting with the fingers and progressing along the forearms. A sponge should be used rather than a brush to prevent damage to the skin. Arms should be held upright to allow water and soap to drip toward the elbows thus preventing recontamination of the hands and fingers. The length of time the scrub is performed should proceed according to the recommendations for the antiseptic being used. Chlorhexidine or an iodophor is recommended for the scrub solution. When using chlorhexidine, a 2% solution is considered only slightly less effective than a 4% and is significantly less irritating to the skin; 2% is thus the preferred concentration. Chlorhexidine solutions of greater than 1% concentration can cause significant eye damage so care must be taken to avoid eye contamination. A 5 minute scrub has been shown to be as effective as a 10 minute scrub and

2–3 minute scrubs have been shown to be as effective in many situations as 5 minute scrubs. A 1–2 minute scrub with chlorhexidine or an iodophor followed by application of an alcohol-based solution has been shown to be as effective as a 5 minute scrub. If an alcohol-based surgical scrub is being used the hands and forearms should be washed with soap and water first, dried thoroughly and then the alcohol solution applied. Quaternary ammonium compounds are not advised as surgical scrubs due to their limited spectrum of activity.

Aseptic preparation of the patient

Skin

Surgical site infection is present when more than 10^5 microorganisms are present per gram of tissue; however, if foreign material is present, then fewer organisms are needed to cause an infection. Most surgical infections are caused by the patient's own bacteria that are introduced into the surgical site from the skin, membranes, or hollow viscera (primarily the gut, but any hollow organ can potentially be a source of infection) during the surgical procedure.

Hair or fur should be clipped immediately before the procedure rather than in advance since advance shaving has been associated with an increased incidence of infection. A wide area should be clipped. In the case of wounds or a surgical exploratory celiotomy or thoracotomy the clip should be wide enough to ensure adequate preparation has been performed in case drains or feeding tubes need to be placed away from the primary surgical site. In traumatic wounds this clip should extend at least 5 cm circumferentially beyond the known extent of the wound. In other situations such as vascular catheter insertion sites, care should be taken to ensure that fur is clipped from the area immediately around the site, and that no fur can contact the catheter or insertion site during or after placement.

Gross contamination should be removed prior to using any antiseptic. In heavily contaminated wounds this may require the use of large volumes of tap water. Tap water has not been shown to increase infection rates or interfere with wound healing. Once this has been completed a surgical prep with an antiseptic should be performed (see Chapter 55, Care of Indwelling Device Insertion Sites; Protocol 55.1). In surgical patients this prep should be performed using sterile gauze in a sterile bowl, sterile saline, and personnel should be wearing a cap and mask. Concentric circles should be used starting from the location of the incision and working outward toward the periphery. There have been very few studies examining the effects of using different antiseptics on both surgical site colonization and surgical site infec-

tion. Chlorhexidine 2% solution is the most commonly recommended antiseptic. It does not have as good *in vitro* effectiveness as 10% povidone-iodine; however, it has better *in vivo* effectiveness, especially against *Staphylococci*, as well as a longer residual effect. In addition, iodine-based compounds may cause a hypersensitivity reaction in healthcare personnel.

Eyes

Sterile preparation before ophthalmic surgery requires treating the tissue surrounding the eye as well as the eye itself. To perform a sterile preparation around the eye, commercially prepared povidone-iodine swabs should be used. These swabs are soaked with a 10% povidone-iodine solution. Detergents must not be used since they can cause breakdown of the epithelium and alkaline burns. Alcohol in or around the eye is extremely irritating to tissues. Chlorhexidine will cause the proteins in the cornea to coagulate and will produce an alkali burn to the eye.

For irrigation of the cornea, conjunctiva, and palpebral fornices, a commercially prepared povidone-iodine 5% solution is available. The solution should be left in contact for 2 minutes and flushed with sterile saline in a bulb syringe. Irrigation of an eye with a corneal ulcer or intraocular irrigation requires use of specific additive-free products. Quaternary ammonium compounds are contraindicated since they can cause epithelial disruption. Generally a balanced salt solution is used.

Antiseptic treatment of wounds

The ideal antiseptic is effective without having significant cytotoxicity so as not to interfere with wound healing (see Table 56.2). Little evidence is available

Table 56.2 Properties of an ideal antiseptic

- Broad spectrum of activity
- Rapid onset of action and rapid kill
- Minimal likelihood of organism developing resistance
- Not affected by presence of organic material
- Residual effect
- Nontoxic to patient and user
- Easy to use
- Economical
- Environmentally friendly

Modified from Rutala WA, Weber DJ, Healthcare Infection Control Practices Advisory Committee, CDC Guideline for Disinfection and Sterilization of Healthcare Facilities, 2008.

regarding cytotoxicity of antiseptics *in vivo*, and published studies contain conflicting information. As a general rule wounds do not need to be irrigated with antiseptics. Antiseptics may have detrimental effects and no benefits have been seen when an antiseptic is used to irrigate a wound as compared to irrigation with 0.9% saline.

Infected wounds and chronic, nonhealing wounds appear to benefit most from the use of antiseptics. All antiseptics have the potential to be cytotoxic if used incorrectly, so close attention must be paid to ensure the appropriate dilution and formulation is being used on the patient. Chlorhexidine and povidone-iodine have been the most oft-studied antiseptics, and chlorhexidine appears to be the most effective antiseptic to use in infected and chronic nonhealing wounds. Although there are significant negative effects on fibroblasts by both antiseptics in vitro, no negative impact on wound healing has been demonstrable in vivo. At concentrations of 0.5% or 1% chlorhexidine has been shown to have more bactericidal effect than povidone-iodine and longer residual effect of up to 6 hours. Chlorhexidine at 0.05% has been shown to have 100% bacterial kill and no toxic effects on wound healing. In addition it did not make any difference whether the chlorhexidine was diluted in sterile water, 0.9% sodium chloride, or lactated Ringer's solution. Based on this it would appear that chlorhexidine at 0.5% should be used if it is felt an antiseptic is indicated for treating an infected or chronic nonhealing wound.

Newer compounds such as cadexomer iodine and some silver compounds definitively enhance healing and appear to be useful in the treatment of chronic wounds.

Hydrogen peroxide should be reserved for at most a one-time initial irrigation of dirty wounds. At a 3% concentration it does not appear to have detrimental *in vivo* effects on wound healing but it is a very ineffective antiseptic. It should never be delivered to wounds under pressure since its foaming action can force debris between tissue planes, enlarging the wound and causing accumulation of gas in tissues.

Mouth

Patients receiving long-term mechanical ventilation are at risk for developing oral lesions and ventilator-associated pneumonia (VAP). Aspiration of oropharyngeal microflora has been shown to be a major cause of VAP. Oral rinsing two to four times daily for 30 seconds with chlorhexidine solution at concentrations of 0.05% to 0.2% has been shown to effectively reduce the incidence of oral lesions and to delay the onset of pneumonia. See Chapter 25, Artificial Airway Management, for more information about oral care in patients with artificial airways.

Bacterial resistance to antiseptics and disinfectants

Intrinsic resistance

Bacteria can have natural resistance to antiseptics and disinfectants, and they can develop resistance to these chemicals in the same way they develop resistance to antibiotics. Gram-negative bacteria, mycobacteria, and spores have natural resistance. This is primarily due to the presence of a complex cell wall and the inherent difficulty in penetrating the membrane of the organism. Occasionally the organism has intrinsic properties that allow it to avoid the antiseptic's action. This intrinsic resistance often means antiseptics are ineffective at concentrations that are safe to be used in patients. Staphylococci occasionally have a natural resistance to antiseptics, which appears to be secondary to the presence of a protective slime around some strains.

Methicillin-resistant *Staphylococcus aureus* can be resistant to phenols and quaternary ammonium compounds. *Pseudomonas aeruginosa* are often resistant to antiseptics due to the structure of their outer membrane. More information about these resistant bacteria is found in Chapter 54, Minimizing Nosocomial Infection.

Biofilms

Pseudomonas and *Serratia marcescens* can rapidly develop resistance to chlorhexidine by forming a biofilm. A similar problem has been noted with povidone-iodine. A **biofilm** is a large number of bacteria covered in an extracellular material that have strongly adhered to the surface of an object. Bacteria inside biofilms are 1,000 times more resistant to antimicrobial agents than when they are not in biofilms. Because of the fact that *Pseudomonas* and *Serratia marascens* can develop a rapid resistance to chlorhexidine, the common practice of having containers of gauze squares soaking in chlorhexidine should not be permitted. Nor should large multiuse containers of chlorhexidine-based ointment be used.

Summary

Proper selection and use of antiseptics, disinfectants, and sterilization are crucial to the prevention of nosocomial infection. Chlorhexidine is currently the antiseptic documented to have the broadest spectrum of activity and least toxicity. Disinfectants should be chosen for their specific activities against target organisms. New antiseptics are constantly being developed to overcome microbial resistance and reduce toxicity.

Recommended reading

Boyce JM, Pittet D. Guideline for hand hygiene in health-care settings. 2002. CDC 51(RR16):1–44.

Chlebicki MP, Safdar N. Topical chlorhexidine for prevention of ventilator-associated pneumonia. Crit Care Med 2007;35: 595–602.

Fernandez R, Griffiths R. Water for wound cleansing. Cochrane Database Syst Rev 2008;(1):CD003861.

Fossum TW. Preparation of the operative site. In Small Animal Surgery, 2nd ed. St Louis, MO: Mosby, 2002:23–27.

Gould CV, Umscheid CA, Rajender K, et al. 2009. CDC Guidelines for prevention of catheter-associated urinary tract infections.

Lambrechts NE, Hurter K, Picard JA, et al. A prospective comparison between stabilized glutaraldehyde and chlorhexidine gluconate for preoperative skin prep antisepsis in dogs. Vet Surg 2004;33: 636–643.

Larson EL, Aiello AE, Lyle C, et al. Assessment of two hand hygiene regimens for intensive care unit personnel. Crit Care Med 2001; 29:944–951.

Lozier S, Pope E, Berg J. Effects of four preparations of 0.05% chlorhexidine diacetate on wound healing in dogs. Vet Surg 1992; 21:107–112.

Mangram AJ, Horan TC, Pearson ML, et al. Guideline for prevention of surgical site infection. Infect Control Hosp Epidemiol 1999;20(4): 250–278.

Mathews KA, Binnington AG. Wound management using honey. Compend Contin Educ Pract Vet 2002;24:53–60.

Mathews KA, Brooks MJ, Valliant AE. A prospective study of intravenous catheter contamination. J Vet Emerg Crit Care 1996;6: 33–43.

McDonnell G, Russell AD. Antiseptics and disinfectants: activity, action and resistance. Clin Microbiol Rev 1999;12:147–179.

O'Grady NP, Alexander M, Dellinger EP, et al. CDC guidelines for the prevention of intravascular catheter-related infections, 2002. CDC 51(RR10):1–26.

Osuna DJ, DeYoung DJ, Walker RL. Comparison of three skin preparation techniques, part 2: clinical trial in 100 dogs. Vet Surg 1990; 19:20–23.

Parienti J, du Cheyron D, Ramakers M, et al. Alcoholic povidone-iodine to prevent central venous catheter colonization: A randomized unit-crossover study. Crit Care Med 2004;32:708–713.

Rutala WA, Weber DJ. Healthcare Infection Control Practices Advisory Committee, CDC Guideline for disinfection and sterilization of healthcare facilities, 2008.

Sanchez IR, Swaim SF, Nusbaum KE, et al. Effects of chlorhexidine diacetate and povidone-iodine on wound healing in dogs. Vet Surg 1988;17:291–295.

Seim HB. Sterilization and disinfection. In Small Animal Surgery, 2nd ed. St Louis, MO: Mosby, 2002:7–10.

Seim HB, Fossum TW. Principles of asepsis. In Small Animal Surgery, 2nd ed. St Louis, MO: Mosby, 2002:1–6.

Stubbs WP, Bellah JR, Vermaas-Hekman D, et al. Chlorhexidine gluconate versus chloroxylenol for preoperative skin preparation in dogs. Vet Surg 1996;25:487–494.

57

Personnel precautions for patients with zoonotic disease

Megan Patterson Melcher and Christopher G. Byers

One of the risks inherent in the field of veterinary medicine is the possibility of contracting a zoonotic disease, or zoonosis. Zoonosis (from the Greek "zoo" meaning animal and "nosos" meaning illness) is defined as a disease of animals transmissible to humans. With today's environment of H1N1 influenza ("swine" flu), anthrax mailings, and bioterrorist threats, zoonotic diseases have increasingly become an area of concern and study.

Due to the unique proximity of animals and humans in veterinary hospitals, the risk of zoonotic pathogen transmission is higher than that for the general population. This chapter will cover types of zoonoses that small animal emergency and critical care personnel may encounter, methods of transmission, prevention measures, and resultant legal and public health issues.

With more than 250 zoonotic organisms known to cause human disease, it is not possible to cover the full spectrum in this chapter. Rather, this chapter will address zoonotic pathogens specifically known to be transmissible from dogs and cats to humans and therefore may potentially be seen in a small animal emergency and critical care hospital. The veterinary professional should remember there are far more zoonoses encountered in large animal and exotic/special species veterinary work.

Types of zoonotic diseases and transmission

Zoonoses are communicable diseases in which the causative agent is passed or carried from an animal to a human either directly or indirectly via fomites or vectors.

The offending organisms may be viruses, bacteria, fungi, or parasites. See Table 57.1 for a listing of most of the known pathogens associated with dogs and cats.

Transmission

If an animal is ill with or potentially carrying one of these pathogens, they represent the first step in the Center for Disease Control's (CDC) three necessary steps for disease transmission[1]:

1. A source of infection: This may include clinically ill animals, asymptomatic carriers, unaffected reservoirs, or fomites.
2. A susceptible host: Susceptibility typically depends on multiple factors, including the immunocompetance of the host, the virulence of the pathogen, and the success of the transmission. Physical susceptibility (i.e., nonintact skin, loss of cough reflex, or gastric acid reduction) or immunological susceptibility (i.e., immunocompromised individuals, people with underlying disease, pregnant women, and unvaccinated people) may increase a host's risk of disease.
3. A method of transmission: This may be via direct contact (such as ingestion, cutaneous, percutaneous, or mucous membranes contact), contact with fomites, aerosol transmission (on mucous membranes or on nonintact skin or inhaled), or vector-borne (insects on the animal or insects or rodents that enter the hospital).

Advanced Monitoring and Procedures for Small Animal Emergency and Critical Care, First Edition. Edited by Jamie M. Burkitt Creedon, Harold Davis.
© 2012 John Wiley & Sons, Inc. Published 2012 by John Wiley & Sons, Inc.

Table 57.1 Pathogens associated with dogs and cats

Disease	Method of transmission to humans	Disease	Method of transmission To humans
Acariasis (mange) *Sarcoptes scabiei, Notoedres cati*, others	Contact with skin (may be nonintact or intact)	Bartonellosis (cat scratch fever) *Bartonella henslae*	Contact with nonintact skin, via inoculation (bite or scratch), vector
Blastomycosis *Blastomyces dermatidis*	Via inoculation (bite, accidental needle stick)	Bordatellosis (kennel cough) *Bordatella bronchiseptica*	Aerosol
Brucellosis *Brucella melitensis, B. abortus, B. suis, B. canis*	Aerosol, contact with nonintact skin	Campylobacteriosis *Campylobacter jejuni, C. fetus, C. coli*	Fecal-oral contact
Chlamydiosis (mammalian) *Chlamydiophila abortus, C. felis*	Aerosol, contact with eyes	Coccidiomycosis *Coccidiodes immitis, C. posadasii*	Aerosol, via inoculation (bite)
Cryptococcosis *Cryptococcus neoformans*	Aerosol	Cryptosporidiosis *Cryptosporidium parvum*	Fecal-oral contact
Dermatophytosis (ringworm) *Microsporum sp., Trichophyton sp., Epidermophyton sp.*	Contact with skin (may be nonintact or intact)	Dipylidium (tapeworm) *Dipylidium caninum*	Vector
Echinococcus *Echinococcus granulosus. E. mulitocularis*	Fecal-oral contact	Erlichiosis, Anaplasmosis *Erlichia spp., Anaplasma spp.*	Vector
Giardiasis *Giardia intestinalis, G. lamblia*	Fecal-oral contact	Cutaneous larval migrans (hookworm) *Ancyclostoma sp.*	Contact with skin (may be nonintact or intact)
Visceral, Ocular, Neuro larval migrans (roundworm) *Toxocara canis, T. cati*	Contact with skin (may be nonintact or intact)	Leishmaniasis *Leishmania spp.*	Vector
Leptospirosis *Leptospira spp.*	Contact with nonintact skin or mucus membranes, aerosol	Listeriosis *Listeria monocytogenes*	Contact with skin (may be nonintact or intact)
Pasturellosis *Pasturella multocida*	Via inoculation (bite or scratch)	Plague *Yersinia pestis*	Vector, contact with nonintact skin, aerosol
Q fever *Coxiella burnettii*	Contact via ingestion, aerosol, vector	Rabies Lyssavirus	Contact with nonintact skin, via inoculation (bite, scratch)
Salmonellosis *Salmonella spp.*	Fecal-oral contact	Sporotrichosis *Sporothirix schenkii*	Contact with nonintact skin
Staphylococcosis *Staphylococcus spp.*	Contact with nonintact skin, aerosol	Streptococcosis *Streptococcus spp.*	Contact with nonintact skin, aerosol
Toxoplasmosis *Toxoplasma gondii*	Fecal-oral contact	Tularemia *Francisella tularensis*	Inoculation (bite, scratch), aerosol, vector

Bacterial zoonoses

Bacterial diseases are some of the most common zoonotic pathogens seen in small animal hospitals. Most, such as kennel cough (*Bordatella bronchiseptica*) and leptospirosis (*Leptospira interrogans*), will be instantly recognizable to today's veterinary personnel.

Bordatellosis

Bordatella bronchiseptica is a gram-negative bacterium that primarily causes tracheobronchitis in dogs. The patient will often have a harsh, honking cough ("kennel cough"). Bordatellosis has also been increasingly identified as a cause of upper respiratory disease in cats.[2] Studies have shown the bacterium is transmissible between cats and dogs, cats and humans, and dogs and humans.[3–5] The pathogen spreads via aerosol transmission. Any patient with suspected bordatellosis should be isolated, and the staff should follow protective measures against aerosolized pathogens. Immunocompromised individuals and people with pre-existing respiratory disease are most at risk for contracting bordatellosis. The disease usually involves the respiratory tract but has been associated with endocarditis, peritonitis, meningitis, and wound infections in people.[6]

Brucellosis

Brucellosis is caused by the gram-negative bacterium *Brucella canis* in dogs. This disease may be transmitted to humans through contamination of nonintact skin with infective vaginal secretions, placental tissue, semen, and sometimes urine and blood. Presenting signs in dogs may include spontaneous abortion, epidydimitis, orchitis, scrotal dermatitis, and/or scrotal necrosis in intact males. Discospondylitis and uveitis in dogs of either sex has also been documented.[7] In people, clinical illness may manifest after a 1- to 2-month incubation period. Symptoms are often flulike and include fever, sweating, headaches, back pain, weakness, orchitis/epidydimitis in males, and spontaneous abortion in women. In rare cases, brucellosis has been linked to sacroiliitis, hepatic disease, endocarditis, colitis, and meningitis.[7] The disease has been reportedly transmissible between human mothers and babies in contaminated breast milk.[8] Brucellosis is on the CDC's nationally notifiable disease list for people in the United States.[9]

Bartonellosis

Bartonellosis, commonly known as "cat scratch fever," is caused by the gram-negative bacterium *Bartonella henslae* (less commonly *B. clarridgeiae*). The disease is transmitted to people primarily through cat bites or scratches, but may also be transmitted via flea or tick vector, from a dog bite or scratch, or from saliva contact with nonintact skin. The feline carrier presenting to a small animal clinic will typically be a young kitten, feral, or stray cat, and is most often a subclinical carrier, since disease in cats is uncommon. If the organism does cause clinical signs in cats, these signs are usually mild and self-limiting, and may include pyrexia, uveitis, and lymphadenomegaly. Human disease is also mild in immunocompetent individuals. Symptoms may include papules/pustules at inoculation site that may progress to nonhealing wounds with regional lymphadenomegaly, fever, headache, and general malaise. There has been a reported human case of optic neuritis stemming from an infection with *B. henslae*.[10] Fatalities have been reported in immunocompromised individuals from infections progressing to bacteremia, meningitis, and hepatitis.[10]

Leptospirosis

Leptospirosis may be caused by any of several serovars of the gram-negative spirochete *Leptospira interrogans*. The pathogen may be transmitted via contact between infected urine or tissue and mucous membranes and/or nonintact skin. Clinical disease is seen primarily in dogs. Cats are susceptible to infection, and though they seldom develop clinical symptoms, they may still transmit the disease. The patient with leptospirosis may present with a variety of signs, as the infection may be peracute, acute, subacute, or chronic. The peracute form of the disease results in sudden death with few or no clinical signs. In the acute form, dogs may have pyrexia, icterus, myalgia, vomiting, diarrhea, and peripheral vascular collapse. The subacute form may cause pyrexia, anorexia, vomiting, dehydration, polydipsia, and often severe renal failure marked by oliguria or anuria. The chronic form is frequently characterized by pyrexia and renal and/or hepatic failure. The majority of cases seen in animal hospitals are subacute and chronic. In people, leptospirosis may range from asymptomatic infections to flulike illness with fever, headache, myalgia, nausea, vomiting, diarrhea, abdominal pain, rash, conjunctivitis, and conjunctival hemorrhage. The most severe form of leptospirosis in people is known as "Weil's disease." It is caused by the serovar *L. icterohemorrhagiae* and results in icterus due to hepatocellular dysfunction and renal failure from tubular damage. This form has a 20%–40% mortality rate in immunocompromised people.[11] Rarely, leptospirosis infections in people may cause neurologic, respiratory, and cardiac manifestations.[12] The leptospirosis vaccine may protect dogs from clinical illness, but vaccinated dogs are still able to acquire the pathogen and shed it in their urine.[13] According to the World Organization for Animal Health (OIE), leptospirosis is a nationally notifiable disease for animals in the United States, but not, as yet, for people.[14]

Plague

Plague is caused by the gram-negative bacterium *Yersina pestis*. In the United States, rodents are the primary reservoir (rats, squirrels, and prairie dogs) and cats are typically infected by fleas or ingestion of the aforementioned rodents. People may contract the disease through contact between blood or purulent exudates and nonintact skin or via aerosols from cats with the pneumonic form. Dogs may contract the pathogen, but infection is often subclinical or may result in mild pyrexia and lymphadenomegaly. No human cases have ever been linked to infected dogs. In cats and people, plague may present in one of its three classic forms: bubonic, septicemic, and pneumonic. Bubonic plague is associated with fever, dehydration, lymphadenomegaly, and hyperesthesia. This form is usually acquired by cats ingesting infected rodents and causes regional lymph nodes (submandibular, cervical, and retropharyngeal) to abcessate (buboes) and drain. Septicemic plague may progress from the bubonic form but is not always associated with bubo formation. In this form, the bacteria spread through the blood or lymphatic system to any organ in the body; the lungs and spleen are most commonly affected in cats and people. Clinical signs are due to septic shock and include fever, anorexia, vomiting, diarrhea, tachycardia, weak pulses, hypotension, cold extremities, disseminated intravascular coagulopathy (DIC), and leukocytosis. This form is usually rapidly fatal. Pneumonic plague may be secondary to the bubonic or septicemic forms or may be primarily contracted from aerosolized plague bacteria. Cats do not typically contract primary pneumonic plague but have been implicated in the aerosol transmission of pneumonic plague to people.[15] Clinical signs may include fever, cough, hemoptysis, and respiratory distress. Since 1977, the CDC has reported 23 human cases of plague associated with aerosolized pneumonic plague droplets from infected cats. A quarter of the cases were in veterinary staff.[16] Plague has caused millions of human fatalities through the ages, and is a nationally notifiable disease for humans and animals in the United States.[9,14]

Staphylococcal infections

Staphylococci (staph) are gram-positive bacteria whose principle habitats are the skin and mucous membranes of mammals and birds. Most staphylococci cause no disease to animals; however, all species are potentially pathogenic. Staph may cause a number of different diseases in dogs, cats, and humans, including skin infections, pneumonia, and bacteremia. Of particular concern to small animal veterinary personnel is methicillin-resistant *Staphylococcus aureus* (MRSA). This is a nosocomial and/or community-acquired human pathogen reportedly transmissible between small animals and people.[17] As of yet, it appears MRSA infections in dogs have been cases of "reverse zoonosis" that are acquired from humans as opposed to the other way around.[17] In a 2009 study, veterinary personnel were found to be the primary source of nosocomial MRSA infections in small animal hospitals.[18] Transmission is via direct contact, fomites, or aerosolization depending on the disease process; in one reported case a person acquired a staph endocarditis from a dog bite wound.[19] MRSA is a nationally notifiable disease for humans in the United States.[9]

Tularemia

Tularemia is caused by the gram-negative bacterium *Francisella tularensis*. This disease is endemic in temperate regions of the world where rodents and rabbits are the primary reservoirs. In small animal medicine, cats are the primary source of zoonotic infection. Transmission is commonly via bites or scratches but may also be contracted from aerosolized particles and vectors. Cats may present with a myriad of clinical signs including pyrexia, lymphadenomegaly, splenomegaly, hepatomegaly, oral ulcers, icterus, and panleukopenia. Dogs appear to be relatively resistant to infection. In humans, clinical disease causes flulike symptoms with fever, headache, and general malaise. The infection may develop into either of the two main syndromes: ulceroglandular or typhoidal. In the ulceroglandular form, ulcerative skin lesions develop at the inoculation site, with regional lymphadenomegaly. The typhoidal form may present as systemic with diarrhea, vomiting, and abdominal pain; or as pneumonic with fever, cough, hemoptysis, and chest pain. Tularemia is nationally notifiable for animals and humans.[9,14]

Fungal zoonoses

Fungal organisms comprise an important category of potential zoonotic infection. Commonly seen fungal infections in small animal veterinary hospitals include blastomycosis, coccidiomycosis, dermatophytosis, and sporotrichosis.

Blastomycosis

Blastomycosis is a systemic mycotic infection caused by the fungus *Blastomyces dermatitidis*. This organism is endemic to many areas of the United States including the Mississippi, Ohio, and Missouri river valleys, and the Mid-Atlantic States.[20] Most human infections are directly from the environment as they are for dogs and cats; however, transmission has been documented in the veterinary field via inoculation from contaminated sharps during fine needle aspirates, necropsies, and from the bite of an infected dog.[10] Patients that present clinically ill with blastomycosis commonly have clinical signs from inhaling infective spores. These may include weight loss, cough, dyspnea, anorexia, skin lesions, ocular disease, and lameness. A patient presenting with uveitis and concurrent skin or respiratory disease in an endemic region should raise marked suspicion for blastomycosis.[20] In people, blastomycosis also affects the lungs and may cause fever, chills, sweating, chest pain, coughing, and difficulty breathing. The fungus may also spread systemically affecting skin, bones, meninges, and the genitourinary tract.[10]

Coccidiomycosis

Coccidiomycosis is a fungal disease caused by the organism *Coccidiodes immitis* or *C. posadasii*. This fungus is primarily found in soil in the southwestern United States where it may cause the disease known as "valley fever." The fungus develops airborne spores during rainy seasons in otherwise arid areas. These spores may be inhaled and cause clinical disease. In dogs, the fungus typically causes mild lower respiratory disease characterized by coughing, pyrexia, anorexia, and weight loss. In more severely infected patients, the disease may become disseminated and cause pyrexia, lameness, anorexia, lymphadenomegaly, draining skin lesions, and even seizures, blindness, and death.[21] In cats, the disseminated form with its concurrent skin lesions is much more common and includes symptoms of weight loss, fever, and inappetance, and occasionally involves respiratory distress.[21] Zoonotic cases of coccidiomycosis have primarily involved veterinary personnel. Cases have involved transmission during a necropsy of an animal with disseminated disease[21] and via a bite from a cat also with the disseminated form of the disease.[22] There is also a potential for transmission of the fungus from bandage material placed on draining wounds infected with *Coccidiodes* spp. The bandage may act as a warm, moist substrate for development of the infective aerosolized spores.[21] Coccidiomycosis in people is similar to that seen in dogs and cats. There are three main forms of the disease: pulmonary, disseminated, and cutaneous. The disease is usually mild in healthy people and may result in flulike symptoms. In immunocompromised patients, the pulmonary form may cause pneumonia and lung

nodules, and the disseminated form may cause skin ulcers, bone lesions, heart inflammation, joint pain, meningitis, and death.[23]

Dermatophytosis

Dermatophytosis, often referred to as ringworm, is a fungal dermatological disease caused by species of *Microsporum canis* or *Trichophyton sulphureum*. Transmission to people is usually through contact between nonintact skin and lesions of infected animals, though even contact between intact skin and asymptomatic carriers may transmit the fungus. The disease has widely varying signs and imperfect diagnostic tests; therefore, personnel should follow precautions in dealing with any animal evincing dermatologic disease. The fungus attacks the hair follicle, and clinical signs often include alopecia, scaling, and crusting. Some animals may have the classic ringlike lesion, but the disease may look like almost any other dermatological disease affecting cats and dogs. Cats are the primary species of concern with regard to zoonotic transmission. People often develop the ring lesions with circular alopecia, scaling, crusting, and ulceration.[24] The disease may be more serious in immunocompromised individuals.

Sporotrichosis

Sporotrichosis is caused by the fungus *Sporothrix schenckii*, which is found in soil throughout the world. Transmission typically occurs via inoculation with the fungus, and in dogs (particularly hunting or free-roaming dogs) is thought to arise from skin penetration with contaminated thorns or wood splinters.[25] In cats, transmission is commonly via scratches or bites from other cats and is seen most often in intact males that are outdoors.[25] The dog with sporotrichosis will typically have the cutaneous or cutaneolymphatic form. Clinical signs of the cutaneous form include nodules in the dermal and subcutaneous layers of the trunk and head that may be ulcerated. Those with the cutaneolymphatic form will have nodules on the distal part of a limb that progress along lymphatic vessels and is associated with regional lymphadenomegaly. In cats, nodules will occur in areas where inoculation occurred and typically resemble nonhealing abscesses and may progress to necrosis of the surrounding area. The organism may become systemic in cats and spread to many organs. Veterinary personnel are most at risk from cats, as the fungus replicates easily and is present in large numbers in ulcerated nodule exudates, as well as in other body tissues and feces.[26] Most infections in people present as ulcerative, cutaneous lesions with purulent discharge and localized lymphadenomegaly. Systemic sporotrichosis is a danger to immunocompromised people and has been documented in people with human immunodeficiency virus (HIV), acquired immunodeficiency syndrome (AIDS), alcoholism, diabetes mellitus, and those receiving immunosuppressive medications.[26]

Viral zoonoses

Zoonotic viruses are another subset of diseases to which small animal veterinary personnel are exposed. Within this category, rabies is of paramount concern, but there is growing evidence that influenza may also be transmissible between small animals and humans.

Rabies

Rabies is caused by a *Lyssavirus* in the Rhabdoviridae family. These viruses are found nearly worldwide and all warm-blooded animals are susceptible to infection. Pathogen transmission is nearly always via inoculation with saliva (bite) and/or contact with saliva and nonintact skin or mucous membranes. A rabid patient may have a variety of clinical signs and a bite wound history and may or may not present with one of the classic rabies syndromes of paralytic or furious. Rabies typically starts with the prodromal phase in dogs and cats. This stage is characterized by pyrexia, apprehension, nervousness, anxiety, avoidance of company, and/or radical behavioral changes from the animal's norm. Licking, biting, or scratching at wound site may be present. In dogs, the furious stage of rabies may develop following the prodromal phase and last for up to 7 days. Classic signs include irritability, restlessness, photophobia, ataxia, disorientation, generalized seizures, viciousness, and pica. Death usually occurs during seizure activity.[27] Cats tend to manifest a more classic furious stage with erratic, vicious behavior, tremors, ataxia, and weakness. The patient with paralytic rabies will develop lower motor neuron paralysis spreading from the infected bite wound.[27] The classic clinical sign of paralytic rabies in dogs is a hanging jaw with concurrent ptyalism as the animal loses its ability to close its mouth or swallow. This results in death from respiratory failure within a few days.[27] Cats primarily present with paralysis progressing from the infected bite area and an increase in vocalization with a marked change in voice.[27] In people, rabies manifests in the prodromal stage as fever, headache, pain at the bite site, and agitation. The furious phase includes violent behavior, restlessness, anxiety, and seizures that may result in death.[28] The paralytic stage symptoms include the inability to swallow, progressive paralysis, and death due

to respiratory failure.[28] The mortality rate for rabies in veterinary and human patients is virtually 100%. Rabies is a nationally notifiable disease for animals and humans.[9,14]

Influenza

Influenza viruses from the *Orthomyxoviridae* family are infectious to humans and many species of animals, including dogs and cats. In the 1970s an influenza epidemic in people resulted in the contraction of symptomatic flu in dogs.[29] And in the recent 2009 outbreak of influenza A (H1N1), also known as "swine flu," the American Veterinary Medical Association (AVMA) confirmed clinical disease in 14 cats and three dogs that had been in contact with infected humans.[30] In cats and dogs, influenza may present with coughing, sneezing, nasal and ocular discharge, anorexia, pyrexia, lethargy, and occasionally secondary pneumonia. To date, influenza is considered a "reverse" zoonotic disease with regard to dogs and cats. This means that they contract the disease from humans as opposed to humans contracting the disease from them. However, influenza does pass back and forth between humans and other animals such as pigs and birds, so the risk of zoonotic transmission exists.

Fecal-oral zoonoses

Within zoonotic diseases there is a special subset that is transmitted primarily in fecal matter. These fecally transmitted zoonotic pathogens—*Campylobacter*, *Cryptosporidium*, *Giardia*, *Salmonella*, and *Toxoplasma*—are some of the most common seen in small animal veterinary medicine.

Campylobacter

Campylobacteriosis is caused in dogs, cats, and humans by the gram-negative bacterium *Campylobacter jejuni*. Transmission is primarily fecal-oral in the veterinary setting. Patients will commonly present with symptoms including diarrhea, vomiting, pyrexia, and anorexia. Clinical disease typically lasts about a week and is most common in puppies and kittens less than 6 months old.[31] In people, *C. jejuni* is the most common cause of bacterial diarrhea in the United States with an estimated two million cases a year.[32] The disease causes enteritis with symptoms of fever and malaise, progressing to diarrhea and abdominal pain. The disease is generally self-limiting in healthy adults but has been linked to the development of Guillain-Barre syndrome (GBS) in approximately 1 in 1,000 cases.[32] GBS is an immune mediated myelitis/neuropathy.[32] Another secondary development that has been identified in human *Campylobacter* infections is Reiter's syndrome, which causes tenosynovitis, skin lesions, uveitis, and urethritis in approximately 7% of cases.[32]

Cryptosporidium

Cryptosporidium parvum is a coccidian protozoan that causes intestinal disease in dogs, cats, and humans and is transmitted via the fecal-oral route. Cats with cryptosporidiosis may have diarrhea, weight loss, tenesmus, blood in the stool, and abdominal discomfort. Disease in cats is typically seen in kittens or in immunocompromised or stressed adults.[33] In dogs, *Cryptosporidium* usually only causes disease in young puppies with concurrent parvovirus or distemper.[33] Symptoms include diarrhea, weight loss, and malabsorption. In humans, the majority of people will develop mild, self-limiting diarrhea with the disease. However, cryptosporidiosis is a leading cause of life-threatening chronic diarrhea in immunocompromised patients, such as those with HIV.[33] Of primary concern to the veterinary staff, oocysts present in fecal matter are highly infectious and highly resistant to environmental deactivation, and there is no routinely successful treatment for infections. *Cryptosporidium* is nationally notifiable for humans.[9]

Giardia

Giardia duodenalis is a protozoan parasite transmitted via the fecal-oral passing of infective cysts. Dogs and cats may present as asymptomatic carriers or evince clinical disease with pale, malodorous, steatorrheic stool, and weight loss.[34] Animals with clinical disease are primarily very young puppies and kittens, or adults that are immunocompromised, stressed, or from kennel situations. In humans, *G. duodenalis* is one of the most common intestinal parasites worldwide. The vast majority of cases stem from contaminated water; however, direct transmission via the feces of infected animals is possible. Symptoms in people may include acute gastroenteritis with diarrhea or a more chronic infection with malabsorptive diarrhea, weight loss, and abdominal pain that waxes and wanes.[35] Giardiasis is a nationally notifiable disease for humans.[9]

Salmonella

Salmonella enterica is a gram-negative bacterium with over 2,400 pathogenic serovars that cause primarily intestinal disease. *S. enterica* is a fecal pathogen that may survive for a long time in the environment and be transmitted via the direct fecal-oral path, in contaminated food and water, on fomites, via contact with cat or dog saliva, and even aerosolized in dried airborne particles.[36]

The majority of affected dogs and cats are subclinical carriers, but when illness does present it is typically an acute enterocolitis with pyrexia, anorexia, lethargy, diarrhea with mucus or blood, abdominal pain, and mesenteric lymphadenomegaly.[36] In some cases, clinical infection may result in septicemia, endotoxemia, and localized organ infection such as *Salmonella* pneumonia.[36] In humans, clinical salmonellosis usually follows a 12- to 36-hour incubation period and includes symptoms such as headache, fever, vomiting, diarrhea, abdominal pain, nausea, myalgia, and dehydration. Of special concern is the transmission of highly drug-resistant strains of *S. typhimurium* DT 104, which has been isolated in dogs and cats and was reported as the causative agent in an outbreak of salmonellosis in cats and people at three small veterinary hospitals.[37] Salmonellosis is a nationally notifiable disease for humans.[9]

Toxoplasmosis

Toxoplasmosis is caused by the coccidian protozoa *Toxoplasma gondii*. Domestic cats and other felines are the definitive hosts for this parasite and shed infective oocytes in their feces. All other species, including dogs and humans, are intermediate hosts and the protozoa will encyst and not be transmissible. In the general population, infection is normally from undercooked meat, contaminated water, and, much less frequently, cat feces. In veterinary hospitals, however, cat feces are of primary concern. The *T. gondii* oocyte is not infectious when first excreted. It takes 1–5 days, depending on temperature and humidity, to sporulate into the infective form. Once the oocyte has entered its infective phase, it may remain infectious in the environment for 18 months and is extremely hardy and difficult to eradicate. Most cats start shedding the oocyte approximately 3–10 days after infection and typically shed for 2 weeks. A majority of infected cats will not become clinically ill with toxoplasmosis but may still transmit the disease to people. A cat ill with toxoplasmosis may have varied symptoms, as the parasite potentially affects virtually any organ system. The most common systems affected are pulmonary, nervous, hepatic, pancreatic, cardiac, and ocular. Symptoms may include pyrexia, pancreatitis, hepatitis, encephalitis, polymyositis, pneumonitis, uveitis, chorioretinitis, fading kitten syndrome, vomiting, diarrhea, and anorexia.[38] In dogs, illness is uncommon but may result in a rapidly fatal systemic disease involving the gastrointestinal tract, the respiratory system, the neuromuscular system, and/or the liver.[38] Cats may shed oocytes for up to 2 weeks following initial infection and have been shown to be susceptible to contracting the parasite again after a previous infection. Cats with latent infections may sometimes re-shed oocytes after secondary infections.[38] In people, infection with toxoplasmosis may cause abortion, chorioretinitis, blindness, hydrocephalus, epilepsy, mental retardation, myelitis, paralysis, fever, malaise, myalgia, lymphadenomegaly, and hepatosplenomegaly.[38] A 2003 study proposed a possible link between toxoplasmosis and schizophrenia.[39]

Other zoonoses

Despite the low occurrence of two zoonotic disease categories, a chapter on this subject would not be complete without a mention of both vector-borne zoonoses, such as anaplasmosis (*Anaplasma* spp.), erlichiosis (*Erlichia* spp.), leismaniasis (*Leishmania* spp.), Rocky Mountain spotted fever (*Rickettsia rickettsii*), and Lyme disease (*Borrelia burgdorferii*), as well as diseases from intestinal cestodes, nematodes, and ascarids.

Vector-borne diseases require an insect such as a flea, tick, or mosquito to pass a pathogen from a reservoir species to humans. Most cats and dogs are not definitive hosts for these diseases and so their role in transmission is to bring vectors into close contact with humans. Good insect and rodent control within the hospital and quick response to flea and tick infestation on incoming patients may be preventative.

Intestinal cestodes, nematodes, and ascarids, also known as "worms," are zoonotic disease-causing agents. Some intestinal parasites, such as the cestodes (tapeworms) *Diplidium caninum* and *Echinococcus multiocularis*, are acquired by humans through the ingestion of fleas. In the case of the ascarids and nematodes *Toxocara cati*, *T. canis* (roundworms), *Ancylostoma* spp. (hookworms), and *Strongyloides stercoralis*, transmission may occur through ingestion of infective oocytes or via skin penetration by the larval stage present in contaminated soil. Again, as in the case of vector-borne diseases, rodent and insect control as well as immediate treatment of any animal infested with fleas may be preventative. In the case of soil contamination, removing stool from the outdoor environment quickly may prevent eggs from developing into the infective stage.

Personnel protection

Zoonotic disease prevention starts before the patient enters the hospital. Identification of potential zoonotic risk starts with knowledge of clinical disease signs and methods of transmission of a given disease. Solid knowledge of disease states may allow the technician or receptionist to identify possible zoonoses based on an animal's symptoms, history, geographic region, and other risk factors, such as age, underlying illness, and proximity to certain high-risk areas or wildlife. The best case scenario is identification over the phone and isolation of the incoming animal before it enters the building. More commonly, rapid isolation of the patient in an examination room once the risk is identified and limitation of personnel contact are instrumental in reducing the likelihood of disease transmission. Signs should be posted to notify other personnel and clients that an infectious disease may be present and what precautions to take.

Hand hygiene

The single most important precaution veterinary personnel may take to prevent the transmission of zoonotic disease is good hand hygiene. Washing with regular soap and water removes debris and is effective in reducing the number of organisms on the skin. The added use of antimicrobial soaps and hand cleansers kills or prevents the replication of many viruses and bacteria. The use of gel, liquid, or cloth hand sanitizers is appropriate in most clinical situations; however, before and after eating, before and after using the restroom, or when hands are visibly soiled, hands should be washed with soap and running water. The proper procedure for hand washing is seen in Chapter 54, Protocol 54.1. Soap should be liquid or foam-based and not bar soap, as the latter may serve as a reservoir for bacterial growth. Soap dispensers should be the type that can be loaded with disposable soap containers and/or be emptied completely, cleaned, and disinfected before being refilled to prevent the colonization of the dispensers with pathogens. When used, hand sanitizers should be rubbed into hands until dry. These procedures are further detailed in Chapter 54, Minimizing Nosocomial Infections.

Veterinary personnel should not wear long fingernails, particularly artificial nails, as they may inhibit adequate hand hygiene.[40] Rings may also harbor organisms that are not killed during hand washing and should be removed during procedures and hand washing. The longer the fingernails and the more rings a technician wears, the greater the surface area for germs to grow. Artificial nails provide dark, moist areas that are particularly inviting to organisms, and rings may trap moisture and provide the same. According to a study published by the CDC in 2000, 16 deaths of human neonates from *Pseudomonas aeroginosa* were attributed to nurses with artificial nails and long, natural nails.[41]

Barrier protection

Barrier protection is another protective measure veterinary personnel should take to prevent the transmission of zoonotic diseases. The most important and regularly used barrier are gloves. Gloves should be worn when handling any animal with unknown history or vaccination status and when handling feces, blood, or other bodily fluids, including during venipuncture and aspiration procedures. They should also be worn when cleaning litter boxes or any surface in possible contact with bodily tissues or fluids, and when handling soiled bedding or any animal with blood or bodily fluid on it. Gloves should be removed immediately after use without touching the external surfaces. Gloves should be removed from the wrist and pulled inside out to prevent hand contamination. Hands should be washed immediately after removing gloves, as there may be small glove defects and/or hands may have been contaminated during glove removal.

Body protection

Disposable or washable gowns, such as surgery gowns, may be worn when holding or restraining a potentially infectious patient or whenever there is a risk of bodily contact with pathogens. Permeable gowns are typically used, but waterproof gowns should be used in cases where there is a risk of contamination with large volumes of bodily fluids. Any time a barrier gown is worn, gloves should also be worn. Gowns should be used for only one patient at a time and must be removed without touching the contaminated outer surface. To do this, untie the gown with gloved hands, pull away from the body by grasping the chest, again with gloved hands, pull down cuffs on each arm and slide gown off arms and away from the body. Then remove the gloves and wash hands thoroughly in case of accidental contamination. If bodily fluid penetrates a semi-permeable gown, remove the gown and contaminated clothing, and shower immediately.

Foot protection

Foot covers and foot baths are useful in reducing the transmission of pathogens on shoes. Disposable surgical booties may be worn and removed just as with gloves to avoid hand contamination. Foot baths are typically composed of a 10% hypochlorite (bleach) solution and should be used when entering and exiting a designated isolation area. Further information on disinfecting foot baths may be found in Chapter 56, Antiseptics, Disinfectants, and Sterilization.

Facial protection

As discussed earlier in this chapter, some pathogens may be transmitted via aerosolization. Facial protection, such as surgical masks, face shields, or goggles, should be worn to protect the mucous membranes of the eyes, nose, and mouth against splashes or when performing procedures that may cause aerosolization of pathogens. Procedures such as dental cleanings, wound flushing, abscess draining, nebulization and coupage, suction, lavage, and necropsy have a high risk of this. In addition, avoid performing resuscitation by breathing into a patient's mouth, nose, or endotracheal tube; rather, one should always use an Ambu® bag or mechanical ventilator. According to the Compendium of Veterinary Standard Precautions for Zoonotic Disease Prevention in Veterinary Personnel,[42] surgical face masks provide adequate protection during most veterinary procedures, including those previously listed. Respiratory protection using particulate respirators is not commonly used in small animal veterinary practice but may have a place if certain diseases such as *Coxiella burnettii*, the causative agent of "Q fever," become more prevalent. Information on respiratory protection and different types of respirators is available through the department of Occupational Safety and Health Administration (OSHA).[43]

Bite and scratch prevention

As many zoonotic pathogens are transmitted through bites or scratches, it is important to prevent these in the veterinary hospital. Knowledge of aggressive tendencies in patients is key to preventing personnel injury. A complete patient history at the time the animal presents to the hospital and comprehensive medical records allow veterinary staff to be forewarned when handling a potentially aggressive animal. Proper restraint by trained staff, including the use of muzzles, heavy gloves, and sedation, all may play an instrumental part in injury prevention.

High-risk procedures

There are certain procedures in veterinary hospitals that require full barrier protection. Birth, cesarean sections, and abortions are all considered high-risk events, as some extremely virulent zoonotic diseases may be passed in birthing tissue and fluids. Necropsies are also high-risk procedures, particularly due to the use of saws and drills that may aerosolize zoonotic pathogens. Respiratory protection should be used if any power tools are used on a potentially zoonotic cadaver.

Isolation

Patients with potentially contagious zoonotic diseases should be isolated from other patients, the visiting public, and all personnel except those essential to their care. If possible, these patients should enter the facility via a separate entrance directly into an isolation ward or a dedicated exam room. If a separate entrance is not available, the patient should be transported directly through the waiting room by personnel wearing barrier protection. Cats and small dogs should be transported in a carrier, and larger dogs on a gurney or stretcher. The animal should be moved into a designated isolation area as soon as possible, and this area should have a separate entrance from the main patient care area; furthermore, only personnel needed for patient care should enter the isolation area. Personnel entry should be restricted and monitored, and a record of all staff that have contact with the patient must be made. Signs must be posted at the entrance to the isolation area to alert staff to the zoonotic disease potential, to notify them of necessary precautions to take, and to warn away other staff. The isolation area should have its own ventilation system to prevent the aerosolization of pathogens to the rest of the hospital.

Disinfecting after a patient leaves

After a confirmed or potentially zoonotic patient has left the designated isolation area, the location should be fully cleaned and disinfected to prevent pathogens from living in the environment. Cleaning a potentially contaminated area involves general removal of large waste and debris; ideally a filtered, central vacuum unit should be used to clean an area and remove potentially aerosolized pathogens. If this is not possible, personnel should take all recommended precautions against aerosolized pathogens. After removal of large debris, the area should be cleaned with a disinfectant shown to be effective against the particular pathogen. No one disinfectant is effective against every pathogen. Table 57.2 lists a number of classes of disinfectants and their efficacy against different pathogens. More information is available in Chapter 54, Antiseptics, Disinfectants, and Sterilization. These products should be used according to manufacturer's instructions for maximum efficacy. In dealing with potentially contaminated bedding, the fabric should initially be shaken gently over a contained area such as a garbage bag to dislodge potentially overlooked debris and gross fecal matter. Full barrier protection, particularly gloves, should be worn in dealing with all bedding. The bedding should be washed with regular laundry detergent and dried normally. To prevent cross-contamination, dirty and clean laundry should be kept separate, but there is no other special precaution recommended with zoonotic patient laundry.[42] Litter boxes should be emptied into a closed garbage container as soon as they are soiled.

Again, the use of disposable litter boxes is ideal, but if regular litter boxes are used, they may be cleaned and disinfected the same way as the overall environment. Food and water bowls may be washed normally with dish detergent if nondisposable ones are used. If a bodily fluid from a potential zoonosis is spilled, it should be sprayed with disinfectant and wiped up with absorbent material. All contaminated refuse should be bagged within the isolation area using gloves, and then rebagged in a second garbage bag outside the isolation area using a clean pair of gloves. The bags should be transported out of the hospital to an external garbage area immediately. Medical waste, including sharps and deceased animals, should be handled according to OSHA blood-borne pathogen standards.[43] It should be reiterated that no handling, transporting, or cleaning of an area with potential zoonotic contamination should be done without full barrier protection: gloves and gowns at a minimum, and shoe covers, masks, goggles, face shields, and/or respirators depending on the suspected pathogen.

Needlestick prevention

Many diseases are transmissible via needlestick injuries. One should rigorously follow safety guidelines when dealing with all sharps. The primary way to prevent needlesticks is never to recap a needle. Dispose of used needles and syringes in a puncture-proof sharps container. If it is necessary to recap a needle, use the one-handed scoop method or a tool, such as a hemostat, to hold the needle cap away from your hand. The one-handed scoop method involves the following: place the cap on a horizontal surface such as a treatment table, hold the syringe, slide the needle into the cap, lift the plunger side of the syringe upward to angle the cap toward the table surface, and press down to tighten on a hard surface. Scalpels come with disposable handles and blades and these are ideal when dealing with potential zoonoses. If a scalpel blade must be removed from a handle, use a hemostat to grasp the blade at its base with the sharp edge facing away from that hand and gently work the blade up and off with constant light pressure and wiggling.

Vector control

Vector control is another important way to minimize the potential exposure to zoonotic pathogens. Insects and rodents are attracted to veterinary hospitals and are common vectors of zoonotic disease. Proper facility cleanliness, food storage, prevention of standing water, and blocking points of entry are necessary to

Table 57.2 Disinfectants and their efficacy against various pathogens

Disinfectant	Effective against	Variable/limited Effective against	Not effective against
Alcohols (isopropyl)	Bacteria Mycobacteria Enveloped viruses Fungi	Non-enveloped viruses	Spores
Biguinides (chlorhexadine)	Bacteria	Mycobacteria Viruses Fungi	Spores
Hypochlorites (bleach)	Bacteria Mycobacteria Viruses Fungi	Spores	
Iodine compounds	Bacteria Enveloped viruses Fungi	Mycobacteria Non-enveloped viruses Spores	
Oxidizing agents (hydrogen peroxide)	Bacteria Mycobacteria Viruses	Spores Fungi	
Phenols	Bacteria Enveloped viruses	Mycobacteria Non-enveloped viruses Fungi	
Quaternary ammonium compounds	Gram-positive bacteria	Gram-negative bacteria Mycobacteria Enveloped viruses Fungi	Nonenveloped viruses Spores

prevent potential vectors from entering the hospital. If an animal carrying fleas or ticks enters the hospital, it should be separated from other patients and immediately treated with the appropriate and safe insecticidal medication(s). Personnel working with it should wear protective clothing.

Client education

Client education is instrumental in the prevention of zoonotic disease transmission. Veterinary personnel should take an active role in informing clients of the importance of prophylactic vaccination against diseases such as rabies, bordatellosis, borreliosis (Lyme disease), and leptospirosis. Control of ecto- and endoparasites is also an important preventative measure, as is prohibi-

tion of predation on reservoir species. All of these steps protect not only the client, but also veterinary personnel who may encounter the client's pet.

Vaccination

Prophylactic vaccination of veterinary personnel is another method of prevention. The CDC's advisory committee on immunization practices recommends that all veterinary personnel who have contact with animals should be vaccinated against rabies. Pre-exposure prophylaxis is a series of three injections that offer protection against unknown rabies exposure or when postexposure vaccination is delayed. Rabies titers should be checked every 2 years and boostered if the titer is too low to offer protection.

Documenting exposure

In case of possible exposure to a zoonotic disease, a veterinary hospital must have a protocol for documenting and responding to the incident. Most hospitals have reporting procedures for bites or other injuries, and these may be readily altered to include contact with possible zoonotic pathogens. This written documentation (Fig. 57.1) should include a list of all personnel involved, specifics of the incident (including the date, time, and location), information on the animal involved, any medical treatment sought, any agencies notified, and follow-up.

Staff training

All of the above-mentioned methods and guidelines for prevention of zoonotic disease transmission hinge on

Potential Zoonotic Disease Exposure

Date(s) of potential exposure:_____ Time(s) of potential exposure:_____
Location of potential exposure: _____ Employee name:_____
Date of birth:_____ Occupation:_____ Other individual(s) involved in exposure: _____
_____
Date/time exposure reported to supervisor:_____ Supervisor name(s):_____

Type of exposure:_____ Body part exposed:_____
Suspected zoonotic pathogen:_____ Animal's name:_____
Species:_____ Breed:_____ Age:_____ Animal's outcome (home,
euthanized, other):_____ If animal belongs to a client, client information (name, address,
telephone number):_____
Witness(es):_____
 How did the exposure occur (describe in detail):_____
_____
_____
_____
_____

Treatment sought?:_____Date/time treatment sought:_____
Type of treatment given:_____
Date/time treatment given:_____ Name of hospital/clinic/physician that treated
employee:_____ Address:_____
Telephone number: _____ Employee admitted to hospital?: _____
Paramedics called?: _____ Employee transported by ambulance?: _____
Notes: _____
_____
_____
_____

Zoonotic pathogen exposure confirmed?:_____ Employee notified?_____
Other personnel notified?:_____ Client notified?:_____
Hospital/clinic/physician notified?_____ Federal agencies notified (CDC, OSHA, DHHS, other)
State/local agencies notified (health department, agriculture, veterinary, other)?: _____
_____

Outcome of potential exposure:_____
Corrective action taken to prevent further exposure events: _____
_____
Notes: _____
_____
Employee signature:_____ Date: _____
Supervisor signature: _____ Date: _____

Figure 57.1 Example reporting form for potential zoonotic disease exposure.

veterinary personnel being aware of them. Staff training is of paramount importance in every step of zoonotic disease prevention. Frequent training and evaluation in addition to written hospital guidelines should be in place so staff are knowledgeable in the prevention of zoonotic disease transmission. In addition, hospitals must keep personnel food storage separate from patient food and medicine storage, and prohibit eating, drinking, or smoking in patient care areas.

High-risk personnel

There is a subset of veterinary personnel who are of particular concern with regard to zoonotic disease transmission. Immunocompromised individuals, such as those with HIV, diabetes mellitus, asplenia, and some congenital abnormalities, as well as pregnant women and those receiving immunosuppressive medications, are at increased risk for contracting zoonotic diseases and experiencing much more severe symptoms. These staff members must be aware of the dangers involved when handling patients, particularly high-risk animals such as ferals, strays, those with unknown vaccination histories, puppies and kittens under 3 months of age, animals consuming raw diets, and those with known zoonotic diseases. Ideally, an immunocompromised staff member should alert his or her supervisor so that policies may be enacted to minimize their risks. These individuals should also notify their personal physician of the zoonotic risks involved with their employment so familiarity with symptoms and proactive monitoring may be established. Pregnant women face a unique immunocompromised situation. Pregnancy suppresses the body's cell-mediated immunity and may increase a women's risk for contracting certain zoonotic diseases.[44]

Legal and public health issues

With the potential of zoonotic disease transmission present in veterinary medicine, legal issues have arisen and will continue to arise. This is a newly evolving field of inquiry as the liability issues involved have yet to be definitively established. In most cases, veterinary personnel who contract a zoonotic disease from a patient while at work are covered under workers' compensation regulations and state workers' occupational disease acts. However, with the increasing focus on zoonotic disease risks, liability will become of paramount concern. In 1986, a veterinarian was successfully sued for failure to provide a safe workplace in a case involving the death of a kennel worker from leptospirosis.[45] This case highlights the potential legal issues still to be resolved. With

regard to client risk, the legal ramifications of zoonotic diseases are still evolving. Veterinarians and veterinary staff have an ethical obligation to notify owners of potential zoonotic disease and to advise them to seek information from their personal physicians. There have been malpractice claims filed against veterinarians for human injury and exposure to rabid or potentially rabid animals,[46] and such may be the future avenue of legal proceedings for zoonotic diseases.

In terms of public health and zoonotic disease, there are varying guidelines in most states and within the federal government defining which diseases must be reported and to whom. In response to the multiple and often confusing regulations, the National Academy of Sciences (NAS) presented a 2005 report calling for the establishment of a federal-level, centralized coordinating system for animal health oversight.[47] This body would organize animal health data for industry, local, state, and federal agencies. Such an oversight body may have facilitated the earlier recognition of West Nile virus (WNV) in people. In the 1999 outbreak, physicians were misdiagnosing WNV patients with Guillain-Barre syndrome, meningitis, encephalitis, and aspiration pneumonia.[48] However, a veterinary pathologist at the Bronx Zoo linked the human and animal outbreaks based on the deaths of crows and other birds, allowing identification of WNV as the cause of human illness.[49] A federal oversight body may prevent similar scenarios in the future.

Conclusion

It is unrealistic to believe that taking rigorous personnel precautions may eradicate all risk of zoonotic disease. The goal of any infection prevention protocol is to substantially lower the risk of disease transmission. In small animal veterinary medicine, the emergency and critical care staff are going to encounter patients with zoonotic diseases. By instituting the procedures outlined in this chapter and expanding knowledge of zoonotic diseases, personnel and hospitals may protect themselves, their clients, the public, and their patients against these pathogens.

References

1. Siegel JD, Rhinehart E, Jackson M, Chiarello L. Guideline for isolation precautions: preventing transmission of infective agents in healthcare setting. 2007. Available through the Centers for Disease Control (CDC) at www.cdc.gov. Accessed April 14, 2010.
2. Hoskins JD, Williams J, Roy AF, Peters JC, McDonough P. Isolation and characterization of *Bordatella bronchiseptica* from cats in southern Louisiana. Veterinary Immunology and Immunopathology 1998;65:173–176.

3. Binns SH, Speakman AJ, Dawsons S, Bennett M, Gaskell RM, Hart CA. The use of pulsed-field gel electrophoresis to examine the epidemiology of *Bordatella bronchiseptica* isolated from cats and other species. Epidemiology and Infection 1998;120:201–208.

4. Dworkin MS, Sullivan PS, Buskin SE, Harrington RD, Oliffe J, MacArthur RD, Lopes CE. *Bordatella bronchiseptica* infection in human immunodeficiency virus-infected patients. Clinical Infection and Disease 1999;28:1095–1099.

5. Bordatella bronchiseptica: Material Safety Data Sheet (MSDS). 2001. Public Health Agency of Canada. WWW.publichealth.gc.ca. Accessed October 19, 2010.

6. Winters JL, O'Connor WN, Broughton RA, Noonan JA. *Bordatella bronchiseptica* pneumonia in a patient with Down syndrome: a case report and review. Pediatrics 1992;89(6)1262–1265.

7. Greene CE, Carmichael LE. Canine brucellosis. In Infectious Diseases of the Dog and Cat, 3rd ed. St. Louis, MO: Saunders Elsevier, 2006:369–381.

8. Brucellosis. www.cdc.gov. Accessed October 19, 2010

9. Nationally Notifiable Infectious Diseases, United States 2010. www.cdc.gov. Accessed April 21, 2010.

10. Weese JS, Peregrine AS, Armstrong J. Occupational health and safety in small animal veterinary practice: part I nonparasitic zoonotic diseases. Canadian Veterinary Journal 2002;43(8): 631–636.

11. Park SK, Lee SH, Kang SK, Kim KJ, Kim MC, Kim KW, Chang NH. Leptospirosis in Chonbuk Province of Korea in 1987: a study of 93 patients. American Journal of Tropical Medicine and Hygiene 1989;41(3):345–351.

12. Levett PN. Leptospirosis. Clinical Microbiology Review 2001;14:296–326.

13. Feigin RD, Anderson DC. Human leptospirosis from immunized dogs. Annals of Internal Medicine 1973;79(6):777–785.

14. World Organization for Animal Health. OIE listed diseases. www.oie.int. Accessed April 14, 2010.

15. Macy D. Plague. In Greene CE, ed. Infectious Diseases of the Dog and Cat, 3rd ed. St. Louis, MO: Saunders Elsevier, 2006: 439–446.

16. Gage KL, Dennis DT, Orloski KA, Ettested P, Brown TL, Reynolds PJ, Pape WJ, Fritz CL, Carter LG, Stein JD. Cases of cat-associated human plague in the Western US, 1977–1998. Clinical Infectious Disease 2000;(30):893–900.

17. Kruth SA. Gram-negative bacterial infections. In Infectious Diseases of the Dog and Cat, 3rd ed. St. Louis, MO: Saunders Elsevier, 2006:320–330.

18. Walther B, Wieler LH, Friedrich AW, Kohn B, Bronnberg L, Lubke-Becker A. *Staphylococcus aureus* and MRSA colonization rates in a small animal hospital: associated with nosocomial infections. Berliner und Munchener tierarztliche Wochenschrift 2009;122(5–6):178–185.

19. Bradshaw SE. Endocarditis due to *Staphylococcus aureus* after a minor dog bite. Southern Medical Journal 2003;96:407–409.

20. Legendre AM. Blastomycosis. In Infectious Diseases of the Dog and Cat, 3rd ed. St. Louis, MO: Saunders Elsevier, 2006:569–576.

21. Greene, RT. Coccidiomycosis and paracoccidiomycosis. In Infectious Diseases of the Dog and Cat, 3rd ed. St. Louis, MO: Saunders Elsevier, 2006:598–608.

22. Giadici A, Saubolle M. Transmission of coccidiomycosis to a human via a cat bite. Journal of Clinical Microbiology 2009;47(2):505–506.

23. James WD, Berger TG, Elston DM. Andrew's Diseases of the Skin: Clinical Dermatology. St. Louis, MO: Saunders Elsevier, 2005.

24. Greene CE, Levy JK. Immunocompromised people and shared human and animal zoonoses, sapronoses, and arthroponoses. In Infectious Diseases of the Dog and Cat, 3rd ed. St. Louis, MO: Saunders Elsevier, 2006: 1051–1068.

25. Rosser EJ, Dunstan RW. Sporotrichosis. In Infectious Diseases of the Dog and Cat, 3rd ed. St. Louis, MO: Saunders Elsevier, 2006:608–612.

26. Dunstan RW, Langham RF, Reimann DA, Wakenell PS. Feline sporotrichosis: a report of five cases with transmission to humans. Journal of the American Academy of Dermatology 1986;15:37.

27. Greene CE, Rupprecht CE. Rabies and other lyssavirus infections. In Infectious Diseases of the Dog and Cat, 3rd ed. St. Louis, MO: Saunders Elsevier, 2006:167–183.

28. Rabies. World Health Organization. www.who.int. Accessed April 14, 2010.

29. Chang CP, New AG, Taylor JF, Chiang HS. Influenza virus isolations from dogs during a human epidemic in Taiwan. International Journal of Zoonoses 1976;3:61–64.

30. 2009 H1N1 Flu virus outbreak. American Veterinary Medical Association Public Health. www.avma.org. Accessed April 14, 2010.

31. Moore, JE. Campylobacter. Veterinary Research 2005;36(3): 351–382.

32. Murray PR, Rosenthal KS, Kobayashi GS, Pfaller MA. *Campylobacter* and *Helicobacter*. In Medical Microbiology. St. Louis, MO: Mosby, 2005:251–257.

33. Barr SC. Cryptosporidiosis and cyclosporiasis. In Infectious Diseases of the Dog and Cat, 3rd ed. St. Louis, MO: Saunders Elsevier, 2006:785–793.

34. Barr SC, Bowman DD. Giardiasis in dogs and cats. Compendium of Continuing Education for the Practicing Veterinarian 1994;16(5):603–614.

35. Giardiasis. www.cdc.gov. Accessed October 20, 2010.

36. Greene CE. Salmonellosis. In Infectious Diseases of the Dog and Cat, 3rd ed. St. Louis, MO: Saunders Elsevier, 2006:355–360.

37. Outbreaks of multi-drug resistant *Salmonella typhimurium* associated with veterinary facilities-Idaho, Minnesota, and Washington. Morbidity and Mortality Weekly Report 50:701–704. www.cdc.gov. Accessed April 14, 2010.

38. Dubey JP, Lappin MR. Toxoplasmosis and neosporosis. In Infectious Diseases of the Dog and Cat, 3rd ed. St. Louis, MO: Saunders Elsevier, 2006:754–775.

39. Torrey EF, Yolken RH. *Toxoplasma gondii* and schizophrenia. Emerging Infectious Diseases 2003;9(11):1375–1380.

40. Pottinger J, Burns S, Manske C. Bacterial carriage by artificial nails. American Journal of Infection Control 1989;17:340–344.

41. Moolenaar RL, Crutcher M, San Joaquin VH, Sewell LV, Hutwagner LC, Carson LA, Robison DA, Smithee LM, Jarvis WR. A prolonged outbreak of *Pseudomonas aeroginosa* in a neonatal intensive care unit: did staff fingernails play a role in disease transmission? Infection Control and Hospital Epidemiology 2000;21:80–85.

42. National Association of State Public Health Veterinarians' Veterinary Infection Control Committee. Compendium of Veterinary Standard Precautions for Zoonotic Disease Prevention in Veterinary Personnel. Journal of the American Veterinary Medical Association 2008;233(3):415–428.

43. U.S. Department of Labor, Occupational Health and Safety Administration. Occupational safety and health standards: toxic and hazardous substances 1910.1030: blood borne pathogens. www.osha.gov. Accessed April 21, 2010.

44. Moore DM, Davis YM, Kaczmarek RG. An overview of occupational hazards among veterinarians, with particular reference to

pregnant women. American Industrial Hygiene Association Journal 1993;54:113–120.

45. Fiala J. CDC study: DVM fail lepto safety practices. DVM Newsmagazine, November 1, 2006.

46. Babcock S, Marsh AE, Lin J, Scott J. Legal implications of zoonoses for clinical veterinarians. Journal of the American Veterinary Medical Association 2008;233(10):1556–1562.

47. National Academy of Sciences. Animal Health at the Crossroads: Preventing, Detecting, and Diagnosing Animal Diseases. Washington: National Academy Press, 2005.

48. Asnis DS, Conetta R, Teizeira AA, Waldman G, Sampson BA. The West Nile outbreak of 1999 in New York: the Flushing Hospital experience. Clinical Infectious Disease 2000;30:413–418.

49. U.S. Government Accountability Office. West Nile outbreak: lessons for public health preparedness. Washington: The Office. GAO/HEHS-00-180. Available at www.gao.gov. Accessed April 14, 2010.

SECTION IX

Specific nursing considerations

SECTION IX

58

Drug administration

Jane Quandt and Elizabeth Olmstead

The patient that undergoes treatment and monitoring in the intensive care unit (ICU) setting receives numerous drug therapies. How these therapies are administered is crucial to the success of the treatment and the well-being of the animal.

Treatment sheet orders

All patients in the ICU should have an order sheet (Figure 58.1A, B) that delineates the treatment requested, the dose, the route of administration, and frequency of administration. The order sheet is also the place to note any the potential interaction that may occur between drugs. For example, a dog on a constant rate infusion of diazepam should not receive an intravenous (IV) antibiotic through the same IV line as the diazepam. Diazepam is incompatible with other drugs and would form precipitates (small particles) in the line. The written order for the treatment drugs should match the label from the pharmacy in that it is the same name, be it generic or a trade name; for example, Torbugesic[R] is the trade name of butorphanol. The name on the order sheet and the name on the drug when it is received from the pharmacy should be one or the other or both names to avoid confusion. When a treatment is administered to the animal, the initials of the person giving the medication should be placed next to the treatment time. When questions arise, initialed treatments allow for tracking of the individual responsible for the action.

Medical records

All administered medications should be clearly noted in the medical record, whether it is paper or electronic. Any

known allergies or adverse drug reactions should be flagged with either a red sticker on the outside of the paper record or an electronic warning on computer records. This indicator is vital to prevent the administration of a drug or a blood product to which the patient has reacted in the past. Either a prominent note should be made on the treatment sheet or a sign should be posted on the patient's cage so that everyone in contact with that patient is made aware of the patient's drug sensitivities.

The pharmacy should also be a source of safeguards against drug administration error. Pharmacy personnel should check medication requests for accuracy of dosing and administration route. To prevent accidental overdose, single drug doses should be dispensed, each in its own labeled syringe, unless the medication comes in a multiuse vial or container.

It is common in veterinary medicine to use extra-label drugs. Extra-label drug use is the use of an approved drug in a way that is not in accordance with the approved manufacturer's instructions. Animals have diseases that require treatment with agents that have been registered for use only in human patients. The Animal Medicinal Drug Use Clarification Act explains extra-label drug use. It states that a veterinarian must be involved; that only FDA-approved drugs are to be used; that a client–veterinarian relationship must exist; that the drug is for therapeutic use only; and that there are to be no residues that may present a risk to public health. When using an extra-label drug, it is important to fully document the dose, route, administration times, disease being treated, and any withdrawal times. It is not a requirement that the client be told it is an extra-label use of a drug.

Advanced Monitoring and Procedures for Small Animal Emergency and Critical Care, First Edition. Edited by Jamie M. Burkitt Creedon, Harold Davis.
© 2012 John Wiley & Sons, Inc. Published 2012 by John Wiley & Sons, Inc.

SMALL ANIMAL INTENSIVE CARE
TREATMENT SHEET
UNIVERSITY OF MINNESOTA
VETERINARY MEDICAL CENTER

Date: _____

PLACE PATIENT LABEL HERE

Clinician: _____   Beeper: _____
                               Home: _____

Student: _____   Beeper: _____
(Full name)   Home: _____

Resuscitation: Full   CPR   DNR
Visitation: Yes   No

Problem List:	Weight: Kg. Scale:
	Special Instructions:
	Patient Status: A B

Plan:	Updated Results/Problem List:
AUS ☐ Surgery ☐	
CBC ☐ CT ☐	
Chem. ☐ MRI ☐	
Coag. ☐ Other:	
UA ☐	
Endoscopy ☐	

Clinician's Signature: _____ **Date:** _____

(a) VMC #80.1 (Rev. 6/o8)   ICU Treatment Sheet

Figure 58.1a ICU order sheet. Used with permission by the University of Minnesota Veterinary Medical Center

Routes of drug administration

The route of drug administration must be appropriate to prevent serious adverse effects or even death. Drugs can be given by various routes, but deviation from an established safe route could lead to severe complications, including death. The route of administration should be specified in the order sheet, and the drug must be verified as having been administered in the manner requested. When using a multiuse vial the top of the vial should be cleaned with an alcohol swab prior to insertion of the needle to prevent possible contamina-tion of the bottle. In the same regard, prior to drug administration into an IV catheter port the site should be cleaned with an alcohol pad. For convenience, the swabs should be kept in multiple locations throughout the ICU room.

The most common route of drug and fluid adminis-tration in the ICU setting is via an indwelling IV cath-eter. Many of the medications given in the ICU can be delivered through the Y-port of the IV fluid line. Com-patibility with the fluid and additives must be estab-lished prior to drug administration through any IV port. When using the same fluid line for incompatible

	Freq	12p	1p	2p	3p	4p	5p	6p	7p	8p	9p	10p	11p	12a
Temp														
Pulse														
Resp. Rate														
MM color														
Lung sounds R/L		╱	╱	╱	╱	╱	╱	╱	╱	╱	╱	╱	╱	╱
PCV/TP		╱	╱	╱	╱	╱	╱	╱	╱	╱	╱	╱	╱	╱
Glucose														
Azostick														
Weight (kg)/scale														
Pain Assessment (1–5)														
Medications & Treatments	Freq	12p	1p	2p	3p	4p	5p	6p	7p	8p	9p	10p	11p	12a
Water														
Diet Orders														
Amount Eaten														
Defecation/Vomit														
Exercise														
Urine Output — Measure														
Estimate														
FLUIDS														
Type #1														
Rate ml/hr														
Type #2														
Rate ml/hr														
Type #3														
Rate ml/hr														
(b) Initials														

Figure 58.1b ICU order sheet.

drugs, the line must be flushed between the administrations. The flushing can be done with 0.9% NaCl or the fluid pump on the line can be allowed to run for 10 minutes before administering the second drug, to allow time for the first drug to be moved through the line. Incompatibilities may range from immediate precipitation (formation of particles) to an undetectable but potentially dangerous pH change. A compatibility chart of commonly used drugs in the ICU can be found in Table 58.1.

In an effort to minimize errors one person should be responsible for setting up the fluids. When a patient is initially set up on IV fluids the tubing should be purged of air by filling the line with fluid; this is done to prevent air embolus. Only one person should be responsible for the addition of fluid additives to avoid the potential of exceeding the ordered concentration.

Certain drugs such as mannitol or blood products may require the use of an in-line filter to prevent the infusion of crystals, particulate matter, or clots. Microfilters of 150–170 μm pore size are commonly used with blood products to remove clots, larger red blood cells, and platelet aggregates. Finer filters with 18–40 μm pore size can be used with drugs such as mannitol to remove microaggregates and crystals. Crystals can be seen as small white precipitates in the IV line or as a cloudiness in the IV line. The use of filters with blood products prevents the possible infusion and formation of emboli. Drug crystals can be irritating to the vein. Filters should be changed if they become occluded or with each new

Table 58.1 Drug compatibility chart

Compatibility Chart	Aminophylline	Ampicillin	Atropine	Butorphanol	Calcium Gluconate	Cefazolin Sodium	Dexamethasone SP	Diazepam	Diltiazem	Diphenhydramine	Dobutamine	Dopamine	Doxycycline	Epinephrine	Famotidine	Fentanyl	Furosemide	Heparin	Hydromorphone	Insulin	Ketamine	Lactated Ringers soln	Lidocaine HCl	Magnesium Sulfate	Mannitol	Metoclopramide HCl	Metronidazole	Midazolam	Morphine	Multivitamins	Ondansetron	Pentobarbital Sodium	Phenobarbitol	Potassium Chloride	Potassium Phosphate	Propofol	Ranitidine	Sodium Bicarbonate	Sodium Chloride	Trimethoprim-Sulfamethoxazole	Unasyn
Aminophylline	C				C	C	C		?	C	×	C	C	×	C		C	C	C	×		C	C	C		C	C	C	×		×	C	C	C	C	C	C	C	C		C
Ampicillin	C	C			?			?	?			×		×	C		C	C	C	C		×	?			×	?	C	C		×	C	C	C	C	C	?	×	C	C	C
Atropine			C	C						C						C	C	C	?				?	C		C	C	C	C	C	C	C	C	C	C	?	C	C	C	C	
Butorphanol			C	C	C					C	C		C	C	C	C	C	C	C				C	C		C		C	C		C	×		C	C	C	C	C	C	C	
Calcium Gluconate	C	?		C	C	×	C				C	C		C		C	C	C					C	C		C	C	C	C			×	C	C	?		×	×	C		
Cefazolin Sodium	C				×	C		C		C	C						C	C	C				C	C		×	C	×	C				C	C		C	×	C	C		×
Dexamethasone SP	C				C		C	?		?						C	C	C	?							C		C	C		C			C		×	C	C	C	C	
Diazepam		?					?	C	×	C	×					C	×	?	×	×	×	?					C				C			×		×	?	?	?	C	×
Diltiazem	?	?				C		×	C	C		C	C	C	C	C	×	C	C			C	C	C		C	C	C	C		C	C	C	C	C	×	C	?	C	C	
Diphenhydramine	C		C	C		C	?	C	C	C	C	C	C	C	C	C	×	×	C			C	C	C		C	C	×	C	C	C	C	C	C	C	×	C	×	C	C	C
Dobutamine	×		C	C	C	C		×		C	C	C		C	C	C	×	×	C	×		C	C	×	?	C	×	×	C	C	C	C	C	C	×	×	C	×	C	×	×
Dopamine	C	×			C				C	C	C	C		C	C	C	C	C	C			?	C	C	C	?	×		C		C	C		C	×		?	×	C	C	C
Doxycycline	C			C					C	C			C	C		C	C	C	C	C		C	C			C			C	×	C			C		C	C	C	C	C	C
Epinephrine	×	×			C	C			C	C	C	C	C	C	C	C	×	×	C	C		C	×	C		C	C	C	C		×	C	×	C	C	C	C	C	C	C	C
Famotidine	C	×		C					C	C	C	C		C	C	C	×	×	C	C		C	C	C		C	C	×	×		×	×	C	C	C	C	C	C	C	C	C
Fentanyl	C	C	C	C	C		C	C	C	C	C	C	C	C	C	C	×	C	C	C		C	C	C		C	C	C	×		×	C	×	C	C	C	C	C	C	C	C
Furosemide	C	C	C	C	C	C	C	×	×	C	×	×	×	×	×	×	C	×	C	C		C	C	C	C	×	C	×	×		×	C	C	×	×	×	C	C	C	C	C
Heparin	C	?		C	C	C		?	C	?	×	×		×	×	×	×	C	?			?	C	C		C	C	C	C		×	C	C	C	×	×	?	C	C	C	C
Hydromorphone	C	C	C	C		?	?	?	C	C	C	×	C	C	C	C	C	C	C	C		C	C	C	C	C	C	C	C		C	C	×	C	×	C	C	×	×	C	C
Insulin	×	C	C	C	?	C	?	?	C	C	×	×	C	C	C	C	C	C	C	C	×	C	C	C		C	C	C	×	C	×	C	×	C	C	C	C	C	×	C	C

Ketamine								x													c		c					c	c							c			c			
Lactated Ringers soln	c	c			c	c		?		c	c	c	?	c		c	c	?	c			c	c	c		c	c	x	c	c	c	c	c	c			c	?		c		c
Lidocaine HCl	c	x			c	x	c		c	c	c	c		x	c		c	c		c	c	c	c			c			c			c		c		c	c	x	c			
Magnesium Sulfate		c			c	c					x		c		c	c		c	c	c		c		c		c	c		c		c			c	c	c		x	c	c		
Mannitol												c					c								c	c					c			x		c		c	c			
Metoclopramide HCl	c	x	c	c	x		c		c	c		?			c	c	x	c		c		c	c	c	c	c		c	c	c	c			c	c	c	c	x	c			
Metronidazole	c	?				c			c			x						c	c			c		c			c	c	c	c									c			
Midazolam	c	x	c	c	c	c	x		c	c	x			c	c	c	x	c	c	c	c	x				c	c	c	c		c	x		c		?	x	x	c	x		
Morphine	x	c	c	c		c	c		c	c	c	c	c	c	c	c	x	x	c		c	c	c	c		c	c	c	c	c	c	x	x	c		c	c	x	c	c		c
Multivitamins		c				c			c				x									c				c	c		c	c								?	c			
Ondansetron	x	x	c			c	c		c	c		c	c		c	c	x	c	c			c		c	c	c		c	c		c			c			c	x	c			x
Pentobarbital Sodium	c		c	x		x				x						x			c			c	c					x	x			c				c	x	c				
Phenobarbitol	c		c		c					x						x		c	x	x		c							x				c			c	x	c	c			
Potassium Chloride	c	c	c	c	c	c	c	x	c	c	x	c		c	c	c	c	c				c	c	c	x	c		c	c		c			c		c	c	c	c			
Potassium Phosphate					?				c	x	x				c									c		c									c							
Propofol	c	c	?	c	c	c	c	x		c	c	c	c	c	c	c	c	c	c		c		c	c	c	c		?	c			c	c	c		c	c	c	c			
Ranitidine	c	?	c			x	c	?	c	c	c	c	c	c		c	c	c	c			c	c			c		x	c		c	x	x	c		c	c		c			
Sodium Bicarbonate	c	x	c		x		c		?		x	x		x	c	c	c	c	x	c		?	x	x	c	x		x	x	?	x	x	c	c		c		c	c			x
Sodium Chloride	c	c		c	c	c	c	?	c	c	c	c	c	c	c	c	c	c	c	c	c		c	c	c	c	c	c	c	c	c		c	c		c	c	c	c	?		c
Trimethoprim-Sulfamethoxazole								c	c									c	c			c		c				x	c										?	c		
Unasyn	c	c							x			x			c			c		c		c							c		x							x	c			c

Sources: Plumb, Donald C., *Veterinary Drug Handbook*, 4th edition, PharmaVet Publishing, 2002; Trissel, Lawrence A., *Handbook of Injectable Drugs*, 11th edition, American Society of Health System Pharmacists, 2001; Trissel, Lawrence A., *Pocket Guide to Injectable Drugs*, American Society of Health System Pharmacists, 1998. C = compatible; x = incompatible; ? = conditional.

BISHOP BURTON COLLEGE

Case Study 58.1   A 4-year-old 6.8 kg domestic shorthair (DSH) male castrated (MC) cat was presented to the ICU for recovery following emergency surgery for a suspected liner foreign body. At surgery a single enterotomy was performed at the distal jejunum to remove a string foreign body. The GI tract was deemed to be healthy. Closure was done in a routine manner. The cat was stable through the surgical procedure with blood pressure, heart rate, respiratory rate, mucous membrane color, body temperature, and pulse oximetry monitored every 5 minutes. Fluid therapy was to continue with Plasma-Lyte 148^R with KCl added at 20 ml/hr IV in the ICU. The ICU technician hung the bag of Plasma-Lyte 148^R with the administration set attached into the fluid pump. A CRI dose of metoclopramide had yet to be added to the fluid bag and therefore the line had not been filled with fluid. Unknowingly, the surgeon hooked the administration set to the cat's IV port, set the drip rate and started the fluid administration pump. Approximately 10 minutes later, the cat suffered a sudden cardiac arrest. The cat was taken from the cage and placed in left lateral recumbency on a central table; cardiopulmonary cerebral resuscitation (CPCR) was initiated. The cat was immediately intubated and external cardiac compressions were instituted. An IV dose of atropine at 0.02 mg/kg was given followed by an IV dose of epinephrine at 0.02 mg/kg. Resuscitation attempts continued for 10 minutes, with ventilation at 20 breaths per minute and cardiac compressions 100 times per minute. Red fluid was seen flowing up into the endotracheal tube and resuscitation efforts were discontinued. It was determined that when the fluid therapy was begun, the administration set had not been purged of air; when the fluid pump was started; the air in the set was given as a bolus to the cat via the IV catheter. This resulted in a fatal air embolism. A standard IV administration set either 60 drops per ml or 10 drops per ml contains 10 ml of air. The drip set and extension line used in this case had an air volume of 24 ml.

The actual cause of death is entrapment of air in the right ventricular outflow tract leading to outflow obstruction and increased venous pressure due to an air lock and decreased myocardial contractility.[1,2] The lesson of this case underscores the importance of having only one person responsible for setting up and instituting fluid therapy in the patient.

syringe drug or bag of blood product. Frequent changing of the filter will assure its proper filtering function.

Drug delivery: Venous access

When an IV catheter is used for fluid or drug administration, the catheter must be verified to be in the vein and patent. Though catheters are generally flushed each time the patient is disconnected from fluids, patency can be difficult to assess due to bandages that are in place for catheter protection and support. Since catheters may not spontaneously bleed back when aspirated, palpation of the vessel that is being flushed may be necessary to ensure patency. If the flush is given in a pulsatile fashion, the fluid can be felt traversing the vein. Fluid that diffuses into the surrounding tissue, resulting in tissue swelling, may be due to a catheter that is extravascular.

In the neonate or very small patient, an **intraosseous (IO)** catheter may be used. Intraosseous catheterization provides rapid access to the central circulatory system.[3] Intraosseous catheterization should not be performed if there are skeletal abnormalities, overlying skin or wound infections, abscess over the bone, bone fractures, or sepsis. The bony sites most commonly used include the flat medial surface of the proximal tibia, tibial tuberosity, trochanteric fossa of the femur, wing of ilium, ischium, and the greater tubercle of the humerus. If more than one hole is placed through a bone cortex, extravasation of fluid or medication into the subcutaneous tissue may occur. When administering fluids intraosseously, observe for fluid extravasation; if it occurs, the needle should be removed and another bone site chosen. A bone should not be reused for 12–24 hours after perforation of a cortex.[3] If the needle is correctly placed and fluid does not flow freely, rotate the needle 90°–180° to move the beveled edge away from the inner core. A standard administration set is used to deliver fluids. The IO needle or catheter is secured by placing a tape butterfly around the hub and then suturing it to the skin. The entrance area should be covered and wrapped as with an IV catheter. The needle should be protected from breakage or bending. The fluid rate in IO needles 18–25 gauge is limited to 11 ml/min with gravity flow and 24 ml/min with 300 mmHg pressure.[3] It is suggested that an intraosseous needle or catheter can remain in place for 72 hours if aseptic catheter maintenance is performed.[3] The risk factors for osteomyelitis are sepsis and catheter use that persists for several days. Substances that can be infused via an intraosseous needle or catheter include blood and blood products, crystalloid and colloid fluids, amino acids, dextrose, aminophylline, antisera, antitoxins, atropine, aureomycin, calcium gluconate, cefoxitin, dexamethasone, diazepam, digitalis, diphenhydramine hydrochloride, dobutamine, dopamine, epinephrine, insulin, morphine, penicillin, procaine hydrochloride, radiopaque dyes, streptomycin, sulfadiazine, sulfathiazole, thiopental sodium 5%, and vitamins.[3] The use of alkaline or hypertonic solutions results in edema, pyknotic marrow nuclei, and decreased cellularity. The changes will spontaneously resolve within 4–6 weeks.

Drug delivery: Enteral

Feeding tubes

Critically ill patients often have indwelling nasogastric (NG), nasoesophageal (NE), or gastrostomy tubes. These ports can be used to administer medications that are labeled to be given orally. When dealing with a fractious patient that makes administration of oral medication impossible, most oral medications can be crushed and dissolved in water to administer through the enteral feeding tube. An oral medication that has a film coating or is a sustained release preparation should not be crushed, as this will change the rate of delivery of the drug, usually resulting in a more rapid uptake and possible overdose. Many oral medications can be administered via NE, NG, or gastrotomy tube; it is important to confirm how the oral medication is to be given prior to administration. Enteral medications should not be delivered via jejunal feeding tubes, as many of these drugs require the acidity of the stomach to allow their absorption. Oral vitamins could be given via a jejunal tube. Sucralfate is often used to coat the esophagus that has been injured by the presence of an esophageal foreign body; therefore, it must be given via the oral cavity. It is necessary to flush with a volume of water adequate to fill the feeding tube after drug administration to prevent the tube from clogging. If clogging of the tube should occur, first try to aspirate the tube with a 6 or 12 cc syringe. If aspiration does not clear the tube, it may cleared by flushing the tube with an acidic brown soda such as Coca-Cola^R. It is advisable to use a 1 cc syringe for the purpose.

Oral medications

Oral medication should be given only to those patients that are capable of active swallowing. Active swallowing is necessary to prevent aspiration or possible erosion of the esophagus. A caustic medication that is not properly swallowed can remain within the lumen of the esophagus. When a patient is allowed food and is eating it is usually best to give oral medication in some type of food, which may ease administration of the medication. If a patient is not allowed food, it may be helpful to follow the oral medication with a dose of water that is delivered via a small syringe. This helps to ensure that the medication is swallowed and decreases the likelihood of its adherence to the esophagus, where it could potentially cause esophagitis or stricture. Timing of oral medication administration in relationship to feeding can be important. Certain medications should be given with food, prior to feeding, or on an empty stomach. Medication administration should be avoided with certain types of food; for example, the antibiotic doxycycline is not to be administered with dairy products.

Sucralfate is commonly given to treat GI ulcers and esophagitis. It is an orally administered agent, frequently given as a slurry, as the pill will readily dissolve in a syringe of water. Sucralfate may interfere with the absorption of other oral medications such as fluroquinolones, fat-soluble vitamins, digoxin, and tetracyclines, and therefore dosing should be separated by at least 2 hours. Sucralfate is most effective in an acidic environment; therefore, an oral H_2 blocker should be given 30–60 minutes after the administration of sucralfate. The best effect will be seen if the sucralfate is given on an empty stomach, 1 hour prior to feeding or 2 hours after feeding.[4]

Activated charcoal is used as an absorbent in the acutely poisoned patient. Charcoal is administered orally, and some patients will eat the charcoal if it is mixed with a small amount of baby food, cheese, or canned pet food. This mixing technique makes administration easier and potentially cleaner than using a dose syringe. If the patient will not readily eat the charcoal mixture, then the liquid charcoal is given via a dose syringe orally. If the animal will not tolerate an oral dosing syringe, an NG tube can be placed for administration. The NG tube is placed in the same manner as for feeding. The tube length is measured to the last rib to ensure placement in the stomach. The nostril is numbed with a drop of viscous 2% oral topical lidocaine solution Qualitest^R. The tube is gently passed through the ventral nasal meatus; as the animal swallows it is threaded down the esophagus into the stomach. Proper tube placement is verified via a lateral radiograph of the thorax. The charcoal is then administrated through the NG tube. Due to the viscosity of charcoal suspension, it may require dilution with water to allow passage through the NG tube. Following administration of the charcoal, the NG tube can be removed or drawn back to the appropriate NE location for continued treatment. If the charcoal is given too rapidly, it can induce emesis and increase the risk for aspiration. The administration of charcoal should be separated by at least 3 hours from other orally administered agents.

Drug delivery: Subcutaneous route

The **subcutaneous (SC)** route is commonly used for insulin, famotidine, and metoclopramide. When giving a SC medication after entry under the skin the needle should be aspirated to ensure it is not in a vessel and still under the skin. Doses of SC medication are checked after injection to ensure that the site is not wet. If there is question as to whether the medication was administered or went through the skin, the clinician should verify and determine whether redosing should be performed. When administering a SC medication it is best to administer the dose between the shoulder blades with the skin tented. If the area between the shoulder blades is not available due to trauma, bandage, skin infection, or scarring, the SC dose is administered where an appropriate skin tent can be obtained. In general when performing SC drug administration it is best to use a small gauge needle such as a 25 gauge to avoid leakage of the agent out of a larger skin puncture. If a large volume of medication or fluid needs to be delivered, a larger gauge needle such as an 18–20 gauge may be used in order to deliver the volume in a timely manner. Note that some fluid may leak from the skin hole.

Drug delivery: Intramuscular route

Intramuscular (IM) injection can be used for the administration of agents such as analgesics and insulin. The commonly used muscles for the site of injection are the epaxial, biceps femoris, semitendinosus, or the triceps. The gauge and length of the needle are important to ensure that the medication is properly deposited in the muscle belly and not in the fat or fascial plane, which could diminish drug absorption or result in delayed adsorption.

Insulin can be given IV or IM for the treatment of the unregulated diabetic. Once the critical state resolves, long-term insulin therapy is usually initiated; long-term insulin therapy is generally administered by the SC route.

Furosemide can be given as a single IV or IM injection or as a constant rate infusion (CRI) in the treatment of renal failure, heart failure, and pulmonary edema.

Constant rate infusion

A CRI consists of a calculated volume of medication at a specific concentration that is added to a set volume and type of fluid for continuous delivery. A CRI can increase the efficacy of a drug because it delivers a steady dose of the agent, which can help maintain steady plasma concentration and enhance safety through slower delivery. A CRI may be used to deliver antibiotics, long-term analgesics, or even sedative drugs for animals that require longer-term sedation or anesthesia. The drugs can be given either mixed in the daily fluids with the fluid bag clearly labeled with the type, amount, and rate the additive is to be administered or via a separate syringe pump or fluid bag.

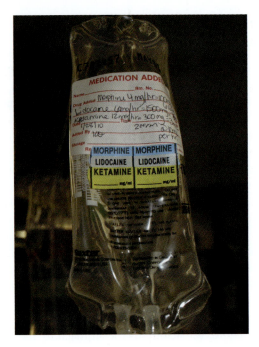

Figure 58.2 A morphine, ketamine, and lidocaine CRI. The drug label should include drug concentration and rate of delivery. It should be initialed by the individual that made up the CRI.

Table 58.2 Metoclopramide constant rate infusion

	<u>2.03</u> mls 5 of mg/ml metoclopramide
Have been added to	<u>1,000</u> mls of fluid.
Delivered at a constant infusion of	<u>100</u> ml/hour it will give <u>1</u> mg/kg/day.
There is	<u>0.010</u> mg/ml metoclopramide.

The drug label on the fluid bag should be large and easy to see (Fig. 58.2). The label is to alert personnel that the bag has an additive, and therefore these fluids should not be used to give a fluid bolus to the patient. A fluid bolus from a bag containing an additive could be unsafe and potentially lethal, such as a fluid bolus containing KCl. It may be safer for certain agents to be given via a separate fluid bag or a syringe pump. The separate bag or syringe pump will allow for a more accurate rate of delivery and easier monitoring, and avoid potential under- or overdosing when fluid rates are changed. Accurate and obvious labeling is fundamental for all medications delivered by CRI. When labeling, the volume of diluent should be listed in case there is a question as to concentration; listing the quantity of diluent allows calculations to be verified (Table 58.2).

When insulin is given as a CRI, it should be infused through an administration line separate from the fluid therapy line. This separation of insulin from the fluids allows for adjustments to be made in the insulin dose without alterations in the fluid therapy rate. Regular insulin adsorbs to the surfaces of IV infusion tubing and filters. Insulin adsorption to the administration equipment can lead to a 20%–30% decrease in its potency. The adsorption process is instantaneous, with most insulin adsorption occurring within the first 30–60 minutes. To saturate binding sites and therefore deliver a more predictable dose when giving an IV infusion, run 50 ml of the insulin-containing solution through the IV tubing, discard this volume, and then begin the infusion.[5]

Drugs such as diazepam are used as a CRI to treat severe seizure disorders. This light-sensitive drug may adhere to the plastic tubing of the IV line and also should not be stored in plastic syringes long-term. It has been found that 10 mg of diazepam in a 2 ml volume can be stored in a polypropylene-polyethylene syringe for 4 hours; longer term storage in a syringe results in absorption of the drug to the plastic surface, which deceases the amount of drug available.[6] The propylene glycol in diazepam is incompatible with most other fluids, and therefore the drug requires a dedicated delivery system. Do not administer if a precipitate forms and does not clear.[7] Diazepam is irritating to veins and should be given only IV via a large central vein. It is suggested that high-dose dextrose, 7.5% or greater, is also best delivered by a central vein due to its hypertonicity. In addition it is recommended that drugs or agents that have an osmolality greater than 600 mOsm/L be infused via a large or central vein to avoid the possible complication of vein irritation or phlebitis that may occur if small peripheral veins are used. Light-sensitive drugs are generally stored in brown bottles and therefore should be protected from the light if they are being delivered as a CRI.

The hyperosmotic agent mannitol is commonly used for treatment of head trauma, renal failure, and glaucoma. Warming of the fluid line decreases the likelihood that the mannitol will recrystallize. Mannitol should be administered with a filter to prevent precipitates from being introduced intravenously. The filter should be changed with every separate dose syringe. Drawing up a 1-hour volume and the use of a syringe pump are recommended to prevent crystallization of the mannitol and to ensure appropriate changing of the filter. Sodium or potassium chloride can cause mannitol to precipitate out of solution if the mannitol concentration is 20% or greater.[8] Due to its hyperosmotic nature it is best to administer mannitol through a large central vein catheter.

Metoclopramide is commonly given as a CRI within the animal's regular IV fluid therapy. Metoclopramide is light-sensitive and therefore the fluid bag should have a covering to prevent light interaction. It is compatible with 5% dextrose in water, 0.9% NaCl, 2.5% dextrose in 0.45% NaCl, Ringer's, and lactated Ringer's solutions (LRS).

Intravenous nutritional support

Total parenteral nutrition (TPN) is administered through a central venous catheter that is specifically designated for TPN. The catheter is placed using aseptic technique into the jugular, medial, or lateral saphenous veins and advanced to a central position. TPN is hyperosmolar; therefore, a central vein is needed for administration. If a central catheter cannot be obtained, partial parenteral nutrition (PPN), which has a lower osmolality, can be provided by use of a peripheral venous catheter. This catheter should also be placed in a sterile manner. Once administration of PPN or TPN has begun, the administration IV line is never disconnected until the bag is empty. The bag travels everywhere with the patient to ensure sterility. If the patient is going to a visiting room the fluid pump can be placed on a mobile IV pole to allow the administration to continue. If the bag must be removed from the fluid pump, the line back flow of blood is prevented by clamping the roller clamp of the line and by clamping the t-port at the catheter. No other products should be given via this administration line or catheter in order to maintain sterility and decrease the potential for bacterial contamination.

Fluid additives

Additives are commonly added to fluids. The additive put in the fluid bag should be noted on the bag label. The label should note the amount of additive added; if it is an electrolyte, the final electrolyte concentration per liter should also be listed.

Additives commonly given to patients in the ICU include potassium salts such as potassium chloride (KCl) or potassium phosphate (KPO$_4$). Potassium must be diluted as noted on the bottle and given slowly when administered intravenously. Undiluted and rapid IV administration may result in a fatal hyperkalemia. The rate of IV potassium chloride should not exceed 0.5 mEq/kg/hr. The potassium chloride can be added to and is compatible with commonly used IV replacement fluids. The fluid bag should be clearly labeled that it contains potassium and the concentration of the potassium. It is best to have a consistent method for noting the concentration, such that all measurements of potassium are denoted as per liter volume regardless of the bag volume. For example, to a 1000 ml bag of LRS with 4 mEq already present is added 16 mEq of KCl; the final concentration would be noted as 20 mEq/L KCl total on the bag label. In some patients there is a deficiency in potassium and phosphate, making the use of KPO_4 warranted. KPO_4 must also be diluted prior to IV administration, and is compatible with dextrose in water and 0.9% NaCl.[9] As with KCl, KPO_4 should not be delivered at a rate greater than 0.5 mEq K+/kg/hr. KCl and KPO_4 can be combined within the same fluid bag as long as the concentration of each potassium source is labeled and the appropriate rate of administration for the combined volume is listed on the order sheet.

Calcium gluconate or calcium chloride 10% are used to treat hypocalcemia. Calcium should be given slowly intravenously over a 10-minute period and the ECG monitored during the infusion to watch for the development of bradycardia. If bradycardia develops, the calcium infusion should be slowed or stopped temporarily. Calcium chloride is extremely caustic if administered extravascularly. Calcium gluconate can be given subcutaneously if diluted with an equal volume of 0.9% NaCl.[10]

Sodium bicarbonate is used to treat metabolic acidosis. A calculated dose is given slowly intravenously; an initial bolus dose can be given over 20–30 minutes with the remainder of the dose given over the next several hours. It can be given with fluids such as 5% dextrose in water, 2.5% dextrose in 0.45% NaCl, Ringer's solution with dextrose, and 0.9% NaCl.[11]

Agents used to treat specific toxicities

N-acetylcysteine (NAC) is considered the treatment of choice for acetaminophen toxicity.[12] The recommended regimen for use of NAC is an initial dose of 140 mg/kg IV up to 280 mg/kg if the toxicosis is severe, followed by 70 mg/kg every 6 hours for seven additional treatments. NAC may cause nausea and vomiting when given orally. Hypotension and bronchospasm can occur with rapid IV administration. Phlebitis occurs with perivascular leaks. It is best given as an IV infusion of a 5% solution, made by diluting 10%–20% NAC in 5% dextrose or 0.9% NaCl, over 30–60 minutes through a 0.2-μm filter.[12]

Fomepizole 4-methylpyrazole (4-MP) is used to treat ethylene glycol poisoning. Once the agent is reconstituted it should be used within 72 hours; it can be stored at room temperature. The reconstituted solution can be further diluted with 5% dextrose in water or 0.9% NaCl. The agent is given intravenously.[13]

Vitamin K_1 is used in the treatment of anticoagulant rodenticide toxicities. Oral absorption is enhanced when given with fatty foods or by giving canned dog food with the vitamin K. IV administration is not recommended due to the potential for anaphylactoid reactions, and IM injections may result in bleeding. An initial SC dose is usually given and then oral long-term therapy is instituted. When giving the SC dose, use a small gauge needle and administer at multiple sites.[14]

Pralidoxime chloride (2-PAM) is used to treat organophosphate poisoning. It works best as an antidote when used in combination with atropine. It can be given as IM or slow IV injection initially, with subsequent IM or SC doses.[15]

Antibiotics

Antibiotics that must be diluted prior to administration should have the dilution instructions listed on the bottle. It is important to note concentration, date, and time of reconstitution, as the shelf life can vary with different concentrations; this is also important for medications that come with a vial of diluent for dilution. Not all staff in the hospital may be clear on the procedure for dilution of that particular medication and may dilute the drug to a different concentration. How the dilution was prepared and how the antibiotic was given must be recorded. The antibiotic ampicillin at a dilution of 100 mg/ml has a shelf life of 30 minutes before degradation of the product. The antibiotic ampicillin sodium/sulbactam sodium, Unasyn®, diluted to 30 mg/ml has a refrigerated storage time of 72 hours.

Amikacin sulfate should be used cautiously—if at all—with the loop diuretics such as furosemide or osmotic diuretics such as mannitol, as there may be in increase in the nephrotoxic or ototoxic effect of the amikacin.[16] The concern for nephrotoxic and ototoxic effects will also hold true for the other aminoglycoside, gentamicin sulfate.

Enrofloxacin is used extra-label as an IV injection. It is diluted 1:1 with 0.9% NaCl for slow IV administration over 10–45 minutes. The injectable form of enrofloxacin must not be mixed with or come in contact with any magnesium-containing solution such as Normosol and Plasmalyte, as microprecipitants may form and lodge in the patient's lung leading to morbidity and mortality. Enrofloxacin should be used cautiously in cats, as doses higher than 15 mg/kg have been associated with ocular toxicity and subsequent blindness.[17]

Metronidazole is commonly used to treat anaerobic bacterial infections. Accurate dosing is important, as neurologic toxicity may result in dogs that receive a high dose either acutely or long-term. An aluminum hub needle should not be used with this drug, as the aluminum can cause a reddish-brown discoloration of the solution.[18]

Inotropes and vasoactive agents

Inotropes and vasopressor agents may be necessary for the treatment of hypotension. Dobutamine and dopamine are commonly used. If the hypotension is severe and does not respond to initial treatments, vasopressor agents such as norepinephrine, epinephrine, phenylephrine, and vasopressin may be used. Dobutamine when diluted for administration should be used within 24 hours. The diluent can be 5% dextrose in water or 0.9% NaCl. Dobutamine is compatible with 0.9% NaCl, dextrose–0.9% NaCl combinations, and LRS, and is administered as a CRI.[19]

Dopamine is also administered as a CRI. It is commonly diluted with 5% dextrose in water, 0.9% NaCl, or LRS and should be used within 24 hours. Solutions that are pink-, yellow-, brown-, or purple-tinged indicate decomposition of the drug and should be discarded.[20]

Phenylephrine is used treat severe hypotension via its alpha-adrenergic effects. It is given intravenously via CRI and is diluted in 0.9% saline or 5% dextrose in water. It should not be used if the solution is brown or contains a precipitate. Phenylephrine is compatible with the standard IV fluids.[21]

Additional agents used to treat hypotension include norepinephrine and vasopressin. Both are compatible with standard IV crystalloid fluids. They are commonly diluted in 0.9% NaCl to ease administration. As with other inotropes and vasopressors, it is recommended that each agent be in a separate bag or syringe to allow for independent adjustment of individual doses.

Nitroprusside sodium is used intravenously to treat severe hypertension. When using this agent, blood pressure must be monitored diligently to prevent severe hypotension. Excessive doses, prolonged therapy greater than 3 days, or severe hepatic or renal insufficiency may lead to profound hypotension or cyanogen or thiocyanate toxicity. Nitroprusside powder is diluted in 5% dextrose in water and protected from light by covering the fluid bag. The solution may have a slight brownish tint, which is normal. Discard the product if the fluid is blue, dark red, or green in color. Once reconstituted, the nitroprusside solution will be stable for 24 hours. Nitroprusside should be given intravenously in a dedicated line, and extravasation should be avoided. An infusion pump is recommended for delivery, to avoid a sudden bolus of the agent.[22]

Analgesics and anesthetics

Animals that require mechanical ventilation often need heavy sedation or light anesthesia to tolerate the endotracheal tube. Pentobarbital sodium is commonly used in long-term ventilator patients. An initial IV loading dose is used to induce anesthesia followed by a CRI for maintenance. Pentobarbital can be diluted in 5% dextrose in water solutions, Ringer's, LRS, or 0.9% NaCl.

Propofol is also commonly used to help maintain ventilator patients or to treat refractory seizure conditions. Propofol is an IV anesthetic agent. It can be given as an IV bolus or as a CRI to maintain anesthesia. Propofol does not contain any antibacterial agent and has the potential to become bacterially contaminated. It should probably not be used beyond 24 hours once the bottle has been opened. Cats may develop Heinz body anemia from long-term use of propofol.[23] The product should not be used if the emulsion has separated. Propofol is compatible with the commonly used IV replacement and maintenance fluids, and can be injected into a running IV line. When used as a CRI, propofol is best delivered via syringe pump to assure an accurate delivery rate. A new formulation of propofol has recently become available, PropoFlo 28TM by Abbott. The preservative benzyl alcohol is added, allowing a shelf life of 28 days. This product is only labeled for IV use in the dog and should not be used in the cat. Benzyl alcohol is potentially toxic to the cat due to the cat's lack of adequate glucuronic acid conjugation.

> **Case Study 58.2** A 4-year-old DSH MC was presented for upper airway dyspnea and retropharyngeal swelling. The cat developed cyanosis. He had a right arytenoidectomy and a temporary tracheostomy tube placed to improve ventilation and oxygenation. While in ICU the cat had several episodes of difficult breathing through the tracheostomy tube; each time the cat received IV propofol to facilitate removal of the tracheostomy tube in order for it to be cleaned of mucous plugs. As the cat improved the tracheostomy tube was removed for short periods of time; in order to reinsert the tube, IV propofol was used. The cat was in the ICU and received multiple doses of propofol over a 7-day period. On the seventh day a routine CBC showed a hematocrit (HCT) of 14% and 25%–50% Heinz bodies. On presentation the HCT was 40%; this was a significant anemia that required treatment with a packed RBC infusion. The packed RBC infusion improved the HCT to 19%, and the cat recovered. It is important when sedating on multiple days to be aware of the possible consequences that sedative and anesthetic drugs may have. This may be species-related or age-related, as older or debilitated animals will take longer to metabolize drugs, resulting in a possible prolonged effect.

Lidocaine is used to treat cardiac arrhythmias and as an analgesic. When used as a CRI, an initial loading dose is administered to achieve an effective plasma concentration, which is then maintained with the CRI. Lidocaine should be used cautiously in cats due to a high risk of adverse

Medical Error/Incident Form

Purpose: To document medication errors to develop systems or policies to reduce or prevent recurrence
Used by: Any VMC Clinician, student or staff member
Reviewed by: Director of Pharmacy. Associate Director of Pharmacy. Veterinary Medical Center Pharmacy and Therapeutics Committee.
                  Medical Director. Director of Patient Services

Reported by: _____ Date reported: _____ Phone#: _____

Date/Time of Incident: _____ VMC Cast #: _____

Brief Description of Error/Incident: _____

_____

_____

Service Area in which error was made (no names please): _____

Patient Type: _____Outpatient   ____ Inpatient Wards   ____Inpatient ICU   ____Prep for Discharge

Species: _____   Drug name: _____   # of doses administered incorrectly _____

Type of Error: ___ Verbal Miscommunication   ____ Prescribing   ____ Dispensing/Labeling

                        ___ Misadministration   ____ Wrong patient/case # _____

Error made by: ____DVM Student   ____ Tech Student   ___CVT   ____ Pharmacist

                   ____ Pharmacy Tech   ____ Pharm Tech Student   ___DVM   ____ Other: ____

Severity of Error:

____1) As expected, no harm noted to patient, no treatment required to remedy
____2) Potentially could have caused prolonged therapy or morbidity; but no additional treatment required
____3) Caused prolonged therapy and/or minor morbidity
____4) Caused apparent significant morbidity
____5) Apparent cause of mortality or resulted in euthanasia

Signature of reporter: _____

Pharmacist's Investigation and Analysis, including financial impact to VMC (Note: If error by pharmacist, investigation
to be performed by alternate:)

Figure 58.3 Incident-error form. Used with permission by the University of Minnesota Veterinary Medical Center

events.[24] Lidocaine has the potential to be toxic, with clinical signs of ataxia, nystagmus, depression, vomiting, seizures, bradycardia, and hypotension. Lidocaine is compatible with the commonly used IV replacement fluids.

The fluid bag should be properly labeled as containing lidocaine. The lidocaine solution containing epinephrine should not be infused intravenously; this product is used for local analgesia application, and IV use of this product could lead to cardiac arrhythmias.[25]

Chemotherapeutic agents

Many chemotherapeutics are given intravenously or even subcutaneously. Patients are given IV fluids to help maintain renal perfusion. Cisplatin, streptozoticin, L-spar, pamidronate, and dicarbizine are all commonly used chemotherapeutic agents for the treatment of osteocarcoma. Gloves should be worn when handling and administering these compounds. Gloves should also be worn when handling any bodily fluids from these patients.

Drug overdose

When a drug is inadvertently overdosed, an incident form should be completed and the doctor immediately notified of the event (Fig. 58.3). The incident form is used not to place blame but to track errors within the hospital and to improve and refine protocols. The patient's vital signs should be assessed to gather baseline data and to evaluate patient stability in the event an overdose leads to a reaction. If the drug is capable of being reversed, the patient's clinician will determine if reversal is warranted. Reversal agents include naloxone for opioids, flumazanil for benzodiazepines, and atipamazole for the alpha-2 agonists. The possible side effects of the overdosed drug should be investigated. If the overdose is severe and leads to increased length of hospitalization, higher costs, or the death of the patient, the hospital director should be informed. The owners should be made aware of the situation.

Case Study 58.3 A male intact Akita was seen for a several-month history of collapse and paralysis. A neurological exam was performed. A test for myasthenia gravis was performed. The dog received IV Tensilon[R] (edrophonium) and the response was noted. The dog immediately improved and was able to move freely. This was considered a positive test for myasthenia gravis, and the dog then received IM neostigmine for treatment. At the time of neostigmine administration, it was noted by technicians involved with the case that the amount of drug seemed to be a large volume. The drug was given, even though there was concern about the amount of drug. The dog subsequently seizured, vomited, and defecated but seemed to recover. Vomiting persisted; treatment with IV and IM atropine was not effective. The dog developed cyanosis and dyspnea. Thoracaic radiographs reveled aspiration pneumonia. The dog required mechanical ventilation to treat hypercarbia and hypoxemia. The dog became hypotensive and developed acute respiratory distress syndrome. The dog's condition worsened and he went into cardiac arrest and died. It was later determined that the neostigmine was inadvertently administered at 10 times the recommended dosage. It is important to question drug doses that seem to be wrong either in amount, in type, in route of delivery, or for the species. If there is any doubt as to the validity of a drug administration, the clinician in charge of the case should be notified and the proper dosing information verified.

The medical therapies that are required in an ICU situation can vary with each patient. The patient treatment sheet should have clear instructions as to dosage and routes of administration. It is vital to be aware of all drug interactions and affects of those medications in that patient. Mistakes can be made by anyone; if there is a question regarding a drug, a dose, or route of administration, it is better to investigate rather than make an error. Record keeping is instrumental to the successful treatment and well-being of the patient in ICU.

References

1. Ober CP, Spotswood TC, Hancock R. Fatal venous air embolism in a cat with retropharyngeal diverticulum. Veterinary Radiology & Ultrasound 2006;47:153–157.
2. Walsh VP, Machon RG, Munday JS, Broome CJ. Suspected fatal venous air embolism during anaesthesia in a Pomeranian dog with pulmonary calcification. Clinical Communication. New Zealand Veterinary Journal 2005;53:359–362.
3. Otto CM, Kaufman GM, Crowe DT. Intraosseous infusion of fluids and therpeautics. The Compendium of Continuing Education Small Animal 1989;11:412–430.
4. Plumb DC. Sucralfate In: Plumb DC, ed. Plumb's Veterinary Drug Handbook, 6th ed. Ames: Blackwell Publishing, 2008: 843–844.
5. Plumb DC. Insulin. In: Plumb DC, ed. Plumb's Veterinary Drug Handbook, 6th ed. Ames: Blackwell Publishing, 2008: 479–484.
6. Trissel LA. Dizepam. In: Trissel LA, ed. Handbook on Injectable Drugs, 9th ed. Bethesda: American Society of Health-Systems Pharmacists Product Development Office, 1996:333–341.
7. Plumb DC. Diazepam. In: Plumb DC, ed. Plumb's Veterinary Drug Handbook, 6th ed. Ames: Blackwell Publishing, 2008: 275–278.
8. Plumb DC. Mannitol. In: Plumb DC, ed. Plumb's Veterinary Drug Handbook, 6th ed. Ames: Blackwell Publishing, 2008:55–556.
9. Plumb DC. Potassium. In: Plumb DC, ed. Plumb's Veterinary Drug Handbook, 6th ed. Ames: Blackwell Publishing, 2008: 731–732.
10. Plumb DC. Calcium. In: Plumb DC, ed. Plumb's Veterinary Drug Handbook, 6th ed. Ames: Blackwell Publishing, 2008:125–129.
11. Plumb DC. Sodium bicarbonate. In: Plumb DC, ed. Plumb's Veterinary Handbook, 6th ed. Ames: Blackwell Publishing, 2008: 822–824.
12. Rahilly L, Mandell DC. Methemoglobinemia. In: Silverstein DC, Hopper K, eds. Small Animal Critical Care Medicine. St Louis: Saunders, 2009:374–378.
13. Plumb DC. Fomepizole. In: Plumb DC, ed. Plumb's Veterinary Drug Handbook, 6th ed. Ames: Blackwell Publishing, 2008: 410–411.
14. Plumb DC. Phytonadione. In: Plumb DC, ed. Plumb's Veterinary Drug Handbook, 6th ed. Ames: Blackwell Publishing, 2008: 734–736.
15. Plumb DC. Pralidoxime chloride. In: Plumb DC, ed. Plumb's Veterinary Drug Handbook, 6th ed. Ames: Blackwell Publishing, 2008:750–751.
16. Plumb DC. Amikacin sulfate. In: Plumb DC, ed. Plumb's Veterinary Drug Handbook, 6th ed. Ames: Blackwell Publishing, 2008: 32–35.
17. Plumb DC. Enrofloxacin. In: Plumb DC, ed. Plumb's Veterinary Drug Handbook, 6th ed. Ames: Blackwell Publishing, 2008: 342–345.
18. Plumb DC. Metronidazole. In: Plumb DC, ed. Plumb's Veterinary Drug Handbook, 6th ed. Ames: Blackwell Publishing, 2008: 610–613.
19. Plumb DC. Dobutamine HCl. In: Plumb DC, ed. Plumb's Veterinary Drug Handbook, 6th ed. Ames: Blackwell Publishing, 2008: 316–317.

20. Plumb DC. Dopamine HCl. In: Plumb DC, ed. Plumb's Veterinary Drug Handbook, 6th ed. Ames: Blackwell Publishing, 2008: 321–323.

21. Plumb DC. Phenylephrine HCl. In: Plumb DC, ed. Plumb's Veterinary Drug Handbook, 6th ed. Ames: Blackwell Publishing, 2008:724–726.

22. Plumb DC. Nitroprusside sodium. In: Plumb DC, ed. Plumb's Veterinary Drug Handbook, 6th ed. Ames: Blackwell Publishing, 2008:659–661.

23. Andress JL, Day TK, Day DG. The effects of consecutive day propofol anesthesia on feline red blood cells. Veterinary Surgery 1995;24:277–282.

24. Pypendop BH, Ilkiw JE. Assessement of the hemodynamic effects of lidocaine administered IV in isoflurane anesthetized cats. Am J Vet Res 2005;66:661–668.

25. Plumb DC. Lidocaine HCl. In: Plumb DC, ed. Plumb's Veterinary Drug Handbook, 6th ed. Ames: Blackwell Publishing, 2008: 536–538.

59

Administration of biological products

Jennifer E. Prittie

The administration of biologic products to veterinary patients has become common practice in the intensive care unit (ICU). Indications include treatment of anemia, coagulopathy, immune-mediated disease, hypoalbuminemia, snake envenomation, and various toxicities. While these products can have a positive impact on morbidity and mortality in selected candidates, their use is not without risk. Adverse transfusion-related events include acute allergy, delayed hypersensitivity, disease transmission, volume overload, acute respiratory distress, and immunosuppression. Detrimental effects can be minimized through thoughtful selection of candidate and product, appropriate administration practices, and careful monitoring to ensure early recognition of transfusion reactions. This chapter reviews indications for available products, recommended administration protocols, and patient troubleshooting. Biologic products rarely utilized in the small animal ICU (i.e., vaccines with or without bacterins, bacterial extracts or toxoids, erythropoietin, and arsenic compounds) are beyond the scope of this chapter and will therefore not be discussed.

Red blood cell (RBC) products

Red blood cell transfusions are indicated for treatment of anemia caused by hemorrhage, hemolysis, or ineffective erythropoeisis. The decision to administer a RBC product is based on patient hematocrit (HCT), Hb level, and, most importantly, on clinical signs. Clinical indications for treatment of anemia include weakness or fatigue, dull mentation, tachycardia, tachypnea, and bounding femoral pulses that cannot be attributed to another etiology.

The primary goal of a RBC transfusion is improved oxygen delivery to the peripheral tissues. However, a threshold HCT or Hb level below which a RBC transfusion is indicated is not clearly established. Tolerance to anemia varies with comorbid factors and the quantity and rapidity of blood loss. Furthermore, there is ongoing controversy regarding the *in vivo* efficacy of transfused RBCs.[1]

Human investigators have documented reduced in-hospital morbidity and mortality with restricted transfusion practices (maintaining the hemoglobin concentration between 7 and 9 g/dL) when compared with more liberal transfusion of RBCs (to maintain hemoglobin concentration >10 g/dl).[2] The lack of benefit and potential harm of transfused RBCs is postulated to result from storage effects on RBC viability and immunomodulating and/or proinflammatory properties of transfused cells. Storage of product for > 15 days results in RBC morphologic alterations that adversely affect capillary navigation and result in compromised microvascular flow; loss of the enzyme 2,3 diphosphoglyconate (2,3-DPG), which normally facilitates oxygen unloading; and generation of proinflammatory cytokines and complement (storage lesion).[3–5] Transfusion-related immunomodulation (TRIM) is associated with biologically active lipids or WBCs in stored blood, and results in downregulation of the recipient's immune function and increased risk of infection.[6–8]

Adverse reactions

Reported adverse reactions to transfusion with RBCs in veterinary patients are broadly categorized as immune or nonimmune in origin (see **Table 59.1**).

Advanced Monitoring and Procedures for Small Animal Emergency and Critical Care, First Edition. Edited by Jamie M. Burkitt Creedon, Harold Davis.
© 2012 John Wiley & Sons, Inc. Published 2012 by John Wiley & Sons, Inc.

Immune-mediated reactions (hypersensitivities) are the most common adverse reactions associated with administration of any biologic product; a detailed review of these reaction types is therefore indicated.

Hypersensitivity

Biologic products contain white blood cells (WBCs), RBCs, hemoglobin (Hb), platelets, clotting factors, albumin, immunoglobulins, and/or animal-derived lipids. These constituents may act as antigens in the recipient animal and result in hypersensitivity reactions. Hypersensitivity is particularly likely following infusion of foreign protein due to protein's high antigenicity, and upon repeat exposure to an antigenic product (i.e., after prior sensitization). Previous exposure to a foreign substance primes the body's immune system, and the body's secondary (called "anamnestic") response involves recruitment of preformed antibodies and augmentation of the original humoral immune response.[9] Types I, II, and III hypersensitivity reactions are frequently reported following administration of biologic products (see Table **59.2**).

Type I hypersensitivity and febrile transfusion reactions

Type I hypersensitivity reactions are also termed acute hypersensitivity, allergy, or anaphylaxis. This type of reaction is mediated through recipient IgE antibodies. Donor antigen cross-links two IgE molecules on recipient mast cells, leading to mast cell degranulation and systemic release of inflammatory mediators.

Mild allergic reactions and leukocyte and platelet sensitivity reactions, which result from binding of recipient antibodies to donor WBCs or platelets, are the most common adverse transfusion-related events in veterinary patients.[10–12] The latter reaction type is termed a "febrile nonhemolytic transfusion reaction" and is associated with a temperature increase of at least 1°C during transfusion.[12]

Table 59.1 Transfusion reactions

Acute Immunologic	Acute Nonimmunologic
Acute hemolysis	Hemolysis from physical damage/contamination
Leukocyte/platelet sensitivity (febrile)	Embolism (air, clot)
Allergy	Sepsis
Transfusion-related lung injury	Volume overload
	Dilutional coagulopathy
Delayed Immunologic	Hypothermia
Delayed hemolysis	Citrate toxicity
Serum sickness	Hyperammonemia
Post-transfusion purpura	
Neonatal isoerythrolysis	**Delayed Nonimmunologic**
Immunosuppression	Infectious disease transmission

Table 59.2 Classification of hypersensitivity reactions

Immune reaction	Mechanism	Clinical Manifestations	Timing
Type I (IgE-mediated)	Binding of antigen-IgE complex with mast cells and release of inflammatory mediators	Fever, facial swelling, pruritus, urticaria, vomiting, diarrhea, anaphylaxis	Minutes to hours
Type II (cytotoxic) AHTR	Interaction between specific IgG or IgM antibodies and red cell-surface antigens	Intravascular hemolysis: Fever, vomiting, dyspnea, hypotension, hemoglobinemia/uria Extravascular hemolysis: Fever, jaundice, decline in PCV	Minutes to hours
Type II (Cytotoxic) DHTR	Interaction between specific IgG antibodies and red cell-surface antigens	Extravascular hemolysis: Hyperbilirubinemia/bilirubinuria, decline in PCV	3–21 days post- transfusion
Type III (Immune complex); serum sickness	Deposition of antigen-antibody complexes in tissues with complement activation and inflammation	Fever, vasculitis, arthralgia, myalgia, lymphadenopathy, glomerulonephritis	1–3 weeks

AHTR, acute hemolytic transfusion reaction; DHTR, delayed hemolytic transfusion reaction.

Table 59.3 Therapies for acute transfusion reactions

Type of reaction	Therapeutic considerations
Acute hemolysis	• Intravascular volume expansion (isotonic crystalloids, 20 ml/kg IV ± nonprotein colloids, 5 ml/kg IV to effect) • Oxygen, bronchodilators for acute respiratory distress (Terbutaline, 0.01 mg/kg SQ B-QID) • Dexamethasone sodium phosphate, 0.125–0.5 mg/kg IV
Allergy	• Diphenhydramine, 2–4 mg/kg IM • ± Dexamethasone sodium phosphate, 0.125–0.5 mg/kg IV
Anaphylactic/ anaphylactoid reaction	• Diphenhydramine, 2–4 mg/kg IM • Dexamethasone sodium phosphate, 0.125–0.5 mg/kg IV • Epinephrine (1:1000), 0.01 mg/kg SQ, IV • Intravascular volume expansion • Vasopressors as needed: Norepinephrine, 0.25–2 µg/kg/minute
Citrate toxicity	Calcium gluconate (10%), 50–150 mg/kg IV administered slowly with EKG monitoring; discontinue if bradycardia develops
Volume overload	Furosemide, 2–4 mg/kg IV; oxygen therapy
Dilutional coagulopathy	Frozen or fresh frozen plasma, 10–20 ml/kg IV until coagulopathy resolved

Clinical signs of allergy are typically mild and include fever, facial swelling, urticaria, pruritus, vomiting, and diarrhea. Much less commonly patients may exhibit hemodynamic collapse and acute respiratory distress; these clinical signs characterize anaphylaxis. A clinically identical reaction that involves complement-mediated mast cell degranulation without the participation of antibodies is an anaphylactoid reaction. While true type I hypersensitivity reactions require previous antigen exposure (sensitization to the antigen), anaphylactoid reactions do not.[1]

Management of allergic reactions involves stopping the product infusion and parenteral administration of antihistamines (see **Table 59.3**). Often the transfusion can be reinstituted with careful monitoring. Signs of anaphylactic shock require aggressive intravenous (IV) fluid resuscitation, IV glucocorticoid administration, and potentially treatment with epinephrine.

Type II hypersensitivity

Administration of blood to a genetically dissimilar recipient of the same species (an allogenic transfusion) can result in an immune response directed at donor RBC surface antigens. This immune response (type II hypersensitivity) results in RBC destruction (hemoly-sis). Two main categories of hemolysis exist: extravascular and intravascular. Extravascular RBC destruction is mediated by the mononuclear-phagocytic system and results in decreased life expectancy of transfused cells but no significant clinical patient decline. Acute intravascular hemolysis is the most dangerous RBC product hypersensitivity reaction and occurs secondary to donor-recipient incompatibility or previous sensitization (in dogs). Prior sensitization is not necessary in feline patients because of the presence of naturally occurring alloantibiodies to RBC surface antigens. Intravascular hemolysis can culminate in disseminated intravascular coagulation (DIC), multiple organ failure (MOF), and death.[9,10]

Clinical signs of acute intravascular hemolysis include vomiting, pyrexia, tachycardia and tachypnea, severe hypotension, and seizures. Hemoglobinemia/uria may also ensue, which can help to differentiate this reaction type from extravascular hemolysis or from a type I hypersensitivity reaction (see Fig. 59.1).[9]

If acute intravascular hemolysis is suspected, the transfusion is terminated and the patient treated aggressively for shock as needed with intravenous fluids, inotropes and/or vasopressors (see Table 59.3). Monitoring for MOF (e.g., respiratory distress, oliguria, coagulopathy) is essential. Additionally, careful inspection of the

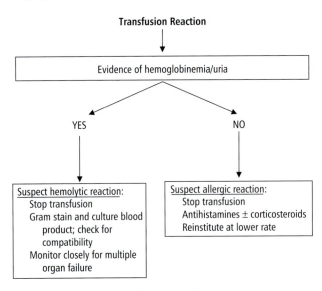

Figure 59.1 Evaluation of acute transfusion reactions.

product for signs of contamination (e.g., product discoloration) or donor-recipient incompatibility (e.g., type A blood administered to a type B cat) is warranted.

Type III hypersensitivity

Type III hypersensitivity, or serum sickness, is characterized by donor antigen interacting with recipient antibodies and formation of immune complexes within the intravascular space. Subsequent systemic deposition of these immune complexes may result in vasculitus, synovitis, arthalgia, myalgia, fever, lymphadenopathy, neuritis, and glomerulonephritis.[9] Clinical signs of serum sickness typically follow antigen exposure by 1–3 weeks. The treatment for serum sickness is largely supportive. Plasmapheresis may be considered for severe cases.

Transfusion-related lung injury

Documented in human transfusion recipients is transfusion-related lung injury (TRALI). This syndrome is characterized by acute dyspnea associated with non-cardiogenic pulmonary edema, and typically occurs within 6 hours of transfusion initiation.[13] The mechanism of lung injury is complex and incompletely elucidated, but probably involves antibodies in donor blood reacting to recipient WBCs (antibody hypothesis) and/or biologically active lipids in stored cellular blood components, known as biologic response modifiers (BRMs). These BRMs activate neutrophils in the lungs that have been "primed" by the underlying patient condition (two-event hypothesis).[14,15] In human patients, TRALI is the leading cause of transfusion-related deaths.[13,15] To the author's knowledge, this syndrome has yet to be documented in veterinary patients.

Nonimmunologic transfusion reactions

Acute nonimmunologic transfusion reactions include hemolysis secondary to inappropriately high flow rates or pressures, circulatory overload, bacterial contamination, air embolization, or pulmonary embolism secondary to inappropriate product filtration.[11] Additionally, massive transfusion (i.e., replacement of a patient's blood volume in less than 24 hours) may result in hypothermia, dilutional coagulopathy, and/or chelation of recipient calcium by donor product anticoagulant (citrate).[16] Citrate toxicity causes hypocalcemic tetany. Hyperammonemia can result from administration of outdated blood products, because ammonia levels in stored blood rise with time.[17] Clinical signs of ammonia accumulation include ataxia, dementia, head pressing, circling, and seizures.

Acute reaction in cats

Reports of transfusion reactions in cats are limited and occur in <10% of transfusion recipients, and typically adverse events (i.e., fever, facial pruritus, vomiting, ptyalism, volume overload) are acute and mild.[20,21] Acute intravascular hemolysis is uncommon, but has been documented in type B cats receiving blood from type A donors.[22]

Acute reactions in dogs

Adverse transfusion-related events in canine recipients have been more commonly reported (3%-40% of recipients), but as with feline recipients, most reactions are mild. Documented reactions include acute hypersensitivity or febrile reactions (92%), and acute (3.2%) and delayed (5%-20%) hemolysis.[16,19]

Tranfusion protocol

Prior to transfusion initiation, close product inspection is warranted. Bacterial contamination can result in purple or brown discoloration of the blood product from deoxygenation, formation of methemoglobin, and/or RBC hemolysis. Careful review of the label will ensure that the correct product type, quantity, species, blood type, and donor are selected. Expired blood products lack *in vivo* efficacy and may cause harm; these should be discarded.

RBC products

Blood products transfused for provision of RBCs include fresh whole blood, stored whole blood, packed RBCs (pRBCs), pRBCs in additive solution, and leukocyte-reduced pRBCs (see **Table 59.4**). Fresh whole blood (WB) is composed of RBCs, leukocytes, platelets, coagu-

Table 59.4 Available red blood cell products

Product	Preparation/Storage	Contents	Indications	Dose
Fresh whole blood	Transfused within 6–8 hours of collection	RBCs, WBCs, platelets, coagulation and plasma proteins	Hemorrhage from trauma or coagulopathy, DIC, severe thrombocytopenia	20 ml/kg raises PCV 10%
Stored whole blood	Stored at 1–6°C in plastic bags, Shelf life 3–4 weeks	RBCs, WBCs, plasma proteins, coagulation factors V and VIII, and platelets decrease with storage	Hypovolemic anemia	20 ml/kg
Packed RBCs	Stored at 1–6°C in plastic bags, Shelf life 3–4 weeks (questionable efficacy after 15 days)	RBCs	Anemia without coagulopathy, concern of volume overload	10 ml/kg raises PCV 10%
Packed RBCs with additive	Stored at 1–6°C with Erythro-Sol, Shelf life ≥ 37 days	RBCs with 100 ml of additive solution	Anemia without coagulopathy, concern of volume overload	10 ml/kg
Leuko-reduced packed RBCs	Stored at 1–6°C in plastic bags, Shelf life 3–4 weeks	RBCs	Anemia, concern of volume overload, history of febrile nonhemolytic transfusion reaction	10 ml/kg

DIC, disseminated intravascular coagulation; PCV, packed cell volume; RBC, red blood cell; WBC, white blood cell.

lation factors, and all other plasma constituents. It is administered within 6–8 hours of collection, ideally immediately. Stored WB is kept longer than 6–8 hours and contains RBCs, plasma proteins, and coagulation factors II, VII, IX and X. Labile coagulation proteins V and VIII and platelets decrease with storage. Indications for WB transfusion are significant hemorrhage associated with either decreased number or function of clotting factors or thrombocytopenia/pathy (fresh WB only).

Packed RBCs contain concentrated RBCs and a small amount of plasma. The PCV of pRBCs is approximately 80%. Additive solution and leukoreduction preserve RBC viability and function and decrease the incidence of FNHTR, respectively. Use of concentrated RBCs limits volume administered to the patient, and this is the blood component of choice for anemia without coagulopathy in patients at risk for volume overload (e.g., history of cardiac or renal disease). RBC products are stored at 1–6°C in plastic bags (see Table 59.4). Shelf life varies with additive solution (see **Table 59.5**).

Plasma products

Plasma products readily available to the veterinarian practitioner include fresh plasma, fresh frozen and stored frozen plasma, and cryoprecipitate. Fresh, fresh frozen, and stored frozen plasma contain coagulation

Table 59.5 Anticoagulant-preservative solutions

Solution	Species	Dilution	Shelf life
Heparin	Dog/cat	625U/50 ml	Immediate
3.8% Sodium citrate	Dog/cat	1 ml/9 ml blood	Immediate
ACD	Dog/cat	1 ml/7–9 ml blood	21 days, dog 30 days, cat
CPDA-1	Dog/cat	1 ml/7 ml blood	20 days, dog 35 days, cat
Additive solutions	Dog	100 ml/250 ml pRBCs	37–42 days

ACD, acid-citrate-dextrose preservative; CPDA-1, citrate-phosphate-dextrose-adenine preservative.

factors, plasma proteins, and all other plasma constituents; plasma is considered "fresh frozen" when stored for up to 1 year at <-18°C (see **Table 59.6**). These products are indicated for treatment of inherited or acquired coagulopathy resulting in clinically significant bleeding, or in preparation for invasive procedures in coagulopathic patients. Cryoprecipitate has similar storage requirements and shelf life comparable to other plasma

Table 59.6 Available plasma and platelet products

Product	Collection/Storage	Contents	Indications	Dose
Fresh frozen plasma (FFP)	Harvested < 6 hrs of blood collection, stored at <-18°C, shelf life 1 yr	Coagulation and plasma proteins, immunoglobulins	Coagulopathy associated with clotting factor deficiency or dysfunction	10–20 ml/kg
Stored frozen plasma	Harvested > 6 hrs of blood collection, stored at <-18°C, shelf life 5 yr	Coagulation factors II, VII, IX, X, plasma proteins, and immunoglobulins	Same as above but amount coagulation factor VIII and vWF deficient for treatment of hemophilia A or vWD	10–20 ml/kg
Cryoprecipitate	Harvested from partial thaw FFP, stored at <-18°C, shelf life 1 yr	Concentrated amount of coagulation factor VIII, vWF, and fibrinogen	vWD, hemophilia A, hypofibrinogemia	1 unit/10 kg
Platelet-rich plasma	Prepared from fresh whole blood by centrifugation, stored at 20–24°C in plastic bags under continuous agitation	Platelets, smaller amounts coagulation and plasma proteins, immunoglobulins	Severe hemorrhage from thrombocytopenia/ thrombocytopathia	Platelets collected from 1 unit whole blood/10 kg
Frozen platelet concentrate	Collected from single donor via plasmapharesis, preserved in DMSO	Platelets, small amounts FFP	Severe hemorrhage from thrombocytopenia/ thrombocytopathia	1 unit/10 kg

vWF, vonWillebrand's disease; vWF, vonWillebrand's factor.

products, and is the component of choice for patients with hemophilia A or von Willebrand's disease.[18]

Other blood products produced from fractionation of plasma are platelet-rich plasma and platelet concentrate (PC) (see Table 59.6). A 6% DMSO-stabilized frozen PC is available (frozen canine platelet concentrate, Animal Blood Services International, Stockbridge, MI).

Investigators have recently demonstrated an inability of platelets in this product to aggregate normally *in vitro* following thaw.[23] There are no data evaluating the *in vivo* efficacy of this product. As platelet products are difficult to store and labile in serum, and studies documenting the efficacy of available products in veterinary patients are limited, prophylactic platelet transfusion is not recommended at this time. However, platelet transfusion may be beneficial for cessation of major bleeding in patients with severe thrombocytopenia (e.g., bone marrow dysfunction, immune-mediated thrombocytopenia) and/or platelet function defects (e.g., uremia, drug therapy, ehrlichiosis, and von Willebrand's disease).[24,25]

Preparation/administration

RBC products are refrigerated to maintain RBC viability and retard bacterial growth. While warming is not necessary, they are frequently warmed to room temperature before administration to avoid patient hypothermia. Warming techniques include the use of a commercially available blood warmer or dilution (for pRBCs) with warm 0.9% NaCl solution. Dilution volume of saline for pRBC products depends on additive or preservative solution used (see Table 59.5). Excessive dilution may result in volume overload in susceptible patients.

Frozen plasma products (with the exception of cryoprecipitate) do not require dilution and are thawed in a water bath gradually warming the bath to 98.6°F (37°C) before administration. Cryoprecipitate is thawed similarly and diluted with 0.9% NaCl solution. Excessive handling or rapid thaw of the fragile plasma bag may result in damage to product components. The plasma product is covered with a plastic bag while thawing to avoid contamination from the water. Frozen PC preserved in DMSO is thawed at room temperature a and gently swirled every 5 minutes during the thawing process.[23] Warming of any blood product to greater than 98.6°F (37°C) may lead to cell lysis, fibrinogen precipitation, and degradation of serum coagulation factors and proteins.[18,24] Once ready for administration, a hang-time limited to 4–6 hours will decrease risk of bacterial colonization.[18,24] If the patient requires administration of the transfusion over more than 4–6 hours (e.g., because of risk of volume overload) the product may be split prior to dilution into a transfer bag and the remainder refrigerated until needed.

Blood products are most commonly administered intravenously. The intraosseous route is appropriate when vascular access is unavailable (e.g., neonates and exotic pets). When administering RBC products intravenously, the diameter of the catheter must be considered. Catheter lumens smaller than 23 gauge may impede flow and increase the risk of RBC lysis. Blood products may be administered through certain commercial infusion pumps. Contact with manufacturers prior to pump use for transfusion purposes is advisable. In emergency situations, blood delivery can be hastened by an external pressure device. Pressure should be exerted evenly over the bag and limited to 300 mmHg.[18,26]

Administration of RBC and plasma transfusions through a dedicated IV line is recommended, and only 0.9% NaCl is utilized for dilution purposes. Fluids containing calcium (i.e, lactated Ringer's solution) may inactivate citrate anticoagulant and result in clot formation when added to the transfusion product. Hypotonic or dextrose-containing solutions administered concurrently with a blood product may result in lysis of the infused RBCs. An in-line blood administration filter (170 μm to 220 μm) is also recommended to capture any debris or blood clots that may result in embolism. For smaller-volume infusions, use of an 18 μm filter attached to intravenous tubing (i.e., minivolume extension set) is an acceptable alternative.[18,24,26]

Initial dose

RBC products are generally transfused to attain a PCV 20%-30% in small animal patients. This "target" PCV, however, will vary with disease and comorbid factors. The volume of WB or pRBCs required to achieve this approximate goal can be calculated utilizing **Equation 59.1**.

$$Kg \times \begin{matrix} 90\,(dogs) \\ or \\ 70\,(cats) \end{matrix} \times \frac{Desired\ PCV - Recipient\ PCV}{Donor\ PCV}$$

$$(59.1)$$

As a general guideline, 2 ml/kg of whole blood raises the PCV 1% and 1 ml/kg of pRBCs raises the PCV 1% (see Table 59.4). These guidelines are not specific and may underestimate the amount of blood required for transfusion. The recommended starting dose for frozen plasma products is 10–20 ml/kg (see Table 59.5). These products are redosed in coagulopathic patients until hemorrhage is controlled. The reader can refer to Table 59.5 for recommended initial doses of other available plasma products.[24]

Monitoring

Prior to administration of any blood product, baseline vitals from the recipient are obtained, including attitude, mucous membrane color, capillary refill time (CRT), heart rate (HR), respiratory rate (RR) and effort, pulse rate and quality, and temperature. These baseline measurements are obtained to allow for comparison with vitals taken during the transfusion process and to aid in detection of a transfusion reaction. The transfusion administration rate is started at 50% of the total calculated rate for the first 30 minutes of the transfusion. During this time, the recipient's vitals and clinical status are monitored every 15 minutes for any change (see **Fig. 59.2**). Changes in vital signs may indicate a transfusion reaction (see Table 59.2). If there are no signs of reaction within 30 minutes of initiation, the rate is increased to 75% of the total calculated rate and the recipient vitals are obtained after 15 minutes at the increased rate. The full transfusion rate is instituted if the recipient demonstrates no reaction after 45 minutes of product administration. Patient monitoring is continued every 30 minutes until completion of the transfusion.

If a sign of reaction is observed at any point during the transfusion, the transfusion must be stopped and a veterinarian notified immediately of the change. The recipient will be evaluated to determine the type of reaction taking place (see Table 59.2 and Fig. 59.1) and the veterinarian will determine the proper course of action (see Table 59.3).

Concentrated human albumin (HA) solution

Albumin is the major osmotically active protein in the body and is responsible for 80% for the plasma colloid osmotic pressure (COP) and preservation of intravascular volume (see Chapter 51, Osmolality and Colloid Osmotic Pressure, for more information). Albumin's additional roles include maintenance of endothelial integrity, mediation of coagulation, scavenging of toxic compounds, transportation of exogenous and endogenous substances, and inhibition of oxidative injury. Hypoalbuminemia is common in critically ill patients with systemic inflammation, and is due to fluid shifts from the intravascular space to the interstitium, gastrointestinal and renal losses, and decreased production. The consequences of hypoalbuminemia in this patient population include enteral feeding intolerance, hypercoagulability, poor wound healing, and MOF. Additionally, serum albumin concentration is inversely related to mortality in both human and veterinary patients.[27–29]

Despite the well-documented detrimental effects of hypoalbuminemia, the merits of albumin transfusion in critically ill patients remain unclear. Studies evaluating

Date:	Technician Initiating Transfusion:								
	Transfusion Product:								
	Donor/Unit ID:								
	Product Volume:								
	Full rate: 1/2 rate: 3/4 rate:								
	Start Time: End Time:								
	Total Volume of Transfusion:								
	Pre PCV TS Post PCV TS								

If there is a significant change in vitals at ANY time please notify the DVM.									
Time	Time Increment	Time due	Actual time done	RR	HR	Rate of Infusion	Temp	Rate ml/hr	Volume infused
Pre transfusion	0								
If no change with 15 minute vitals, continue at 1/2 transfusion rate									
15 minutes post start	15								
If no change with 30 minute vitals, increase to 3/4 tranfusion rate									
30 minutes post start	15								
If no change with 45 minute vitals, increase to full tranfusion rate.									
45 minutes post start	15								
60 minutes post start	15								
75 minutes post start	15								
90 minutes post start	15								
120 minutes post start	30								
150 minutes post start	30								
180 minutes post start	30								
240 minutes post start	60								
300 minutes post start	60								
360 minutes post start	60								
Transfusion must be completed within 6 hours or discard remainder of blood									

Figure 59.2 Example blood product tranfusion log.

the safety and efficacy of transfusion with albumin products have met with conflicting results, and a survival benefit associated with its administration has yet to be documented in any specific patient population.[30–32] Correction of underlying cause of hypoalbuminemia, use of nonprotein colloids to support COP and maintain intravascular volume, and provision of nutrition remain fundamental goals of treatment in all sick patients. Supplementation of albumin may be prudent in select patients with severe ongoing fluid losses and resultant intravascular volume depletion or significant peripheral and organ edema and associated organ dysfunction.

Currently, the only readily available source of species-specific albumin is plasma transfusion, administration of which may be limited by cost, availability, and the potential for volume overload. An alternative and more effective means of affecting serum albumin concentration is infusion of a concentrated HA solution, produced from fractionation of human plasma (albumin (human) 25%, Octapharma USA, Hoboken, NJ). However, while pharmaceutical HA does increase albumin concentration, this product has no proven survival advantage and is associated with significant complications in veterinary patients.[33–35] The most clinically relevant adverse effects are related to the highly antigenic nature of HA. As a foreign protein, HA elicits immune responses in both critically ill and healthy dogs. Anti-HA IgG antibodies have been demonstrated in some dogs with no prior exposure to HA and in most dogs following a single HA infusion (typically 2–6 weeks after transfusion).[36]

Adverse reactions

Reported acute reactions in canine HA recipients include mild type 1 hypersensitivities and, less commonly, hemodynamic collapse and signs of hypovolemic shock that characterize anaphylactic/anaphylactoid responses.[34,35,37] These reactions are documented following both initial and repeat exposure to HA. More recently, occurrence of serum sickness has been documented in canine HA recipients.[35] Facial and peripheral edema, vomiting and inappetance, urticaria, joint effusion and lameness, acute renal failure, and death several days to weeks following HA infusion are reported. The more severe clinical signs attributable to serum sickness occur in healthy dogs. This dichotomy may be related to immunocompetence and normal serum albumin concentrations in these recipients.[36]

Transfusion protocol

Risk assessment, careful recipient selection, familiarization with available HA products, and close patient mon-

itoring are paramount to safe administration of HA. Reasonable goals for HA administration are to increase serum albumin to 2.0–2.5 g/dL and COP to 14–20 mmHg, respectively.

Preparation/administration

Prior to administration, the product is inspected for turbidity or discoloration and, if present, discarded. Human albumin is administered within 4 hours of opening the vial to decrease potential of bacterial contamination. A vented delivery set may be used as HA is supplied in a glass vial, or the contents can be aseptically transferred to a buretrol for administration. Transfusion filters are routinely used with HA to filter macroaggregates that may form in solution, but according to the package insert, a filter is not required. The product may be directly administered or diluted with crystalloids.[33,35]

Dose

Dosages are based on either a calculated albumin deficit or an extrapolated empirical dosage of 2–5 ml of 25% HA per kg. Albumin deficit can be estimated using **Equation 59.2.**

$$10 \times (\text{serum albumin desired} - \text{serum albumin of patient})$$
$$\times \text{body weight (kg)} \times 0.3 = \text{albumin deficit}$$

$$(59.2)$$

Monitoring

Baseline vitals are obtained prior to HA administration, and frequent monitoring of perfusion parameters, including CRT, HR, pulse rate and quality, RR and effort, and temperature, is required throughout transfusion. Infusion rates are typically started at a decreased rate and slowly increased to full rate if no sign of reaction occurs (see Fig. 59.1). Signs of acute reaction warrant cessation of transfusion or decrease of transfusion rate. Emergency management of hypersensitivity reactions is outlined in Table 59.2. Due to the hyperoncotic nature of HA solution, volume overload may complicate therapy, and close monitoring of respiratory parameters and volume status (e.g., central venous pressure measurements) is also indicated.

After HA administration, re-evaluation of the patient's interstitial edema status, serum albumin concentration, and/or COP will determine transfusion efficacy. While significant ongoing protein losses may interfere with reaching target albumin level, repeat administration of this foreign protein is ill-advised. Implementation of nonprotein colloid therapy and nutritional support are recommended to maintain plasma COP following HA transfusion.

Lyophilized canine albumin (5g), manufactured by Animal Blood Resources International, may become available in the near future, and will likely decrease the incidence of severe hypersensitivity reactions in dogs. The reader is referred to the manufacturer to check product availability and obtain information regarding dosage and administration protocols (canine albumin, Animal Blood Resources International).

Human intravenous immunoglobulin (hIVIG)

Human intravenous immunoglobulin (hIVIG) is fractionated from plasma pooled from 1,000–10,000 blood donors. This product is comprised of at least 90% biologically active IgG and smaller amounts of IgE, IgA, IgM, and IgD. The immunomodulating properties of hIVIG have proven beneficial in a variety of human immune-mediated disorders, including systemic lupus erythematosus, myasthenia gravis, pure RBC aplasia, immune-mediated neutropenia, vasculitis, and toxic epidermal necrolysis.[38,39]

The mechanisms of action of hIVIG are complex but are postulated to include phagocyte Fc receptor blockade and resultant decreased phagocytic activity of mononuclear cells, modulation of T-cell function (inhibition of cytotoxic T cells), and attenuation of complement-mediated damage and proinflammatory cytokines.[38]

Commercially available hIVIG has been utilized with some success in dogs and cats affected with immune-mediated hemolytic anemia (IMHA), immune-mediated thrombocytopenia (ITP), myasthenia gravis, sudden acquired retinal degeneration syndrome (SARDS), myelofibrosis, erythema multiforme, and a variety of other immune-mediated dermatologic disorders (i.e., toxic epidermal necrolysis, Stevens-Johnson syndrome).[40–43]

Adverse Reactions

Adverse effects in human patients following IVIG administration are uncommon, affecting <5% of patients, and are typically limited to fever and malaise. More serious effects reported include hypotension during infusion, renal failure, aseptic meningitis, hemolytic anemia, thromboembolic events, and anaphylaxis in patients with IgA deficiency. Volume overload and resultant pulmonary edema and TRALI have also been reported.[38]

Similarly, complications associated with hIVIG administration in veterinary patients are infrequently reported. Dogs with IMHA treated with this product have developed transient thrombocytopenia and thromboembolism, but these findings may be unrelated to

IVIG and instead associated with the patients' underlying diseases.[40,43] Vomiting was reported following infusion of hIVIG in a healthy dog.[43] Other potential adverse effects are related to the product's hyperoncotic nature (i.e., volume overload, especially in patients with underlying cardiovascular disease) and antigenicity, which may result in acute or delayed hypersensitivity reactions. The potential for sensitization in veterinary patients has been postulated. This may preclude safe repeat infusion of this product in individual patients.

Transfusion protocol

Preparation/administration

Lyophilized hIVIG products can be stored at room temperature for up to 24 months prior to rehydration.[44] A variety of diluents may be used for reconstitution; these vary with product and manufacturer, but include sterile water, 0.9% NaCl, and 5% dextrose (Gammagard S/D package insert, Baxter Healthcare Corporation, Westlake Village, CA; Sandoglobulin® immune globulin intravenous (human) package insert, Novartis Pharmaceuticals, East Hanover, NJ). Rehydration is recommended over 15–20 minutes, and gentle handling of the product during this process is advisable to prevent foaming. Refrigeration is required following reconstitution, and the product must be administered within 24 hours to reduce risk of contamination.[44]

Immunoglobulin is administered via a designated peripheral or central venous catheter. Most hIVIG manufacturers advocate the use of an in-line filter during transfusion; filter size recommendations vary.[d,e] The product is administered at room temperature for optimal patient comfort.[44]

Dose

The optimal dose of hIVIG in veterinary patients is unknown. Historical doses of hIVIG in animals range from 0.5 to 1.5 g/kg.[40–43] In five dogs with ITP, a low-dose therapy (0.28–0.34 g/kg) was utilized and deemed efficacious.[41]

Monitoring

An infusion period of 6–12 hours is recommended in human patients to ensure safe delivery, and hang times of 4–8 hours are reported in veterinary patients.[40–44] In all species, transfusion is initiated at a slow rate (0.01 ml/kg/min) and gradually increased every 30–60 minutes to a maintenance rate not to exceed 0.08 ml/kg/min. Fluid-sensitive patients may not tolerate high fluid rates. Frequent monitoring during administration should include: CRT, HR, pulse rate and quality, RR and effort, and temperature (see Fig. 59.1). Signs of acute hypersensitivity warrant prompt, temporary cessation of the infusion and antihistamine administration (see Tables 59.2 and 59.3). Most patients tolerate reinstitution and completion of the transfusion at a slower infusion rate.

Specific immunoglobulin therapy

Very few small animal toxicities exist for which a specific antidote can be provided. Three such toxicities are poisonous snake envenomation, tetanus, and digitalis glycoside overdose. In each case, the antidote provided is specific immunoglobulin(s) that target(s) the toxicant, limiting host toxicity via immunomodulation.

Snake envenomation

Approximately 20 species of snakes native to the United States are venomous. Most small animal envenomations occur in the southwestern part of the country, and are attributable to Crotalidae species, or pit vipers (i.e., rattlesnakes, cottonmouths, and copperheads). Of the pit vipers, the Eastern diamondback rattlesnake is responsible for the majority of human fatalities annually. Less frequently, envenomations are due to Elapidae (i.e., coral snakes).[45–47]

Snake venom consists of mixtures of enzymatic proteins (i.e., hylauronidase, collagenase, proteases, and phospholipases) that cause local tissue injury and vasculitis, enhancing spread of the venom. Other proteins and enzymes, including fibrinolysins and thrombin-like enzymes, result in defibrination (depletion of fibrinogen and fibrin) and friable clot formation, respectively. The end result is coagulopathy characterized by bleeding propensity. Victims of snake bites are also at risk for renal failure and for neurotoxicity associated with neuromuscular blockade, the latter typically caused by Elapidae envenomation. Lethality following envenomation is associated with the smaller low-molecular-weight polypeptides in the venom that result in increased capillary permeability, intravascular volume depletion from third spacing of fluids, and hypovolemic shock.[45,46,48]

While supportive measures such as administration of intravenous fluids, analgesics, and antibiotics (for documented concurrent bacterial infection) are the standard of care for victims of snake bites, administration of antivenom plays the most important role in morbidity and mortality reduction in many of these animals. A mortality reduction of 36% was observed comparing dogs that were treated with antivenom with those who were not in one study.[49] The two products that thatmost frequently utilized for treatment of rattlesnake bites in human patients are antivenin (Crotalidae) polyvalent (ACP) (Fort Dodge Animal Health, Overland Park, KS) and Crotalidae Polyvalent Immune Fab antivenom

Table 59.7 Comparison of crotalid antivenoms

Property	ACP	FabAv
Source	Horse	Sheep
Immunoglobulin	IgG	Fab fragment
Potency	+	+++
Antigenicity	+++	+
Initial Dose	10–50 ml (1–5 vials)	4–6 vials
Clearance/need for repeat administration	+	+++
Approximate Cost	$250/vial	$3,500/vial
Licensure	Human, animal	Human

ACP, antivenin (Crotalidae) polyvalent; FabAV, Crotalidae Polyvalent Immune Fab (ovine).

(FabAV) (ovine, Protherics, Nashville, TN)[47] (see **Table 59.7**). ACP is an antiserum comprised of equine gammaglobulins. This product is rich in antibodies that target the venoms of all endemic pit viper species, but in addition contains allergenic equine protein contaminant. Fab antivenom has approximately five times the potency of ACP, and is more efficacious than ACP for treatment of crotalid-induced neurotoxicity.[47,50] Furthermore, FabAV is less allergenic than is ACP, as it is pure Fab immunoglobulin and as such contains less contaminant than does ACP antivenom.[47,50,51] A potential drawback to FabAV is its shorter half-life, which may allow for recurrence of the effects of unneutralized venom and necessitate repeat dosing.[51,52] While a multicenter trial evaluating the efficacy of FabAV in veterinary patients is under way, ACP is currently the only product licensed for use in animals in the western hemisphere.

Adverse effects

Adverse effects associated with antivenom therapy are uncommon, and most are related to patient hypersensitivity to foreign proteins in the antiserum. Mild, self-limiting type 1 hypersensitivity reactions have a reported prevalence of 14%-56% and 4% in humans and dogs, respectively.[47, 51–55] In two reports of rattlesnake envenomation in dogs, ACP therapy resulted in type 1 hypersensitivity in 1/22 and 0/23 patients, respectively.[54,55] Clinical signs referable to allergy in affected dogs were limited to facial swelling and pruritus. Anaphylaxis has not been reported in veterinary patients. The reported incidence of serum sickness in human snake bite victims treated with ACP or FabAV is 18%-86% and 16%, respectively.[47] A single case of serum sickness resulting from ACP administration to a dog following *Crotalus adamanteus* envenomation has been reported.[56] The dog developed fever, anorexia, lethargy, and generalized pitting edema 3 days after ACP therapy. The dog made a full recovery.

An antivenom formulated from hyperimmune equine serum (IgG) is also available for small animal victims of systemic elapid snake envenomation.[57] Similar acute and/or delayed hypersensitivity reactions may complicate therapy with this antivenom, with one fatal acute anaphylactic reaction reported in a canine patient following initial exposure to the product.[58]

Protocol

Antivenom therapy is recommended for victims of snake bites with worsening local injury, clinically significant coagulopathy, or systemic signs of shock. The recommended initial dosage of antivenom varies with bite size and amount of venom injected, time elapsed since envenomation, severity of clinical signs, and patient size.

Preparation/administration

Skin testing for prediction of allergic response may be performed by injecting a 1:10 dilution of antivenom at 0.02 ml subcutaneously. A positive reaction, manifested by a wheal surrounded by erythema, occurs within 30 minutes.[59] A negative skin test, however, does not guarantee a severe reaction will not take place, and the time it takes to perform the test delays prompt administration of the antivenom (the sooner the product is administered, the more effective it is).[48,59] Therefore, routine skin testing is not recommended.

Antivenom is reconstituted with the provided diluent. It should be swirled but not shaken, and the vial warmed to body temperature to facilitate reconstitution, which usually takes between 10 and 15 minutes.[48] The reconstituted antivenom is diluted at a ratio of one vial to 100–250 ml of isotonic crystalloids, adjusting the volume to prevent fluid overload in at-risk patients.[59] The initial dosage is administered intravenously over 30 minutes.

Dose

The suggested starting dose ranges from 10 to 50 ml (one to five vials). Redosing depending on product and clinical efficacy may be necessary. Antivenom is costly and financial constraints may need to be considered before administration.[48]

Monitoring

Careful patient monitoring during infusion is paramount for early detection of allergy or anaphylaxis, and emergency drugs including epinephrine, antihistamines, and corticosteroids should be readily available while monitoring for a reaction. Frequent measurement of

tissue swelling and reassessment of coagulation status will help determine the need for antivenom redosing. The dose may be repeated as needed every 2 hours for clinically significant coagulopathy or if local swelling worsens despite therapy.[45]

Tetanus

Tetanus is an acute toxigenic illness that occurs subsequent to infection with the spore-forming bacillus *Clostridium tetani*. In dogs and cats, the source of the infection is typically a contaminated penetrating wound, and clinical signs of illness occur 5–10 days following inoculation of the organism.

Clostridium tetani spores produce two toxins, tetanolysin and tetanospasmin, the latter of which is responsible for the neurologic signs associated with infection. The toxin travels up peripheral nerves and hematologically to the central nervous system and inhibits the release of the inhibitory neurotransmitters gamma-aminobutyric acid (GABA) and glycine. Loss of neuronal inhibition of skeletal muscle and autonomic dysfunction ensue.

Clinical signs associated with infection include severe muscle rigidity and cranial nerve deficits (i.e., facial muscle spasms [risus sardonicus], lockjaw [trismus], third eyelid protrusion, and dysphagia). Additionally, disinhibition of the sympathetic nervous system and excessive catecholamine levels may result in tachycardia and hypertension.[60,61]

Specific immunoglobulins that target tetanospasmin in the blood are a mainstay of therapy. Two products exist for treatment of tetanus in dogs, cats, and humans: equine antitetanus serum (ATS) (Professional Biological Company, Denver, CO) and human tetanus immune globulin (TIG) (Bayer Corporation, Elkhart, IN).[61,62] As both are comprised of foreign proteins, hypersensitivity reactions are possible during and following administration.

Protocol

Recommended antitoxin dosage varies widely from 100 to 1,000 units/kg with a maximal dosage of 20,000 units. Antitoxin may be administered intravenously (ATS), intramuscularly (ATS, TIG), or subcutaneously (ATS). Other reported dosing regimens include 1,000 units at the wound site or 1–10 units intrathecally. However, intrathecal administration has been shown to increase morbidity and mortality in human patients and is not currently recommended.[61]

Patients receiving antitoxin are monitored closely for signs of acute hypersensitivity, and emergency drugs (see Table 59.2) should be readily available.

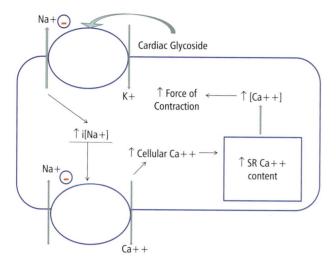

Figure 59.3 Mechanism of action of cardiac glycosides. Cardiac glycosides inhibit the cardiac Na+/K+ATPase pump. This inhibition leads to an accumulation of intracellular Na$^+$, decreased Na$^+$, Ca^{2+} exchange and a resultant increase in intracellular Ca^{2+}. Higher intracellular Ca^{2+} concentration leads to increased force of ventricular contraction.

Digibind

Digitalis glycosides (i.e., digoxin) are frequently prescribed by practitioners for cardiovascular disease in veterinary patients. These agents exert positive inotropic effects via dose-dependent inhibition of the cardiac Na-K-ATPase pump, and subsequent increased intracellular calcium and force of cardiac contraction (see **Fig. 59.3**). Antiarrhythmic effects are mediated through an increase in parasympathetic tone and include decreased sinus rate, depressed impulse conduction through the AV node, prolonged AV refractory period, and decreased automaticity of specialized atrial fibers. These effects make glycosides appropriate agents for management of supraventricular tachycardias and systolic dysfunction.

These agents, however, have low therapeutic to toxic ratios, and inadvertent overdose can be fatal. Extracardiac effects associated with digitalis glycoside toxicity are common, and include depression and inappetance, nausea, vomiting, and diarrhea. More importantly, overdose can result in a variety of cardiac conduction disturbances (i.e., atrioventricular block and bundle branch block), atrial and ventricular arrhythmias, and life-threatening hyperkalemia and resultant cardiac dysrhythmias.

Treatment of toxicity may include gastric decontamination, IV fluid therapy, administration of cardioprotective drugs (i.e., calcium and antiarrhythmic agents), and cardiac pacing. Additionally, in cases of life-threatening toxicosis in human patients and sporadically in veteri-

nary case reports, digoxin-specific antibody is administered. [63-67]

Digibind (Digoxin Immune Fab (ovine), GlaxoSmithKline, Research Triangle Park, NC) is ovine-derived, digoxin-specific Fab antibody fragment with a reported efficacy of >80% in patients with refractory, life-threatening digitalis glycoside toxicity.[65]

Adverse reactions

Potential side effects associated with this therapy are infrequently reported in human reviews, but include allergic reactions (<1%), severe acute hypokalemia from reversal of pump paralysis (4%), and exacerbation of congestive heart failure.[63-66] No detrimental effects have been reported in the few veterinary cases to which this therapy has been applied. However, the foreign nature of the Fab fragments (ovine-derived) imparts the potential for more serious allergic or anaphylactic reactions, and repeat dosing is currently not recommended in veterinary patients.

Protocol

Preparation/administration

Digibind is diluted with isotonic saline and administered through a 0.22 μm filter.[64,67] It may be bolused in emergency situations; however, an infusion over 1–2 hours is recommended when possible.[64]

Dose

Determination of appropriate Digibind dose is based on the digoxin body load (DBL), which is estimated by either the serum concentration or the amount ingested.[64] The serum digoxin concentration obtained 8 hours after the last dose is incorporated into Equation 59.3, where *V = volume of distribution in dogs (5.6 L/kg for digoxin and 0.56 L/kg of digitoxin).

$$\text{DBL} = \frac{\text{Serum glycoside concentration (ng/ml)} \times {}^*V \times \text{body weight (kg)}}{1000} \quad (59.3)$$

The dose of Digibind is then calculated utilizing Equation 59.4, where *DBL = digoxin body load (see Eq. 59.3).[64,67]

$$\frac{{}^*\text{DBL}}{0.6 \text{ mg/vial}} = \# \text{ of vials} \quad (59.4)$$

Alternatively, if the amount of digoxin ingested is known, this information can be utilized to determine Fab dosing. Approximately 0.6 mg of digoxin is neutralized for every 40 mg vial of Fab administered.[67] For acute ingestion, 40 mg of Digibind is administered for every 1 mg of digoxin consumed.[67] If the DBL is unknown, an empirical Fab dose of 80 mg is suggested.[64]

Thrombolytic agents

Endothelial injury, alterations in blood flow, and hyper-coagulable states increase the risk for thrombosis (clot formation). These risk factors (known together as Virchow's triad) are associated with many conditions common to critically ill veterinary patients, including but not limited to sepsis, systemic inflammatory response syndrome, hyperadrenocorticism, diabetes mellitus, cardiomyopathy, neoplasia, protein-losing nephropathy or enteropathy, immune-mediated hemolytic anemia, bite wounds, snake envenomation, polytrauma, heat stroke, and burns. The end results of thrombosis are maldistribution of blood flow (which may cause signs of shock), tissue ischemia, and hypoxia.

The fibrinolytic system is responsible for clot dissolution through the formation of the enzyme plasmin. Plasmin is derived from the inactive proenzyme plasminogen via the action of the body's plasminogen activators. Once generated, plasmin is responsible for fibrinolysis (fibrin degradation and subsequent clot lysis) (see **Fig. 59.4**).

Thrombolytic agents augment fibrinolysis via conversion of plasminogen to plasmin, and have been utilized for treatment of thrombi in both human and veterinary patients.

Indications for thrombolytic agents in human patients include massive pulmonary embolism complicated by right heart failure and/or hypotension, and > 50% obstruction of a major pulmonary artery. Contraindications include acute myocardial infarction, intracranial hemorrhage, head trauma, and ischemic stroke.[68–71]

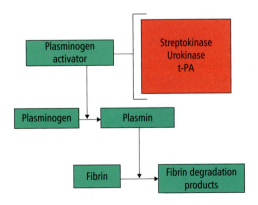

Figure 59.4 Initiation of fibrinolysis.

Specific indications and contraindications are not established for veterinary patients.

Despite lack of established indications, thrombolytic agents have been utilized in dogs and cats with clots of the arterial and venous circulation. No survival advantage has been documented associated with their administration, and reported adverse effects, including fever, hyperkalemia, significant hemorrhage, and acute death are common.[72–76]

Products

Available agents include streptokinase, urokinase-type plasminogen activator (u-PA), and tissue-type plasminogen activator (t-PA).

Streptokinase

Streptokinase is a bacterial protein produced by hemolytic species of *Streptococci* that indirectly activates plasminogen to plasmin. Because of its bacterial origin, this protein can elicit an immune response in the recipient, particularly in patients with previous β-hemolytic *Streptococci* infection. Circulating antibodies to streptokinase limit the efficacy of the agent (necessitating a loading dose initially) and may result in hypersensitivity reactions. Reported signs in human patients include pruritus, rash, and hypotension and bradycardia more commonly following rapid infusion and thought to be associated with histamine and/or bradykinin release. Additional detrimental effects associated with streptokinase administration are systemic hemorrhage due to activation of fibrin-bound (thrombus-associated) AND circulating plasminogen, and ischemia-reperfusion injury when blood flow to ischemic areas is re-established. Reperfusion of such areas leads to systemic release of reactive oxygen species, metabolic acidosis, and hyperkalemia.

Tissue plasminogen activator

Tissue plasminogen activator is secreted by endothelial cells and circulates in the blood. Human recombinant t-PA is derived from mammalian cell tissue culture, and hypersensitivity reactions are possible in veterinary patients, as are systemic bleeding and reperfusion injury. However, as t-PA is more specific for thrombus-associated plasminogen (as opposed to circulating plasminogen), severe hemorrhage is less likely than with streptokinase.

Urokinase

Urokinase is found in the urine and produced from human neonatal kidney cells in tissue culture. This enzyme has clot specificity in between that of streptokinase and t-PA. This product has been infrequently administered to veterinary patients and carries risks similar to other thrombolytic agents.

Protocol

The patient receiving thrombolytic therapy requires intensive monitoring and nursing care. The most common complication of these agents is hemorrhage, which may manifest as a dropping PCV in association with hematuria, gastrointestinal or oral mucosal bleeding, bleeding from catheter insertion sites, dyspnea, or changes in neurologic status.[71] Catheter-associated bleeding may be subtle and go undetected until a substantial volume of blood is lost, as hemorrhage can migrate down fascial planes or be covered by catheter wraps.[73] Direct manual pressure may be applied to a hemorrhaging catheter site, and bleeding patients may require therapy with blood components. Frequent assessment of mucous membrane color and CRT, RR and effort, HR, pulse quality, blood pressure, and temperature can aid in detection of ongoing bleeding. Metabolic acidosis and electrolyte abnormalities such as hyperkalemia associated with tissue reperfusion are common complications of thrombolytic therapy and depending on severity can be fatal. Continuous ECG monitoring is indicated as rising serum potassium causes a progression of ECG changes. Narrow, peaked or "tented" T-waves, flattening and disappearance of the P waves, and widening of the QRS complexes typify the cardiotoxicity associated with progressive hyperkalemia. Tachypnea is nonspecific and may indicate a metabolic acidosis with secondary respiratory compensation, pain, pulmonary thromboembolism, or hemorrhage. Allergic reactions and anaphylaxis are not well documented in the veterinary patient, but result in pruritus, rash, and fever in humans.[68]

Conclusions

Most veterinarians would consider biologic products as an essential component of their armamentarium. These agents are indicated for a variety of clinical syndromes in critically ill patients but do carry significant risks. Safe administration of biologic products involves appropriate patient selection, awareness of associated adverse effects and timely interventions if an untoward reaction is suspected. Implementation of evidence-based guidelines and standardized hospital protocols for administration of these products are recommended.

References

1. Prittie J. Triggers for use, optimal dosing, and problems associated with red cell transfusions. Veterinary Clinic Small Anim 2003; 33: 1261–1275.
2. Hebert P, Yetsir E, Marin C, et al. A multicenter, randomized, controlled clinical trial of transfusion requirements in critical care. N Engl J Med 1999; 340(6): 409–417.
3. Hebert P, Tnmouth A, and Corwin H. Controversies in RBC transfusion in the critically ill. Chest 2007; 131: 1583–1590.
4. Marik R and Sibbald W. Effects of stored-blood transfusion on oxygen delivery in patients with sepsis. JAMA 1993; 269: 3024–3029.
5. Napolitano L and Corwin H. Efficacy of red blood cell transfusion in the critically ill. Crit Care Clin 2004; 20; 255–268.
6. Hill G, Frawley W, Griffith K, et al. Allogeneic blood transfusion increases the risk of postoperative bacterial infection: a meta-analysis. J of Trauma 2003; 54: 908–914.
7. Vincent J, Baron J, Reinhart K, et al. ABC (Anemia and blood transfusion in critical care) investigators. Anemia and blood transfusion in critically ill patients. JAMA 2002; 288(12): 1499–1507.
8. Gunst M and Minei J. Transfusion of blood products and nosocomial infection in surgical patients. Curr Opin Crit Care 2007; 13: 428–432.
9. Tizard I. 1992. Hypersensitivity reactions. In Veterinary Immunology: An Introduction pp. 335–370. W.B. Saunders Company.
10. Bracker K and Drellich S. Transfusion reactions. Comp Cont Ed 2005; 27(7) : 500–512.
11. Harrell K and Kristensen A. Canine transfusion reactions and their management. Vet Clin North Am Small Anim Pract 1995; 25: 1333–1364.
12. Kleinman S, Chan P and Robillard P. Risks associated with transfusion of cellular blood components in Canada. Transfus Med Rev 2003; 17(2): 120–162.
13. Silliman C, Boshkov K, Mehdizadehkashi Z, et al. Transfusion-related acute lung injury: epidemiology and a prospective analysis of etiologic factors. Blood 2003; 101: 454–462.
14. Sachs U. Pathophysiology of TRALI: current concepts. Intens Care Med 2007; 33(Suppl 1): S3-S11.
15. Boshkov L. Transfusion-related acute lung injury and the ICU. Crit Care Clin 2005: 21; 479–495.
16. Jutkowitz L Rozanski E, Moreau J, et al. Massive transfusion in dogs: 15 cases (1997–2001). J Am Vet Med Assoc 2002; 220: 1664–1669.
17. Waddel L, Holt D, Hughes D, et al. The effect of storage on ammonia concentration in canine packed red blood cells. J Vet Emerg Crit Care 2001; 11: 23–26.
18. Hohenhaus A. 2006. Blood transfusion and blood substitutes. In Dibartola: Fluid, Electrolytes, and Acid-Base Disorders In Small Animal Practice pp. 567–583. Elsevier Inc.
19. Harrell K, Rarrow J, and Kristensen A. Canine transfusion reactions, part II: Revention and treatment. Comp Cont Ed 1997; 19(2): 193–201.
20. Klaser D, Reine N, and Hohenhaus A. Red blood cell transfusions in cats: 126 cases (1999). J Am Vet Med Assoc 2005; 226: 920–923.
21. Weingart C, Giger U, and Kohn B. Whole blood transfusions in 91 cats: a clinical evaluation. J Fel Med and Surg 2004; 6: 139–148.
22. Giger U and Akol K. Acute hemolytic transfusion reaction in an abyssinian cat with blood type B. J Vet Int Med 1990; 4: 315–316.
23. Guillaumin J, Jandrey K, Norris J et al. Analysis of a commercial dimethyl-sulfoxide-stabilized frozen canine platelet concentrate by turbidimetric aggregometry. J Vet Emerg Crit Care 2010; 20(6): 571–577.
24. Haldane S, Roberts J, Marks S, et al. Transfusion medicine. Comp Cont Ed 2004; 26(7): 502–519.

25. Abrams-Ogg A. Triggers for prophylactic use of platelet transfusions and optimal dosing in thrombocytopenic dogs and cats. Vet Clin Small Anim 2005; 33: 1401–1418.

26. Lewis, Heitkemper, Dirksen, et al. Medical-Surgical Nursing 2007. Section XI (31). St. Louis, Mosby-Elsevier.

27. Mazzaferro E, Rudloff E, and Kirby R. The role of albumin replacement in the critically ill veterinary patient. J Vet Emer Crit Care 2002; 12(2): 113–124.

28. Vincent J, Dubois M, Navickis R, et al. Hypoalbuminemia in acute illness: is there a rationale for intervention. A meta-analysis of cohort studies and controlled trials. Ann of Surg 2003; 237(3): 319–334.

29. Michel K. Prognostic value of clinical nutritional assessment in canine patients. J Vet Emer Crit Care 1993; 3(2): 96–103.

30. Wilkes M and Navackis R. Patient survival after human albumin administration: a neta-analysis of randomized, controlled trials. Ann of Intern Med 2001; 135: 149–164.

31. Cochrane Injuries Group Albumin Reviewers. Human albumin administration in critically ill patients: systematic review of randomized controlled trials. Br Med J 1998; 317: 235–240.

32. SAFE study investigators. A comparison of albumin and saline for fluid resuscitation in the intensive care unit. N Engl J Med 2004; 350(22): 2247–2256.

33. Trow A, Rozanski E, deLaforcade, et al. Evaluation of use of human albumin in critically ill dogs: 73 cases (2003–2006). J Am Vet Med Assoc 2008; 233(4): 607–612.

34. Cohn L, Kerl M, Lenox C, et al. Response of healthy dogs to infusions of human serum albumin. Am J Vet Res 2007; 68(6): 657–663.

35. Francis A, Martin L, Haldorson G, et al. Adverse reactions suggestive of type III hypersensitivity in six healthy dogs given human albumin. J Am Vet Med Assoc 2007; 230(6): 873–879.

36. Martin L, Luther T, Alpe D, et al. Serum antibodies against human albumin in critically ill and healthy dogs. J Am Vet Med Assoc 2008; 232(7): 1004–1009.

37. Mathews K and Barry M. The use of 25% human serum albumin: outcome and efficacy in raising serum albumin and systemic blood pressure in critically ill dogs and cats. J Vet Emer Crit Care 2005; 15(2): 110–118.

38. Mackay I and Rosen F. Immunomodulation of autoimmune and inflammatory diseases with intravenous immune globulin. N Engl J Med 2001; 345(10): 747–755.

39. Knezevic-Maramica and Kruskall M. Intravenous immune globulins: an update for clinicians. Transf 2003; 43: 1460–1480.

40. Kellerman D and Bruyette D. Intravenous human immunoglobulin for the treatment of immune-mediated hemolytic anemia in 13 dogs. J Vet Intern Med 1997; 11: 327–332.

41. Bianco D, Armstrong P, and Washabau R. Treatment of severe immune-mediated thrombocytopenia with human IV immunoglobulin in 5 dogs. J Vet Intern Med 2007; 21: 694–699.

42. Byrne K and Giger U. Use of human immunoglobulin for treatment of severe erythema multiforme in a cat. J Am Vet Med Assoc 2002; 220(2): 197–201.

43. Scott-Moncrieff J and Reagan W. Human intravenous immunoglobulin therapy. Sem Vet Med and Surg (Sm Anim) 1997; 12(3): 178–185.

44. Murphy E, Martin S, & Valine-Patterson J. Developing practice guidelines for the administration of intravenous immunoglobulin. Journ of Infusn Nurs 2005; 28(4): 265–272.

45. Najman L and Seshadri R. Rattlesnake envenomation. Comp Cont Ed 2007; 29(3): 166–177.

46. Juckett G and Hancox J. Venomous snakebites in the United States: management review and update. Am Fam Phys 2002; 66(1): 30–38.

47. Gold B, Dart R, and Barish R. Bites of venomous snakes. N Engl J Med 2002; 347(5): 347–356.

48. Peterson M. Snake bite: pit vipers. Clin Tech Small Anim Pract 2006; 21: 174–182.

49. Schaer M. Eastern diamondback rattlesnake envenomation of 20 dogs. Comp Cont Ed; 6(11): 997–1006.

50. Consroe R, Egan N, Russel F, et al. Comparison of a new ovin antigen binding fragment (Fab) antivenin for United States Crotalidae with the commercial antivenin for protection against venom-induced lethality in mice. Am J Trop Med Hyg 1995; 53: 507–510.

51. Dart R, Seifert s, Boyer L, et al. A randomized multicenter trial of crotalidea polyvalent immune Fab (ovine) antivenom for the treatment of crotaline snakebit in the United States. Arch Intern Med 2001; 161: 2030–2036.

52. Dart R and McNally J. Efficacy, safety, and use of snake antivenoms in the United States. Ann Emerg Med 2001; 37: 181–188.

53. Jurkovich G, Luterman A, McCullar K, et al. Complications of crotalidae antivenin therapy. J Trauma 1988; 28: 1032–1037.

54. Willey J and Schaer M. Eastern diamondback rattlesnake (Crotalus adamanteus) envenomation of dogs: 31 cases (1982–2002). J Am Anim Hosp Assoc 2005; 41: 22–33.

55. Hackett T, Wingfield W, Mazzaferro E, et al. Clinical findings associated with prairie rattlesnake bites in dogs: 100 cases (198–1998). J Am Vet Med Assoc 2002; 220(11): 1675–680.

56. Berdoulay P, Schaer M, and Starr J. Serum sickness in a dog associated with antivenin therapy for snake bit caused by Crotalus adamanteus. J Vet Emerg Crit Care 2005; 15(3): 206–212.

57. Heller J, Mellor D, Hodgson J, et al. Elapid snake envenomation in dogs in New South Wales: a review. Aust Vet J 2007; 85(11): 469–479.

58. Kremer K and Schaer M. Coral snake (Micrurus Fulvius Fulvius) envenomation in 5 dogs: present and earlier findings. J Vet Emer Crit Care 1995; 5(1): 9–15.

59. Peterson M. Snake bite: coral snakes. Clin Tech Small Anim Pract 2006; 21: 183.

60. Loose N and Carey S. A dog with generalized muscle stiffness. Vet Med 2004; 99(1): 1089–1097.

61. Linnenbrink T and McMichael M. Tetanus: Pathophysiology, clinical signs, diagnosis, and update on new treatment modalities. J Vet Emerg Crit Care 2006; 16(3): 199–207.

62. Coleman ES. Clostridial neurotoxins: tetanus and botulism. Comp Cont Ed 1998; 20(10): 1089–1097.

63. Smith T, Butler V, Haber E, et al. Treatment of life-threatening digitalis intoxication with digoxin-specific Fab antibody fragments. N Engl J Med 1982; 307: 1357–1362.

64. Martiny S, Phelps S, and Massey K. Treatment of severe digitalis intoxication with digoxin-specific antibody fragments: a clinical review. Crit Care Med 1988; 16(6): 629–635.

65. Lapostolle Frederic, Borron S, Verdier C, et al. Digoxin-specific Fab fragments as single first-line therapy in digitalis poisoning. Crit Care Med 2008; 36: 3014–3018.

66. Antman E, Wenger T, Butler V, et al. Treatment of 150 cases of life-threatening digitalis intoxication with digoxin-specific Fab antibody fragments. Circ 1990; 81: 1744–1752.

67. Senior D, Feist E, Stuart L, et al. Treatment of acute digoxin toxicosis with digoxin immune Fab (ovine). JVIM 1991; 5(5): 302–303.

68. Jaffe A. Thrombolytic therapy. 1994 In The Pharmacologic Approach to the Critically Ill Patient pp. 347–364. Williams & Wilkins.

69. Whelan M and O'Toole T. The use of thrombolytic agents. Comp Cont Ed 2007; 29(8): 476–81.

70. Menon V, Harrington R, Hochman J, et al. Thrombolysis and adjunctive therapy in acute myocardial infarction: The seventh ACCP conference on antithrombotic and thrombolytic therapy. Chest 2004; 126(S3): 549S-575S.

71. Thompson M, Scott-Moncrieff C, and Hogan D. Thrombolytic therapy in dogs and cats. J Vet Emerg Crit Care 2001; 11(2): 111–121.

72. Killingsworth C, Eryster G, Adams T, et al. Streptokinase treatment of cats with experimentally induced aortic thrombosis. Am J Vet Res 1986; 47(6): 1351–1359.

73. Moore K, Morris N, Dhupa N, et al. Retrospective study of streptokinase administration in 46 cats with arterial thromboembolism. J Vet Emerg Crit Care 2000; 10: 245–257.

74. Ramsey C, Burney, Macintire D, et al. Use of streptokinase in four dogs with thrombosis. J Am Vet Med Assoc 1996; 209(4): 780–785.

75. Tater K, Drellich S, and Beck K. Management of femoral artery thrombosis in an immature dog. J Vet Emerg Crit Care 2005; 15(1): 52–59.

76. Whelan MF, O'Toole T, Chan D, et al. Retrospective evaluation ofurokinase use in cats with arterial thromboembolism. J Vet Emerg Crit Care 2005; 15(S8).

60

Blood glucose monitoring and glycemic control

Erica L. Reineke

In animals, blood glucose concentration is maintained within a very narrow range due to a dynamic balance between production, storage, and release of glucose. Quantitively, glucose is the most abundant carbohydrate that exists in the circulation and serves as the principal fuel for peripheral tissues except during prolonged fasting.[1] Glucose comes from intestinal absorption through digestion of carbohydrates, from breakdown of glycogen, or from production of glucose via precursors such as lactate, pyruvate, amino acids and glycerol. When blood glucose concentration rises, the anabolic hormone insulin is secreted from the β–cells in the pancreas.[2] Ultimately, the effect of insulin is to lower blood glucose concentration by causing increased transport of glucose into cells where it is used to form energy or stored in the form of glycogen. In addition, insulin also decreases the production of additional glucose by inhibiting gluconeogenesis and glycogenolysis. When hypoglycemia develops, there is increased secretion of the counter-regulatory hormones: glucagon, catecholamines, cortisol, and growth hormone. These hormones increase blood glucose concentration though inhibition of peripheral glucose utilization, increasing hepatic glycogenolysis and gluconeogenesis, and inhibition of insulin secretion. The maintenance of a normal blood glucose concentration depends on appropriate hormone secretion in response to changing blood glucose concentrations in addition to normal hepatic glycogen synthesis, glycogenolysis, and gluconeogenesis.[2] Abnormalities in any of these physiologic functions can lead to either high or low blood glucose levels.

Abnormalities in glucose homeostasis

Abnormalities in glucose homeostasis (low or high blood glucose concentrations) occur commonly in the small animal patient. Normal blood glucose concentrations vary from 53–117 mg/dL (2.9 to 6.5 mmol/L) in the resting state in dogs and 57–131 mg/dL (3.1 to 7.2 mmol/L) in cats.[3] The appearance of clinical signs related to altered blood glucose depends not only on the absolute glucose concentration, but also on the duration, degree, but rate of decline or rise of glucose.

Hypoglycemia

Hypoglycemia occurs when the blood glucose concentration reaches <50 mg/dl in both dogs and cats. Clinical signs of hypoglycemia primarily manifest as cerebral dysfunction including behavioral changes, ataxia, collapse, seizures, stupor and coma.[4–6] These clinical signs occur because the brain, unlike most other tissues in the body, has an obligatory need for glucose for the production of ATP.[7] The brain has limited glycogen stores; therefore, it relies on hepatic glycogen breakdown to supply the glucose it requires for normal function. Other clinical signs of hypoglycemia which may occur in the small animal patient, such as pacing, vocalizing, restlessness, shaking and trembling, likely result from activation of the adrenergic system in response to impending hypoglycemia.[5]

When neuroglycopenia, or hypoglycemia of the central nervous system occurs, the reduction in cerebral ATP production results in dysfunction of the

Advanced Monitoring and Procedures for Small Animal Emergency and Critical Care, First Edition. Edited by Jamie M. Burkitt Creedon, Harold Davis.
© 2012 John Wiley & Sons, Inc. Published 2012 by John Wiley & Sons, Inc.

membrane-associated Na-K-ATPase pumps. The result of this pump failure is cell swelling and release of excitatory neurotransmitters such as glutamate and aspartate, which ultimately results in the clinical signs associated with cerebral dysfunction. Severe and prolonged hypoglycemia can lead to neuronal cell death.[8,9] Therefore, early recognition and emergency treatment of hypoglycemia is essential to prevent permanent neuronal damage.

Hypoglycemia may occur in the small animal patient due to decreased production of glucose by the body or increased utilization. Common causes of hypoglycemia include juvenile and toy breed hypoglycemia, insulinoma or iatrogenic insulin overdose, hepatic failure, sepsis, and xylitol ingestion.

Hyperglycemia

Hyperglycemia is considered to be present when the blood glucose concentration exceeds 117 mg/dl in dogs. In cats, hyperglycemia is less well defined but is usually considered to be present when the blood glucose concentration exceeds 130 mg/dl. When only mild elevations in blood glucose concentration occur, clinical signs are generally absent. However, with severe elevations in blood glucose concentrations, clinical signs can include increased thirst and urination, dehydration, alterations in mental status, and coma.

Since glucose contributes to the osmolality of the blood, it is capable of causing the movement of water between body compartments. Hyperglycemia results in fluid shifting from the intracellular compartment into the intravascular space resulting in cellular shrinkage.[10] Once the glucose concentration in the blood exceeds the renal transport maximum, glucosuria will occur. The result is an osmotic diuresis, which may potentiate dehydration and hypovolemia in animals who are unable to drink water to compensate for these fluid losses.[11] In addition, chronic hyperglycemia and hyperosmolality induces the formation of osmotically active idiogenic osmoles in the brain. The purpose of idiogenic osmoles is to protect the brain against cerebral dehydration by preventing water movement from the brain into the blood.[12]

In addition to its effects on water distribution in the body, hyperglycemia can also contribute to the suppression of the immune system. Hyperglycemia has been found to inhibit cytokine release from macrophages and to impair phagocytosis and free radical production from leukocytes.[13,14] Finally, hyperglycemia can contribute to an overall proinflammatory and prothrombotic state through release of pro-inflammatory cytokines and activation of the coagulation system.[13,14]

Documented causes of hyperglycemia in veterinary patients include diabetes mellitus, hyperadrenocorticism, acromegaly, stress, and pancreatitis. There are also iatrogenic causes such as the administration of glucose-containing fluids, parenteral nutrition, and administering medications such as glucocorticoids. In addition, hyperglycemia has been also documented to occur in critically ill animals including those with head trauma, sepsis, and congestive heart failure.[15–18]

Hyperglycemia that occurs secondary to critical illness in nondiabetic patients has been termed stress hyperglycemia or diabetes of injury. Stress hyperglycemia likely results from a combination of low or normal insulin concentrations, increased counter-regulatory hormone secretion, peripheral tissue insulin resistance, and deranged hepatic autoregulatory mechanisms.[14] Initially, this was considered to be an adaptive response of the body during illness or injury to maintain an energy supply to non-insulin dependent tissues such as the brain and immune system.[19] However, a large body of evidence in the human medical literature suggests that even moderate hyperglycemia can contribute to both morbidity and mortality in critically ill humans with severe brain injury, trauma, burns, sepsis, myocardial infarction and stroke.[20–26]

Although hyperglycemia has been documented to occur in critically ill veterinary patients, its effect on outcome is less well defined. In a study of dogs and cats sustaining head trauma, hyperglycemia at admission was associated with worse neurologic disease but not outcome.[15] However, in a study evaluating dogs and cats presenting to an emergency service with congestive heart failure, hyperglycemia at admission was associated with a worse outcome.[18] Critically ill cats admitted to an intensive care unit were found to have a higher median blood glucose concentration (183 mg/dL, range 51–321 mg/dL) than healthy controls and found to have similar hormonal derangements as critically ill humans.[27] Similarly, in a subsequent study, 16% of critically ill dogs admitted to an intensive care unit were found to have hyperglycemia. In this study, nonsurvivors had significantly higher blood glucose concentrations than survivors. Interestingly, those dogs that developed hyperglycemia during hospitalization had a longer length of hospitalization and more septic complications.[17]

In conclusion, current veterinary research suggests that hyperglycemia is occurring in critically ill veterinary patients. However, further clinical research is needed to determine whether these elevations in blood glucose actually have detrimental consequences in our patients or whether hyperglycemia is just a reflection of disease severity.

Blood glucose monitoring

As derangements in blood glucose concentration are common, blood glucose measurements and serial blood glucose monitoring should be performed on all critically ill patients. For patients presenting on an emergency basis, a blood glucose measurement should be performed at the time of presentation to the veterinary hospital, especially if clinical signs such as altered mental status, seizures, or coma are present. Hospitalized patients should have blood glucose measurements performed at least once daily or more often depending on the underlying disease process or administration of therapies, such as dextrose containing fluids or insulin, which are known to affect blood glucose concentration.

The method by which glucose is measured and the type of blood drawn (arterial, venous, or capillary) may lead to differing blood glucose measurements. Therefore, it is important to become familiar with the various methods available to measure blood glucose concentration and possible confounding issues a veterinary technician and clinician might encounter.

Blood glucose measurements can be performed on whole blood, serum, or plasma. Glucose measurements performed on plasma or serum are approximately 12%-13% higher than whole blood measurements.[28] This is because the water content of red blood cells (73%) is less than that of plasma (93%), and because glucose is freely diffusible between plasma and erythrocytes; the greater the water content of plasma means that the glucose concentration per unit volume is higher.[28] In addition, as the water content of whole blood is the sum of plasma water and red blood cell water, glucose concentration will strongly depend on the hematocrit of the sample. For example, in severe anemia, whole blood glucose and plasma glucose concentration will be nearly equal. With rising hematocrits, the disparity between whole blood and plasma glucose concentration increases.[29,30] For the most part, the differences in glucose concentration between plasma and whole blood are minor (<20% difference) and will typically not affect clinical decision making. However, in human medicine, to avoid any potential clinical misinterpretation, it has been suggested that only glucose concentration in plasma be reported. The current recommendation is to apply the constant factor of 1.11 for the conversion between concentration of glucose in blood and the equivalent concentration in plasma.[31] No similar recommendations currently exist in veterinary medicine.

Measured glucose concentration may also vary depending on the location of the blood drawn. For example, venous blood samples will give slightly lower results than capillary samples. However, in fasting subjects the glucose values obtained in arterial, capillary, and venous samples are practically the same. It is only after meals when glucose uptake by the periphery may be rapid, which results in arterial and capillary glucose samples possibly exceeding venous samples.[28]

Glucose concentration, if not measured immediately, will decrease after blood collection due to ongoing glycolysis by red blood cells and leukocytes. This may lead to an artifactual lower blood glucose measurement.[29] Addition of preservatives, such as sodium fluoride, may help to avoid or delay this loss.[28] Another option for avoiding artifactually low blood glucose measurements is to promptly separate plasma from the cellular components in blood and measure the glucose concentration of the plasma.

Methods of measuring glucose concentration

Glucose measurements are based on one of three enzymes systems—glucose oxidase, glucose-1-dehydrogenase, or hexokinase—which cause glucose conversion.[29,32] These enzymatic reactions are either colorimetrically detected through reflectance or absorbance photometry, or amperometrically (electrochemical) detected. For example, glucose oxidase catalyzed reactions result in the production of gluconic acid and hydrogen peroxide. In colorimetric detection systems, hydrogen peroxide reacts with various hydrogen donors to produce a color change that is proportional to glucose concentration. This color change is measured using a reflectance photometer that converts the reflected light to an electronic signal for digital display.[33] Amperometric detection systems utilize the glucose oxidase or glucose-1-dehydrogenase enzymes. In amperometric measuring devices, an electrical current is produced from the reaction that is directly measured. Finally, for systems utilizing the enzyme hexokinase, NADH reacts with a dye to produce a color change detected by the machine.[33]

Instruments used to measure glucose

Blood glucose measurements are typically performed either in a central laboratory or cage-side using portable devices. As pathologic changes in blood glucose concentration require immediate intervention, blood glucose measuring devices need to provide rapid and accurate results. Unfortunately, central laboratory measurements of blood glucose concentration take too long to obtain to be clinically useful. Therefore, cage-side glucose measuring devices are typically used in the clinical setting. In addition to providing rapid results, these cage-side portable blood glucose measuring devices also use minimal amounts of blood thereby helping to limit anemia that may result from frequent blood sampling.

Common instruments currently used to rapidly evaluate blood glucose concentration in small animals include portable blood glucose meters (PBGM) and point-of-care (POC) analyzers such as the I-stat (Abbott Point of Care Inc., Princeton, NJ) and the NOVA Stat Profile (NOVA Biomedical, Waltham, MA). Point-of-care refers to any laboratory test performed outside a clinical laboratory by nonlaboratory personnel.[34]

Due to the unacceptable time delay in laboratory glucose measurements, PBGM devices and POC analyzers such as the I-stat and NOVA stat profile are extremely useful in the management of critically ill small animal patients. However, it is important for the veterinarian and technician to understand and recognize potential interferences that may exist with glucose measurements obtained by these devices, particularly with PBGMs.

Table 60.1 Variables that may affect blood glucose measurements obtained with PBGM

Variable	Affect on Glucose Measurement
Hematocrit:	
• Increased Hemotocrit (polycythemia or dehydration)	Decreases
• Decreased Hematocrit (anemia)	Increases
Drugs:	
• Dopamine	Increases
• Mannitol	Increases
• Acetaminophen	Increases
Oxygen Tension (pO$_2$)	
• Hyperoxia (paO2 > 100 mmHg)	Decreases
• Hypoxia	Increases
Small Sample Size (<3 ʋl)	Decreases

Portable blood glucose meters

Many PBGMs are available from different manufacturers to measure blood glucose concentration. These devices were originally developed to allow for self-monitoring of glucose by humans with diabetes mellitus. The benefits of glucose measurements provided by PBGM include rapid results, ease of use, minimal blood requirements, and cost-effectiveness. Portable blood glucose meters use test strips that consist of an enzyme-impregnated reagent pad that is either sponge-like or covered with a mesh or membrane. When a drop of blood is applied to the surface, plasma soaks through into the reagent layer and red cells are retained on the surface.[35] Depending on the particular device, it may use colorimetric or amperometric detection systems to measure glucose concentration.

The accuracy of PBGMs has been extensively evaluated in the human literature. In several human studies, large variations in the accuracy of different PBGMs in different glycemic ranges have been found.[36–38] Other factors such as hematocrit, inadequate sample volume, drugs, partial pressure of oxygen (pO$_2$), and user error have also been documented to affect the accuracy of glucose measurements obtained with PBGMs.[33,39–41] User errors most commonly cited to affect the accuracy of blood glucose measurements obtained by PBGMs include failure to maintain the meter properly, incorrect techniques or operating procedures, or failure to follow instructions for meter use. Table 60.1 is a summary of some of the variables that may affect blood glucose measurements obtained by PBGMs.

Increases in hematocrit decrease glucose measurements and vice versa. In PBGMs, this may be caused by

mechanical impedance of plasma diffusion into the reagent layer of the strip at higher hematocrits, resulting in slower diffusion of glucose and hence lower glucose measurements are obtained.[42] In patients with anemia, artifactually increased blood glucose measurements may be obtained, which may result in masking hypoglycemia.

Substances such as drugs may also affect glucose measurements obtained by PBGMs. In a study published in 2000 evaluating the effect of 30 different commonly used drugs on glucose concentration measured by seven different PBGMs, the investigators found that ascorbic acid (vitamin C), acetaminophen, dopamine, and mannitol were all found to interfere with glucose measurements. Acetaminophen increased glucose measurements on several PBGMs.[43] This effect may be clinically relevant in small animals when acetaminophen ingestion can lead to hepatic failure and hypoglycemia. Dopamine falsely increased glucose measurements in some devices primarily at high drug concentrations, as did the drug mannitol.[43]

Partial pressure of oxygen, pH, and temperature have also been evaluated to determine their effects on blood glucose concentration obtained with PBGMs. When oxygen tension is high (PaO$_2$ > 100 mmHg) investigators have found falsely lowered glucose readings in glucose oxidase systems.[44] This may be relevant in patients receiving high concentrations of supplemental oxygen, such as those under general anesthesia. Conversely, lower oxygen tensions (PaO$_2$ < 40 mmHg) had a negligible effect on glucose concentration. Blood pH, on the other hand, has not been shown to be a major source of error at a pH range of 6.8–7.84.[45–46] Finally, some data suggests that cold temperatures may adversely affect the accuracy of glucose measurements.[47–48]

Multiple studies evaluating 15 different PBGMs have been published in the veterinary literature.[49–52] Some of these PBGMs have since been replaced by newer models, prompting a recent study evaluating six different PBGMs. In this study, the investigators evaluated blood samples from normal dogs, dogs with diabetes mellitus, and dogs that had a variety of medical conditions including insulinoma. The investigators found that in general the glucose measurements obtained by most of the PBGMs were lower than laboratory measurements, and this effect was more pronounced in the hyperglycemic range. In contrast, results obtained by the AlphaTrak (Abbott Laboratories, Abbott Park, IL) did not consistently provide results that were either higher or lower than the laboratory values. In almost all cases, even though the blood glucose measurements obtained by the PBGMs were different from the reference laboratory values, they were unlikely to adversely affect clinical decision making.[52]

In conclusion, despite pitfalls that may be encountered when using PBGMs, they will continue to be a valuable tool to measure blood glucose concentration in the veterinary setting. To prevent possible user error, it is important to always follow the manufacturer's instructions on maintenance and calibration of the device. In addition, whenever a new PBGM is obtained by a veterinary hospital, blood glucose results should be compared with laboratory measurements to ascertain whether these results are consistently higher or lower than expected. Finally, if a patient is identified as hypoglycemic on a PBGM, the veterinary clinician should be notified; however, treatment may be recommend only if the patient is exhibiting clinical signs consistent with low blood glucose. Alternatively, a comparison laboratory measurement of blood glucose concentration should be obtained.[52]

Point of care analyzers

The use of POC analyzers is becoming increasingly common in veterinary clinical practice. Similar to PBGMs, these analyzers require minimal amounts of blood, and results are rapid. The i-STAT is the only POC analyzer that has been evaluated in dogs thus far.[51] The i-STAT measures glucose amperometrically through the glucose oxidation reaction. In a study published in 2000, investigators found that the i-STAT provided accurate glucose concentration results that varied from the reference method by only 15% and did not result in altered clinical decisions.[51]

To the author's knowledge, the accuracy of the NOVA Stat Profile in measuring glucose concentration has not yet been evaluated in small animal patients. However, this device has been validated for use in human patients and is likely to provide results consistent with laboratory methods. The NOVA Stat Profile uses an electrode that is covered by a three-layered membrane in which glucose oxidase is immobilized. As glucose flows through the membrane, it reacts with glucose oxidase, resulting in the generation of hydrogen peroxide. The instrument is calibrated using an aqueous glucose standard solution.[35] Similar to measurements obtained by PBGMs, hematocrit may affect glucose values obtained by this method.[53]

Newer glucose monitoring devices

Recently, continuous glucose monitoring systems that measure interstitial glucose concentration have received intense interest in both human and veterinary medicine as an attractive method by which to monitor blood glucose concentration. Interstitial glucose concentration has been extensively studied and found to mimic blood glucose in a variety of species including rats, rabbits, dogs, and humans.[54] This knowledge has led to the development of a continuous glucose monitoring system (CGMS) that measures interstitial glucose concentration within the subcutaneous space. The CGMS has been approved by the U.S. Food and Drug Administration (FDA) for use in human diabetic patients and has resulted in significant improvements in glycemic control.[55]

The Medtronic MiniMed™ CGMS® Gold (Medtronic Diabetes, Northridge, CA) consists of a recording device and a flexible electrode glucose sensor. The sensor is implanted in the subcutaneous space via a spring-loaded insertion device and is connected to a small monitor (170 g) that can be worn by the patient or placed in a cage. The sensor contains an electrode covered by a glucose diffusion limiting membrane. When glucose flows onto the membrane in the electrode, it is oxidized to hydrogen peroxide by glucose oxidase. Glucose is then determined amperometrically for glucose concentrations between 40 and 400 mg/dL. The CGMS measures interstitial glucose concentrations every 10 seconds, and an average value is recorded by the device every 5 minutes. Because changes in blood glucose are related to changes in interstitial glucose, the CGMS can be used to estimate blood glucose from the interstitial measurements. To obtain this estimate, the CGMS must be calibrated with at least three blood glucose measurements during a 24-hour period.

Since its development, the CGMS has been used in clinically normal animals, as well as in diabetic dogs and cats.[56-58] In 1999, Rebrin et al. found that subcutaneous interstitial glucose sensing accurately mimics plasma glucose irrespective of changes in plasma insulin in experimental dogs. However, in this same study, it was shown that rapid changes in blood glucose result in slower changes in interstitial glucose, with a time delay between changes in blood glucose and interstitial glucose typically less than 10 minutes.[54] Clinical veterinary studies have since been performed to evaluate the accuracy of the CGMS in stable diabetic dogs and cats. The investigators found that there was significant correlation (dogs, r = 0.81; cats, r = 0.82) between the CGMS device and blood glucose concentration.[57,58] A final veterinary study evaluated the use of the CGMS in diabetic keto-acidotic dogs and cats. The results of this study also found that the CGMS provides clinically accurate estimates of blood glucose concentration and that these measurements were not affected by tissue perfusion (based on Doppler blood pressure measurements, blood lactate concentration, and rectal-axillary temperature gradients), body condition score, or degree of ketosis.[59]

Newer real-time and wireless devices, such as the Medtronic MiniMed™ Guardian® Real-Time CGMS (Medtronic Diabetes, Northridge, CA), DexCom™ Seven® System (DexCom Inc., San Diego, CA) and Abbott Freestyle Navigator® System (Abbott Laboratories, Abbott Park, IL), have since been developed that allow clinicians to identify fluctuations in blood glucose as they are occurring in the patient. These real-time devices allow the clinician to avoid placing multiple catheters for blood sampling or performing repeated venipuncture to measure blood glucose, both of which can contribute to morbidity in the patient by contributing to patient stress, catheter complications, and even anemia in small animal patients. The addition of alarms that can notify veterinary technicians of either dangerously high or low glucose excursions make these devices even more clinically useful. These newer generations of CGMS devices are currently being investigated for use in clinical veterinary patients at several veterinary teaching hospitals. In the future, these noninvasive glucose monitoring devices may replace portable blood glucose meters as the main method by which glucose is monitored, especially in critically ill patients receiving insulin infusions that require frequent monitoring of blood glucose concentration.

The author's experience with the Medtronic Minimed™ Guardian RT™ CGMS device is that it is both reliable and useful for monitoring blood glucose concentration in hospitalized patients. Compared with intermittent glucose monitoring, continuous monitoring of blood glucose concentration may help to identify rapid changes that may be missed in patients in which blood glucose is measured intermittently. This may be important in diabetic patients that are having blood glucose curves performed in order to evaluate insulin dose. In addition, stress associated with repeated handling for venipuncture, especially in cats, can contribute to patient discomfort and elevations in blood glucose that could confuse the clinical picture. The CGMS devices are also extremely useful in patients in which repeated phlebotomy is either contraindicated due to underlying disease or cannot be performed.

Several disadvantages of the CGMS include the initial cost for the device, the cost of the sensors, and the need to obtain blood glucose measurements for calibrations. Another potential disadvantage of the interstitial glucose monitoring system is the time delay for rapid changes in blood glucose concentration to be reflected in the interstitial space. Therefore, data obtained from these devices should be interpreted cautiously when large changes in blood glucose concentration are suspected. In these situations, evaluating blood glucose trends over time may be more clinically useful.

Placement of the CGMS in dogs and cats is a simple process. Figure 60.1 shows the placement of the Guardian RT™ device in a patient for glucose monitoring. First, a small area of hair is clipped, usually just caudal to the shoulder blades. The area should not be cleaned with alcohol, as this may interfere with the adherence of the sensor. The sensor is then placed into the spring-loaded insertion device. The insertion device is placed against the patient's skin and the sensor is discharged. The transmitter is then attached to the sensor and both are covered with a clear adherent bandage. After a 2-hour initialization period, the CGMS device will begin to continuously display estimates of blood glucose concentration once it has been calibrated with data from a blood glucose measurement. The CGMS will then need to be recalibrated every 8 hours with either a portable blood glucose meter or point-of-care analyzer measurement of blood glucose. If there is any concern that inaccurate estimates of blood glucose are being obtained by the CGMS (either extremely high or low readings), the patient's blood glucose should be checked with the device being used for calibration. If this measurement is different from the CGMS readings, the CGMS should be recalibrated with this new glucose measurement. If the problem persists, the sensor should be removed and replaced.

Glycemic control

Glycemic control implies the maintenance of blood glucose within a clinically acceptable range. This is achieved through the administration of dextrose, insulin,

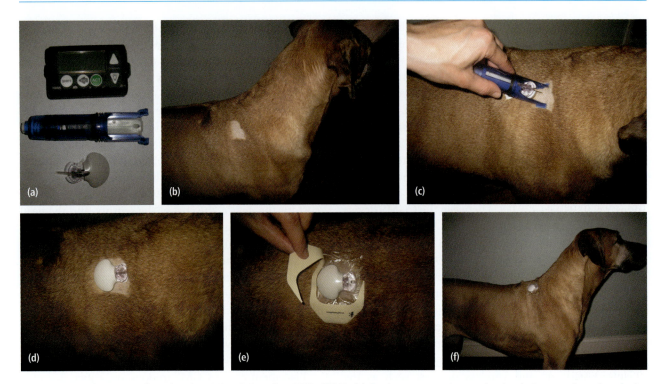

Figure 60.1 Placement of Medtronic Minimed Guardian RT™ CGMS. (a) Equipment: monitor, spring-loaded sensor insertion device for accurate placement, blood glucose sensor with transducer attached, (b) small area of clipped fur just caudal to the scapula, (c) using the spring-loaded device for sensor insertion, (d) sensor with transducer attached, (e) clear adherent dressing being placed over sensor and transducer, (f) dog wearing sensor with transducer attached.

or medications known to raise or lower blood glucose concentration. Patients in whom interventions are required to maintain clinically acceptable blood glucose concentrations should have frequent blood glucose monitoring performed to avoid complications associated with hypo- and hyperglycemia. Frequent monitoring is particularly important in the short- and long-term management of diabetic patients, in which glycemic control is achieved through adjustments in insulin therapy.

The benefits of glycemic control in human patients with diabetes mellitus include a reduction in mortality as well as a reduction in diabetes-related complications such as blindness, kidney failure, and heart failure.[60] In addition to its value in patients with diabetes mellitus, glycemic control with insulin therapy in also utilized in critically ill humans who develop hyperglycemia during hospitalization.[61-63] Currently, the use of insulin therapy to control critical illness associated hyperglycemia has yet to be evaluated in veterinary medicine.

Treatment of hyperglycemia

The treatment of hyperglycemia in veterinary medicine depends on the underlying disease process contributing to the elevation of blood glucose. For example, stress hyperglycemia in cats associated with patient struggling can result in blood glucose as high as 613 mg/dL with or without glucosuria.[63] Since stress hyperglycemia can last 90–120 minutes, one should wait at least 3 hours before retesting or instituting treatment for hyperglycemia.

Hyperglycemia caused by diabetes mellitus requires administration of the hormone insulin. Insulin will promote peripheral glucose uptake, inhibit lipolysis and release of free fatty acids, and decrease glycogenolysis and increase glycogenesis.[2] Insulin is available in several forms with differing durations of action. Typically, regular insulin, in which the duration of action is approximately 3–8 hours when given intramuscularly or 1–4 hours when given intravenously, is administered during hospitalization until the patient is eating and drinking. Regular insulin is usually administered either intravenously as a constant rate infusion or intramuscularly. Other newer, short-acting insulins, such as lispro (Humalog®, Eli Lilly) and aspart (Novolog®, Nova Nordisk) are currently being used in humans for treatment of diabetes mellitus. The benefits of these newer insulin analogues include a faster onset of action and a shorter duration of action, allowing for finer control of blood glucose. A clinical study evaluating the use of lispro in the treatment of diabetic ketoacidotic dogs is currently under way; however, the use of these newer insulin analogues cannot be recommended at this time.

Insulin may also be used to treat persistent hyperglycemia that results from veterinarian directed interventions. Both the administration of dextrose-containing fluids such as parenteral nutrition and the administration of medications that are known to affect blood glucose concentration such as vasopressors or steroids can cause hyperglycemia.

When the presence of hyperglycemia cannot be explained by either diabetes mellitus or veterinarian-directed interventions, the patient should be re-evaluated by either the veterinary technician or doctor for worsening of the underlying disease condition or the development of complications. This may involve performing a physical examination, hemodynamic monitoring, and diagnostic tests. In addition, persistent hyperglycemia needs to be definitively established prior to initiating insulin therapy.

Intravenous insulin constant-rate infusion

Table 60.2 is an example of an intravenous (IV) insulin infusion chart. The infusion is prepared by adding

Table 60.2 Constant rate infusion of regular insulin

Blood Glucose Concentration (mg/dL)	Rate of Administration of Insulin Solution (ml/hr)*	% Dextrose Added to Maintenance Intravenous Fluids**
>250	10	None
200–250	7	2.5%
150–200	5	2.5%
100–150	5	5%
<100	Stop insulin infusion	5%

*Solution comprised of regular insulin at a dose of 2.2 U/kg for dogs, or 1.1 U/kg for cats, added to 250 ml 0.9% NaCl or lactated Ringer's solution. Adjustments to rate of insulin therapy are made based on measurements of blood glucose concentration.

**These intravenous fluids are administered separately and in addition to the insulin infusion when needed to compensate for ongoing losses, dehydration, and to maintain intravascular volume in the patient.

Adapted from Macintire DK. Treatment of diabetic ketoacidosis in dogs by continuous low-dose intravenous infusion of insulin. J Am Vet Med Assoc 1993;202:1266–1272.

regular insulin (2.2 U/kg for dogs, 1.1 U/kg for cats) to 250 mL of 0.9% NaCl. It is initially administered at a rate of 10 mL/hr in a line separate from that used for fluid therapy.[65] At least 50 mL of the insulin-containing fluids should be run through the drip set prior to administering it to the patient because insulin readily adheres to plastic and glass.

Generally, the placement of two separate IV catheters is recommended: one catheter for insulin and an additional catheter for IV fluids and blood sampling. Separate catheters are recommended in order to avoid starting and stopping the insulin infusion during blood sampling for glucose monitoring. In addition, if IV fluids containing dextrose are being administered, blood sampling for glucose monitoring should be done from a separate catheter to avoid falsely elevated blood glucose measurements that may occur from contamination with dextrose containing fluids. A multiple lumen catheter, either placed centrally or peripherally, may also be used. The most distal lumen of the central catheter is typically reserved for blood sampling. A separate peripheral catheter, in addition to the central catheter, should be maintained for the administration of dextrose-containing IV fluids. This is to avoid contamination of the blood sample being obtained for glucose monitoring with the dextrose-containing IV fluids that may artificially elevate the glucose concentration. If the maintenance of a separate peripheral catheter is not possible or the administration of greater than 5% dextrose solutions necessitates fluid administration through the central catheter (see section on treatment of hypoglycemia below), a large presample should be obtained (5–10 mL of blood) prior to checking the blood glucose. If there is any question about the measured blood glucose concentration (i.e., suspicion of a falsely elevated blood glucose) even with the larger presample, direct venipuncture for blood glucose measurement should be obtained for comparison.

Blood glucose concentration should be monitored every 1–2 hours, and changes in insulin rate should be made based on each glucose measurement when insulin is administered intravenously. IV insulin is typically administered until the patient can be switched to a longer-acting insulin product in patients with diabetes mellitus or when insulin administration is no longer needed to maintain glycemic control.

Intramuscular insulin techniques

When given intramuscularly, regular insulin can be administered hourly or less frequently depending on the technique chosen. The hourly technique involves the intramuscular (IM) administration of regular insulin and measurement of blood glucose concentration every hour. The usual initial dose for the IM insulin protocol is 0.2 U/kg of regular insulin. After one hour, the blood glucose concentration is checked, and if it exceeds 250 mg/dL, 0.1 U/kg regular insulin is administered intramuscularly. This protocol is repeated on an hourly basis as long as the blood glucose concentration exceeds 250 mg/dL. Once the blood glucose drops below 250 mg/dL, regular insulin is administered intramuscularly every 4–6 hours or subcutaneously every 8 hours if the hydration status is adequate. In patients with diabetic ketoacidosis, a 2.5%–5% dextrose-containing infusion (see Fig. 60.2 for instructions on calculating a dextrose infusion) is initiated at this time.[66] Once the blood glucose concentration has reached an acceptable clinical range, blood glucose is monitored less frequently. The goal of insulin therapy is to cause a gradual decline in the blood glucose concentration, preferably at a rate of about 50 to 75 mg/dL/hour.[67] Subcutaneous administration of insulin is not recommended in the initial treatment of critically ill diabetic patients, as dehydration can lead to erratic absorption of insulin.

In contrast to the hourly administration of regular insulin, regular insulin (0.25 U/kg) can be administered intramuscularly every 4–6 hours. This is less labor-intensive compared with the hourly administration of regular insulin. Following the first dose of insulin, blood glucose is checked hourly but then the frequency of blood glucose monitoring can be decreased depending on the duration of insulin action. An hourly decline of 50 mg/dL in the blood glucose concentration is ideal. If the blood glucose is dropping too rapidly, the veterinarian should be notified and subsequent insulin dosages may be decreased.

Initiation of longer-acting insulin

Once the patient is eating and drinking, longer acting insulin therapy is often instituted for glycemic control. Several intermediate-acting and long-acting insulin products are available for use, including neutral protamine hagedorn (NPH), purified porcine insulin zinc, protamine zinc insulin (PZI), and glargine insulin.

Purified porcine insulin zinc (Vetsulin®, Intervet/Schering Plough Animal Health) is the only FDA-approved insulin for use in both dogs and cats. Glargine insulin (Lantus, Aventis Pharmaceuticals, Bridgewater, NJ) is one of the newer insulin analogues being used in the diabetic management of companion animals. This insulin was introduced in 2001 and marketed as a long-acting peakless insulin for use in humans. Glargine's use in diabetic cats has been investigated, and initial reports suggest that it is safe and effective in the management

Desired Strength of Solution = Amount of Dextrose Needed (ml)
50% Dextrose   Volume of Infusion (ml)

Consider making 1 L of a 2.5% Dextrose solution
1. Convert percentage to decimals

2. $\dfrac{0.025 \text{ Dextrose}}{0.50 \text{ Dextrose}} = \dfrac{X \text{ ml}}{1000 \text{ ml}}$

   0.025 (1000 ml) = 0.50 (X ml)
   X = 50 ml of 50% Dextrose

3. Add 50 ml of 50% dextrose to 950 ml (If you do not remove the 50 ml from the total volume, the solution will be slightly less than 2.5% dextrose)

Consider making 500 ml of a 5% dextrose solution
1. Convert percentages to decimals

2. $\dfrac{0.05 \text{ Dextrose}}{0.50 \text{ Dextrose}} = \dfrac{X \text{ ml}}{500 \text{ ml}}$

   0.05 (500 ml) = 0.50 (X ml)
   X = 50 ml of 50% dextrose

3. Add 50 ml of 50% dextrose to 450 ml

Figure 60.2 Calculation of a percent dextrose solution using 50% dextrose.

of diabetes mellitus.[69] Table 60.3 lists available insulin products and current initial insulin dose recommendations in dogs and cats.

Specific considerations when administering insulin

Insulin is commercially available in 40, 100, and 500 U/mL concentrations, which are designated U-40, U-100, and U-500, respectively.[68] Depending on the concentration of the insulin being administered, there are specific syringes, also labeled U-40, U-100, and U-500, that should be used. For example, glargine insulin should be administered only with a U-100 syringe. It is important to always check that the label on the insulin syringe matches the concentration of the insulin being administered.

Insulin syringes are also available in different sizes including 1 mL, 1/2 mL and 3/10 mL with different gauge needles. Lines on the insulin syringes are units. For example, the 1 mL insulin syringes are generally marked with a line for every two units, that is, 2, 4, 6, 8. The 1/2-mL syringe is marked with a line for every unit. The 3/10-mL syringe is marked with lines for every 1/2 or 1 unit.

Insulin should always be stored in a refrigerator, as freezing and heat inactivate insulin in the bottle. The exception to this rule is glargine, which may be stored

Table 60.3 Insulin types and initial dose recommendations

Insulin	Concentration	Recommended Initial Dose	
		Dog	Cat
NPH	U-100[a]	0.25–0.5 U/kg every 12 hours	1 unit/cat every 12 hours
Porcine Zinc (Lente)	U-40[b]	0.5 U/kg every 12 hours	1–2 U/cat or 0.25–0.5 U/kg every 12 hours[c]
PZI	U-40[b]	Not recommended	0.4 U/kg or 1 U/cat every 12 hours
Glargine	U-100[a]	No currently recommended dose[d]	0.25–0.5 U/kg every 12–24 hours

[a]U-100: 100 units/ml.

[b]U-40: 40 units/ml.

[c]A recommended starting dose is 0.25 U/kg twice daily if the blood glucose concentration is between 216 and 342 mg/dL, and 0.5 U/kg twice daily if the blood glucose concentration is >360 mg/dL. Alternatively, a dose of 1 U/cat twice daily for cats weighing less than 4 kg and 1.5–2.0 U/cat twice daily for cats weighing > 4 kg can be used to initiate therapy.

[d]Only one study evaluating the effect of glargine in diabetic dogs currently exists in the veterinary literature. These dogs were given glargine (0.05–0.1 U/kg) concurrently with NPH insulin (Mori A, Sako T, Lee P, et al. Comparison of time-action profiles of insulin glargine and NPH insulin in normal and diabetic dogs. Vet Res Commun (2008) 32: 563–573).

at room temperature once opened. Unopened glargine should be stored in the refrigerator. Once opened, whether refrigerated or not, glargine should be discarded after 28 days according to the manufacturer. Currently, it has also been a common recommendation that other insulin preparations be discarded after 1 month. However, many veterinarians allow use of an opened bottle of insulin that is refrigerated for up to 3 months before discarding. However, if clinical signs recur in a previously well-controlled diabetic patient, loss of activity of the insulin could be the cause, and the insulin bottle should be replaced.

Prior to drawing insulin up in an insulin syringe, the bottle should be gently rolled between the palms of the hands (15–20 times) to allow for uniform resuspension of the insulin within the liquid. Failure to mix the insulin properly could decrease its effectiveness. It is important not to shake the insulin bottle, as this could create small air bubbles within the vial leading to inaccurate dosing.

Always administer the type of insulin as designated by the treatment orders. In other words, Vetsulin® should not be substituted for NPH as each insulin product will have a different duration of action and effect in each individual patient.

Glucose monitoring

When insulin is administered in the treatment of hyperglycemia, blood glucose concentration is monitored closely to prevent rapid changes in blood glucose and hypoglycemia. When a rapid decline in blood glucose

occurs in patients with chronic hyperglcemia, cerebral edema may result. This is due to the development of active idiogenic osmoles within the brain. These idiogenic osmoles are eliminated slowly, and a rapid reduction in serum osmolality establishes an osmotic gradient across the blood brain barrier leading to cerebral edema.[12]

During the treatment of a patient with hyperglycemia, the patient should be observed closely for neurologic signs, such as changes in mentation and seizure activity, which could indicate cerebral edema or hypoglycemia. If neurologic signs develop, a blood glucose concentration is typically checked to rule out hypoglycemia. If the patient is not hypoglycemic and the neurologic signs are attributed to a rapid drop in blood glucose concentration, mannitol may be administered (0.5–1 g/kg intravenously over 20–30 minutes) to decrease cerebral edema.

Treatment of hypoglycemia

Acute hypoglycemia requires immediate therapy because the longer the hypoglycemic episode lasts, the greater the potential for irreversible brain damage. Patients who are presented on an emergency basis or who develop clinical signs attributable to hypoglycemia during hospitalization are often treated with an IV bolus of 50% dextrose (0.25–0.5 g/kg). 50% Dextrose is very hypertonic and ideally it is diluted to less than 10% with sterile water. This dose of dextrose is often repeated as indicated by serial blood glucose measurements or until clinical signs are resolved. Dextrose and dextrose-containing fluids should never be given subcutaneously.

Following a bolus of dextrose, the patient may be placed on a constant rate infusion of 2.5%–5% dextrose in crystalloid solutions. To make 1 L of a 2.5% dextrose solution, 50 mL of 50% dextrose can be added to 950 mL of fluids (total volume of 1 L). To make 1 L of a 5% dextrose infusion, 100 mL of 50% dextrose is added to a 900 mL of fluid (remove 100 mL of fluids from a 1 L bag). See Figure 60.2 for instructions on how to calculate a percentage dextrose infusion.

Both 2.5% and 5% dextrose infusions may be administered through a peripheral venous catheter. However, when higher concentrations of dextrose (>5% solution) are needed to maintain a normal blood glucose, higher concentrations of dextrose (>5% solution) may be administered through a central line. This is because glucose infusions greater than 5% are extremely irritating to the vascular endothelium and may result in thrombophlebitis.[71] Therefore, administering higher concentrations of dextrose solutions in a larger vein will help to decrease the incidence of thrombophlebitis. Alternatively, rather than increasing the concentration of the dextrose infusion, the rate (mL/hour) of dextrose administration may be increased. This will allow for increased delivery of dextrose to the patient. Finally, 5% dextrose in water (D5W) may also be administered intravenously to supplement dextrose but should be given cautiously, as profound hyponatremia can develop if large volumes are administered. The goal of glucose supplementation is usually to maintain the blood glucose concentration within the normal physiologic range, as hyperglycemia can have deleterious consequences.

In addition to IV dextrose supplementation, hypoglycemic patients are often fed as soon as possible, which will also help to increase the blood glucose. However, feeding may not be recommended in patients with hypotension, low body temperature, vomiting, or other conditions in which feeding may be contraindicated.

If seizure activity is present in a patient with low blood glucose and does not resolve despite attaining euglycemia, anticonvulsant therapy such as diazepam (0.25–0.5 mg/kg), midazolam (0.2 mg/kg), or phenobarbital (2.0–4.0 mg/kg) should be administered intravenously.[72] Severe hypoglycemia and prolonged seizure activity can result in cerebral edema. Treatment for cerebral edema involves oxygen administration, elevation of the head 15–30° above the horizontal plane, and administration of hypertonic agents (see Chapter 61, Care of the Patient with Intracranial Disease).[73] Hypertonic agents such as mannitol and hypertonic saline do not cross an intact blood brain barrier and thus reduce cerebral edema by osmotically drawing water out of the brain. Common doses are as follows: mannitol 0.5–1 g/kg IV or 7.5% NaCl 3–5 mL/kg IV over 15–20 minutes.

Hypoglycemia caused by insulinomas can be very challenging to treat. Dextrose administration in these patients can trigger tumor secretion of insulin and rebound hypoglycemia. Therefore, several other medications are available in the treatment of insulinoma with the effect of raising the blood glucose concentration by increasing endogenous glucose production. The steroid dexamethasone (0.5 mg/kg IV every 12–24 hours) is given to increase hepatic gluconeogenesis and glycogenolysis as well as inhibit peripheral glucose uptake.[74] A constant rate infusion of the hormone glucagon with concurrent dextrose infusion is an additional treatment for insulinoma-associated hypoglycemia.[75,76] Glucagon should be reconstituted with the provided diluent and added to 1 L of 0.9% NaCl resulting in a solution with a glucagon concentration of 1 μg/mL. This medication is usually started at a dose of 5 ng/kg/min and the infusion dose may be increased as needed up to 20 ng/kg/min to maintain blood glucose concentration greater than 60 mg/dL.[74,75] A syringe or IV fluid pump should be used to allow for accurate dosing of this medication. This medication cannot be given orally. Finally, the drug diazoxide, which inhibits insulin release and stimulates hepatic release of glucose via gluconeogenesis, is also potentially useful for treatment of hypoglycemia in dogs with insulinoma. In addition to the above-listed effect, diazoxide also causes adrenomedullary release of epinephrine, which increases insulin resistance at the level of the insulin receptor. The dose ranges from 10 to 40 mg/kg/day orally and is generally titrated as indicated by the blood glucose concentration.[74] The most common side effect seen with use of this drug is gastrointestinal upset including diarrhea, vomiting, and anorexia, which may be minimized by administering this medication with food.[76]

Blood glucose should be monitored closely, at least every 2 hours if not more frequently, in all patients following a hypoglycemic episode until it can be established that the primary cause has been resolved or effectively controlled. Any animal that presents with symptomatic hypoglycemia should be hospitalized until it is eating and drinking normally.

Conclusion

Blood glucose monitoring is an important aspect in the management of emergent and critically ill companion animals. The prompt recognition and treatment of both hyperglycemia and hypoglycemia is essential for the veterinary technician. There are a number of ways to measure blood glucose concentration in veterinary patients; however, portable blood glucose meters and point-of-care analyzers are most commonly used to quickly measure blood glucose concentration cage-side in the hospital. Newer glucose monitoring devices are now available that allow for continuous glucose monitoring using interstitial glucose measurements. These noninvasive devices allow for minute-to-minute monitoring of blood glucose concentration potentially allowing for quicker detection and treatment of aberrations in blood glucose concentration. Glycemic control in critically ill patients is achieved in most patients with the use of either insulin and/or dextrose. It is extremely important for both veterinary clinicians and technicians to understand the clinical indications for their use as well as how to safely and effectively administer these medications to our patients.

References

1. Burrin JM, Price CP. Measurement of blood glucose. Ann Clin Biochem 1985;22:327–342.
2. Arthur C Guyton and John E. Hall. 1996. Textbook of Medical Physiology, 9th ed. Philadelphia: W.B. Saunders.
3. Willard MD, Tvedten H, Turnwald GH. Small animal clinical diagnosis by laboratory methods, 3rd ed. Philadelphia: W.B. Saunders, 1999: 371.
4. Walters PC, Drobatz KJ. Hypoglycemia. Compendium: Continuing Education for veterinarians 1992;9:1150–1159.
5. Whitley NT, Drobatz KJ, Panciera DL. Insulin overdose in dogs and cats: 7 cases (1986–1993). J Am Vet Med Assoc 1997;211(3): 326–330.
6. Kraje AC. Hypoglycemia and irreversible neurologic complications in a cat with insulinoma. J Am Vet Med Assoc 2003;223(6): 812–814.
7. Boyle PJ. Alteration in brain glucose metabolism induced by hypoglycemia in man. Diabetologia 40:S69, 1997.
8. Cheol H, Bum KS, Young LE, et al. Regional differences of glutamate induced swelling in culture rat brain astrocytes. Life Sci 2004;76:573–583.
9. Bergles DE, Jahr CE. Synaptic activation of glutamate transporters in hippocampal astrocytes. Neuron 1997;19:1297–1308.
10. Wellman ML, Dibartola SP, and Kohn CW. 2000. Applied physiology of body fluids in dogs and cats. In Fluid, Electrolyte and Acid-Base Disorders in Small Animal Practice, edited by Stephen DiBartola, pp. 3–26. St. Louis: Saunders Elsevier.
11. Panciera DL. 2000. Fluid therapy in endocrine and metabolic disorders. In Fluid, Electrolyte and Acid-Base Disorders in Small Animal Practice, edited by Stephen DiBartola, pp. 478–489. St. Louis: Saunders Elsevier.
12. Arieff AI, Kleeman CR. Studies on mechanisms of cerebral edema in diabetic comas: effects of hyperglycemia and rapid lowering of plasma glucose in normal rabbits. J Clin Invest 1973; 52:571.
13. Marik, PE, Raghavan M. Stress-hyperglycemia, insulin and immunomodulation in sepsis. Inten Care Med 2004;30: 748–756.
14. Mizock BA. Alterations in fuel metabolism in critical illness: hyperglycemia. Best Pract Res Clin En. 2001;15(4):533–551.
15. Syring RS, Otto CM, Drobatz KJ. Hyperglycemia in dogs and cats with head trauma: 122 cases (1997–1999). J Am Vet Med Assoc. 2001;218(7):1124–1129.
16. Hardie EM, Rawlings CA, George JW. Plasma-glucose concentrations in dogs and cats before and after surgery: comparison of healthy animals and animals with sepsis. Am Vet Res. 1985;46(8):1700–1704.
17. Torre DM, deLaforcade AM, Chan DL. Incidence and clinical relevance of hyperglycemia in critically ill dogs. J Vet Intern Med. 2007;21(5):971–975.
18. Brady CA, Hughes D, Drobatz KJ. Association of hyponatremia and hyperglycemia with outcome in dogs with congestive heart failure. J Vet Emerg Crit Care. 2004;14(3):177–182.
19. Langouche L, Van den Berghe G. Glucose metabolism and insulin therapy. Crit Care Clin 2006;22(1):119–129.
20. Rovlias A, Kotsou S. The influence of hyperglycemia on neurological outcome in patients with severe head injury. Neurosurgery 2000;46:335–342.
21. Jeremitsky E, Omert LA, Dunham CM, et al. Association of hyperglycemia with increased mortality after severe brain injury. J Trauma 2005;58:47–50.
22. Laird AM, Miller PR, Kilgo PD, et al. Relationship of early hyperglycemia to mortality in trauma patients. J Trauma 2004;56: 1058–1062.
23. Gore DC, Chinkes D, Heggers J, et al. Association of hyperglycemia with increased mortality after severe burn injury. J Trauma 2001;51:540–544.
24. Bochicchio GV, Sung J, Joshi M, et al. Persistent hyperglycemia is predictive of outcome in critically ill trauma patients. J Trauma 2005;58:921–924.
25. Capes SE, Hunt D, Malmberg K, et al. Stress hyperglycemia and increased risk of death after myocardial infarction in patients with and without diabetes: a systematic overview. Lancet 2000;355:773–778.
26. Capes SE, Hunt D, Malmberg K, et al. Stress hyperglycemia and prognosis of stroke in nondiabetic and diabetic patients: a systematic overview. Stroke 2001;32:2426–2432.
27. Chan DL, Freeman LM, Rozanski EA, et al. Alterations in carbohydrate metabolism in critically ill cats. J Vet Emerg Crit Care 2006;16(2)(S1):S7–S13.
28. Burrin JM, Price CP. Measurement of blood glucose. Ann Clin Biochem 1995;22:327–342.
29. Steven L. Stockham and Michael A. Scott. 2008. Fundamentals of Veterinary Clinical Pathology, 2nd ed. Ames, IA: Blackwell Publishing.
30. Brunkhorst FM, Wahl HG. Blood glucose measurements in the critically ill: more than just a blood draw. Critical Care 2006;10(6):178–179.
31. Orazio PD, Burnett RW, Fogh-Anderson N, et al. Approved IFC recommendation on reporting results for blood glucose. Clin Chem Lab Med 2006;44(12):1486–1490.
32. Price C. Point-of-care testing in diabetes mellitus. Clin Chem Med 2003;41:1213–1219.
33. Dungan K, Chapman J, Braithwaite SS, et al. Glucose measurement: confounding issues in setting targets for inpatient management. Diabetes Care 2007;30(2):403–409.
34. G.J. Kost, Guideline for point of care testing: improving patient outcomes. Am J Clin Pathol 1995;104: S111–S127.
35. Weiner K. Whole blood glucose: what are we actually measuring? Ann Clin Biochem 1995;32:1–8.
36. Brunner GA, Ellmerer M, Sendlhofer G, et al. Validation of home blood glucose meters with respect to clinical and analytical approaches. Diabetes Care 1998;21:585–590.

37. Chan JC, Wong RY, Cheung CK, et al. Accuracy, precision and user-acceptibility of self blood glucose monitoring machines. Diabetes Res Clin Pract 1997;36:91–104.

38. Trajonoski Z, Brunner GA, Gfrerer RJ, et al. Accuracy of home blood glucose meters during hypoglycemia. Diabetes Care 1996;19:1412–1415.

39. Chmielewski SA. Advances and strategies for glucose monitoring. Am J Clin Pathol 1995:104(suppl):59–71.

40. Arens S, Moons V, Meuleman P, et al. Evaluation of Glucocard Memory 2 and Accutrend sensor blood glucose meters. Clin Chem Lab Med 1998;36:47–52.

41. Devresse K, Leroux-Roels G. Laboratory assessment of five glucose meters designed for self-monitoring of blood glucose concentration. Eur J Clin Chem Clin Biochem 1993;31: 829–837.

42. Dacombe CM, Dalton RG, Goldie DJ, et al. Effect of packed cell volume on blood glucose estimations. Arch Dis Child 1981;56:789–791.

43. Tang Z, Xiaogu D, Louie R, Kost GJ. Effects of drugs on glucose measurements with handheld glucose meters and a portable glucose analyzer. Am J Clin Pathol 2000;113:75–86.

44. Tang Z, Louie RF, Payes M, et al. Oxygen effects on glucose measurements with a reference analyzer and three handheld meters. Diabetes Technol Ther 2000;2:349–362.

45. Kost GJ, Vu HT, Inn M, et al. Multicenter study of whole-blood creatinine, total carbon dioxide content, and chemistry profiling for laboratory and point-of-care testing in critical care in the United States. Crit Care Med 2000;28:2379–2389.

46. Tang Z, Du X, Louie RF, Kost GJ. Effects of pH on glucose measurements with handheld glucose meters and a portable glucose analyzer for point-of-care testing. Arch Pathol Lab Med 2000;124:577–582.

47. Oberg D, Ostenson CG. Performance of glucose dehydrogenase- and glucose oxidase-based blood glucose meters at high altitude and low temperature (letter). Diabetes Care 2005;28:1261.

48. Haupt A, Berg B, Paschen P, et al. The effects of skin temperature and testing site on blood glucose measurements taken by a modern blood glucose monitoring device. Diabetes Technol Ther 2005;7:597–601.

49. Wess G, Reusch C. Evaluation of five portable blood glucose meters for use in dogs. J Am Vet Med Assoc 2000;216(2): 203–209.

50. Wess G, Reusch C. Assessment of five portable blood glucose meters for use in cats. Am J Vet Res 2000;61(12):1587–1592.

51. Cohn LA, McCaw DL, Tate DJ, Johnson JC. Assessment of five portable blood glucose meters, a point-of-care analyzer, and color test strips for measuring blood glucose concentration in dogs. J Am Vet Med Assoc 2000;216(2):198–202.

52. Cohen LA, Nelson RW, Kass PH, et al. Evaluation of six portable blood glucose meters for measuring blood glucose concentration in dogs. J Am Vet Med Assoc 2009;235(3):276–280.

53. Fogh-Anderson N, Wimberly PD, Thode J, Siggaard-Anderson O. Direct reading glucose electrodes detect the molality of glucose in plasma and whole blood. Clin Chim Acta 1990; 189:33–38.

54. Rebrin K, Steil G, Van Antwerp W, et al. Subcutaneous glucose predicts plasma glucose independent of insulin: implications for continuous monitoring. Am J Physiol 1999;277: E561–E571.

55. Bode BW, Gross TM, Thornton KR. Continuous glucose monitoring used to adjust diabetes therapy improved glycosylated hemoglobin: a pilot study. Diab Res Clin Prac 1999; 46: 183–190.

56. Wiedmeyer CE, Johnson PJ, Cohn L, et al. Evaluation of a continuous glucose monitoring system for use in dogs, cats and horses. J Am Vet Med Assoc 2003;223(7):987–992.

57. Davison LJ, Slater LA, Herrtage ME, et al. Evaluation of a continuous glucose monitoring system in diabetic dogs. J Small Anim Prac 2003;44:435–442.

58. Ristic J, Herrtage ME, Walti-Lauger SM, et al. Evaluation of a continous glucose monitoring system in cats with diabetes mellitus. J Fel Med Surg 2005;7:153–162.

59. Reineke EL, Fletcher DJ, King L, et al. The accuracy of a continuous glucose monitoring system (CGMS) in diabetic ketoacidotic dogs and cats (abstract). J Vet Emerg Crit Care 2006;S2: S16–S17.

60. Diabetes Control and Complications Trial Research Group. The effect of intensive treatment of diabetes on the development and progression of long-term complications in insulin-dependent diabetes mellitus. N Engl J Med 1993;329:977–986.

61. Van den Berghe G, Wouters P, Weekers F, et al. Intensive insulin therapy in critically ill patients. N Engl J Med 2001;345: 1359–1367.

62. Van den Berghe G, Wilmer A, Hermans G, et al. Intensive insulin therapy in the medical ICU. N Engl J Med 2006;354: 449–461.

63. Krinsley JS. Effect of an intensive glucose management protocol on the mortality of critically ill adult patients. Mayo Clin Proc 2004;79:992–1000.

64. Rand JS, Kinnaird E, Baglioni A, et al. Acute stress hyperglycemia in cats is associated with struggling and increased concentrations of lactate and norepinephrine. J Vet Int Med 2002;16(2): 123–132.

65. Macintire DK. Treatment of diabetic ketoacidosis in dogs by continuous low-dose intravenous infusion of insulin. J Am Vet Med Assoc 1993;202(8):1266–1270.

66. Chastain CB, Nichols CE. Low-dose intramuscular insulin therapy for diabetic ketoacidosis in dogs. J Am Vet Med Assoc 1981;178(6):561–564.

67. Nelson R.W. Disorders of the endocrine pancreas. In: Nelson RW, Couto CG, eds. Small Animal Internal Medicine. 3rd ed. St. Louis, MO: Mosby Elsevier, 2009:764–809.

68. Haycock P: Insulin absorption: understanding the variables. Clin Diabetes 1986;4:98.

69. Weaver KE, Rozanski EA, Mahoney OM, et al. Use of glargine and lente insulins in cats with diabetes mellitus. J Vet Int Med 2006;20:234–238.

70. Donald C. Plumb. 2002. Veterinary Drug Handbook, 4th ed. Ames: Iowa State University Press.

71. Hessov Ib, Bojsen-Moller M, Melsen F. Experimental infusion thrombophlebitis. Inten Care Med 1979, 5:79–81.

72. Syring RS. Assessment and treatment of central nervous system abnormalities in the emergency patient. Vet Clin Small Anim 2005;35:343–358.

73. Steiner JM, Bruyette DS. Canine insulinoma. Comp Cont Ed 1996;18:13–16.

74. Fischer JR, Smith SA, Harkin KR. Glucagon constant-rate infusion: a novel strategy for the management of hyperinsulinemic-hypoglycemic crisis in the dog. J Am Anim Hosp Assoc 2000;36:27–32.

75. Smith SA, Harkin KR, Fischer JR. Glucagon constant rate infusion for hyperinsulinemic hypoglycemic crisis with neuroglycopenia in 6 dogs. J Vet Int Med 2000;14:344.

76. Donald C. Plumb. 2002. Veterinary Drug Handbook, 4th ed. Ames: Iowa State UniversityPress.

61

Care of the patient with intracranial disease

Marie K. Holowaychuk and Sara M. Ostenkamp

Introduction

Animals with intracranial disease may have any one of a number of underlying disorders such as traumatic brain injury, idiopathic epilepsy, meningitis, encephalitis, or neoplasia. Signs associated with the disease will vary and the patients will differ in terms of the intensity of the nursing care they require. For example, one patient may be a dog hospitalized for observation following cluster seizures, while another may be a cat recovering from a craniotomy to remove a brain tumor. Regardless of the underlying disease or severity of signs, the goal for all patients with intracranial disease is to preserve their brain function. This is achieved by ensuring adequate cerebral blood flow (CBF) by maintaining a normal cerebral perfusion pressure (CPP) of 50–60 mmHg.[1] In the normal or uninjured brain, pressure autoregulation maintains a constant CBF despite a wide range of mean arterial blood pressures (MAP; 50–150 mmHg).[1] When MAP is maintained within that range and CPP increases, cerebral blood vessels constrict to decrease overall cerebral blood volume and intracranial pressure (ICP). However, as MAP decreases to below 50 mmHg, CBF decreases and is dependent on MAP.[1] In addition to MAP, CPP is affected by changes in ICP (see Eq. 61.1). Elevations in ICP will decrease CPP, thereby resulting in worsening of brain function.[1] Henceforth, the aim in all patients hospitalized for intracranial disease is to ensure stability of cardiovascular parameters, namely, blood pressure, and most importantly, to prevent elevations in ICP.

$$CPP = MAP - ICP \qquad (61.1)$$

ICP may increase for many reasons including the underlying disease process itself. For example, masses such as tumors or abscesses, cerebral edema or hemorrhage following a traumatic injury, or hydrocephalus due to a congenital malformation are all space-occupying lesions that may cause elevations in ICP. Because a rigid nonexpandable skull surrounds the brain, if there are pathologic increases in intracranial tissue or fluid, the ICP will increase because of the additional intracranial volume (see Fig. 61.1).[2] If surgery is not an option to remove the structural abnormality contributing to the increase in intracranial volume, other treatments must be employed. These may include the administration of steroids to reduce tumor-associated inflammation in patients with neoplasia or to reduce the production of cerebrospinal fluid (CSF) in patients with hydrocephalus. Alternatively, mannitol or hypertonic saline may be given to decrease ICP (see Box 61.1). Ultimately, the goal with these treatments is to reduce intracranial tissue or fluid volume.

Intracranial volume and thus ICP can also be increased due to physiologic increases in blood volume. These physiologic alterations can be monitored and addressed by veterinary technicians, in an attempt to prevent increases in ICP. For example, increases in venous blood volume may occur due to jugular venous obstruction, a head-down position, or increases in central venous pressure.[2] Therefore, in order to decrease ICP, it is important that patients with intracranial disease be carefully positioned so as not to place pressure on the jugular veins or increase blood flow to the head. Additionally, increases in arterial blood volume and subsequently ICP can occur due to systemic hypertension, hypoventilation,

Advanced Monitoring and Procedures for Small Animal Emergency and Critical Care, First Edition. Edited by Jamie M. Burkitt Creedon, Harold Davis.
© 2012 John Wiley & Sons, Inc. Published 2012 by John Wiley & Sons, Inc.

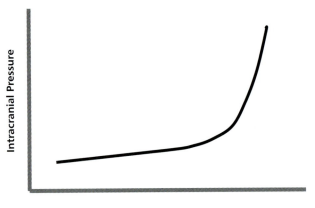

Figure 61.1 Relationship between intracranial pressure (ICP) and volume. At low intracranial volumes, increases in intracranial volume produce minimal changes in ICP. However, small increases in intracranial volume will eventually cause dramatic increases in ICP.

hypoxemia, or increases in cerebral metabolic rate due to seizures, agitation, or elevations in body temperature.[2] Thus, it is imperative that patients with intracranial disease maintain normal blood pressure, ventilation, and oxygenation, and that seizures are treated quickly and any temperature elevations are eliminated. Clearly, the veterinary technician has the very important task of monitoring for changes that may lead to ICP elevations and, if possible, preventing some of the physiologic changes that may lead to increases in ICP.

Because these physiologic changes can occur very quickly, resulting in rapid deteriorations in a patient's status, animals with intracranial disease must be constantly and closely monitored. Therefore, it is imperative that these patients receive 24-hour monitoring. This ensures that nursing care and appropriate monitoring will be provided continuously, so that changes in a patient's status can be detected quickly and treated appropriately. Many of the monitoring devices or treatment modalities required for patients with intracranial disease are available only at 24-hour or specialty hospitals. For these reasons, in order to provide the best care possible, it is recommended that patients with intracranial disease be transferred to a facility capable of providing 24-hour monitoring and nursing care.

Serial neurologic examinations

Patients with intracranial disease require constant monitoring, including serial neurologic examinations. Because the patient's condition can change very quickly, it is important that the neurologic status is assessed fre-

Box 61.1 Medications

Mannitol
Mechanism of action
- Increases the osmotic gradient between the vasculature and brain causing fluid to move out of the brain and into the blood

Storage
- Room temperature for lower concentrations
- Incubator for higher concentrations (>15%) to avoid crystal formation
- Bottles stored at room temperature can be heated in warm water bath or incubator, but should be body temperature upon administration

Administration
Dose
- 0.25–1 gram/kg IV[22]
- Give slowly via a syringe pump or slow push (over 15–20 minutes)
- Can be repeated every 4–6 hours as needed

Draw up using a filter needle (Monoject filter needle, Kendall Healthcare (Covidien), Mansfield, MA) or administer with an in-line filter (Hemonate filter, Gesco International, San Antonio, TX)

Administer in a dedicated line (i.e., do not mix with other medications)

Monitor
- Urine output
- Electrolytes
- Respiratory rate and effort (risk of fluid overload and pulmonary edema)
- Blood pressure

Hypertonic saline (NaCl 7%)
Mechanism of action
Increases the osmolality of the blood to cause water to shift from the brain into the intravascular space

Administration
Dose
- 4 mL/kg bolus over 5–10 minutes[11,23]
- Typically drawn into a syringe and administered via syringe pump or slow push

Monitor
- Urine output
- Electrolytes (sodium and chloride)
- Respiratory rate and effort (risk of fluid overload)

Cautions
- Repeated doses can cause local vascular irritation (preferably give via a central line)
- Fast administration may cause bronchoconstriction and vasodilation
- Can cause hypernatremia and hyperchloremia

quently in order to detect changes as they arise. The veterinary technician should contact a clinician immediately if the patient's neurologic status is deteriorating, or if the results of the neurologic examination are difficult to interpret. Neurologic examination findings will vary depending on the severity of the intracranial disease and may include mild to pronounced neurologic deficits. It is very important that the veterinary technician coming on shift immediately assess any patients with intracranial disease in order to obtain a baseline from which to compare subsequent examinations. If an initial examination is not performed, observations by the veterinary technician may be assumed to be "normal" for that patient when in fact they may have progressed from previous evaluations. Such a circumstance could result in a devastating failure to detect deterioration in a patient's status in a timely manner.

The patient should be assessed frequently to determine its level of consciousness, pupillary light reflexes, pupil size, posture, and reflexes (see Box 61.2). Almost all patients with intracranial disease will have an abnormal level of consciousness that will vary from a mildly altered mentation to a coma. If the patient is sedated, it may be difficult to assess its level of consciousness. Regardless, patients receiving sedative medications should be intermittently "woken up" (i.e., sedation

briefly stopped) to enable proper assessment of their mentation and level of consciousness (see Box 61.3). Normally, patients with mild intracranial disease will still have periods of alertness and responsiveness to their environment. As the severity of intracranial disease progresses, patients will become increasingly altered and less capable of responding to their environment. Additionally, some patients will exhibit an inappropriate response to environmental stimuli, such as excessive vocalization. Patients that progress to a stuporous or semi-comatose state will be less responsive to visual or auditory stimuli in their environment until they are responsive only to painful (i.e., noxious) stimuli. Finally, an animal that is comatose is unresponsive to all environmental stimuli including repeated noxious stimuli.[3]

It is important when assessing patients with intracranial disease never to assume that a patient is "sleeping" and for that reason not assess its mentation. A patient that has otherwise been responsive to environmental stimuli may progress into a semi-comatose to comatose state, and if one assumes the patient is "sleeping," the patient's condition may continue to deteriorate without intervention. Therefore, patients should always be awakened every 1–2 hours if they appear to be sleeping, in order to properly assess their level of consciousness and ensure that it is not deteriorating.

It is also important that pupillary light reflexes and pupil size be assessed in patients with intracranial disease on a frequent basis. A pupillary light reflex (PLR) is tested by shining a bright light into the pupil and assessing for constriction of the pupil (direct reflex).[3] The opposite pupil should constrict at the same time (consensual reflex). It is not necessary to assess the consensual reflex if the direct PLR is present in both eyes.[3] Generally, a critically ill patient with mild elevations in ICP will have normal pupillary light reflexes that will progress to slow or completely unresponsive pupils in patients with moderate to severe elevations in ICP.[4] In addition to alterations in the pupillary light reflex, patients with moderate to severe elevations in ICP will also exhibit changes in their pupil size. While patients with mild elevations in ICP will have normal to slightly

---

Box 61.2 Serial neurologic examinations

Normal Findings
- Alert and responsive to the environment
- Normal pupillary light reflex
- Normal pupil size bilaterally
- Normal gait and normal spinal reflexes

Mild Intracranial Disease
- Depressed or inappropriate mentation
- Slow pupillary light reflexes
- Normal pupil size bilaterally
- Paresis

Moderate Intracranial Disease
- Stuporous/semi-comatose but responsive to noxious (i.e., painful) stimuli
- Absent pupillary light reflex
- Miotic (i.e., pinpoint) pupils
- Recumbency +/− extensor rigidity of the forelimbs

Severe Intracranial Disease
- Comatose and unresponsive to noxious stimuli
- Absent pupillary light reflex
- Mydriatic (i.e., dilated) pupils
- Recumbent +/− loss of muscle tone and spinal reflexes
- Loss of facial sensation or gag reflex

Box 61.3 Assessing mentation and level of consciousness

Normal: alert and responsive to the environment
Altered: abnormal or decreased response to environmental stimuli
Stuporous/semi-comatose: responsive only to painful stimuli
Comatose: unresponsive to painful stimuli

miotic (i.e., constricted) pupils, patients with moderate to severe elevations in ICP will have progressively altered pupil sizes ranging from miotic or pinpoint pupils to unilateral or bilateral mydriatic (i.e., dilated) pupils that are completely unresponsive to light.[4] Miotic or mydriatic pupils in a patient with intracranial disease and previously normal-sized pupils represents an emergency and a clinician should be contacted immediately.

Ideally, patients with intracranial disease that are not sedated should have their posture and reflexes assessed frequently. Patients with mild intracranial disease will exhibit a normal posture, gait, and reflexes. As the severity of intracranial disease worsens, patients will exhibit varying degrees of paresis (weakness) progressing to full recumbency.[4] Additionally, patients may exhibit other abnormalities including circling, a head tilt, decerebellate rigidity, or decerebrate rigidity. Decerebellate rigidity is characterized by opisthotonus (extension of the head and neck), with the forelimbs extended.[3] Animals exhibiting decerebellate rigidity also typically have flexed hips and normal mentation. In contrast, patients with decerebrate rigidity have a stuporous or comatose mentation that is associated with opisthotonus and extension of all limbs.[3] Finally, a patient with severe intracranial disease may have a complete loss of muscle tone and decreased to absent spinal reflexes. The simplest spinal reflex to test in patients with intracranial disease is the withdrawal reflex. This reflex is elicited by applying a noxious stimulus to the tested limb by pinching the nail bed or toe with fingers or a hemostat.[3] The normal reflex is contraction of the flexor muscles and withdrawal of the tested limb.

Cranial nerve reflexes should also be assessed, the easiest of which include the gag reflex and facial sensation. To assess the gag reflex, stimulate the pharynx with a finger to elicit a gag.[3] An absent gag reflex may be due to excessive sedation if the patient is receiving sedatives; however, in the absence of sedating medications, loss of the gag reflex represents severe intracranial disease. The loss of a gag reflex is especially concerning because it puts the patient at risk for aspiration since the patient cannot normally swallow and protect its airway. Therefore, if the patient is noted to have lost its gag reflex, a clinician should be contacted immediately and endotracheal intubation considered. Facial sensation is assessed by touching the medial or lateral canthus of the eye to cause a blink (palpebral reflex), stimulating the nasal mucosa with a pen or hemostats to cause withdrawal of the head, or pinching the skin of the face with a hemostat and observing for a blink or facial twitch on that side.[3] Loss of facial sensation also indicates severe intracranial disease, and if it is a new finding, the clinician should be contacted immediately.

While it would seem that a patient with intracranial disease is "stable" and its condition is unlikely to change, indeed patients with intracranial disease can deteriorate rapidly and without warning. Therefore, the importance of frequent and thorough neurologic examinations cannot be stressed enough, with the goal of detecting subtle changes in a patient's neurologic status before they have progressed to a state in which the changes are irreversible.

Nursing care

Managing hospitalized patients with intracranial disease requires intensive monitoring and special attention to the animal's comfort. A substantial component of nursing care for patients with intracranial disease is avoiding further brain injury as a result of increased ICP. Superior nursing care of these patients relies primarily on the ideal setup of the patient's cage or kennel to reduce the risk of further brain injury. By selecting a cage that is free from unnecessary stimulation but easily visible for constant monitoring, veterinary technicians can quickly recognize any change in a patient's mentation that may be indicative of an increase in ICP. Whether the patient is active or recumbent will also guide the arrangement of the animal's cage or kennel. Appropriate bedding should be selected that provides adequate cushioning, allows the patient to be kept clean, and optimizes the comfort of the patient.

The cage location for a dog or cat with intracranial disease can play a major role in reducing unnecessary stimulation. Environmental stressors can induce an unsafe and prolonged increase in ICP. Ideally, these patients should be placed in a location free from loud noises, such as barking dogs. Avoid selecting a cage in an area with heavy foot traffic, and place signs on or near the cage alerting staff to keep loud noises at a minimum. If auditory stimulation cannot be minimized simply by cage location, cotton can be placed in the patient's ears if tolerated. To avoid misinterpretation of decreased response to auditory stimuli or sending the animal home with cotton in its ears, always put white tape on the patient's head and write "cotton in ears" on the tape (see Fig. 61.2).

Visual and tactile stimulation should also be reduced. Select a cage far away from bright lights in a darker corner of the intensive care unit. A cage isolated from others can reduce the number of veterinary technicians, doctors, and other animals passing by that could disturb the patient. Reduce tactile stimulation by clustering treatments together, which will minimize the frequency of entering the cage or kennel throughout the day. For example, treatments such as examination of PLRs,

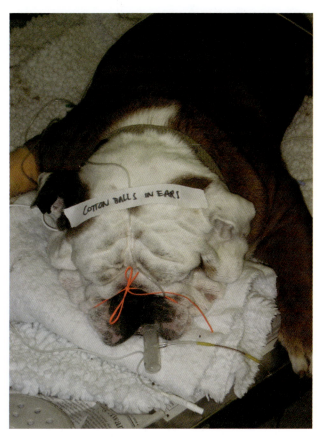

Figure 61.2 A bulldog is intubated following treatment for cluster seizures and has cotton in his ears to prevent auditory stimulation.

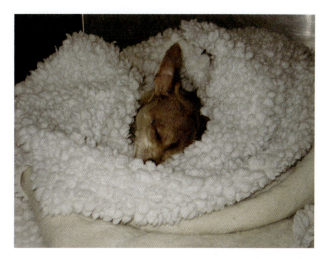

Figure 61.3 A chihuahua with vestibular disease is surrounded by padding and blankets to prevent it from injuring itself when it rolls.

auscultation, and venipuncture can be conducted when the patient is due to be turned.

While reduction of stressors is important in cage selection, it is also important to keep in mind that the patient needs to be monitored closely. Veterinary technicians should be able to identify any change in the animal's level of consciousness, as this is one of the first signs of an increase in ICP.[5] Other parameters such as the patient's respiratory rate and character, blood pressure, heart rate and rhythm, pulse oximetry, end-tidal CO_2, and body temperature can all be monitored without disturbing the patient and can provide additional indications that a patient's condition is changing. Patients with intracranial disease are also prone to have seizures and therefore must be in a location in which they can be readily monitored and accessed quickly if necessary. Additionally, it is important that clinician orders are already available in the event that the patient experiences a seizure, so that the animal can be treated immediately rather than after the clinician is called.

The safety and comfort of patients with intracranial disease are controlled by a carefully designed cage or kennel. Depending on the particular disease affecting the patient, the animal may be active or recumbent. Active or moving patients, such as those with vestibular signs that are circling or rolling, or animals experiencing generalized seizures will benefit from a cage that is heavily padded on all sides. A cradle can also be made using rolled towels or foam padding on either side of smaller dogs and cats, to protect them from injury (see Fig. 61.3). Keep in mind that a patient surrounded by extra bedding or moving excessively may develop hyperthermia; therefore, more frequent monitoring of body temperature may be warranted in these patients. A patient who continuously circles in the kennel or cage should not have any unnecessary fluid lines or monitoring cords in their path. Coiled intravenous fluid administration sets prevent lines from lying on the cage floor and getting tangled, and can be mounted to the ceiling of the cage (see Fig. 61.4).

Recumbent patients are those who are stuporous or comatose, heavily medicated, sedated for mechanical ventilation, or recovering from surgery. These animals require more padding, such as a thick mattress, to limit pressure on joints and prevent the formation of decubital ulcers. Nonambulatory patients should ideally be kept in sternal recumbency or, if lateral, should be turned frequently (every 4–6 hours) to prevent atelectasis of the dependent lung.[6] Patients in sternal recumbency should still have their rear limbs or hips rotated. Passive range of motion and massage of the limbs should

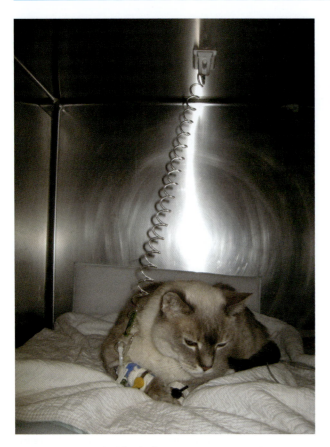

Figure 61.4 A coiled fluid administration set is used on a cat to prevent tangling of the fluid lines with excessive movement or circling.

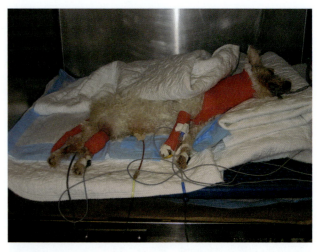

Figure 61.5 A Maltese recovers after being hit by a car and sustaining head and cervical trauma. Note that the dog is positioned on a 30° incline to help prevent elevations in ICP or aspiration.

be performed to reduce edema and stimulate blood flow to the extremities. See Chapter 46, Nursing Care of the Long-Term Anesthetized Patient, for more information regarding how to perform passive range of motion. It is also important to keep these inactive patients clean by frequently checking for urine and providing bedding that can wick away urine to prevent urine scald. Intermittent urinary catheterization or placement of an indwelling catheter may be necessary in patients that are unable to void on their own and when bladder expression is not possible or contraindicated.

Another concern for the recumbent patient with intracranial disease is the positioning of the patient's body. By using slanted grates or boards, or additional towels and bedding, the patient's forelimbs and head should be elevated at a 30° angle at all times (see Fig. 61.5). This positioning maximizes CSF outflow and cerebral venous drainage, thus alleviating risks of ICP elevation.[7,8] Additionally, many of the comatose or sedated patients have a loss of protective reflexes, such

as a gag reflex. Positioning the patient on an incline may reduce the risk of aspiration if the patient vomits or regurgitates.[9] When placing the patient's cranial end in this elevated position, obstruction of the jugular veins should be prevented. This can be accomplished most easily by placing extra blankets or bedding under the patient's forelimbs, neck, and head to angle the cranial portion of the body on an incline. It is important that incline does not exceed 30°, as excessive head elevation will decrease cerebral blood flow and thus decrease CPP.[2]

Ensure that the bedding is not placed only under the neck, as this may occlude jugular blood flow. Occlusion for venipuncture or catheterization or the placement of pressure bandages should also be avoided.

Often patients with intracranial disease receive oxygen therapy for treatment of hypoxemia. However, it is important to be cautious regarding the route of oxygen supplementation. Although administration of oxygen via nasal cannulae is relatively easy, it is imperative not to stress the animal or cause it to sneeze during cannula placement, as this may lead to elevations in the patient's ICP and deterioration of the neurologic status.[10] For that reason, clinicians may elect to provide oxygen supplementation via flow-by, facemask, or oxygen cages or hoods.

Veterinary technicians are also relied on for the assessment of pain in patients with intracranial disease. Patients most likely to exhibit pain due to their intracranial disease are those with traumatic brain injury.

Unfortunately, assessment for pain in all patients with intracranial disease can be difficult given that patients are often heavily medicated, sedated, or exhibiting inappropriate mentation. Still, this is an important task for the veterinary technician because pain or anxiety that is untreated may lead to elevations in ICP that can worsen the patient's condition.[2] Therefore, if the patient exhibits any signs associated with pain, a clinician should be notified immediately so that appropriate analgesics can be administered. Fentanyl, a short-acting opioid, is typically the drug of choice because it provides immediate effective analgesia and can be titrated to effect.[11] Additionally, because it is short-acting, the infusion may be discontinued if assessment of neurologic function is required. Similarly, its effects can be reversed with naloxone if immediate evaluation of the neurologic status is desired.

It is also frequently the task of the veterinary technician to provide nutrition to patients with intracranial disease. While even the most neurologically abnormal patients can maintain a good appetite, it is important not to offer food or water to all patients with intracranial disease. Prior to doing so, the patient should be placed in sternal recumbency if it is not able sit or stand on its own. Additionally, a gag reflex should be tested to ensure that the patient is able to swallow. Next, a small amount of water can be offered via bowl or syringe, to ensure that the patient is able to drink normally and does not cough. If the patient is able to drink water, food may be offered. After feeding, if a patient remains laterally recumbent, it is recommended that they remain elevated on a 30° incline to prevent aspiration.

Fluid therapy is also required in the patient with intracranial disease to ensure normovolemia and normal blood pressure and to minimize electrolyte abnormalities.[3] Fluids are typically administered intravenously at a maintenance rate unless the patient has abnormal ongoing losses such as with a fever. Additionally, animals receiving steroids may be polyuric and have higher fluid requirements. Similarly, patients that have received mannitol or hypertonic saline will also have increased fluid requirements. Fluids should be administered until the patient is able to eat and drink its recommended maintenance requirements. The adequacy of fluid administration can be determined by monitoring daily body weight or urine output (normal should be 1–2 mL/kg/hr) in patients with indwelling urinary catheters.

Patient monitoring

It is extremely important to monitor patients with intracranial disease closely to ensure that blood pressure, oxygenation, ventilation, and temperature are normal.

Because alterations in these findings can contribute to further brain injury in these patients, it is important that any abnormalities be treated immediately. Blood pressure should be measured regularly in patients with intracranial disease, especially those patients with moderate to severe intracranial disease. Hypotension as indicated by a systolic blood pressure (SBP) < 100 mmHg or a MAP < 80 mmHg is dangerous because it may lead to decreased cerebral perfusion in patients with elevated ICP.[12] The patient's normal response to a decrease in cerebral perfusion is to vasodilate its cerebral vessels, which can lead to an increase in ICP. Likewise, elevations in blood pressure such as a MAP > 120 mmHg are undesirable because it can lead to reflex cerebral vasoconstriction, thus decreasing cerebral perfusion.[12] If blood pressure measurements are outside the normal range (SBP < 100 mmHg or 120 mmHg < MAP < 80 mmHg), the veterinary technician should contact a clinician immediately.

In patients with severe intracranial disease, a Cushing's reflex may occur as a near-death event. This includes systemic hypertension that occurs as the patient mounts a final effort to maintain cerebral perfusion in the face of an elevated ICP.[2] The patient's heart rate may decrease dramatically in response to the hypertension. Thus, bradycardia in conjunction with systemic hypertension represents a life-threatening emergency in a patient with intracranial disease, and the clinician should be contacted immediately.

Pulse oximetry should also be performed regularly to assess oxygenation in patients with intracranial disease. Because hypoxemia can hasten the progression of brain damage, if an SpO_2 < 95% is detected, a clinician should be notified.[12] If the patient is intubated or has a nasal cannula in place, an end tidal carbon dioxide ($ETCO_2$) monitor can be applied to provide a noninvasive method of measuring ventilation. $ETCO_2$ correlates with $PaCO_2$; therefore, an elevation in $ETCO_2$ > 50 mmHg is suggestive of hypoventilation. Hypoventilation can have serious consequences in patients with intracranial disease, as it may lead to cerebral vasodilation and elevations in ICP. Therefore, if increased $ETCO_2$ is noted, the clinician should be contacted as manual or mechanical ventilation may be indicated.

Arterial blood gas (ABG) monitoring is another method by which the patient's oxygenation and ventilation can be assessed. An ABG is especially helpful in patients with intracranial disease that are stuporous or comatose or have an abnormal respiratory pattern. A PaO_2 < 80 mmHg indicates hypoxemia, and if this is seen, oxygen supplementation should be provided. Likewise, an ideal $PaCO_2$ is in the low end of the normal range. A $PaCO_2$ > 50 mmHg indicates hypoventilation and is of concern in a patient with a stuporous or comatose mentation. If the hypoventilation persists, a clinician should be contacted because the patient may require manual or mechanical ventilation. Should an animal need to be intubated for manual or mechanical ventilation, it is imperative that the intubation occur quickly, in order to avoid coughing or gagging that may further increase the patient's ICP.[3] Once the patient is intubated and manually ventilated, continuous monitoring of CO_2 via ABG or ETCO2 is crucial. Overventilation of patients with intracranial disease can be detrimental, as decreases in $PaCO_2$ to < 25 mmHg will cause cerebral vasoconstriction and reduced CPP.[13] In an emergent situation, hyperventilation can be used to reduce ICP by reducing cerebral blood flow; however, if the patient is stable and being maintained with manual or mechanical ventilation, a target of 35–45 mmHg for $PaCO_2$ should be the goal.[2]

It is also important in patients with intracranial disease to maintain body temperature within the normal range. Patients with traumatic brain injury or those undergoing intracranial surgery can have impaired thermoregulation.[3] Ideally, temperature should be monitored continuously in the recumbent patient with the placement of a rectal probe, and appropriate measures to maintain the temperature in the normal range should be employed. Hyperthermia is associated with a poor outcome in patients with intracranial disease, as it may increase cerebral blood flow and lead to elevations in ICP.[14] As such, steps should be taken to externally cool patients with intracranial disease and elevated body temperatures. Hypothermia decreases the cerebral metabolic rate and is thought to be neuroprotective; however, controlled hypothermia is not routinely practiced in veterinary medicine and is not recommended at this time.

Because most patients with intracranial disease are not highly mobile, and because their condition can change from moment to moment, continuous ECG monitoring is beneficial and recommended. Not only can changes in heart rate be detected quickly, but the ECG can also be monitored for arrhythmias such as ventricular premature contractions (VPCs), ventricular tachycardia, sinus tachycardia, sinus bradycardia, or AV block, all of which can be seen in patients with intracranial disease.

In addition to monitoring the cardiovascular and respiratory systems, patients with intracranial disease should also have their electrolytes, lactate, and blood glucose monitored regularly. Hyperlactatemia is often detected in patients with intracranial disease. Causes for hyperlactatemia in patients with intracranial disease include hypoperfusion, hypoxemia, and seizures or tremors.[15] Hyperlactatemia has also been associated

with some forms of neoplasia and seems to occur frequently in dogs with brain tumors, the mechanism of which is unknown at this time.[16] Blood glucose should also be monitored frequently to ensure that the patient is not hypoglycemic, as this will confound a patient's neurologic signs and put them at risk for seizures. Additionally, hyperglycemia has been documented in dogs and cats with head trauma and the degree of hyperglycemia was associated with the severity of head trauma.[17] Hyperglycemia has also been associated with increased mortality rates and poorer neurologic outcomes in experimental animal models and clinically in people.[18,19] If hypo- or hyperglycemia is noted in a patient with intracranial disease, the clinician should be contacted immediately to determine whether treatment is indicated.

Advanced monitoring techniques

Electrophysiologic techniques such as electroencephalography (EEG) are available primarily at teaching institutions and specialty hospitals. EEG provides a graphic recording of the electrical activity of the brain and is helpful for determining the presence and type of cerebral disease.[20] The amount of voltage, speed of activity, and presence or absence of "spikes" (very fast activity) indicates inflammatory or degenerative changes and seizure activity.[20] The EEG can change over time with progression or resolution of the disease; therefore, patients are sometimes monitored continuously (see Fig. 61.6). The EEG varies with the level of consciousness, and drugs such as sedatives, tranquilizers, and anesthetic agents can also alter results.[20]

ICP monitoring is used frequently in human hospitals but only rarely in the clinical veterinary setting. Available methods for ICP monitoring include the use of an

---

Box 61.4 Desired parameters for monitoring patients with intracranial disease

Blood pressure	80 mmHg < MAP < 110 mmHg
Pulse oximetry	SpO_2 > 95%
Heart rate	Within normal limits for the species and size of the patient
Respiratory rate	10–20 breaths per minute
Temperature	37–38°C (98.5–100.5°F)
Blood glucose	80–120 mg/dL (4.4–6.6 mmol/L)
Blood gases	PaO_2 > 80 mmHg, 35 mmHg < $PaCO_2$ < 45 mmHg
End-tidal CO2	ETCO2 40–50 mmHg

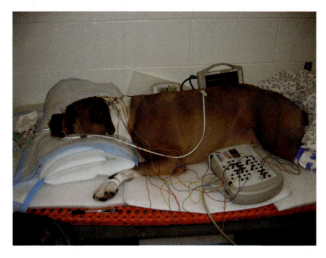

Figure 61.6 A boxer is continuously monitored with an EEG while undergoing mechanical ventilation.

intracranial bolt or screw attached to a fluid-filled system with a pressure transducer or a fiberoptic transducer.[21] Measurement of ICP may be useful in patients in which neurologic signs cannot be used to detect deterioration or improvement in neurologic status due to the loss of other observable neurologic functions or because the patient is sedated or anesthetized.[21] Complications of ICP monitor placement include focal edema, hemorrhage, parenchymal injury, and infection.[21] Due to limited experience with ICP placement in veterinary patients and the associated complications that can occur, ICP monitoring is rarely used.

Summary

- The goal for all patients with intracranial disease is to protect brain function by preserving cerebral perfusion and preventing elevations in ICP.
- Steps must be taken to ensure that temperature, oxygenation, ventilation, and blood pressure are maintained within the normal range and that pain, agitation, and seizure activity are treated expeditiously.
- Patients with intracranial disease can deteriorate rapidly; therefore, continuous monitoring by veterinary technicians at a 24-hour hospital is recommended.
- Serial neurologic examinations including assessment of the level of consciousness, pupillary light reflex, pupil size, posture, spinal reflexes, and cranial nerves is recommended.
- Veterinary technicians must ensure that patients with intracranial disease are housed in an environment

that has minimal visual and tactile stimuli but that enables continuous monitoring and easy access if emergency treatment is required.
- Patient comfort is imperative and may necessitate the use of a padded cage and thick bedding to prevent further injury.
- Patients with intracranial disease should be positioned on an incline with minimal pressure on the jugular veins to reduce ICP and prevent aspiration.
- Patients with intracranial disease require intensive care that often includes fluid therapy, nutritional support, oxygen supplementation, passive range of motion of the limbs, and pain management.
- Monitoring of blood gas values, electrolytes, and blood glucose is important as abnormalities can worsen the prognosis of patients with intracranial disease.

References

1. Bagley RS. 1996. Pathophysiological sequelae of intracranial disease. Veterinary Clinics of North America Small Animal Practice. 26:711–733.
2. Bershad EM, Humphreis III WE, Suarez JI. 2008. Intracranial hypertension. Seminars in Neurology. 28(5):690–702.
3. Platt SR and Olby NJ. 2004. BSAVA Manual of Canine and Feline Neurology, 3rd ed. Quedgeley: British Small Animal Veterinary Association.
4. Platt SR, Simona ST, McDonnell JJ. 2001. The prognostic value of the modified Glasgow coma scale in head trauma in dogs. Journal of Veterinary Internal Medicine. 15:581–584.
5. LeJeune M and Howard-Fain T. 2002. Caring for patients with increased intracranial pressure. Nursing. 32(11):2–5.
6. Cooper SJ. 2004. Methods to prevent ventilator-associated lung injury: a summary. Intensive and Critical Care Nursing. 20(6):358–365.
7. Frank JI. 1993. Management of intracranial hypertension. Medical Clinics of North America. 77(1):61–76.
8. Winkelman C. 2000. Effect of backrest position on intracranial and cerebral perfusion pressures in traumatically brain-injured adults. American Journal of Critical Care. 9(6):373–380.
9. Hess DR. 2005. Patient positioning and ventilator-associated pneumonia. Respiratory Care. 50(7):892–898.
10. Holowaychuk MK, Hansen BD, Marks SL, Hanel RM, Mariani CL. 2007. Head trauma. Standards of Care: Emergency and Critical Care Medicine. 9(6):1–8.
11. Armitage-Chan EA, Wetmore LA, Chan DL. 2007. Anesthetic management of the head trauma patient. Journal of Veterinary Emergency and Critical Care. 17(1):5–14.
12. Bratton SL, Chestnut RM, Ghajar J, McConnell Hammond FF, Harris OA, Hartl R, Manley GT, Nemecek A, Newell DW, Rosenthal G, Schouten J, Shutter L, Timmons SD, Ullman JS, Videtta W, Wilberger JE, Wright DW. 2007. Guidelines for the management of severe traumatic brain injury. I. Blood pressure and oxygenation. Journal of neurotrauma. 24(Suppl 1):S7-S13.
13. Muizelaar JP, Marmarou A, Ward JD, Kontos HA, Choi SC, Becker DP, Gruemer H, Young HF. 1991. Adverse effects of prolonged hyperventilation in patients with severe head injury. Journal of Neurosurgery. 75(5):731–739.

14. Oliveira-Filho J, Ezzeddine MA, Segal AZ, Buonanno FS, Chang Y, Ogilvy CS, Rordorf G, Schwamm LH, Koroshetz WJ, McDonald CT. 2001. Fever in subarachnoid hemorrhage: relationship to vasospasm and outcome. Neurology 56(10):1299–1304.

15. Pang DS and Boysen S. 2007. Lactate in veterinary critical care: pathophysiology and management. Journal of the American Animal Hospital Association. 43:270–279.

16. Sullivan LA, Campbell VL, Klopp LS, Rao S. 2009. Blood lactate concentrations in anesthetized dogs with intracranial disease. Journal of Veterinary Internal Medicine 23:488–492.

17. Syring RS, Otto CM, Drobatz KJ. 2001. Hyperglycemia in dogs and cats with head trauma: 122 cases (1997–1999). Journal of the American Veterinary Medical Assoication. 218:1124–1129.

18. Capes SE, Hunt D, Malmberg K, Pthak P, Gerstein HC. 2001. Stress hyperglycemia and prognosis of stroke in nondiabetic and diabetic patients: a systematic review. Stroke. 32(10): 2426–2432.

19. Rovlias A and Kotsou S. 2000. The influence of hyperglycemia on neurological outcome in patients with severe head injury. Neurosurgery 46(2):335–342.

20. Lorenz MD and Kornegay JN. 2004. Handbook of Veterinary Neurology, 4th ed. St. Louis, MO: Saunders.

21. Bonagura JD. 2000. Kirk's Current Veterinary Therapy XIII Small Animal Practice. Philadelphia: Saunders.

22. Plumb DC. 2008. Veterinary Drug Handbook, 6th ed. Ames: Blackwell Publishing.

23. Macintire DK, Drobatz KJ, Haskins SC, Saxon WD. 2005. Manual of Small Animal Emergency and Critical Care Medicine. Philadelphia: Lippincott Williams & Wilkins.

62

Care of the environmentally injured animal

Michael S. Lagutchik and Adrian Ford

This chapter will discuss care and management of dogs and cats with various environmental injuries. Specific injuries to be discussed include burns, cold-induced injury (frostbite and hypothermia), heat-induced injury, nonsurgical management of open wounds and necrotic tissues, and presurgical care of open fractures. The chapter will emphasize the specialized nursing guidelines that are critical to improve the likelihood of successful outcome.

Burn injury

Burn injuries are typically caused by environmental factors (e.g., fires, scalding water, motor vehicle mufflers, stoves, caustic chemicals) or iatrogenic factors (e.g., heat lamps, electric heating pads). While uncommon, these injuries can not only cause severe pain and complicated local wounds, but also result in serious metabolic abnormalities and systemic infection that can lead to life-threatening compromise. Burn injury management is labor-intensive and time-consuming; however, it is the quality of nursing care that often makes the difference between a successful outcome and severe complications or death.

Initial patient triage and evaluation

Be prepared to provide emergency therapy to establish an airway and provide supplemental oxygen therapy if the patient was exposed to smoke inhalation injury and has developed airway or pulmonary edema. Be prepared to perform cardiopulmonary-cerebral resuscitation if cardiac, respiratory, or cardiopulmonary arrest has occurred.

Burn evaluation

It is important to determine the severity of the burn once the patient has been resuscitated and stabilized. General characteristics of the wound that are important to examine include color, texture, presence or absence of pain, moistness, and extent of swelling, if present. These characteristics are summarized in Box 62.1.[1]

Box 62.1 Burn wound characteristics

Superficial burn: Skin is red and painful, similar to sunburn, involving the outer layer of the epidermis.

Superficial partial-thickness burn: Skin has a red or mottled appearance, with epidermal sloughing, fluid leakage, swelling, and extreme hypersensitivity (pain), involving the epidermis and variable amounts of dermis. Hair should not easily pull out.

Deep partial-thickness burn: Skin is black or yellow-white and hair follicles are destroyed. Skin surface is dry. These burns are generally less painful, as nerve endings are destroyed. If any hair remains, it will pull out easily.

Full-thickness burn: Skin is black, dry, and leathery. These burns have destroyed the epidermis and dermis and expose underlying connective tissue, muscle, and bone. Any eschar that forms is painless.

Total body surface area burn estimation

Estimate the percentage of the total body surface area (TBSA) that is burned by adding the estimated percent of burn from each of the following body areas:[1]

1. Head and neck (H&N): 9%
2. Chest (C): 18%

Advanced Monitoring and Procedures for Small Animal Emergency and Critical Care, First Edition. Edited by Jamie M. Burkitt Creedon, Harold Davis.
© 2012 John Wiley & Sons, Inc. Published 2012 by John Wiley & Sons, Inc.

3.   Abdomen (A): 18%
4.   Each forelimb (L FL, R FL): 9%
5.   Each hindlimb (L HL, R HL): 18%

$$TBSA = H/N + C + A + L\,FL + R\,FL + L\,HL + R\,HL$$
(62.1)

For example, the estimated TBSA burn for a dog with burns to the chest and abdomen and left forelimb would be 18% (chest) + 18% (abdomen) + 9% (L FL) = 45%.

The percentage TBSA is important in assessing severity, anticipating problems, and determining prognosis. Patients with TBSA >20% often have severe metabolic problems (e.g., hypovolemic shock, albumin and electrolyte losses, acidoses, renal failure); patients with TBSA >50% have a poor prognosis.[1,2] Any discussion of prognosis must take into consideration not only the TBSA but also the severity of the burn.[2] Note that initial evaluation of the severity of the burn wound may be inaccurate, as wounds often progress over a period of 3–7 days before completely manifesting ultimate severity.

General patient management recommendations

Monitor and treat for complications related to burn injury, to include shock, fluid losses, respiratory problems, and electrolyte abnormalities. Stabilize the patient first. Manage pain using appropriate analgesics; monitor pain using a pain scoring system (see Chapter 42, Pain Recognition and Management) every 4–6 hours initially.

Cool the burned skin using cool water (7–18°C [45–65°F]) by immersion, application of compresses, or gentle spray for at least 30 minutes.[2] Do not apply ice to any burned skin, as the vasoconstriction it causes may impede wound healing and may worsen the extent of tissue damage. Measure the patient's rectal or esophageal temperature frequently to monitor for and prevent patient hypothermia.

Minimize potential contamination of burned skin. It is important to physically handle these patients properly every time, even more so than is done for critically ill patients. Hands must be washed thoroughly every time before handling burn patients. Clean exam gloves may be worn for superficial burns and superficial partial-thickness burns; sterile surgical gloves must be worn when handling deep partial-thickness burns and full-thickness burns. Generally, it is not necessary to don barrier protection (e.g., disposable gowns, face masks, head cover) for superficial or superficial partial-thickness burns; however, be sure that these wounds are not contacted by things such as personal clothing, stethoscopes, or other instruments or monitors. It is recommended to don barrier protection when handling deep partial-thickness burns and full-thickness burns and to wear sterile gloves when handling wounds directly. To reduce the risk of cross-contamination, gloves should be changed and hands should be washed before handling other burn wounds and invasive devices on the same patient.

Provide excellent nursing care. Turn or rotate the patient every 4 hours if recumbent, and perform passive range of motion (PROM) exercises of all limbs except burned limbs every 4 hours. Provide soft, padded bedding. Prevent urine scalding and fecal soiling; consider indwelling or intermittent urethral catheterization according to hospital policy. Provide nutrition, ideally as voluntary intake by the patient; consider assisted enteral or parenteral nutrition if the patient is inappetant or nutritional intake is not adequate.

Follow strict aseptic technique when placing invasive devices (e.g., IV [intravenous] catheters, urethral catheters) and use at least clean examination gloves whenever handling patients and especially when manipulating catheters, adapters, fluid lines, and other equipment. Unless absolutely necessary, do not place invasive devices through burned skin. Provide antibiotic coverage as directed by the attending veterinarian. Note that severe infection and sepsis are major concerns due to loss of protective skin barrier; however, systemic antibiotics are generally not recommended unless the patient is immunocompromised, has pneumonia or acute lung injury, or is septic or suspected of being septic.[1,2] Proper management of the burn wound is the best way to reduce the chance of infection.

Burn wound management recommendations
(see Protocol 62.1)

Depending on severity and extent of burn, the patient may require daily heavy sedation or general anesthesia to allow debridement and management. Even though burn patients may appear stable when awake, extreme care must be taken to monitor burn patients adequately during sedation or anesthesia to avoid complications. The level of monitoring provided should be as for any critically ill surgical patient.

Superficial or superficial partial-thickness burns are generally managed with daily cool water lavage, followed by topical silver sulfadiazine (SSD) cream application until healed or the wound worsens.[1] Deep partial-thickness and full-thickness burns need varying degrees of daily wound debridement. This may be accomplished by use of conservative debridement, chemical debridement, or surgical debridement.

Conservative debridement of deep partial-thickness and full-thickness burns involves hydrotherapy using

Protocol 62.1 Management of burn wounds

1. Provide heavy sedation or general anesthesia to allow debridement and management, as directed by the attending veterinarian.
2. *Superficial or superficial partial-thickness burns*
   a. Perform daily cool water lavage.
   b. Apply topical silver sulfadiazine cream.
3. *Deep partial-thickness and full-thickness burns*
   a. Perform daily wound debridement as directed by the attending veterinarian using conservative debridement or chemical debridement.
      i. Conservative debridement: Perform hydrotherapy using sterile saline lavage under light pressure or application of a wet-to-dry saline dressing under a light bandage for several hours, followed by removal of obvious necrotic or dead tissue using aseptic technique.
      ii. Enzymatic debridement: Apply a topical agent containing enzymes that degrade and loosen necrotic tissue.
4. *Protect burn wounds*
   a. Apply silver sulfadiazine cream, or other agent as directed by the attending veterinarian, in a thin layer directly on the wound.
   b. Apply a light protective bandage if the burn area is amenable to application.

sterile saline lavage under light pressure or application of a wet-to-dry saline dressing under a light bandage for several hours, followed by removal of obvious necrotic or dead tissue using aseptic technique.[1] Enzymatic debridement may be performed using a topical agent containing enzymes that degrade and loosen necrotic tissue. Surgical debridement may be necessary in very deep or widespread wounds to more aggressively remove necrotic tissue.

Topical medication and bandaging are the next steps in burn wound management. Following debridement, a topical agent is applied. The most commonly used agent is SSD cream. This agent has antimicrobial properties against a wide range of bacterial agents and limited fungal agents, and stimulates re-epithelialization of wounds. SSD is applied in a thin layer directly on the wound and either covered by a nonadherent dressing (if the wound area is bandaged) or left uncovered (if bandaging is not permissible due to wound size or location). Other agents used topically include aloe vera and unpasteurized honey. While there are some benefits to these products, SSD offers the simplest alternative and is recommended by these authors.

Burn wounds are generally bandaged if the burn area is amenable to application (i.e., the bandage can be placed without increasing patient discomfort, the burn area is relatively small, and the bandage will not increase the potential for wound injury). Any bandage applied must be applied correctly and not cause chafing or mechanical movement. If there is any doubt about whether to bandage a burn wound or not, it is better to leave the wound unbandaged. A brief discussion of bandage application is found in Protocol 62.5 below and the section in this chapter on managing open and necrotic wounds. In most cases, a wet-to-wet bandage is recommended to keep wounds moist and to improve comfort. Bandages must be changed at least daily; more frequent changes may be necessary if wound exudate is excessive or the bandage becomes soiled.

Superficial and superficial partial-thickness wounds generally heal within 3 weeks.[1] Deep partial-thickness and full-thickness burns generally require surgical closure at some point once a healthy granulation bed has formed. The timing of closure of open burn wounds depends on many factors (e.g., wound size and severity, wound location).

In summary, patients with burn wounds require intensive management, with utmost attention to minimizing contamination and supportive care. The keys to proper nursing care include daily wound care and bandaging, prevention of wound contamination and cross-contamination, adequate analgesia, and general supportive nursing care. The more severe the burn wound, the more intense the nursing care required, and the more likely that excellent nursing care will make the difference between positive outcome and failure.

Cold-induced injury

Cold-induced injuries include local or regional injuries (e.g., frostbite of an extremity) and generalized hypothermia (whole-body cold injury). Hypothermia is very common in veterinary practice. Frostbite, however, is uncommon in dogs and cats and tends to be related to geographic location (i.e., freezing climates) and use of the animal (e.g., as sled dogs).

Nonfreezing injuries

Nonfreezing injuries typically involve the extremities, occur despite the tissue not actually freezing, and are commonly due to prolonged cold exposure. In people, common terms to describe these types of injuries are "chillblains" and "immersion foot" or "trench foot"; similar terms are not used in veterinary medicine. With nonfreezing injuries, extremities (ear pinnae, paws, tail tip, scrotum) are exposed to cold temperatures above freezing for prolonged periods (>12 hours), causing intense erythema of the skin, pain, and pruritus. If skin is exposed to damp conditions or submerged and exposed to cold, tissue edema and maceration may also develop.

Management of nonfreezing cold injuries

Treatment of nonfreezing cold injuries involves removing the animal from the cold environment and passively warming the affected tissues slowly. Passive warming of nonfreezing injuries can be accomplished by moving the patient to a warm room (e.g., a hospital) and gently wrapping the patient or affected body part in warm blankets or towels.

Freezing injury

Freezing injury, or "frostbite," is the development of cold injury in which tissues actually become frozen, with crystallization (ice formation) of tissue and cell water. Frostbite is seen at environmental temperatures below 0°C (32°F) and primarily affects the distal extremities, ears, nose, scrotum, and tail. Frostbite varies in severity from superficial (1st degree frostbite) to deep injury (4th degree frostbite).

Clinical signs of freezing injury

Clinical signs of superficial frostbite (1st and 2nd degree frostbite) include a gray to white, waxy appearance of affected skin; blistering of affected skin may be present with 2nd degree frostbite. Clinical signs of deep frostbite (3rd and 4th degree frostbite) include involvement of the entire epidermis, but no subcutaneous tissues (3rd degree) to involvement of subcutaneous tissues, to possibly include muscle and bone (4th degree frostbite). Tissues affected with deep frostbite may be black and friable. In all cases of frostbite, pain may be intense, especially during rewarming of tissues.

Management of patients with freezing injury

(see Protocol 62.2)

Treatment of frostbite involves rapid warming of affected tissues, overall patient management (e.g., treatment of whole-body hypothermia, trauma, or shock as appropriate), analgesia, and protection of affected tissues.[3] Affected tissues may be warmed by immersion in a water bath that is 40–43°C (104–108°F) for at least 20 minutes or until thawing has occurred[3] or by wrapping the affected tissue with warm, wet towels for 15–20 minutes, changing the towels every 5 minutes. Do not use dry heat to warm tissues, and never rub or massage the tissues, as further injury may occur. Provide systemic analgesia, as frostbite is extremely painful. Protect the affected tissues by applying loose protective bandages, minimizing movement (confine to a cage), and

---

Protocol 62.2 Management of freezing injury (frostbite)

1. Treat whole-body hypothermia, trauma, or shock as directed by the attending veterinarian (see Protocol 62.3).
2. Provide systemic analgesia as directed by the attending veterinarian.
3. Warm frozen tissues gently and slowly, using one of two methods:
   a. Immerse in a water bath that is 40.3–42.6°C (104–108°F) for at least 20 minutes or until thawing has occurred.
   b. Wrap with warm, wet towels for 15–20 minutes, changing the towels every 5 minutes.
   c. Do not use dry heat or rub or massage tissues to warm tissues.
4. Protect affected tissues
   a. Apply loose protective bandages.
   b. Minimize movement (confine to a cage).
   c. Apply an Elizabethan collar to prevent self-trauma.
5. Aseptically aspirate large blisters that develop.
6. Manage open, infected, or necrotic wounds as described elsewhere in this text.

---

applying an Elizabethan collar to the patient to prevent self-trauma. In most cases, antibiotic use is not recommended.[3] Aseptically aspirate large blisters that develop.[3] In some cases, open wounds, infected wounds, or necrotic wounds may develop in tissue that was frostbitten.

Hypothermia

Hypothermia is defined as a core body temperature that is below normal, and is subdivided into primary and secondary hypothermia.[4] Core temperature refers to the temperature of the blood in the pulmonary artery, and is the "gold standard" for measurement of true body temperature. In veterinary patients, rectal or esophageal temperature measurements are more practical, even though they may be lower than core temperature in many instances. Primary hypothermia is caused by exposure to low environmental temperatures; secondary hypothermia has multifactorial causes, including low body temperature due to trauma, toxicity, underlying illness, anesthesia and surgery, and other factors. This differentiation is important, as patients with primary hypothermia can apparently tolerate much more severe hypothermia than patients with secondary hypothermia,[4] and adverse effects due to hypothermia have been reported in patients with secondary hypothermia at significantly closer-to-normal temperatures than patients with primary hypothermia.[4] Regardless of the type of hypothermia, the mechanisms that lead to hypothermia are excessive heat loss, decreased heat production, or both. According to a revised classification scheme,[4] primary hypothermia is classified as mild (32.5–37.5°C [90–99°F]), moderate (28.0–32.5°C [82–90°F]), severe (20.2–28.0°C [68–82°F]), or profound (<20.2°C [68°F]). Using this same scheme, secondary hypothermia is classified as mild (37.0–37.5°C [98–99.9°F]), moderate (35.8–37.0°C [96–98°F]), severe (33.6–35.8°C [92–96°F]), or profound (<33.6°C [92°F]).

Complications related to hypothermia

Hypothermia can cause many types of complications. The duration and severity of hypothermia, type of hypothermia (primary or secondary), and the patient's ability to adapt directly affect which complications develop and how severe those complications become. It is most important for the healthcare worker to recognize the potential problems rather than specific temperatures at which to expect these problems.

Glucose, electrolyte, and venous blood gas measurements should be performed at least every 6–12 hours initially. Hyperglycemia is common in mild and moderate hypothermia; specific measures to reduce blood sugar are seldom necessary. Hypoglycemia can develop in severely hypothermic patients, and dextrose supplementation may be necessary. Hypokalemia is common in mild to moderate hypothermia, and supplementation is necessary. Hyperkalemia is reported in severe hypothermia; specific measures may be necessary (e.g., insulin-dextrose administration, bicarbonate administration) if potassium is >7–8 mmol/L. Metabolic and respiratory acidosis are reported in most types and degrees of hypothermia; these typically correct with fluid therapy and patient warming.

Hemostatic defects are common. Patients are commonly in a hypocoagulable state with prolonged clotting times. Platelet abnormalities are also noted. Patients with mild hypothermia typically have increased platelet aggregation, whereas patients with severe hypothermia have decreased platelet aggregation. Serial platelet counts and coagulation testing should be performed on admission and every 6–12 hours after admission until patients are stable, to screen for abnormalities.

Tachycardia and hypertension are common in mild to moderate hypothermia. As hypothermia worsens, bradycardia and hypotension develop, and other cardiac arrhythmias may develop. For these reasons, continuous electrocardiography (ECG) and blood pressure monitoring is recommended until the patient is stabilized. It is recommended[3] to avoid giving drugs, to include anti-arrhythmic agents, until the body temperature is >30–

32°C (86–90.3°F), as drugs are believed ineffective at temperatures below this.

Technicians must be aware that measures to correct hypothermia can actually cause complications to develop, such as "afterdrop" and "rewarming shock";[4,5] thus, careful warming and close monitoring are essential when managing hypothermic patients. "Afterdrop" is the continued decrease in the patient's core temperature as warming is provided and is due to the return of cold peripheral blood to the central circulation. To prevent "afterdrop," it is important to warm the patient's trunk (chest and abdomen), not the extremities. "Rewarming shock" develops with excessively rapid warming and is due to the sudden development of systemic vasodilatation. This vasodilatation causes hypotension at a time when the circulatory system may not be able to react. The systemic hypotension is aggravated by the increased metabolic demand that develops as hypothermic patients are rewarmed, which increases the demand for perfusion. To prevent or reduce "rewarming shock," IV fluid therapy must be provided and assessment of volume status (e.g., serial body weight measurement, central venous pressure [CVP], clinical signs of hydration), systemic blood pressure, and tissue perfusion (e.g., evaluation of capillary refill time [CRT], lactate clearance, change in mentation, urine output) must be monitored carefully. Other possible problems associated with warming a hypothermic patient are due to changes in regional blood flow (e.g., development of cerebral edema, cerebral ischemia), reperfusion of tissue beds (e.g., development of systemic reperfusion injury, pancreatitis), and other factors (e.g., pneumonia, pulmonary edema, acute respiratory distress syndrome [ARDS]).[4]

Management of patients with hypothermia
(see Protocol 62.3)

Hypothermic patients must be warmed rapidly but carefully, and with anticipation for possible complications. Additionally, cardiovascular support (principally IV fluid therapy), management of coexisting problems, and prevention of rewarming complications are necessary.[5] The recommended rate of rewarming is to increase the core body temperature by 0.06–0.13°C (2–4°F) per hour.[4-6]

Rewarming can be by passive surface warming, active surface warming, active core warming, or a combination of these.[4] Passive surface warming involves the use of external wraps, typically blankets or towels, to prevent heat loss while the animal "self-generates" heat; this method is typically effective for patients with mild hypothermia and adequate blood volume. Active surface warming involves the use of externally applied heat

Protocol 62.3 Management of hypothermia

1. Warm rapidly but carefully.
    a. Increase the body temperature by 0.06–0.13°C (2–4°F) per hour.
    b. Warm to a temperature of 37.2°C (98.5°F) and then cease use of all warming methods except passive warming.

    Mild hypothermia, adequate blood volume: Warm using passive surface warming (wrap patient in blankets or towels; hospitalize in warm environment).
    Moderate-to-severe hypothermia; mild hypothermia with inadequate blood volume

    a. Warm using active surface warming (use of externally applied heat sources such as forced-air devices, warm water bottles, heating pads or lamps, or dryers).
    b. Apply heat to the thorax and abdomen, and not the extremities.
    c. Perform passive warming as above.

    Severe-to-profound hypothermia

    a. Warm using active core warming (heat inhaled air provided by endotracheal tube, warm peritoneal or pleural lavage, warm IV fluids, and urinary bladder and rectal lavage with warm fluids).
    b. Perform active and passive warming as above.
2. Provide cardiovascular support
    a. Provide IV fluids at relatively moderate rates (2–3 times maintenance rates, or 2–10 mL/kg/h) until normothermic.
    b. Once resuscitated and stabilized, provide continued IV fluids as directed by the attending veterinarian.
    c. Provide oxygen supplementation for severe to profound hypothermia to reduce risk of cardiac arrhythmias.
3. Anticipate and manage complications
    a. Perform continuous ECG monitoring, and treat arrhythmias as directed by the attending veterinarian, but do not treat until body temperature is 30–32°C (86–90.3°F).
    b. Monitor for glucose, electrolyte, and acid-base abnormalities every 6–12 hours.
    c. Monitor platelet count and coagulation parameters every 6–12 hours.
    d. Provide analgesia as directed by the attending veterinarian.
    e. Perform continuous or intermittent blood pressure monitoring, lactate clearance, continuous or intermittent CVP measurement, serial body weight, changes in mentation, and urine output to monitor for "rewarming shock."
    f. Perform continuous temperature measurement, to monitor for correction of hypothermia and "afterdrop."

sources, such as forced-air devices, warm water bottles, heating pads or lamps, or dryers, to provide heat to offset the patient's inability to generate heat; this method is recommended for patients with all types and severity of hypothermia. With active surface warming, especially in cats,[4] it is important to provide IV volume support to maintain normotension and to prevent shock. When using this method, apply heat to the thorax and abdomen, and not the extremities, as this avoids peripheral vasodilatation and prevents the decreased thermoregulatory response seen when extremities are warmed, both of which contribute to persistent hypothermia and "afterdrop."[4] Active core warming involves the more aggressive use of heat provided centrally to rapidly increase core temperature, using methods such as heating inhaled air provided by endotracheal tube, warm peritoneal or pleural lavage, warmed IV fluids, and urinary bladder and rectal lavage with warmed fluids. This method is typically reserved for severe or profound hypothermia; of these, warming IV fluids to no more than 42.6°C (108°F) is easy to do (run the IV administration set tubing through a bowl of warm water, microwave the bag of crystalloid fluid before use, or use commercial fluid warmers), effective, and least prone to complications. The temperature of IV fluids should not exceed 42.6°C (108°F) to avoid injury to cellular components of the peripheral blood. The current recommendation[4–6] is to warm hypothermic patients to a temperature of 37.2°C (98.5°F) and then cease use of all warming methods except passive warming, while providing blood volume support (i.e., IV fluids) at relatively moderate rates to avoid volume overload (10–15 mL/kg/h) that is possible in hypothermic patients being rewarmed.[4,6]

In summary, patients with cold-induced injuries require intensive management, with utmost attention to rapidly but carefully rewarming the patient while minimizing complications and providing supportive care. The keys to proper nursing care include targeted rewarming of the trunk, adequate IV fluid therapy, and intensive monitoring.

Heat-induced injury

Heat-induced injury, primarily seen in dogs, develops when there is an increase in core body temperature as a result of exertion, exposure to increased environmental temperature and humidity, or both. The subsequent hyperthermia exceeds the capability of the patient to compensate. There are three types of heat-induced injury based on the severity of the resulting injury. In people, these are described as heat cramps, heat exhaustion or prostration, and heat stroke. In veterinary patients, heat-induced injury is better described as being mild (heat stress), moderate (heat exhaustion), or severe (heat stroke).[6,7]

Classification of heat-induced injuries

Heat stress is characterized by development of excessive thirst, discomfort associated with physical activity, and sodium and chloride abnormalities, but with controlled panting (i.e., the patient can control or reduce panting when exposed to a noxious inhalant such as alcohol).[6] Generally, treatment of heat stress involves removing the patient from the source of heat, stopping exercise, and cooling by use of fans or movement to an air-conditioned area. Close monitoring for several hours is necessary to ensure heat stress does not progress and that rebound hypothermia does not develop. Key parameters to monitor, in addition to frequent body temperature measurement, include changes in mentation, development of petecchiae or ecchymoses, hematuria, weakness or collapse, clinical signs of shock (e.g., tachypnea, tachycardia, weak pulse quality, pale mucous membranes), and anxiety or restlessness.

Heat exhaustion is present when the signs of heat stress are present, as well as weakness, anxiety, and uncontrolled panting (i.e., the patient cannot reduce panting when exposed to a noxious inhalant).[6] Generally, treatment of heat exhaustion is the same as for heat stress, but more aggressive measures of cooling are often necessary. The patient must be removed from the source of heat and all activity must be stopped. Cooling by use of fans or movement to an air-conditioned area should be done if possible. The hallmark treatment for moderate and severe heat injuries is to thoroughly soak the hair coat to the skin to reduce core body temperature. Close monitoring for several hours as stated for heat stress is necessary to ensure heat exhaustion does not progress and that rebound hypothermia does not develop.

Heat stroke is present when signs of heat exhaustion are present, coupled with varying degrees of central nervous system (CNS) abnormalities (encephalopathy). The most common CNS abnormalities include changes in mentation and level of consciousness (e.g., obtunded, stupor, coma), seizures, abnormal pupil size, cortical blindness, head tremors, and ataxia.[7] Heat stroke is a life-threatening condition. It is characterized by a severe increase in core temperature and widespread, multiple organ injury with risk of progression to multiple organ dysfunction syndrome (MODS). No specific body temperature defines heat stroke in veterinary patients; however, temperatures as low as 41.3°C (105.8°F) have been associated with pathology.[8] Laboratory studies using animals have established that heat directly induces tissue injury and that the severity of tissue injury and

cell death is a function of the degree and duration of hyperthermia.[9] Veterinary technicians must be prepared to rapidly recognize and treat heat stroke, because the severity of organ injury related to heat injury is directly related to the length of time the patient is hyperthermic. Retrospective veterinary studies report multiple serious complications and high fatality rates in heat stroke patients despite proper treatment.[10] These cases are challenging and require intensive treatment and monitoring. With aggressive medical therapy and intensive nursing care, many of these patients will successfully recover.

Causes of heat stroke

Heat stroke can be caused by a rise in core body temperature due to physical activity or endogenous sources (exertional heat stroke) or due to exposure to increased ambient temperature or exogenous sources (classical or environmental heat stroke).[9] A retrospective study[10] conducted at a veterinary teaching hospital found large and brachycephalic breeds were more likely than smaller breeds to present for heat stroke. Additionally, the mean environmental temperature on the days when animals presented with heat stroke was significantly increased when compared with average temperatures.[10] In veterinary patients, the cause of heat stroke is often a combination of exertional and environmental factors, to include high ambient temperatures, confinement in unventilated or poorly ventilated areas, and high ambient humidity.

Fundamental management concepts

The paramount treatment objective is to decrease body temperature in a controlled way as quickly as possible and support the cardiovascular system. Poor outcomes result from prolonged hyperthermia.[11] Continuous core body temperature monitoring must be performed until body temperature has remained normal without temperature support for 2 hours. Thereafter, these authors recommend that temperature be measured continuously or at least every 4 hours. A myriad of concurrent problems may be present or develop; these must be anticipated and monitored for closely.[12]

Initial management considerations

Triage of the heat stroke patient is similar for other types of injury or illness, but with emphasis on assessing mentation, airway and breathing, circulation, and body temperature. Patients typically present with obtundation or stupor; however, heat stroke patients can be alert and responsive, stuporous, or comatose. Patients presenting in stupor or coma are in imminent danger of death. Some heat stroke patients present actively seizuring.[7]

The triaging technician should examine the airway by visual inspection if necessary, and evaluate inhalation and exhalation sounds at the upper and lower airway. The respiratory system is an important component in thermal regulation for two primary reasons: (1) exhaled gases are a source of heat loss, and (2) increases in the work of breathing can contribute to increased body temperature. A common source of hyperthermia is partial or intermittent airway obstruction. The obstruction can be due to anatomical conditions or foreign objects. Conditions such as elongated soft palate, stenotic nares, everted laryngeal saccules, narrow trachea, or laryngeal paralysis are predisposing factors to heat injury.[13]

Anticipate that in a state of hyperthermia, the patient's initial physiological response will be to move blood to the surface vessels to maximize conductive cooling. The initial phase will generally include renal and splanchnic vasoconstriction, peripheral vasodilatation, and an increased cardiac output.[14] Over time, if the body temperature remains high, splanchnic and renal vasoconstriction will eventually fail, creating conditions favorable for venous pooling and hypovolemia or distributive shock.[13] Staff should monitor continuous ECG, blood pressure, mucous membrane color, and capillary refill time. Any abnormalities should be reported to the attending veterinarian immediately.

Although pulmonary artery temperature measurement is the gold standard for evaluating core body temperature, rectal temperature compares well and can be performed with little risk or expense. Note that rectal temperature may lag behind core body temperature by up to 15 minutes.[15] Heat stroke patients may therefore be hypothermic, hyperthermic, or normothermic on presentation, based on cooling measures initiated by the owner or handler and length of time since onset of heat stroke.[7]

Emergency management of hyperthermic patients (see Protocol 62.4)

Emergency interventions must be performed immediately to optimize outcome.[6,12] If the patient is apneic or is not breathing adequately, the patient must be intubated and intermittent manual or mechanical positive pressure ventilation provided.[16] It is important to note that if the patient is intubated, the airway must be protected during the cooling phase, as an open endotracheal tube presents a route for aspiration of running water. Supplemental oxygen therapy is necessary by routine means until normoxemia is confirmed with the patient breathing room air. The method of oxygen delivery used should not interfere with cooling efforts during the initial phase of care. Oxygen cages and oxygen masks can create increased humidity and prevent maximal heat dissipation. Nasal oxygen delivery methods are often most successful.

Patients presenting with heat stroke with a rectal temperature >40.9°C (105°F) require emergency cooling measures. Numerous cooling methods are described in human and veterinary literature; no one technique has been shown to be superior or ideal.[8] In many cases, a combination of cooling methods is necessary. The rate of cooling should be as rapid as possible until the body temperature is 40.9°C (105°F).[6] The most practical, most expedient, and most rapid method to reduce body temperature is to soak the patient to the skin with room-temperature ("tepid") water.[7] The patient can be placed under running tepid water in a well-drained tub or run or submerged partially in a tub of tepid water. The key is to soak the entire patient as rapidly as possible, and to soak through the hair coat to soak the skin thoroughly.

The value of IV fluids in patient cooling and support cannot be overstated. Unless there are specific contraindications, IV fluid therapy using room-temperature fluids should be initiated for all heat stroke patients.[7] For conduction to maximize heat dissipation, adequate circulating blood and plasma volume are required.[9] Additionally, IV administration of room-temperature fluids reduces core body temperature.

Additional cooling methods can be used to supplement wetting the skin thoroughly and using room-temperature IV fluids. Fans can be directed on the patient to facilitate surface cooling, remembering that it is essential that the skin be thoroughly wet for fans to be effective. Further, to effectively use conduction to dissipate heat from the patient, the ambient temperature of the treatment room should be reduced to maximize the temperature gradient between ambient environment and body.[9] In most instances, however, this is not practical in a timely manner. Finally, some human studies suggest that cooling of carotid arteries (e.g., by ice packs placed over the neck) induces vasodilatation, which may increase cerebral perfusion.[18] Future veterinary studies may reveal positive therapeutic modalities that include advanced brain hypothermia.

Note that cold IV fluids, ice-water baths, and surface cooling with ice water or ice packs are contraindicated because they cause peripheral vasoconstriction with sustained increase in core temperature; cause shivering, generates more internal heat; and promote capillary sludging, which contributes to coagulopathy. Similarly, placing isopropyl alcohol on the footpads is commonly done, but is generally ineffective because the paw pads have such a small surface area. Wetting a large percentage of the pet's surface area to the skin with alcohol is required for adequate cooling, which, while potentially increasing conductive heat dissipation and

Protocol 62.4 Management of heat-induced injury

1. Triage the patient as for other types of injury or illness: carefully assess mentation, airway and breathing, circulation, and body temperature.
   a. Establish and protect the airway if apneic.
   b. Provide supplemental oxygen therapy.
   c. Establish at least one IV catheter and resuscitate from shock and persistent hypotension.
2. Emergently cool the patient if rectal temperature is >40.9°C (105°F), cooling as rapidly as possible until the body temperature is 40.9°C (105°F).
   a. Soak the patient to the skin with copious amounts of room-temperature ("tepid") water.
   b. Administer room-temperature IV fluids at rates necessary to combat shock or persistent hypotension.
   c. Direct fans on the patient to facilitate surface cooling.
   d. Reduce the room temperature, if possible.
   e. Do *not* use cold IV fluids, ice-water baths, or surface cooling with ice water or ice packs.
3. Reduce the rate of cooling once the patient's body temperature is <40.9°C (105°F) to avoid rebound hypothermia.
   a. Cease cooling with water and dry the hair/skin.
   b. Remove fans.
   c. Return room temperature to normal.
4. Provide supportive warming once the patient's temperature has been reduced to 39.8°C (103°F).
   a. All active cooling efforts must cease.
   b. Continue temperature monitoring.
   c. Actively warm the patient to prevent rebound hypothermia if temperature is at or below 38°C (100°F).
5. Monitor for and treat concurrent problems.
   a. Monitor blood pressures, lactate clearance, urine output, mentation, and other measures of perfusion to check for shock hypotension. Continue IV fluid therapy as directed by the attending veterinarian.
   b. Monitor blood glucose and venous blood gas analyses every 6–12 hours. Maintain normoglycemia with supplemental dextrose.
   c. Monitor arterial blood gas analysis or pulse oximetry and capnography to assess oxygenation and ventilation. IV fluids should be supplemented with dextrose as needed to maintain normoglycemia.
   d. Monitor for occult or active bleeding and petecchiae and ecchymoses; perform coagulation tests every 6–12 hours and serial CBCs every 12–24 hours to screen for thrombocytopenia and coagulopathies.
   e. Monitor the ECG continuously to detect cardiac arrhythmias, especially ventricular arrhythmias. Provide specific anti-arrhythmic therapy as directed for hemodynamically unstable patients.
   f. Monitor for vomiting and diarrhea, provide excellent nursing care to maintain patient hygiene, provide gastro-intestinal protectants as directed, and provide enteral or parenteral nutrition as directed.
   g. Monitor urine output hourly and assess creatinine every 12–24 hours. Place and maintain urethral catheters as directed.
   h. Monitor respiratory rate hourly, perform thoracic auscultation at least every 4 hours, and perform thoracic radiographs if pulmonary edema or other abnormalities are suspected. Perform arterial blood gas analysis or pulse oximetry and capnography every 4–6 hours initially, then as needed, to assess oxygenation and ventilation. Consider mechanical ventilation if the patient cannot oxygenate or ventilate adequately.
   i. Monitor mentation and level of consciousness, vision, gait, and postural responses, and monitor for seizures.

promoting evaporative cooling, is not worth the risk of combustion.[7]

Once the patient's body temperature is <40.9°C (105°F), the rate of cooling can be reduced to avoid rebound hypothermia. Ancillary cooling measures can be removed (e.g., remove fans, return room temperature to normal), and the patient's skin can be dried. Supportive warming is necessary once the patient's temperature has been reduced to 39.8°C (103°F). At this point, all cooling efforts must cease, continuous temperature monitoring must continue, and the attending technician should be prepared to actively warm the patient to prevent an excessive drop in body temperature ("rebound hypothermia") from aggressive cooling measures.[13] Although warming a patient with a temperature of 39.8°C (103°F) may seem counterintuitive, the nursing team should anticipate a period of rebound hypothermia. Additionally, the delay between rectal temperature and true core temperature probably means that the true core temperature may be lower.[15]

Monitor for and treat concurrent problems

Patients with heat stroke often present in shock and may develop sustained hypotension. IV fluid therapy should be continued not only to cool the patient but also to maintain adequate tissue perfusion. In some cases, fresh-frozen plasma or albumin transfusions may be indicated to treat concurrent problems such as disseminated intravascular coagulation or hypoalbuminemia. Continuous or intermittent blood pressure measurement, lactate clearance, clinical assessment of perfusion, and assessment of volume status should be monitored over time.

Glucose, acid-base, and electrolyte abnormalities are common, due to shock and reduced tissue perfusion. Blood glucose measurement and venous blood gas analyses, to include measurement of blood lactate concentration, are necessary, generally at intervals of every 6–12 hours, depending on the severity of the derangements. If concurrent pulmonary abnormalities are present, arterial blood gas analysis (or surrogates such as pulse oximetry and capnography) may be necessary to optimally assess oxygenation and ventilation. IV fluids should be supplemented with dextrose as needed to maintain normoglycemia.

Heat stroke patients are at an increased risk for developing hypercoagulable and consumptive coagulopathic states (e.g., disseminated intravascular coagulation [DIC]).[7] Thus, the technician should be prepared to run the full spectrum of coagulation testing.[8] In many cases, thrombocytopenia will develop in the first 24 hours; technicians should observe for clinical signs of this (e.g., petecchiae, ecchymoses) as well as perform serial complete blood counts (CBCs) at least daily. Additionally, careful monitoring for signs of clotting abnormalities (e.g., hematoma formation, intracavitary bleeding, epistaxis, hematuria) is necessary throughout the hospital stay,[17] and coagulation testing should be considered every 6–12 hours until the patient is stabilized. It is common for these patients to receive blood component therapy.[8]

Heat stroke patients are at increased risk for development of cardiac arrhythmias, especially ventricular arrhythmias. Continuous or intermittent ECG monitoring is necessary to identify arrhythmias. Specific anti-arrhythmic therapy may be indicated if the patient develops hemodynamic instability due to the arrhythmia.

Patients suffering from heat stroke often will have concurrent vomiting and diarrhea. In some cases, the diarrhea will be hemorrhagic.[8] Hemorrhagic diarrhea is common and can create husbandry challenges. Hygiene is critical, and bedding should be changed as needed, long hair shaved, tails wrapped, and patients bathed. Gastrointestinal protection agents may be administered.[17] Nutritional support may be necessary during the hospital stay, to include enteral or parenteral feeding.[8]

Renal insufficiency may develop. The full spectrum of urine laboratory testing will probably be ordered. The technician should anticipate placing a urinary catheter with a closed collection system to monitor adequacy of urine output. Urine production should be maintained at 1–2 mL/kg/hour. If the patient fails to produce urine at target rates, the veterinarian should be notified.[7]

As heat stroke often induces multiple organ dysfunction syndrome (MODS), careful monitoring of the respiratory system is necessary. During initial resuscitation and for the next 12 hours, the respiratory rate should be monitored hourly, thoracic auscultation should be performed at least every 4 hours, and thoracic radiographs should be performed if pulmonary edema is suspected. Arterial blood gas analysis or surrogates should be performed as needed to assess oxygenation and ventilation, as discussed above. Mechanical ventilation may be necessary if the patient cannot oxygenate or ventilate adequately.

Generally, CNS abnormalities resolve with mild or moderate cases of heat stroke. However, severe heat stroke may cause cerebral edema and necrosis, and thus careful monitoring is necessary. Cortical blindness usually resolves, but may take several days. Persistence of altered mentation, ataxia, tremors, or seizures strongly suggest increased intracranial pressure; specific therapy may be necessary (e.g., mannitol infusion).

In summary, patients with heat injury require intensive management, with utmost attention to rapid reduction in body temperature. The keys to proper nursing care include rapid targeted temperature reduction using thorough soaking of the skin with tepid water, cessation of cooling measures at an appropriate temperature to prevent rebound hypothermia, and intensive monitoring and supportive care to minimize development of myriad potential complications.

Open wounds/necrotic tissue

Patients with wounds are frequently presented for veterinary care. Wounds commonly result from animal bites, motor vehicle trauma, or other trauma. In most cases, traumatic wounds can be classified as contaminated or dirty/infected wounds; the difference is based on how long the wound existed before presentation. Contaminated wounds generally are considered those <6 hours old, and dirty/infected wounds are considered those >6 hours old and generally with obvious exudates or infection.[19] Wounds are often noted in conjunction with potentially life-threatening injuries; thus, in all patients presenting with wounds, a detailed systematic triage examination and a careful search for—and management of—more severe concurrent injuries must take precedence over management of wounds. In all instances, wound care follows resuscitation and stabilization of the patient.

Considerations in wound management

The primary goal in wound management is to create a healthy wound bed, one that has adequate blood supply to support repair, and without contamination or necrotic tissue that will impede healing and increase the risk of infection.[19,20] Unless simple and small, many wounds will require frequent evaluation, generally at least once daily, based on location, extent, severity, and other factors. Many wounds will need to be managed as open wounds (although protected by bandages until smaller) before definitive surgical repair. The steps in daily wound evaluation are to assess the response to or need for antibiotics, debride dying or necrotic tissues and lavage the wound, assess for surgical closure, and protect the wound.[19]

Initial wound management recommendations[19,20] (see Protocol 62.5)

Provide effective analgesia or anesthesia based on wound severity, location, and other factors. Apply sterile

---

Protocol 62.5 Management of open or necrotic wounds

1. Triage the patient first for life-threatening problems.
   a. Provide appropriate resuscitation and stabilization before focusing on wounds.
   b. Apply direct pressure followed by a temporary pressure bandage to stop active hemorrhage at wound sites.
2. Manage potential local and systemic infection.
   a. Collect and submit samples for microbial culture and sensitivity testing, preferably before antibiotic therapy is started.
   b. Initiate antibiotic therapy as directed by the attending veterinarian within the first 6 hours of the wound's development, or as soon as possible thereafter.
   c. Culture the wound if obvious infection develops during any phase of wound management, if the wound fails to heal normally, or if systemic signs of infection develop.
3. Provide initial wound management.
   a. Provide effective analgesia or anesthesia based on wound severity, location, and other factors, as directed by the attending veterinarian.
   b. Apply sterile water-soluble lubricant to the wound bed and then clip the hair generously around the wound.
   c. Gently cleanse the skin around the wound, but not the wound bed, with surgical scrub.
   d. Gently lavage the lubricant and gross contaminants from the wound using sterile saline or lactated Ringer's solution (LRS).
   e. Debride grossly necrotic tissues and nonviable tissue carefully using aseptic technique and sharp dissection in accordance with hospital policy.
      i. Do not mass ligate tissues or use cautery excessively.
      ii. Do not damage, transect, or ligate major blood vessels (unless actively hemorrhaging) or nerves, as these are crucial to maintain effective blood flow and innervation distally.
   f. Lavage the wound to remove particulate debris and reduce bacterial contamination.
      i. Thoroughly lavage the wound bed with at least 1 L for this final lavage
      ii. Lavage under pressure, using a lavage pressure of 7–8 mmHg: use a 16-gauge hypodermic needle attached to an IV administration set attached to a 1 L bag of saline pressurized to 300 mmHg using a pressure cuff.
   g. Bandage the wound.
      i. Apply a primary layer to provide mechanical debridement initially, using a wet-to-dry bandage, consisting of sterile gauze sponges saturated with sterile saline, gently wrung to eliminate excessive moisture, and applied directly to the wound.
      ii. Apply several dry gauze sponges over the primary layer.
      iii. Apply a secondary layer over the primary layer, using cast padding or roll cotton +/- splints to provide support.
      iv. Apply a tertiary layer of nonadherent conforming bandage (e.g., VetWrap®), adhesive bandage (e.g., Elastikon®), or both, using light compression.
4. Provide daily wound care, using appropriate analgesia, sedation, or anesthesia.
   a. Change bandages at least once daily, but more frequently if heavy discharge is present or the bandage is soiled or partially removed by the patient.
   b. Lavage the wound as above at every bandage change.
   c. Debride the wound as above at every bandage change.
   d. Apply a new bandage as above; however, change the primary layer to a nonadherent dressing once a healthy granulation bed is formed.

water-soluble lubricant to the wound bed and then clip the hair generously around the wound. Gently cleanse the skin around the wound, but not the wound bed, with surgical scrub. Gently lavage the lubricant and gross contaminants from the wound using sterile saline or lactated Ringer's solution (LRS); do not use tap water except in very grossly contaminated wounds with large amounts of debris, in which case it may be more expedient to flush the wound with warm water under gentle pressure initially. The goal of this initial lavage is to remove gross contaminants and reduce the bacterial burden.

The next step is to debride grossly necrotic tissues and nonviable tissue carefully using aseptic technique and sharp dissection in accordance with hospital policy. Do not mass ligate tissues or use cautery excessively, as this usually leads to necrosis of these tissues and serves as a bed for infection. Use caution not to damage, transect, or ligate major blood vessels (unless actively hemorrhaging) or nerves, as these are crucial to maintain effective blood flow and innervation distally.

Lavage of the wound is necessary to remove particulate debris and reduce bacterial contamination. Thoroughly lavage the wound bed with copious amounts of sterile saline or LRS; use at least 1 L for this final lavage—remember the adage, "The solution to pollution is dilution." Use lavage under pressure. Most authors recommend a that a lavage pressure of 7–8 mmHg be used; less pressure will not allow adequate lavage, and greater pressure drives bacteria into deeper spaces and causes tissue disruption and edema that may impede healing.[21] Commercially available lavage devices are available. However, a simple device that has been shown to generate the ideal pressure uses a 16-gauge hypodermic needle attached to an IV administration set attached to a 1 L bag of saline pressurized to 300 mmHg using a pressure cuff.[21] Other techniques commonly used (syringes and needles, lavage bottles and needles) have actually been shown to either generate too little or too much pressure, and should not be used.[21] The use of antibiotics or disinfectants in the lavage solution is controversial; follow hospital policy as to whether or not to add these agents and concentrations to be used if added. In most cases, simple saline or LRS lavage is most important.

Bandaging recommendations

In nearly all cases, open wounds should be bandaged[19] to protect the wound from contamination and support the wound while it heals. The primary layer is the dressing that actually contacts the open wound. When mechanical debridement is desired (i.e., in most wounds after initial management has been performed, with varying degrees of contamination or infection), an adherent dressing is used. Once a healthy granulation bed has formed, convert to a nonadherent dressing. The most common adherent dressing is a wet-to-dry bandage, consisting of sterile gauze sponges that are saturated with sterile saline, gently wrung to eliminate excessive moisture, and then applied directly to the wound. Over the wet dressing, several dry gauze sponges are applied. In large wounds, laparotomy sponges may be optimal to cover more wound bed. The dry gauze "wicks" moisture and contaminants and exudate from the wound while the moist gauze provides some debridement by the mechanical action of the gauze on the wound bed. The most common nonadherent dressing is a semi-occlusive cotton pad (e.g., Telfa®, Kendall Healthcare) that retains moisture against the wound bed and wicks exudate from the surface of the wound. The attending veterinarian will direct use of topical medications on the wound bed. Commonly used agents include SSD ointment or triple-antibiotic ointment. Sugar and honey have been used in grossly contaminated wounds with positive effects.[20]

The secondary layer is applied over the primary layer. Most commonly, rolled cast padding or roll cotton is used to provide support. Splints can be included in the secondary layer, if used. The tertiary layer typically consists of nonadherent conforming bandage (e.g., VetWrap®, 3M, St. Paul, MN), adhesive bandage (e.g., Elastikon®, Johnson & Johnson, New Brunswick, NJ), or both. This layer holds the dressing and secondary layer in place, provides additional support, and provides more durable protection of the underlying layers. In most cases, the tertiary layer is applied just tight enough to hold the bandage in place, and without compression.

After initial placement, bandages are changed at least once daily. More frequent bandage changes may be necessary if the wound has a heavy discharge or the bandage becomes soiled or partially removed by the patient. Once wound discharge is reduced and a healthy granulation bed has formed, bandage changes become less frequent, generally every 2–3 days.

Antibiotic use in patients with open or necrotic wounds

Systemic antibiotic use will be at the discretion of the attending veterinarian. In many cases of contaminated wounds, with proper management, the wound can be converted to clean-contaminated, and systemic antibiotics may not be indicated. In most cases of dirty/infected wounds, antibiotics are clearly indicated for several days. Wound cultures are indicated at admission if the patient presents with a dirty/infected wound, if obvious infection develops during any phase of wound management, if the wound fails to heal normally, or if systemic signs of infection develop.

In summary, patients with open or necrotic wounds require careful management, especially during initial wound care. The keys to proper nursing care include thorough wound lavage, removal of gross contaminants, microbial culture and sensitivity, appropriate antibiotic use, and wound protection using carefully applied bandages. Daily wound care and debridement are critical to the long-term wound healing, and are the key areas where excellent nursing care will make the difference between positive outcome and failure.

Open fractures

Fractured bones and dislocated joints are generally not considered life-threatening emergencies. However, open fractures, in which the skin and subcutaneous tissues overlying a fracture are injured and expose fracture ends and fragments to external contamination, pose a very real risk of increasing morbidity and mortality because they provide access to microbial organisms that can cause local infection (i.e., osteomyelitis, cellulitis) and serve as a nidus of infection for systemic infection. Thus, proper management of open fractures is an important part of the overall management of trauma patients. Early and proper management of open fractures is critical, and open fractures should be treated as a medical emergency, once more pressing problems are addressed.

Causes of open fractures

The majority of open fractures are caused by motor vehicle trauma. However, gunshot injury, entrapment injury, and blunt trauma from non-motor vehicle causes are also common. It is important to recognize that the forces involved in trauma that cause fractures are intense, and probably have caused trauma to more-critical organ systems. Thus, addressing the overall patient for life-threatening injuries takes precedence over open fractures.

Initial nursing interventions

(see Protocol 62.6)

Technicians must address life-threatening problems first, using the standard approach to trauma management presented elsewhere. While fractures, especially open fractures, are generally obvious and attract intense attention, skilled technicians will focus on the "ABCs" of initial trauma patient management. While evaluating the entire patient and initiating life-saving therapy, it is wise to protect the open fracture site, as follows.[22] Do not attempt to reduce bone(s) protruding at fracture

---

Protocol 62.6 Management of open fractures

1. Address life-threatening problems first!
   a. Use a standardized approach to trauma management.
   b. Focus on the "ABCs" of initial trauma patient management.
   c. Protect the open fracture site.
      i. Do not attempt to reduce bone(s) protruding at the fracture site.
      ii. Remove any large gross contaminants from the wound (e.g., leaves, rocks, stick fragments), but do not attempt to clip the hair or cleanse the wound at this point.
      iii. Cover the fracture and wound with sterile nonadherent dressing and apply a light bandage.
2. Prevent bacterial infection, provide analgesia, and promote normal healing pending surgical fracture repair.
   a. Culture open fracture sites as soon as possible after presentation and before antibiotic use if possible.
   b. Administer antibiotics as directed by the attending veterinarian.
   c. Never withhold antibiotic therapy in any patient with an open fracture.
   d. Provide appropriate analgesia; reassess pain every 4–6 hours using a pain scoring system.
   e. Manage soft tissue injuries over the fracture site appropriately (see Protocol 62.5).
3. Manage orthopedic injuries.
   a. Immobilize the fracture if directed to do so, to minimize pain, improve function, and prevent further injury to the neurovascular bundle and bone. Use a spoon splint, lateral plastic splint, or Robert-Jones bandage.
   b. If an immobilizing device is not applied, apply a sterile wet-to-dry bandage to open fractures (see Protocol 62.5). Change bandages at least once daily, based on degree of strike-through, soiling, or loosening.
4. Monitor patients with open fractures.
   a. Focus on the overall status of the patient.
   b. Recognize common complications due to open fractures.
      i. Assess pain frequently and provide appropriate analgesia.
      ii. Base continued antibiotic use on the initial culture and sensitivity results.
      iii. Monitor the open fracture site at least daily for evidence of local infection, and monitor the patient frequently for evidence of systemic infection.
      iv. Assess adequacy of immobilization, if applied, and monitor for complications of immobilizing devices (e.g., chafing, distal swelling, pain, skin wounds, tissue maceration).

sites, as this "drags" contamination to the fracture site and may cause injury to the neurovascular bundle. Immediately remove any large gross contaminants from the wound (e.g., leaves, rocks, stick fragments), but do not attempt to clip the hair or cleanse the wound at this point. Cover the fracture and wound with sterile non-adherent dressing and apply a light bandage. This bandage should not be placed in an attempt to stabilize or immobilize the fracture at this time; it is simply to protect the open wounds and exposed bone from further contamination during initial patient resuscitation.

Specific management recommendations for open fractures

Patients with open fractures generally will require surgical correction of the fracture, either on site or after referral for definitive care. Either way, the specific management recommendations are the same, as follows,[20,22] with the overriding aims to prevent bacterial infection and promote normal healing. Culture open fracture sites as soon as possible after presentation and before antibiotic use if possible. Studies have shown that the majority of open fractures are infected on admission and that in the majority of cases, the organism cultured on admission is the same organism involved in later infections.[22] Administer antibiotics as directed, focusing on use of IV antibiotics based on likely contaminants. Never withhold antibiotic therapy in any patient with an open fracture. Address pain with appropriate analgesic therapy (often initiated at presentation); reassess pain every 4–6 hours using a pain scoring system. Manage soft tissue injuries over the fracture site appropriately, as proper management of the wound contributes to a successful outcome. Follow the recommendations provided earlier in this chapter for wounds and necrotic tissue. Manage orthopedic injuries. Once the wound has been treated, the focus shifts to management of the actual fracture.

In most situations, immediate definitive fracture repair will be delayed until the patient is stabilized and/or transferred for definitive repair. If possible, immobilize the fracture to minimize pain, improve function, and prevent further injury to the neurovascular bundle and bone. Several options are available, including the use of spoon splints, lateral plastic splints, or Robert-Jones bandages. Follow hospital policy and directions of the attending veterinarian as to whether to apply some type of immobilizing device. In most cases, it is better to leave the fracture alone rather than to incorrectly apply an immobilizing device. If an immobilizing device is not applied, apply a sterile wet-to-dry bandage to open fractures, as described earlier in this chapter. Always use a wet dressing over open fractures, as it is important to keep soft tissues and bones

moist for optimal healing. Change bandages at least once daily, based on degree of strike-through, soiling, or loosening.

Monitoring of patients with open fractures

Monitor the patient, focusing on the overall status of the patient. Specific monitoring related to the open fracture involves recognizing common complications due to open fractures. Assess pain frequently and provide appropriate analgesia. Base continued antibiotic use on the initial culture and sensitivity results. Monitor the open fracture site at least daily for evidence of local infection, and monitor the patient frequently for evidence of systemic infection. Assess adequacy of immobilization, if applied, and monitor for complications of immobilizing devices (e.g., chafing, distal swelling, pain, skin wounds, tissue maceration).

In summary, patients with open fractures require careful management, with utmost attention to identifying and treating life-threatening problems first. The keys to proper nursing care include protecting the wound and immobilizing the fracture initially, followed by appropriate antibiotic therapy, effective analgesia, daily wound care, fracture immobilization if appropriate, and supportive care pending definitive fracture repair.

References

1. Garzotto CK. Thermal burn injuries. In: Silverstein DC, Hopper K, eds. Small Animal Critical Care Medicine. St. Louis, MO: Saunders/Elsevier, 2009:683–686.
2. Mathews K. Burn injury and smoke inhalation. In: Mathews K, ed. Veterinary Emergency and Critical Care Manual. Guelph, Ontario, Canada: Lifelearn, 2006:682–689.
3. Mathews K. Accidental hypothermia. In: Mathews K, ed. Veterinary Emergency and Critical Care Manual. Guelph, Ontario, Canada: Lifelearn, 2006:291–296.
4. Oncken AK, Kirby R, Rudloff E. Hypothermia in critically ill dogs and cats. Comp Cont Edu Pract Vet 2001;23:506–521.
5. Todd J, Powell LL. Hypothermia. In: Silverstein DC, Hopper K, eds. Small Animal Critical Care Medicine. St. Louis, MO: Saunders/Elsevier, 2009:720–722.
6. Mathews K. Hyperthermia, heat stroke, malignant hyperthermia. In: Mathews K, ed. Veterinary Emergency and Critical Care Manual. Guelph, Ontario, Canada: Lifelearn, 2006:297–303.
7. Drobatz KJ. Heat stroke. In: Silverstein DC, Hopper K, eds. Small Animal Critical Care Medicine. St. Louis, MO: Saunders/Elsevier, 2009:723–726.
8. Smarick SD. Heatstroke: keeping them alive. In Proceedings. 14th Int Vet Emerg Crit Care Symp 2009:167–170.
9. Bouchama A, Dehbi M, Chaves-Carballo E. Cooling and hemodynamic management in heatstroke: practical recommendations. Critical Care [serial online]. 05/12/07;11 (issue 3):R54. Available at: www.ccforum.com/content/11/3/R54. Accessed May 15, 2010.
10. Bruchim Y, Klement E, Saragusty J, et al. Heat stroke in dogs: a retrospective study of 54 cases (1999–2004) and analysis of risk factors for death. J Vet Intern Med 2008;1:38–46.

11. Harker J, Gibson P. Heat-stroke: a review of rapid cooling techniques. Intensive Crit Care Nursing 1995;11:198–202.

12. Flournoy WS, Macintire DK, Wohl JS. Heat stroke in dogs: clinical signs, treatment, prognosis, and prevention. Comp Cont Edu Pract Vet 2003;25:422–431.

13. Tabor B. Heatstroke in dogs. *Vet Tech* 2007;28. Available at: www.vettechjournal.com. Accessed May 31, 2010.

14. Casa DJ. Exercise in heat. I. fundamentals of thermal physiology, performance implications, and dehydration. J Athlet Train 1999;34: 246–252.

15. Hoedemaekers CW, Ezzahti M, Gerritsen M, et al. (2007) Comparison of cooling methods to induce and maintain normo- and hypothermia in intensive care unit patients: a prospective intervention study. *Critical Care* [serial online]. 08/24/07;11 (issue 4):R91. Available at: www.ccforum.com/content/11/R91. Accessed May 15, 2010.

16. Shawver D, Battaglia A. Mechanical ventilation. In: Battaglia A, ed. Small Animal Emergency and Critical Care: A Manual for the Veterinary Technician. Ithaca, NY: WB Saunders Co, 2000: 100–107.

17. McMichael M. Heatstroke. In: Cann CC, Hunsberger S, eds. Handbook of Veterinary Emergency Protocols: Dog and Cat. Jackson, WY: Teton NewMedia, 2008:228–230.

18. Thulesius O. Thermal reactions of blood vessels in vascular stroke and heatstroke. Med Principles Practice 2006;15:316–321.

19. Garzotto CK. Wound management. In: Silverstein DC, Hopper K, eds. Small Animal Critical Care Medicine. St. Louis, MO: Saunders/Elsevier, 2009:676–682.

20. Halling K. Wounds and open fractures. In: Mathews K, ed. Veterinary Emergency and Critical Care Manual. Guelph, Ontario, Canada: Lifelearn, 2006;702–708.

21. Gall TT and Monnet E. Evaluation of fluid pressures of common wound-flushing techniques. Am J Vet Res 2010;71: 1384–1386.

22. Tillson MD. Open fracture management. Vet Clin North Am Small Anim Pract 1995;1093–1110.

63

Safe handling and care of patients exposed to radioactive and antineoplastic agents

Michael S. Kent and Paul Primas

The safe handling and care of patients exposed to either radioactive or chemotherapeutic agents is essential. These patients present a particular challenge in that they may need extensive and intensive nursing care and have the potential to endanger the very people providing that care if proper precautions are not taken. Further, how to best protect oneself is not always straightforward. Multiple studies have shown that improper handling of the agents and patients treated can result in exposure of the nursing staff. This can carry a serious health risk for caregivers. In order to decrease this risk, procedures and protocols should be established at each practice using or caring for patients exposed to these agents. It is important that staff at each facility have knowledge of federal, state, and local regulations when developing such a plan. Exposure to these agents can occur during chemotherapy drug or radiopharmaceutical preparation or administration, or when handling an exposed or treated patient or waste from that patient. Limiting contamination of areas where drugs are stored and prepared and where these patients are treated and cared for is essential in maintaining a safe work environment. General radiation safety is also extremely important when using radiation to diagnose or treat patients; this includes the use of diagnostic x-ray machines. This chapter is divided into two parts covering radiation and chemotherapy safety.

Radiation

Definitions and terms

Radiation is energy that travels as waves or in the form of high energy particles. Radiation is only damaging to cells if it is ionizing, meaning that it has the ability to break bonds or liberate bound electrons from molecules within cells. X-rays, beta particles, gamma rays, electrons, and photons are all different types of ionizing radiation that are used in veterinary medicine for diagnostic and therapeutic purposes.

The unit of absorbed dose for radiation is the gray (Gy), which is defined as joule/kg. This unit does not take into account the biological damage potential, which varies with different types of radiation. For example, 10 Gy of alpha particles or neutrons will cause more severe damage to cells than will 10 Gy of electromagnetic radiation. To help account for this variability, units of rem (roentgen equivalent in man) or sieverts (Sv; 1 Sv = 100 rem) are used. These units of absorbed dose take into account a factor assigned to different types of radiation based on the severity of their biological effects on humans.

The curie (Ci) and the bequerel (Bq) are units of activity for a radioactive substance. A bequerel is the SI unit for radioactivity and is defined as 1 disintegration/second. The curie is defined as the approximate activity of 1 gram of the isotope ^{226}Ra (radium) and is equal to 3.7×10^{10} disintegrations/second. Generally, mCi doses of a radiopharmaceutical are used for imaging or therapeutic purposes.

Dose limits

The Nuclear Regulatory Commission (NRC) is the body charged with regulating nuclear materials used for medical reasons within the United States.[1] By special agreement with contract states, licensing a facility to use

---

Advanced Monitoring and Procedures for Small Animal Emergency and Critical Care, First Edition. Edited by Jamie M. Burkitt Creedon, Harold Davis.
© 2012 John Wiley & Sons, Inc. Published 2012 by John Wiley & Sons, Inc.

Table 63.1 Annual dose limits for whole body exposure (adapted from NRC Regulations [10 CFR] PART 20, Standards for protection against radiation)

Adult: occupation dose limit	5 rems (0.05 Sv)
Member of the public	0.1 rem (1 mSv)
Minors (under 18 years of age): occupational dose limit	0.5 rems (0.005 Sv)
Embryos/fetus: for mother who is a radiation worker	0.5 rem (5 mSv) over term of pregnancy

Table 63.2 Commonly used radiopharmaceuticals used in veterinary medicine and their corresponding half-lives

Radionucleotide	Approximate Physical Half-life ($t^{1/2}$)
Technesium-99M (^{99m}Tc)	6 hours
Iodine 125 (^{125}I)	59 days
Iodine 131 (^{131}I)	8 days
Samarium 153 (^{153}Sm)	1.93 days

radioactive substances may also be delegated to the state government. The NRC has set maximum limits of radiation exposure for humans. These limits are different for the public, radiation workers, fetuses, and other groups (see Table 63.1).[2] These differences are based on the relative risk of each group. For example, fetuses are more sensitive to radiation damage than adults, particularly during the first 3 months of gestation, so they have a relatively low legal limit for exposure. The general public is also to be protected from increased exposure as compared with radiation workers.

A stochastic effect is a side effect that can occur at any dose exposure, but whose risk increases as the dose increases. The risk of developing cancer after radiation exposure is one example of this. Compared with someone who was not exposed, exposure to even low doses of radiation increases the risk of developing cancer later in life. However, the increased risk of developing cancer with low-level exposure, on the order received treating and handling radioactive patients when proper precautions are taken, is difficult to quantify but is probably very low.

Radiopharmaceuticals

Veterinary uses

A radiopharmaceutical is a radioactive drug that is used either to diagnose or treat disease. The radiopharmaceuticals most commonly used in veterinary medicine are technetium-99 (^{99m}TC) and iodine-131 (^{131}I), although others such as samarium-153 (^{153}Sm) and phosphorus-32 (^{32}P) have also been used.[3–6] Technesium is used in diagnostic radiology and has a relatively short half-life. When bound to pertechnetate it is most commonly used for the diagnosis of portosystemic shunts and thyroid disorders. When bound to methylene diphosphonate (MDP) it is taken up by osteoblasts and can be used to identify active areas of bone remodeling and is therefore commonly used to help identify patients with osteosarcoma or other cancers with bone metastasis.[7–9] ^{131}I is

most commonly used to treat hyperthyroidism in cats and occasionally to treat thyroid carcinomas in either dogs or cats.[10–12] Table 63.2 lists the most commonly used radiopharmaceuticals and their half-lives.

Concept of half-life

How long a particular radiopharmaceutical is actively emitting radiation is based on the physical half-life ($t^{1/2}$) of the particular isotope. The physical half-life is defined as the amount of time required for the radioactivity to decrease by half and is constant for each isotope. In general after 10 half-lives an element is considered no longer radioactive. This is the reason that if a patient dies directly after receiving a radiopharmaceutical, their body must be stored in a shielded freezer designated for this purpose and is not released for 10 half-lives. In the case of ^{131}I this would be approximately 80 days.

The biological half-life is defined as the amount of time for a patient to eliminate one half of the activity of the compound from the body. Most agents are excreted in the urine and/or feces. When a radiopharmaceutical is given to a patient, the length of time the patient is actively giving off radiation is based on both the physical half-life of the element and the biological half-life. Combining these terms gives you the effective half-life, which can be variable between patients due to variation in the biological half-life between individuals.

Radiation protection

As with patients who are exposed to x-rays for diagnostic imaging (radiographs or computed tomography scans), patients receiving external beam radiation therapy are not radioactive and do not present a risk of exposure to caregivers. This is in contrast to patients who receive a radiopharmaceutical agent resulting in residual radioactive material being present in their bodies, leading to risk for anyone who comes in contact with them, their blood or other body fluids such as urine, or their feces. These patients also have the potential to contaminate the environment, which could also place their owners or caregivers at risk for exposure to radiation.

The most basic concept of radiation protection is to limit exposure as much as possible. This concept should be applied to anyone potentially coming into contact with any form of radiation. The term "ALARA" (as low as reasonably achievable) is a mainstay of radiation protection and should be closely adhered to. In order to limit one's exposure when working with radiation or with a radioactive patient, the three main factors to keep in mind are time, distance, and shielding. Limiting the amount of contact time with a patient will decrease the amount of dose that the caregiver absorbs. Since radiation dose falls off as the distance squared, increasing the distance from a patient substantially decreases the dose received. For example, if a person is 2 meters away from a patient who is radioactive, that person will receive one quarter of the dose that would have been received if he or she were standing one 1 meter away. Shielding the radioactive source or patient will also greatly reduce potential exposure. For all of these reasons patients treated with a radiopharmaceutical are housed separately from other patients and kept out of commonly entered areas. This can be difficult if the patient is ill, however, particularly in the first few days after being treated.

External beam radiation protection

One potential source of exposure to radiation occurs while taking radiographs. While it is a well-established fact that one should never place any part of one's body in the primary beam while holding a patient for radiographs, exposure may still be received from scatter radiation. Whenever possible everyone but the patient should leave the room when a radiograph is being made. Chemical sedation and the use of restraint devices such as sand bags can be used to limit the need to have someone in the room. In some states it is not permissible to be in the room while a radiograph is being taken. Regardless of the law, every attempt should be made to limit exposure if someone is holding an animal during this procedure. With critically ill patients it may at times be impractical to sedate or restrain the patient appropriately for radiographs without having one or more people holding the animal. To decrease the time of exposure, careful technique should be used to decrease the number of repeat radiographs that are needed. Wearing lead gloves will not prevent exposure of one's hands if they are in the primary beam, and the field should be properly collimated so that no one has any body part within the primary beam. Additionally, lead gowns, gloves, and thyroid shields will largely protect you from scatter radiation and should be worn. No one person should be

designated to regularly hold animals for radiographs; this task should be shared among trained individuals, thus limiting the exposure to any one person. Lastly, anyone taking radiographs should have received training in the proper use of equipment and the steps that can be taken to reduce the risk of exposure. Anyone taking radiographs should be properly monitored using a radiation detection device (dosimeter) to ensure that he or she is not receiving too large of a cumulative dose. Radiation detection badges are usually checked monthly or quarterly and reports are to be made available to the individual so he or she is aware of what exposure may have been received.

Radionucleotide safety

Any facility using a radionucleotide will have a designated radiation safety officer and a radiation safety plan as part of their licensing requirements. This plan will detail how long a patient needs to be held after exposure and safety procedures. If a treated patient is brought into a practice for care other than where it was initially treated, the facility should be contacted and notified. Each treating facility will have a plan in place for handling radioactive patients and should be familiar with local rules and regulations. The length of time after exposure for which there is a concern for people working with the animal or its blood depends on the particular radionucleotide. For technesium there is little concern of exposure after 48 hours, while patients treated with ^{131}I this can present a hazard for a month or more. It should be remembered that their blood, urine, and feces are also radioactive. These patients should be isolated, their cages labeled as radioactive, and contact minimized until it is determined if they still present a hazard. Minimal precautions to be taken include wearing gloves, gowns, plastic shoe covers, and a face shield when coming in contact with these patients. Cages should not be hosed to limit the risk of aerosolizing and spreading radioactive material present in excreta. Geiger-Muller counters can be used to measure electron or photon radiation directly from the surface of a patient or from areas that may have become contaminated. These detectors generally give readouts in counts per minute or milliroentgen (mR) per hour.

In a patient treated with ^{131}I, a Geiger counter can be placed over their thyroid area and over any waste or bodily fluids to check for radioactivity. To see if the work environment is contaminated, wipe tests should be done. Wipe tests are done by taking swabs of the cage, counters, floors, and other areas where a radiation patient was present and placing the wipes in a scintillation counter. Wipe tests are generally part of any radiation safety plan for a facility using radionucleotides. Remember that once an area is contaminated, it may take up to 10 physical half-lives for the area to be safe unless proper decontamination procedures are followed. All waste from animals should be kept separately and checked for radioactivity. It should be stored properly and shielded until it is no longer radioactive before disposal. As the local legal requirements vary for radioactive waste disposal, the treating facility should be consulted regarding waste disposal or withholding times before any animal waste is disposed of in municipal trash.

Although generally not required as part of routine employee monitoring, if there is concern that an exposure might have taken place, a bioassay test can be performed to see if an employee has absorbed any radionucleotide. This procedure requires specialized equipment. It is a noninvasive test where a gamma counter is placed near the neck area to see if a person is emitting gamma rays from absorbed radionucleotide that may have accumulated in the thyroid.

Chemotherapy

According to American Society of Health-System Pharmacists, a drug should be considered hazardous if it is genotoxic, carcinogenic, teratogenic, and/or could lead to decreased fertility or cause serious organ or other toxicities at low doses in experimental animals.[13] Drugs that are classified as chemotherapuetic or antineoplastic agents fall into at least one of these categories and should be handled with care. Drugs for which there are no data regarding these potential toxicities such as new or investigational drugs should also be handled as hazardous materials.

As there is little information available as to a safe level of exposure to any one particular drug or chemical, it is always safest to limit exposure to as low as is reasonably achievable. In a sense it is the same concept as presented for radiological hazards earlier in this chapter.

The risk of exposure to a hazardous agent is based on the properties of the drug itself and the amount to which one is exposed. Exposure can occur by drugs being inhaled (if they are aerosolized), absorbed through the skin, or ingested. Sources of exposure to hazardous chemicals for the nursing staff can occur during transport and handling of chemotherapy drug vials, drug preparation, administration, handling of the patients themselves after receiving a cytotoxic drug, handling of animal waste, and from working in an environment that has become contaminated by any of the above.[14]

There are multiple studies of healthcare workers that show residual drug in their urine.[15,16] In addition, chromosomal changes consistent with exposure to mutagens have been found in people who regularly work with chemotherapy drugs.[17,18] As with radiation the additional risk of developing cancer after exposure to low levels of chemotherapy is poorly understood.

Limiting exposure

The Occupational Health and Safety Administration states that sound practices require that a Hazardous Safety and Drug plan be developed at institutions where hazardous drugs are used to minimize the risk to employees.[19]

All chemotherapeutic drugs should be mixed in a biological safety hood. Minimally, a class II laminar flow biological safety cabinet should be used.[15,19] A pharmacy isolator may be preferable, as it has been shown that the area directly outside laminar flow hoods can routinely become contaminated.[20,21] The use of a closed drug delivery system such as the PhaSeal™ system (Carmel Pharma AB, Göteborg, Sweden) while administering chemotherapy can also decrease the risk of exposure and avoid contamination of the work environment.[15,22] Proper training in the use of a closed system is important to help avoid accidents leading to contamination.[23] When spill of a chemotherapeutic drug does occur, a chemotherapy spill kit should be maintained to help with containment and decontamination. Several kits are commercially available.

One of the most important ways to protect oneself from exposure to patient or environmental chemotherapy hazards is by wearing gloves.[14] It is very important to use gloves designed for the particular agents being used. Glove thickness and length are also important in protecting the wearer from exposure. Specially manufactured chemotherapy gloves should be worn whenever mixing or administering drugs or when handling patients who have received chemotherapy. Chemotherapy gloves can be made from several different materials, including latex, neoprene, and nitrile. Ideally, they should extend to cover a gown at the wrist so no skin is exposed. These gloves must undergo testing by the manufacturer to ensure that they are not permeable to chemotherapy agents. Examination gloves in general are not sufficient to protect from exposure.

The disposal of contaminated materials and waste from chemotherapy preparation and administration and from patients exposed to chemotherapy is regulated by federal (Environment Protection Agency), state, and local regulation, and an institutional plan should be developed to ensure that any facility using these hazardous drugs is in compliance. In general all needles and other sharps should be disposed of in a separate, appropriately labeled chemotherapy designated sharps container. Needles should not be removed, recapped, or broken off from syringes that come in contact with hazardous chemicals and blood or bodily fluids from patients exposed to chemotherapy agents. Further, syringes should never be reused.

It has been recommended that bedding contaminated with blood, urine, feces, or other bodily fluids from patients treated with chemotherapy be treated as potentially hazardous for at least 48 hours after treatment. Soiled bedding should be stored separately from other laundry and prewashed and then washed a second time with regular laundry. The laundry bag should either be disposed of as chemotherapy waste or washed with the bedding if it is reusable.

Checking for environmental contamination with hazardous drugs is not easily done, as there are no commercially available wipe tests. This means that in order to minimize exposure several basic steps should be taken. Work areas where hazardous drugs are prepared or used should be clearly labeled with appropriate signage. No eating, drinking, smoking, applying of cosmetics, or other activities of this type should be done in an area where hazardous drugs are used or where patients treated with these drugs are housed.

Personnel who are pregnant, believe they might be pregnant, are actively trying to conceive, or are breast feeding should avoid any chemotherapy agents and the area in which they are administered. As this may require reassignment of duties or changes in job descriptions, labor laws should be followed, but minimally the employee should be made aware of potential risks to her fetus if she is exposed to chemotherapeutic agents. Proper handling of all hazardous drugs for preparation, transport, and administration should be carried out as outlined elsewhere in this chapter. The work areas and patient handling areas should be regularly cleaned.

Chemotherapeutic drugs are most commonly used to treat dogs and cats with cancer, although some of these same agents have also been used to treat inflammatory and autoimmune diseases such as granulomatous meningoencephalitis (GME) and autoimmune hemolytic anemia (AIHA). To ensure that all personnel know with which patients they need to take extra precautions, cages of patients treated with hazardous drugs should be clearly labeled.

Chemotherapy elimination

How long a drug is present in a patient after it is dosed depends on many factors, including properties of the drug itself, its metabolism, and individual patient and species characteristics. For most cytotoxic drugs full pharmacokinetic information is not available in veterinary patients. One study showed that vincristine, viblastine, cyclophosphamide, and doxorubicin could all be detected in dog urine after infusion.[24] Another study looked at residual drugs in dog urine after they were treated with several commonly used chemotherapy drugs including cyclophosphamide, doxorubicin, vinblastine, and vincristine. After oral cyclophosphamide dosing there was no detectable drug in the urine after one day. With vincristine and vinblastine low levels of drug were detectable for up to 7 days post-treatment. Doxorubicin still had low but detectable levels of drug at 3 weeks after administration.[25] In a separate study these same investigators found that most serum samples contained little to no detectable drug by 7 days after treatment.[26] These results indicate that care should be taken when handling chemotherapy patients for up to several weeks after treatment.

References

1. Nuclear Regulatory Commission: Our Governing Legislation (http://www.nrc.gov/about-nrc/governing-laws.html). Accessed December 31, 2010.
2. Nuclear Regulatory Commission: NRC Regulations (10 CFR) Part 20, Standard for Protection against Radiation. Accessed December 31, 2010.
3. Moe L, Boysen M, Aas M, et al. Maxillectomy and targeted radionuclide therapy with ^{153}Sm-EDTMP in a recurrent canine osteosarcoma. Journal of Small Animal Practice 1996;37:241–246.
4. Lattimer JC, Corwin LA, Jr., Stapleton J, et al. Clinical and clinicopathologic response of canine bone tumor patients to treatment with samarium-153-EDTMP [see comments]. Journal of Nuclear Medicine 1990;31:1316–1325.
5. Shapiro W, Turrel J. Management of pleural effusion secondary to metastatic adenocarcinoma in a dog. J Am Vet Med Assoc 1988;192:530–532.
6. Smith M, Turrel JM. Radiophosphorus (32P) treatment of bone marrow disorders in dogs: 11 cases (1970–1987). J Am Vet Med Assoc 1989;194:98–102.
7. Berg J, Lamb CR, O'Callaghan MW. Bone scintigraphy in the initial evaluation of dogs with primary bone tumors. Journal of the American Veterinary Medical Association 1990;196:917–920.
8. Forrest LJ, Thrall DE. Bone scintigraphy for metastasis detection in canine osteosarcoma. Veterinary Radiology & Ultrasound 1994;35:124–130.
9. Jankowski M, Steyn P, Lana S, et al. Nuclear scanning with 99mTc-HDP for the initial evaluation of osseous metastasis in canine osteosarcoma. Veterinary and Comparative Oncology 2003;1:152–158.
10. Turrel JM, McEntee MC, Burke BP, et al. Sodium iodide I 131 treatment of dogs with nonresectable thyroid tumors: 39 cases (1990–2003). J Am Vet Med Assoc 2006;229:542–548.
11. Adams WH, Walker MA, Daniel GB, et al. Treatment of differentiated thyroid carcinoma in 7 dogs utilizing 131I. Veterinary Radiology & Ultrasound 1995;36:417–424.
12. Chun R, Garrett LD, Sargeant J, et al. Predictors of response to radioiodine therapy in hyperthyroid cats. Vet Radiol Ultrasound 2002;43:587–591.

13. ASHP technical assistance bulletin on handling cytotoxic and hazardous drugs. Am J Hosp Pharm 1990;47:1033–1049.

14. NIOSH Publication No. 2004–165: Preventing Occupational Exposure to Antineoplastic and Other Hazardous Drugs in Health Care Settings In: Health NIfOSa, ed., 2004.

15. Wick C, Slawson MH, Jorgenson JA, et al. Using a closed-system protective device to reduce personnel exposure to antineoplastic agents. Am J Health Syst Pharm 2003;60:2314–2320.

16. Sessink PJ, de Roos JH, Pierik FH, et al. Occupational exposure of animal caretakers to cyclophosphamide. J Occup Med 1993;35: 47–52.

17. Connor TH. Hazardous anticancer drugs in health care: environmental exposure assessment. Ann N Y Acad Sci 2006;1076: 615–623.

18. Sessink PJ, Cerna M, Rossner P, et al. Urinary cyclophosphamide excretion and chromosomal aberrations in peripheral blood lymphocytes after occupational exposure to antineoplastic agents. Mutat Res 1994;309:193–199.

19. United States Department of Labor: Occupational Safety & Health Administration. Controlling Occupational Exposure to Hazardous Drugs. OSHA Technical Manual, VI: chapter 2.

20. Bigelow S, Schulz H, Dobish R, et al. Antineoplastic agent workplace contamination study: the Alberta Cancer Board Pharmacy perspective Phase III. J Oncol Pharm Pract 2009;15:157–160.

21. Connor TH, Anderson RW, Sessink PJ, et al. Surface contamination with antineoplastic agents in six cancer treatment centers in Canada and the United States. Am J Health Syst Pharm 1999;56: 1427–1432.

22. Connor TH, Anderson RW, Sessink PJ, et al. Effectiveness of a closed-system device in containing surface contamination with cyclophosphamide and ifosfamide in an i.v. admixture area. Am J Health Syst Pharm 2002;59:68–72.

23. Kandel-Tschiederer B, Kessler M, Schwietzer A, et al. Reduction of workplace contamination with platinum-containing cytostatic drugs in a veterinary hospital by introduction of a closed system. Vet Rec 2010;166:822–825.

24. Hamscher G, Mohring SA, Knobloch A, et al. Determination of drug residues in urine of dogs receiving anti-cancer chemotherapy by liquid chromatography-electrospray ionization–tandem mass spectrometry: is there an environmental or occupational risk? J Anal Toxicol 2010;34:142–148.

25. Knobloch A, Mohring SA, Eberle N, et al. Cytotoxic drug residues in urine of dogs receiving anticancer chemotherapy. J Vet Intern Med 2010;24:384–390.

26. Knobloch A, Mohring SA, Eberle N, et al. Drug residues in serum of dogs receiving anticancer chemotherapy. J Vet Intern Med 2010;24:379–383.

64

Medical charting

Karl E. Jandrey and Sharon Fornes

Veterinary medical records serve several purposes. There are four main reasons to maintain accurate and up-to-date medical records.

1. **A medical record is a legal document of patient care.** As a legal document, a complete medical record can be used in court as a representation of the treatment that was planned and completed on an animal. If the record is incomplete or is in error, the courts may rule in favor of the client even if no negligence can be proven from the record.[1] The components of a complete medical record will be discussed later in the chapter.

2. **The medical record makes the path of patient care obvious to all readers.** A primary function of the medical record is to document the path of patient care and the thought process behind it. To this extent, a complete medical record should detail all patient data and the assessment of those data. This patient-centered information leads to the unique and particular diagnostic and therapeutic path. For example, the reader of a medical record should be able to easily identify whether a patient's data are within normal reference intervals, whether a trend is improving over time, which procedures were performed on the patient, and the results of a particular intervention. A properly executed and comprehensive medical record will facilitate the development of future diagnostic or therapeutic plans for the ongoing treatment of the animal.

3. **The medical record allows for the documentation of all communication between veterinary staff and clients.** Whether it documents communication between the animal's owner and the staff at the practice or within the practice itself, the medical record is an essential tool to maximize continuity of care. By facilitating effective communication, medical records ensure that all doctors and associated hospital staff members involved in the patient's care are aware of the treatment plan. If documented correctly, a medical record can thereby allow for consistent and accurate standardization of patient care.[2]

4. **The medical record allows for documentation for research or publication.**[2] Along with the legal implications of medical records, the importance of a complete and comprehensive medical record is underscored by its use in clinical research. Medical records provide data from which case reports or research papers may be written. Missing medical record information can grossly diminish the impact of a research publication by reducing the amount of usable data, which then may function to reduce the sample size. To avoid this, the medical record should present its information in a clear and concise format that allows research personnel to obtain the information quickly.

Medical record documentation

Because a medical record is frequently referenced, an accurate and clearly written record is of the utmost importance. Taking care to appropriately document data

Advanced Monitoring and Procedures for Small Animal Emergency and Critical Care, First Edition. Edited by Jamie M. Burkitt Creedon, Harold Davis.
© 2012 John Wiley & Sons, Inc. Published 2012 by John Wiley & Sons, Inc.

can greatly facilitate the clarity and accuracy of a medical record. There are seven components to proper medical record documentation.

1. **Documentation of authorization for patient care.** Authorization for patient care is necessary before treatment of the animal can commence. It is of great importance to ensure that appropriate forms have been signed and that witnessed oral consent is documented.[3] These consent forms for each visit/procedure can be placed in the plans and progress notes of the complete medical record.

2. **Timely documentation of information in the record.** This functions to better ensure accurate recollection of the data. It is important to time- and date-stamp any entry if possible. For example, if the animal is unstable, information that was obtained in the initial excitement of an emergency presentation may be recalled with less clarity hours later. Any history and pertinent information should be recorded in the appropriate place in the chart when it becomes possible. Alternatively, an assistant can document information as it unfolds if his or her participation is not essential to the emergency interventions ongoing for the patient.

3. **Clear indication of the person who performed a task or treatment.** This is usually accomplished by documentation of the person's initials on the record or treatment sheet. The purpose to initial the records will allow for questions to be directed to the appropriate parties.

4. **Legible handwriting.** Legibility of the record is essential to prevent misinterpretation. If one cannot write legibly, one should consider typed or computerized medical records.

5. **Appropriate notation of corrections to the record.** Care should be taken if a correction in a medical record is required. To overwrite, scratch out, erase, black out with a marker, or use correction fluid or tape are inappropriate methods for correction. The appropriate method of correction is to initial and draw a single line through the entry that was created in error. The correction should then be written and initialed near the entry that was replaced. The use of any method other than the accepted convention could be considered as tampering with the record and may be used against the veterinary healthcare team in a court of law.[1,3]

6. **Use of proper writing implements.** Permanent ink should be used to make entries in the handwritten medical record. There is controversy about the appropriate color of ink to use. Local regulation and clinic preferences (standard operating procedures [SOPs]) may have some variation. The following are arguments for the exclusive use of black pen in a medical record:[4] better reproduction on a photocopier, better contrast on white paper, and the tendency to be more permanent. However, an advantage of blue ink over black ink is to provide contrast to the black ink of preprinted forms. With blue ink, new entries on preprinted forms may be more easily distinguished.

7. **Use of acronyms and abbreviations.** Acronyms and abbreviations used in the clinic should be standardized. Confusion may arise, for example, in determining whether "mm" refers to millimeters or mucous membranes. The Academy of Veterinary Technician Anesthetists (www.avta-vts.org) has a published list of acceptable abbreviations. The development of a list of acceptable abbreviations for each individual hospital could also be helpful to avoid miscommunication between staff members. Beware, however, that records are often shared between facilities. Other facilities may not understand a particular hospital's abbreviation standards unless provided with a key.

Medical record organization

A standardized medical record organization is important for many reasons. During a patient's stay in a veterinary hospital, much data is collected and assessed daily. If these data are consistently written in the same format, information retrieval is timely and accurate. This may help in legal cases, to evaluate therapeutic goals, and to use the medical record for clinical research. Data are most useful and clinical efficiency is maximized when information is placed in a consistent location.

An organized medical record is most commonly formatted in a chronological order. Reverse chronological order (last visit on top and the first visit on the bottom) is a common method for assembly of the medical record.[5]

Medical records can also be organized by section (e.g., financial, authorization forms, treatment sheets, pharmacy, laboratory, plans, and progress notes). The creation of sections within a patient record facilitates quicker reference in a large comprehensive medical record.

Medical record format

There are two common formats used for the documentation of medical records: the conventional method and the Problem-Oriented Medical Record (POMR). The conventional method documents information as it is obtained. It may be less time-consuming than the POMR and tends to be used in general practice. The POMR records patient data according to the patient's problem. POMRs are often used in academic and specialty practices to clearly document and transmit the logical forward-thinking approach that is required for patients with complicated disease processes. POMRs are also used as effective teaching tools because they allow the reader to readily uncover the thought process of the writer. However, though POMR records are very organized and detailed, a disadvantage is that they may be more time-consuming to produce.[3]

Components of a complete medical record

A complete medical record should include a thorough and accurate daily description of all data obtained for a particular patient, the assessment of these data, and a discussion of the resultant plan (which is comprised of diagnostic, therapeutic, and client education components). The complete medical record should include nine components:

1. Client information
2. Patient information
3. Presenting complaint
4. History (from both the client as well as other prior medical records)
5. Physical examination
6. Problem lists
7. Progress notes
8. Communication log
9. Comments

Client information

This area of the medical record is devoted to the client where all pertinent information about the animal owner(s) is kept. All contact information (physical and mailing addresses, electronic contact, landline and mobile telephone numbers, and special notations) about the animal owners should be placed here. These listed people are the legal guardians of the animal and permit access to this information. Those not listed in this are unable to access patient information under privacy and confidentiality agreements. Although these are not commonplace in veterinary medicine, patient confidentiality must be respected by the hospital and all members of its staff. Release of patient information to a third party must be approved by the client.

Patient information

The patient data is recorded here and includes the signalment (age, breed, sex, birth date). Pedigree or individual medical information (allergies, behavioral) can be placed here.

Presenting complaint

The presenting complaint is recorded by the reception or medical records staff when the appointment is made. This is the information in the words of the client that transmits the reason for which they seek veterinary medical care.

History

A comprehensive history is obtained from the client on the initial visit and is updated periodically as the animals' health status changes. A history needs to be taken every time an animal presents for a new illness (known as the history of the presenting illness [HPI]). Past pertinent history (PPH) can be helpful in determining onset of the problem or relationship to the HPI.

Physical examination

A physical examination may be completed one or multiple times daily and should be documented at least once daily throughout the animal's hospitalization. All the body systems should be examined and documented properly to ensure and prove that they were examined.

Problem lists

Problem lists enumerate the conditions being managed during a hospitalization period. In a problem list, "problems" can be created, resolved, combined with other problems and renamed, or inactivated at any time. This provides the veterinarian with a means of obtaining an overview of all problems that the animal may have had and whether they were addressed or resolved, without the requirement to examine the entire record.[3]

A master problem list (Fig. 64.1) is often created and placed on the first page of the patient record. The master problem list is a summary of all the problems for which the patient has been examined. This includes the date the problem was identified, as well as when it was resolved (if applicable). It functions as a quick glance into the patient's medical history and can thereby facilitate a focused search, much like a table of contents.

Progress notes

Progress notes are the daily SOAP (see the italicized words defined below that form the acronym) of the patient. Each day for each problem, an entry is created that contains the data relevant to that problem. *Subjective* and *objective* data are placed in this section and should include the information gained from diagnostics

	VETERINARY MEDICAL TEACHING HOSPITAL UNIVERSITY OF CALIFORNIA, DAVIS		
NUMBER	PROBLEM	DATE ENTERED	DATE RESOLVED

D2760 (12/90) Form #48-R **MASTER PROBLEM LIST**

Figure 64.1 Master problem list is a summary of all the problems for which the patient has been examined.

and therapeutic interventions, as well as the new physical examination or any physiologic measurements. A patient's response to treatments is also recorded in this section. A differentiation is made in human medicine between the information that comes from the patient (subjective) and that measured in analysis (objective). In veterinary medicine, the information given by the client may be treated as subjective. However, historical data from a client can be measured and clearly objective; therefore, "data" is a more proper term. The SOAP would therefore be referred to as the DAP. An *assessment* follows the data and should include information pertinent to the patient's prognosis. The purpose of the assessment is to refine and document the new thoughts of the clinician. Based on the assessment of all the previous data, a new *plan* is created. This plan must discuss at least one of three distinct areas of focus: diagnostic plans, therapeutic plans, and/or client education plans.

Communication log

The communication log is the section of the POMR that contains the information about any and all contact between members of the hospital staff with the client and/or referring veterinarian(s). This includes detailed phone calls, e-mails, text messages, or client visits. Proper documentation also includes reference to client education, date, time, names, and content of the communication. In a referral hospital, the names, contact information, and addresses of the primary care provider (PCP) and, if applicable, referring DVM (RDVM) should also be on the record.

The information found in the communication log is often equally as important as the daily SOAP. As this information is not likely to be organized in any other area of the POMR, the communication log should be carefully and comprehensively documented. Electronic medical records may be finalized and locked with a time and date stamp. However, communications logs should not be locked. Added information via telephone communication may arrive without attachment to a hospital visit and, therefore, no daily POMR. This message may be added into the record in chronological order when the record is not locked. Information from delayed diagnostic tests can be recorded back to the visit to which they pertain. This communication is essential to provide continuity for the patient's medical and surgical treatment data since it may alter the assessment of the patient problem.

Comments

The comments section is the part of a complete medical record designed for other miscellaneous details. Often an additional page or pages are available if there was insufficient room in the space provided on a medical record or form. In some computerized medical record systems, this is the only other editable section to which information can be added once the medical record is finalized and locked.

Other additions to the patient record

Examples of additions to the patient record when applicable include: medications (particularly drug sensitivity), pertinent patient information such as aggressive/caution, special needs, mentation, appetite, food intake, visual analog pain scales, body conditioning score, and lab results. Other additions may include warning labels placed on the outside of the medical record or in the header of the computerized medical record. Alternatively, these may be addenda to the plans and progress notes for hospitalized patients that are included in the description of patient observations.

Clinician order sheets and treatment/flow sheets

In addition to details about patient data, future treatment and diagnostic plans, and client education, a medical record should include clinician order sheets and treatment/flow sheets. These function to help ensure quality and continuity of care for the veterinary patient. They are part of the progress notes since pertinent data from these are abstracted into the computerized medical record. In paper medical records, these sheets are inserted chronologically to accompany the daily DAP. The following section will focus on the information found in order sheets and flow sheets, and it will highlight appropriate methods to notate findings and interpret information.

Clinician orders

Many hospitals combine the clinician's orders with patient observation or flow sheets. Order sheets can be simple for wards patients that are stable (Fig. 64.2) or they can be elaborate depending on the level of intensive care delivered (Fig. 64.3). In all cases, the appropriate treatment, diagnostic, and monitoring plans should be legibly written for clear documentation.

Treatment sheets

Treatment sheets are the part of the medical record that contain recorded data collected throughout the animal's hospitalization. Treatment sheets (Fig. 64.4) can be as simple as recording observations and the treatments provided to an animal. The preferred format is to write in the medical order using a clear format. For example:

Figure 64.2 An example of a clinicians' order form. The clinician writes the patient orders noting the drug, dosage, route and time; other therapies or procedures may be included. The time the treatment was given is circled.

VETERINARY MEDICAL TEACHING HOSPITAL
UNIVERSITY OF CALIFORNIA, DAVIS

CLINICIAN: _____

PHONE # _____ PGR: _____

STUDENT: _____

PHONE # : _____ PGR: _____

SAICU - CLINICIAN ORDERS - ENTRIES MUST BE SIGNED AND UPDATED TWICE DAILY

DATE _____ TIME _____ AM / PM

FLUIDS /MEDS / TREATMENTS	DOSAGE	ROUTE	START TIME

Monitor:

Observation q ____ hr (mentation; breathing rate; breathing effort)

☐ Vital signs q ____ hr (observations plus: heart rate; auscult heart & lungs; mucous membr color & CRT)

Temp q ___ hr ECG q ____ hr Doppler BP q ____ hr Dinamap BP q ___ hr Direct BP q ___ hr CVP q ___ hr

Pulse Oxim q ___ hr Urine output q ___ hr _____ q ___ hr _____ q ___ hr _____ q ___ hr

Laboratory:

☐ ICU panel 1 q ___ hr Art/Ven (oximetry, blood gases; electrolytes; glucose; lactate)

☐ ICU panel 2 q ___ hr (panel 1 plus osmolality; colloid osmotic pressure)

☐ PCV/TS q ___ hr ☐ Lactate q ___ hr ☐ Vet-test BUN q ___ hr ☐ Urine Sp Gr q ___ hr

☐ ACT q ___ hr ☐ Glucom q ___ hr ☐ Vet-test Creat q ___ hr ☐ Urine dipstick q ___ hr

☐ COP q ___ hr ☐ ABL glucose q ___ hr ☐ ABL electrolytes q ___ hr ☐ Urine electrolytes q ___ hr

☐ Osmolality q ___ hr ☐ ABL blood gas q ___ hr ☐ _____ q ___ hr ☐ _____ q ___ hr

General nursing care:

Standard care: Weigh q 24 hrs; indwelling catheter care as per protocol; heparin lock unused catheters

☐ Recumbent care: Standard care + resposition and physical therapy q 4 hrs

☐ Comatose patient care: Recumbent care + oral & eye care as per protocol

☐ _____ q ___ hr ☐ _____ q ___ hr ☐ _____ q ___ hr

Nutrition:

☐ NPO ☐ NPO except oral meds ☐ No food, water ad lib ☐ No food, offer _____ ml water q ___ hr

☐ Water ad lib; feed _____ of _____ q ___ hr ☐ TPN: _____ as per protocol; goal: _____

       (amount of food) (type of food)   (formula)   (daily Kcals)

Contingencies (change/cancel any default contingenies?)

_____

CPR status: ☐ Full CPR ☐ Closed-chest CPR ☐ No CPR Signature: _____

Form #38SRevised 12/23/04

Figure 64.3 An intensive care unit (ICU) clinicians' order form. Space is provided for writing medications and treatments. A portion of the order form contains prompts and check boxes for ordering monitoring, laboratory and general nursing care. An area is included for writing contingency orders for example, *if the heart rate is greater than 180 bpm, then call the doctor.*

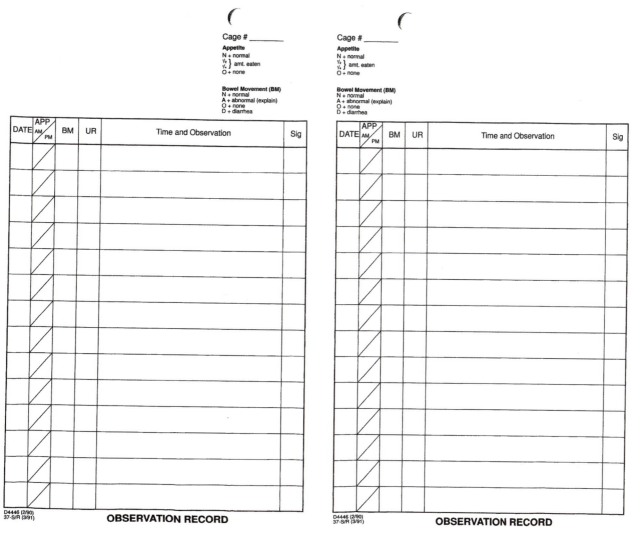

Figure 64.4 A patient observation form. The form is used by the technician to record his/hers nursing notes. An area is included to document appetite, urination, defecation and technician initials.

"lactated Ringer's solution qs 20 mEq/L at 120ml/hr IV" or "Famotidine 10 mg IV q12h."

Daily patient flow sheets

Patient daily flow sheets may be complicated, multipage treatment sheets that give detailed information in areas of subsections of the document outlining treatments, monitoring, and observations (Fig. 64.5a–e). Though the format of these flow sheets is often tailored to the purpose and individual clinic, completed treatment sheets are considered part of the patient's medical record and must contain basic information.

Patient identification

First, the patient's basic identification must be found on each page of all forms on the flow sheet (Fig. 64.5a) as

well as every piece of the medical record. This enables a page that becomes detached from the record to be easily returned to the record. The date should also be included on each page, and a time may be appropriate for certain entries.

Patient weight

The patient flow sheet should include the patient's weight at presentation as well as daily updates (Fig. 64.5a). This is important to determine effective pharmaceutical treatment and the assessment of need for other treatments. A patient's weight may also be used to calculate the charges for care provided. Recording of weight may be delayed until certain initial interventions required for more life-threatening conditions are completed.

VETERINARY MEDICAL TEACHING HOSPITAL
UNIVERSITY OF CALIFORNIA, DAVIS

S.A. ICU FLOWSHEET

Date:		Admission Date:	
1° Clinician:		Pager:	Phone:
ICU Clinician:		Pager:	Phone:
Student:		Pager:	Phone:

Major Problems:

DAILY TREATMENTS	DAY	SWING	GRAVEYARD
WEIGHT (kg)			
INTENSIVIST NURSE			
INTENSIVIST NURSE			
INTENSIVIST NURSE			

CPR: ☐ FULL CPR   ☐ CC/CPR   ☐ D.N.R

Discharge Information

Date:

Time:

Ward/cage:

SHIFT SUMMARY

DAY SHIFT:

SWING SHIFT:

GRAVEYARD SHIFT:

CATHETER INSERT DATE:	CATHETER INSERT DATE:	CATHETER INSERT DATE:	CATHETER INSERT DATE:	CATHETER INSERT DATE:
CATH. INSERTED/INITIALS	CATH. INSERTED/INITIALS	CATH. INSERTED/INITIALS	CATH. INSERTED/INITIALS	CATH. INSERTED/INITIALS
LOCATION:	LOCATION:	LOCATION:	LOCATION:	LOCATION:
SIZE: TYPE:	SIZE: TYPE:	SIZE: TYPE:	SIZE: TYPE:	SIZE: TYPE:
SITE COND.:	SITE COND.:	SITE COND.:	SITE COND.:	SITE COND.:
ASPIRATES: YES NO	ASPIRATES: YES NO	ASPIRATES: YES NO	ASPIRATES: YES NO	ASPIRATES: YES NO
FLUSHES: GOOD FAIR POOR	FLUSHES: GOOD FAIR POOR	FLUSHES: GOOD FAIR POOR	FLUSHES: GOOD FAIR POOR	FLUSHES: GOOD FAIR POOR
AMT. EXPOSED: IN/CM	AMT. EXPOSED: IN/CM	AMT. EXPOSED: IN/CM	AMT. EXPOSED: IN/CM	AMT. EXPOSED: IN/CM
IV CATH CARE DUE:	IV CATH CARE DUE:	IV CATH CARE DUE:	IV CATH CARE DUE:	IV CATH CARE DUE:

Figure 64.5a The first page of a multipage ICU flow sheet. The page includes an area for patient, clinician and caregiver (veterinary technician) identification. An area is included for the veterinary technician to write an end of shift patient summary. The purpose of the summary is to briefly discuss the highlights of the shift. Catheter care information is documented at the bottom of the flow chart.

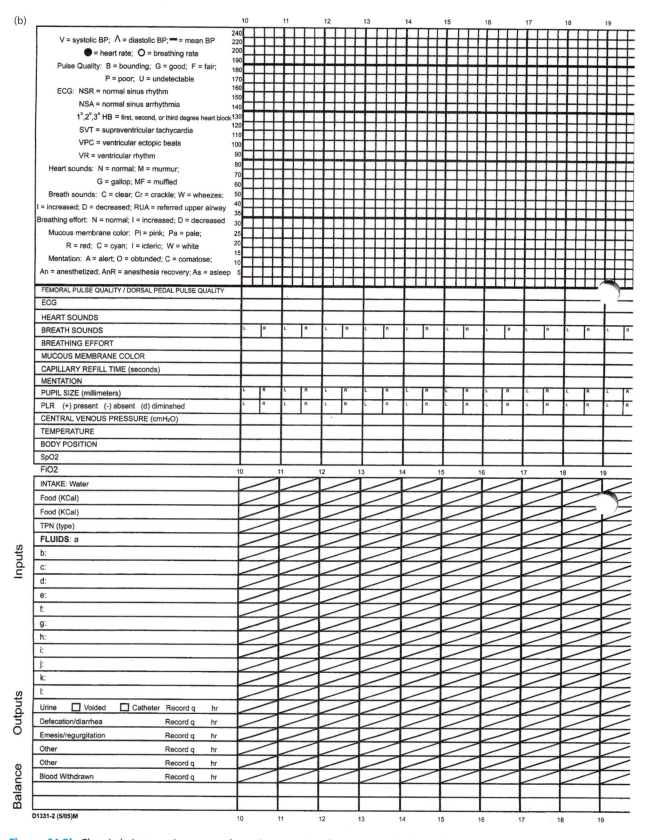

Figure 64.5b The vital signs section covers the various monitored parameters for the cardiovascular, respiratory, and neurological systems. The graphic section facilitates easy monitoring of trends. The input section contains space for documenting food, water, and IV fluids. The output section contains space for documenting urine, defecation, vomitus, and blood. Both input and output sections allow for keeping a running total of ins and outs.

ICU LABORATORY

TIME																
PCV (%)																
TP (Gm/dl)																
Plasma color																
Plasma transparency																
Arterial/Venous																
Body temperature (C/F)																
Inspired oxygen (%)																
Hemoglobin (Gm/dl)																
Oxyhemoglobin (%)																
Methemoglobin (%)																
Carboxyhemoglobin (%)																
Oxygen content (ml/dl)																
Potassium (mEq/L)																
Sodium (mEq/L)																
Calcium(ionized) (mM/L)																
Chloride (mEq/L)																
Glucose (mg/dl)																
Lactate (mM/L)																
pH tc (units)																
PCO2tc (mmHg)																
PO2tc (mmHg)																
A-a pO2 (mmHg)																
SBE c (mEq/L)																
HCO3c (mEq/L)																
COP (mm Hg)																
Osmolality (mOsm/Kg)																
Creatinine (Vet-test)																
BUN (Vet-test)																
Azostick																
Glucometer																
Activ Clotting Time (sec)																
Urinalysis Time																
Collection method																
Color																
Transparency																
Specific Gravity																
Osmolality (mOsm/Kg)																
Sodium (mEq/L)																
Potassium (mEq/L)																
Chloride (mEq/L)																
Protein																
pH																
Blood																
Ketones																
Bilirubin																
Glucose																

Figure 64.5c The lab section of a patient flow.

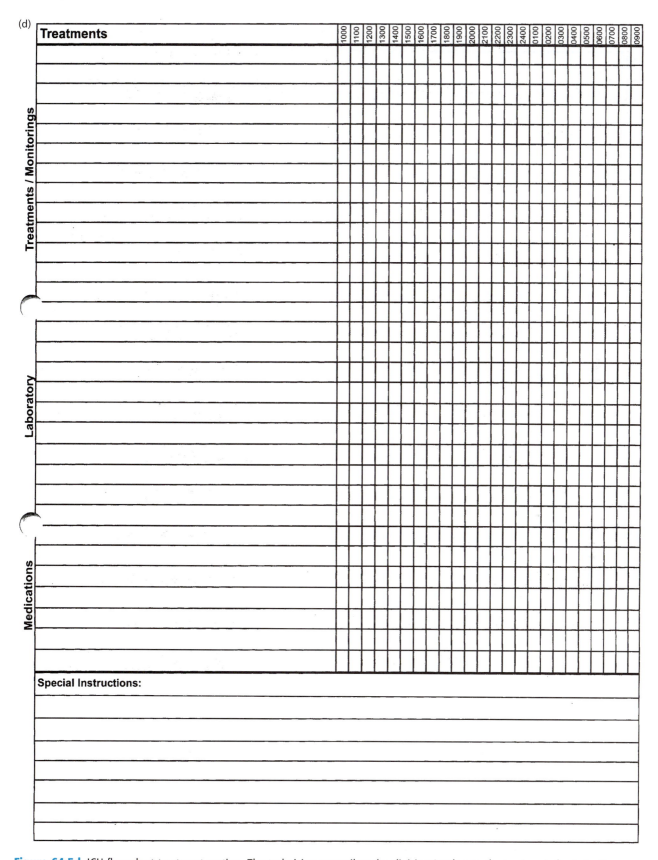

Figure 64.5d ICU flow chart treatment section. The technician transcribes the clinicians' orders to the treatment sheet. Sections are provided for treatments/monitoring, laboratory, medications and special instructions. The time the treatment was given is circled.

(e)

Controlled Drug Record						
Drug	Mg	Route	CRI/Bolus	Time	Source	Name

Controlled Drug Record						
Drug	Mg	Route	CRI/Bolus	Time	Source	Name

Observations

Figure 64.5e Controlled drug log and observation page of an ICU flow chart. The controlled drug section allows for documentation of controlled drug administration. Nursing notes are written in the observation section. Adhesive strips are used to attach ECG strips to the patient flow chart.

Nutritional considerations

What is to be fed and the frequency to offer food is essential. The volume in cups/cans or weight in grams should be noted for both the amount offered as well as the amount ingested. Special dietary needs and feeding instructions should be clear, especially if using various enteral feeding tubes or parenteral nutrition. In addition, nutritional considerations should be notated on the record. The patient that has no oral administration of food or medication should be labeled NPO (*non per os*). This is important for animals that are going to be anesthetized because preanesthetic protocol may require the removal of food from the animal at a certain time. Therefore, this information should be easily distinguished on a record so that the animal can undergo anesthesia at the intended time. If a hospitalized animal is to be fed or given water, the amount type of food and appetite or water consumption should be notated on the record (Fig. 64.5b). Some methods to indicate appetite are a number scale (0–5), where other methods use +/– symbols to indicate whether an animal ate/drank or did not eat/drink. Notation of the patient's nutritional considerations is important on two levels. First, the more nutritional information included in the record, the more fully will the staff understand the individual patient's eating preferences. Second, because some owners may bring the patient's own food or favorite treats to the hospital to encourage appetite, providing a record of nutrition will allow the hospital staff to tally and keep watch on the patient's ingested calorie content. Ideally, the exact calorie content ingested should be documented.

Laboratory measurements

The data obtained from patient-side laboratory evaluation should be placed in the appropriate section of the medical record and flow sheet (Fig. 64.5c). This notation in the record may be the only area it is recorded since some point-of-care machines do not have hard-copy printouts of these data.

Patient treatments and observations

Medications

The "rights" of pharmacotherapy include right drug, right patient, right time interval, and right route. Accurate notation of pharmacologic information into the flow sheet (Fig. 64.5d) plays a major role in ensuring the correct method of administration of a drug. Medications and treatment regimens should be recorded in the sheet exactly as the veterinarian prescribed.[6] Standardized orders require all medications to be written in the exact amount of drug in milligrams administered. It is preferred to write the total dosage in milligrams (mg) with the appropriate time interval and not just a dose per body weight (mg/kg). Drug volumes should not be used due to the varying concentrations of preparations between manufacturers. It is expected that the veterinarian who prescribes the medication will write the order clearly (e.g., ampicillin 250 mg IV q8h). An order in total dose such as "250 mg" is much clearer than "22 mg/kg" because drugs dosed in milligram/kilogram (mg/kg) are also subject to computational error. Before being written in the medical record or delivered to the patient, any clarifications should be addressed to the clinician who wrote the order. In some hospitals, the time for the treatment to be completed is indicated on the treatment sheet by an open circle. When the treatment is completed, the time at which it was delivered is written in the circle. Alternatively, some hospitals prefer the treatment order to be written as a number on the hour at which treatment should be delivered. When the treatment is completed, the number is then circled indicating completion. A hospital standard for consistency in format of the orders should be followed.

As part of the medication section, special legal considerations and maintenance of a controlled drugs log is essential. All controlled drugs administered to patients must be noted in both the patient record and in the controlled drug log (Fig. 64.5e). Some facilities have a drug log created at the time of dispensation by the use of automated dispensing equipment. This log will be proof required during audits by the Drug Enforcement Agency (DEA) or the state veterinary board. This should include patient information as well as the amount and route of the drug administered. The starting volume and remainder in a multiuse vials are also recorded.

Fluids

Accurate fluid orders include many specific parameters. The type of fluid, dose and concentration, rate (per unit time), additive solutions or medications, and total hourly/daily tallies should be clearly indicated to ensure adherence (Fig. 64.5b). The complete measurement of fluid input can be compared with all net fluid output over time to direct adjustments in fluid treatment orders. Whether the fluids were administered via intravenous (IV) or subcutaneous bolus with or without the use of a fluid pump should be noted. Daily catheter evaluations should also be noted (Fig. 64.5a). How often the catheter was checked (q24h at a minimum or as indicated) and by whom is also part of the fluid orders. Any information regarding the catheter replacement (date, personnel, anatomic site, catheter size and length) is also helpful for optimal patient care as well as troubleshooting in the event of a catheter mishap. Annotate the removal of the old catheter and the site of placement of the new catheter (including gauge, length, amount exposed, vessel quality, and whether it aspirates or can be flushed easily). Other information to include on the record regarding a new catheter placement is: the date of placement, the initials of the person who placed the catheter, site (i.e., left rear limb, lateral saphenous vein, or right jugular vein), and catheter size (e.g., 22g 1 ½ inch over the needle catheter or 5fr, 10 cm guide wire, double lumen catheter). Notations of the patient's hydration status as measured by skin turgor, tear film, mucous membranes, and/or ocular position will help to gauge efficacy of therapy.

Body systems evaluations

The veterinarian uses the information found in the flow sheets to assess the response to treatment, to plan the next daily treatment, diagnostic, and monitoring plans, as well as to predict recovery of the animal. The body systems used for evaluation include: cardiovascular, respiratory, neurologic, and urinary (Fig. 64.5b). These body systems have parameters the veterinary technician can evaluate and notate in the medical record. Typically, data from individual body systems are organized in the medical record in proximity to one another. This arrangement facilitates evaluation by the caregivers to organize constellations of data into a more global perspective of the patient's status.

Cardiovascular system

Initial or serial vital measurements (e.g., temperature [temp], heart rate [hr], pulse rate [pr], respiratory rate [rr]) must be included in the patient flow sheet. These will help assess whether a particular treatment is successful and sufficient. For example, a flow sheet should include the following pieces of information necessary for the understanding of the patients' perfusion: heart rate/pulse rate, pulse quality, mentation, extremity temperature, mucous membrane color, and capillary refill time. Using these parameters, poor distal perfusion may be assessed in shock, where the rectal-extremity (interdigital) temperature difference may be large (>4°C [9°F]) due to peripheral vasoconstriction. Similarly, pale mucous membranes with a slow capillary refill time, tachycardia, weak femoral pulses, and decreased mentation are all signs of poor perfusion. Normal capillary refill time (CRT) should be approximately <2 seconds. Conversely, an extremely rapid CRT accompanied by bright pink or red mucous membranes may indicate vasodilation.[7,8] Electrocardiogram interpretations or

rhythm strips should be part of this portion of the medical record.

Respiratory system

Important parameters to annotate in the section devoted to the pulmonary system are respiratory rate, effort (apparent ease, origin of effort [e.g., thorax vs. abdomen]), associated sound (type of sound, origin, volume change in reference to phase of respiration), or irregularities in respiratory pattern.

Nervous system

Upon initial presentation or triage of the animal, observations of the patient's level of consciousness and response to the surroundings is essential to the examining veterinarian.[7] The mentation of an animal may range from alert to obtunded to stuporus to comatose. In the daily flow sheet, the writer must mention the level of consciousness and any behavioral changes in the patient. Changes in level of mentation are important markers or improvement or decline in health status. Behavior may also give an indication that there may be some neurologic changes in the animal. The animal may circle, head-press, or become aggressive or withdrawn. Modifications of these mental states should be interpreted in light of the treatments given as well as in postoperative states after anesthesia or pain control has been administered.[6,7]

Urinary system

Some animals have preference for the substrate on which to eliminate or respond to special commands taught by the owners. These unique data should be annotated in the area related to the urinary system. Any urinary catheter, as is the case with an IV catheter, should have information regarding the date of placement (and by whom), catheter type and frequency of care, and any problems with it (e.g., leaking). The amount of urine production (hourly/daily) is important to note in milliliters whether obtained as an estimates from voided urination or specific amounts measured from the urinary collection systems. Collected urine samples may be weighed and subtracted from the weight of hospital bedding to estimate the urine output (UOP) as closely as possible. Normal UOP is 1–2 mL/kg/hour. Volumes more or less than this need to be addressed by the clinician once discovered. An Elizabethan collar may also be required to prevent premature removal of the catheter by the patient. This should also be notated on the record to ensure that nursing personnel keep the collar on the patient until the urinary catheter is removed.

Patient privacy

Although there are strict regulations and laws in place to protect the identification of human patients in both verbal and research communications, veterinary medicine does not have a global policy for client/patient privacy.[9] Veterinary caregivers should be sensitive to client/patient privacy especially with the advent and growth of social networking sites. Written, photographic, and verbal confidentiality should be maintained for clients and patients. Client consent forms for the use of patient images and data are used to avoid inappropriate use against the clients' wishes. There may be local or regional confidentiality agreements. Be aware of the laws regarding the patient and client confidentiality. Obtain a client release[3] for anything that you may need to disclose to a third party.

Conclusions

The most accepted charting methods are those that are found to be user-friendly. The choice of charting method lies within the judgment of each clinic. For example, the use of a 24-hour clock may be preferred to a 12-hour a.m./p.m. clock. Despite the fact that a 24-hour clock is best used to avoid any confusion in a hospital where 24-hour service is provided, most people are not comfortable with this method. Internal standardization within a practice enables clear and precise communication among the veterinary healthcare team.

Storage of records may vary by area. State veterinary medical boards have mandated the minimum length of time that records must be maintained. When records are purged, security must be maintained due to the confidential information therein. Shredding of documents is an acceptable and preferred method of securely purging medical records. Many companies provide this service when a large number of medical records is culled.

Standards and guidelines of veterinary medical record keeping can be found at the local, state, and national veterinary associations. The following are some suggested associations where the salient details can be found: American Veterinary Medical Association (AVMA, www.avma.org), American Animal Hospital Association (AAHA, www.aahanet.org), state Veterinary Medical Boards (VMB; e.g., for California, go to www.vmb.ca.gov), and the Veterinary Emergency and Critical Care Society (VECCS, www.veccs.org).

References

1. Aiken TD. Ethics in nursing. In: Aiken TD, Legal, Ethical, and Political Issues in Nursing. 2nd ed. Philadelphia: F. A. Davis, 2004:109.
2. Chavis SA, Hutton JL, Bassert JM. Medical records. In: McCurnin DM, Bassert JM, Clinical Textbook for the Veterinary Technicians, 5th ed. Philadelphia: WB Saunders, 2002:814–816.
3. Goebel RA. Recordkeeping, business transactions, and clinic adminstration. In: Pratt PW, ed. Principles and Practice of Veterinary Technology. St. Louis, MO: Mosby, 1998:44.
4. Babcock SL, Pfeiffer C. Laws and regulations concerning the confidentiality of veterinarian-client communication, J Am Vet Am Assoc, 2006;229:3365–3369.
5. Hackett TB., Physical examination. In: Silverstein, DC, Hopper K, Small Animal Critical Care Medicine, St. Louis: Saunders Elsevier, 2009:2–5.
6. Rockett J, Lattanzio C, Anderson K. Veterinary technician practice model and documentation. In: Patient Assessment, Intervention and Documentation for the Veterinary Technician, Clifton Park, NY: Delmar, 2009:3–17.
7. Pattengale P. Task 3.03 filing. In: Pattengale P, Tasks for the Veterinary Assistant, Philadelphia: Lippincott Williams & Wilkins, 2005:41.
8. Crowe DT. Patient triage. In: Silverstein, DC, Hopper K, Small Animal Critical Care Medicine. St. Louis, MO: Saunders Elsevier, 2009:5–7.
9. LSU Law Center's Medical and Public Health Law Site, Website. Photoreduction of Records. Available at http://biotech.law.lsu.edu/books/aspen/Aspen-Photored.html. Accessed March 8, 2009.

65

Compassion fatigue: healing with a heart

Katherine Dobbs

Veterinary medicine is often more than just a career; it is a calling. It attracts compassionate, caring individuals who want to help those animals that are ill and injured. By the very nature of companion animal medicine, veterinary professionals find themselves helping pet owners and families through the suffering and sorrow as well. Yet veterinary professionals do this work of caring for others in emotional and physical pain at a cost to themselves: the "cost of caring," otherwise known as compassion fatigue.[1] Nowhere is this truer than in emergency critical care.

Compassion is being aware of another's suffering, but also feeling compelled to help relieve this suffering. Veterinary professionals see the need of animals in pain or discomfort, and feel obliged to act. Fatigue is simply the process of becoming weary or exhausted while delivering this care. Compassion fatigue has been called the "hurt of the heart," something anyone in the veterinary profession may suffer at any point along his or her career. The veterinary professional is a target for compassion fatigue because the profession attracts people with compassion. Without compassion, there would be no compassion fatigue; yet this ability to be compassionate is a basic element of the veterinary professional. A professional with no compassion would not be able to deliver the highest quality care to those animals in need.

The veterinary professional may not be aware of this condition of compassion fatigue, even while suffering from its effect. It can create issues within relationships both at home and at work. Compassion fatigue can lead to physical illness that prevents the veterinary professional from feeling well and doing his or her best work.

Compassion fatigue also has negative effects on the business of veterinary medicine within an organization or practice. Individuals on the team with compassion fatigue can experience mental weariness and have difficulty concentrating, which can make them prone to accidents including medical mistakes. The increased physical illnesses experienced by these team members will lead to a higher rate of absenteeism, and the overwhelming effects of compassion fatigue can lead to turnover in the practice and attrition in the profession. These organizational symptoms can lead to a management nightmare, plus they negatively affect the bottom-line profitability of the practice. In the veterinary profession overall, it is likely that compassion fatigue both personal and organizational contributes to the ever-increasing rates of attrition. Although many will say they are leaving the profession due to lack of financial rewards, it may be because the emotional satisfaction is now lacking for them personally; it is no longer worth the paycheck to endure the hardships.

From the perspective of the individual, there are recognized causes of compassion fatigue that can make a person more susceptible:

Causes of compassion fatigue[2]

Placing needs of others before your own

Caregivers typically care for others better than they care for themselves. The irony is that the less they take care of themselves, the less they can take care of others, including the pets and families that sustain the veterinary profession.

Advanced Monitoring and Procedures for Small Animal Emergency and Critical Care, First Edition. Edited by Jamie M. Burkitt Creedon, Harold Davis.
© 2012 John Wiley & Sons, Inc. Published 2012 by John Wiley & Sons, Inc.

Unresolved past trauma and pain

A veterinary professional may be more prone to compassion fatigue because of incidents or situations from his or her past. One theory suggests that those who already suffer from compassion fatigue tend to move into the helping professions. These people may have taken on the role of caretaker for others at a young age before beginning their professional life, and sought out a profession that allowed them to remain in the caregiver role.

Lack of healthy life coping skills

Resiliency is necessary for a person to bounce back from negative situations in his or her personal and professional life. Those who do not have the needed coping skills will suffer more quickly and more deeply when faced with professional challenges. They may not possess the coping skills to recover fast or fully.

Lack of self-awareness that limits growth

In order for the veterinary professional to grow in his or her personal and/or professional life, he or she must possess self-awareness. This includes an ability to identify strengths and weaknesses, set realistic goals, and possess the initiative and fortitude to obtain these goals.

Giving care to others under stress

This defines any care giving profession, although in veterinary medicine there are two levels of care that may not be present in most nursing equivalents; the patient animal receiving direct care, which is unable to express itself with words, and the pet owner, who is speaking on behalf of the animal. The pet owner needs to be educated and convinced of the veterinary professional's good intentions in order for him or her to trust the veterinary team with their pet. This adds a second dimension of complexity to the veterinary profession.

Lack of personal boundaries

Often, caregivers in general do not set up personal boundaries because they want to be all things to all people. They may have trouble saying "no," both in their personal and professional lives, so that their boundaries are never protected and they allow themselves to become overextended. This makes them susceptible to compassion fatigue, and at the same time can lead to feelings of guilt, which can be a dangerous combination.

Inability to communicate needs

Caregivers tend to ignore or hide their own needs, or express them in negative ways when the dam breaks.

Then their attempts at communication manifest as whining, angry outbursts, excessive complaining, and the like. This can damage their personal and professional relationships, as well as their ability to have a positive outlook on life.

In order to diagnosis individual compassion fatigue, the symptoms must be revealed and recognized.

Symptoms of compassion fatigue[2]

Bottled-up emotions

Often, veterinary professionals lack the space, time, or inclination to release their emotions, particularly during their work day. Instead they stuff these feelings down inside until they are filled up and overflowing with emotion. Eventually, they will burst, and this may be in their workplace or their home, making innocent bystanders the victims. In general compassion fatigue manifests itself at home by causing the person to become withdrawn, have a decreased interest in intimacy, experience mistrust, and become isolated from friends, with a definite impact on parenting by causing projection of anger or blame and intolerance.

Impulse to rescue anyone (or anything) in need

Many veterinary professionals have a house full of rescued pets and can certainly relate to this impulse. It can happen in the personal life of the person as well, when he or she attracts those people who are needy; the desire to "fix" goes beyond animals at times.

Isolation from others

Veterinary professionals may feel themselves drawing back from people at work or at home, wanting to be alone in the midst of their negative swirl of emotions. Others may tire of their countless stories of death and misery from the work day, and may pull away from the veterinary professional. This creates a wall separating them from those who want to help.

Sadness and apathy

It may be easy enough for someone to recognize when he or she feels sad, but less obvious and more dangerous can be apathy. This is when it hurts too much to care anymore. This can be particularly harmful in the practice setting, when the veterinary professional may no longer be able to deliver the empathic client service and team support that is so necessary in the profession. It has been demonstrated that apathy or remaining emotionally detached from patients (and clients) is not an effective coping strategy; stress and emotional exhaustion will still occur.

Need to voice excessive complaints about management and coworkers

Displaced emotions can result in anger or dissatisfaction that manifests itself as complaints about those surrounding the affected veterinary professional. This can put the person's career or position at risk and in general makes the person difficult to work with or employ.

Lack of interest in self-care practices

Often, veterinary professionals understand what they need to do to take care of themselves, but they lack the interest or motivation to really do the things that are necessary. These are typically the things that could help them the most in fighting compassion fatigue. They include measures such as eating right, getting enough rest, and exercising regularly.

Recurring nightmare and flashbacks

If a veterinary professional is having bad dreams about work when asleep, or reliving particularly bad moments or events when awake, this could be a sure sign that he or she is reaching an emotional limit.

Persistent physical ailments

Veterinary professionals may have nagging ailments that don't ever seem to disappear, such as headaches, stomachaches, or backaches. The illness may not be enough to keep them home from work most days, but they make it more difficult to get through the work day and do their best work. When veterinary professionals do reach their limit, this is when compassion fatigue can result in higher absenteeism as they decide not to even try to face the daily struggle either for physical or emotional reasons.

Difficulty concentrating, mentally tired

Carrying all of that emotional baggage can wear a person out mentally, making it more difficult to stay on task or complete tasks.

Prone to accidents

This diverted mental energy increases the risk of making mistakes, both medical and physical. Compassion fatigue can result in clinical errors that could cost a patient its life.

When individuals on the team are affected by compassion fatigue, there will be symptoms present in the organization overall.

Symptoms of organizational compassion fatigue[2]

Excessive amount of worker's compensation claims

Individuals with compassion fatigue often have difficulty concentrating and are mentally tired, leading them to be prone to accidents. When those accidents happen on the clock, they become worker's compensation claims. Spikes in the number of injuries due to animal restraint in particular can be a red flag for the presence of organizational compassion fatigue; it is not likely that all of a sudden the team forgot how to restrain.

High absenteeism, turnover

When individuals with compassion fatigue experience those chronic physical ailments such as stomachaches, headaches, and other frequent maladies, their absences lead to higher absenteeism overall in the organization. When the physical stress becomes too much, the veterinary professional will look for a way to escape. He or she will consider moving on to another facility, or another profession altogether.

Changes in coworkers' relationships

As individuals with compassion fatigue begin to isolate themselves, they put a strain on their relationships with others in the practice. At a time when coworkers need each other more than ever, it is easier and safer for the affected person (or people) to hide his or her pain and avoid interaction altogether.

Inability for teams to work well together, and inability to complete assigned tasks

Sadness and apathy in affected team members make it difficult for the team to work together and accomplish its goals. If each person does not believe in the end result and put forth his or her fair share of effort, the team fizzles and the job is not accomplished. Difficulty concentrating makes it that much harder for each person to handle his or her share of the work load and complete it to the level of quality desired.

Team challenges rules and regulations, and displays lack of flexibility

That impulse of the employee to rescue anything in need is particularly difficult to police. Practices find they need policies in place to address abandoned animals, stray animals brought in by good Samaritans, and employees who want to adopt animals and use their employee privileges or discounts to provide medical care to these pets that would have otherwise been euthanized by their family of origin. The battles can become fierce over the right thing to do both morally for the animal, and practically for the business.

Aggressive behavior among teammates

Those team members who are bottling up their emotions will eventually explode, and the others around them at the time may be the victims of this undesirable if not aggressive behavior. The innocent bystander wonders what set off the affected person's explosion, without understanding that the perpetrator had been bottling up feelings for weeks or months.

Unhealthy competition among teammates

If an incentive program is dropped into a mix of individuals affected by compassion fatigue, the competition will be fierce with more negative results than positive.

Rampant rumors and gossip

When team members resort to voicing excessive complaints about their team members and supervisors in general, it is easy for them to complain in private to their allies, thus creating gossip and rumors as their unhappiness spreads through the team.

Constant changes in practice policies

As the management team tries in vain to put out all the "fires" that are sparking from the emotional contagion in the practice, they will rapidly change policies to try to fix the problems, with little or no success because the team also lacks flexibility and challenges the rules and regulations. The vicious cycle has begun, or continues to whirl.

Organizational compassion fatigue may present in other ways as well, including an increase in the percent of accounts receivable in a practice. The practice owner or members of management may feel powerless to provide the level of care they know they can deliver, because their clients may not be able to afford the care. So they let bills climb and invoices go unpaid or slowly paid, and therefore bear the financial burden of wanting to provide caregiving at any cost, and with this increased cost to the practice.

Diagnostic tools

To assess and monitor an individual's level of compassion satisfaction in his or her caregiving career, and his or her risk of burnout and compassion fatigue, the Professional Quality of Life Scale (ProQOL V) was developed by B. Hudnall Stamm. This is widely recognized as the "golden standard" or most accurate way of measur-

ing compassion fatigue (also known as secondary trauma), compassion satisfaction, and burnout. Completing this test helps to assess where the veterinary professional is in regards to these job factors. An individual can take this test at frequent intervals, perhaps monthly or quarterly, to monitor how well he or she is dealing with the realities of doing the work of a veterinary professional in emergency critical care medicine. This testing can also be initiated by the practice management in order to continue awareness and improve diagnosis in a timely manner.

The phases of becoming a caregiver

With increased awareness, the veterinary professional can come to recognize that compassion fatigue is a hazard inherent to the veterinary workplace, and learn ways to minimize or cope with compassion fatigue. The organization as a whole can contribute to this awareness of compassion fatigue, and develop an action plan to overcome compassion fatigue. To begin, it can be helpful to understand how the animal caregiver becomes introduced to this work of caring. Often, the veterinary professional experiences a calling to help animals from the time he or she is young. This desire to provide care and comfort helps the professional obtain the education and experience needed to enter veterinary medicine. In the beginning, the veterinary professional is motivated and enthused to provide this care, and often the difficulties of the job are not apparent at first. However, as reality sinks in that there will be long hours, difficult cases, and emotional strife, the enthusiasm dampens. Veterinary professionals can experience emotions they were not expecting, such as anger and frustration. Physically and mentally these people begin to falter, or come to the realization that they must find a balance between the effort exerted at work on those animals that need care and the effort of taking care of themselves. This can be as simple as getting enough rest and proper nutrition, so they have the physical stamina to do the job. It can also be as complex as finding time to meet personal emotional needs by enjoying sources of satisfaction outside of veterinary medicine. If this balance is not achieved, the veterinary professional may choose to leave the profession altogether, feeling overwhelmed by the realities of the job they dreamed of for many years or perhaps a lifetime.

Stressors and satisfiers

As emergency critical care team members, there are numerous reasons to experience stress at work, but at the same time there is also satisfaction from the work done in these challenging workplaces. Robert G. Roop performed a survey of the veterinary profession (Humane Society of the U.S., 2003–2004) called the Compassion Satisfaction and Fatigue Survey. The survey was completed by veterinarians, technicians and assistants, office staff and managers to identify the top stressors and satisfiers for each of these three categories of professionals. Veterinarians responded that their top three stressors are difficult and noncompliant clients, not enough time (specifically to devote to patient care), and discussing/disputing fees. The top three satisfiers identified by veterinarians included helping/healing animals, thankful clients, and working as a team. When examined side by side, it is apparent that as a stressor is reduced a corresponding satisfier is increased; reducing the number of difficult and noncompliant clients leads to more thankful clients.

Technicians and assistants identified their top three stressors as difficult or noncompliant clients, problems with coworkers, and not enough time (again, specifically to devote to patient care). Their top three satisfiers include helping/healing animals, working as a team, and thankful clients. Again, reducing the number of problems with coworkers would increase the satisfaction of working as a team, so the balance is tipped in a favorable direction. For the remainder of the support staff, front office and practice management, the top three stressors are difficult or noncompliant clients, time demands, and disputes over fees/billing. The top three satisfiers include thankful clients, daily contact with animals, and helping/healing animals. These results illustrate that while the front office and practice management members are the farthest removed from the animals and delivery of patient care, they are involved in veterinary medicine because of their desire to be a part of the health care team. Overall, the results of this survey also point to the conclusion that an increase in client communication and satisfaction efforts will increase the satisfaction gained from thankful clients, while in turn reducing the number of difficult and noncompliant clients for the entire veterinary practice team. Since difficult and noncompliant clients are the top stressor for every position in the practice, devoting time to this topic would be beneficial for the practice overall and the team members individually.

When the author of this survey decided to investigate compassion fatigue, it was soon apparent that the compassion satisfaction elements had to be considered as well. When looking at all the stressors apparent in the veterinary profession, there had to be sources of satisfaction that helped to balance these stressors and motivate the veterinary professional to report to work each day.

In essence, it was determined that compassion satisfaction acts as an antidote to compassion fatigue. In order to minimize and cope with compassion fatigue in our profession of veterinary medicine, we need to focus on increasing those sources of satisfaction.

Compassion fatigue versus burnout

Burnout is another word that is commonly used in the veterinary profession. It often describes the veterinary professional's feelings on a particularly tough day in practice, or perhaps in the midst of a string of tough days. Burnout has been defined in many publications, and the central concept is that burnout involves the veterinary professional's interaction with the work environment. This work environment includes the location of the facility, the nature of the professional's commute, the work hours and level of pay, the type of equipment and facilities provided, and the nature of the team and management, among other factors. The compassion fatigue and satisfaction survey also measured the veterinary team members' risk of burnout, and the results suggest that veterinary professionals are at low risk for burnout. The low burnout risk is attributed to the presence of the compassion satisfiers, the good things about the work that keep veterinary professionals coming back every day. More often than not, when a colleague claims that he or she is feeling "burned out," it is actually an expression of compassion fatigue. It is important to discern compassion fatigue from burnout in order identify, prevent, and minimize compassion fatigue.

The conditions of burnout and compassion fatigue have also been contrasted by members of the medical profession. While burnout involves the elements of the work environment, compassion fatigue involves the interaction between the clinician and the patient, and in the case of the veterinary professional, the client or pet owner. While the factors of the work environment can be changed, particularly at a different place of employment, compassion fatigue runs deeper. Simply put, burnout is more associated with *where* the veterinary professional works; if the job is left behind, the burnout may also be left behind. However, compassion fatigue is more associated with the work the veterinary professional does and the level of emotional care giving provided, and it will follow that professional wherever he or she goes as long as he or she remains in a caregiving role. Whenever the veterinary professional is exposed to relationships with clients and patients, compassion fatigue will be a factor. This is important to realize. Many times a veterinary professional will leave behind a position in one practice, only to experience the same emotional exhaustion (i.e., compassion fatigue) with added new sources of stress at a new practice. At this point, he or she may request his or her job back at their previous practice. This boomerang effect indicates that the veterinary professional is likely experiencing compassion fatigue and has been unsuccessful at outrunning its effects.

The three-pronged approach

There is a shared responsibility when it comes to monitoring and minimizing compassion fatigue. One perspective has been called the "three-pronged approach." It emphasizes the need for the organization to care for the staff, the need for colleagues within the profession to support each other, and the responsibility of the individual caregiver to care for him- or herself. A fourth prong can be considered an overarching concept, and that is the responsibility of the profession as a whole to recognize and manage compassion fatigue in the industry.

There are methods that can be used to create and maintain a healthy workplace, which satisfies this first prong in this approach. Patricia Smith, founder of the Compassion Fatigue Awareness Project, provides us with a template to creating a healthy practice called the Eight Laws Governing a Healthy Workplace.[2] These laws can help define a way for the veterinary professional and the entire profession of veterinary medicine to prevent or minimize compassion fatigue within the business setting of veterinary medicine.

1. **Take a break.** Oftentimes veterinary professionals are so focused on their patients and the practice that they ignore their break and lunch times. Management should insist that these breaks are taken; likewise, individuals should make it a priority. It is also beneficial to find a true place of respite, for these breaks to provide a change of scenery. This could be as simple as a picnic table outside on the back lawn, or as fancy as a gazebo within a memorial garden for the staff. Indoors, of course, a break room is nice, and perhaps the room can be decorated to represent a complete change of scenery. Be creative, and get the team involved in designing a special place just for them. When it comes to providing respite from the stressful events that can lead to compassion fatigue, there should be a place and time where it is safe to discuss the effects that these incidents have upon the team. This can be take the form of routine Morbidity and Mortality (M&M) rounds where difficult cases are re-examined and emotions are

expressed, or there could be memorial services for special patients at which everyone gets a chance for closure. Too often the veterinary professional must run straight from one catastrophe to the next patient that needs help, so there is no chance for closure. Again, the team should be involved in how they want to express their emotions and discuss difficult cases.

2. **Take or make opportunities for continuing education.** Most veterinary professionals understand that continuing education is important for the practice of veterinary medicine. The field is ever-changing, and the professional must stay on top of new advances in medicine. It is important to realize that continuing education (CE) can also help to prevent and combat compassion fatigue. It is one of those compassion satisfiers that is so needed, and it benefits the practice because everyone gains from a knowledgeable and skilled team. Everyone should be included in CE, from the reception staff to the kennel help and each position in between. These CE opportunities can be in-house seminars taught by the practice team members, or can be presented by outside sources. They can be online courses or Web seminars, or journals and text books. The opportunities are endless, so a type of CE can be found that is appropriate for all team members and types of practices. Remember that when team members are sent to an outside conference, if the practice is investing money in their education, they should be prepared to come back and teach others what they have learned.

3. **Take advantage of self-care benefits.** Caregivers are encouraged to fight compassion fatigue by caring for themselves, and the practice can help them make a commitment to this process. Health insurance benefits are often the first thing that comes to mind, but it also needs to be determined if the employer is going to offer mental health benefits or an Employee Assistance Program (EAP). Personal issues undoubtedly affect professional behavior and success, and the practice can help to keep employees emotionally healthy by providing these benefits. Even taking advantage of time off benefits is important for self-care. Many practices have moved to a system of paid time off or PTO, so that there is no explanation needed when time off is requested. This can be beneficial when a team member is sick physically, or weary mentally, and he or she no longer has to explain or pretend to be sick. There are other initiatives the practice may choose to take such as providing exercise or wellness

equipment in-house or offering discounts to local fitness facilities. Additional preventive health initiatives can be suggested and provided by health insurance providers. These can include wellness programs to help employees lose weight, stop smoking, or simply take better care of themselves.

4. **Locate or request tools for the job.** When a job needs to be performed, the proper tools to accomplish the task must be provided. This includes the training to get the job done. The employer should not expect a technician to run a CBC without the proper equipment and instructions, nor should they expect a front office team to communicate with other practices without a telephone and fax machine and phone numbers. Some tools involve equipment, supplies, and inventory, but some tools are less tangible, such as the time and authority to complete the assigned task. This is particularly true if the individual is involved in management or supervision. The upper management or practice owner may need to provide the motivation, mentoring, education, and resources to help others manage the team and the practice operations.

5. **Monitor and report workload.** There can be multiple levels of management in an organization, depending on the size and structure of the facility. The person who monitors the workload of the individual should be the supervisor closest to this employee. For example, a technician supervisor monitors the workloads of each technician, while the hospital manager monitors the workloads of the team supervisors. Workload can be documented and monitored using a Project Log that details what is on an employee's ongoing to-do list. This can help the employee avoid becoming overwhelmed or overcommitted. An employee may need to request scheduled designated "administrative time" to work on and complete the projects he or she needs to get done. It is often unrealistic for the leaders to expect a team member to complete an extra project during the spare moments in between main duties, yet often that is just what is asked. Team members should learn to recognize when they have become overloaded, and should prevent this from happening as much as possible in the future. The team member should be sure to reach agreement with the manager when it comes to accepting deadlines, and get his or her help in reprioritizing the projects on the list according to what the practice needs; this can often fluctuate. The management team is important in helping each person, the entire team, and the practice overall resist compassion fatigue.

Yet management is also in a position of susceptibility when it comes to compassion fatigue on a personal level. In fact, those managers who have "come up" within the veterinary profession often face a special set of circumstances. If they began as technicians, as many have, they used to have daily contact with animals that they helped and healed, which provided a great amount of satisfaction. Now as a member of management, they have less time with the pets, more time with difficult clients, more time with problems among coworkers, and less time enjoying the team atmosphere. This creates an intense situation that leads to a distinct type of management compassion fatigue, yet the organization depends on these people to manage the business and the team. They must maintain a precarious balance, dealing with their own compassion fatigue as well as helping the team members deal with theirs. When creating a plan to prevent and minimize compassion fatigue, the managers' dual roles must be taken into consideration as well.

6. **Create and maintain relationships.** In the Compassion Satisfaction and Fatigue survey it was determined that working as a team is a satisfier for many veterinary professionals. It is important to foster good team relations for many different reasons relating to the business as a whole and to the veterinary professional as an individual. Leaders should lead the way by being first to participate in activities during staff meetings and team events. Although they may not seem fun on paper, many of these activities are great ways to have a good time and learn a valuable lesson together as a team. On a more personal level, the practice can implement a Buddy System where team members encourage and monitor each other in their self-care efforts. This Buddy System can be initiated by either the team or the management of a practice.

7. **Push open or walk through the "open doors."** An open door policy sounds good for many reasons, yet it can be difficult to achieve. While the manager needs to be available for employee needs, he or she also needs to have uninterrupted time to accomplish management tasks. Nonemergent issues may have to wait until a more appropriate time. The manager is trying his or her best to maintain accessibility and efficiency in the business of management just as everyone else is doing with their daily tasks. If the veterinary team knows when there is a better time they can approach management, yet understand the system for intervening in a crisis or emergency situation, then everyone will find balance. During group meetings, an open door policy means everyone

should feel free to participate in open communication and encourage their teammates to do the same. The team can also take advantage of submitting anonymous suggestions to management in a safe way such as a confidential suggestion box.

8. **Acknowledge and express grief.** In medicine, a patient death is often accompanied by a debriefing process for the staff present. This can involve outside counselors and resources brought in for the employees. However, in veterinary medicine, the team can experience a string of crises and deaths without so much as a mention of this reality; the team members often must suppress their emotions in order to move on to other patients and clients that need them and require their full attention. Ignoring these feelings and the difficult circumstances we face daily in veterinary medicine can be dangerous in the long run, and it is beneficial to prevent this "blanket of silence" that so often pervades veterinary practices. Each team can work together to invent what works for their individual practice.

Perhaps the practice can implement an Immediate Debriefing Form that provides a place to briefly describe the incident, list the employees present, note the attending doctor or lead technician who is responsible for reporting the incident, and provide notice of any employee who needs the management to follow up and ascertain their emotional well-being at a later time. On a personal level, it is beneficial for a team member to debrief with someone who has a similar base of experience and can understand the situation within the first 24–72 hours following an incident. This type of intervention is often called Critical Incident Debriefing. During the debriefing conversation it should become clear that the situation itself has led to the death, rather than the team members themselves. At the same time, it is beneficial to discuss what was done, and could be done better next time. This puts the focus on the future, and helps the team learn from the past if possible.

It is also important to help the team realize when the situation may have involved difficult choices made by the pet owner. There could have even been a dollar limit that the client had to spend on their pet, and the care was therefore too expensive for the family. It is particularly difficult for the veterinary team to know they can help, yet lack the permission to proceed due to financial restraints. When the patient's family must make a choice, there are times when the team may not agree with the decision. Yet it is that pet owner's choice to decide to pursue diagnostics, continue treatment, or provide his or her pet with humane euthanasia. In the emergency critical care setting, these choices must be made many times a day, and the cumulative effects of the results of these choices can wear on the veterinary team. Team members must realize that they cannot judge or let their personal feelings cloud the situation, because they cannot speak for that family or that pet owner. It can be difficult for veterinary professionals to understand the decisions an owner is facing in the life of his or her family and pet. It is the veterinary team's duty to provide what care is allowed for the pet, and respect the pet owner's choices and decisions along the way.

If there are ways to improve the team's response in an emergency situation, then this should be discussed without placing blame or becoming defensive. The team is faced with learning opportunities every day, and they will continue to improve how they care for pets if they recognize these opportunities when they present themselves. At times, this moment of learning is simply to understand that there was nothing different that could have been done to change the outcome for that pet or that family. The team must be mindful that "success" is often seen by them as the recovery of the pet, yet "success" in the minds of the family could be as simple or as complex as humane euthanasia when that is their choice. It is not the team's choice to make, nor is it their blame to carry.

When it comes to satisfying the second prong of the "three-pronged approach," veterinary professionals helping to support their colleagues, it is important to realize that no one is alone; every veterinary professional is susceptible to compassion fatigue, and most will suffer its effects at some point during his or her career. Information gained on compassion fatigue can help team members provide this support. When an employee is experiencing the more difficult phases of care giving—when his or her enthusiasm has dampened and he or she begins to feel overwhelmed—an attentive colleague can intervene and lend a listening ear. Following a traumatic scenario, colleagues can check in with each other, both validating the presence of negative emotions and offering support to each other. There are even many small ways through which colleagues can improve the environment for themselves and each other, such as remembering basic politeness and gratitude.

The third prong is self-care, and each team member must be responsible for him- or herself. It is necessary to provide the body with its needs such as rest, nutrition, and protection. It is also necessary to maintain good mental or emotional health. Some basics of self-care include acknowledging needs and wants, clarifying goals, creating a sustainable plan, and finding balance. This balance should include hobbies outside veterinary medicine and scheduling special time to enjoy interesting activities. To start, identify five things that must be done every day, such as shower, eat, or go to work. Then, the veterinary professional adds five more things that would energize him- or herself. To help answer this, the veterinary professional can determine what he or she would do with a complete day off, with no work, no chores, and no errands. The fun activities could include visiting with a friend, reading for pleasure, taking a walk in nature, and so on. Then each week or two, the veterinary professional can add one of these new self-energizing ideas to his or her routine. The professional should stick to this plan and see how it feels to be caring for him- or herself for a change.

Another simple thing that can help is called a "role-shedding ritual." When it is time to clock out and step out the door, the veterinary professional can designate a literal or figurative ritual that will help him or her to transition from work mode to home mode. Some people already do this without really thinking of it as a role-shedding ritual. It can involve changing out of scrubs and into street clothes before leaving work, listening to music or audio books in the car, stopping by the park to take a quick walk, or even putting a little note or picture on the outside of the garage door that serves as a reminder that now it is time to enjoy being home.

Professionals in emergency critical care in particular often have patients they are leaving behind when they clock out and go home. This can make it particularly difficult for a caregiver to disengage and get his or her mind off of work. It can help to follow an organized process when wrapping things up at the end of a shift. After determining what needs to be finished or delegated and what can wait until tomorrow, there can be a routine that signals the end of the workday. There is someone else in charge of the patients, so the veterinary professional can remind him- or herself of this and feel comfortable leaving the practice and the patients under the care of others. Focus on the positive outcomes of the day, rather than the one or two negative moments, letting the satisfiers far outweigh the stressors.

Creating a compassionate culture

There have been factors identified that relate to compassion fatigue among healthcare workers in particular. These include inadequate professional training, poor mentoring, low staffing, and an organizational culture that does not encourage, value, and recognize exemplary displays of compassion. It is believed that if employees do not feel respected and appreciated for their efforts, and if they do not feel cared about by those who have responsibility for them, it will be more difficult for them to establish and maintain a truly caring environment for patients.

As these factors leading to compassion fatigue among healthcare workers are examined, it is clear that there are plenty of ways to help the veterinary professional move through and out of the fog of compassion fatigue. Professional training should be provided from an employee's first day, and colleagues should never stop encouraging each other to continue their learning and growing. Mentoring is perhaps the most important task that can be used for individuals to support each other and the profession, yet it requires sensitivity to know which employees need mentoring and how they can be best served. It also requires time to create personal bonds, set professional boundaries, and develop trust so that employees are open and responsive to being mentored by other members of the team. Low staffing is a reality for many practices, and the unexpected loss of an employee often leads to filling in that space using the "warm body" technique. This is avoidable if the management team continually accepts resumes and applications for all positions even when there is no opening, and conducts ongoing interviews to line up the best candidates for when an opening occurs. If the management has established open communication with each team member, the management is also better prepared to know when an employee may be reaching a personal or professional goal that will take him or her from the practice (e.g., graduating school, completing certification) or to realize when an employee is struggling and thus when involuntary termination is unavoidable. Employee loss should never be a surprise, in most cases. If it is, then the management is not projecting employee needs very far into the future, and they are not forming successful relationships with team members.

Organizational culture is so important to minimizing the effects of organizational compassion fatigue. The management team (including practice owners and all levels of supervision) must encourage, value, and recognize exemplary displays of compassion by the employees. This could be extra time spent with a grieving client in the examination room, staying late to provide patient care that is necessary, or supporting a teammate through a difficult case. The practice leadership must be careful not to assume this is unprofitable "down time" or just employees "riding the clock," when instead it may be the extension of compassion that really needs to be displayed by the team members. Management should freely use the word "compassion" as often as possible when describing activities that they are praising, as this will help the team members make the connection that it is this display of compassion that is being recognized and rewarded. Managers in general find it is easy to focus on the problem or trouble employees who constantly need guidance and counseling. However, those employees

Box 65.1 The Caregiver's Bill of Rights, by Patricia Smith

As a caregiver, I have the right . . .
   . . . to be respected for the work I choose to do.
   . . . to take pride in my work and know that I am making a difference.
   . . . to garner appreciation and validation for the care I give others.
   . . . to receive adequate pay for my job as a professional caregiver.
   . . . to discern my personal boundaries and have others respect my choices.
   . . . to seek assistance from others, if and when it is necessary.
   . . . to take time off to re-energize myself.
   . . . to socialize, maintain my interests, and sustain a balanced lifestyle.
   . . . to my own feelings, including negative emotions such as anger, sadness, and frustration.
   . . . to express my thoughts and feelings to appropriate people at appropriate times.
   . . . to convey hope to those in my care.
   . . . to believe those in my care will prosper in mind, body, and spirit as a result of my caregiving.

who probably deserve the support of management the most are those who need to see real proof of how much they are respected and appreciated. This goes beyond tangible rewards and "employee of the month" plagues to words and actions that provide employees the feeling that they are cared about. This is where that personal bond is so important.

There is no greater gift we can give as veterinary professionals than providing care for animals that are sick and injured, and that find themselves in our care within an emergency critical care facility. You have devoted your career, and often your life, to these special souls who cannot speak for themselves, and often your payment of puppy breath and kitten kisses, wagging tails and bright eyes, far exceeds any type of monetary value. While doing your important work, remember to take care of yourself so that these animals can continue to call on you during their time of need. Maintain your compassion, work to overcome your fatigue, and remain an essential part of the world of veterinary medicine.

References

1. Figley CR, Roop RG. The costs of caring. In: Figley CR, Roop RG, Compassion Fatigue in the Animal-Care Community. Washington: The Humane Society of the United States, 2006:1–6.
2. Smith P. Part I: What is compassion fatigue? In: Healthy Caregiving: A Guide to Recognizing and Managing Compassion Fatigue, Presenter's Guide Level 1. Patricia Smith, 2008:23–53.

Recommended reading

Compassion Fatigue Awareness Project, with discussion forum, at http://compassionfatigue.org.
Dobbs, Katherine. Blog and articles at www.katherinedobbs.com.
Figley, CR and Roop RG. *Compassion Fatigue in the Animal-Care Community*. The Humane Society of the United States, 2006.
Life stress test at http://www.cliving.org/lifstrstst.htm.
Professional Quality of Life information at http://www.proqol.org/Home_Page.html.
Professional Quality of Life V Test at http://www.proqol.org/ProQol_Test.html.
Smith, Patricia. *Healthy Caregiving: A Guide to Recognizing and Managing Compassion Fatigue, Student Guide Level 1*. Published by the author, 2008.
Smith, Patricia. *To Weep for a Stranger*. Published by the author, 2009.

Index

Note: Pages followed by "b" indicate boxes; "f," figures; "p," protocols; and "t," tables.

Advanced Monitoring and Procedures for Small Animal Emergency and Critical Care, First Edition. Edited by Jamie M. Burkitt Creedon, Harold Davis.
© 2012 John Wiley & Sons, Inc. Published 2012 by John Wiley & Sons, Inc.